a LANGE medical book

CURRENT Diagnosis & Treatment in Orthopedics

Fourth Edition

Edited by

Harry B. Skinner, MD, PhD
Professor and Chairman
Department of Orthopaedic Surgery
University of California, Irvine
Irvine, California

Lange Medical Books/McGraw-Hill
Medical Publishing Division

New York Chicago San Francisco Lisbon London Madrid Mexico City
Milan New Delhi San Juan Seoul Singapore Sydney Toronto

The McGraw-Hill Companies

Current Diagnosis & Treatment in Orthopedics, Fourth Edition

ISBN: 0-07-143833-5 (Domestic)
ISSN: 1081-0056

7 8 9 0 IBT/IBT 1 9 8 7 6 5 4 3 2 1

Notice

Medicine is an ever-changing science. As new research and clinical experience broaden our knowledge, changes in treatment and drug therapy are required. The authors and the publisher of this work have checked with sources believed to be reliable in their efforts to provide information that is complete and generally in accord with the standards accepted at the time of publication. However, in view of the possibility of human error or changes in medical sciences, neither the authors nor the publisher nor any other party who has been involved in the preparation or publication of this work warrants that the information contained herein is in every respect accurate or complete, and they disclaim all responsibility for any errors or omissions or for the results obtained from use of the information contained in this work. Readers are encouraged to confirm the information contained herein with other sources. For example and in particular, readers are advised to check the product information sheet included in the package of each drug they plan to administer to be certain that the information contained in this work is accurate and that changes have not been made in the recommended dose or in the contraindications for administration. This recommendation is of particular importance in connection with new or infrequently used drugs.

This book was set in Garamond by Silverchair Science + Communications, Inc.
The editors were Hilarie Surrena, Christie Naglieri, and Regina Y. Brown.
The production supervisor was Catherine Saggese.
The index was prepared by Ann Blum.
The cover designer was Mary McKeon.
IBT Global was printer and binder.

This book is printed on acid-free paper.

INTERNATIONAL EDITION ISBN 0-07-110451-8

Contents

Authors

Juan F. Agudelo, MD
Resident, Department of Orthopedic Surgery, University of Colorado School of Medicine, Oakland, California
Musculoskeletal Trauma Surgery

Michael S. Bednar, MD
Associate Professor, Department of Orthopaedic Surgery and Rehabilitation, Loyola University Medical Center, Maywood, Illinois
Mbednar@lumc.edu
Hand Surgery

Nitin N. Bhatia, MD
Assistant Clinical Professor; Chief, Spine Service; Director, The UC Irvine Spine Center, Department of Orthopaedic Surgery, University of California, Irvine, Medical Center, Orange, California
bhatian@uci.edu
Disorders, Diseases, and Injuries of the Spine

Vincent J. Caiozzo, PhD
Professor, Department of Orthopaedic Surgery, School of Medicine, University of California, Irvine
vjcaiozz@uci.edu
Basic Science in Orthopedic Surgery

Loretta B. Chou, MD
Assistant Professor, Division of Orthopaedic Surgery, Stanford University School of Medicine, Stanford, California
lchou@stanford.edu
Foot & Ankle Surgery

Ranjan Gupta, MD
Associate Professor, Department of Orthopaedic Surgery, Center for Biomedical Engineering, University of California, Irvine
ranjang@uci.edu
Basic Science in Orthopedic Surgery; Adult Reconstructive Surgery

Bang H. Hoang, MD
Assistant Professor, Department of Orthopaedic Surgery, School of Medicine, University of California, Irvine
Musculoskeletal Oncology

Serena S. Hu, MD
Professor of Clinical Orthopaedics, Department of Orthopaedic Surgery, University of California, San Francisco
Hus@orthosurg.ucsf.edu
Disorder, Diseases, & Injuries of the Spine

Lee D. Kaplan, MD
Sports Medicine

Mary Ann E. Keenan, MD
Chief, Neuro-Orthopaedics Surgery, Department of Orthopaedic Surgery, University of Pennsylvania School of Medicine, Philadelphia
maryann.keenan@uphs.upenn.edu
Rehabilitation

Terry R. Light, MD
Dr. William M. Scholl Professor and Chairman, Department of Orthopaedic Surgery and Rehabilitation, Loyola University Medical Center, Maywood, Illinois
tlight@lumc.edu
Hand Surgery

Jeffrey Mann, MD
Alta-Bates Summit Medical Center, Oakland, California
Jeffmann@msn.com
Foot & Ankle Surgery

Patrick J. McMahon, MD
Assistant Professor, Divisions of Sports Medicine, and Shoulder and Elbow Surgery, Department of Orthopedic Surgery, University of Pittsburgh School of Medicine, Pittsburgh, Pennsylvania
mcmahonp@msx.upmc.edu
Sports Medicine

Samir Mehta, MD
Administrative Chief Resident; Instructor, Department of Orthopaedic Surgery, University of Pennsylvania, Philadelphia
Samir.mehta@uphs.upenn.edu
Rehabilitation

Robert S. Namba, MD
Associate Clinical Professor of Orthopaedic Surgery, University of California, Irvine, School of Medicine; Attending Surgeon, Southern California Permanente Medical Group, Anaheim, California
Robert.s.namba@kp.org
Adult Reconstructive Surgery

Anand Parekh, MRCS
Research Fellow, Department of Orthopedic Surgery, University of Colorado School of Medicine, Denver Colorado, Denver Health Medical Center, Denver, Colorado
Anand.parekh@dhha.org
Musculoskeletal Trauma Surgery

George T. Rab , MD
Ben Ali Shriners Professor of Pediatric Orthopedics, Chair, Department of Orthopedic Surgery, Chief, Division of Pediatric Orthopedics, University of California, Davis, School of Medicine; Consulting Physician, Shriners Hospitals for Children, Northern California
George.rab@ucdmc.ucdavis.edu
Pediatric Orthopedic Surgery

R. Lor Randall, MD, FACS
Associate Professor, Director, Sarcoma Services Chief, SARC Lab, Huntsman Cancer Institute and Primary Children's Medical Center, University of Utah, Salt Lake City, Utah
Musculoskeletal Oncology

Steven D. K. Ross, MD
Clinical Professor, Department of Orthopaedic Surgery, University of California, Irvine, College of Medicine, Orange, California
Sdross@uci.edu
Foot & Ankle Surgery

John R. Shank, MD
Private Practice, Colorado Springs, Colorado
johnrshank@yahoo.com
Musculoskeletal Trauma Surgery

Harry B. Skinner, MD, PhD
Professor and Chairman, Department of Orthopaedic Surgery, University of California, Irvine
hskinner@uci.edu
Basic Science in Orthopedic Surgery; General Considerations in Orthopedic Surgery; Sports Medicine; Adult Reconstructive Surgery; Orthopedic Infections

Douglas G. Smith, MD
Harborview Medical Center, Department of Orthopedics and Sports Medicine, Seattle, Washington
dgsmith@u.washington.edu
Amputations

Wade R. Smith, MD
Associate Professor of Orthopedic Surgery, University of Colorado School of Medicine, Denver, Colorado; Director of Orthopedic Surgery, Denver Health Medical Center, Denver, Colorado
Wsmith@dhha.org
Musculoskeletal Trauma Surgery

Robert K-B Tay, MD
Assistant Professor in Residence, Department of Orthopaedic Surgery, University of California, San Francisco
tayb@orthosurg.ucsf.edu
Disorder, Diseases, & Injuries of the Spine

Clifford B. Tribus, MD
Associate Professor, Division of Orthopedics, University of Wisconsin School of Medicine, Madison, Wisconsin
tribus@surgery.wisc.edu
Disorder, Diseases, & Injuries of the Spine

Scott C. Wilson, MD
Assistant Professor of Orthopedic Surgery, Tulane University School of Medicine, New Orleans, Louisiana
mshinn@Tulane.edu
Orthopedic Infections

Preface

This *Current Diagnosis and Treatment in Orthopedics* is the Fourth Edition of the orthopedic surgery contribution to the Lange Current Series of books. It is surprising to realize that it has been 10 years since the first edition of this book. The goal of this book has not changed. It is intended to fill a need for a ready source of up-to-date information on disorders and diseases treated by orthopedic surgeons and related physicians. The format in this edition is unchanged from previous: there is emphasis on the major diagnostic features of disease states, the natural history of the disease where appropriate, the work-up required for definitive diagnosis, and, finally, definitive treatment. The book focuses on orthopedic conditions, de-emphasizing the treatment of the patient from a general medical viewpoint, except when it pertains to the orthopedic problem under consideration. Importantly, pathophysiology, epidemiology, and pathology are included when they assist in arriving at a definitive diagnosis or an understanding of the treatment of the diseases or condition. In many conditions, such as infection or neoplasm, it is extremely important to understand the pathophysiology because the disease may be encountered at various time points in the progression of the disease.

This edition of the *Current Diagnosis and Treatment in Orthopedics* is truly current.

The entire book has been updated in its references to include only those references since 2000, except in cases where classic articles are necessary to refer back to major advances in understanding or treatment, or in situations where there has been little change in the sub-specialization in orthopedics, such as rehabilitation. These selected references to the older literature represent landmarks in the advancement of the understanding of orthopedic diseases and conditions, and serve as useful sources of the fundamental basis for understanding these diseases and conditions.

INTENDED AUDIENCE

The unique format of the Lange series textbooks allows readers of many levels of understanding to derive benefit from the information.

Students will find that the book encompasses virtually all aspects of orthopedics that they will encounter in classes and as sub-interns in major teaching institutions. Residents and house officers can use the book as a ready reference covering the majority of disorders and conditions in emergency and elective orthopedic surgery. Despite its small size, it is truly comprehensive. Because of the organization of the book on a sub-specialty basis, review of individual chapters will provide house officers rotating on sub-specialty orthopedic services with an excellent basis for further in-depth study.

For emergency room physicians, especially those with medical backgrounds, the text provides an excellent resource in managing orthopedic problems seen on an emergent basis. Similarly, family practice, pediatricians, general practitioners, and internists will find the book particularly helpful in the referral decision process, and as a resource to explain disorders to patients. Finally, practicing orthopedic surgeons, particularly those in sub-specialties of orthopedics, will find the book a helpful resource in reassuring them that their treatment in areas outside their sub-specialty interest is current and up-to-date.

ORGANIZATION

The book is structured similarly to the structure of orthopedic surgery. Natural sub-specialization has occurred in orthopedic surgery over the years, which has resulted in some overlap in anatomic areas. This has resulted in the book having some overlap and some artificial division of subjects. Because of the primarily sub-specialization structure, the reader is encouraged to read entire chapters, or for more discrete topics, go directly to the index for information. For example, the house officer rotating on the pediatric orthopedic service would find reading the pediatric chapter to be a prudent method of developing a baseline knowledge in pediatric orthopedic surgery. Knee problems however, might be best approached by looking in the sports medicine chapter, or in the adult reconstruction chapter, since these areas overlap, mostly in age of patient.

The first chapter serves as a basis for the rest of the book because it summarizes current basic information that is fundamental in the understanding of orthopedic surgery. Chapter Two introduces aspects of interest in the perioper-

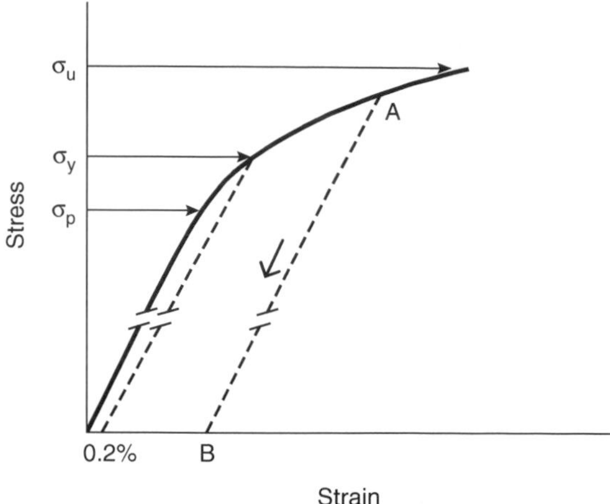

Figure 1–1. A generalized stress–strain diagram illustrating the mechanical properties of a material subjected to stress. The proportional limit (σ_p) of a material is the stress at which permanent or plastic deformation begins. Because the proportional limit is difficult to measure accurately for some materials, a 0.2% strain offset line parallel to the linear region of the curve is constructed. The stress corresponding to this line is defined as the yield stress (σ_y). If stress is removed after the initiation of plastic deformation (point A), only the elastic deformation denoted by the linear portion of the stress–strain curve is recovered. The ultimate tensile strength (σ_u) is the maximal stress that a material can withstand in a single application before it fails.

discussions pertain to the stress–strain curve, although differing terminology in the load-elongation curve is noted parenthetically.

The initial linear or elastic portion of the stress–strain curve (see Figure 1–1) depicts the amount of stress a material can withstand before permanently deforming. The slope of this line is termed the **modulus of elasticity** (stiffness) of the material. A high modulus of elasticity indicates that the material is difficult to deform, whereas a low modulus indicates that the material is more pliable. The modulus of elasticity is an excellent basis on which different materials can be compared. When materials such as those used in implants are compared, however, it is important to remember that the modulus of elasticity is a property only of the material itself and not of the structure. Implant stiffness in bending—or, more correctly, flexural rigidity—is a function both of material elastic modulus and of design geometry.

The **proportional limit,** or σ_p, of a material is the stress at which permanent or plastic deformation begins. The proportional limit, however, is difficult to measure accurately for some materials. Therefore, a 0.2% strain offset line parallel to the linear region of the curve is constructed, as shown in Figure 1–1. The stress corresponding to this line is defined as the **yield stress,** or σ_y. If stress is removed after the initiation of plastic deformation (point A in Figure 1–1), only the elastic deformation denoted by the linear portion of the stress–strain curve is recovered. The **ultimate tensile strength** (failure load), or σ_u, is the maximal stress that a material can withstand in a single application before it fails.

When subjected to repeated loading in a physiologic environment, a material may fail at stresses well below the ultimate tensile strength. The **fatigue curve,** or **S-N curve,** demonstrates the behavior of a metal during cyclic loading and is shown in Figure 1–2. Generally, as the number of cycles (**N**) increases, the amount of applied stress (**S**) that the metal can withstand before failure decreases. The **endurance limit** of a material is the maximal stress below which fatigue failure will never occur regardless of the number of cycles. Fatigue failure will occur if the combination of local peak stresses and number of loading cycles at that stress are excessive. Although most materials exhibit a lower stress at failure with cyclic loading, some do not, such as pyrolytic carbon, making it appropriate for high-cycle applications such as heart valves. Environmental conditions strongly influence fatigue behavior. The physiologic environment, which is corrosive, can significantly reduce the number of cycles to failure and the endurance limit of a material.

Materials can be evaluated in terms of ductility, toughness, viscoelasticity, friction, lubrication, and wear.

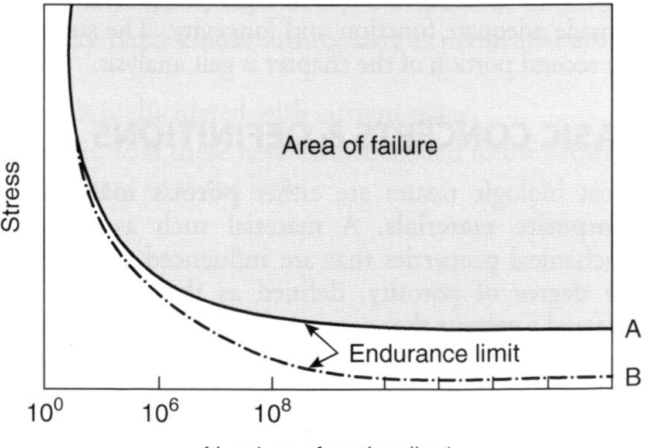

Figure 1–2. A generalized diagram comparing two fatigue curves, or S-N curves, for the same material. Curve A illustrates the material's endurance limit in a noncorrosive environment, and curve B illustrates its endurance limit in a corrosive environment. The body is an example of a corrosive environment for implant materials.

These properties are introduced here, and many of them are explored in detail in subsequent sections.

Ductility is defined as the amount of deformation that a material undergoes before failure and is characterized in terms of total strain. A brittle material will fail with minimal strain caused by propagation of a crack because the yield stress is higher than the tensile stress. A ductile material, however, will fail only after markedly increased strain and decreased cross-sectional area. Polymethylmethacrylate (PMMA, a polymer) and ceramics are brittle materials, whereas metals exhibit relatively more ductility. Environmental conditions, especially changes in temperature, can alter the ductility of materials.

Toughness is defined as the energy imparted to a material to cause it to fracture and is measured by the total area under the stress–strain curve.

Because all biologic tissues are viscoelastic in nature, a thorough understanding of **viscoelasticity** is essential. A viscoelastic material is one that exhibits different properties when loaded at different strain rates. Thus, its mechanical properties are time-dependent. Bone, for example, absorbs more energy at fast loading rates, such as in high-speed motor vehicle accidents, than at slow loading rates, such as in recreational snow skiing.

Viscoelastic materials have three important properties: hysteresis, creep, and stress relaxation. When a viscoelastic material is subjected to cyclic loading, the stress–strain relationship during the loading process differs from that during the unloading process (Figure 1–3). This difference in stress–strain response is termed **hysteresis.** The deviation between loading and unloading processes depends on the degree of viscous behavior. The area between the two curves is a measure of the energy lost by internal friction during the loading process. **Creep,** which is also called **cold flow** and observed in polyethylene components, is defined as a deformation that occurs in a material under constant stress. Some deformation is permanent, persisting even when the stress is released. The decrease in stress associated with a constant strain over time is a result of **stress relaxation,** a phenomenon evident, for example, in the loosening of fracture fixation plates. The time necessary to attain creep, or stress relaxation equilibrium, is an inherent property of the material.

Friction refers to the resistance between two bodies when one slides over the other. Friction is greatest at slow rates and decreases with faster rates. This is because the surface asperities (peaks) tend to adhere to one another more strongly at slower rates. Mechanisms of **lubrication** reduce the friction between two surfaces. Several lubrication mechanisms are present in articular cartilage to overcome friction processes in normal joint motion. Similarly, mechanisms are present in polyethylene-metal articulations to overcome friction in joint replacements.

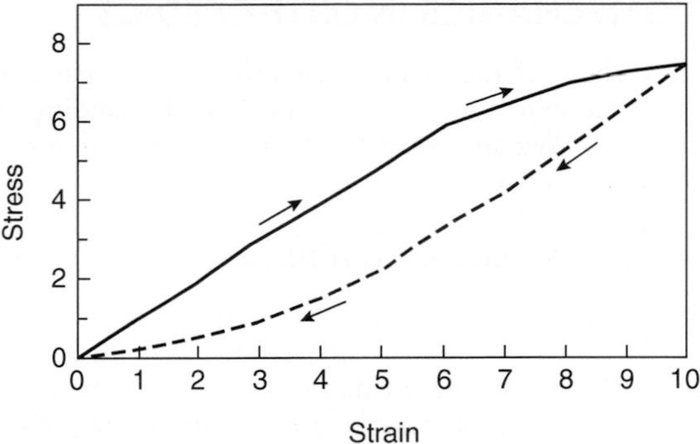

Figure 1–3. When a viscoelastic material is subjected to cyclic loading, the stress–strain curve during the loading process (solid lines) differs from that during the unloading process (dotted lines). This difference in stress–strain response is called **hysteresis.** The area between the two curves is a measure of the energy lost by internal friction during the loading process.

Wear can occur from friction and is defined as the removal of surface material by mechanical motion. Wear is always observed between two moving surfaces, but lubrication mechanisms act to reduce the detrimental effects of excessive wear. Three types of wear mechanisms are apparent in normal and prosthetic joint motion: abrasive, adhesive, and three-body wear. **Abrasive wear** is the generation of material particles from a softer surface when it moves against a rougher, harder surface. An example of the product of abrasive wear is sawdust, which results from the movement of sandpaper against a wood surface. The amount of wear depends on factors such as contact stress, hardness, and finish of the bearing surfaces.

Adhesive wear results when a thin film of material is transferred from one bearing surface to the other. In prosthetic joints, the transfer film can be either polyethylene or the passivated (corrosion-resistant) layer of metal. Regardless of the material, wear occurs in the surface that loses the transfer film. If the particles from the transfer film are shed from the other surface as well, they behave as a third body and also result in wear.

Three-body wear occurs when another particle is located between two bearing surfaces. Cement particles act as third bodies in prosthetic joints. Implant designers continue to search for compatible substances that reduce friction at articulating surfaces and thereby reduce the amount of wear debris generated. Wear of polyethylene is the dominant problem in total joint replacement today because the wear debris generated is biologically active and leads to osteolysis.

BIOMECHANICS IN ORTHOPEDICS

An analysis of the factors that influence normal and prosthetic joint function requires an understanding of free-body diagrams as well as the concepts of force, moment, and equilibrium.

Force, Moment, & Equilibrium

Forces and moments are vector quantities—that is, they are described by point of application, magnitude, and direction. A force represents the action of one body on another. The action may be applied directly (eg, via a push or a pull) or from a distance (eg, via gravity). A normal tensile or compressive force is applied perpendicular to a surface, whereas a shear force is applied parallel to a surface. A force that is applied eccentrically produces a moment.

The force generated by gravity on an object acts at the center of gravity. An object that is symmetric has its center of gravity in the geometrically centered position, whereas an object that is asymmetric has its center of gravity closer to its "heavier" end. The center of gravity for the human body is the resultant of the individual centers of gravity from each segment of the body. Therefore, as the body segments move, the center of gravity changes accordingly and may even lie outside the body in extreme positions, such as encountered in gymnastics. A moment is defined as the product of the quantity of force and the perpendicular distance between the line of action of the force and the center of rotation. A moment usually results in a rotation of the object about a fixed axis.

Newton's first law states that a body (or object) is in equilibrium if the sum of the forces and moments acting on the body are balanced; therefore, the sum of forces and moments for each direction must equal zero. The concept of equilibrium is important in understanding and determining force–body interactions, such as the increased joint reaction force occurring in an extended arm because of an external weight and such as the increased joint reaction force occurring in the hip at a specific moment during walking.

Free-Body Diagrams

A free-body diagram can be used schematically to represent all the forces and moments acting on a joint. The concepts of equilibrium can be extended to determine joint reaction or muscle forces for different conditions, as demonstrated in the following two examples.

Example 1: Determine the force on the abductor muscle of a person's hip joint (the abductor force, or F_{AB}) and the joint reaction force (the F_J) when the person is standing on one leg. The weight of the trunk,

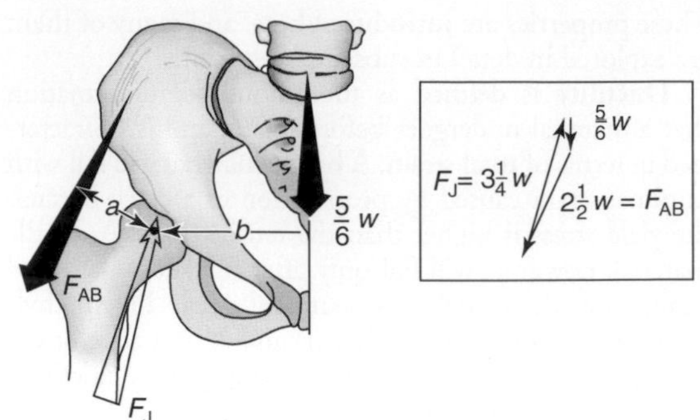

Figure 1–4. A free body diagram and force triangle illustrating the method for determining the force of the abductor muscle of a person's hip joint (F_{AB}) and the joint reaction force (F_J) when the person is standing on one leg and the total weight (w) of the person is known. See the discussion of example 1 in the text.

both arms, and one leg is 5/6 of the total weight (w) of the person. As illustrated in Figure 1–4, this weight will tend to rotate the body about the femoral head and is counteracted by the pull of the abductor muscles on the pelvis. The necessary equation to solve for F_{AB} is as follows:

$$F_{AB} \times a = \frac{B}{nw} \times b$$

In solving the equation, assume that a = 5 cm and that b = 15 cm.

After this equation is solved, two of the three forces are known. The remaining force (the F_J) can be determined from a force triangle (see Figure 1–4) because, according to Newton's first law, the sum of forces must equal zero.

Example 2: Determine the force on a person's deltoid muscle (the deltoid force, or F_D) and the force of the joint acting about the shoulder (F_J) when the person holds a metal weight (w) at arm's length (Figure 1–5). The weight of the arm is ignored because only the increase in forces about the shoulder caused by the metal weight is to be determined. F_D is determined by summing the moments about the joint center. The necessary equation is as follows:

$$F_D \times a = w \times b$$

In solving the equation, assume that a = 5 cm and that b = 60 cm.

After this equation is solved, an F_J of 1150 N is determined using a force triangle (see Figure 1–5).

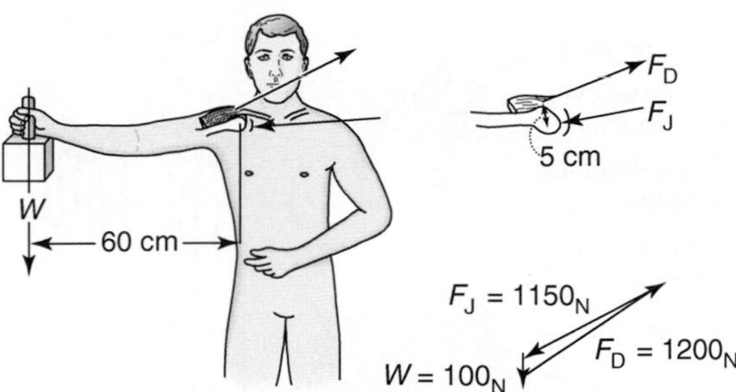

Figure 1–5. A free body diagram and force triangle illustrating the method for determining the force of a person's deltoid muscle (F_D) and the force of the joint acting about the shoulder (F_J) when the person holds a metal weight (w) at arm's length. See the discussion of example 2 in the text.

Moments of Inertia

The orientation of the bone's or implant's cross-sectional area with respect to the applied principal load also greatly influences the biomechanical performance. Bending and torsion occur in long bones and are important considerations in the design of implants. In general, the farther that material mass is distributed from the axis of bending or torsion while still retaining structural integrity, the more resistant the structure will be to bending or torsion. The **area moment of inertia** is a mathematical expression for resistance to bending, and the **polar moment of inertia** is a mathematical expression for resistance to torsion. Both types of moment of inertia relate the cross-sectional geometry and orientation of the object with respect to the applied axial load. The larger the area moment of inertia or the polar moment of inertia, the less likely the material will fail. Figure 1–6 summarizes the area moments of inertia for representative shapes important to orthopedic surgery. Creating an open slot in an object will significantly decrease the polar moment of inertia of the object.

Knowledge of moments of inertia is important for understanding mechanical behavior in relation to object geometry. For instance, the length of the long bones predisposes them to high bending moments. Their tubular shape helps them resist bending in all directions, however. This resistance to bending is attributable to the large area moment of inertia because the majority of bone tissue is distributed away from the neutral axis. The concept of moment of inertia is crucial in the design of implants that are exposed to excessive bending and torsional stresses.

Hills BA: Boundary lubrication in vivo. Proc Inst Mech Eng [H] 2000;214:83. [PMID: 10718053]

BIOLOGIC TISSUES IN ORTHOPEDICS

The functions of the musculoskeletal system are to provide support for the body, to protect the vital organs, and to facilitate easy movement of joints. The bone, articular cartilage, tendon, ligament, nerve, and muscle all interact to fulfill these functions. The musculoskeletal tissues are integrally specialized to perform their duties and have excellent regenerative and reparative processes. They also adapt and undergo compositional changes in response to increased or decreased stress states. Specialized components of the musculoskeletal system, such as the intervertebral disk, are particularly suited for supporting large stress loads while resisting movement.

Bones

Bones are dynamic tissues that serve a variety of functions and have the ability to remodel to changes in internal and external stimuli. Bones provide support for the trunk and extremities, provide attachment to ligaments and tendons, protect vital organs, and act as a mineral and iron reservoir for the maintenance of homeostasis.

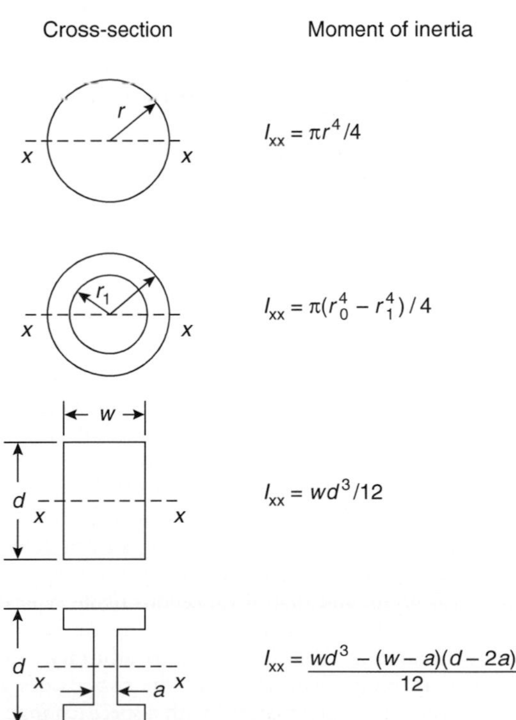

Figure 1–6. Summary of the area moments of inertia for representative shapes important to orthopedic surgery.

A. Structural Composition

Bone is a composite consisting of two types of material. The first material is an organic extracellular matrix that contains collagen, accounts for approximately 30–35% of the dry weight of bone, and is responsible for providing flexibility and resilience to the bone. The second material consists primarily of calcium and phosphorous salts, especially hydroxyapatite [$Ca_{10}(PO_4)_6(OH)_2$], accounts for approximately 65–70% of the dry weight of bone, and contributes to the hardness and rigidity of the bone. Microscopically, bone can be classified as either woven or lamellar.

Woven bone, which is also called **primary bone,** is characterized by a random arrangement of cells and collagen. Because of its relatively disoriented composition, woven bone demonstrates isotropic mechanical characteristics, with similar properties observed regardless of the direction of applied stress. Woven bone is associated with periods of rapid formation, such as the initial stages of fracture repair or biologic implant fixation. Woven bone, which has a low mineral content, remodels to lamellar bone.

Lamellar bone is a slower forming, mature bone that is characterized by an orderly cellular distribution and regular orientation of collagen fibers (Figure 1–7). The lamellae can be parallel to one another or concentrically organized around a vascular canal called a **Haversian system** or **osteon.** At the periphery of each osteon is a cement line, a narrow area containing ground substance primarily composed of glycosaminoglycans. Neither the canaliculi nor the collagen fibers cross the cement line. Biomechanically, the cement line is the weakest link in the microstructure of bone. The organized structure of lamellar bone makes it anisotropic, as seen in the fact that it is stronger during axial loading than it is during transverse, or shear, loading.

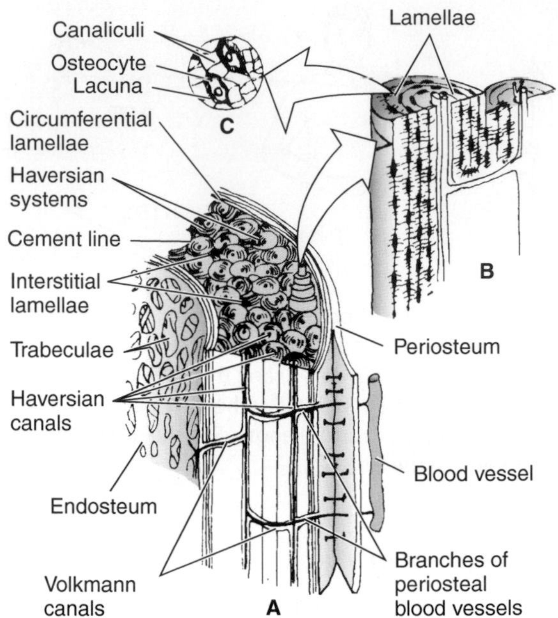

Figure 1–7. The structure of bone. **A:** A section of the diaphysis of a long bone, depicted without inner marrow. Each osteon is bounded by a cement line. **B:** Each osteon consists of lamellae, concentric rings composed of mineral matrix surrounding the Haversian canal. **C:** Along the boundaries of the lamellae are small cavities known as lacunae, each of which contains a single osteocyte. Radiating from the lacunae are tiny canals, or canaliculi, into which the cytoplasmic processes of the osteocytes extend. (Reproduced, with permission, from Nordin M, Frankel VH: Biomechanics of bone. In: Nordin M, Frankel VH, eds: *Basic Biomechanics of the Musculoskeletal System.* Lea & Febiger, 1989.)

Bone can be classified macroscopically as cortical tissue and cancellous (trabecular) tissue. Both types are morphologically lamellar bone. Cortical tissue relies on osteons for cell communication. Because trabecular width is small, however, the canaliculi can communicate directly with blood vessels in the medullary canal. The basic differences between cortical tissue and cancellous tissue relate to porosity and apparent density. The porosity of cortical tissue typically ranges from 5% to 30%, and that of cancellous tissue ranges from 30% to 90%. The apparent density of cortical tissue is approximately 1.8 g/cm, and that of cancellous tissue typically ranges from 0.1 to 1.0 g/cm. The distinction between cortical tissue and cancellous tissue is arbitrary, however, and in biomechanical terms, the two tissues are often considered as one material with a specific range in porosity and density.

The organization of cortical and cancellous tissue in bone allows for adaptation to function. Cortical tissue always surrounds cancellous tissue, but the relative quantity of each type of tissue varies with the functional requirements of the bone. In long bones, the cortical tissue of the diaphysis is arranged as a hollow cylinder to best resist bending. The metaphyseal region of the long bones flares to increase the bone volume and surface area in a manner that minimizes the stress of joint contact. The cancellous tissue in this region provides an intricate network that distributes weight-bearing forces and joint reaction forces into the bulk of the bone tissue.

B. Biomechanical Behavior

The mechanical properties of cortical bone differ from those of cancellous bone. Cortical bone is stiffer than cancellous bone. Cortical bone fractures in vivo when the strain exceeds 2%, but cancellous bone does not until the strain exceeds 75%. The larger capacity for energy storage (area under the stress–strain curve) of cancellous bone is a function of porosity. Despite different stiffness values for cortical and cancellous bone, the following axiom is valid for all bone tissue: Because the compressive strength of the tissue is proportional to the square of the apparent density, and the elastic modulus or material stiffness of the tissue is proportional to the cube of the apparent density, any increase in porosity, as occurs with aging, will decrease the apparent density of bone, which, in turn, will decrease the compressive strength and elastic modulus of bone.

Variations in the strength and stiffness of bone also result from specimen orientation (longitudinal versus transverse) and loading configuration (tensile, compressive, or shear). Generally, the strength and stiffness of bone are greatest in the direction of the common load application (longitudinally for long bones). With regard to orientation, cortical bone (Figure 1–8) is strongest in the longitudinal direction. With regard to loading configuration, cortical bone is strongest in compression and weakest in shear.

Tensile loading is the application of equal and opposite forces (loads) outward from the surface. Maximal stresses are in a plane perpendicular to the load application and result in elongation of the material. Microscopic studies show that the tensile failure in bones with Haversian systems is caused by debonding of the cement lines and pullout of the osteons. Bones with a large percentage of cancellous tissue demonstrate trabecular fracture with tensile loading.

The converse of tensile loading is **compressive loading,** which is defined as the application of equal and opposite forces toward the surface. Under compression, a material shortens and widens. Microscopic studies show that compressive failure occurs by oblique cracking of the osteons in cortical bone and of the trabeculae in cancellous bone. Vertebral fractures, especially associated with osteoporosis, are associated with compressive loading.

The application of either a tensile load or a compressive load produces a shear stress in the material. **Shear loading** is the application of a load parallel to a surface, and the deformation is angular. Clinical studies show that shear fractures are most common to regions with a large percentage of cancellous bone, such as the tibial plateau.

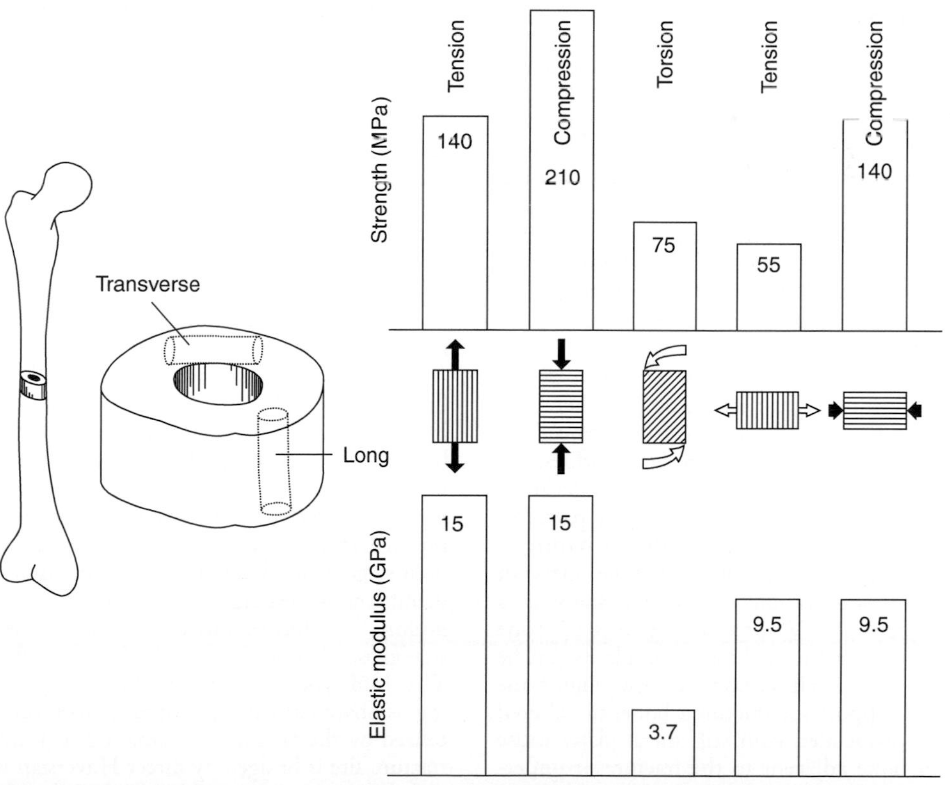

Figure 1–8. The effects of specimen orientation and loading configuration on the strength and elastic modulus of cortical bone from the diaphyseal region of a long bone.

Bone is a viscoelastic material, and its mechanical behavior is therefore influenced by strain rate. Bones are approximately 50% stiffer at high strain rates than at low strain rates, and the load to failure nearly doubles at high strain rates. The result is a doubling of the stored energy at high strain rates. Clinical studies show that the loading rate influences the fracture pattern and the associated soft-tissue damage. Low strain rates, characterized by little stored energy, result in undisplaced fractures and no associated soft-tissue damage. High strain rates, however, are associated with massive damage to the bone and soft tissue owing to the marked increase in stored energy.

Bone fractures can be produced either from a single load that exceeds the ultimate tensile strength of the bone or from repeated loading that leads to fatigue failure. Because bone is self-repairing, fatigue fracture occurs only when the rate of microdamage resulting from repeated loading exceeds the intrinsic repair rate of the bone. Fatigue fractures are most common during strenuous activity when the muscles have become fatigued and are therefore unable to store energy adequately and absorb the stress imposed on the bone. When the muscles are fatigued, the bone is required to carry the increased stress.

C. Remodeling Mechanisms

Bone has the ability to alter its size, shape, and structure in response to mechanical demands. According to Wolff's law regarding bone remodeling in response to stress, bone resorption occurs with decreased stress, bone hypertrophy occurs with increased stress, and the planes of increased stress follow the principal trabecular orientation. Thus, bone remodeling occurs under a variety of circumstances that alter the normal stress patterns. Clinically, altered stress patterns resulting from fixation devices or joint prostheses have caused concern about effects on the long-term bone architecture.

Bone mass and body weight are positively correlated, especially for weight-bearing bones. Therefore, immobilization or weightlessness (as experienced by astronauts) decreases the strength and stiffness of bone. The subsequent loss in bone mass results from the alteration or absence of normal stress patterns. Bone mass, however, is regained with the return of normal stress patterns. The loss of bone mass in response to immobilization or weightlessness is a direct consequence of Wolff's law. Associated bone resorption in response to orthopedic implants can be deleterious to bone healing, however. Although bone plates provide support for fractured bone, the altered stress patterns associated with stiff metal plates cause resorption of bone adjacent to the fracture or underneath the plate. Therefore, removal of the plate may precipitate another fracture. Resorption of bone is also reported in total hip and knee replacements. This is particularly common with larger diameter noncemented femoral stems, which have an increased moment of inertia and thus have less flexibility than do smaller diameter cemented stems.

The resorption of bone in response to a stiff implant, which alters the stress pattern the bone carries, is termed **stress shielding.** The degree of stress shielding does not depend on the absolute flexibility of the prosthesis but, rather, on the amount of reduced flexibility in the implant in relation to the flexibility of the bone. Clinically, stress shielding could also be detrimental to the longevity of implant fixation. In an effort to reduce stress shielding, designers of implants are using materials with a degree of flexural rigidity that approximates the flexibility of bone.

D. Healing Mechanisms

The fracture healing process involves five stages: impact, inflammation, soft callus formation, hard callus formation, and remodeling. Impact begins with the initiation of the fracture and continues until energy has completely dissipated. The inflammation stage is characterized by hematoma formation at the fracture site, bone necrosis at the ends of the fragments, and an inflammatory infiltrate. Granulation tissue gradually replaces the hematoma, fibroblasts produce collagen, and osteoclasts begin to remove necrotic bone. The subsidence of pain and swelling marks the initiation of the third, or soft callus, stage. This stage is characterized by increased vascularity and abundant new cartilage formation. The end of the soft callus stage is associated with fibrous or cartilaginous tissue uniting the fragments. During the fourth, or hard callus, stage, the callus converts to woven bone and appears clinically healed. The final stage of the healing process involves slow remodeling from woven to lamellar bone and reconstruction of the medullary canal.

Three types of fracture healing are described. The first type, endochondral fracture healing, is characterized by an initial phase of cartilage formation, followed by the formation of new bone on the calcified cartilage template. The second type, membranous fracture healing, is characterized by bone formation from direct mesenchymal tissue without an intervening cartilaginous stage. Combinations of endochondral healing and membranous healing are typical of normal fracture healing. The former process is observed between fracture gaps, whereas the latter is observed subperiosteally. The third type of fracture healing, primary bone healing, is observed with rigid internal fixation and characterized by the absence of visible callus formation. The fracture site is bridged by direct Haversian remodeling, and there are no discernible histologic stages of inflammation or soft and hard callus formation.

Articular Cartilage

Articular cartilage is primarily avascular and has an abnormally small cellular density. The chief functions of articular cartilage are to distribute joint loads over a large area and to allow relative movement of the joint surfaces with minimal friction and wear.

A. Structural Composition

Articular cartilage is composed of chondrocytes and an organic matrix. The chondrocytes account for less than 10% of the tissue volume, and they manufacture, secrete, and maintain the organic component of the cellular matrix. The organic matrix is a dense network of type II collagen in a concentrated proteoglycan solution. Collagen accounts for 10–30% of the organic matrix; proteoglycan accounts for 3–10%; and water, inorganic salts, and matrix proteins account for the remaining 60–87%.

The basic collagen unit consists of tropocollagen molecules, which form covalent cross-links between collagen molecules to increase the tensile strength of the fibrils. The most important mechanical properties of the collagen fiber are tensile strength and stiffness. Fiber resistance to compression is relatively ineffective because the large ratio of length to diameter (slenderness ratio) predisposes the fibers to buckling. The anisotropic nature of cartilage is thought to be related to several factors, including variations in fiber arrangements within the planes parallel to the articular surface, the collagen fiber cross-link density, and the collagen–proteoglycan interactions.

The mechanical properties of the cartilage are attributed to the inhomogeneous distribution of collagen fibrils (Figure 1–9). The superficial tangential zone contains sheets of fine, densely packed collagen fibers that are randomly woven in planes parallel to the articular surface. The middle zone contains randomly oriented and homogeneously dispersed fibers that are widely spaced to account for increased matrix content. Finally, the deep zone contains larger, radially oriented collagen fiber bundles that eventually cross the tidemark, enter the calcified cartilage, and anchor the tissue to the underlying bone.

Proteoglycans are monomers that consist of a protein core with glycosaminoglycan units (either keratan sulfate or chondroitin sulfate units) covalently bound to the core. Proteoglycan aggregation promotes immobilization of the proteoglycans within the collagen network and adds structural rigidity to the matrix. There are numerous age-related changes in the structure and composition of the proteoglycan matrix, including the following: a decrease in proteoglycan content from approximately 7% at birth to half that by adulthood, an increase in protein content with maturity, a dramatic drop in the ratio of chondroitin sulfate to keratan sulfate with aging, and a decrease in water content as proteoglycan subunits become smaller with aging. The overall effect is that the cartilage stiffens. The development of osteoarthritis is associated with dramatic changes in cartilage metabolism. Initially, there is increased proteoglycan synthesis, and the water content of osteoarthritic cartilage is actually increased.

The water content of normal cartilage permits the diffusion of gases, nutrients, and waste products between the chondrocytes and the nutrient-rich synovial fluid. The water is primarily concentrated (80%) near the articular surface and decreases in a linear fashion with increasing depth, such that the deep zone is 65% water. The location and movement of water are important in controlling mechanical function and lubrication properties of the cartilage.

Zones

Superficial tangential (10–20%)

Middle (40–60%)

Deep (30%)

Calcified cartilage

Articular surface

Tidemark

Subchondral bone

Cancellous bone

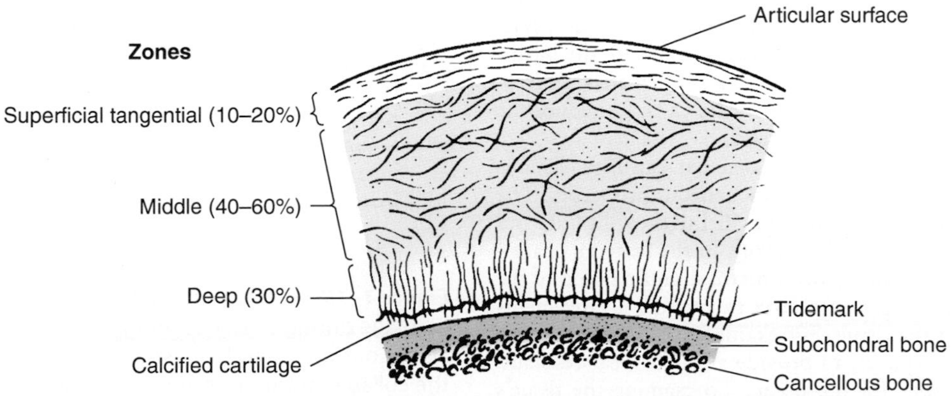

Figure 1–9. **Orientation of the collagen fiber network in the three zones of the articular cartilage.** (Modified and reproduced, with permission, from Mow VC et al: Biomechanics of articular cartilage. In: Nordin M, Frankel VH, eds: *Basic Biomechanics of the Musculoskeletal System.* Lea & Febiger, 1989.)

Important structural interactions occur between proteoglycans and collagen fibers in cartilage. A small percentage of the proteoglycans may serve as a bonding agent between the collagen fibrils that span distances too great for the maintenance or formation of cross-links. These structural interactions are thought to provide strong mechanical interactions. In essence, the proteoglycans and collagen fibers interact to form a porous, composite, fiber-reinforced matrix, possessing all the essential mechanical characteristics of a solid that is swollen with water and able to resist the stresses and strains of joint lubrication.

B. Biomechanical Behavior

The biomechanical behavior of articular cartilage is best understood when the cartilage is considered as a viscoelastic and composite material consisting of a fluid phase and a solid phase. The compressive behavior of cartilage is primarily caused by the flow of interstitial fluid, whereas the shear behavior of cartilage is primarily caused by the motion of collagen fibers and proteoglycans. The creep behavior of cartilage is characterized by the exudation of interstitial fluid, which occurs with compressive loading. The applied surface load is balanced by the compressive stress developed within the collagen–proteoglycan matrix and the frictional drag generated by the flow of the interstitial fluid during exudation. Typically, human cartilage takes 4–16 hours to reach creep equilibrium, and the amount of creep is inversely proportional to the square of the tissue thickness.

Similar to creep, stress relaxation is the response of the tissue to compressive forces on the articular surface. An initial compressive phase, characterized by increased stress, is associated with fluid exudation. In the subsequent relaxation phase, stress decay is associated with fluid redistribution within the porous collagen–proteoglycan matrix. The rate of stress relaxation is used to determine the permeability coefficient of the tissue, and the equilibrium stress is used to measure the intrinsic compressive modulus of the solid matrix. Microstructural changes in osteoarthritic cartilage reduce the compressive stiffness of cartilage.

Under uniaxial tension, articular cartilage demonstrates anisotropic and inhomogeneous properties. The tissue is stronger and stiffer parallel to the split lines and in superficial regions. Variations in the material characteristics are a result of the structural organization of the collagen–proteoglycan matrix in layering arrangements throughout the tissue. For example, the superficial tangential zone appears to provide a tough, wear-resistant, protective zone for the tissue. To examine the tissue's intrinsic response to tension, the biphasic viscoelastic effects of the tissue must be negated. This can be achieved by testing the tissue at low strain rates or by performing incremental testing and allowing for stress relaxation equilibrium to be achieved before continuing. The tissue tends to stiffen with increasing strain. Typically, specimens are pulled to the failure point at a displacement rate of 0.5 cm/min.

The shape of the stress–strain curve (Figure 1–10) can be described in morphologic changes of the collagen fibers: (1) the toe region designates collagen fiber pullout, (2) the linear region designates stretching of the aligned collagen fibers, and (3) failure is the point at which all of the collagen fibers have ruptured. The tensile properties of the tissue are thus changed by an alteration of the molecular structure of collagen, an alteration in the organization of the fibers within the collagenous network, or a change in collagen fiber cross-linking. For this reason, disruption of the collagen network may be a key factor in the initial development of osteoarthritis.

When the cartilage is tested in pure shear under infinitesimal strain conditions, no pressure gradients or volume changes are observed within the tissue as they are during tension or compression conditions. Thus, the viscoelastic shear properties of cartilage can be determined in a steady-state dynamic shear experiment. Cartilage shear stiffness is a function of collagen content or collagen–proteoglycan interaction. Increased collagen content reduces frictional dissipation of the load, and this in turn results in increased shear loading.

C. Lubrication Mechanisms

Sophisticated lubrication processes are responsible for the minimal wear of normal cartilage under large and

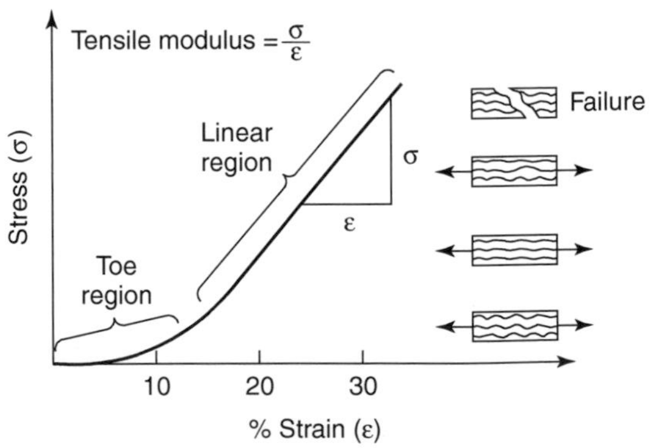

Figure 1–10. A stress–strain diagram for articular cartilage during tensile loading. The schematic representations on the right illustrate the orientation of the collagen fibrils in response to loading. (Reproduced, with permission, from Mow VC et al: Biomechanics of articular cartilage. In Nordin M, Frankel VH, eds: *Basic Biomechanics of the Musculoskeletal System.* Lea & Febiger, 1989.)

varied joint stresses. Four types of lubrication mechanisms are related to articular cartilage: boundary, fluid film, mixed, and self-lubrication. These mechanisms are inherent properties of the composition of the tissue with respect to water content and collagen–proteoglycan matrix orientation. Normal joints display all of the lubrication mechanisms just mentioned, whereas artificial joints are thought primarily to display elastohydrodynamic and boundary lubrication mechanisms.

The boundary mechanism protects the joint from surface-to-surface wear by means of an adsorbed lubricant. This mechanism, which depends chiefly on the chemical properties of the lubricant, is most important under severe loading conditions when contact surfaces must sustain high loads.

The fluid film mechanism relies on a thin layer of lubricant that causes greater surface separation. The load on the joint surface is supported by the pressure on the film. Fluid film lubrication occurs with rigid (squeeze-film or hydrodynamic) bodies as well as with deformable (elastohydrodynamic) bodies. When two rigid surfaces are nonparallel and move tangentially with respect to each other, the pressure generated by the lubricant in the gap between the two surfaces is sufficient to raise one surface above the other. Moreover, when two rigid surfaces are parallel and move perpendicular to each other, the pressure generated by the lubricant is sufficient to keep the surfaces separated. This squeeze-film or hydrodynamic lubrication mechanism is able to carry high loads for short durations. When the squeeze-film mechanism generates a pressure great enough to deform the surface and thereby increase the amount of bearing surface area, elastohydrodynamic lubrication mechanisms begin to make the necessary adjustments. Increased bearing surface area allows less lubricant to escape from between the surfaces, decreasing the stress and increasing the duration associated with motion.

The mixed lubrication mechanism is a combination of the boundary and fluid film mechanisms. Boundary lubrication is essential in areas of asperity contact, and fluid film lubrication is present in areas of no contact. Therefore, most of the friction is generated in the boundary lubricated areas, whereas most of the load is carried by the fluid film.

Self-lubrication, or weeping, relies on the exudation of fluid in front of and beneath the surface of the rotating joint. Once the area of peak stress passes a given point, the cartilage reabsorbs the fluid and returns to its original dimensions. This lubrication mechanism results from the inhomogeneous character of the collagen and water distribution throughout the cartilage. When the pressure rises and strains are low, the tissue is most permeable and a large amount of water is exuded in front of the leading contact edge of the joint. As the joint advances, the load increases in the region of expelled fluid and the increased pressure and strains decrease the tissue permeability to fluid. This prevents the fluid on the articular surface from returning to the cartilage. As the contact surface moves past the point of contact, the pressure and strains are again low and the tissue permeability is increased, resulting in the return of fluid to the cartilage in preparation for the cycle to start again.

Synovial fluid is a key component in the lubrication process in joints. It is non-Newtonian, indicating that the resistance to flow increases more slowly than the flow of the fluid. Joint fluid in normal joints, abnormal joints, and artificial joints is different. Hence, different mechanisms of lubrication come into play in each situation with implications for joint surface damage and artificial joint wear.

D. Wear Mechanisms

Wear is the removal of material from a surface and is caused by the mechanical action of two surfaces in contact. The principal types of wear experienced in articular cartilage are interface wear and fatigue wear.

Interface wear occurs when bearing surfaces come into direct contact with no lubricating film separating them. This type of wear may be found in an impaired or degenerated synovial joint. When ultrastructural surface defects in articular cartilage result in softer tissue with increased permeability, the fluid from the lubricant film may easily leak through the cartilage surface, thereby increasing the probability of direct contact between asperities. There are two forms of interface wear: adhesive wear, which occurs when surface fragments adhere to one another and are torn from the surface during sliding, and abrasive wear, which occurs when a soft material is scraped by a harder one.

Fatigue wear results from the accumulation of microscopic damage within the bearing material under repetitive stress. In the cartilage, three mechanisms are primarily responsible for fatigue wear. First, repetitive stress on the collagen–proteoglycan matrix can disrupt the collagen fibers, the proteoglycan molecules, or the interface between the two. In this case, cartilage fatigue is caused by the tensile failure of the collagen network, and proteoglycan changes could be considered part of the accumulated tissue damage. Second, repetitive and massive exudation and inhibition of interstitial fluid may cause a proteoglycan washout from the cartilage matrix near the articular surface. This results in decreased stiffness and increased tissue permeability. Third, during synovial joint impact loading, insufficient time for internal fluid redistribution to relieve high stress in the compacted region may result in tissue damage.

Numerous structural defects of the articular cartilage are caused or exacerbated by wear and damage. For example, fibrillations (splitting of the articular surface) are associated with wear and will eventually extend the full thickness of the cartilage. Destructive smooth-surface thinning is apparent when layers erode rather than split. In these and other types of surface damage of the cartilage, more than a single wear mechanism is likely to be responsible.

Several biomechanical hypotheses cover cartilage degradation. Factors associated with progressive failure of the tissue include the magnitude of imposed stress, the total number of sustained stress peaks, changes in the intrinsic molecular and microscopic structure of the collagen–proteoglycan matrix, and changes in the intrinsic mechanical property of the tissue. Failure-initiating mechanisms include a loosening of the collagen network, which allows for abnormal expansion of the proteoglycan matrix and swelling of the tissue, and a decrease in cartilage stiffness, which is accompanied by an increase in tissue permeability.

Biomechanically, conditions that cause excessive stress concentrations may result in increased tissue damage or wear. Joint surface incongruity, such as the incongruity of the hip joint in patients who had Perthes disease during childhood, can result in abnormally small contact areas, which are associated with increased stress and increased tissue damage. Moreover, the presence of high contact pressures between the articular surfaces, such as that seen in patients with a shallow acetabulum (acetabular dysplasia), can reduce the probability of fluid film lubrication, allow for continued tissue damage, and also increase the risk of early degenerative arthritis.

Tendons & Ligaments

Tendons and ligaments are similar both structurally and biomechanically and differ only in function. Tendons attach muscle to bone; transmit loads from the muscle to the bone, which results in joint motion; and allow the muscle belly to remain an optimal distance from the joint on which it acts. Ligaments attach bone to bone, augment mechanical stability of the joint, guide joint motion, and prevent excessive joint displacement.

A. Structural Composition

Both the tendons and the ligaments are parallel-fibered collagenous tissues that are sparsely vascularized. They contain relatively few fibroblasts (constituting approximately 20% of their volume) and an abundant extracellular matrix. The matrix consists of approximately 70% water and 30% collagen, ground substance, and elastin.

The fibroblasts secrete a precursor of collagen, procollagen, which is cleaved extracellularly to form type I collagen. Cross-links between collagen molecules provide strength to the tissue. The arrangement of the collagen fibers determines tissue function. In tendons, a parallel arrangement of the collagen fibers provides the tissues with the ability to sustain high uniaxial tensile loads. In ligaments, the nearly parallel fibers, which are intimately interlaced with one another, provide the ability to sustain loads in one predominant direction but allow for carrying small tensile loads in other directions.

Tendons and ligaments are surrounded by loose areolar connective tissue. The paratenon forms a protective sheath around the tissue and enhances gliding. At places where the tendons are subjected to large friction forces, a parietal synovial membrane is found just beneath the paratenon and additionally facilitates gliding. Each individual fiber bundle is bound by the endotenon. At the musculotendinous junction, the endotenon continues into the perimysium. At the tendoosseous junction, the collagen fibers of the endotenon continue into the bone as perforating fibers (Sharpey fibers) and become continuous with the periosteum.

Tendons and connective tissues of the musculotendinous junction help determine the mechanical characteristics of whole muscle during contraction and passive extension. The muscle cells are extensively involuted and folded at the junction to provide maximal surface area for attachment, thereby allowing for greater fixation and transmission of forces. The sarcomeres directly adjacent to the junction of fast contracting muscles are shortened in length. This may represent an adaptation to decrease the force intensity within the junction. A complex intracellular and extracellular transmitting membrane consisting of a glycoprotein links the contractile intracellular proteins to the extracellular protein connective tissue.

The tendon insertions and ligament insertions to the bone are structurally similar. The collagen fibers from the tissue intermesh with fibrocartilage. The fibrocartilage gradually becomes mineralized, and this mineralized cartilage merges with cortical bone. These transition zones produce a gradual alteration in the mechanical properties of the tissue, resulting in a decreased stress concentration effect at the insertion of the tendon or ligament to the bone.

B. Mechanical Behavior

Tendons and ligaments are viscoelastic structures that have specific mechanical properties related to their function and composition. Tendons are strong enough to sustain high tensile forces resulting from muscle contraction during joint motion, but they are also sufficiently flexible to angulate around bone surfaces, to change the final direction of muscle pull. Ligaments are pliant and flexible enough to allow natural movements of the bones they connect; however, they are strong, are

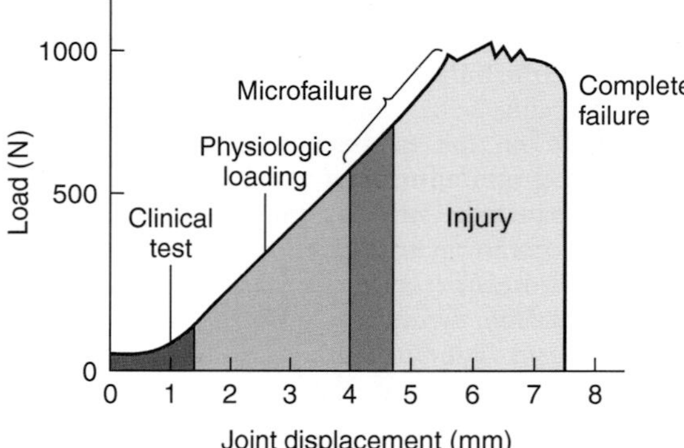

Figure 1–11. **The load-elongation curve for progressive failure of the anterior cruciate ligament.** (Reproduced, with permission, from Carlstedt CA, Nordin M: Biomechanics of tendons and ligaments. In: Nordin M, Frankel VH, eds: *Basic Biomechanics of the Musculoskeletal System.* Lea & Febiger, 1989.)

not extensible, and offer suitable resistance to applied forces and large joint movements. Because tendons and ligaments are viscoelastic structures, the injury they sustain is affected by the rate of loading as well as the amount of the stress load. The stress–strain and load-elongation curves for ligaments and tendons, like those for articular cartilage, have several regions that characterize the tissue behavior.

Figure 1–11 shows the load-elongation curve for progressive failure of the anterior cruciate ligament. Like the curve in Figure 1–10, the curve in Figure 1–11 has a toe region (correlating with the region labeled clinical test, when the anterior drawer test was administered) and a linear region preceding the failure region. In Figure 1–11, the curve in the toe region represents large elongations with small changes in load. This pattern is thought to reflect the straightening of the wavy, relaxed collagen fibers with increased loads. Within the linear region, the collagen fibers continue to become more parallel in orientation as physiologic loading proceeds. At the end of the linear region, small force reductions can be observed in the load-deformation curve. These dips are caused by the early sequential failure of a few maximally stretched fiber bundles. The final region represents major failure of fiber bundles in an unpredictable manner. Complete failure occurs rapidly, and the load-supporting ability of the tissue is substantially reduced.

The mechanical behavior characteristics of the anterior cruciate ligament differ somewhat from those of soft tissues that contain a high proportion of elastin fibers. These tissues can elongate up to 50% before stiffness markedly increases. After 50% elongation, however, the stiffness increases greatly with increased loading, and failure is abrupt with minimal further elongation. Load-elongation curves for several soft tissues are shown in Figure 1–12.

The viscoelastic behavior of ligaments is best exemplified in the bone-ligament-bone complex. Anterior

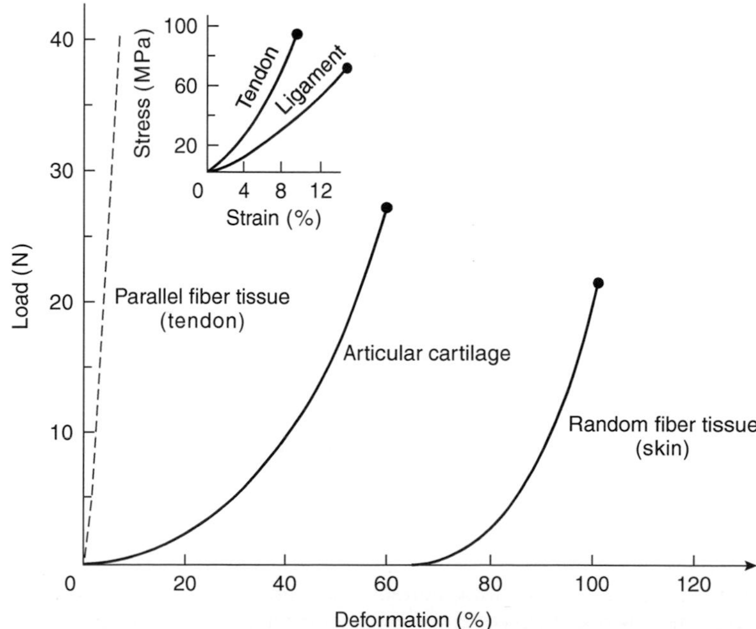

Figure 1–12. Load-elongation curves for several soft tissues. The range in mechanical properties of the tissues is attributable to collagen fiber orientation and interaction with the extracellular matrix.

cruciate ligaments in primate knee specimens were tested in tension to failure at both slow and fast loading rates to determine the viscoelastic nature of the bone-ligament-bone complex. At slow loading rates the bony insertion of the ligament was the weakest link, and an avulsion resulted. At fast loading rates, the ligament was the weakest link, and a midsubstance rupture generally was found. At slow rates, the load to failure was decreased by 20% and the stored energy was decreased by 30% in comparison with results with fast rates. The stiffness of the bone-ligament-bone complex was relatively unaffected by strain rate, however. Increased strain rates demonstrated a greater increase in strength for bone as compared with ligaments.

The mechanical properties of ligaments are closely related to the number and quality of the cross-links within the collagen fibers. Therefore, any process that affects collagen formation or maturation directly influences the properties of the ligaments. As aging continues, the number and the quality of cross-links increase, thereby increasing the tensile strength of the tissue. Moreover, the diameter of the collagen fibril increases with age. As aging progresses, however, collagen reaches a mechanical plateau, after which point tensile strength and stiffness decrease. There is also a decrease in the tissue collagen content, and this contributes to the continued decline in the mechanical properties of the tissue.

Tendons and ligaments remodel in response to mechanical demand. Physical training increases the tensile strength of the tendons and the ligament-bone interface, whereas immobilization decreases tensile strength. Even if the tissue maintains a relatively constant cross-sectional area during immobilization, the increased tissue metabolism results in proportionately more immature collagen and a decrease in the amount and quality of cross-links between molecules. Investigators who studied ligaments that were immobilized for 8 weeks and control ligaments found that the previously immobilized ligaments required 12 months of reconditioning before they demonstrated strength and stiffness values comparable to those of the control ligaments.

Studies of nonsteroidal antiinflammatory drugs (NSAIDs) such as indomethacin demonstrated that treatment results in increases in the proportion of insoluble collagen and the total collagen content in tissue. It also leads to increased tensile strength, which is probably attributable to increased collagen molecule cross-links. Therefore, short-term NSAID therapy may increase the rate of biomechanical restoration of the tendons and ligaments.

C. Injury Mechanisms

Tendons and ligaments are subjected to less than a third of their ultimate stress during normal physiologic loading. The maximal physiologic strain ranges from 2% to 5%. Several factors lead to tissue injury, however. When tendons and ligaments are subjected to stresses that exceed the physiologic range, microfailure of collagen bundles occurs before the yield point of the tissue is reached. When the yield point is reached, the tissue undergoes gross failure and the joint simultaneously becomes displaced. The amount of force produced by the maximal contraction of the muscle results in a maximal tensile stress in the tendon. The extent of tendon injury is influenced by the amount of tendon cross-sectional area compared with that for muscle. The larger the muscle cross-sectional area, the higher the magnitude of the force produced by the contraction and thus the greater the tensile load transmitted through the tendon.

Clinically, ligament injuries are characterized according to degree of severity. First-degree sprains are typified by minimal pain and demonstrate no detectable joint instability despite microfailure of collagen fibers. Second-degree sprains cause severe pain and demonstrate minimal joint instability. This instability is most likely masked by muscle activity, however. Therefore, testing must be performed with the patient under anesthesia for proper evaluation. Second-degree sprains are characterized by partial ligament rupture and progressive failure of the collagen fibers, with the result that ligament strength and stiffness decrease by 50%. Third-degree sprains cause severe pain during the course of the injury and minimal pain afterward. The joint is completely unstable. Most collagen fibers have ruptured, but a few may remain intact, giving the ligament the appearance of continuity even though it is incapable of supporting loads. Abnormally high stress on the articular cartilage results if pressure is exerted on a joint that is unstable owing to ligament or joint capsule rupture.

D. Healing Mechanisms

During tendon and ligament healing and repair, fibroblastic infiltration from the adjacent tissues is essential. The healing events are initiated by an inflammatory response, which is characterized by polymorphonuclear cell infiltration, capillary budding, and fluid exudation and continues during the first 3 days following the injury. After 4 days, fibroplasia occurs and is accompanied by the significant accumulation of fibroblasts. Within 3 weeks, a mass of granulation tissue surrounds the damaged tissue. During the next week, collagen fibers become longitudinally oriented. During the next 3 months, the individual collagen fibers form bundles identical to the original bundles.

Sutured tendons heal with a progressive penetration of connective tissue from the outside. The deposited collagen fibers become progressively oriented until eventually they form tendon fibers like the original ones. This orientation of collagen fibers is essential because the tensile strength of repaired tendon depends on collagen content and orientation. If tendon is sutured during the first 7–10 days of healing, the strength of the suture maintains the fixation until adequate callus forms.

Tendon mobilization during healing is important to avoid adhesion of the tendon to adjacent tissue, particularly in cases involving the flexor tendons of the hand. Motion can be passive to prevent adhesion and at the same time to prevent putting excessive tensile stress on the suture line. The gliding properties of flexor tendons that were mobilized are consistently superior to those of flexor tendons that were immobilized during the healing process.

Direct apposition of the surfaces of a divided ligament provides the most favorable conditions for healing because it minimizes scar formation, accelerates repair, hastens collagenization, and comes closer to restoring normal ligamentous tissue. Care must be taken during the repair of ligaments to avoid subsequent common problems with healing, however. For instance, divided and immobilized ligaments heal with a fibrous tissue gap between the two ends, whereas sutured ligaments unite without a fibrous tissue gap. If excessive tension is placed on a suture, necrosis and failure to heal are observed. Unsutured ligaments can retract, shorten, and become atrophic, however, making repair difficult 2 weeks following the injury. In spite of this, many ligaments are not routinely repaired in orthopedic surgery.

The anterior cruciate ligament is often severely damaged in cases of midsubstance rupture and generally does not fare well following repair. The ligament is intraarticular, with synovial fluid tending to disrupt the repair. Instability of the knee also tends to place excessive stress on the repair unless the knee is immobilized, which leads to joint stiffness and muscle atrophy.

Bellucci G, Seedhom BB: Tensile fatigue behaviour of articular cartilage. Biorheology 2002;39:193. [PMID: 12082282]

Ding M: Age variations in the properties of human tibial trabecular bone and cartilage. Acta Orthop Scand 2000;292:1. [PMID: 10951715]

Ding M et al: Mutual associations among microstructural, physical and mechanical properties of human cancellous bone. J Bone Joint Surg Br 2002;84:900. [PMID: 12211688]

Fung YCB: *Biomechanics: Mechanical Properties of Living Tissues.* Springer-Verlag, 1981.

Jay GD et al: Lubricating ability of aspirated synovial fluid from emergency department patients with knee joint synovitis. J Rheumatol 2004;31:557. [PMID: 14994405]

Kjaer M: Role of extracellular matrix in adaptation of tendon and skeletal muscle to mechanical loading. Physiol Rev 2004;84:649. [PMID: 15044685]

Kopperdahl DL et al: Quantitative computed tomography estimates of the mechanical properties of human vertebral trabecular bone. J Orthop Res 2002;20:801.

Mazzuco D, Spector M: The role of joint fluid in the tribology of total joint arthroplasty. Clin Orthop 2004;429:17. [PMID: 15577461]

Mountney J et al: Tensile strength of the medial patellofemoral ligament before and after repair or reconstruction. J Bone Joint Surg Br 2005;87:36. [PMID: 15686235]

Mow VC, Guo XE: Mechano-electrochemical properties of articular cartilage: Their inhomogeneities and anisotropies. Annu Rev Biomed Eng 2002;4:175. [PMID:12117756]

Musgrave DS et al: Gene therapy and tissue engineering in orthopedic surgery. J Am Acad Orthop Surg 2002;10:6. [PMID: 11809046]

Shinar H et al: Mapping the fiber orientation in articular cartilage at rest and under pressure studied by 2H double quantum filtered MRI. Magn Reson Med 2002;48:322. [PMID: 12210941]

Silva MJ et al: Recent progress in flexor tendon healing. J Orthop Sci 2002;7:508. [PMID: 12181670]

Silver FH, Bradica G, Tria A: Viscoelastic behavior of osteoarthritic cartilage. Connect Tissue Res 2001;42:223. [PMID: 11913493]

Vanwanseele B et al: Knee cartilage of spinal cord-injured patients displays progressive thinning in the absence of normal joint loading and movement. Arthritis Rheum 2002; 46:2073. [PMID: 12209511]

Wu JZ, Herzog W: Elastic anisotropy of articular cartilage is associated with the microstructures of collagen fibers and chondrocytes. J Biomech 2002;35:931. [PMID: 12052395]

Skeletal Muscle

Skeletal muscles perform a wide variety of mechanical and biologic functions. From a mechanical perspective, it is obvious that skeletal muscles generate force and length changes. The generation of force and length change gives rise to the production of mechanical work and power. Less obvious is the fact that skeletal muscles are often subjected to so-called lengthening or eccentric contractions. During these types of contractions, muscles may act as so-called dynamic joint stabilizers and may store energy. From a biologic perspective, skeletal muscles are believed to secrete various growth factors such as insulin-like growth factor 1 (IGF-1), which is thought to play an important autocrine/paracrine role in regulating muscle fiber size. Additionally, it has been proposed that skeletal muscles play a key role in maintaining the health of motor neurons.

A. Skeletal Muscle Structure

1. Macroscopic anatomy—Figure 1–13 provides both a macroscopic and microscopic perspective of the structure of skeletal muscle. From a macroscopic perspective, skeletal muscles are composed of tens of thousands of individual muscle fibers (muscle cells). Muscles that are involved in fine motor control usually contain a small number of muscle fibers compared with those muscles involved in activities requiring the generation of large forces and power outputs. Muscle fibers are usually found in so-called bundles that are also referred to as **fascicles.** Each fascicle typically contains approximately 10–30 muscle fibers that are encased in a connective tissue sheath known as the **endomysium.**

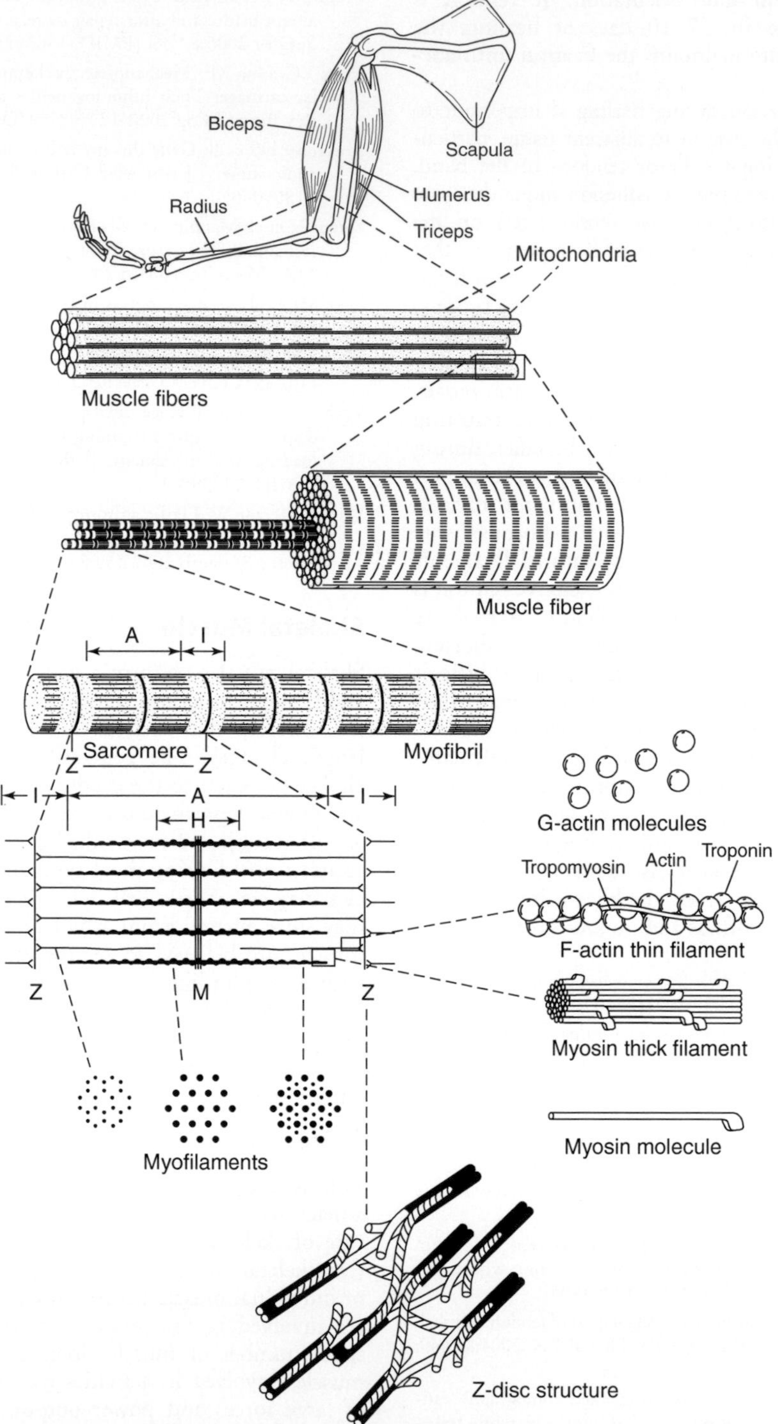

Figure 1–13. Overview of macroscopic and microscopic structure of skeletal muscle. (Reprinted, with permission, from McMahon TA: *Muscles, Reflexes, and Locomotion.* Princeton University Press, 1984.)

From an architectural perspective, muscles are often classified on the basis of the orientations of the muscle fibers' longitudinal axes relative to that of the entire muscle. For instance, **longitudinal** muscles are composed of muscle fibers whose longitudinal axis runs parallel to that of the whole muscle. Good examples of this type of architecture are the rectus abdominis and the sartorius muscles. In **fusiform** muscles, the fibers run parallel to the longitudinal axis throughout most of the muscle, but they taper at the ends of the muscle. The soleus and brachioradialis muscles are typical of this architecture. Muscles can also exhibit a so-called **pennate** (unipennate, bipennate) architecture whereby the longitudinal axis of the individual muscle fibers runs diagonal to that of the whole muscle. A good example of a bipennate muscle is the gastrocnemius muscle. The muscle fibers of **angular** or **fan-shaped** muscles radiate from a narrow attachment at one end and fan out, resulting in a broad attachment at the other end as is seen in muscles like the pectoralis major.

Consistent with the theme of structure–function relationships, muscle architecture can be an important determinant of the mechanical properties of skeletal muscle. For instance, fusiform muscles typically have longer muscle fibers than bipennate muscles. Functionally, this means that a fusiform muscle should be able to generate greater shortening velocities and muscle length excursions at the whole muscle level. In contrast, muscles with a pennate or bipennate architecture have shorter fibers, but the fibers are packed in such a manner that a larger number of muscle fibers are in parallel to one another, resulting in a larger physiologic cross-sectional area. Hence, the pennate muscle has a greater capacity for generating force.

2. Molecular anatomy of the myofibril—The structure of skeletal muscle at the molecular level is quite complex (see Figure 1–13). Each muscle fiber is made up of thousands of so-called **myofibrils** that are arranged in parallel to one another. Each myofibril has a cross-sectional area of approximately 1 μm^2. Hence, a muscle fiber with a cross-sectional area of approximately 1000 μm^2 would contain approximately 1000 myofibrils. Typically, the cross-sectional area of a muscle fiber can range from approximately 1000 to 7000 μm^2. Each myofibril consists of a repeating series of striations that are caused by the arrangement of so-called **sarcomeres** in series. Each sarcomere is approximately 2–3 μm in length. Sarcomeres are often referred to as the contractile units of skeletal muscle.

In a general sense, sarcomeres consist of Z-lines, thin filaments, and thick filaments. The interdigitation of thick and thin filaments along with the presence of Z-lines is primarily responsible for the striation pattern of skeletal muscle. As shown in Figure 1–14, the Z-lines are dense thin structures that are found in the middle of the so-called I-band. In reality, each Z-line represents an anchor point to which thin filaments are attached. By definition, the collection of proteins between each Z-line is known as a sarcomere. Hence, the I-band represents a region where no overlap occurs of the thin filaments (by thick filaments), yielding a relatively light band. The A-band is composed of the thick filament and is strongly birefringent, producing a dark band on microscopic inspection. By definition, the length of the A-band is equivalent to the length of the thick filament. Normally, the thick and thin filaments partially overlap, and as a result a lighter region occurs in the middle of the A-band known as the H-zone.

Changes in sarcomere length and, as a result, muscle fiber length are caused by the sliding of the thick and thin filaments relative to one another. In its most simplistic sense, this model states that contraction takes place not because of changes in the individual lengths of thick and thin filaments, but rather by the sliding of thin filaments past thick filaments. This model of contraction is known as the **sliding-filament hypothesis.** The changes in striation patterns during shortening contractions played a central role in developing the sliding-filament hypothesis. In this context, Table 1–1 summarizes the changes in the striation pattern that occur during isometric, shortening (isotonic), and lengthening (eccentric) contractions.

3. Molecular anatomy of the sarcomere—As shown in Figure 1–14 and in Table 1–2, the overall structure of the sarcomere became quite complex as more sophisticated techniques for studying skeletal muscle evolved. On a basic level, the sarcomeric proteins and those associated with the sarcomere can be placed into four different categories: (1) contractile; (2) regulatory contractile; (3) structural; and (4) costameric.

As shown in Table 1–2, the primary contractile proteins are simply **actin** and **myosin.** These are referred to as contractile proteins, given their central role in the contractile process. Individual monomers of actin bind to one another to form so-called actin filaments. In contrast, the thick filament is composed primarily of myosin heavy-chain molecules packed in an antiparallel arrangement. A more detailed description of myosin is provided later. Regulatory contractile proteins are defined as those that turn the contractile apparatus on or off and those that can modulate the activity of the myosin heavy chain. In skeletal muscle, the regulatory contractile proteins involved in turning the contractile apparatus on or off are associated exclusively with the actin filament, and these proteins include **tropomyosin, troponin-T, troponin-I,** and **troponin-C.** Collectively, the thin filament is composed of the actin filament and these (ie, tropomyosin, troponin-T, troponin-I, and troponin-C) regulatory contractile proteins. Other regulatory contractile proteins are associated with the myosin heavy chain, and these are referred to collectively as **myosin light**

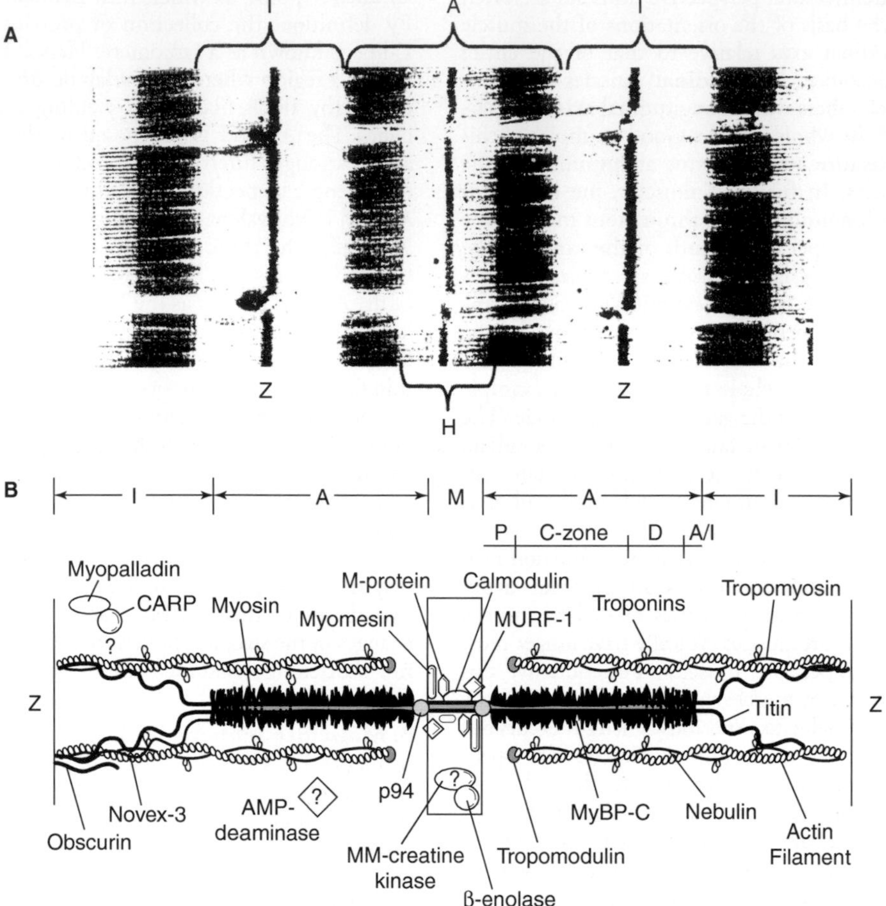

Figure 1–14. Striation pattern and various proteins associated with sarcomere. Electron micrograph of sarcomeres is shown in (**A**). A schematic illustration of the various structures and proteins of the sarcomere is shown in (**B**). p94 = muscle-specific calpain. MURF-1 = muscle ring finger-1, which is believed to be part of the ubiquitin-proteosome complex involved in protein degradation. MyBP-C = myosin-binding protein-C, otherwise known as C-protein. CARP = cardiac adriamycin-responsive protein. (A reproduced, with permission, from Aidley DJ: *The Physiology of Excitable Cells.* Cambridge University Press, 1998. B reproduced, with permission, from Clark KA et al: Striated muscle cytoarchitecture: An intricate web of form and function. Ann Rev Cell Dev Biol 2002;18:637.) Also, see Table 1–2.

Table 1–1. Effect of different types of contractions on the various bands, zones, lines, and length.

Type of Contraction	Z-line	I-band	A-band	H-zone	M-line	Sarcomere Length
Isometric	↔	↔	↔	↔	↔	↔
Shortening (isotonic)	↔	↓	↔	↓	↔	↓
Lengthening (eccentric)	↔	↑	↔	↑	↔	↑

↔ = no change in length; ↑ = increase in length; ↓ = decrease in length.

Table 1–2. Overview of proteins involved with the sarcomere and cytoskeletal-extracellular matrix interactions.

Classes and Types of Sarcomeric Proteins	Molecular Wt (kDa)	Location	Function
Contractile proteins			
Myosin heavy chain	~200	Thick filament	Molecular motor; binds to actin; generates force and length change
Actin	~42	Thin filament	Binds myosin and translates force and/or length changes
Regulatory contractile proteins			
Tropomyosin	~37	Thin filament	Regulates interaction between actin and myosin; stabilizes thin filament
Troponin-T	~30	Thin filament	Couples troponin complex to actin?
Troponin-I	~22	Thin filament	Influences position of tropomyosin
Troponin-C	~18	Thin filament	Binds Ca^{+2}, influences position of tropomyosin
Myosin light chain-1	~22	Thick filament	Influences V_{max}?
Myosin light chain-2	~20	Thick filament	Influences tension–pCa^{+2} relationship
Myosin light chain-3	~18	Thick filament	Influences V_{max}
Structural proteins			
Associated with thin filament			
CapZ-α, CapZ-β	~36, ~32	Z-line	Caps free end of actin, regulates actin filament length; binds to α-actinin
Tropomodulin	~40	Thin filament	Caps pointed end of actin filament
Nebulin	~600–900	I-band	Anchors actin to Z-line; molecular ruler of actin filament length?
Associated with thick filament			
Myosin binding protein-C	~140	Thick filament	Binds to lever arm and rod region of MHC; titin binding site
Myomesin	~185	M-line	Binds to myosin and titin; may play role in linking myosin and titin
MurF-1	~40	M-line	May play key role in degradation
Calpain-3; p94		M-line	Binds to titin
Titin	~3000–4000	Spans A–I bands	Molecular spring? Sarcomere template?
Associated with Z-line			
α-Actinin	~97	Z-line	Major protein of Z-line
LIM	~23	Z-line	Binds α-actinin, zyxin, β-spectrin
FATZ	~32	Z-line	Binds calcineurin to Z-line
Intermediate filaments			
Desmin	~53	Z-line	Longitudinal and lateral alignment of sarcomeres
Skelemin	~200	M-band	M-line integrity
Vimentin	~53	Z-line	Periodicity of Z-lines
Costameric proteins			
Ankyrin	17–440	Costamere	Localization
α-Dystrobrevin	~87	Costamere	Membrane stabilization; transmembrane signaling involved with NOS
α/β-Dystroglycan	~156, 43	Costamere	Prevents injury to sarcolemma
Dystrophin	427	Costamere	Stabilizes cytoskeleton and sarcolemma
α-Fodrin	85	Costamere	Attachment of cytoskeleton to ECM; signaling
Integrins	~90 and 150	Costamere	Stabilization of cytoskeleton
α-Sarcoglycan	~240	Costamere	Binds dystrophin and α-dystrobrevin; associated with NOS
α/β-Spectrin	~250	Costamere	Stabilization of sarcomere
Syntrophins	~57–60	Costamere	NOS?
Talin	~235	Costamere/MTJ	Role in stabilizing link between muscle fiber and tendon fibrils?
Vinculin	116 ~130	Costamere/MTJ	Role in stabilizing link between muscle fiber and tendon fibrils?

MHC = myosin heavy drain; LIM = cysteine-rich double zinc finger motifs that mediate protein binding; FATC = filamin, α-actinin and telethonin-associated Z-line protein; NOS = nitric oxide synthase; ECM = extracellular matrix.

chains (MLCs) because of their relatively low molecular weight. These MLCs may possibly be involved in regulating the kinetics of crossbridge cycling.

Structural and costameric proteins play several essential roles. First, electron micrographs (see Figure 1–14) demonstrate that sarcomeres are organized in a very orderly fashion such that the Z-lines of adjoining sarcomeres appear to be in register with one another. As noted in Table 1–2, key intermediate filaments like **desmin** and **vimentin** are believed to play key roles in aligning the Z-line of one sarcomere with that of another. Other proteins like **synemin** are also thought to be involved in the alignment of sarcomeres. Structural proteins also play a key role in developing a mechanical linkage between sarcomeres and the extracellular matrix. These sites of connectivity between the sarcomere, cell membrane, and extracellular matrix are referred to as **costameres** (see section 5. Molecular anatomy of the connection between the cytoskeleton and the extracellular matrix).

4. Molecular anatomy of myosin molecule—Although the term *myosin molecule* is often used, in reality the myosin molecule is a hexameric structure composed of two myosin heavy chains, two so-called essential light chains (MLC_1 or MLC_3), and two regulatory light chains (MLC_2). The term *heavy* or *light* is used in reference to the molecular weights of each of these proteins. Each myosin heavy chain is composed of a rod region, lever arm (also known as S_2), and a globular head (also known as S_1). The rod region plays an important role in the packing of individual myosin heavy chains into thick filaments. The globular head contains the key functional domains of this molecular motor. Within the globular head (Figure 1–15) are domains that contain (1) the actin-binding site, (2) the nucleotide (adenosine triphosphate [ATP])-binding site, and (3) the enzymatic (adenosine triphosphatase [ATPase]) properties responsible for converting chemical energy in the form of ATP into mechanical work and heat. The essential and regulatory light chains are bound to the so-called lever arm or S_2 region (see Figure 1–15). Each globular head has bound to it one essential and one regulatory light chain. Mutations of some of these domains (eg, the actin-binding site) are thought to play roles in diseases such as familial hypertrophic cardiomyopathy. As noted earlier, the light chains are thought to play modulatory roles in regulating the kinetics of the crossbridge cycle.

The complexity of the myosin molecule is further complicated by the presence of isoforms for both the myosin heavy and light chains. Although it has long been recognized that muscles could be classified as **slow** or **fast twitch** (based on twitch properties), the importance of myosin heavy-chain isoforms has only been intensely studied during the past 20 years. In many smaller adult mammals (eg, mice, rats, rabbits), four myosin heavy-chains isoforms are identified and classified as **slow Type I, fast Type IIA, fast Type IIX,** and **fast Type IIB** (in order of increasing ATPase activities and associated maximal shortening velocities). In adult humans, the slow Type I, fast Type IIA, and fast Type IIX myosin heavy-chain isoforms are expressed. This scheme of classifying myosin heavy-chain isoforms forms the basis for the nomenclature typically used to identify different muscle fiber types. Hence, a slow Type I muscle fiber would exclusively express the slow Type I myosin heavy-chain isoform.

Note that there are isoforms for myosin heavy chains, myosin light chains, tropomyosin, troponin-T, troponin-I, and troponin-C. Hence, by mixing and matching these contractile and regulatory contractile proteins, the complexity that can arise in the design of sarcomeres becomes readily apparent.

The sequence of the crossbridge cycle is shown in Figure 1–15. First, myosin is detached from actin. Second, the head of the myosin heavy chain is attached to actin and releases Pi, leading to the power stroke (change in position of head between Figure 1–15B and 1–15C). Following completion of the power stroke, adenosine diphosphate (ADP) is released, and subsequently ATP binds to the nucleotide-binding site (Figure 1–15D, E). The hydrolysis of ATP ultimately leads to the globular head of the myosin heavy chain returning to its original position. The magnitude of crossbridge cycling that occurs during a single contraction is enormous and can approach rates equivalent to 10^{17}–10^{18} crossbridge cycles per gram of muscle per second.

In thinking about the plasticity of the sarcomere and its constituent proteins, note that mechanical unloading and denervation lead to a decrease in the number of sarcomeres in parallel. From a functional perspective, this leads to a decrease in the capacity to produce force. In contrast, resistance training leads to an increase in the number of sarcomeres in parallel, and, as a consequence, increased capacity to produce force.

Factors such as mechanical unloading (eg, as accompanies cast immobilization) and altered thyroid hormone status produce shifts in the contractile and regulatory contractile protein isoform profiles such that they become faster. For instance, cast immobilization may lead to a transition from the slow type I to the fast type IIX myosin heavy-chain isoform. From a functional perspective, this will lead to an increase in maximal shortening velocity. Although it is commonly thought that strength training is an effective tool for increasing sprint speed, note that this will produce fast-to-slow transitions in myosin heavy-chain isoform expression.

5. Molecular anatomy of the connection between the cytoskeleton and the extracellular matrix—Costameres are important structures that link the cytoskeleton of skeletal muscle with the extracellular matrix

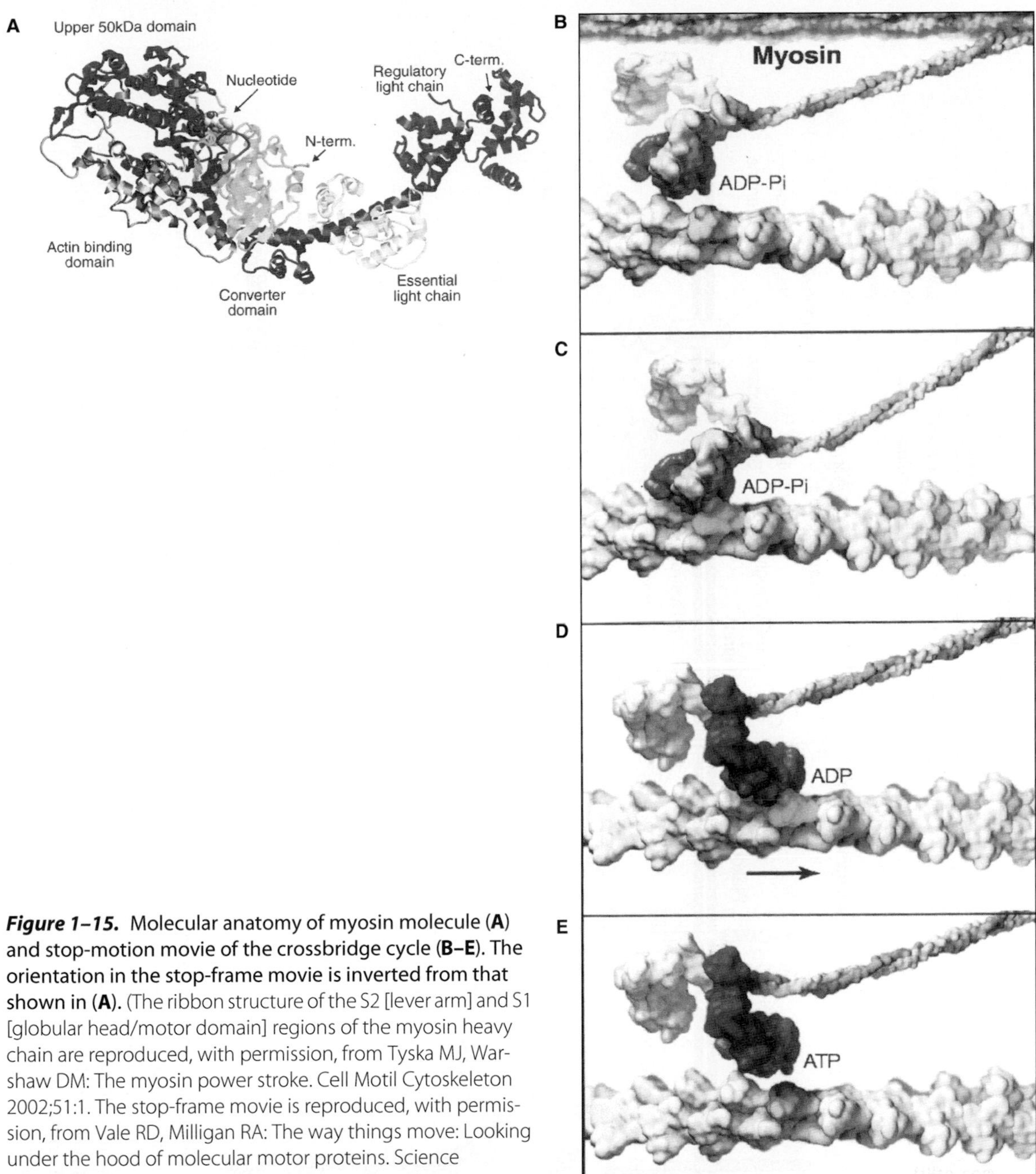

Figure 1–15. Molecular anatomy of myosin molecule (**A**) and stop-motion movie of the crossbridge cycle (**B–E**). The orientation in the stop-frame movie is inverted from that shown in (**A**). (The ribbon structure of the S2 [lever arm] and S1 [globular head/motor domain] regions of the myosin heavy chain are reproduced, with permission, from Tyska MJ, Warshaw DM: The myosin power stroke. Cell Motil Cytoskeleton 2002;51:1. The stop-frame movie is reproduced, with permission, from Vale RD, Milligan RA: The way things move: Looking under the hood of molecular motor proteins. Science 2000;288:88.)

(Figure 1–16). Currently, it is believed that the costameres serve at least three different functions: (1) aligning the sarcolemma with the cytoskeleton; (2) maintaining membrane integrity during different types of contractions, preventing injury to the sarcolemma; and (3) possibly playing a role in the lateral transmission of force. From a structural perspective, costameres are found aligned with the Z- and M-lines. This linkage occurs as a result of so-called intermediate filaments. Note that mutations in the costameric structure are

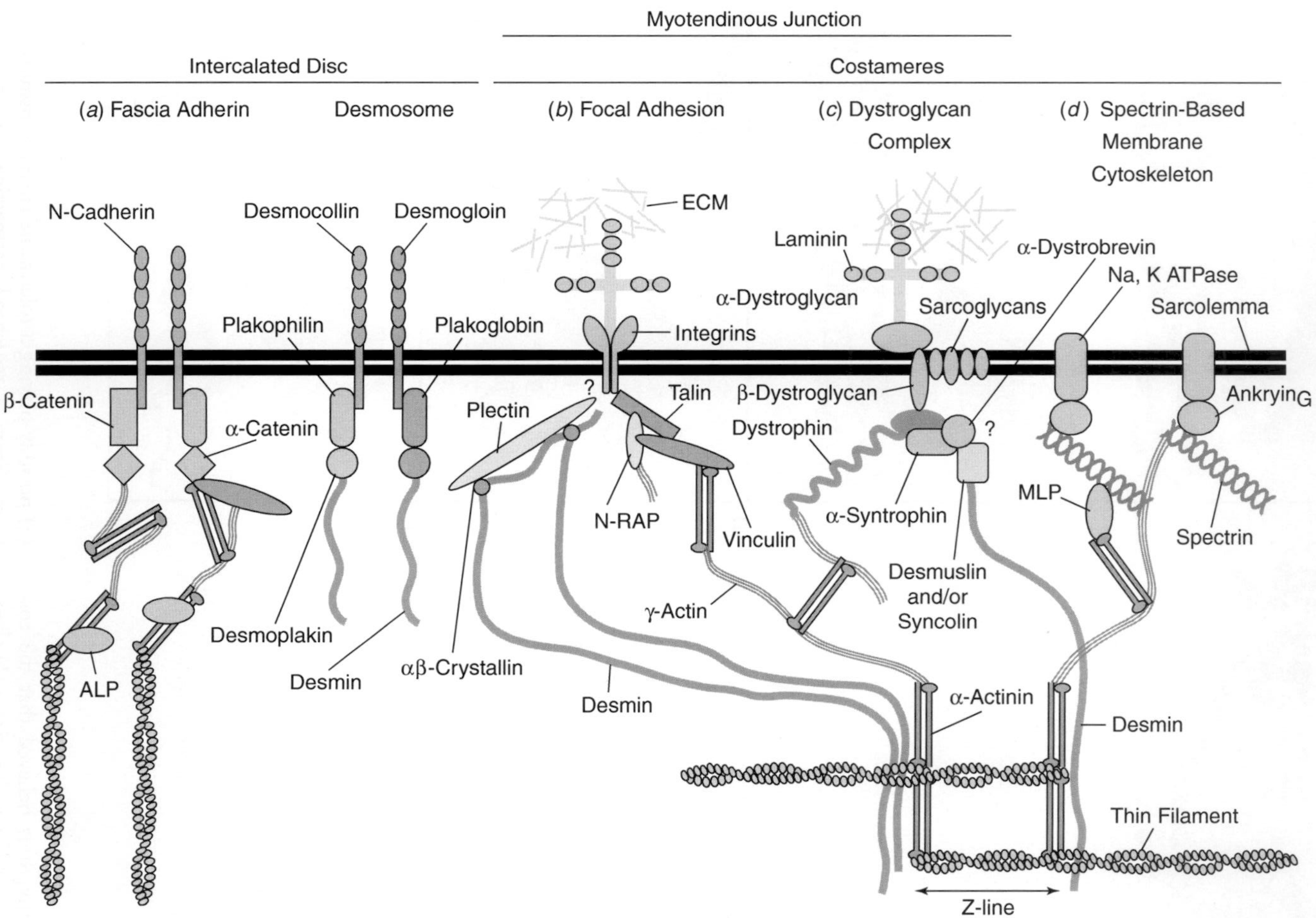

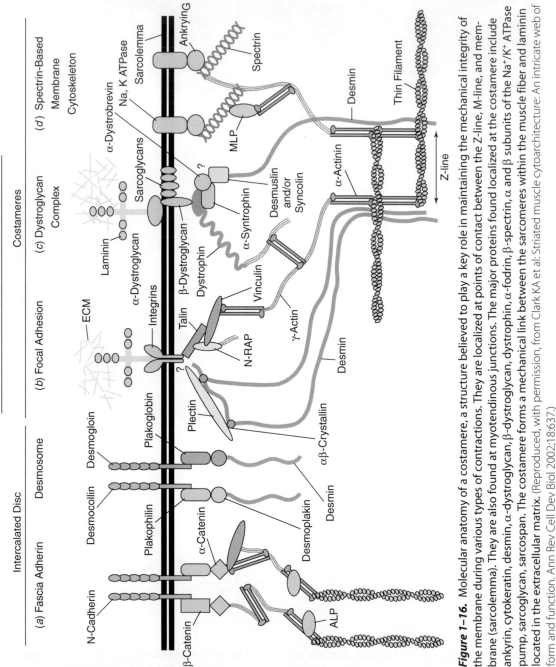

Figure 1–16. **Molecular anatomy of a costamere, a structure believed to play a key role in maintaining the mechanical integrity of the membrane during various types of contractions. They are localized at points of contact between the Z-line, M-line, and membrane (sarcolemma). They are also found at myotendinous junctions. The major proteins found localized at the costamere include ankyrin, cytokeratin, desmin, α-dystroglycan, β-dystroglycan, dystrophin, α-fodrin, β-spectrin, α and β subunits of the Na^+/K^+ ATPase pump, sarcoglycan, sarcospan. The costamere forms a mechanical link between the sarcomeres within the muscle fiber and laminin located in the extracellular matrix.** (Reproduced, with permission, from Clark KA et al: Striated muscle cytoarchitecture: An intricate web of form and function. Ann Rev Cell Dev Biol 2002;18:637.)

thought to be involved in some of the muscular dystrophies. Additionally, these structures may play an important role in protecting muscle fibers from eccentrically induced muscle damage.

6. The on-and-off switch of the molecular motor: Excitation-contraction coupling—From a mechanical perspective, all of the sarcomeres must become activated in a synchronous fashion. An asynchronous activation of sarcomeres would lead to large heterogeneities in sarcomere length along the length of a muscle fiber with some sarcomeres actively shortening, whereas the nonactivated sarcomeres would be lengthened. The net result might be a contraction, whereby there is little overall shortening of the muscle fiber. The synchronous activation of all sarcomeres requires an elaborate reticulum that functionally couples the depolarization of the sarcolemma (cell membrane) with activation of the sarcomere. The coupling between excitation and contraction involves extensive invaginations of the sarcolemma known as **transverse tubules** (T-tubules), which are associated with the **sarcoplasmic reticulum.** The sarcoplasmic reticulum is a network of membranes wrapped around the myofibrils, containing a large store of Ca^{2+}. When a skeletal muscle fiber is excited, the depolarization of the sarcolemma is propagated into the T-tubules. Excitation of the T-tubules then leads to the release of Ca^{2+} from the ends of the sarcoplasmic reticulum via so-called **Ca^{2+} release channels** (also known as ryanodine receptors). The Ca^{2+} quickly diffuses into the space occupied by the sarcomere, binding to troponin-C. This then causes tropomyosin to rotate about the longitudinal axis of the actin filament, uncovering the myosin binding sites of each actin molecule. The globular head of the myosin heavy chain attaches to this binding site and goes through its power stroke, leading to the production of force or length change. Simply stated it is the binding of Ca^{2+} to troponin-C that turns on the contractile apparatus.

The contractile activity of the sarcomere is turned off by resequestering Ca^{2+} back into the sarcoplasmic reticulum via **Ca^{2+} ATPase pumps** located along the length of the sarcoplasmic reticulum. The dissociation of Ca^{2+} from troponin-C causes tropomyosin to rotate back into its original position, once again covering up or blocking the myosin-binding sites of each actin molecule. In this manner, the globular head of the myosin heavy chain is prevented from binding to actin, leading to decay in force production and causing the muscle to relax.

As mentioned earlier, there are a number of isoforms for the contractile and regulatory contractile proteins. Isoforms are also identified for the Ca^{2+} release channels and Ca^{2+} ATPase pumps of the sarcoplasmic reticulum. These different isoforms play a key role in determining the rate of activation (ie, the release of Ca^{2+}) and relaxation (resequestration of Ca^{2+}). Mechanical unloading of skeletal muscle typically leads to an increased expression of the fast isoforms of the Ca^{2+} release channels, whereas reloading or strength training produces the opposite effect.

B. Skeletal Muscle Function

In a general sense, the mechanical activity of skeletal muscle depends on two factors: the pattern of stimulation and the extent of loading. The most basic unit of contractile response is known as a twitch. Simply stated, a twitch is the mechanical response of skeletal muscle to a single brief stimulus (Figure 1–17). This single stimulus leads to a single pulse of Ca^{2+} released from the sarcoplasmic reticulum. This single pulse of Ca^{2+} is nonsaturating, meaning that it binds to only some of the troponin-C molecules. In turn, this causes only some of the tropomyosin molecules to rotate about the longitudinal axis of the actin filament, uncovering only some of the myosin-binding sites. From a mechanical perspective, this leads to a submaximal force transient called a **twitch** (see Figure 1–17A). The Ca^{2+} is quickly resequestered by the sarcoplasmic reticulum, and force returns to resting levels.

The amount of Ca^{2+} released by the sarcoplasmic reticulum can be modulated by the pattern of stimulation. If a muscle is repetitively stimulated but with long durations between each stimulus, then the mechanical response will appear as a series of individual twitches, and the force produced will be submaximal. If the muscle is stimulated using a moderate frequency, however, then the mechanical response caused by one stimulus will fuse with that of the second stimulus, leading to a mechanical response known as **tetanus,** and the amplitude depends on the balance between Ca^{2+} release and resequestration. A greater frequency of stimulation leads to a greater release of Ca^{2+} and production of force (Figure 1–17B). Tetanus has two types: one in which partial relaxation occurs between each stimulus (unfused) and another in which no discernible relaxation happens between stimuli (fused) (Figure 1–17B). During fused tetanus, all of the Ca^{2+}-binding sites of troponin-C are saturated, causing all of the myosin-binding sites to be exposed. This results in the greatest production of force.

As noted earlier, the loading of skeletal muscle also plays a key role in determining the mechanical response. For instance, if a muscle contracts against an immovable object, the muscle does not shorten, and hence muscle length remains constant. This type of contraction is referred to as **an isometric contraction** (iso = same; metros = length), and it is under these loading conditions that the muscle produces maximal force. If a muscle contracts against a load that is submaximal (ie, less than the maximal force the muscle can generate), then the muscle shortens. This type of contraction is often

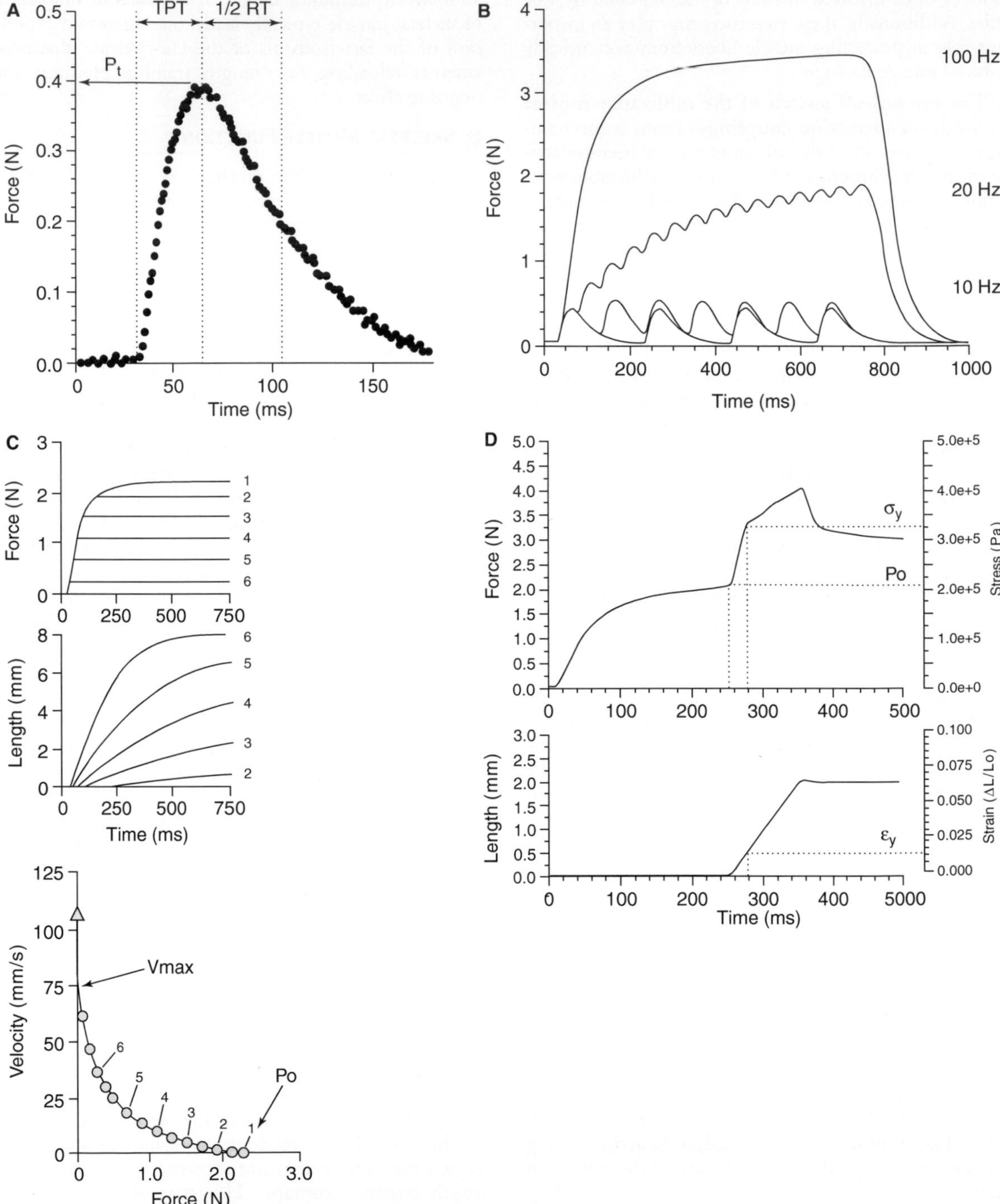

Figure 1–17. Various mechanical measurements that are typically made. The kinetics of a twitch are shown in (**A**). P_t = maximal twitch tension; TPT = time-to-peak tension; $^1/_2$ *RT* = one-half relaxation time. The importance of stimulation frequency in regulating the release of Ca^{2+} from the sarcoplasmic reticulum and ultimately force production is shown in (**B**). Methods used to determine the force–velocity relationship are shown in (**C**). V_{max} = maximal shortening velocity; P_o = maximal isometric tension. The mechanical response of a fully activated muscle to a strain of approximately 6% is shown in (**D**). σ = yield stress; ε = yield strain.

referred to as either a **shortening** or an **isotonic contraction.** Muscles not only work under these types of loading conditions, but they work almost as often under conditions in which the muscle is activated and forcibly lengthened. These types of contractions are known as **lengthening** or **eccentric contractions.**

1. Conceptual framework of factors that determine muscle function—From an orthopedics perspective, it would be beneficial to have a framework that would include the key factors that determine the mechanical function of skeletal muscle. Such a framework is laid out in Figure 1–18 and revolves around the context of net mechanical work. In a general context, the net mechanical work produced by skeletal muscle during cyclic length changes (eg, cyclic sinusoidal length changes) is determined by those factors that determine the positive amount of work produced during the shortening phase and those factors that determine the amount of mechanical work done on relengthening the muscle (ie, negative work).

The four determinants of the amount of positive work that can be produced during the shortening phase are (1) the length–tension relationship, (2) the rate of activation, (3) the force–velocity relationship in the shortening domain, and (4) the rate of relaxation. Two factors determine the amount of work done on the muscle during lengthening: (1) the force–velocity relationship in the lengthening domain and (2) the passive stiffness of the muscle. From an engineering perspective, each of these factors can be thought of as representing design constraints, one of which is static (the length–tension relationship) and others are dynamic. The term *static* in reference to the length–tension relationship implies that the basic dimensions of the sarcomere (and hence length–tension relationship) do not appear to be malleable. In contrast, the other factors can all be altered by factors influencing the mechanical loading of skeletal muscle (eg, immobilization), innervation (partial/complete denervation), and hormonal milieu (eg, thyroid, steroids).

2. Length–tension relationship—The amount of force a muscle can generate depends on muscle length; this length–tension relationship is shown in Figure 1–19. Typically, three regions of the length–tension relationship are described. The ascending limb extends from a sarcomere length of approximately 1.3–2.0 μm. In this region,

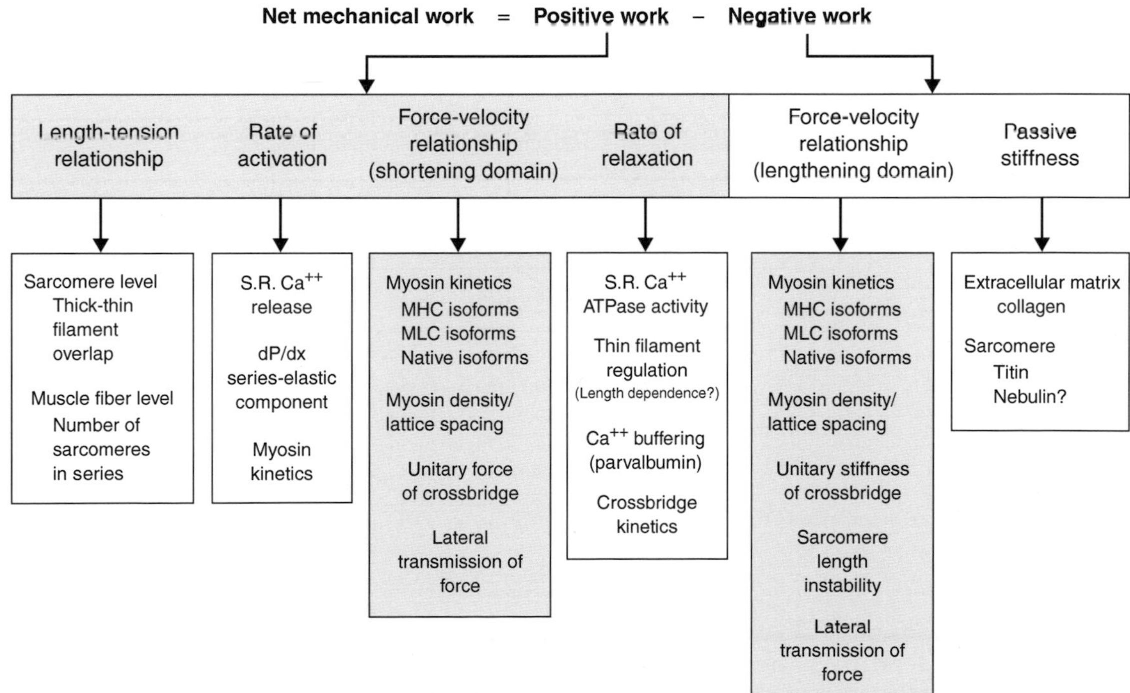

Figure 1–18. Various factors that limit the production of mechanical work and power. S.R. = sarcoplasmic reticulum. *dP/dx* = stiffness of series elastic component. MHC = myosin heavy chain. MLC = myosin light chain. (Modified, with permission, from Caiozzo VJ: Phenotypic plasticity of skeletal muscle: Mechanical consequences. Muscle Nerve 2002;26:740.)

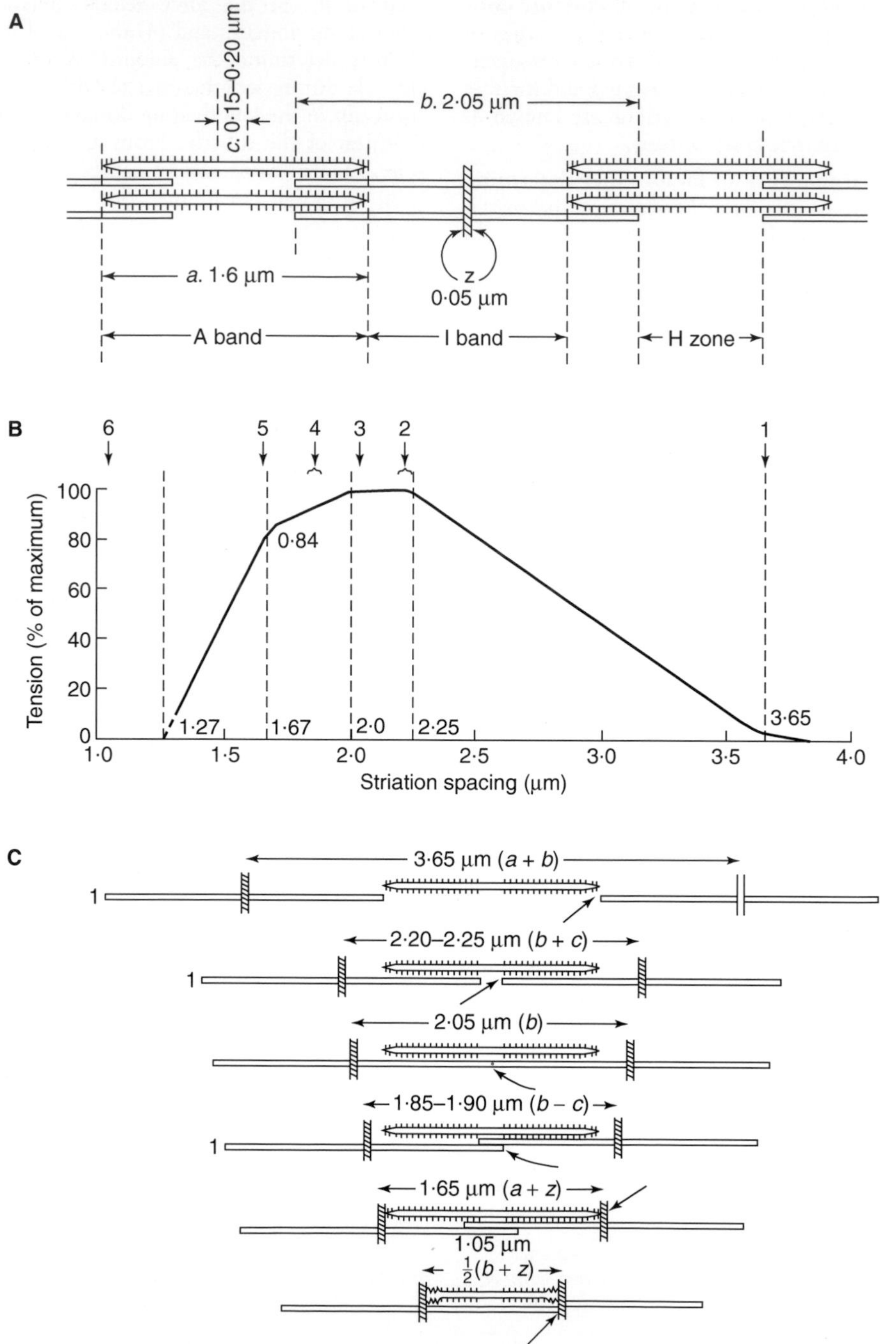

Figure 1–19. **Length–tension relationship.** (Reproduced, with permission, from Gordon AM et al: The variation in isometric tension with sarcomere length in vertebrate muscle fibres. J Physiol 1966;184:170.)

the amount of isometric tension increases in direct proportion to the increase in sarcomere length. The plateau region extends from approximately 2.0 to 2.5 μm in mammalian fibers, and in this range there is an optimal overlap between the thick and thin filaments. Beyond a sarcomere length of 2.5 μm, the isometric force that can be produced decreases as a linear function of increases in sarcomere length, reflecting a progressive decrease in overlap between the thick and thin filaments.

The length–tension relationship of the sarcomere is thought to represent a static design criteria, implying that it does not change with various types of interventions such as mechanical unloading. However, it is well known that muscles immobilized in a lengthened position increase the number of sarcomeres in series, leading to the longitudinal growth of the fiber. In contrast, immobilization in a shortened position reduces the number of sarcomeres in series and results in a shorter muscle fiber. Hence, such manipulations have the potential for influencing the overall length–tension relationships of muscle fibers and whole muscles. Clearly, contractures may have a large effect on the number of sarcomeres in series and result in various clinical complications such as equinus contractures.

3. Force–velocity relationship in the shortening domain—When a muscle contracts against a light load, it is able to shorten at a relatively high velocity. However, when a muscle contracts against a heavy load, it shortens at a relatively slow velocity. The relationship between the force and shortening velocity is shown in Figure 1–17C and reveals that the force–velocity relationship in the shortening domain can be described by a rectangular hyperbola. Importantly, the shape and dimensions of this relationship depend on the types of contractile protein isoforms and how they are packaged. As noted earlier, **maximal shortening velocity** is primarily determined by the types of myosin heavy-chain isoforms present in the muscle fiber. For instance, a muscle fiber that expresses only the slow type I myosin heavy chain has a much slower V_{max} than one that expresses only the fast type IIX or IIB myosin heavy-chain isoforms. V_{max} does not depend on the cross-sectional area of the muscle fiber. The **maximal isometric tension** that a muscle can produce, often referred to as P_o, is largely independent of myosin heavy-chain isoforms but is heavily dependent on the number of sarcomeres in parallel (ie, cross-sectional area). Hence, in an individual who has marked atrophy, P_o would be expected to be significantly reduced but V_{max} would be unchanged. In this context, the force–velocity relationship can be referred to as a dynamic design criterion, meaning that changes in either cross-sectional area or myosin heavy-chain isoform expression can alter the shape and dimensions of this relationship. Importantly, this relationship represents a design criterion because the muscle can only operate on or below the force–velocity relationship.

The product of force × velocity is mechanical power. Hence, the force–velocity relationship also defines the maximal amount of mechanical power that can be produced under any given loading condition. This has important implications for a wide variety of movements.

4. Force–velocity relationship in the lengthening domain—When a muscle is maximally activated and then forcibly lengthened, the tension that can be generated is much greater than that observed under isometric conditions. However, at velocities beyond a relatively low lengthening velocity, tension does not rise any further. This is shown in Figure 1–20. Although muscles commonly perform lengthening contractions, our understanding of the factors that determine the shape of the force–velocity relationship in the lengthening domain is relatively poor. The shape and dimensions of the force–velocity relationship in the lengthening domain are much more complicated than these same dimensions in the shortening domain. In the shortening domain, the force–velocity relationship can be described by a planar curve with the axes of force and velocity. In the lengthening domain, the relationship is three-dimensional, dependent on force, velocity, and time.

An example of the response of skeletal muscle to a lengthening contraction is shown in Figure 1–17D. Note that the muscle is stimulated, and force is allowed to move onto its isometric plateau. A constant-velocity

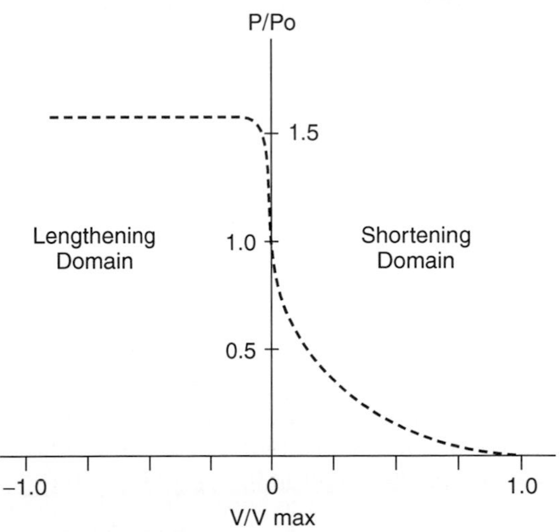

Figure 1–20. Force–velocity relationship in both the shortening and lengthening domains. (Reproduced, with permission, from Caiozzo VJ: Phenotypic plasticity of skeletal muscle: Mechanical consequences. Muscle Nerve 2002;26:740.)

stretch is then imposed on the muscle, and tension rises rapidly. However, at a strain of approximately 1–2%, a sudden change occurs in the rise in tension such that the slope decreases dramatically. The initial force response is often referred to as short-range stiffness. Note that both before and after the yield, force is constantly changing but the velocity of lengthening remains constant. This demonstrates the complexity of understanding the force–velocity relationship in the lengthening domain.

From a functional perspective, the force–velocity relationship in the lengthening domain is important because it determines the amount of work done on relengthening a muscle that is either fully or partially activated. Additionally, muscles are thought to act as dynamic joint stabilizers, so it might be hypothesized that stiffer muscles might better protect joints and ligaments (ie, anterior cruciate ligament) that are susceptible to injury. Newer studies show that mechanical unloading dramatically reduces both the stiffness and elastic modulus of skeletal muscle. The loss of elastic modulus occurs either because of a decrease in crossbridge density or to changes in the unitary stiffness of crossbridges.

5. Passive stiffness of skeletal muscle—The passive stiffness of skeletal muscle is influenced by both sarcomeric and extracellular matrix proteins. **Titin** is the largest known protein identified to date, and it attaches the thick filaments to the Z-line. Within the titin molecule is a unique region, the PEVK region, that functions like a molecular spring. The term *PEVK* refers to the abundance of proline (P), glutamate (E), valine (V), and leucine (K) found in this region. The passive tension of skeletal muscle fibers during stretch may, in part, be caused by the properties of titin. Newer evidence suggests that titin also acts as a molecular blueprint for the organization and structure of the sarcomere, and that titin may play a key role in regulating mechanosensitivity and mechanotransduction in skeletal muscle. For instance, titin contains a kinase domain near the M-line, and this appears to play a prime role in regulating the response of skeletal muscle to increased/decreased mechanical loading by providing a signaling bridge between the sarcomere and nucleus. Newer data suggest that mechanical unloading of skeletal muscle (especially slow type I fibers) results in a loss of titin relative to other myofibrillar proteins such as myosin, but it does not produce shifts in the types of titin isoforms. This, in turn, is believed to impact the passive stiffness of skeletal muscle, but it should be emphasized that the loss in stiffness associated with mechanical unloading is relatively small.

Although the extracellular matrix (ECM) is composed of a number of proteins, the major constituents are collagen and laminin. Fifteen different collagens are identified to date, and the most prevalent types found in skeletal muscle are types I and III. Type I collagen is more common in slow skeletal muscle, whereas type III is more abundant in fast skeletal muscles. Type I and III collagens are each composed of three individual chains that are arranged in a triple helical fashion. Type I collagen is composed of two $\alpha 1$ chains and one $\alpha 2$ chain. In contrast, type III is composed of three $\alpha 1$ chains. Each of the different types of chains (eg, I$\alpha 1$) is a product of its own specific gene. From a mechanical perspective, type I collagen is known to have a high tensile strength, whereas type III is more compliant.

Skeletal muscle fibers can be exposed to a variety of forces (eg, normal and shear stress) and strains (normal and shear strain). In a simplistic sense, isometric contractions are associated with high stresses and no strain. Alternatively, passive stresses can be imposed on a skeletal muscle fiber that result in stretch, producing a given amount of strain (relative change in length). To date, the scientific community only has a basic understanding of the effects of different loading conditions on the collagen content of skeletal muscle and associated regulatory pathways. Several studies show that mechanical unloading via hindlimb suspension results in a downregulation of the expression of type I and III collagens. In contrast, the responses of collagen genes/proteins to chronic stretch have not been studied in any detail, yet knowledge in this area may have important clinical ramifications. For instance, orthopedic surgeons commonly use distraction osteogenesis (Ilizarov procedure) as a method to correct limb length deformities. Unfortunately, such procedures (ie, distraction osteogenesis) often result in complications like equinus contractures, which are hypothesized to occur in skeletal muscle because of a proliferation of collagen content.

Anderson JB et al: Physiology: Postprandial cardiac hypertrophy in pythons. Nature 2005;434(7029):37.

Caiozzo VJ: Phenotypic plasticity of skeletal muscle: Mechanical consequences. Muscle Nerve 2002;26:740. [PMID: 12451599]

Clark KA et al: Striated muscle cytoarchitecture: An intricate web of form and function. Ann Rev Cell Dev Biol 2002;18:637. [PMID: 12142273]

Gordon AM et al: The variation in isometric tension with sarcomere length in vertebrate muscle fibres. J Physiol 1966;184:170. [PMID: 5921536]

Tyska MJ, Warshaw DM. The myosin power stroke. Cell Motil Cytoskeleton 2002;51:1. [PMID: 11810692]

Vale RD, Milligan RA. The way things move: Looking under the hood of molecular motor proteins. Science 2000;288:88. [PMID: 10753125]

Intervertebral Disks

The intervertebral disks sustain and distribute loads and also prevent excessive motion of the spine. An individual's intervertebral disks account for 20–33% of his or her spinal column height. The disks are subjected to high stresses during normal daily activity, and stress may double during increased activity, lifting, or trauma. Whether intervertebral disk failure occurs depends on loading rate and stress distribution.

A. Structural Composition

Each intervertebral disk has a nucleus pulposus surrounded by a thick capsule called the annulus fibrosus (Figure 1–21). End-plates composed of hyaline cartilage separate the intervertebral disk from the vertebral body. The unique interplay of the nucleus pulposus, annulus fibrosus, and end-plates accounts for the ability of the disk to withstand compressive, rotational, and shear forces. It is likely that hedgehog genes and the bone morphogenetic protein (BMP) inhibitors, including Pax-1, sonic hedgehog, Indian hedgehog, and Noggin genes, are key factors involved with intervertebral disc formation.

The nucleus pulposus lies in the center of the intervertebral disk, except in the lumbar spine, where it lies slightly posterior, at the junction of the middle and posterior thirds of the sagittal diameter. The nucleus pulposus is composed of a loose network of fine fibrous strands in a gelatinous matrix that contains water-binding glycosaminoglycans. The number of glycosaminoglycans decreases with age, thereby decreasing the hydration of the nucleus pulposus.

The annulus fibrosus is the ringlike outer portion of the disk and consists of fibrocartilage and fibrous tissue. The fibrocartilage is in a series of concentric laminated bands. In the first band, the collagen fibers are principally oriented at a 30-degree angle in one direction; in the second band, they are oriented at a 30-degree angle in the opposite direction; and the pattern continues (Figure 1–21A), with the result that the annular fibers form an intricate crisscross arrangement (Figure 1–21B). Centrally, the collagen fibers of the annulus fibrosus are attached to the cartilaginous end plates. Peripherally, the fibers are attached to the bone of the vertebral body by Sharpey fibers.

B. Biomechanical Behavior

The interaction between the nucleus pulposus and the annulus fibrosus accounts for the mechanical behavior of the intervertebral disk. The mechanical properties of the disk are viscoelastic and therefore depend on the loading rate and duration.

During compressive loading, the stress is transferred from the vertebral end plates to the intervertebral disk. With compression, pressure increases in the nucleus pulposus, and the fluid exerts hydrostatic pressure on the annulus fibrosus. As a result, the central portion of the vertebral end plates are pushed away from one another, and the annular bands are pushed radially outward. The bulging annular bands develop tensile stress in all directions, the optimal orientation for maximal mechanical strength for the collagen fibers.

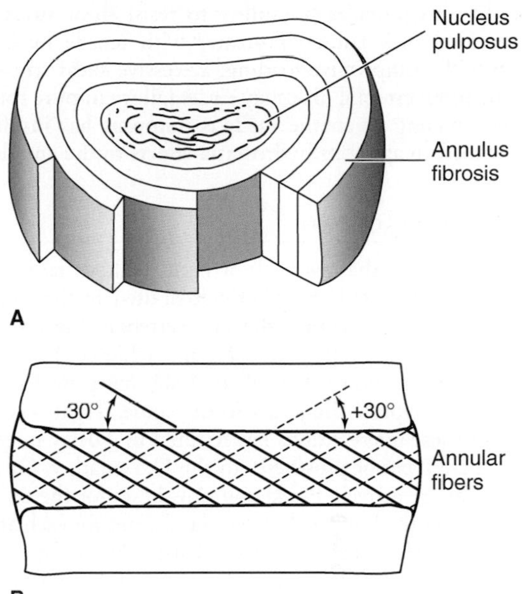

Figure 1–21. The intervertebral disk consists of a nucleus pulposus surrounded by the annulus fibrosus. In the first band of the annulus fibrosus, the collagen fibers are principally oriented at a 30-degree angle in one direction; in the second band, they are oriented at a 30-degree angle in the opposite direction; and the pattern continues (**A**), with the result that the annular fibers form an intricate crisscross arrangement (**B**). (Reproduced, with permission, from White AA, Panjabi MM: *Clinical Biomechanics of the Spine.* Lippincott, 1978.)

When the nucleus pulposus ages, its hydration decreases and its hydrostatic properties change. The load-transferring mechanism of the disk is greatly altered if sufficient hydrostatic pressure does not develop. In this situation, the annulus fibrosus transfers the stress to the periphery of the intervertebral disk; however, the fibers are subjected to compressive stress, which is not the optimal loading orientation for collagen fibers. This situation could lead to inadequate stress transfer from successive vertebral bodies, and this in turn could result in compression fractures of the vertebral bodies.

The nucleus pulposus has no effect during tensile loading of the intervertebral disk. Tensile loads are supported by tensile and shear stresses in the annulus fibrosus. The orientation of the collagen fibers of the annulus fibrosus provides no ability to resist shear stresses. Therefore, disk failure is greater with tensile loading than with compressive loading. Excessive shear stresses in the intervertebral disk may cause failure in pure rotational loading when the nucleus pulposus has insufficient load to apply its hydrostatic effects to the annulus fibrosus.

C. Disc Replacement

Pain located in the low back or neck, without radiation to the extremities, is frequently attributed to the structures in the area, namely the intervertebral disk and/or the facet joints. The relief of pain achieved by joint replacement in other areas of the body has provided an impetus to replace the joints in the spine. Tight regulation of these interventions has resulted in a delay in getting these types of prostheses to the U.S. market. Other countries are actively marketing prostheses for the cervical disc and the lumbar disc. Several designs for each area are now in clinical studies in the United States. In addition to pain relief, these prostheses offer the maintenance of at least some motion in the disc space, compared to fusion. Some of these replacements are metal on metal; others are designed like a traditional joint replacement with a polyethylene bearing component. The efficacy of these devices remains to be seen, especially when compared to the potential complications that might ensue.

Bass EC et al: Biaxial testing of human annulus fibrosus and its implications for a constitutive formulation. Ann Biomed Eng 2004;32:1231. [PMID: 15493511]

Carl A et al: New developments in nucleus pulposus replacement technology. Spine J 2004;4(Suppl 6):325S. [PMID:15541685]

Dipaola CP et al: Molecular signaling in intervertebral disk development. J Orthop Res 2005;23:1112. [PMID: 15936916]

Kumaresan S et al: Contribution of disc degeneration to osteophyte formation in the cervical spine: A biomechanical investigation. J Orthop Res 2001;19:977. [PMID: 11562150]

Kurtz SM et al: Analysis of a retrieved polyethylene total disc replacement component. Spine J 2005;5:344. [PMID: 15863092]

Lee SH et al: In vitro measurement of pressure in intervertebral discs and annulus fibrosus with and without annular tears during discography. Spine J 2004;4:614. [PMID: 15541691]

Simunic DI, Broom ND, Robertson PA: Biomechanical factors influencing nuclear disruption of the intervertebral disc. Spine 2001;26:1223. [PMID: 11389387]

Zigler JE: Lumbar spine arthroplasty using the ProDisc II. Spine J 2004;4(Suppl 6):260S. [PMID: 15541675]

Peripheral Nerves

Peripheral nerves are heterogeneous composite structures comprised of multiple cell types including neurons, Schwann cells, macrophages, and fibroblasts. The primary function of peripheral nerves is the propagation of action potentials. To improve the speed of action potential propagation (ie, nerve conduction velocity) without increasing the diameter of the axon, the Schwann cell, the primary glial cell of the peripheral nervous system, forms a myelin sheath around the axon to insulate the axon and reduce dissipation of the action potential.

A. Structural Composition

The peripheral nerve is composed of motor, sensory, and sympathetic nerve fibers. Such fibers can be either myelinated or unmyelinated. The average diameter of myelinated fibers is 2–22 μm, and unmyelinated axons are 0.4–1.25 μm. Surrounding the individual myelinated nerve fibers or the group of unmyelinated nerve fibers is the endoneurium, a collection of thin collagen strands that provides adequate nourishment and protects the individual axons. Multiple nerve fibers collect to form a group of fibers called a *fascicle.* Such fascicles are bound and encircled by the perineurium, a collection of a connective tissue sheath composed of perineurial cells. The perineurium is the major contributor to the nerve's tensile integrity and strength and is also the blood–nerve barrier. Several fascicles may be arranged into a group fascicle surrounded by connective tissue, termed the internal or interfascicular epineurium. The connective tissue that surrounds the periphery of the entire nerve is called the external or extrafascicular epineurium. The primary function of this connective tissue structure is to nourish and protect the fascicles. Fascicular patterns are divided into the following three types: monofascicular, oligofascicular, and polyfascicular. Monofascicular patterns consist of one large fascicle, whereas oligofascicular patterns consist of a few fascicles; polyfascicular patterns consist of many fascicles of varying sizes that can be arranged with or without groupings of fascicles. Nerves found in the upper arm are routinely polyfascicular. In its course from the upper arm to the fingertips, a peripheral nerve undergoes changes from polyfascicular pattern in the upper arm, oligofascicular in the elbow region, and monofascicular in the hand and fingers. For example, the ulnar nerve is polyfascicular as it exits the brachial plexus until just before the elbow, at which point it becomes oligofascicular. After the division into the motor branch at the wrist, the pattern is monofascicular. These patterns may help determine which type of nerve repair is appropriate for a particular nerve injury. In surgical nerve repair, proper identification of fascicular arrangement is crucial to achieving a successful outcome. Peripheral nerves are extensively vascularized with separate yet interconnected microvascular systems in the epineurium, perineurium, and endoneurium. The vascular pattern of the peripheral nerve is characterized by longitudinally oriented groups of vessels, with a great number of communicating anastomoses. The vasculature is composed of an intrinsic vascular system consisting of vascular plexa in the epineurium, perineurium, and endoneurium and an extrinsic system derived from closely associated vessels running with the nerve. From a surgical perspective, the role of the intraneural microvascular system is vital in regard to the effects of chronic irritation, compression, mobilization, stretching, and transection. If considering a group fascicular or fascicular repair technique, the effects of intraneural vascular damage secondary to surgical manipulation need to be considered.

B. Role of Myelin Sheath

One of the primary functions of a myelin sheath is to provide faster, more efficient transmission of the nerve impulse. Myelin itself acts as an insulator around the axon, reducing the dissipation of the action potential into the surrounding medium as it propagates through the axon. There are discontinuities in the myelin sheath along the nerve fiber that are known as nodes of Ranvier and contain high concentrations of voltage-gated sodium channels. The arrival of an action potential at a node depolarizes the membrane, opening the sodium channels to induce a massive influx of sodium ions into the axon. This generates an electrical pulse that is propagated down the axon to the next node of Ranvier, a process termed *saltatory conduction.* Saltatory conduction allows not only for an increased speed of nerve impulse transmission, but also reduces the energy requirement as well. Myelin is not just a conduit for conduction, however. Several myelinopathies, including type I Charcot-Marie-Tooth disease and multiple sclerosis, feature axonal pathology secondary to myelin dysfunction. Although the reciprocal relationship between neurons and glial cells is maintained, many of the clinical manifestations of these diseases are directly related to secondary axonal loss rather than to primary myelin dysfunction. Furthermore, mice with mutations in genes that encode the myelin-specific proteins myelin-associated glycoprotein (MAG), proteolipid protein (PLP), and ciliary neurotrophic factor (CNTF) exhibit evidence of axonal degeneration. MAG localizes to the periaxonal membrane and has a similar structure to members of the immunoglobulin family that participate in cell adhesion. MAG-deficient mice seem to develop apparently normal myelin sheaths and appear phenotypically normal. However, the caliber of myelinated axons decreases, and by 8 months functional contact between the axon and myelin is disrupted and the axons undergo a degenerative process similar to many human peripheral neuropathies. PLP is the major protein constituent of central nervous system myelin. PLP-deficient mice initially appear phenotypically normal and exhibit only minor myelin abnormalities, but they eventually develop behavioral motor abnormalities resulting from ongoing swelling and degeneration of small-diameter myelinated axons. CNTF is a neurotrophic factor that plays an important role in the neural response to injury. Adult CNTF-null mutant mice exhibit a progressive atrophy and degeneration of large-diameter motor neurons, in addition to disruption of the axon–Schwann cell communication network in the paranodal region, resulting in a small reduction in muscle strength. This evidence suggests a functional role for myelin in regulating the maturation, maintenance, and viability of myelinated axons.

Myelin is formed from the extension of the plasma membrane of Schwann cells. Myelin is unique in its high lipid-to-protein ratio, including high contents of galactosphingolipids and saturated long-chain fatty acids. For myelin to achieve its insulating properties, nonconducting structures as well as aqueous cytosolic molecules must be removed. Myelin excludes much of its conductive extracellular and cytoplasmic material by fusing large surfaces of the cytoplasmic leaflets of its plasma membrane, forming a morphological structure called the major dense line. The apposing exoplasmic surfaces of the plasma membrane also fuse to form intraperiod lines. Schmidt-Lanterman incisures are cytoplasmic channels that extend from the internal limit to the external limit of the major dense line. These channels facilitate communication between the axon and Schwann cell body and assure adequate nutritional supply within the regions of compacted myelin.

Gupta R et al: Schwann cells up-regulate vascular endothelial growth factor secondary to chronic nerve compression injury. Muscle Nerve 2005;31(4):452. [PMID: 15685607]

Rowshan K et al: Current surgical techniques in nerve repair. Operative Techniques in Orthopaedics 2004;14(3):163.

Rummler LS et al: The anatomy and biochemistry of myelin and myelination. Operative Techniques in Orthopaedics 2004;14(3): 146.

IMPLANT MATERIALS IN ORTHOPEDICS

The body is a harsh chemical environment for foreign materials. An implanted material can have its mechanical and biologic properties significantly altered by body fluids. Degradation mechanisms, such as corrosion or leaching, can be accelerated by ion concentrations and pH changes in body fluids. The body's response to an implant can range from a benign to a chronic inflammatory reaction, with the degree of biologic response largely dependent on the implanted material. For optimal performance in physiologic environments, implant materials should have suitable mechanical strength, biocompatibility, and structural biostability. As the field of biomaterials science developed, various classification schemes for implantable materials were proposed, including schemes based on chemical composition and biologic response.

Implant materials can be classified as biotolerant, bioinert, and bioactive. **Biotolerant materials,** such as stainless steel and PMMA, are usually characterized by a thin fibrous tissue layer along the bone-implant interface. The fibrous tissue layer develops in part as a result of leaching processes that produce chemicals that irritate the surrounding tissues. **Bioinert materials,** such as cobalt-based alloys, titanium, and aluminum oxide, are characterized by direct bone contact, or osseointegration, at the interface under favorable mechanical conditions. Osseointegration is achieved because the material surface is chemically nonreactive to the surrounding tissues and body fluids. **Bioactive materials,** such as calcium phosphate ceramics, particularly hydroxyapatite, have a bone-implant interface characterized by direct chemical bonding of the implant with surrounding bone. This chemical bond is believed to be caused by the presence of free calcium and phosphate ion groups at the implant surface. The calcium phosphate materials can be used as implants or coatings. Other bioactive materials are the growth factors, which are finding application in stimulating desired responses from connective tissues.

Minimizing the local and systemic response to an implanted material through improved biocompatibility is only one engineering concern for reconstructive implant surgery. A prosthetic implant must appropriately transfer stress at the bone-implant surface to ensure long-term implant stability. Nonphysiologic stress transfer may cause pressure necrosis or resorption at the bone-implant interface. Necrotic and resorbed bone may lead to implant loosening and migration, thus compromising implant longevity. Polyethylene wear particles are linked to osteolysis, also compromising implant longevity. Moreover, it is essential that materials have properties capable of sustaining the cyclic forces to which the implant will be subjected. For example, if the material properties are not adequate for load sharing, the implant may fail because of fracture. If the geometry and material properties of the implant make it too rigid in comparison with the bone, then stress shielding of the bone is likely to occur, making bone resorption and implant loosening inevitable.

In addition to acceptable biocompatibility characteristics, biomaterials must demonstrate material properties suitable for their desired use. Materials used to manufacture total joint replacement systems must demonstrate a yield stress that is greater than the stress expected from joint forces but must also have a flexural rigidity that will not result in unacceptable amounts of stress shielding of the bone. General stress–strain curves for the classes of materials allow for the comparison of material properties (Figure 1–22). For instance, ceramics are characterized by a high elastic modulus but are extremely brittle. In contrast with ceramics, metals have a lower elastic modulus but demonstrate increased ductility.

The most commonly used biomaterial combinations for orthopedic joint replacement are metals and metal

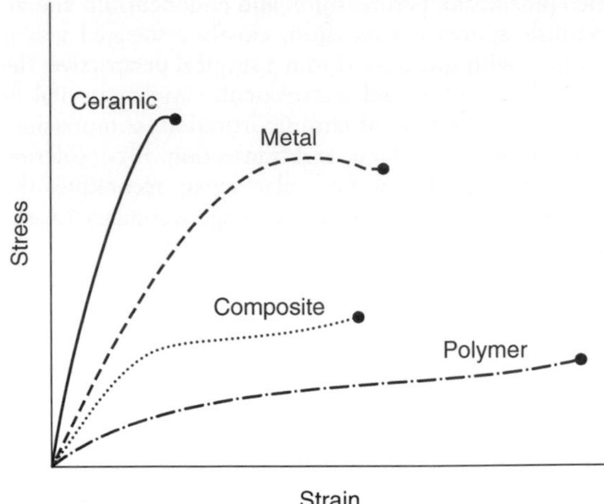

Figure 1–22. Representative stress–strain curves for the classes of materials used in orthopedic implants.

alloys articulating with ultrahigh-molecular-weight polyethylene (UHMWPE). Stainless steel, an iron-based alloy, was used in Charnley's original hip prosthesis and is the material most commonly used for internal fixation plates, rods, and screws. Advances in materials science have produced stronger cobalt-based and titanium-based alloys. The wear resistance of cobalt-based alloys makes them desirable for applications involving articulating surfaces. Titanium-based alloys, which have a modulus of elasticity closer to that of bone than the other metal alloys do, are currently being manufactured as femoral hip stems to reduce the effects of stress shielding.

Polymers and ceramics are also important classes of materials for orthopedic implant applications. UHMWPE has a low coefficient of friction, making it ideal for an articulating surface. PMMA is used as a grouting agent in total joint arthroplasty to provide immediate fixation of total joint components to the skeleton. Porous-coated components require ingrowth of tissue to the porous coating over a period of weeks or months to obtain stability. Aluminum oxide and zirconium oxide have gained popularity as materials for ceramic femoral heads because of their high wear resistance and low coefficient of friction. Finally, calcium phosphate ceramics, particularly hydroxyapatite, are used in monolithic form as an augmentation material for metaphyseal bone defects and as a coating on metal devices for total joint arthroplasty.

Metals

The suitability of a metal component for maintaining longevity of a total joint replacement depends on the design of the implant and the biocompatibility, strength, wear, and corrosion characteristics of the metal. Materials scientists can improve on one or several of the characteristics of a metal alloy by varying the composition or by using different manufacturing processes.

An understanding of the terminology used to describe the strength and stiffness characteristics of a metal is essential in making informed decisions about the different metal alloys. The most important characteristics are elastic modulus, yield stress, ultimate tensile stress, and fatigue stress. As discussed at the beginning of this chapter, these properties can be determined from stress–strain curves and fatigue curves. The composition specifications and mechanical characteristics of all metals and their alloys used for orthopedic implants were standardized by the American Society for Testing and Materials (ASTM).

The grain size, inclusion content, and surface porosity influence the strength characteristics of a metal. In general, the larger the grain size, the lower the tensile and fatigue strength at fracture. Excessive inclusions or a high surface porosity weakens the metal by acting as stress risers and by providing areas for crevice corrosion. Manufacturing processes can be used to control these factors. For example, heating metal to a temperature near its melting point increases the grain size, whereas forging processes decreases the grain size.

Corrosion is a chemical reaction process that weakens the metal. Three types of corrosion are prevalent in implant materials: fatigue, galvanic, and crevice corrosion. Although all metals corrode in the physiologic environment, the severity of corrosion is determined by the chemical composition of the metal. Stainless steel corrodes more readily than either cobalt-based or titanium-based alloys. The chromium and molybdenum content of both stainless steel and cobalt-based alloys produces a corrosion-resistant surface layer. Titanium-based alloys have an adherent oxide passive film layer that provides their corrosion resistance.

The surfaces of all metallic implants are passivated (made passive to corrosion) with nitric acid to form an oxide surface layer that increases corrosion resistance. **Fatigue corrosion** may occur, however, if this passive film layer on the implant surface was scratched or cracked and does not self-passivate in vivo. The ability to self-passivate may be hindered by wear processes or micromovement between modular components, a process called *fretting*. Once corrosion begins, the implant weakens and will fail at a stress level below the endurance limit of the metal.

Galvanic corrosion occurs when an electric current is established between two metals that have different chemical or metallurgic compositions. Some differences arise from manufacturing processes and may be subtle, as in the difference between annealed bone plates and cold-worked screws made of stainless steel. Other differences that lead to galvanic corrosion arise from the close contact of two different metals in an implant, such as a titanium alloy femoral stem in contact with a cobalt alloy head. An evaluation of retrieved mixed metal femoral hip components consisting of a cobalt-chromium modular head on a titanium alloy stem demonstrated some degree of corrosion in the majority of the components. Further evaluation determined that corrosion occurred in all components that were implanted for longer than 40 months. The long-term clinical significance of the presence of corrosion caused by femoral component modularity is unknown. To avoid catastrophic galvanic corrosion, however, stainless steels should never be used with either cobalt-based or titanium-based alloys.

Crevice corrosion generally occurs when the fluid in contact with a metal becomes stagnant, resulting in a local oxygen depletion and a subsequent decrease in pH in relation to the rest of the implant. This form of corrosion is most prevalent underneath bone plates at the screw-plate junction. The mechanism of crevice corrosion, however, is apparent in point or structural defects in a metal. Corrosion of a defect results in progressive deepening of the defect, leading to the development of large stress concentrations and catastrophic failure of the implant.

A. Iron-Based Alloys

There are four major groups of iron-based alloys or stainless steels, classified according to their microstructure. The group III (austenitic) stainless steels, which are labeled 316 and 316L, are used for orthopedic implants. The difference between 316 and 316L is that the latter contains a smaller percentage of carbon. Lowering the carbon content increases the corrosion resistance. Among the various elements contained in 316 and 316L stainless steels is molybdenum, which hardens the passive layer and increases pitting corrosion resistance.

Iron-based alloys have a wide range of mechanical properties (Table 1–3) that make them desirable for implant applications. Despite composition modifications, stainless steels are susceptible to corrosion inside the body, however. Therefore, they are most appropriate for temporary devices such as bone plates, bone screws, hip nails, and intramedullary nails.

Corrosion of stainless steels occurs for one of several reasons. The most common reason is incorrect metal composition, which increases the chance that galvanic corrosion processes will occur. Molybdenum is added to these metals to increase corrosion resistance; however, too much molybdenum can embrittle the alloy. Chromium carbide may form between the grain boundaries and result in grain boundary corrosion. This phenomenon is referred to as **sensitization.**

Table 1–3. Minimum mechanical requirements for metal implant materials, as standardized by the American Society for Testing and Materials (ASTM).

Material Type	ASTM Number	Ultimate Elastic Modulus (GPa)	0.2% Offset Tensile Strength (MPa)	Yield Strength (MPa)	Elongation (%)	Reduction of Area (%)
Iron-based alloys						
Annealed stainless steel 316	F55-82	200	515	205	40	—
Annealed stainless steel 316L	F55-82	200	480	170	40	—
Cold-worked stainless steel 316 and 316L	F55-82	200	860	690	12	—
Cobalt-based alloys						
Cast Co-Cr-Mo alloy	F75-87	250	655	450	8	8
Wrought Co-Ni-Cr-Mo alloy	F562-84	240	793–1000	241–448	50	65
Titanium and titanium-based alloys						
Unalloyed titanium	F67-89	105	240–550	170–483	15–24	25–30
Cast Ti-6Al-4V alloy	F1108-88	110	860	858	8	14
Wrought Ti-6Al-4V ELI alloy	F136-84	110	860–896	795–827	10	25

Another reason for corrosion is mismatch of implant components, especially when bone plates and screws are used, because even implants manufactured by the same company in different lots can be susceptible to corrosion processes caused by compositional differences. Crevice corrosion can occur at the junction of the screw with the bone plate and develops from local changes in pH and oxygen concentration that may result from slightly different manufacturing processes of the components.

Leaving plates and screws used to fix fractures in younger patients increases the risk of slow progressive corrosion over the years. Failure of the plate resulting from corrosion processes may also lead to bone fracture because stress shielding invariably occurs under the plate. Titanium alloy plates and rods are gaining popularity because of their corrosion resistance and lower elastic modulus, properties that lower the degree of stress shielding.

B. Cobalt-Based Alloys

The mechanical properties that make cobalt-based alloys suitable for load-bearing implant applications are summarized in Table 1–3. Among the elements contained in these alloys is molybdenum, which is added to produce finer grains and thereby results in higher strength. The cobalt-based alloys are characterized by high fatigue resistance and high ultimate tensile strength levels, properties that make them appropriate for applications requiring a long service life and ability to resist fracture. The high wear resistance of these alloys also makes them desirable for load-bearing and articulating surface applications. Cobalt-chromium alloys are primarily used for components in total joint implants.

Despite the advantages of cobalt-based alloys, some reported cases show that surface porosities act as stress risers and lead to premature fatigue failure. Hot isostatic pressing (HIP)—a process that involves simultaneously applying both heat and pressure to consolidate powder into a solid form—was adapted to significantly reduce surface porosity in cast metals. After this process is performed, the material must be heat treated to attain maximal benefit. When performed properly, HIP increases the fatigue resistance, static strength characteristics, and corrosion resistance of cobalt-based alloys. Unfortunately, the heat treatment necessary to apply porous coatings, such as beads, obviates much of the benefit of HIPing.

C. Titanium and Zirconium Alloys

Commercially pure titanium and titanium-based alloys are metals of low density (4.5 g/cm^3) and have chemical properties suitable for implant applications. Zirconium is in the same group in the periodic table. Both metals form an adherent, highly stable oxide surface layer that makes them extremely resistant to corrosion and chemically nonreactive to the surrounding tissues.

The mechanical properties of titanium and titanium-based alloys are summarized in Table 1–3. The elastic modulus value for titanium-based alloys is approximately 110 GPa, which is approximately half the value for iron-based or cobalt-based alloys but is still at least five times greater than the value for bone. Zirconium, when alloyed with niobium (2.5%) and oxygen (0.11%), has a modulus of 97.9 GPa. The higher the impurity content of the metal, the higher the strength and brittleness. Titanium and zirconium can be alloyed together and in combination with a variety of other metals, including niobium, tantalum, molybdenum, and iron. Because of their low density, these alloys have superior specific strength (strength per density) over all other metals. Titanium has poor shear strength and wear resistance, however, making it unsuitable for applications involving articulating surfaces. It also exhibits notch sensitivity, which means that a small flaw or crack on the surface, such as might occur with mechanical damage, can cause a tremendous reduction in strength and increase the susceptibility to fracture.

New manufacturing techniques are attempting to improve titanium-based alloys as bearing surfaces. Nitrogen ion implantation techniques were evaluated for their ability to increase the wear resistance and surface hardness of the alloys. The ion implantation process embeds elemental nitrogen ions in the surface, which causes distortions or strains within the crystal lattice of the metal and results in increased surface microhardness. The results are not adequate to allow titanium or its alloys to be used as bearing surfaces. However, an oxidized zirconium alloy (ASTM F2384) has produced a bearing surface that is showing promise in clinical trials for the last several years. In vitro studies show that the increased surface hardness from the oxide layer significantly improves the wear resistance of the treated implant. The surface oxide layer is very thin (approximately 0.004 mm) but extremely adherent.

Polymers

Polymers have a wide range of properties attributable to variations in their chemical composition, structure, and manufacturing process, which make them suitable for several different implant applications. The choice of polymer for application is dictated by the effect of the physiologic environment on the stability of the material. Some polymers, such as PMMA, leach toxic substances into the surrounding tissues. Conversely, other polymers, such as silicone, absorb fluids from the body, and this absorption alters the mechanical properties. Despite the possible consequences of polymer implantation, the use of polymers as implant materials has been successful.

All polymers are composed of long chains of repeating units. These units may form linear, cross-linked, or branched chains. The individual chains may be organized in an orderly crystalline form having parallel or folded chains, or they may have an amorphous structure or a mixed structure. The molecular weight, chemical composition, degree of crystallinity, size and polarity of side groups, and degree of cross-linking determine the mechanical properties of the polymer. In general, as the molecular weight and crystallinity increase, the tensile strength and the resistance to cracking increase. The crystallinity is decreased by copolymerization, branching of chains, and large side groups.

A. Ultrahigh-Molecular-Weight Polyethylene

UHMWPE possesses an array of properties, including high abrasion resistance, low friction, high impact strength, excellent toughness, low density, ease of fabrication, biocompatibility, and biostability, that makes it an attractive material for use in fabricating bearing surfaces for total joint replacements. UHMWPE is the material of choice for the liner of acetabular cups in total hip arthroplasties, the tibial insert, patellar components in total knee arthroplasties, and other load-bearing interfaces. The clinical performance of these components for nearly three decades has been excellent; however, there are concerns about the long-term wear of these devices. The concern is not only that the materials will wear out, but also that the wear debris generated will evoke an undesirable biologic reaction. It is known that particles in the submicron size undergo phagocytosis, resulting in a variety of biologic reactions. The reactions can include granulomatous lesions, osteolysis, and bone resorption. The phenomenon of wear of UHMWPE in total joint replacement is widely regarded as one of the most challenging problems in contemporary orthopedics.

A variety of factors influence the wear of polyethylene. These include the nature or quality of the starting material; the degree of cross-linking, strength, and toughness of the material; the manufacturing technique; the thickness of the polyethylene; the component sterilization conditions; and the storage environment and age of the component. The composition and physical properties of the starting materials used in the fabrication of UHMWPE components—in particular, molecular weight—have a profound effect on the material's performance. It is widely agreed that low-molecular-weight impurities and a high crystallinity are detrimental to the clinical performance. Increased crystallinity causes less resistance to crack initiation, crack propagation, and oxidation-enhanced wear.

UHMWPE is either machined from ram-extruded bar stock or compression molded directly from the starting powder. Ram extrusion is a two-step process in which the starting powder is first heated and pressurized in a polymerizing chamber followed by extrusion of bar stock. The second step, usually performed by the implant manufacturer, is the machining of the component with a precision cutting tool. By contrast, direct compression molding is a one-step process. A preshaped component and premeasured volume of starting powder are placed into a heated mold, and the component is then formed under pressure. Each manufacturing process has its own unique characteristics and problems. Some engineers believe that compression-molded components, although more expensive to produce, result in products with enhanced in vivo wear performance.

In general, as the thickness of the UHMWPE components decreases, the stresses increases, and therefore, the wear also increases. This is because with an increase in thickness, the structural stiffness of the component increases, even when the value of the modulus of elasticity of the material remains unchanged. This effect has resulted in a recommendation for the minimal thickness of acetabular liners of approximately 5–6 mm and tibial inserts of 7–8 mm.

Several manufacturers choose gamma irradiation for sterilizing UHMWPE components at doses between 25,000 and 40,000 Gy. Gamma radiation causes both cross-linking and chain fission and is the major contributor to subsequent surface and subsurface oxidative degradation of the components. Other manufacturers choose surface sterilization techniques, such as ethylene oxide, or one of the several plasma techniques, which have no effect on the bulk properties of the polyethylene. There is considerable literature on the effect of a number of variables associated with sterilization, packaging, and aging of polyethylene on the in vivo and in vitro physical and mechanical properties. These include the method of sterilization, sterilization dosage, packaging atmosphere, and aging conditions. For example, irradiation and storage in an inert atmosphere reduces the oxidative degradation before implantation. Because of this volume of work, no consensus has yet emerged on these effects. As noted, gamma sterilization, particularly in air, causes significant reduction of the various mechanical characteristics that are related to the subsequent wear and performance of the material. These parameters include crystallinity, melting temperature, oxidation strength, tensile properties, and density.

Irradiation of polyethylene at much higher doses (50,000–150,000 Gy) followed by an annealing process results in a cross-linked polyethylene with different properties. Early hip simulator wear studies indicate that this cross-linked polyethylene has very low wear rates and superior wear properties compared with conventional polyethylene. Early clinical trials seem to confirm a reduction in wear rates but not to the magnitude predicted by the wear simulator studies.

B. Polymethylmethacrylate

Self-curing PMMA, commonly used as a grouting agent, is often called the weak link in total joint arthroplasty. Compared with cortical bone, bone cement has a lower elastic modulus and significantly inferior mechanical strength properties. The tensile strength of PMMA is similar to that of cancellous bone. The low modulus of elasticity allows for gradual transfer of stress from implant to bone. Mechanically, PMMA is weakest in shear loading and strongest in compression loading configurations.

Implant design and cementing technique must compensate for weakness in tension, to avoid catastrophic failure of the cement. The poor fatigue strength of PMMA can be attributed primarily to porosity. Studies show that PMMA porosity is increased and fatigue strength is further decreased by mixing the cement with chilled monomer, rather than with monomer at room temperature. Therefore, if chilled monomer must be used, it is crucial to use porosity reduction techniques, such as centrifugation or vacuum mixing, concurrently. The fatigue strength of PMMA is also decreased by the presence of inclusions, such as bone chips and blood.

Aside from the inherent mechanical weakness of PMMA, the polymerization process causes local and systemic biologic effects. Locally, adjacent tissues can become necrotic because of the extreme heat of polymerization, which can generate temperatures approaching 100° C. Systemically, the leaching of monomer during the curing process may cause hypotension.

The fatigue properties of PMMA manufactured by different companies vary because of intrinsic compositional differences, such as the size of the polymer beads, the addition of copolymers, and the presence of additives and radiopacifiers. In a study of the fatigue life of five commonly used bone cements (CMW, LVC, Palacos R, Simplex P, and Zimmer Regular), investigators prepared each cement in the manner suggested by its manufacturer. They found that Palacos R and Simplex P had equivalent fatigue strengths and that these two products had significantly greater fatigue strengths than the other three products. For each product, investigators compared the fatigue life of a regular sample with that of a sample that had undergone a process to reduce its porosity. In the case of each product, a reduction in the cement's porosity increased its fatigue life. Moreover, when investigators centrifuged two packages of Simplex P mixed with chilled monomer for 60 s, they found a fivefold increase in the fatigue properties of this cement.

Antibiotics were added to bone cement at the time of surgery for years to reduce the risk of infection or to treat infection. Heat-stable antibiotics that are eluted from the bone cement inhibit antibiotic growth for variable periods from days to weeks. To obtain more uniform formulations, manufacturers have now obtained permission from the Food and Drug Administration

(FDA) to make the bone cement with premixed antibiotics. Studies show that the fatigue strength of the cement is not reduced with these additions.

Ceramics

Ceramics are wear resistant and strong in compression, but they are extremely brittle and susceptible to cracking. Ceramic materials must be carefully chosen for specific implant applications because chemical composition affects the mechanical properties and biologic responses of each ceramic. For instance, in calcium phosphate ceramics, an alteration in the ratio of calcium to phosphorous can significantly alter the in vivo dissolution rate of the ceramic.

The mechanical properties of ceramics depend on grain size, porosity, density, and crystallinity. Strength is normally improved with increased density, increased crystallinity, and decreased porosity. The hardness and wettability of ceramics and the fact that ceramics can be polished to smooth surfaces make them ideal candidates for bearing surfaces. Nevertheless, for a ceramic implant to be reliable, its design must avoid sharp corners and notches, to overcome the predictable mechanical flaws of the material.

A. Aluminum Oxide

The catastrophic effects of implant loosening associated with polyethylene wear debris led to interest in using other materials at the articulating surface. The use of aluminum oxide (Al_2O_3) was explored because it is a highly biocompatible material with high frictional resistance. In fact, the coefficient of friction for alumina-on-alumina articulations is approximately 2.3 times less than the coefficient for metal-on-polyethylene articulations. Studies show that alumina-on-alumina articulations demonstrate approximately 5000 times less wear than metal-on-polyethylene articulations do under experimental loading conditions.

In clinical practice, all-alumina acetabular components have not performed well, probably because of loosening caused by the modulus mismatch between aluminum oxide and bone. Designs to circumvent this problem have fixed an alumina bearing component inside a metal ingrowth cup, so the bone can grow into a porous metal surface. Ceramic-on-polyethylene articulations show clinical promise, however. Aluminum oxide has excellent wear characteristics, and any ceramic wear debris that does accumulate at the interface may be less bioreactive than polyethylene or PMMA wear debris. Alumina-on-alumina articulations demonstrate very low wear rates when clinically applied with a metal shell for attachment to acetabular bone. Although the alumina wear rates are low, problems have occurred because of placement of the components, allowing impingement and abrasion of the neck of the femoral component.

Despite the excellent wear and friction characteristics of aluminum oxide, its fracture toughness and tensile strength are relatively low. The fracture rate of alumina is low but significant. In one series, the authors reported 13 failures out of 5500 implantations over 25 years (0.23%), and disturbingly, they were unable to attribute some of the fractures to any rational explanation. Fracture can be a result of microstructural flaws, which are statistical in nature. The elastic modulus of aluminum oxide is approximately 20 times greater than that of cortical bone. Increased grain size decreases strength and a large grain size is linked to reported cases of catastrophic wear. Careful regulation of manufacturing processes is necessary to obtain reliable aluminum oxide implants with small grain size, high density, high purity, adequate strength, and adequate component size. With these caveats, these alumina-on-alumina implants may have a role in hip replacement in younger patients because of their reduced rate of particulate wear production. The high strength and hardness of alumina also recommend it for use with polyethylene bearings.

B. Zirconium Oxide

Zirconium oxide (Zirconia) temporarily became an attractive material for highly loaded joint replacement applications. Pure zirconium oxide can be maintained in a metastable, tetragonal crystal structure with fine grain structure, with the addition of a stabilizing oxide, such as yttrium oxide (Y_2O_3).

In comparison with aluminum oxide, zirconium oxide exhibits increased fracture toughness, increased bending strength, and decreased elastic modulus. Moreover, Zirconia-to-polyethylene articulations demonstrate favorable wear characteristics compared with alumina-to-polyethylene articulations in vitro. Because the mechanical and wear properties of zirconium oxide are superior to those of aluminum oxide, it is possible to manufacture smaller femoral heads for low-friction total hip arthroplasty. However, several studies show an increase in the monoclinic phase of Zirconia over time in vivo, calling into question the long-term biostability of the material. Further, the phase change was associated with an increase in surface roughness and wear rates of polyethylene bearing surfaces. Other problems have plagued proponents of Zirconia as a bearing material. Catastrophic failure was seen in a high proportion of Zirconia heads produced in a tunnel kiln in Europe, which were shown on retrieval to have high (21–68%) monoclinic phase present. Zirconia femoral heads may need significant research to demonstrate safety and regain consumer confidence. Although still available in some markets, Zirconia femoral heads may have a very limited place in the orthopedic market.

C. HYDROXYAPATITE

Calcium phosphate ceramics, classified as polycrystalline ceramics, have a material structure derived from individual crystals that become fused at the grain boundaries during high-temperature sintering processes.

Tribasic calcium phosphate [$Ca_{10}(PO_4)_6(OH)_2$], which is commonly called **hydroxyapatite,** is a geologic mineral that closely resembles the natural mineral in vertebrate bone tissue. Tribasic calcium phosphate should not be confused with other calcium phosphate ceramics, especially tricalcium phosphate [$Ca_3(PO_4)_2$], which is chemically similar to hydroxyapatite but is not a natural bone mineral.

Bulk hydroxyapatite (HA) is manufactured from a starting powder, and the manufacturing process consists of compression molding and subsequent sintering. Macroporous ceramics can be obtained by combining the starting mixture with hydrogen peroxide. Otherwise, a dense structure with a small percentage of micropores results. Dense HA ceramics have a compressive strength greater than that of cortical bone; however, their tensile strength is approximately 2.5 times less than their compressive strength. Small reductions in density can significantly reduce tensile characteristics of the ceramic. Bulk HA can also be formed with a very uniform pore structure by the chemical conversion of calcium carbonate coral structures. This material can be used to augment bone graft in cancellous bone areas.

Although the static mechanical properties of bulk HA are good, the resistance to fatigue failure is low in physiologic conditions, as is common with sintered ceramics and particularly bioactive ceramics. Therefore, bulk HA is not suitable for applications requiring mechanical loading. Bulk HA is used successfully in clinical practice as a bone graft substitute to fill defects associated with fractures or as a bone graft extender for fractures or fusions. A composite prosthesis made by plasma spraying thin (approximately 50 μm) coatings of HA or other calcium phosphate compounds onto a metal substrate was developed and is able to withstand the physiologic stresses imposed on it while providing an osteoconductive surface to achieve optimal bone apposition and ingrowth. These coatings can be applied by other means including chemical deposition from solution. Generally, HA coatings do not provide adequate fixation of bone when applied to smooth metal surfaces, and they require a roughened or porous surface for long-term fixation. Experimental results indicate that HA stimulates more extensive and uniform growth of bone into a porous-surfaced femoral stem or acetabular cup and probably aids bone growth across gaps between implants and surrounding bone. The durability of the fixation of the prosthesis to bone may be related to the quality and durability of the coating. HA coatings on ingrowth/ongrowth surfaces is probably not needed in the primary procedure but is considered by many surgeons to be helpful in the revision procedure, to obtain more reliable bone ingrowth.

Several formulations of an injectable hydroxyapatite are now available for minimally invasive surgery. These materials are similar to PMMA in that the setting process is a chemical reaction that yields the final product, in this case hydroxyapatite, or a similar calcium phosphate compound.

D. PYROLYTIC CARBON

Carbon occurs naturally in many forms, each having different structures, material properties, and uses. Coal is an example of carbon in its amorphous form with no crystalline structure. Graphite has an organized crystalline structure, in which carbon atoms are arranged in two-dimensional hexagonal sheets tightly joined by strong covalent bonds. Diamond is a third form of carbon having a three-dimensional cubic crystal structure with increased atomic bonds.

Pyrolytic carbon is a manufactured material formed by the pyrolysis, or heating, of gaseous hydrocarbons, causing them to decompose to a stable gas and carbon. The resulting pyrolytic carbon is usually deposited on a graphite substrate in a turbostratic, two-dimensional crystalline structure with a high concentration of three-dimensional diamond cross-link bonding. In general, the physical properties of pyrolytic carbon fall between those of graphite and diamond. The form of pyrolytic carbon used as a surgical implant material has a very fine grain structure (approximately 50 Å), and isotropic physical and mechanical properties. Pyrolytic carbon is chemically inert and resistant to wear and mechanical fatigue with a fatigue strength at 10^9 cycles close to its failure strength. It also has a high fracture strength, and low elasticity modulus (21–26 GPa), which falls within the range of moduli reported for cortical bone. Its biocompatibility is well documented and has been confirmed clinically in extensive use in cardiovascular implants for more than 30 years. Pyrolytic carbon has also proved to be extremely biocompatible in both osseous and soft tissues.

Pyrolytic carbon was evaluated in cardiovascular, dental, soft-tissue, and orthopedic implants. It is the material of choice for the construction of mechanical artificial heart valves. The human heart beats on an average of 100,000 times per day, or 35 million times per year. The carbon-on-carbon pivot systems in heart valves must resist stress and wear each time the heart beats. The history of successful function in heart valve components demonstrates the outstanding wear resistance of the carbon-on-carbon articulation, biocompatibility, high fatigue strength, and structural durability of the pyrolytic carbon material. Pyrolytic carbons were evaluated clinically in orthopedics for replacement of the small bones and joints of the hands and feet. Nonconstrained pyrolytic carbon metacarpophalangeal joint replacements were evaluated in human clinical trials with results at long-term follow-up demonstrating excellent performance of the implants with a 15-year survival rate of more than 70%. The long-term clinical results of the metacarpophalangeal joint arthroplasties verify the biologic and biomechanical compatibility of pyrolytic carbons in a demanding orthopedic application. With FDA approval, these joints are now being marketed for general use.

Baleani M et al: Fatigue strength of PMMA bone cement mixed with gentamicin and barium sulphate vs pure PMMA. Proc Inst Mech Eng (H) 2003;217:9. [PMID: 12578214]

Catledge SA et al: Surface crystalline phases and nanoindentation hardness of explanted femoral heads. J Mater Sci Mater Med 2003;14:863. [PMID: 15348523]

Cook SD et al: Long-term follow-up of pyrolytic carbon metacarpophalangeal implants. J Bone Joint Surg Am 1999;81:635. [PMID: 10360692]

Endo MM et al: Comparative wear and wear debris under three different counterface conditions of crosslinked and non-crosslinked ultra high molecular weight polyethylene. Biomed Mater Eng 2001;11:23. [PMID: 11281576]

Ezzet KA et al: Oxidized zirconium femoral components reduce polyethylene wear in a knee simulator. Clin Orthop 2004; 428.120. [PMID: 15534531]

Food and Drug Administration, HHS: Medical devices; reclassification of polymethylmethacrylate (PMMA) bone cement. Final rule. Fed Regist 2002;67:46852. [PMID: 12125716]

Friedman RJ et al: Current concepts in orthopaedic biomaterials and implant fixation. J Bone Joint Surg Am 1993;75:1086. [PMID: 11132264]

Gott VL, Alejo DE, Cameron DE: Mechanical heart valves: 50 years of evolution. Ann Thorac Surg 2003;76:S2230. [PMID: 14667692]

Hannouche D et al: Fractures of ceramic bearings: History and present status. Clin Orthop 2003;417:19. [PMID: 14646699]

Haraguchi K et al: Phase transformation of a Zirconia ceramic head after total hip arthroplasty. J Bone Joint Surg Br 2001; 83:996. [PMID: 11603539]

Hernigou P, Bahrami T: Zirconia and alumina ceramics in comparison with stainless-steel heads. Polyethylene wear after a minimum ten-year follow-up. J Bone Joint Surg Br 2003; 85:504. [PMID: 12793553]

Jeffers JR, Browne M, Taylor M: Damage accumulation, fatigue and creep behaviour of vacuum mixed bone cement. Biomaterials 2005;26:5532. [PMID: 15860209]

Kurtz SM et al: In vivo degradation of polyethylene liners after gamma sterilization in air. J Bone Joint Surg Am 2005;87: 815. [PMID: 15805212]

Laskin RS: An oxidized Zr ceramic surfaced femoral component for total knee arthroplasty. Clin Orthop 2003;416:191. [PMID: 14646761]

Lewis G, Carroll M: Rheological properties of acrylic bone cement during curing and the role of the size of the powder particles. J Biomed Mater Res 2002;63(2):191. [PMID: 11870653]

Lim TH et al: Biomechanical evaluation of an injectable calcium phosphate cement for vertebroplasty. Spine 2002;27:1297. [PMID: 12065977]

Ma L, Sines G: Fatigue behavior of a pyrolytic carbon. J Biomed Mater Res 2000;51(1):61. [PMID: 10813746]

Mashoof AA et al: Supplementation of autogenous bone graft with coralline hydroxyapatite in posterior spine fusion for idiopathic adolescent scoliosis. Orthopedics 2002;25:1073. [PMID: 12401014]

Masonis JL et al: Zirconia femoral head fractures: A clinical and retrieval analysis. J Arthroplasty 2004;19:898. [PMID: 15483807]

McKellop H et al: Development of an extremely wear-resistant ultra high molecular weight polyethylene for total hip replacements. J Orthop Res 1999;17(2):157. [PMID: 10221831]

Morscher EW, Wirz D: Current state of cement fixation in THR. Acta Orthop Belg 2002;68:1. [PMID: 11915452]

Murphy BP, Prendergast PJ. The relationship between stress, porosity, and nonlinear damage accumulation in acrylic bone cement. J Biomed Mater Res 2002;59:646. [PMID: 11774326]

Oonishi H, Kadoya Y: Wear of high-dose gamma-irradiated polyethylene in total hip replacements. J Orthop Sci 2000;5(3): 223. [PMID: 10982661]

Porter AE et al: Bone bonding to hydroxyapatite and titanium surfaces on femoral stems retrieved from human subjects at autopsy. Biomaterials 2004;25:5199. [PMID: 15109844]

Ries MD et al: Polyethylene wear performance of oxidized zirconium and cobalt-chromium knee components under abrasive conditions. J Bone Joint Surg Am 2002;84(Suppl 2):129. [PMID: 11712832]

Ries MD et al: Relationship between gravimetric wear and particle generation in hip simulators: Conventional compared with cross-linked polyethylene. J Bone Joint Surg Am 2001;83 (Suppl 2, Pt 2):116. [PMID: 11712832]

Sakoda H et al: A comparison of the wear and physical properties of silane cross-linked polyethylene and ultra-high molecular weight polyethylene. J Arthroplasty 2001;16:1018. [PMID: 11740757]

Schulz M et al: Early results of proximal interphalangeal joint replacement with pyrolytic carbon prosthesis (Ascension) idiopathic and post-traumatic arthritis. Handchir Mikrochir Plast Chir 2005;37:26. [PMID: 15744654]

Sharkey PF et al: The bearing surface in total hip arthroplasty: Evolution or revolution. Instr Course Lect 2000;49:41. [PMID: 10829160]

Smith SL, Unsworth A: An in vitro wear study of alumina-alumina total hip prostheses. Proc Inst Mech Eng [H] 2001;215:443. [PMID: 11726044]

Spector BM et al: Wear performance of ultra-high molecular weight polyethylene on oxidized zirconium total knee femoral components. J Bone Joint Surg Am 2001;83(Suppl 2, Pt 2):80. [PMID: 11712839]

Sun L et al: Material fundamentals and clinical performance of plasma-sprayed hydroxyapatite coatings: A review. J Biomed Mater Res 2001;58:570. [PMID: 11505433]

Urban JA et al: Ceramic-on-polyethylene bearing surfaces in total hip arthroplasty. Seventeen to twenty-one-year results. J Bone Joint Surg Am 2001;83:1688. [PMID: 11701792]

Vallo CI: Flexural strength distribution of a PMMA-based bone cement. J Biomed Mater Res 2002;63:226. [PMID: 11870658]

Weisman DL et al: In vitro evaluation of antibiotic elution from polymethylmethacrylate (PMMA) and mechanical assessment of antibiotic-PMMA composites. Vet Surg 2000;29:245. [PMID:10871226]

Yamamoto T et al: Wear analysis of retrieved ceramic-on-ceramic articulations in total hip arthroplasty: Femoral head makes contact with the rim of the socket outside of the bearing surface. J Biomed Mater Res B Appl Biomater 2005;73:301. [PMID: 15742373]

GROWTH FACTORS

Biology

Growth factors hold great promise for the treatment of a variety of musculoskeletal conditions. The response of bone to structural damage is nearly unique in biology. The vast majority of tissues, when traumatized, heal with a fibrous scar, the cells and structure of which are not normal and are unable to assume fully the function of the tissue. In contrast, bone, the cornea, and the liver are capable of true cellular, morphologic, and functional regeneration. The initial phase of bone healing is characterized by an inflammatory response in consolidation of the hematoma within the fracture site. This is followed by the proliferation of periosteal, endosteal, and marrow stromal cells adjacent to the site, and recruitment of undifferentiated mesenchymal cells from nearby soft tissues. These cells and their progeny differentiate to become chondroblasts, chondrocytes, osteoblasts, and osteocytes. The cartilage formed is eventually replaced by bone, and the early woven bone is remodeled to a more mature lamellar structure.

Growth factors are polypeptides that serve as signaling agents for cells. These local proteins bind to specific receptors, occasionally with the assistance of extracellular binding proteins, to stimulate or inhibit functions inside the cell during development and throughout an organism's life. For example, growth/differentiation factor-5 (GDF-5) is essential for normal appendicular skeletal and joint development in humans. GDF-5 acts at two stages of skeletal development and by two distinct mechanisms: (1) promoting the initial stages of chondrogenesis by promoting cell adhesion and (2) increasing the size of the skeletal elements by increasing proliferation within the epiphyseal cartilage adjacent to its expression within the joint interzone. The discovery of these substances revolutionized the field of cell biology by revealing the mechanisms of regulation of cell activities. Growth factors are present in plasma or tissues, in concentrations measured in billionths of a gram; yet, they are the principal effectors of critical cellular functions, such as cell proliferation, matrix synthesis, and tissue differentiation. Cytokines are similar to growth factors because they are receptor-activating locally acting polypeptides. Although cytokines were originally characterized from cells of the hematopoietic and immune cell systems, the distinction is rather artificial because most authors currently consider growth factors to be a subset of cytokines.

Although the same growth factor is often found throughout the body, they are named based on their function and tissue of origin. Several growth-promoting substances are identified in bone matrix and at the site of fracture healing. These growth factors are believed to play a role in the healing process. Among these are the transforming growth factor beta (TGF-β), BMP, fibroblast growth factors (FGF), IGFs, and platelet-derived growth factor (PDGF). These growth factors are produced by osteoblasts and incorporated into the extracellular matrix during bone formation. Small amounts of growth factors can also be trapped systemically from serum and incorporated into the matrix. The present hypothesis is that growth factors are located within the matrix until remodeling or trauma causes solubilization and release of the proteins.

A. Transforming Growth Factor Beta

TGF-βs are a family of dimeric polypeptide growth factors and coded by closely related genes. The family includes at least five molecules known as TGF-β 1–4, and, by itself, it is a member of a superfamily that includes BMPs, activins, and GDFs, among others, that regulate morphogenesis in early development. The broad range of cellular activities regulated by TGF-βs include the proliferation and expression of differentiated phenotypes of many of the cell populations that make up the skeleton. Among these are the mesenchymal precursor cells for chondrocytes, osteoblasts, and osteoclasts. The presence of TGF-βs in normal fracture healing suggests they play a role in the repair process. TGF-βs are secreted in an inactive form requiring acid pH or heat for activation. These dimeric, disulfide bonded molecules mediate their function through receptors that act as serine/threonine kinases. The receptors autophosphorylate, after forming a complex with TGF-β, activate Smad intracellular pathways that translocate to the nucleus and regulate gene transcription. Thus far, eight mammalian Smad proteins are identified. After oligomerization, these proteins enter the nucleus to regulate transcription following assembly with transcriptional cofactors and comodulators. Because articular cartilage has limited potential for repair, TGF-β 1 is used in animal studies for its stimulatory effect on chondrogenesis in periosteal explants.

B. Bone Morphogenetic Protein

Related to the TGF-βs, the bone morphogenic proteins constitute a family of at least 15 growth factors originally identified for their ability to stimulate de novo bone formation. The BMPs are also referred to as osteogenic proteins (OPs); hence, there is some name confusion because BMP-7 is also called OP-1. BMPs are the only growth factors that can stimulate differentiation of mesenchymal stem cells into a chondroblastic (BMP-2) and osteoblastic (BMP-5, -6, and -7) direction. These BMP molecules are also quite effective osteoinductive agents. Noggin and chordin are extracellular binding proteins that alter binding of BMP molecules with their receptors. When implanted, most BMPs can stimulate a cascade of cellular events that closely mimics the process of endochondral ossification in normal fracture healing. Precursor cells are recruited and differentiated into chondrocytes that manufacture cartilage matrix. The cartilage is then gradually replaced by bone as osteoblasts populate the site. Eventually, bone marrow elements fill the newly formed intertrabecular spaces, and the bone remodels. Overexpression of BMP-4 in inflammatory cells is responsible for fibrodysplasia ossificans progressiva.

C. Fibroblast Growth Factors

Fibroblast growth factors are currently a group of eleven polypeptides that were originally discovered on the basis of their mitogenic effect on fibroblasts and have four known receptors. Acid fibroblast growth factor and basic fibroblast growth factor, also termed FGF-1 and FGF-2, respectively, are both implicated in cartilage and bone regulation. Basic FGF is generally more potent than acid FGF. FGFs have a significant proliferative effect on osteoblasts but less effect on protein synthesis. FGFs probably enhance bone formation by increasing the number of cells capable of synthesizing bone collagen. FGFs are also angiogenic factors, which are important for neovascularization during bone healing. A defect in the FGF receptor 3 is implicated as the cause for achondroplasia.

D. Insulin-Like Growth Factor

The pivotal role of IGF in regulating endochondral ossification in skeletal growth suggests that this factor may also participate in endochondral ossification of bone healing. IGF regulates both bone matrix formation and cell replication. Of all the growth factors present in bone matrix, IGF-2 has the highest concentration; however, IGF-1 is four to seven times more potent than IGF-2. IGF-1, also known as somatomedin C, is produced in the liver and by skeletal tissue in response to stimulation with growth hormone. The cells that secrete IGFs also secrete any one of the six IGF-binding proteins that actually regulate the effectiveness of this growth factor.

Both IGF-1 and IGF-2 stimulate preosteoblastic cell replication by increasing the number of cells capable of synthesizing bone matrix. However, their mitogenic effect is less pronounced than those of other growth factors. IGFs also have independent effects on the differentiation of osteoblasts, increasing bone collagen production and inhibiting collagen degradation. Recent studies evaluating the endogenous tissue levels of different growth factors within healing tendon lesions show that there are low endogenous levels of IGF-I. As such, the exogenous administration of IG-1 during the first 2 weeks following injury may provide a therapeutic advantage by bolstering low endogenous tissue levels and thereby enhancing the metabolic response of individual tendon fibroblasts.

E. Platelet-Derived Growth Factor

PDGF was discovered in serum as having a major mitogenic activity responsible for growth of cultured mesenchymal cells. It is a dimeric molecule that exists in two isoforms (A and B). When it is overproduced with some tumors, the protooncogene name is *c-sis*. PDGF is a potent regulator of bone cells and chondrocytes and plays a role in tendon healing.

F. Vascular Endothelial Growth Factor

Vascular endothelial growth factor (VEGF), a potent angiogenic agent, is found in endothelial cells and responsible for the formation of new vasculature. It is involved with the angiogenesis of calcified cartilage and distraction angiogenesis. Although not significantly involved in the formation of normal bone, VEGF is involved with angiogenesis of malignancy. Clinical trials are being performed to evaluate the effectiveness of VEGF therapy into ischemic areas and the role of anti-VEGF therapy for treating malignancy. Studies show that administering autologous platelet-rich clots through the action of VEGF may be beneficial to the treatment of tendon injuries by inducing cell proliferation and promoting the synthesis of angiogenic factors during the healing process.

Applications

Extensive efforts are being made to find methods by which growth factors can be used to stimulate local bone healing and bone formation in a variety of clinical models. The growth factors TGF-β, BMP, IGF-1, and basic FGF are currently the only growth factors that are demonstrated to possess substantial capacity for in vivo bone stimulation. Growth factors are probably best able to exert a stimulatory effect when used in conditions associated with impaired healing. Research has begun to show increasing evidence that growth factors can be used in vivo to stimulate bone healing and bone formation. The growth factors BMP-2 and BMP-7, also known as **osteogenic protein-1 (OP-1),** are in the final stages of pivotal human trials. Issues of the best delivery system are currently being debated from the use of collagen gel/sponge carrier to ex vivo adenoviral-mediated delivery systems.

There are many challenges to the clinical application of growth factors. It is unlikely that cell-signaling molecules act independently of one another or are present in isolation from one another at their sites of action. Although therapeutic measures that employ single agents may be efficacious in some circumstances, it is likely that most clinical applications will require the development of combination or serial treatment regimens. In addition, because the specific actions of growth factors are context dependent, it is critical to distinguish appropriate from inappropriate indications. Considerable effort is directed at altering the method of treating anterior cruciate ligament (ACL) ruptures. Certain growth factors such as TGF-β 1, PDGF-AB, and FGF-2 can alter the biologic functions of human ACL cells in a collagen-glycosaminoglycan (CG) scaffold implanted as a bridge at the site of an ACL rupture. The addition of these selected growth factors to an implantable CG scaffold may actually facilitate ligament healing in the gap between the ruptured ends of the human ACL.

The therapeutic application of growth factors must also accommodate the fact that most factors have a widespread and variable distribution of target cells. A growth factor administered to elicit a desired response from one cell type may also influence other cell types, possibly in unintended or undesirable ways. Finally, in addition to demonstrating acceptable safety profiles and providing a physician-friendly delivery system in the current era of cost consciousness in health care, a growth factor treatment must demonstrate cost effectiveness along with clinical efficacy. Growth factors have many potential orthopedic applications. As challenges are met, it is plausible, if not probable, that growth factors will provide a means of treating patients with a variety of musculoskeletal disorders.

Anitua E et al: Autologous preparations rich in growth factors promote proliferation and induce VEGF and HGF production by human tendon cells in culture J Orthop Res 2005;23(2):281. [PMID: 15779147]

Buxton B et al: Growth/differentiation factor-5 (GDF-5) and skeletal development. J Bone Joint Surg 2001;83A:S23. [PMID: 11263662]

Dahlgren LA et al: Temporal expression of growth factors and matrix molecules in healing tendon lesions. J Orthop Res 2005;23(1):84. [PMID: 15607879]

Meaney Murray M et al: The effect of selected growth factors on human anterior cruciate ligament cell interactions with a three-dimensional collagen-GAG scaffold. J Orthop Res 2003;21:238. [PMID: 12568954]

Miura Y et al: Brief exposure to high-dose transforming growth factor-beta 1 enhances periosteal chondrogenesis in vitro: A preliminary report. J Bone Joint Surg Am 2002;84:793. [PMID: 12004023]

Musgrave DS et al: Gene therapy and tissue engineering in orthopaedic surgery. J Am Acad Orthop Surg 2002;10:6. [PMID: 11809046]

Yoon ST, Boden SD: Osteoinductive molecules in orthopaedics: Basic science and preclinical studies. Clin Orthop 2002;395:33. [PMID: 11937864]

IMPLANT DESIGN & BIOLOGIC ATTACHMENT PROPERTIES

Total joint arthroplasty requires the type of implant materials and design that can support large functional loads. The implant must remain stable and rigid with respect to the bone while sustaining these loads. Adequate interface fixation requires interface micromotion of less than 100 μm or gap spaces less than a fraction of a millimeter. Precise and uniform contact between the device and surrounding bone depends on the skill of the surgeon and the design of the instrumentation with which the site is prepared. The surface area of actual contact is probably small relative to the surface area of the implant. The contact points tend to induce areas of stress concentration rather than distribute the stress evenly. Bone maintains its structural integrity by responding to stress. In areas of stress concentration, bone resorption often occurs. Additionally, fibrous encapsulations of varying thicknesses are commonly found, and these further alter the ability of the implant to distribute stress uniformly. Implant loosening and migration may eventually occur and cause discomfort to the patient, in which case the implant may need to be removed.

Implant Fixation Mechanisms

Several types of implant fixation methods and surface texture designs were investigated to obtain better surgical fit and stress distribution at the implant-bone interface. The methods include the use of a grouting agent, direct bone apposition to the implant surface, bone growth into porous-surfaced implants, and chemical bonding between bone and surface-active ceramic implant coatings.

A. Grouting Agents

PMMA bone cement provides a mechanical interlock between the metal prosthesis and adjacent bone. Bone cement is not an adhesive; therefore, mechanical interlocking depends on the amount of interdigitation of the cement with trabecular bone and the quality of the fixation between the cement and the metal. The most favorable effect of cement fixation is immediate stability of the implant. Bone cement allows for load distribution over a larger area of bone, which reduces stress concentrations that may result in pressure necrosis and remodeling. Despite the early clinical advantages of cement fixation, the long-term results (15–25 years) are not as encouraging. The poor fatigue properties of cement lead to fractures of the cement. These fractures result in altered stress patterns in the bone, eventually leading to bone remodeling and implant loosening. Particulate debris that results from cement fracture is associated with osteolysis and aseptic loosening.

Improvements in the mechanical properties of cement and cementing techniques over the past two to three decades are leading to more promising results regarding the longevity of cemented prostheses. Femoral stems that were implanted with modern cement techniques maintain stability and function beyond 10 years in 95–98% of the cases.

B. Direct Bone Apposition

Optimal osseointegration at the bone-implant interface is affected by the material properties and design of the implant. Implant design encompasses both the surface texture and geometry of the implant. The mechanical properties of the implant-bone interface were investigated with various surface preparations, including smooth finishes, roughened or grit-blasted finishes, and grooved surfaces. Histologically, implants with smooth finishes have interfaces characterized by fibrous encapsulation, whereas implants with grit-blasted finishes have interfaces characterized by areas of direct bone apposition. Numerous studies demonstrated that surface texture is a significant factor in obtaining adequate implant fixation with direct bone apposition methods.

Evaluation of implant materials, including PMMA, commercially pure titanium, aluminum oxide, and low-temperature isotropic pyrolytic carbon with various surface finishes, demonstrated that the implant elastic modulus or surface composition did not significantly affect the interface attachment strength or histologic response. Surface texture significantly affected the interface mechanical properties, however. Implants with grit-blasted surfaces exhibited significantly higher interface attachment strengths than implants with polished surfaces did. Histologically, all implants with grit-blasted surfaces demonstrated areas of direct bone apposition, whereas all implants with polished surfaces demonstrated fibrous encapsulation (Figure 1–23), indicating that bone apposition required textured interface surface for attachment.

C. Porous Ingrowth Attachment

The long-term problems associated with implant fixation with PMMA led to the development the porous coating as a method for permanent biologic fixation of prostheses. It is generally accepted that an implant can achieve stabilization by tissue growth into the surface porous structure if (1) the material is bioinert, (2) there is direct apposition of the bone at the implant interface,

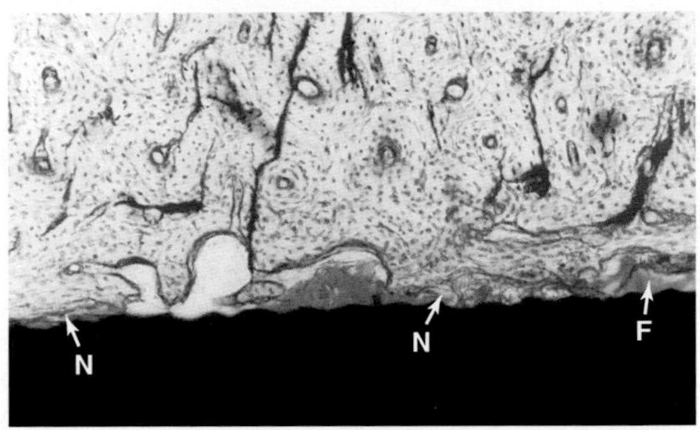

Figure 1–23. Histologic appearance of mechanically tested grit-blasted titanium alloy implants 10 weeks after implantation. Areas of direct bone apposition (N) and minimal fibrous tissue (F) were observed at the implant interface. The undecalcified histologic section was photographed using simultaneous transmitted and reflected illumination (basic fuchsin and toluidine blue stain; original magnification × 160).

(3) there is minimal or no movement at the implant site, and (4) the porous structure has appropriate pore size and morphology.

Porous coatings are effective as a means of biologic fixation because their interface attachment strength of fixation is at least an order of magnitude higher than that of nonporous implants relying on direct bone apposition for fixation.

To maintain optimal bone growth into a porous structure, the pores must be large enough to accommodate the development of bone tissue. Several groups of investigators concluded that a pore size of 100 μm allowed bone ingrowth but that a pore size greater than 150 μm was necessary for osteon formation. Another group investigated the optimal pore size range for cobalt-based alloys by observing the rate of bone ingrowth and time necessary to attain maximal attachment strength. The results indicated that although a pore size range of 50–400 μm obtained the maximal attachment strength in the shortest time, osteon formation was not demonstrated histologically at this range. In addition to a minimal pore size, an effective porous coating must also have appropriate pore morphology. The available porous layer for bone growth must be large enough to accommodate a sufficient quantity of bone to maintain adequate fixation, and a volume fraction porosity of 35–40% is accepted as optimal for effective biologic fixation of an implant with a strongly bonded porous layer. The volume fraction porosity is related to the interconnection pore size, particle interconnectivity, and particle size of the porous coating. Particle interconnectivity is important for ensuring adequate strength within the coating and between the coating and substrate. Too much particle interconnectivity can decrease the interconnection pore size and restrict the amount and type of ingrown tissue, however. A two-layer porous surface creates an interconnected and open porosity that is effective in creating a three-dimensional mechanical interlock of the ingrown bone.

Several different types of porous coatings were evaluated, including the fiber mesh, beaded porous, and irregular plasma-sprayed types. The fiber mesh type of porous coating is composed of wires that are cut and kinked to form the specific shape of the coating. The wires are then bonded to a solid metal substrate of the same metallic alloy through a sintering process in an inert gas environment or vacuum. The porosity obtained with this technique ranges from 40% to 50% with a mean pore size of 270 μm. A void type of porous coating was obtained using a cobalt-based or titanium-based alloy. Magnesium microspheres are mixed with the base alloy by means of an investment casting technique. Under high temperatures, the magnesium evaporates, leaving pores on the surface of the alloy. This technique produces pores with different depths and connectivities. The most frequently studied porous coating is the beaded type. Cobalt-based alloy or titanium metal powder or macrobeads are either gravity compacted or applied with an organic binder onto a substrate. The beads are then sintered to the substrate at a submelting temperature for the base metal. The porosity ranges from 30% to 45% with pore diameters ranging from 100 to 400 μm. Production of another type of porous coating involves plasma-spraying titanium to either a titanium-based or cobalt-based alloy substrate. The plasma-spray technique is further discussed with regard to ceramic coatings (see following section).

The extent to which implants are covered with porous coating varies. On femoral stems, it ranges anywhere from complete coverage to coverage of the proximal third. The extent of porous coating to achieve optimal stability is not determined. Circumferential coverage is preferable, however, to prevent wear debris migration toward the distal portion of the prosthetic stem.

Clinically, the short-term results for porous-coated prostheses are comparable to those for cemented prostheses. Histologically, retrieved human prostheses demonstrated variable amounts of bone ingrowth, ranging from limited to extensive, with large amounts of fibrous tissue (Figure 1–24). Some retrieved prostheses exhibited complete fibrous tissue infiltration into the porous surface. Components with limited bone ingrowth showed fibrous tissue that was oriented in a fashion capable of load transmission. The bone ingrowth and extensive fibrous ingrowth are most likely effective mechanisms for early implant stabilization. A histologic analysis performed on six retrieved, noncemented, porous-coated femoral hip components demonstrated a significant increase in bone ingrowth from 19 to 53 months after implantation. The data showed that human bone remodels slowly and advances appositionally with limited endochondral ossification. Therefore, to achieve reproducible bone ingrowth, the porous coating must be adjacent to cortical bone.

D. Surface Topography and Coatings

Calcium phosphate coatings on metal surfaces were developed to overcome the mechanical problems of the ceramic as well as the biologic shortcomings of the metal. Many composite implants are manufactured to have the mechanical properties of the metal and the biologic properties of the bioactive ceramics. However, evidence is mounting from animal studies suggesting that quantity of ingrowth is approximately 80% dependent on the microscopic surface morphology and only modestly (approximately 20%) dependent on the hydroxyapatite (HA) chemistry. The bone formation is apparently encouraged by a microscopically rough surface, which is routinely produced with a crystalline HA surface coating. Titanium ingrowth was enhanced by acid etching the surface of implants, which changes its microscopic topography. Biological coatings of HA (calcium phosphates) may still enhance the chemistry of the surface, and they are the standard method of inducing ingrowth.

The bond between a metal substrate and a HA coating is critical to the success of a coated prosthesis. The processes and techniques of coating a prosthesis vary, and for this reason not all HA coatings perform equivalently.

A coating thickness of 50 μm is generally accepted as adequate for coverage of nonporous surfaces; thinner coatings are necessary for porous coatings to keep from blocking the pores. Coating thickness >50 μm tend to separate from the substrate and can cause debris that compromises the bearing surfaces. A coating thickness of 25–45 μm does not occlude the pores or alter the mechanical bone ingrowth properties of the porous surface.

Chemical dissolution of an HA surface within the first few months of implantation occurs when coating thicknesses of 15 μm or less are used. Calcium phosphate coatings are applied to substrates by a variety of methods, including dip coating, vacuum deposition, and plasma spraying. In dip coating, the substrate can either be dipped into a suspension of ceramic powder in a carrier or be dipped into a liquid form of glass ceramic. In vacuum deposition, ceramic material is removed from a source and deposited onto the target substrate.

Plasma-spraying methods are used by most manufacturers to apply calcium phosphate coatings to metal surfaces, particularly for load-bearing applications. A plasma or ionized gas is created by passing a gas or mix-

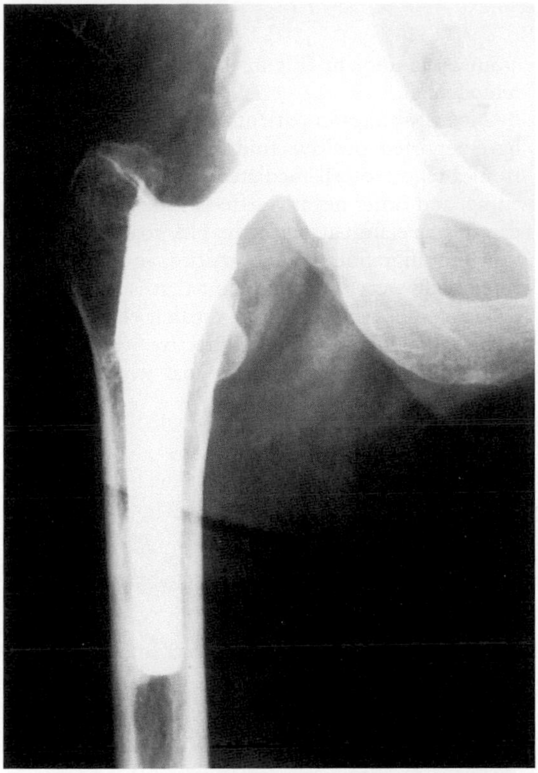

A 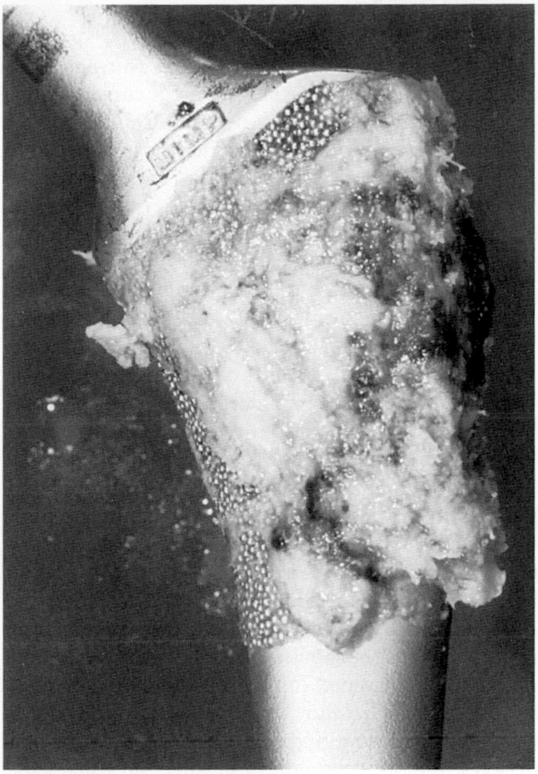 B

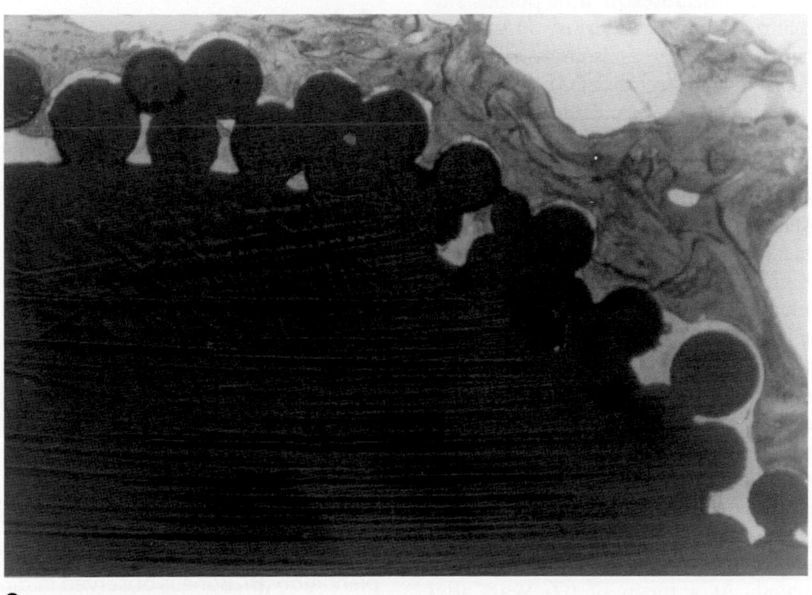

C

Figure 1–24. Four years after implantation, an uncemented porous-coated femoral stem was removed for revision because the patient suffered persistent thigh pain and limp. **A:** The radiograph taken prior to stem removal showed a relatively poor fit, without subsidence but with the presence of nonanatomic remodeling, as evidenced by the so-called pedestal sign. **B:** Gross specimen (posterior aspect) analysis suggested that the component was well fixed, as demonstrated by large amounts of bone. **C:** Histologic examination demonstrated extensive bone ingrowth (basic fuchsin and toluidine blue stain; original magnification × 24).

ture of gases (usually argon or a mixture of nitrogen and hydrogen) through a high-energy, direct current (DC) electric arc struck between two electrodes. Then the coating powder suspended in a carrier gas is introduced into this plasma stream, melted, and propelled onto the substrate target, usually at high velocities. The coating is applied in several layers, each approximately 5–10 μm thick.

Because of the high temperatures necessary for plasma spraying, the ceramic coating material may be chemically or structurally altered from the original ceramic. For this reason, all HA coatings are not identical and may vary among manufacturers in their composition, crystallinity, density, purity, and structure. These differences may affect the surface topography, bioactivity, and bioresorbability of coatings and make it nearly impossible to predict their long-term in vivo behavior. To ensure the correct composition of HA coatings, manufacturers perform a variety of tests, including radiograph diffraction, infrared spectroscopy, scanning electron microscopy, and atomic absorption spectroscopy. Several studies showed that HA-coated implants are superior to uncoated implants in terms of interface attachment strength and bone apposition. In newer research, HA coating improved bone purchase and bone-screw interface strength in healthy and osteopenic animals. Also, the properties of HA-coated implants with larger surface areas (macrotextured or porous surfaces) are superior to the properties of HA-coated implants with smaller surface areas (smooth surfaces). IGF-1, basic fibroblast growth factor (bFGF) and TGF-β 1, alone and in combination, were tested to augment osseointegration and were absorbed onto a carrier of β-tricalcium phosphate (β-TCP). These composites were implanted into a defect around a hydroxyapatite-coated, stainless steel implant in the proximal tibia of rat in a model of revision arthroplasty. Although no growth factor combination significantly enhanced new bone formation or the mechanical strength of the implant, of the growth factors tested, only bFGF had any beneficial effect on the host response to the implant, perhaps by delaying osteoblast differentiation and thereby prolonging osteoclast access to the ceramic.

Clinical experience with HA-coated orthopedic prostheses is limited. Therefore, only short-term studies based on clinical follow-ups and radiographic evaluations exist. In a prospective bilateral total hip replacement study, a titanium prosthesis with and without HA coating was evaluated. At a mean of 6.6 years after implantation, there was no difference in clinical or radiographic results. Similar short-term results were reported for HA-coated, porous, cobalt-chromium primary and revision femoral hip stems. Other findings in early clinical studies of HA-coated porous implants included decreased pain, decreased radiolucent lines around the implant (Figure 1-25), and improved bone remodeling.

Not all studies in patients with HA-coated implants have reported positive findings. In fact, some newer studies reported cell-mediated osteolysis, implant loosening, and other negative effects linked with the degradation or delamination of the HA coating, the generation and migration of HA particles, and the subsequent three-body wear of the implant that is caused by these particles. These findings suggest that changing the surface topology might be an effective way of achieving the same or nearly the same goal with less potential problems.

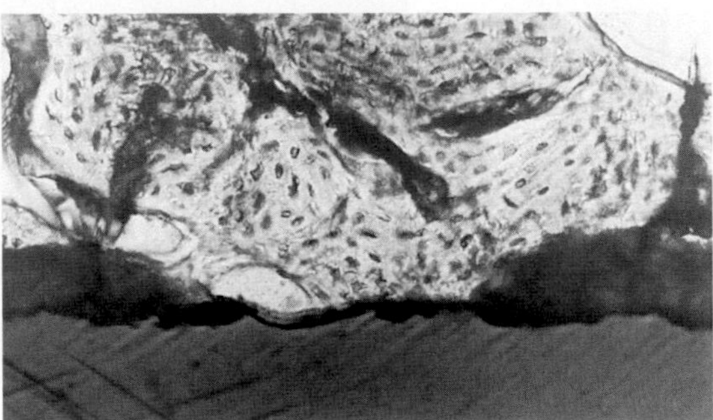

A

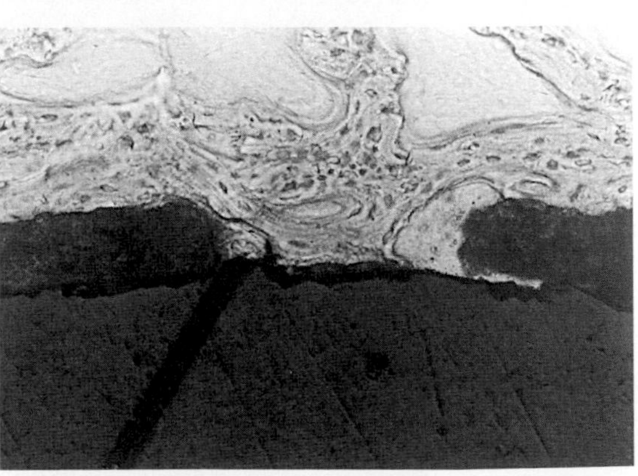

B

Figure 1–25. Histologic appearance of an HA-coated implant with a defect shown at two points in time: at 10 weeks after implantation (**A**) and at 32 weeks after implantation (**B**). Bone is observed in direct apposition to the HA coating and extending continuously from the edge of the HA material into the defect and along the metal substrate. The undecalcified histologic sections were photographed using simultaneous transmitted and reflected illumination (basic fuchsin and toluidine blue stain; original magnification × 160).

Factors That Affect Biologic Attachment

Attachment at the bone-implant interface is affected by the material properties and design of the implant, surgical technique, initial implant stability, and direct contact with the surrounding bone. Initial implant stability and apposition with bone are not always achievable but are vital for implant longevity. Persistent micromotion at the bone-implant interface causes bone resorption and necrosis, which can in turn result in fibrous tissue infiltration at the interface and in implant loosening. Moreover, any initial gap between the implant and surrounding bone may adversely alter the amount of osseointegration and the rate at which it occurs.

A. Motion at the Bone-Implant Interface

Motion of an implant within the surgical site has a primary influence on biologic fixation and implant longevity. Initial implant stability is essential for the early tissue infiltrate within the porous structure to differentiate into bone by either direct bone formation or appositional bone growth. When excessive early movement occurs at the bone-implant interface, bone formation within the pores is inhibited. The majority of research concerning motion at the interface involves porous implants; however, the findings are applicable for press-fit implant systems.

Studies of implants suggest that relative motion of greater than 150 μm at the bone-implant interface prevents bone formation, although a well-ordered fibrous tissue interface was maintained and provided adequate implant attachment. When interface motion was 40 μm, bone ingrowth occurred, but the calcified ingrown bone was not continuous with the surrounding bone. These findings support the concept that in optimal bone growth into porous surfaces or bone apposition onto press-fit surfaces requires little or no initial micromotion at the interface.

In a study of HA coating in a continuous loaded implant model, investigators found that when interface motion led to the formation of a fibrous membrane, the HA coating was able to convert the membrane to bone. Furthermore, pulsed electromagnetic fields accelerated HA osteointegration in trabecular bone.

B. Surgical Fit

The technical difficulties in cutting bone precisely to provide an exact fit around the implant often result in a poor surgical fit. Implant and instrumentation design may also make it difficult to achieve initial implant-bone interface apposition. When a femoral stem is press-fit into the femoral canal, only 10–20% of the prosthesis comes into direct contact with bone.

The effects of interface gaps and poor surgical fit of implants were investigated by numerous groups. In studies of HA-coated prostheses, researchers found that the HA coating does not compensate for improper implant placement or poor surgical technique. The cell populations necessary for bone formation are identical across large interface gaps and in press-fit situations. In large gaps, the rate of gap filling and subsequent ingrowth is delayed, and the quality of bone at the interface may also be reduced. Such studies indicate the potential benefits of robot-controlled surgery, where much better initial apposition can be obtained.

Aldini NN et al: Pedicular fixation in the osteoporotic spine: A pilot in vivo study on long-term ovariectomized sheep. J Orthop Res 2002;20:1217. [PMID: 12472232]

Bach CM et al: No functional impairment after Robodoc total hip arthroplasty: Gait analysis in 25 patients. Acta Orthop Scand 2002;73:386. [PMID: 12358109]

Bobyn JD et al: The optimum pore size for the fixation of porous-surfaced metal implants by the ingrowth of bone. Clin Orthop 1980;150:263. [PMID: 7428231]

Clarke SA et al: The effect of osteogenic growth factors on bone growth into a ceramic filled defect around an implant. J Orthop Res 2004;22:1016. [PMID: 15304274]

DeGroot K et al: Plasma sprayed coatings of hydroxylapatite. J Biomed Mater Res 1987;21:1375.

Fernandez-Pradas JM et al: Characterization of calcium phosphate coatings deposited by Nd-YAG laser ablation at 355 nm: Influence of thickness. Biomaterials 2002;23:1989. [PMID: 11996040]

Freels DB et al: Animal model for evaluation of soft tissue ingrowth into various types of porous coating. Clin Orthop 2002;397: 315. [PMID: 11953623]

Geesink RG: Osteoconductive coatings for total joint arthroplasty. Clin Orthop 2002;395:53. [PMID: 11937866]

Hacking SA et al: Acid-etched microtexture for enhancement of bone growth into porous-coated implants. J Bone Joint Surg Br 2003;85:1182. [PMID: 14653605]

Hacking SA et al: Relative contributions of chemistry and topography to the osseointegration of hydroxyapatite coatings. Clin Orthop 2002;405:24. [PMID: 12461353]

Jinno T et al: Comparison of hydroxyapatite and hydroxyapatite tricalcium-phosphate coatings. J Arthroplasty 2002;17:902. [PMID: 12375251]

Karabatsos B et al: Osseointegration of hydroxyapatite porous-coated femoral implants in a canine model. Clin Orthop 2001;392:442. [PMID: 11716420]

Kim YH et al: Comparison of porous-coated titanium femoral stems with and without hydroxyapatite coating. J Bone Joint Surg Am 2003;85:1682. [PMID: 12954825]

LeGeros RZ: Properties of osteoconductive biomaterials: Calcium phosphates. Clin Orthop 2002;395:81. [PMID: 11937868]

Manso M et al: Biological evaluation of aerosol-gel-derived hydroxyapatite coatings with human mesenchymal stem cells. Biomaterials 2002;23:3985. [PMID: 12162331]

Nevelos JE et al: Wear of HIPed and non-HIPed alumina-alumina hip joints under standard and severe simulator testing conditions. Biomaterials 2001;22:2191. [PMID: 11456058]

Noble PC et al: The anatomic basis of femoral component design. Clin Orthop 1988;235:148. [PMID:3416522]

Paprosky WG, Burnett RS. Extensively porous-coated femoral stems in revision hip arthroplasty: Rationale and results. Am J Orthop 2002;31:471. [PMID: 12216970]

Pilliar RM et al: Observations on the effect of movement on bone ingrowth into porous-surfaced implants. Clin Orthop 1986; 208:108. [PMID: 3720113]

Soballe K et al: Hydroxyapatite coating converts fibrous tissue to bone around loaded implants. J Bone Joint Surg Br 1993; 75:270. [PMID: 8444949]

Thomas KA et al: The effect of surface macrotexture and hydroxylapatite coating on the mechanical strengths and histologic profiles of titanium implant materials. J Biomed Mater Res 1987;21:1395. [PMID: 3429474]

Thomsen MN et al: Robotically-milled bone cavities: A comparison with hand-broaching in different types of cementless hip stems. Acta Orthop Scand 2002;73:379. [PMID: 12358108]

TISSUE RESPONSE TO IMPLANT MATERIALS

The effect of an implanted material on adjacent tissues depends on the amount and type of substance released into the tissues, the histologic response to the material, and the wear and corrosion properties of the material. The type of response to the implant determines the biologic classification of the material.

Biocompatibility

Biotolerant materials, such as stainless steel, PMMA, and UHMWPE, elicit the worst tissue response. When these materials are used, a fibrous tissue layer may form between the bone and the implant. This fibrous layer is generally observable as a radiolucent line on radiographs. Examination with light microscopy shows the presence of numerous macrophages near resorbing adjacent bone and the resulting fibrous tissue that contains macrophages and foreign body giant cells.

PMMA elicits adverse local and systemic effects from the moment of its introduction into the body. At the time of implantation, PMMA causes local tissue necrosis because of the extreme heat of polymerization. During the polymerization process, monomer may leach into the surrounding tissues and cause hypotension. Finally, PMMA fragmentation particles elicit a chronic macrophage response at the implant-bone interface, which can result in progressive osteoclasis and eventual aseptic loosening of the implant. Macrophages are stimulated by cell necrosis, bacteria, and foreign particulate matter. Particulate matter is the primary cause of aseptic loosening in cemented joint arthroplasties. In spite of this, bulk PMMA is well tolerated by the body, whereas particulate PMMA is not.

Bioinert materials, such as titanium and cobalt-chromium alloys, usually cause minimal tissue irritation. With stable implants of either titanium or cobalt-chromium alloys, appositional bone growth or osseointegration occurs. If titanium implants are used in articulating surface applications, however, they have poor wear resistance, and the excessive wear particles behave as biotolerant materials. These particles elicit a chronic macrophage response, which can lead to implant loosening. However, newer animal studies showed that coating titanium implants with autologous osteoblasts accelerates and enhances the osseointegration of these implants and could be a successful biotechnology for future clinical applications.

Bioactive materials, such as calcium phosphate ceramics, offer the best biologic advantage of implant materials. The biocompatibility of the calcium phosphate ceramics is well documented. In response to these implanted ceramics, the body typically responds (1) without local or systemic toxicity, (2) without inflammatory or foreign body reaction, (3) without alteration of natural mineralization processes, (4) with functional integration of bone, and (5) with chemical bonding to bone via natural bone cementing mechanisms. Implant surfaces coated with HA are characterized as being capable of forming direct, intimate bonds with the surrounding bone. The bonding area (approximately 50–200 μm) contains biologic apatite crystals that are highly oriented at the interface with a 10-μm periodicity similar to that of calcified tissue, as determined by electron diffraction studies. The bone apatite crystals are arranged against the implant surface in a palisade fashion, resembling the natural bonding between two bone fragments. The bonding area contains a ground substance that is heavily mineralized, although devoid of collagen fibrils, and is likened to the natural bone cementing substance, which is amorphous in structure, heavily mineralized, and rich in mucopolysaccharides.

One study used animal models to characterize tissue-specific reactions to particles of bone-substitute materials for osteocompatibility. Tested particles included demineralized bone powder (DBP), nonresorbable calcium phosphate (nrCP), PMMA, polyethylene (PE), and resorbable calcium phosphates (rCPs). Although both DBP and nrCP were incorporated into the reactive medullary and cortical bone, DBP also induced enchondral osteogenesis, and nrCP evoked a fibrous reaction. Although PMMA particles were surrounded with a fibrous layer, they did not impair bone healing. PE shards and rCPs were inflammatory and inhibited osseous repair. rCPs, PMMA, and PE shards all generated inflammatory reactions with each particle being surrounded by fibrous tissue and large multinucleated giant cells. DBP showed both osteoinductive as well as osteocompatible properties. Although nrCP was shown to be osteocompatible, rCPs stimulated various degrees of inflammatory responses. PMMA was osteocompatible and did not interfere with the bone healing process. PE was not osteocompatible and generated foreign body reactions in both sites. It is important to distinguish among the osteoinductive, osteocompatible, and inflammatory properties of particles that may be used as bone-substitute materials.

Problems Associated with Maintaining Implant Longevity

Implant loosening, which can result from bone loss that is caused either by stress shielding or by osteolysis, has been a problem associated with total joint arthroplasty since its inception. Periprosthetic osteolysis presents radiographically as diffuse femoral cortical thinning or as a focal cystic lesion.

Although the exact cause of osteolysis is unknown, it is thought to be a result of movement of the implant, primarily at the bearing surface, with generation of wear particles that migrate to the implant-bone interface, where they cause a tissue reaction. Movement at taper joints, or between the implant and bone cement, can cause particulate material. Particulate debris in the 0.1–1.0 μm range are most active in stimulating bone resorption and eventually causing implant loosening. Macrophages play a key role in the osteoclastic process by elaborating cytokines in host defense and in forming precursors for osteoclasts. TNF-α is a key cytokine in the osteolysis process. The prevalence of osteolysis in stable cemented femoral components ranges from 3% to 8%. It appears, however, that osteolysis is observed earlier in patients with stable uncemented components and that the prevalence increases with time in vivo. The prevalence in uncemented systems ranges from 10% to 20% after 2–9 years in vivo. Newer studies suggest that hydrostatic pressure may play a far greater role in the induction of osteolysis than previously thought.

In addition to osteolysis, another problem with total joint implants is the increase in metal ions released into the body. This problem is especially associated with uncemented porous-coated implants. Systemic and long-term effects caused by wear and corrosion are just being discovered. An understanding of the wear and corrosion mechanisms associated with decreasing implant longevity is vital for the development of improved implant designs and material manufacturing methods.

A. Surface Damage of Polyethylene Implants

Osteolysis, loosening, and other complications that reduce implant longevity are attributed to polyethylene wear particles. Careful examination of retrieved polyethylene components demonstrated a variety of modes by which surface damage occurs. These include scratching, burnishing, embedding of debris, pitting (the presence of shallow, irregular surface voids in the surface), surface deformation (permanent deformation on the articulating surface), abrasion (characterized by a tufted or shredded appearance of the polyethylene), and delamination (separation of large, thin surface sheets of polyethylene from implant components).

Fatigue is suggested as the primary mechanism of polyethylene surface damage because the damage was correlated with the length of time since implantation (number of cycles in the fatigue curve shown in Figure 1–2) and with patient weight (applied load or stress in Figure 1–2). Surface damage is noticeably less in acetabular components than in tibial components. The increased polyethylene damage in total knee arthroplasties can be attributed to reduced surface conformity and to compression-tension loading patterns. Nonconformity of articulating components in total knee arthroplasties results in contact stresses that approximate or exceed the yield strength of the polyethylene. Cruciate-retaining designs vary the location of contact over the entire articulating surface, thereby subjecting the implant components to alternating compression-tension contact stresses throughout the loading cycle. This cyclic process could contribute to the beginning and spread of cracks, which may lead to pitting, delamination, and other fatigue failure modes.

The elastic modulus and thickness of the polyethylene are significant predictors of contact stresses large enough to cause surface damage. An increased elastic modulus, as is found with enhanced (Hylamer) polyethylene, raises contact stresses and can be expected to result in increased wear. This is important in component design because the elastic modulus of polyethylene near the surface may increase up to 100% over 10 years in vivo. A reduced level of polyethylene thickness, as is found in metal-backed acetabular and tibial components, can result in increased wear and creep, eventually leading to cracking and separation of the polyethylene from the metal. To avoid the high stresses that cause cracking, acetabular polyethylene thickness should be greater than 6 mm, and tibial polyethylene thickness should be greater than 8 mm. Another concern regarding metal-backed components is that loosening of the metal backing may cause the screws to break and migrate into the polyethylene insert, and this in turn can result in the generation of large amounts of metal and polyethylene wear debris.

The current practice is to try to minimize polyethylene wear debris through the use of highly cross-linked polyethylene for total hip applications, with some trials for total knee applications. The higher contact stresses on knee components is concerning from a materials viewpoint because the cross-linked material has a lower ductility and fatigue strength, although even in this application, early reports are encouraging. Other strategies to reduce particulate wear include alternative bearings, such as ceramic on ceramic, metal on metal, and ceramic on polyethylene, either as bulk ceramic (alumina) or as a surface treatment(oxidized zirconium).

B. Fatigue of Porous-Coated Implants

The primary failure mode of load-bearing orthopedic implants is fatigue. The majority of hip and knee systems have sintered porous coatings to maximize biologic fixation or cement impregnation. The fatigue properties of these porous-coated implants are influenced not only by the sintering treatment but also by a notch effect from the coating.

Sintering affects the fatigue properties of coated implants by altering the microstructure of their metal substrate. With titanium-based alloys, sintering requires that the material be heat treated above the beta phase transition temperature, which reduces the fatigue properties of the material by approximately 40%. When postsintering heat treatments are performed, the fatigue strength of the previously sintered titanium-based alloy increases by 25%. With cobalt-based alloys, sintering does not necessarily result in a reduction of fatigue strength. A dissolution of carbides and an increase in porosity occur, however, when cobalt-based alloys with less than 0.3% carbon are exposed to sintering temperatures. Additionally, with improper cooling, the sintered cobalt-based alloys can develop continuous grain boundary precipitates.

Investigators performed studies to determine the effects of sintering, postsintering heat treatments, and HIP techniques on the fatigue properties of nonporous and porous-coated cobalt-based alloys. They reported that sintered materials exhibited severe porosity and continuous grain boundary precipitates, which resulted in reduced fatigue and tensile strength. HIP eliminated the porosity and grain boundary precipitation resulting from sintering, however. Moreover, HIP of the sintered materials increased the tensile and fatigue properties in implants with or without a porous coating.

Aside from manufacturing processes, which may alter the fatigue properties of the substrate, porous coatings demonstrate a notch effect at the contact regions. These regions are susceptible to the initiation of cracks, which may continue to propagate along surface grain boundaries. This effect is most significant for the titanium-based alloys.

The fatigue properties that are caused by sintering and the notch effect of coating in load-bearing implants can be reduced by the following measures: (1) avoiding the use of porous coating in regions of maximal tensile stress, (2) using an additional heat treatment process on previously sintered titanium-based alloys, and (3) using HIP on previously sintered cobalt-based alloys.

The fatigue properties have to be considered in relation to newer animal studies that evaluated the roles of sex and estrogen therapy on the amount of bone ingrowth into porous cobalt-chromium implants. Histological examination showed significantly more bone ingrowth in areas with cortical bone contact than in areas with cancellous bone contact, with no difference between male and female animals. However, ovariectomized animals showed less overall bone ingrowth than male and female controls, and bone ingrowth in areas with cortical bone contact did not decrease significantly, whereas bone ingrowth in areas with cancellous bone contact was significantly impaired. In another study evaluating osseointegration, osteoblasts from patients older than 60 years were less able to form bone on Ti-6Al-4V implants. Taken together, these data suggest that extensively coated or full-coated porous prostheses are recommended to achieve enough cortical bone contact and ingrowth for postmenopausal patients.

C. Metal Implants: Ion Release, Metal-on-Metal Bearings, and Immunology

Any metal exposed to the physiologic environment will corrode. Corrosion is most evident in fracture fixation devices. Retrieval studies of stainless steel components revealed evidence of pitting and crevice corrosion in approximately 75% of the components.

Apart from potential implant mechanical failure, the clinical significance of corrosion is determined by the type and quantity of metal ion that is released and by the local and systemic effects of ion release. The widespread use of porous coatings on metallic implants and the popularity of metal-on-metal bearing surfaces has raised additional concerns regarding metal ion release. Porous coatings increase the amount of surface area that is exposed to body fluids by a factor of 1.2 to 7.2. Depending on the type and morphology of the porous coating, the increased surface area could increase the corrosion and ion release rates by a factor of 1.2 to 5.2. Unlike the metallic surface of cemented implants, the metallic surface of porous implants is in direct contact with the endosteal bone surface and vasculature, creating an environment in which a cellular response to metallic ions is possible. Another significant source of metal ions in the systemic circulation is the loose prosthesis. Local synovial fluid levels were increased in most prostheses at revision, but examination of blood showed that metal ion concentrations were elevated only in cases involving loose components. The metal-on-metal (MOM) bearing does not directly increase the corrosion area but does produce metal particulate debris that has a very large surface area to volume ratio. This debris then is available to dissolve and put ions into the systemic circulation. Significantly increased levels of implant elements are documented in serum and urine after implantation of these devices. Reference values for two of these elements in blood are cobalt, <0.15 μg/L, and chromium, <0.26 μg/L. Blood cobalt levels are reported to be 5–20 times higher and chromium levels 5–10 times higher than reference levels for MOM bearing total hips.

Released metal ions (Al, Co, Cr, Fe, Mn, Ni, Ti, and V ions) have one of four types of possible effects on the body: metabolic, bacteriologic, immunogenic, or oncogenic. With the possible exception of titanium, the metallic elements used to fabricate implants are either essential or toxic to processes of metabolism. Although it is known that excessive concentrations of essential elements can produce toxic effects, the ultimate fate of the released ions locally, systemically, or in remote organ systems remains to be determined. There is a reported increase in chromosome translocations and aneuploidy in peripheral lymphocytes after MOM hip arthroplasties, but the risk of cancer does not seem to be increased in the few underpowered studies available.

Metal sensitivity induced by metal ion release is not a common problem causing prosthesis loosening. The prevalence of dermal sensitivity in patients with joint replacements is greater than in the general population, and dermal patch testing is not accepted for identifying patients at risk for hypersensitivity to the implant materials. Nickel, chromium, and cobalt (present in cobalt-chromium [Co-Cr] alloy) are the ions most frequently responsible for metal sensitivity reactions. When investigators studied porous-coated hip and knee devices retrieved from patients, they reported the finding of a cellular response in interfacial and interstitial tissues. Although none of the components were removed because of infection and none had shown clinical or radiographic evidence of loosening, the investigators identified an inflammatory infiltrate with accompanying vascular proliferation in 22% of the components. The predominant cell types within the porous coatings were lymphocytes and histiocytes, although giant cells were also present. Several groups reported that delayed hypersensitivity can produce an immunologic reaction in which T cells recognize a metal ion-protein complex, release a variety of lymphokines, and stimulate a mononuclear infiltration. Further research is necessary, however, to determine if an allergic or hypersensitivity response to metal ions is responsible for inflammatory infiltrates. Various tests were proposed to determine if a particular patient is likely to have a sensitivity reaction. However, sensitivity is rare, so routine testing would be expensive and unrewarding, and in the case of a positive history, the surgeon would still be likely to use a component that does not contain the potentially offending elements, such as titanium alloy or zirconium alloy, with ceramic as a femoral head.

MOM bearing surfaces, on the one hand, have the potential to reduce the wear debris problem, but, on the other hand, they are certain to raise levels of circulating ions and raise issues of long-term safety from an organ viewpoint. Hypersensitivity issues may also be increased.

Anissian L et al: Cobalt ions influence proliferation and function of human osteoblast-like cells. Acta Orthop Scand 2002;73:369. [PMID: 12143988]

Berzins A et al: Surface damage in machined ram-extruded and net-shape molded retrieved polyethylene tibial inserts of total knee replacements. J Bone Joint Surg Am 2002;84:1534. [PMID: 12208909]

Brown SR et al: Long-term survival of McKee-Farrar total hip prostheses. Clin Orthop 2002;402:157. [PMID: 12218479]

Cook SD et al: Inflammatory response in retrieved noncemented porous coated implants. Clin Orthop 1991;264:209. [PMID: 1997238]

Cook SD et al: The effect of post-sintering heat treatments on the fatigue properties of porous coated Ti-6Al-4V alloy. J Biomed Mater Res 1988;22:287. [PMID: 3372550]

Dorr LD et al: Histologic, biochemical, and ion analysis of tissue and fluids during total hip arthroplasty. Clin Orthop 1990; 261:82. [PMID: 2173987]

Edwards SA et al: Analysis of polyethylene thickness of tibial components in total knee replacement. J Bone Joint Surg Am 2002;84:369. [PMID: 11886905]

Eid K et al: Tissue reactions to particles of bone-substitute materials in intraosseous and heterotopic sites in rats: Discrimination of osteoinduction, osteocompatibility, and inflammation. J Orthop Res 2001;19:962-9. [PMID: 11562148]

Friberg L et al: *Handbook on the Toxicology of Metals.* Elsevier, 1986.

Frosch KH et al: Autologous osteoblasts enhance osseointegration of porous titanium implants. J Orthop Res 2003;21:213. [PMID: 12568951]

Georgette FS, Davidson JA: The effect of hot isostatic pressing on the fatigue and tensile strength of a cast, porous coated Co-Cr-Mo alloy. J Biomed Mater Res 1986;20:1229. [PMID: 3782180]

Goldberg JR et al: A multicenter retrieval study of the taper interfaces of modular hip prostheses. Clin Orthop 2002;401:149. [PMID: 12151892]

Hallab NJ, Mikecz K, Jacobs JJ: A triple assay technique for the evaluation of metal-induced, delayed-type hypersensitivity responses in patients with or receiving total joint arthroplasty. J Biomed Mater Res 2000;53:480. [PMID: 10984695]

Hallab NJ et al: Immune responses correlate with serum-metal in metal-on-metal hip arthroplasty. J Arthroplasty 2004;19 (Suppl):88. [PMID: 15578560]

Hallab NJ et al: Metal sensitivity in patients with orthopaedic implants. J Bone Joint Surg Am 2001;83:428. [PMID: 11263649]

Huang CH et al: Particle size and morphology of UHMWPE wear debris in failed total knee arthroplasties—A comparison between mobile bearing and fixed bearing knees. J Orthop Res 2002;20:1038. [PMID: 12382971]

Ingrahm E, Fisher J: The role of macrophages in osteolysis of total joint replacement. Biomaterials 2005;26:1271. [PMID: 15475057]

Ladon D et al: Changes in metal levels and chromosome aberrations in the peripheral blood of patients after metal-on-metal hip arthroplasty. J Arthroplasty 2004;19(Suppl):78. [PMID: 15578558]

MacDonald SJ: Can a safe level for metal ions in patients with metal-on-metal total hip arthroplasties be determined? J Arthroplasty 2004;19(Suppl):71. [PMID: 15578557]

Merritt K, Rodrigo JJ: Immune response to synthetic materials. Sensitization of patients receiving orthopaedic implants. Clin Orthop 1996;326:71. [PMID: 8620661]

Muratoglu OK et al: Optical analysis of surface changes on early retrievals of highly cross-linked and conventional polyethylene tibial inserts. J Arthroplasty 2003;18(Suppl 1):42. [PMID: 14560410]

Murray DW, Rushton N: Macrophages stimulate bone resorption when they phagocytose particles. J Bone Joint Surg Br 1990; 72:988.

Rao AR et al: Tibial interface wear in retrieved total knee components and correlations with modular insert motion. J Bone Joint Surg Am 2002;84:1849. [PMID: 12377918]

Santavirta S et al: Alternative materials to improve total hip replacement tribology. Acta Orthop Scand 2003;74:380. [PMID: 14521286]

Shih LY et al: The effects of sex and estrogen therapy on bone ingrowth into porous coated implant. J Orthop Res 2003;21: 1033. [PMID: 14554216]

Shrivastava R et al: Effects of chromium on the immune system. FEMS Immunol Med Microbiol 2002;34:1. [PMID: 12208600]

Skoglund B et al: PMMA particles and pressure—A study of the osteolytic properties of two agents proposed to cause prosthetic loosening. J Orthop Res 21(2):196. [PMID: 12568949]

Wright TM, Bartel DL: The problem of surface damage in polyethylene total knee components. Clin Orthop 1986;205;67. [PMID: 3698394]

Wroblewski BM, Siney PD, Fleming PA: Wear of enhanced ultrahigh molecular-weight polyethylene (Hylamer) in combination with a 22.225 mm diameter zirconia femoral head. J Bone Joint Surg Br 2003;85:376. [PMID: 12729113]

Zhang H et al: The effects of patient age on human osteoblasts' response to Ti-6Al-4V implants in vitro. J Orthop Res 2004; 22:30. [PMID: 14656656]

GAIT ANALYSIS

Harry B. Skinner, MD, PhD

The science of studying human walking is called gait analysis. This science evolved as a means of quantitating the individual components of gait. As measurement techniques were refined to permit the determination of forces, moments, and movements of the human body, these techniques were applied to functions other than walking. Thus, it has been possible to measure the functional demands of wheelchair motion and running, as well as activities as diverse as pitching a baseball. The study of gait analysis was assisted by the development of devices that are able to measure gait in terms of (1) movement in space, (2) metabolic energy consumed during movement, (3) functional patterns of muscles during movement, and (4) forces applied to the ground during movement. Direct measurements of these factors permit the secondary determination of quantities concerning mechanical work, joint moments, and center of pressure, which in turn are helpful in quantifying the function of prostheses and the effects of ataxia. The techniques of gait analysis are applied to other facets of human function. Motion analysis, for example, is applied to elucidate the kinesthetic changes in the spine occurring with fatigue in a study of repetitive lifting.

GAIT CYCLES, PHASES, & EVENTS

For uniformity in the reporting of gait measurements, investigators adopted several definitions concerning gait cycle. One **gait cycle** is defined as the time from initial ground contact of one foot to subsequent ground contact of the same foot. This is then normalized to 100%, with the intervening phases, periods, and events (Figure 1–26) defined on this basis. Ground contact is chosen as the beginning of the cycle because it is easily defined. The duration of the gait cycle varies, depending on the height, weight, and age of the individual whose gait is being analyzed as well as on any pathologic process affecting the individual's movement. Normalization of the gait cycle into percentages facilitates comparison among individuals.

Two **gait phases** are recognized: the stance phase and the swing phase. The normal **stance phase,** when the extremity is on the ground, accounts for approximately 62% of the cycle, and the normal **swing phase** of that extremity accounts for the remainder. The proportions vary with speed. Each phase is divided into periods. The stance phase starts with double-limb support, is followed by single-limb support, and ends with a second period of double-limb support. Each period of double-limb support accounts for an estimated 10% of the gait cycle. The swing phase is divided into early, mid, and late periods, with each period accounting for approximately 13% of the gait cycle. Swing phase for one limb corresponds to stance phase for the opposite limb.

The swing and stance phases are also divided into **gait events** (see Figure 1–26). Terms such as **heel strike** and **toe-off,** which are used to describe the events in the gait cycle, were initially derived from the observation of normal gait. The nomenclature of gait analysis, however, is evolving to take into account the fact that these terms are inadequate in describing the gait of individuals who have joint contractures, joint instability, pain, spasticity, or other conditions that alter the gait so the heel may never strike the floor or the heel and toe may strike simultaneously or depart simultaneously. In gait analysis, the various events are recognized by observation and can be correlated with measurements of the ground reaction force and motion variables. Observation is greatly enhanced through the use of slow-motion photography or video equipment.

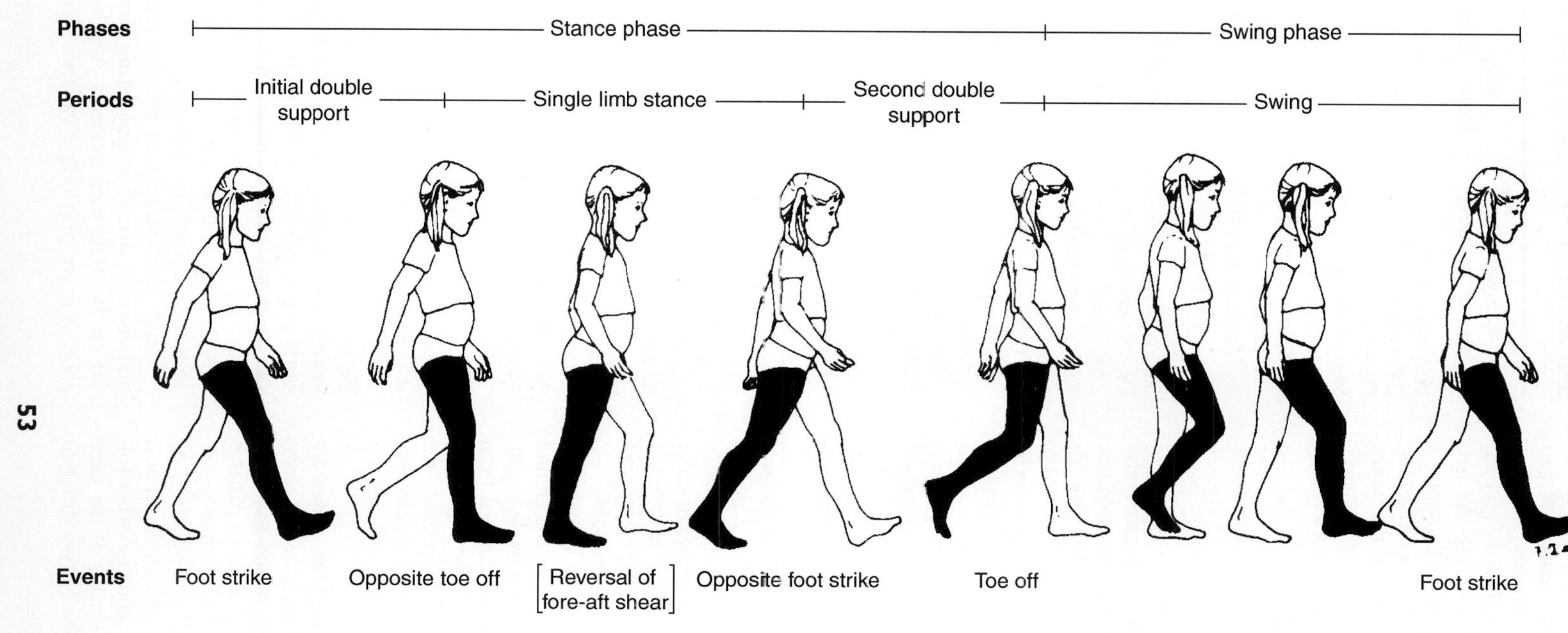

Figure 1–26. The typical normal gait cycle, with the phases, periods, and events of gait shown. (From DH Sutherland.)

GAIT MEASUREMENTS

The quantities measured in a complete analysis of gait include three-dimensional translation, velocity, acceleration for all motion segments, forces exerted on the ground, electromyographic response of muscles during the gait cycle, and metabolic energy consumption. Obviously, a complete gait analysis is an expensive and time-consuming procedure and perhaps not even possible within the endurance limits of some patients studied. A typical gait analysis is problem oriented and focuses on information relevant to the disorder being addressed by the clinician.

Movement during Gait

A. Stride Characteristics

The fundamental data needed for almost any gait analysis are basic measurements termed *stride characteristics.* These are necessary because they form a baseline for interpreting all of the other aspects of gait. The stride characteristic variables are velocity (speed), gait cycle, cadence, stride length, step length, single- and double-limb support time, and swing and stance time.

Velocity of gait is the measure of forward progression of an individual's center of gravity, which is generally located midline and anterior to the sacrum. Velocity is expressed as an average number of meters per minute, although it is obvious that the instantaneous velocity can vary somewhat.

Gait cycle is measured as the number of seconds from the initial ground contact of one foot until the subsequent ground contact of the same foot. **Cadence** is the number of steps per minute (the number of times both feet strike the ground per minute) and is different from the number of strides per minute (the number of times the same foot strikes the ground per minute).

Step length is measured as the distance (number of meters) covered from the time one foot strikes the ground until the opposite foot strikes. It differs from stride length, which is the distance (number of meters) covered from the time one foot strikes the ground to the next time the same foot strikes the ground. In normal individuals, the length of each step is half of the stride length. But in people with pathologic processes that affect gait, the lengths of the two steps are different.

Single-limb and double-limb support times are periods of the gait cycle that can be measured in terms of seconds or in terms of percentage of the gait cycle (Table 1–4 and Figure 1–26). These periods in patients with a painful condition such as an ankle sprain generally differ from periods in normal individuals. Less obvious is the fact that the two double-limb support times (one following left foot strike and the other following right foot strike), which are usually of the same length in normal individuals, may be of two different lengths in patients with pathologic processes that affect gait. **Swing and stance times** can also be measured in terms of seconds or in terms of percentage of gait cycle.

Gait characteristics of normal men and women at free walking speed are shown in Table 1–4, and a sampling of these data for normal children at selected ages is presented in Table 1–5. Gait measurements are generally made at the **free walking speed** for each person because that speed is selected by the person to minimize energy consumption and is therefore considered the optimal gait velocity. Velocities that are slower or faster can be continuously maintained by individuals as long as the metabolic energy consumption remains in the aerobic range. These velocities are more costly in terms of energy expenditure, however.

Stride characteristics are sensitive indicators of diseases and disorders that affect gait. Many variables have a bearing on the stride measurements. Age, height, weight, and shoe wear are physiologic variables that help define the

Table 1–4. Gait characteristics of normal men and women at free walking speed.

Component (Unit of Measure)	Men (Mean ± 1SD)	Women (Mean ± 1SD)
Velocity (m/min)	91 ± 12	74 ± 9
Gait cycle (s)	1.06 ± 0.09	1.03 ± 0.08
Cadence (steps/min)	113 ± 9	117 ± 9
Step length (cm)[a]	78 ± 6	62 ± 5
Stride length (cm)	160	137
Single-limb support[a]		
Time (s)	0.44	0.39
As proportion of gait cycle (%)	40	38
Swing (s)[a]	0.41 ± 0.04	0.39 ± 0.03
Stance (s)[a]	0.65 ± 0.07	0.64 ± 0.06
Lateral motion of the head (cm)	5.9 ± 1.7	4.0 ± 1.1
Vertical motion of the head (cm)		
During right stance	4.8 ± 1.1	4.1 ± 0.9
During left stance	4.9 ± 1.1	4.1 ± 0.9
Hip flexion-extension used (degree)	48 ± 5	40 ± 4
Anteroposterior pelvic tilting (degree)	7.1 ± 2.4	5.5 ± 1.3
Transverse pelvic rotation (degree)	12 ± 4	10 ± 3

[a]Right equals left in normal individuals.

Data adapted, with permission, from Murray MP, Gore DR: Gait patients with hip pain or loss of hip joint motion. In: Black J, Dumbleton JH, eds: *Clinical Biomechanics: A Case History Approach,* Churchill Livingstone, 1981; and from Rancho Los Amigos Hospital data on normal values.

Table 1–5. Gait characteristics of normal children at free walking speeds for selected ages.

Component (Unit of Measure)	1 Year	2 Years	3 Years	4 Years	5 Years
Velocity (m/min)	38.2	43.1	51.3	64.8	68.6
Gait cycle (s)	0.68	0.78	0.77	0.77	0.83
Cadence (steps/min)	175.7	155.8	153.5	153.4	143.5
Step length (cm)[a]	21.6	27.5	32.9	42.3	47.9
Stride length (cm)	43.0	54.9	66.8	84.3	96.5
Single-limb support as proportion of gait cycle (%)[a]	32.1	33.5	34.8	36.5	37.6

[a]Right equals left in normal individuals.

Data adapted, with permission, from Sutherland DH et al: The development of mature gait. J Bone Joint Surg Am 1980;62:336; and from Sutherland DH et al: The development of mature walking. Clin Dev Med 1988;104:1.

basic parameters of velocity, cadence, and gait cycle. Abnormalities resulting from an anatomic change, such as joint replacement, degenerative disease of the lower extremities, or knee fusion, can be demonstrated as nonspecific and asymmetric variations in the stride characteristics. External variables such as those affecting the walking surface (eg, sand, concrete, and ice) can markedly alter stride measurements and must be considered in comparing data from different treatment groups or locations. Data are also sensitive to measurement technique. "Free" walking behavior in a laboratory may be different from that which takes place unobserved on a street and is definitely different from walking on a treadmill. Thus, to eliminate extraneous variables, care must be exercised not only in measuring stride characteristics but also in interpreting them.

B. Motion Analysis

Motion analysis is necessary for the complete characterization of gait. Aside from simply recording motions, quantification of the dynamic range of motion of a joint or body segment is called *kinematics*. Rather than measuring all limb segments, investigators generally focus on motion in certain limb segments and the trunk. Although major displacements of the lower extremities and upper extremities are occurring during gait, the center of mass of the body is only moving approximately 2–4 cm in a mediolateral direction and 2 cm in a superoinferior direction. Simultaneously, pelvic and trunk motion is occurring around the center of mass in a sinusoidal fashion. To conserve angular momentum, the upper extremity moves forward with the contralateral lower extremity.

Motion analysis has benefits and limitations. On the one hand, it provides more information to the clinician than does simple analysis of stride characteristics. For example, although stride analysis may show that the single-limb support time is reduced, motion analysis can clarify whether this is caused by decreased hip or knee motion, weakness of knee or ankle musculature, or some other condition, and it can also permit documentation of the benefit of intervention. On the other hand, motion analysis equipment is expensive, although this is improving, as is the need for human input to the data analysis. It also presents difficulties in defining motion segments accurately and sometimes in measuring relatively small movements. There are problems, for example, in placing the markers to determine mediolateral pelvic rotation or anteroposterior pelvic rotation and in measuring these movements, whereas measuring knee flexion and extension is much easier. Highly sophisticated motion analysis systems were developed to maximize the accuracy and efficiency of these measurements, with a significant improvement. One study was able to discern abnormal tibial motion during gait in ACL-deficient knees.

Motion analysis has taken on new functions with the interest in upper extremity motion, especially in sports. Training problems and injuries in baseball pitching, golf, and racquet sports, among others, can be defined in terms of motions (rotations, displacements, and angular velocities) of the upper extremity joints. For example, world-class tennis players achieve ball velocities of 40–50 meters per second (m/s), with elbow extension and shoulder internal rotation angular velocity peaks of 1510 degrees per second (deg/s) and 2400 deg/s, respectively. Motion analysis can lead to methods of prevention and treatment, as well as improvement in technique.

Energy Consumption during Gait

Energy expenditure results from muscle function and is possible as a direct result of the body's use of food. Steady-state aerobic metabolism is the optimal means of using oxygen to metabolize food, although less efficient anaerobic mechanisms are available. Measurements of oxygen consumption per unit of time can be converted to measurements of energy expenditure or power. An oxygen consumption measurement of 1 L/min is approximately equivalent to an energy consumption measurement of 5 kcal/min.

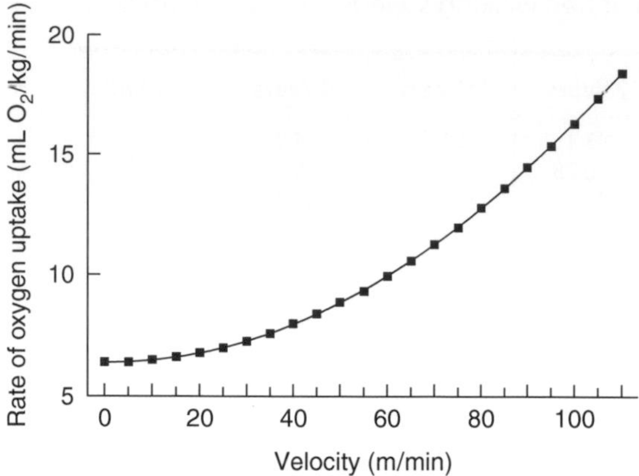

Figure 1–27. Rate of oxygen uptake as a function of velocity.

Energy expenditure per unit of body mass can be expressed per step, per unit of distance, or per unit of time. Most commonly, energy expenditure is measured in terms of **rate of oxygen uptake,** expressed as milliliters of oxygen per kilogram per minute (mL O_2/kg/min), and **net oxygen cost,** expressed as milliliters of oxygen per kilogram per meter (mL O_2/kg/m). Both the rate of oxygen uptake and the net oxygen cost depend on the velocity (*v*) of walking, expressed in terms of m/min. The approximate relations are as follows:

$$\text{Rate of oxygen uptake} = 0.001\,v^2 + 6.0$$

$$\text{Net oxygen cost} = \frac{6.0}{v} + 0.0011\,v$$

The rate of oxygen uptake for normal adults is 11.9 ± 2.3 mL O_2/kg/min, and the net oxygen cost is 0.15 mL O_2/kg/m.

The rate of oxygen uptake increases with the square of the velocity (Figure 1–27). Body mass is obviously important in determining energetics, but location of the mass is even more important. An increase in weight around the center of mass (ie, the waist) is not nearly as energy costly as an increase around the ankles. This is because the center of mass moves at a near constant velocity with relatively small motions. Conversely, the ankles must be accelerated and decelerated constantly during gait, with each acceleration and deceleration requiring energy. When net oxygen cost for normal individuals is expressed as a function of velocity, there is a minimum in the energy consumption curve at approximately 80 m/min (1.3 m/s) at approximately 0.16 mL O_2/kg/m (approximately 1.1 J/kg/m), indicating that this is the most efficient velocity of ambulation (Figure 1–28). Similarly, the most efficient running speed is between 3 and 4 m/s at an energy consumption rate of approximately 3.1 J/kg/m.

Energy expenditure in gait assumes importance when gait efficiency decreases or when the most efficient attainable gait velocity is markedly below normal. Attempts to increase velocity can increase energy costs to the point that sustained ambulation cannot be maintained. This can be seen, for example, in the case of traumatic transfemoral amputation. Although the amputee may ambulate with a net oxygen cost of approximately 0.28 mL O_2/kg/m, which is nearly 100% above normal (0.15 ± 0.02 mL O_2/kg/m), attempts to increase the speed could push the amputee into the anaerobic consumption range and thereby limit the ambulation distance. A similar problem can be seen in the case of a paraplegic who has adequate muscle function to ambulate before gaining weight but finds that the net oxygen cost of increased weight makes wheelchair mobility more energy efficient.

Muscle Function during Gait

Measurement of the function of muscles during gait is helpful in understanding and treating problems associated with cerebral palsy, stroke, poliomyelitis, and other diseases that alter the normal pattern of muscle function. The activity of muscles during gait is determined by **dynamic electromyography** through the use of either surface electrodes or fine-wire electrodes inserted into muscles. Electrical activity generated from these muscles is monitored and recorded in an on-off fashion as a function of the gait cycle. Activity does not necessarily indicate agonistic (contracting) or antagonistic (lengthening) function, but this determination can be made with simultaneous motion analysis. At present, it is not possible to quantify the relationship between electromyographic activity and force.

Normal functioning of the muscles can be presented as a function of the gait cycle and is shown in Figure 1–29.

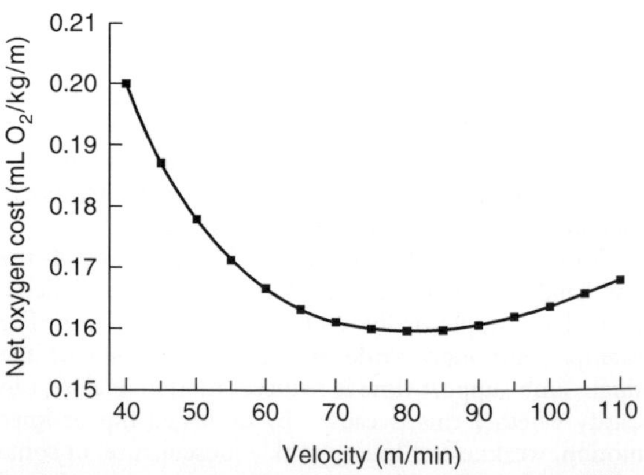

Figure 1–28. Net oxygen cost as a function of velocity.

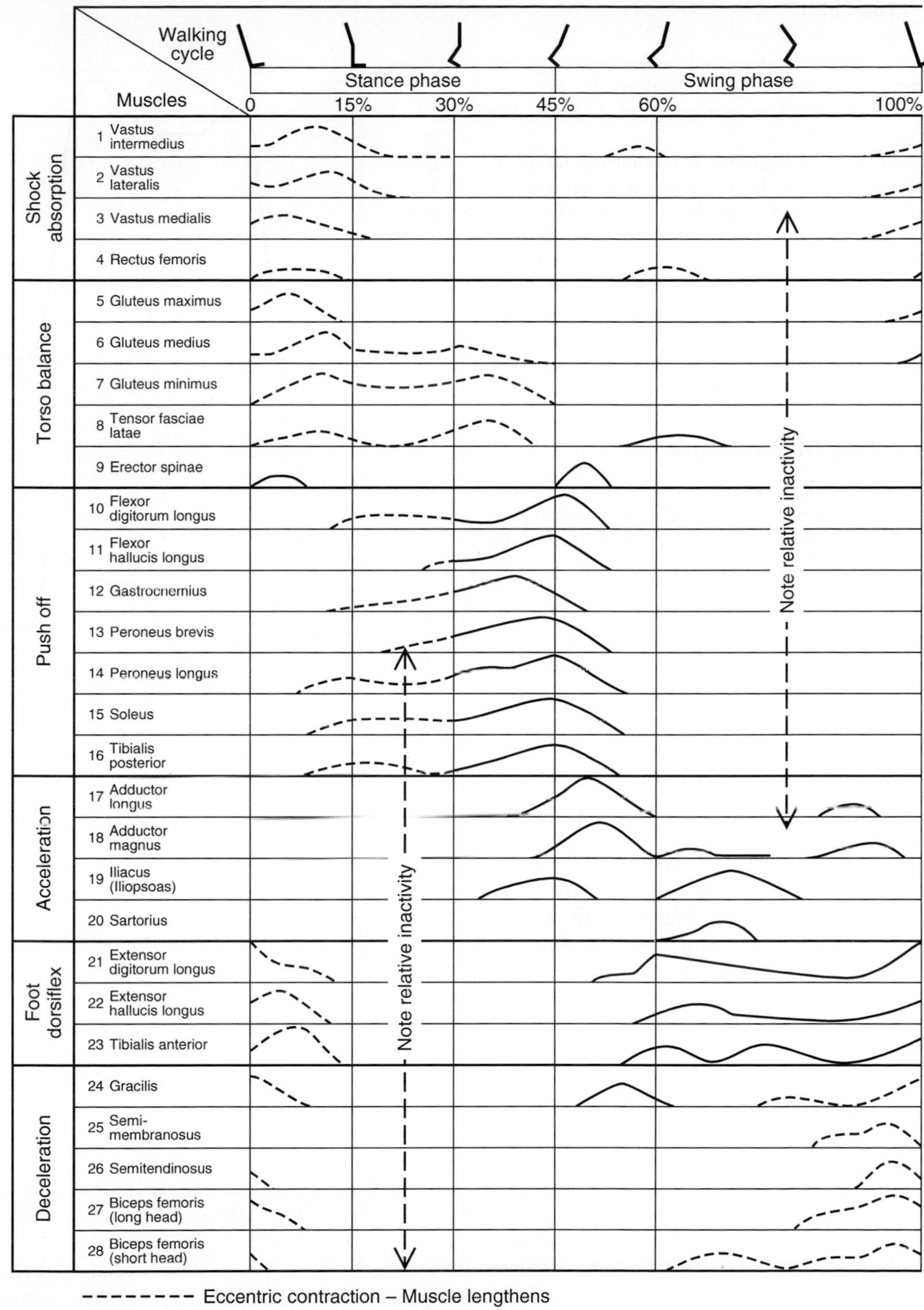

Figure 1–29. **Tabulation of the on-off activity of the major muscles in the lower extremity during gait. Dashed lines show eccentric contraction (muscle lengthens); solid lines show concentric contraction (muscle shortens).** (Reproduced, with permission, from Charles O Bechtel, Los Angeles, CA. American Academy of Orthopaedic Surgeons: *Atlas of Orthotics: Biomechanical Principles and Application.* Mosby, 1975.)

Most muscle activity is generated at the beginning and end of the stance and swing phases of gait because it is necessary at these times to accelerate and decelerate the extremities.

Dynamic electromyography is particularly useful in disorders associated with spasticity, such as cerebral palsy and cerebral vascular accident. In these disorders, the results of functional muscle testing of the patient in the supine position can be markedly different from the results of testing in the upright ambulating position. For example, the tibialis anterior may function normally when the patient is supine, but dynamic electromyography may reveal a varus-deforming force of the hindfoot during ambulation.

Forces during Gait: Kinetics

Forces acting during ambulation arise from gravity, inertia, and ground reaction. At ambulation speeds, viscous drag can be ignored. The **gravitational force** (mass × gravity) must be considered because it causes moments around centers of rotation for limb segments and body segments. The **inertial force** is proportional to the acceleration of the body segment and acts in the opposite direction because it resists acceleration. The **ground reaction force** is a measurement of the load applied to a device such as a force platform and has three components: vertical ground reaction force, fore-aft shear, and mediolateral shear.

Typical curves for the three components of the ground reaction force are shown in Figure 1–30. The dip in the vertical force curve (Figure 1–30A) during the single-limb stance phase of gait occurs because the inertial forces reduce the ground reaction force below body weight. The fore-aft shear (Figure 1–30B) is negative after the heel strike because the foot is pushing the plate anterior. On toe-off, the converse is occurring so the shear force is in the opposite direction. Again, correlation of ground reaction forces to stride characteristics can be beneficial in interpreting gait data. Force platform data show variations with walking speed, shoe wear, and compensatory mechanisms of gait, such as the avoidance of weight bearing on a painful extremity. The components of the ground reaction force in gait can be an indication of dynamic aspects of gait. The vertical ground reaction force tends to increase in magnitude and higher frequency content with increasing velocity and flatten with lower velocity and/or lower extremity pain. Examination of the frequency content especially in the medial-lateral shear component is an indicator of balance control, as in scoliosis. Static measurements provide center of pressure variations, also as a measure of balance control.

More sophisticated force measurement devices were developed to permit measurement of pressure (force per

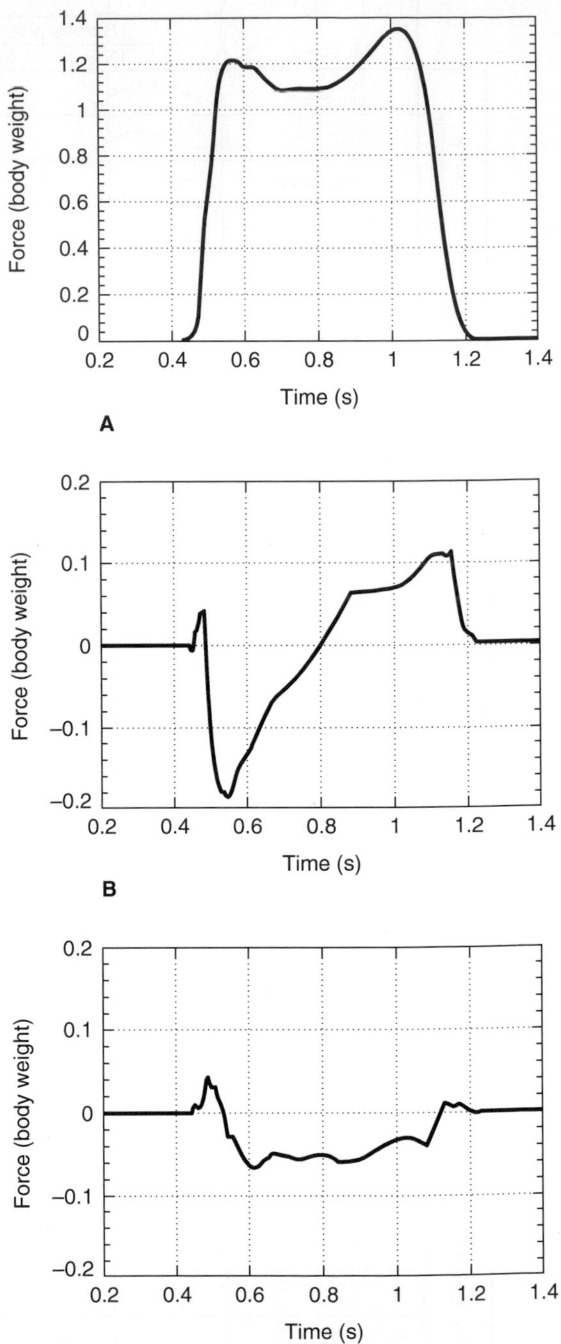

Figure 1–30. The typical ground reaction force for the left foot, shown with its three components. **A:** Vertical force. **B:** Fore-aft shear, which in this plot is negative for heel strike and positive for toe-off. **C:** Mediolateral shear, which in this plot is negative in the lateral direction. (Courtesy of S. Rossi.)

unit area). These devices can yield both in-shoe pressures and pressures applied to the external surface of the shoe by a force platform. Thus discrimination of measures at the 1-cm^2 level is possible, allowing studies of feet of diabetic patients to discern differences shoe wear can have on the risk of skin breakdown.

Andriacchi TP, Alexander EJ: Studies of human locomotion: past, present, future. J Biomech 2000;33:1217. [PMID: 10899330]

Anglin C, Wyss UP: Review of arm motion analysis. Proc Inst Mech Eng (H) 2000;214:541. [PMID: 11109862]

Burdett RG et al: Comparison of mechanical work and metabolic energy consumption during normal gait. J Orthop Res 1983; 1:63. [PMID: 6679577]

Chambers HG, Sutherland DH: A practical guide to gait analysis. J Am Acad Orthop Surg 2002;10:222. [PMID: 12041944]

Fleisig G et al: Kinematics used by world class tennis players to produce high-velocity serves. Sports Biomech 2003;2:51. [PMID: 14658245]

Marshall RN, Elliott BC: Long-axis rotation: The missing link in proximal-to-distal segmental sequencing. J Sports Sci 2000; 18:247. [PMID: 10824641]

Park SS et al: The shoulder in baseball pitching: Biomechanics and related injuries-part 1. Bull Hosp Jt Dis 2002-3;61:68. [PMID:12828383]

Park SS et al: The shoulder in baseball pitching: Biomechanics and related injuries-part 2. Bull Hosp Jt Dis 2002-3;61:80. [PMID: 12828384]

Perry J et al: Functional evaluation of the pes anserinus transfer by electromyography and gait analysis. J Bone Joint Surg Am 1980;62:973. [PMID: 7430186]

Saibene F, Minetti AE: Biomechanical and physiological aspects of legged gait in humans. Eur J Appl Physiol 2003;88:297. [PMID: 12527959]

Sutherland DH et al: The development of mature gait. J Bone Joint Surg Am 1980;62:336. [PMID: 7364807]

ROLE OF GAIT ANALYSIS IN THE MANAGEMENT OF GAIT DISORDERS

Gait analysis was traditionally been a research tool and continues to find its primary use in the research arena. However, the impetus to document the benefit of medical intervention has resulted in a reliance on gait analysis to quantify gains made by surgery or other treatments. There continue to be proponents of gait analysis as a clinical diagnostic tool. New areas in which gait analysis is under investigation include Parkinson's disease, cervical myelopathy, high-heeled gait, and even depression. The publication of normative data permits the definition of pathologic gait and thereby defines a goal in the rehabilitation of a patient with a gait disorder. Analysis in gait laboratories can measure the initial deviation from normal as well as the improvements occurring through the rehabilitation process. Even as gait laboratories assume a more prominent role in evaluation of patients, however, the data generated from research laboratories have already affected clinical practice in a variety of ways.

New techniques of analysis were developed as computer sophistication and availability evolved. Gait is a process with inherent variability, which must be understood and accounted for to maximize its utility. Fractal analysis is one approach and may result in a better description of gait rhythm variations during maturation from childhood to adulthood. Understanding and predicting muscle activation patterns can be accomplished using artificial neural network models. These are particularly exciting because their use may lead to active control of prostheses. Part of the variability of gait arises from differences in body size. Scaling the gait data to body size can reduce intersubject variability and provide a tighter evaluation of abnormality. Identification of "abnormal" gait can be subtle in some cases in view of the variable and voluminous data generated. The common method of evaluation is principal component analysis, which quantifies the deviation of variables from normal. A newer report evaluates variability based on an index that used the squared distance from the mean obtained from joint angle measurements of many subjects. These techniques promise to improve the usefulness of gait analysis in the evaluation and treatment of orthopedic patients.

Gait studies of patients with transfemoral and transtibial amputations resulted in an objective evaluation of ambulatory potential after prosthetic replacement. Early studies demonstrated that amputations at more proximal levels resulted in greater loss of symmetry and increased energy expenditure (Table 1–6). These findings stimulated renewed attempts to maintain amputations at the most distal level. Other studies showed that strengthening the muscles of the residual limb in patients with transtibial amputations resulted in velocities that were improved although still lower than normal. Recent electromyographic studies of gait in transfemoral amputees demonstrated the importance of reattaching biarticular muscles that are transected at the amputation site to bone to maintain their function.

Techniques for gait analysis of amputees also provide the objective means of comparing various prosthetic components, such as the solid ankle cushion heel (SACH) foot, and the multiaxial and uniaxial feet.

Gait analysis is now a common tool in the treatment and evaluation of patients who have cerebral palsy or have suffered from a cerebrovascular accident or head injury. For disorders such as these, gait improvement can be expected for 6 months or more. Studies suggest that the natural history of gait in child and adolescent cerebral palsy is one of deterioration with aging, an important finding when evaluating long-term effects of intervention to improve gait. The use of electromyographic gait data can improve the results of muscle transfers in this group

Table 1–6. Results of free walking gait analysis in patients with transfemoral (TF) and transtibial (TT) amputations.

Cause and Level of Amputation	Velocity (m/min)	Cadence (steps/min)	Stride Length (m)	Gait Cycle (s)	Rate of Oxygen Uptake (mL/kg/min)	Net Oxygen Cost (mL/kg/m)
Traumatic TF amputation	55	86	1.26	1.42	12.7	0.28
Dysvascular TF amputation	36	72	1.00	1.66	12.6	0.35
Traumatic TT amputation	68	98	1.38	1.22	12.4	0.22
Dysvascular TT amputation	45	87	1.02	1.36	11.7	0.26

Data adapted, with permission, from Bagley AM, Skinner HB: Progress in gait analysis in amputees: A special review. Crit Rev Phys Rehabil Med 1991;3:101.

of patients. Knowledge of the activity period of a muscle (swing phase/stance phase) can allow prediction of the effect of transfer of that muscle. Thus, gait analysis is applied to spastic equinovarus feet to determine the efficacy of transfers of tibialis anterior and tibialis posterior. Similarly, gait analysis can be used to evaluate different surgical interventions, such as selective dorsal rhizotomies and orthopedic surgical interventions in spastic diplegic patients, showing improvement in energy cost and gait kinematics with both interventions.

Clinicians can use gait analysis to provide objective clinical data whenever orthotics are prescribed. Gait analysis before and after the application of an orthosis can quantify the effects in an objective manner. In evaluating the results, clinicians should remember that an orthosis that eliminates motion of a joint may improve function by putting the joint in a better position without bringing the patient back to a normal state. With orthotic fitting, lack of motion at a joint such as the ankle results in an increase in energy consumption and an alteration of gait symmetry, compared to normal. But without orthotic fitting, a poor joint position such as ankle equinus may make the gait even more inefficient and asymmetric. Similarly, ankle-foot orthoses (AFOs) thought to work through changes in spastic reflexes are shown with gait studies to be less effective than hinged AFOs in children with cerebral palsy. Other studies also showed that design of orthoses can be evaluated. In hemiplegic stroke patients, the use of a cane or the combination of a cane and an AFO were found to decrease energy consumption significantly.

Gait analysis is also improving surgical decision making. One study allowed experienced clinicians to review videotape and clinical examination data before recommending a treatment plan. After reviewing complete gait data, the same clinicians changed recommendations in 52% of patients. A second study showed 39% of planned surgical procedures on children were deemed unnecessary after gait analysis. Evaluation of a patient's gait before and after a procedure can demonstrate the efficacy of the procedure and assist in postoperative care. A newer study demonstrated that the Van Nes rotational osteotomy allowed ambulation in children with proximal femoral focal deficiency at a more energy efficient rate than children with a Syme amputation. Gait analysis can allow objective comparisons of various procedures. This is primarily applicable, however, to those procedures in which the end point is an improvement of function. For example, walking efficiency as determined by velocity statistically is the same for transfemoral amputation and for proximal tibial replacement for tumor, but below normal for both treatments for age. Such a comparison of therapy choices can aid in the surgical decision process or the informed consent process. Procedures such as joint replacement have pain as the primary indication for surgery, although improvement of function is also a desirable by-product.

The results of surgical procedures such as total knee arthroplasty and total hip arthroplasty depend on a whole host of variables, including the surgeons' experience and the patients' age, preexisting disease, cooperation, and motivation. Clinical evaluation of the results of these procedures is at best crude from a functional viewpoint. For example, evaluation criteria include walking distance and the ability to climb stairs sequentially. Although the application of sophisticated gait analysis techniques to total joint replacement is relatively new, normative data on total knee and total hip replacement surgery have appeared in the literature for some time. These data are shown in Tables 1–7, 1–8, and 1–9. To date, gait analysis is unable to settle controversies that concern prosthesis design and are related to the efficacy of one type of cemented hip prosthesis versus another, the efficacy of cemented versus uncemented hip prostheses. Another controversy is the issue of the efficacy of prostheses that sacrifice the posterior cruciate ligament of the knee versus those that preserve this ligament and whether mobile bearing knee designs

Table 1–7. Results of free walking gait analysis in patients with total knee arthroplasty.

Study[a]	Patient Diagnosis	Time Since Surgery (yr)	Velocity (m/min)	Cadence (steps/min)	Stride Length (m)	Prosthesis Design
(1) Collopy et al (1977)	OA	1	57	100	1.2	Geometric
	RA	1	46	98	0.9	Geometric
(2) Simon et al (1983)	OA	3.3	63	100.6	1.2	Duopatellar
(3) Skinner et al (1983)	OA or RA	Preop	38.9	87.6	0.864	—
	OA or RA	5	46.5	91.5	1.01	Multiple
(4) Skinner et al (1983)	OA or RA	5.5	50.7	91	1.30	Polycentric
(5) Olsson and Barck (1986)	OA	9	62.4	107	1.14	Gunston-Hult
(6) Berman et al (1987)	OA, with normal contralateral knee	1.5	49.6	—	1.07	Total condylar
	OA, with asymptomatic diseased contralateral knee	2.0	35.2	—	0.958	—
	OA in both knees	1.3	54.5	—	1.07	—
(7) Waters et al (1987)	RA	0.9	63	103	1.31	—
(8) Kroll et al (1989)	OA	1.1	64.1	109.7	1.18	—
(9) Steiner, Simon, and Pisciotta (1989)	OA or RA	1.0	69	114	1.18	Total condylar or unicompartmental

[a]References are as follows: (1) Collopy MC et al: Kinesiologic measurements of functional performance before and after geometric total knee replacement. Clin Orthop 1977;126:196. (2) Simon SR et al: Quantitative gait analysis after knee arthroplasty for monoarticular degenerative arthritis. J Bone Joint Surg Am 1983;65:605. (3) Skinner HB et al: Ambulatory function in total knee arthroplasty. South Med J 1983;76:1237. (4) Skinner HB et al: Correlation of gait analysis and clinical evaluation of polycentric total knee arthroplasty. Orthopedics 1983;6:576. (5) Olsson E, Barck A: Correlation between clinical examination and quantitative gait analysis in patients operated upon with the Gunston-Hult knee prosthesis. Scand J Rehab Med 1986;18:101. (6) Berman AT et al: Quantitative gait analysis after unilateral or bilateral total knee replacement. J Bone Joint Surg Am 1987;69:1340. (7) Waters RL et al: The energy cost of walking with arthritis of the hip and knee. Clin Orthop 1987;214:278. (8) Kroll MA et al: The relationship of stride characteristics to pain before and after total knee arthroplasty. Clin Orthop 1989;239:191. (9) Steiner ME, Simon SR, Pisciotta JC: Early changes in gait and maximum knee torque following knee arthroplasty. Clin Orthop 1989;238:174.
OA = osteoarthrosis; RA = rheumatoid arthritis.

Reproduced, with permission, from Skinner HB: Pathokinesiology and total joint arthroplasty. Clin Orthop 1993;288:78.

demonstrate a benefit over nonmobile bearing knee designs. Thus far, variability in the data has prevented demonstration of a clear difference in designs. As advances in prosthesis design and gait analysis continue, improvements in the management of patients with gait disorders will also continue.

Andriacchi TP et al: The influence of total knee replacement design on walking and stair climbing. J Bone Joint Surg Am 1982; 64:1328. [PMID: 7142241]

Bagley AM, Skinner HB: Progress in gait analysis in amputees: A special review. Crit Rev Phys Rehabil Med 1991;3:101.

Chambers HG, Sutherland DH: A practical guide to gait analysis. J Am Acad Orthop Surg 2002;10:222. [PMID: 12041944]

Chau T: A review of analytical techniques for gait data. Part I: Fuzzy, statistical and fractal methods. Gait Posture 2001; 13:49. [PMID: 11166554]

DeLuca PA et al: Alterations in surgical decision making in patients with cerebral palsy based on three-dimensional gait analysis. J Pediatr Orthop 1997;17:608.

Dennis DA et al: Multicenter determination of in vivo kinematics after total knee arthroplasty. Clin Orthop 2003;416:37. [PMID: 14646738]

De Visser E et al: Gait and electromyographic analysis of patients recovering after limb-saving surgery. Clin Biomech 2000;15: 592. [PMID: 10936431]

Gefen A et al: Analysis of muscular fatigue and foot stability during high-heeled gait. Gait Posture 2002;15:56. [PMID: 11809581]

Hesse S et al: Non-velocity-related effects of a rigid double-stopped ankle-foot orthosis on gait and lower limb muscle activity of hemiparetic subjects with an equinovarus deformity. Stroke 1999;30:1855. [PMID: 10471436]

Huang G-F et al: Gait analysis and energy consumption of below-knee amputees wearing three different prosthetic feet. Gait Posture 2000;12:162. [PMID: 10998614]

Table 1–8. Results of free walking gait analysis in patients with total hip arthroplasty.

Study[a]	Patient Diagnosis	Time Since Surgery (yr)	Velocity (m/min)	Cadence (steps/min)	Stride Length (m)	Prosthesis Design
(1) Murray, Brewer, and Zuege (1972)	NA	—	50.0	—	0.98	McKee-Farrar
(2) Stauffer, Smidt, and Wadsworth (1974)	NA	0.5	37.1	80.4	—	Charnley
(3) Murray et al (1975)	OA or RA	2	65	106	1.23	McKee-Farrar
(4) Murray et al (1976)	OA or RA	0.5	62	102	—	Charnley
	OA or RA	0.5	57	102	—	Müller
	OA or RA	0.5	55	100	—	McKee-Farrar
(5) Murray et al (1979)	OA or RA	2	68	110	—	Charnley or Müller
(6) Brown et al (1980)	OA	1	55	101	1.12	—
(7) Olsson, Goldie, and Wykman (1986)	OA or RA	1	53.4*	97.2	1.08	Charnley
	NA	—	48.0*	93	1.00	H.P. Garches
(8) Mattsson, Brostrom, and Linnarsson (1990)	OA	1	80*	—	—	Charnley or H.P. Garches

[a]References are as follows: (1) Murray MP, Brewer BJ, Zuege RC: Kinesiologic measurements of functional performance before and after McKee-Farrar total hip replacement. J Bone Joint Surg Am 1972;54:237. (2) Stauffer RN, Smidt GL, Wadsworth JB: Clinical and biomechanical analysis of gait following Charnley total hip replacement. Clin Orthop 1974;99:70. (3) Murray MP et al: Kinesiology after McKee-Farrar total hip replacement: A two-year follow-up of one hundred cases. J Bone Joint Surg Am 1975;57:337. (4) Murray MP et al: Comparison of functional performance after McKee-Farrar, Charnley, and Müller total hip replacement: A six-month follow-up of one hundred sixty-five cases. Clin Orthop 1976;21:33. (5) Murray MP et al: Comparison of the functional performance of patients with Charnley and Müller total hip replacement. Acta Orthop Scand 1979;50:563. (6) Brown M et al: Walking efficiency before and after total hip replacement. Phys Ther 1980;60:1259. (7) Olsson E, Goldie I, Wykman A: Total hip replacement: A comparison between cemented (Charnley) and noncemented (H.P. Garches) fixation by clinical assessment and objective gait analysis. Scand J Rehab Med 1986;18:107. (8) Mattsson E, Brostrom LA, Linnarsson D: Walking efficiency after cemented and noncemented total hip arthroplasty. Clin Orthop 1990;254:170.

*Asterisk indicates velocity at fast walking speed; otherwise, velocity is at free walking speed.

NA = diagnostic data not available; OA = osteoarthritis; RA = rheumatoid arthritis.

Reproduced, with permission, from Skinner HB: Pathokinesiology and total joint arthroplasty. Clin Orthop 1993;288:78.

Table 1–9. Results of energy consumption analysis during gait in patients with total hip arthroplasty.

Study[a]	Patient Diagnosis	Time Since Surgery (yr)	Velocity (m/min)	Rate of Oxygen Uptake (mL/kg/min)	Net Oxygen Cost (mL/kg/m)
(1) Pugh (1973)	OA	—	—	10.0	0.15
(2) Brown et al (1980)	OA	1	55	11.86	0.22
(3) McBeath, Bahrke, and Balke (1980)	NA	2	64.5	12.13	0.186
(4) Mattsson, Brostrom, and Linnarsson (1990)	OA	1	80*	—	0.221

[a]References are as follows: (1) Pugh LG: The oxygen intake and energy cost of walking before and after unilateral hip replacement with some observations on the use of crutches. J Bone Joint Surg Br 1973;55:742. (2) Brown M et al: Walking efficiency before and after total hip replacement. Phys Ther 1980;60:1259. (3) McBeath AA, Bahrke MS, Balke B: Walking efficiency before and after total hip replacement as determined by oxygen consumption. J Bone Joint Surg Am 1980;62:807. (4) Mattsson E, Brostrom LA, Linnarsson D: Walking efficiency after cemented and noncemented total hip arthroplasty. Clin Orthop 1990;254:170.

*Asterisk indicates velocity at fast walking speed; otherwise, velocity is at free walking speed.

OA = osteoarthritis; NA = diagnostic data not available.

Reproduced, with permission, from Skinner HB: Pathokinesiology and total joint arthroplasty. Clin Orthop 1993;288:78.

Johnson DC et al: The evolution of gait in childhood and adolescent cerebral palsy. J Pediatr Orthop 1997;17:392. [PMID: 9150031]

Kay RM et al: Impact of postoperative gait analysis on orthopedic care. Clin Orthop 2000;372:259. [PMID: 10818985]

Kay RM et al: The effect of preoperative gait analysis on orthopedic decision making. Clin Orthop 2000;372:217. [PMID: 10738430]

Nowak MD et al: Design enhancement of a solid ankle-foot orthosis: Real-time contact pressures evaluation. J Rehabil Res Dev 2000;37:273. [PMID: 10917259]

Pierrynowski MR, Galea V: Enhancing the ability of gait analyses to differentiate between groups: Scaling gait data to body size. Gait Posture 2001;13:193. [PMID: 11323225]

Prentice SD et al: Artificial neural network model for the generation of muscle activation patterns for human locomotion. J Electromyogr Kinesiol 2001;11:19. [PMID: 11166605]

Reitman JS, Postema K, Geertzen JH: Gait analysis in prosthetics: opinions, ideas and conclusions. Prosthet Orthot Int 2002; 26:50. [PMID: 12043926]

Romkes J, Brunner R: Comparison of a dynamic and a hinged ankle-foot orthosis by gait analysis in patients with hemiplegic cerebral palsy. Gait Posture 2002;15:18. [PMID: 11809577]

Sanders JE et al: Effects of changes in cadence, prosthetic componentry, and time on the interface pressures and shear stresses of three trans-tibial amputees. Clin Biomech 2000;15:684. [PMID: 10946102]

Schmalz T et al: Energy expenditure and biomechanical characteristics of lower limb amputee gait: The influence of prosthetic alignment and different prosthetic components. Gait Posture 2002;16:255. [PMID: 12443950]

Simon SR: Quantification of human motion: gait analysis-benefits and limitations to its application to clinical problems. J Biomech 2004;37:1869.

Thomas SS et al: A 2-year follow-up of outcomes following orthopedic surgery or selective dorsal rhizotomy in children with spastic diplegia. J Pediatr Orthop B 2004;13:358. [PMID: 15599225]

Tingley M et al: An index to quantify normality of gait in young children. Gait Posture 2002;16:149. [PMID: 12297256]

REFERENCES

Cristal P et al, eds: *Biological and Biomechanical Performance of Biomaterials.* Elsevier, 1986.

Friberg L et al: *Handbook on the Toxicology of Metals.* Elsevier, 1986.

Fung YCB: *Biomechanics: Mechanical Properties of Living Tissues.* Springer-Verlag, 1981.

Gage JR et al: Instructional course lecture, The American Academy of Orthopaedic Surgeons. Gait Analysis: Principles and applications emphasis on its use in cerebral palsy. J Bone Joint Surg Am 1995;77:1607.

Perry J: *Gait Analysis: Normal and Pathological Function.* Slack, 1992.

Rose J, Gamble JG, eds: *Human Walking,* 2nd ed. Williams & Wilkins, 1994.

General Considerations in Orthopedic Surgery

2

Harry B. Skinner, MD, PhD

Orthopedic surgery encompasses the entire process of caring for the surgical patient, from diagnostic evaluation to the preoperative evaluation and through the postoperative and rehabilitative period. Although the surgical procedure itself is the key step toward helping the patient, the preliminary and follow-up care can determine whether the surgery is successful.

DIAGNOSTIC WORK-UP

History and Physical Exam

Although it may seem obvious, the history and physical exam are still important in the evaluation of the patient. Every office visit is a history and physical exam, whether a new or a return visit. The completeness of the history and physical has assumed new importance in view of the complexities required for compliance with federal regulations. Regulations require that a chief complaint be specified, and this must be clearly defined because it determines the direction for the rest of the history and physical. The history must address the key features of the problem, both to elucidate the medical problem and to cover the subsidiary requirements for billing purposes. The social history and past medical history are similarly important because they change billing codes without necessarily affecting outcome or success of care. The physical again must cover the essentials necessary for diagnosis, and frequently the confirmation of the diagnosis is based on physical exam, but such considerations as skin condition and blood supply must be documented, despite the fact that this process is also part of the surgical evaluation. The next step is imaging and laboratory exams. The most important point here is to use the most cost-effective examination possible while keeping patient safety, satisfaction, and convenience in mind.

Imaging Studies

A. Roentgenography

Roentgenography is still the most cost-effective and most important initial diagnostic test in the orthopedist's armamentarium. Almost every patient should have a radiograph prior to going to a more sophisticated imaging study. Certain situations are obvious; for example, a 68-year-old man with knee pain should have standing, flexed-knee posteroanterior (PA), lateral, and merchant plain film views taken. If those views show normal joint spaces, consideration of intraarticular pathology, such as a degenerative meniscus tear, can be worked up with magnetic resonance imaging (MRI). The normal views usually ordered are as follows:

1. **Neck pain**—No history of trauma, more than 4 weeks' duration.

   Younger than 35 years: anteroposterior (AP) lateral, odontoid

   Older than 35 years: obliques

   History of trauma: flexion/extension laterals (obtain on first visit)

2. **Thoracic spine pain and tenderness**—

   Younger than 40 years, no reason to suspect malignancy: AP and lateral (if history of trauma, or possibility of osteoporosis on first visit, otherwise at 4 weeks).

   Consider cervical (C)-spine as a source of referred pain to thoracic (T)-spine if no tenderness in T-spine.

3. **Lumbar (L)-sacral (S)-spine**—

   Younger than 40 years, no reason to suspect malignancy after 4 weeks duration of the pain. With significant trauma, at first visit, or possible malignancy (ie, weight loss, malaise, fatigue): AP, lateral.

   Add obliques for chronic low back pain (ie, spondylolisthesis).

4. **Hips**—

   AP pelvis, lateral of affected hip.

   Consider lumbar-sacral (L-S) series if pain is in the buttock rather than in the groin.

5. **Knees—**

   Older than 40 years or history of meniscectomy: Rosenberg, lateral, and sunrise films. Merchant views are similar to sunrise. The Rosenberg view is a 10-degree down shot of the PA of the knees while standing at 45 degrees of flexion.

   For other knees: AP, lateral, and sunrise.

   In the child, up to age 16, consider a pelvis film with the complaint of knee pain and negative physical exam referable to the knee.

6. **Femur, tibia, humerus, forearm**—AP and lateral are indicated for trauma, palpable lesions, or suspected tumors.

7. **Ankle**—AP lateral and mortise.

8. **Foot**—AP, lateral, and oblique for routine evaluation.

9. **Shoulder**—AP, axillary, scapular Y, and outlet views.

10. **Elbow**—AP and lateral (true lateral).

11. **Hand/wrist—**

    Hand: PA and lateral.

    Wrist: PA, lateral, and oblique

    For suspected instability: clenched fist PA in radial and ulnar deviation.

Follow-up radiographs are obtained when a change in the radiographic findings is expected. Remember that bone changes occur slowly, so radiographic changes take a comparable length of time. Radiographs are obtained in view of the clinical picture. For example, closed treatment of a distal radius fracture would not be expected to show changes because of healing for a minimum of 2 weeks. However, displacement of the fracture could occur sooner. Hence, radiographs to show displacement might be obtained at 1 week and 2 weeks. If no displacement is observed, the fracture position could be considered stable, and the next films might be obtained at 6 weeks—the earliest time healing might be observed. Similarly, closed treatment of an adult tibia fracture might be followed with radiographs at 2-week intervals, checking for displacement and healing, whereas a tibia fracture treated with an intramedullary rod might be followed at monthly intervals to check for healing.

B. Magnetic Resonance Imaging

This imaging modality is very useful, but like electron beam computed tomography (CT), MRI is sometimes too revealing. This method should be reserved for clarifying a particular problem. Frequently in orthopedics, a bony lesion can be localized with a radiograph or bone scan, which then provides a focus for the MRI. MRI is useful for some bony lesions, such as osteonecrosis, tumors, fatigue fractures, and osteomyelitis. It is also helpful in some soft-tissue problems, such as knee meniscus tears and shoulder rotator cuff tears. MRI should not be used when the diagnosis can be made with a less expensive test. For example, the use of the MRI in knee studies in patients older than 45 years should always be preceded by plain films of the knee, as noted earlier. An MRI of an arthritic knee adds little additional information because the meniscus and anterior cruciate ligament are likely to be damaged from the arthritic process already. However, the MRI can be very helpful in determining soft-tissue extension of tumors or infection.

The advent of new portable MRI units that perform limited studies with more resolution adds a new dimension to their use. These can provide data on the progression of disorders such as rheumatoid arthritis or osteomyelitis in a timely and cost-effective way. The possibility of osteomyelitis in the bones adjacent to ulcers on the foot is easily determined with this test because it shows the changes, typically edema, in the bone with osteomyelitis. A bone scan usually does not have the resolution to distinguish the inflammatory response in the soft tissue from the bony involvement. Osteomyelitis should be treated much differently from a soft-tissue ulcer, which does not affect the bone.

C. Computed Tomography

The CT scan is an extremely important imaging modality for examining bony lesions such as fractures. Frequently, plain films provide some information about the fracture of interest, but the CT scan provides the three-dimensional information that can only otherwise be determined from the integration of the plain films in the surgeon's mind. The CT scan adds significantly to the management of such fractures as tibial plateaus, scapular fractures, ankle fractures, and cervical and lumbar spine fractures, as well as many others. Again, if little information can be gained that cannot be already discerned from the plain films, the CT scan only adds expense and patient inconvenience. The spiral CT makes imaging with this modality less expensive and much more rapid. The CT scan is also now the method of choice for determining whether a pulmonary embolus (PE) has occurred. Again, a CT for this indication is easier on the patient, more accurate, and less invasive than angiography.

D. Technetium-99m Bone Scan

The bone scan finds many uses in orthopedic surgery. Keep in mind that the bone scan labels the osteoblast activity with the radioactive tracer, technetium-99; thus, bone formation activity is recorded and little or no bone resorption activity is noted. Any disorder that results in increased bone formation, therefore, results in a "hot" bone scan. This means that a disorder such as multiple myeloma may not show up on a bone scan because only osteoclastic activity is involved in the majority of lesions. This test is helpful in discerning loose total hip and total knee prostheses, however, even though the findings are nonspecific. It is very helpful in examining probable benign bone lesions because a cold bone scan largely rules out an aggressive process such as a malignancy. The bone scan is also helpful in diagnosing any disorder of unknown origin when there is pain localized to a particular region. A cold bone scan implies that the problem is a soft-tissue one, whereas a hot bone scan points to a region that may benefit from MRI.

Laboratory Exams

The two most important laboratory exams are for C-reactive protein and the erythrocyte sedimentation rate. These two tests indicate whether an inflammatory process, malignancy, or rheumatologic disorder are diagnostic considerations. If these tests are negative, systemic causes of a complaint can frequently be ruled out. In that situation, a more localized disorder should be identified. The next most important test is the complete blood count, which provides the general indication of the patient's health, revealing information about anemia, infectious processes, and so on. The next most useful laboratory test for the orthopedic surgeon is the synovial fluid analysis. This test typically should include a culture and sensitivity. If there is any concern about infection, a cell count, differential, protein, and glucose measurement should be performed. Crystals should be looked for because they indicate chondrocalcinosis or gout. Elevated protein and reduced glucose levels suggest infection. The final factor that should be considered with any major surgery is the patient's nutritional status, which is evaluated with several tests, including lymphocyte count and levels of prealbumin, albumin, and serum iron transferrin.

Educating & Informing Patients & Their Families

Surgical procedures in orthopedics have varying degrees of difficulty and importance, ranging from a relatively simple clawtoe correction to the performance of a multilevel complex spinal fusion. After the decision to employ surgery as a therapeutic modality is made, it is important to help the patient completely understand what to expect before, during, and after surgery. This process, which the legal profession calls **informed consent,** has the more important purpose of ensuring the patient's cooperation and satisfaction.

To comply with the requirements of the legal profession and accrediting organizations, such as the Joint Commission on Accreditation of Healthcare Organizations (JCAHO), the surgeon must provide an explanation of the risks, prognosis, alternatives, and complications that might be encountered. The risks should be reviewed in some detail for the general risks encountered in typical orthopedic surgical procedures. The risks and the complications that occur in surgery are intimately associated and thus must be dealt with together. The alternatives are sometimes straightforward. For example, a patient with an open fracture has a high risk of infection if not adequately treated with irrigation, debridement, and antibiotics. Thus, in such a situation, any reasonable and prudent person would consent to the procedure. The choice between alternatives can become significantly more subtle, however. For example, it is possible that a choice must be made between two different procedures or between a particular procedure and no procedure. In this situation, the surgeon must consider the psychosocial and physical attributes of the patient so as to assist him or her in making this decision. For example, consider men, both 75 years of age, with severe degenerative disease in the right knee noted on radiograph. One individual is now at the point where he cannot play golf, a situation that is reducing his physical exercise and a number of his social outlets. The other individual leads a relatively sedentary lifestyle, seldom walks more than a block, and obtains cardiorespiratory exercise by swimming, an activity in which his knee does not bother him. The surgeon should recommend knee replacement to one individual but not the other. At the same time, both men must be offered the alternatives, which include continued nonsteroidal antiinflammatory medicine, bracing, sleeping medication, and analgesics.

Patients with an active lifestyle are becoming much more concerned about what will happen to them in the postoperative period, including how soon they can safely travel, when they can work, and when they will be fully able to take care of themselves. They are also concerned about what social services are available to help them if they cannot care for themselves fully. The surgeon must be prepared to address these questions and also advise patients with lower extremity or spinal problems about when they will be able to walk. In the same manner, after procedures on the hand or upper extremity, patients must be advised about when they will be able to use the hand. Advising the patient of these situations before surgery can prevent unexpected surprises in the postoperative period.

The patient should also be informed about the range of expectations for ambulation or use of the upper extremity because individuals vary in their response to surgery. For example, patients should be advised that after surgery on the hip or knee, they will need a walker for a few days, move to crutches, and typically be done with the crutches in the range of 2–4 weeks. They will use a cane before 6 weeks and be done with the cane before 3 months. Patients should be cautioned about travel after surgery, particularly with lower extremity injuries, because of the risk of deep venous thrombosis (DVT). In such cases, discourage (for the first 6 weeks) plane trips longer than an hour and extended car trips made without stopping perhaps every 45 minutes. Antiinflammatory medication (to reduce platelet adhesion) or anticoagulants should be recommended if such travel is unavoidable.

A. Explaining the Procedures

An essential part of the patient's presurgical preparation and postsurgical cooperation is knowing what to expect at every step in the process. Nuances become important in the process of explaining the surgical procedures and their implications. For example, scheduling a bunion procedure 2 weeks prior to a patient's participation in her daughter's wedding could upset the patient if she fails to realize that she will be unable to wear the shoes she purchased for the event. Similarly, lifestyle considerations can affect the decision-making process in cases of medial gonarthrosis, in which the choice between a unicompartmental knee replacement and a high tibial osteotomy could be influenced by whether the patient plays tennis and holds a physically strenuous job or, alternatively, whether the patient is sedentary and works behind a desk most of the day.

B. Reviewing the Risks and Possible Complications

Reviewing the perioperative risks is important for all patients and optimally should be done well in advance and then repeated closer to the time of surgery. Some patients require more detailed explanations, particularly if their relatives have undergone surgery in the past and had a problem with anesthesia or a complication such as a PE or infection. Based on the patient's responses to explanations, the health care team members needs to alter their approach to reach a balance between inadequately informing the patient and inducing unnecessary alarm that could make the patient refuse to undergo a procedure judged to be both beneficial and necessary.

Risk is a poorly understood concept in our culture. Some situations are considered to be higher in risk than they actually are. Some risks are understood better than others. It can help the patient to understand if these risks are put in perspective. The risks can be surprisingly high or low but still disturbing to the patient. For example, many people have moved away from California to avoid an earthquake or refuse to fly commercial aircraft because of the risk, not realizing that the risk of death is 10–100 times higher while driving a car (Table 2–1). This lack of understanding of the risk can contribute to significant differences in the perception of liability associated with these activities. For example, the death benefit from a commercial airline accident might reach several million dollars per passenger, whereas death in an automobile accident might have no death benefit at all. Thus, the *perception* of risk is very important and must be clarified in the patient's mind. Similarly, patients can understand and accept having a myocardial infarction after a major surgery because they can clearly see the strain on the heart from the surgery. However, they are not nearly as understanding of a lower extremity paralysis that can result from the epidural anesthetic for that surgery. The explanation of risks must be individualized for each patient. The patient with a previous myocardial infarction is clearly different from the healthy 20-year-old (see Table 2–1). Across-the-board rates of problems do not translate into direct risks for the individual patient.

Table 2–1. Rates of death and complications associated with common activities.

Death or Complication	Percentage
Death (from MI after previous MI)	1
Major bleed (7 days, warfarin, INR 2.65)	0.02
GI ulcer/bleed perforation (naproxen 6 months)	1
Paralysis (from epidural)	0.02
Death (frequent flying professor/year)	0.001
Death (automobile/year)	0.016
Earthquake in California/per year	0.00018

GI = gastrointestinal; INR = international normalized ratio; MI = myocardial infarction.

Although all procedures carry some risks, the incidence and type of risks and complications vary with the surgical procedure as well as with the patient's age and general health. Potential problems are listed and discussed here in alphabetical order.

1. Amputation—The potential problem of amputation is seldom of acute concern except in cases of significant trauma. The topic of amputation can frequently be discussed with the risk of infection because ischemia and infection can increase the risk of amputation.

2. Anesthesia—One of the major risks in orthopedic surgery is associated with anesthesia, not because complications of anesthesia are frequent but because they can be devastating. Death occurs at a rate of approximately 1 in 200,000 patients undergoing elective anesthesia. Other complications include but are not limited to the following: nerve damage and paraplegia from nerve blocks; headaches from dural leaks following use of spinal anesthetics; aspiration of stomach contents;

and cardiac problems, including ischemia and arrhythmias. The surgeon should discuss these problems with the patient only in general terms, allowing the anesthesiologist to provide the most detailed explanations.

3. Arthritis—Virtually any procedure that enters a joint, other than to replace it, has the potential to cause damage to that joint. In some instances, as in an intra-articular fracture, the surgery will likely lessen the risk of arthritis. Even in these instances, the patient should be told that the risk of damage is still real because the joint surface healing will not result in a normal cartilage surface.

4. Blood loss—Patients should be given a reasonably accurate estimate of blood loss as well as the opportunity to donate autologous blood prior to surgery. Designated donor blood is probably not safer but gives the patient who receives it a sense of security. The use of erythropoietin can elevate preoperative hemoglobin (Hgb) levels (usually for patients with Hgb <13) and thereby reduce postoperative homologous blood transfusion needs. Other alternatives include the use of intraoperative blood salvage for reinfusion (OrthoPAT, Antovac). The use of erythropoietin is generally accepted by Jehovah's Witness patients, whereas the autologous reinfusion acceptance is variable. To help minimize blood loss during surgery, the patient's use of nonsteroidal antiinflammatory drugs (NSAIDs) should be discontinued approximately 2 weeks before surgery. Discontinuation of NSAIDs can significantly compromise comfort and incite rheumatoid flares in many patients who rely on these drugs. To minimize the risk, newer COX-II inhibitor NSAIDs may be used as a substitute during this period; no platelet disorders or bleeding time derangement occurs with these drugs because they do not affect platelet function or inhibit thromboxane A_2.

5. Blood vessel damage—Arterial and venous damage take on greater significance as the size of the vessel increases and the arterial supply becomes more calcified with age and vascular disease. Patients generally understand this, but it must be emphasized where appropriate. Hip and knee replacement put unusual strains on the femoral and popliteal vessels, from positioning, and may damage calcified arteries.

6. Deep venous thrombosis/pulmonary embolism—Virtually all lower extremity and spine procedures in orthopedics involve some risk of DVT, which should be explained to the patient. As many as 25% of patients who undergo a relatively high-risk procedure such as total hip arthroplasty have venographically diagnosed DVT. The risk of PE is much less, however, and is in the range of 0.3% for fatal emboli. This rate of fatal PE is approximately a 10-fold increase over the rate of fatal PE in the U.S. population in men older than 65 years. The risks associated with other procedures may be lower. In any case, the patient should be reassured that prevention procedures commensurate with risk will be undertaken.

7. Fracture—Many procedures in orthopedic surgery carry the risk of a bone fracture. Some procedures, such as uncemented hip replacement, present a higher risk for this complication, but virtually any orthopedic procedure could result in fracture of a bone. The patient must be informed of the risk in relation to the probability of the occurrence of such a problem.

8. Infection—The risk of infection in orthopedic surgery ranges from near zero in procedures such as arthroscopy to several percent in open fracture surgery. The problem of infection should be emphasized in proportion to risk. For example, if a diabetic patient is to undergo knee replacement, he or she should not only be assured that all steps will be taken to prevent infection (eg, administration of prophylactic antibiotics, use of ultrafiltration of air, or ultraviolet lights in the operating room) but should also be told of the various techniques that would be considered if infection occurred. These options include debridement, prosthesis removal, gastrocnemius flap, reinsertion, arthrodesis, and amputation. The common use of external fixation devices for fracture care is accompanied by the frequent problems associated with pin care. The patient and family should be informed about the problems caused by percutaneous devices to prevent the presumption that something has gone wrong. Skin problems are frequently associated with infection but may arise from other causes, such as adjacent scars compromising the blood supply to a surgical flap. Older patients and individuals who are smokers, have diabetes, or have wounds on the distal lower extremity are at increased risk. In such cases, the patient may be warned that delayed healing or necrosis of the skin edges may occur.

9. Loss of reduction—Although fracture care continues to improve, displacement of hardware or fracture fragments may necessitate a second procedure. The explanation of this risk should be individualized, based on the type of fracture. Loss of reduction may contribute to delayed union or nonunion of fractures. These problems may occur despite optimal care by the orthopedic surgeon. Poor vascular supply or smoking can be a factor leading to nonunion. The rate of nonunion is site dependent but is only a few percent.

10. Nerve damage—Certain procedures are associated with nerve damage, although the damage is usually minor. For example, medial parapatellar incisions on the knee cause some numbness from cutting the infrapatellar branch of the saphenous nerve. The patient should be informed in advance if some degree of minor nerve damage is anticipated in association with the particular surgical procedure being pursued and should also be informed of the risks of unexpected nerve damage that accompany all surgical procedures.

C. Prognosis

The prognosis of the procedure is intimately related to the procedure. However, certain guidelines may be given. The expected time off work or time away from activities is important to the patient and depend on the patient's occupation, age, and available sick leave. The bank president with more control over her agenda will be able to return to work activities sooner than the day laborer. Driving is an important activity for many people, and limitations placed by a procedure can determine how much postoperative assistance a patient will need.

The patient should be given reasonable expectations about range of motion, strength, possible disability, and when these should return to normal, if at all. Furthermore, walking or writing ability, ability to use a computer keyboard, and the time to expect to be able to do such activities may be appropriate for some patients. Again, these have to be individualized for each patient and determined for each home situation.

D. Keeping the Patient and Family Informed

Immediately before elective surgery, the surgeon can help comfort the patient and family by meeting them in the preoperative area and appearing relaxed, well rested, and positive about the outcome of the surgery. Giving the family a good estimate of the surgery time is important, but they should also be reassured that delays do not necessarily indicate the occurrence of complications that are detrimental to the patient. If the family members wish to be notified about delays, they should be encouraged to leave instructions about where they can be contacted. When surgery is completed and the patient is no longer at risk of untoward accidents such as aspiration during extubation, a member of the surgical team should apprise the family of the outcome. At this time, it is appropriate to emphasize particular concerns to the family, such as the need to continue vigilance for infection in a diabetic patient who has undergone foot surgery.

Johnson BF et al: Relationship between changes in the deep venous system and the development of the postthrombotic syndrome after an acute episode of lower limb deep vein thrombosis. A one- to six-year follow-up. J Vasc Surg 1995;21:307. [PMID: 7853603]

Lilienfeld DE: Decreasing mortality from pulmonary embolism in the United States, 1979–1996. Int J Epidemiol 2000;29:465. [PMID: 10869318]

Lilienfeld DE, Godbold JH: Geographic distribution of pulmonary embolism mortality rates in the United States, 1980 to 1984. Am Heart J 1992;124:1068. [PMID: 1529881]

McKee MD et al: The effect of smoking on clinical outcome and complication rates following Ilizarov reconstruction. J Orthop Trauma 2003;17:663. [PMID: 14600564]

Nosanchuk JS: Quantitative microbiologic study of blood salvaged by intraoperative membrane filtration. Arch Pathol Lab Med 2001;125(9):1204. [PMID: 11520273]

Salvati E et al: Recent advances in venous thromboembolic prophylaxis during and after total hip replacement. J Bone Joint Surg Am 2000;82:252. [PMID: 10682733]

Tamir L et al: Recombinant human erythropoietin reduces allogeneic blood transfusion requirements in patients undergoing major orthopedic surgery. Haematologia (Budap) 2000;30(3): 93. [PMID: 11128112]

Warner C: The use of the orthopaedic perioperative autotransfusion (OrthoPAT) system in total joint replacement surgery. Orthop Nurs 2001;20(6):29. [PMID: 12025800]

SURGICAL MANAGEMENT

Preoperative Care

A. The Team Approach

Inclusion of nurses, residents, anesthesiologists, and other members of the surgical team in the planning process can improve the efficiency and therefore affect the outcome of a surgical procedure. Good estimates of the length of the operative procedure and of the patient's anticipated blood loss and muscle relaxation requirements minimizes the risks from anesthesia and surgery. Reviewing the site of the operation and assessing the need for any special supplies and equipment, such as prostheses, lasers, or fracture tables, also contributes to efficiency and optimal results. Special care must be exercised by all members of the operative team to prevent "wrong side" surgery. It is now a JCAHO standard to have the surgical team "mark" the surgical site.

B. Preparing and Positioning the Patient

Once the patient is in the operating room, every effort should be made to make him or her comfortable. A calm, efficient, and professional demeanor by everyone involved is necessary both before and after anesthesia is induced. If the anesthesiologist indicates that placement of the antithromboembolic hose, intermittent pneumatic compression stockings, or tourniquets will improve efficiency, these can be put in place prior to induction. Placement of arterial lines, central lines, and Foley catheters should be done after the patient is anesthetized, if possible. Location of the operating table must be adjusted to ensure good lighting, optimize the efficiency of the surgeon and staff, and allow for maintenance of surgical sterile technique.

Positioning of the patient is the responsibility of both the surgeon and the anesthesiologist to facilitate the operation and to ensure the patient's safety. A perfectly executed operation can be marred by a nerve palsy that results from the failure to pad a remote area appropriately. If the patient is placed in the lateral decubitus position, the peroneal nerve at the knee and the brachial plexus of the downside shoulder girdle must be protected. During shoulder surgery, the surgeon must take care to avoid stretching the patient's brachial plexus or cervical nerve roots while attempting to maximize the operative field. Similarly, the patient's shoulder should not be abducted past 90 degrees, and joints with contractures should not be forced into unusual positions. These precautions are particularly necessary in treating rheumatoid patients or older osteoporotic patients. Injury to the extremities and loss of lines can be avoided by careful planning and synchronization when positioning patients into the lateral decubitus position or prone position.

C. Use of Antibiotics

Except in cases in which concern about infection requires unambiguous cultures to be obtained, prophylactic antibiotics should be started prior to skin incision. A first- or second-generation cephalosporin antibiotic is considered appropriate for orthopedic procedures.

D. Use of a Tourniquet

A tourniquet can be extremely helpful in some procedures and is practically mandatory for others. The tourniquet stops the flow of blood to and from an extremity. To achieve this, the pneumatic tourniquet is inflated to a pressure that must be significantly higher than the arterial pressure because the pressure is dissipated in the soft tissue underneath the tourniquet.

1. Tourniquet size and placement—The tourniquet should be wide enough for the extremity while still permitting adequate exposure of the extremity. Particularly in cases involving surgery on muscles that cross the elbow or knee, the tourniquet should be placed as proximal as possible to ensure the muscles have adequate stretch to permit full joint motion. When a tourniquet is used on a large extremity with a great deal of adipose tissue, care must be taken to ensure that the tourniquet does not slip distally, which could result in wrinkles in the tourniquet and localized pressure on the skin. Slippage can be prevented by applying 5-cm (2-inch) adhesive tape to the skin in a longitudinal direction below the cast padding placed under the tourniquet.

2. Tourniquet time and pressure—The effects of tourniquets on tissues are a combination of time and pressure on individual structures. Neural and muscle tissue are most sensitive, with deleterious effects arising from direct pressure to structures and from distal ischemia.

Several considerations are involved in the selection of the level of tourniquet pressure. First, the level must be low enough to avoid pressure damage to sensitive neural structures but high enough so the pressure around the arterial supply to the extremity is greater than systolic pressure (Figure 2–1). Second, if the patient's blood pressure is labile, a margin of safety is usually necessary. In a patient with a stable blood pressure, tourniquet pressures of 75 mm Hg above preinduction systolic pressure are typically adequate, although some surgeons use pressures as high as twice systolic. If the tourniquet is on an extremity with a great deal of adipose tissue, higher pressures are necessary to achieve adequate pressure at the artery to stop blood flow. Tourniquets should be calibrated and can be tested with an independent pressure measurement device or alternatively by palpation of the pulse and gradual elevation of pressure until the pulse disappears.

Complications will arise if tourniquets are used at high pressure for too long. The effects can sometimes

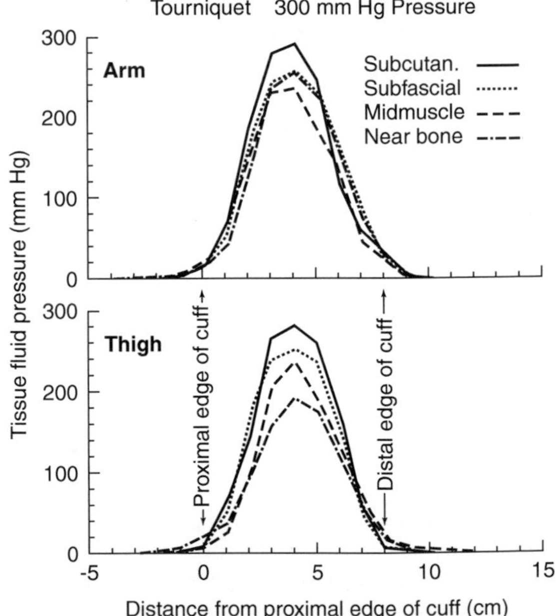

Figure 2–1. Distribution of tissue fluid pressure at four depths beneath pneumatic tourniquet with cuff pressure of 300 mm Hg applied on arms (**top**) and thighs (**bottom**). Values represent means for six limbs on each graph. (Reproduced, with permission, from Hargens AR et al: Local compression patterns beneath pneumatic tourniquets applied to arms and thighs of human cadavers. J Orthop Res 1987;5:247.)

be mitigated by using wider cuffs and curved cuffs, which allow for higher and more uniform pressure below the tourniquet. A rule of thumb is that tourniquet pressures should not be elevated for longer than 2 hours, and less time is preferable. In a canine study of the muscle tissue distal to the tourniquet, investigators found that 90-minute tourniquet times with 5 minutes between reinflation minimized the ischemic damage. This finding points to the need for efficiency in performing surgical procedures under tourniquet. After tourniquet release, reflex hyperemia and edema are frequently encountered, making closure more difficult. Exsanguination with an Esmarch bandage prior to tourniquet inflation facilitates emptying of large veins of the thigh and arm, although it is not recommended to use an Esmarch in trauma cases. Careful exsanguination may help prevent DVT, especially when reinflation of the tourniquet is planned.

Barwell J et al: The effects of early tourniquet release during total knee arthroplasty: A prospective randomized double-blind study. J Bone Joint Surg Br 1997;79:265. [PMID: 9119854]

Classen DC et al: The timing of prophylactic administration of antibiotics and the risk of surgical wound infection. N Engl J Med 1992;326:281. [PMID: 1728731]

Darmanis S, Papanikolaou A, Pavlakis D: Fatal intra-operative pulmonary embolism following application of an Esmarch bandage. Injury. 2002 ;33:761. [PMID: 12379384]

Fernandez AH, Monge V, Garcinuno MA: Surgical antibiotic prophylaxis: effect in postoperative infections. Eur J Epidemiol 2001;17:369. [PMID: 11767963]

Hargens AR et al: Local compression patterns beneath pneumatic tourniquets applied to arms and thighs of human cadavers. J Orthop Res 1987;5:247. [PMID: 3572594]

Idusuyi OB, Morrey BF: Peroneal nerve palsy after total knee arthroplasty. Assessment of predisposing and prognostic factors. J Bone Joint Surg Am 1996;78:177. [PMID: 8609107]

Ostman B et al: Tourniquet-induced ischemia and reperfusion in human skeletal muscle. Clin Orthop 2004;418:260. [PMID: 15043128]

Pedowitz RA et al: The use of lower tourniquet inflation pressures in extremity surgery facilitated by curved and wide tourniquets and an integrated cuff inflation system. Clin Orthop 1993;287:237. [PMID: 8448950]

Sapega AA et al: Optimizing tourniquet application and release times in extremity surgery. J Bone Joint Surg Am 1985;67: 303. [PMID: 3968122]

Wakai A et al: Pneumatic tourniquets in extremity surgery. J Am Acad Orthop Surg 2001;9:345. [PMID: 11575914]

Operative Care

The surgical team should make every effort to work efficiently during the period between the administration of anesthesia and the conclusion of the final steps of preoperative preparation, which may take from 10 to 30 minutes or longer. It is in the best interests of the patient to minimize the time between onset of anesthesia and the beginning of surgery.

A. Incision Sites and Approaches

Although the surgical wound "heals side-to-side, not end-to-end," the incorrect placement or the excessive length of a surgical incision for a given procedure only serves to increase surgical trauma to the patient, slow the healing process, and lengthen the rehabilitation period. If there is any doubt about the surgical incision site, roentgenographic examination should be considered. Use of an image intensifier should be considered in obese patients or in patients with previous surgery and retained hardware.

The incision should be made perpendicular to the skin, generally longitudinally, and with a sharp knife. In tumor biopsies, longitudinal incisions are always made. The approach by the surgeon through the subcutaneous fatty layer is variable and depends on the location on the body. In most areas, sharp dissection with a knife through the subcutaneous tissue to the fascial layer is indicated. In the upper extremity and in areas where cutaneous nerves can be troublesome if injured, blunt dissection is used because cutaneous nerves travel in the fatty tissue. Many surgeons prefer blunt dissection with scissors used to spread tissue perpendicular to the wound. Hemostasis is obtained layer by layer. Subcutaneous fat usually is not dissected from the skin, because this might devascularize it.

Surgeons must be extremely careful with the skin, making sure to avoid crushing it when forceps are used. The skin should never be clamped, nor should it be excessively stretched. A larger incision is much better for the skin than extreme tension. Care of the soft tissues includes keeping them moist, avoiding excessive retraction, and being especially careful of neurovascular bundles. Nerves suffer damage from both traction and compression. Nerve palsies and paresthesias can spoil an otherwise well-performed operation in the eyes of both the surgeon and the patient. Care of the cartilage includes keeping it moist because drying has a deleterious effect.

Surgical approaches that go through internerve planes, such as between the deltoid and the pectoralis major, should be used to avoid denervation of muscles. The splitting of muscles in the surgical approach should also be avoided because splitting is generally more traumatic and more likely to denervate the muscle. This rule does not always apply in tumor surgery because it is important to keep tumor cells in a single compartment.

B. Orthopedic Instruments and Drains

It is mandatory that tools be sharp at all times because the sharpness enables the surgeon to avoid the excessive pressure that creates problems by plunging into the depths of the wound. When an osteotome or elevator is needed, the concurrent use of a hammer is preferred because achieving exact control is possible by the strength and number of hammer taps, whereas control is difficult to achieve by pushing on an osteotome. With drill points and power saws, the sharpness of the instruments should be maintained to reduce necrosis secondary to heating and to facilitate the operation. Unless using a drill guide, the surgeon should start drilling bone in a perpendicular direction even though the final direction may be at some angle to the direction of the bone. This prevents slipping off the desired bone entry point. Holes in long bones are stress concentration sites. Care should be taken to minimize the likelihood and degree of stress concentration by rounding holes and using drill holes to terminate saw cuts (Figure 2–2). When holes were made in bone, especially in the lower extremity, the patient should be advised against torsional loading.

Obtaining hemostasis in bone can be troublesome, and the use of microcrystalline collagen is preferred to bone wax because of the foreign body response. Postoperative bleeding is common from bony surfaces. Despite the traditional use of drains by surgeons, evidence is accumulating that at least for some operations, such as total hip or total knee replacement, wound drainage may not be necessary and may lead to increased blood loss. If drains are used, they should be secured to prevent accidental removal and should be large enough to prevent clogging by clot formation. Drains are generally removed within 48 hours of surgery unless they are used to eliminate dead space.

C. Closure and Dressing

Wound closure should be done quickly and efficiently to minimize total operative and anesthesia time. It should also be accomplished carefully to avoid damage to the skin. When a previous scar is entered, it is sometimes worthwhile to remove scar tissue from the edge of the skin, as well as from the subcutaneous tissue, to provide a more vascular area for healing. Meticulous subcutaneous wound closure is necessary to avoid tension on the skin in many areas on the extremities. Four-throw square knots are important for knot security, especially when plans call for use of continuous passive motion machines or early motion, which may apply repetitive stress to the wound before it heals. Tissue adhesives are an advent in wound closure. One study found no difference between adhesives and sutures for closure of incisions, although the adhesives generally resulted in a more cosmetic wound.

Dressings should be padded with cotton or gauze to discourage the formation of hematomas. Closed wound suction drainage does not change outcome and is associated with a higher infection rate in total knee arthro-

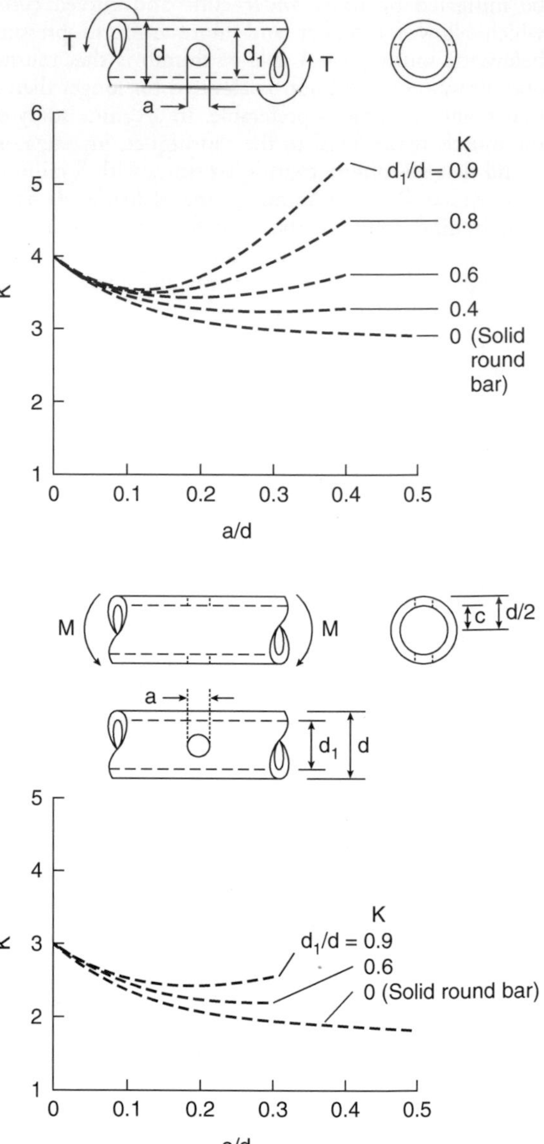

Figure 2–2. Stress concentration factors for torsion (**top**) or bending (**bottom**) of a round bar or tube with a transverse hole, where a = the size of the hole; d = the outside diameter of the tube; d_1 = the inside diameter of the tube; K = the stress concentration factor, defined as the factor by which stress is increased by the hole; M = the bending moment; and T = the torsional load. (Modified and reproduced, with permission, from Peterson RE: *Stress Concentration Factors: Charts and Relations Useful in Making Strength Calculations for Machine Parts and Structural Elements.* Wiley, 1974.)

plasty. Tape should be avoided when possible because it sometimes causes allergic reactions, and also the combination of wound swelling and shear from the tape can lead to blistering and other problems.

Batra EK et al: Influence of surgeon's tying technique on knot security. J Appl Biomater 1993;4:241. [PMID: 10146307]

Brown MD, Brookfield KF: A randomized study of closed wound suction drainage for extensive lumbar spine surgery. Spine 2004;29(10):1066. [PMID: 15131430]

Coulthard P et al: Tissue adhesives for closure of surgical incisions. Cochrane Database Syst Rev 2004;(2):CD004287. [PMID: 15106245]

Kolt JD: Use of adhesive surgical tape with the absorbable continuous subcuticular suture. ANZ J Surg 2003;73(8):626. [PMID: 12887534]

Minnema B et al: Risk factors for surgical site infections following primary total knee arthroplasty. Infect Control Hosp Epidemiol 2004;25:477. [PMID:15242195]

Ong CC, Jacobsen AS, Joseph VT: Comparing wound closure using tissue glue versus subcuticular suture for pediatric surgical incisions: A prospective randomized trial. Pediatr Surg Int 2002; 18:553. Epub accessed June 14, 2002. [PMID: 12415411]

POSTOPERATIVE CARE

Inpatient Care

Postoperative care begins in the postanesthesia room and is the same for both inpatients and outpatients. It is imperative that the orthopedic surgeon takes an active and early role in the treatment of the postoperative patient, including pain management, blood management, and DVT prophylaxis. As soon as practicable, neurologic and vascular evaluation of the operated area should be made. Sensory and motor exam of the pertinent upper or lower extremity nerves should be documented as soon as practical. Early vascular surgery consultation is indicated if pulses are absent or diminished. The wound site should be checked for excessive drainage, and, when appropriate, compartment syndrome should be considered. The general medical condition of the patient, although primarily the concern of the anesthesiologist, should be evaluated to be sure the anesthesiologist is aware of special concerns regarding the individual patient.

During the subsequent postoperative period, orthopedic aspects of care are relatively routine for most procedures. The main responsibility of the orthopedic surgeon is the evaluation of the vascular and neural status of the extremities affected by the surgery, as well as pain control and vigilance for disorders such as DVT or PE. The frequency of postsurgical examinations depends on the clinical setting. Hourly examinations may be necessary in the face of a potential compartment syndrome, although daily examinations are usually adequate. Epidural morphine analgesia may significantly mute or alter the pain picture in a compartment syndrome, making clinical evaluation difficult if not impossible in the immediate postoperative period.

A. Pain Management

Pain management is a major issue in the United States. There is a growing concern that patients are undermedicated for pain control and suffering unnecessarily. The public has embraced this concept, resulting in litigation and disciplinary action by state medical boards for undermedication. Physicians traditionally were seen as being reluctant to prescribe narcotic medication as a result of concerns that they would be disciplined by state medical boards. This concept has lead to a major initiative by the JCAHO to address pain control as a patient "right." JCAHO mandates that pain control be a factor in the total evaluation of the patient and pain evaluation be performed as the fifth vital sign. The scale used is the numeric scale from 0 to 10, similar to the visual analogue scale, with 0 being no pain and 10 being unbearable pain. Acceptable pain levels are defined as 4 and below.

Pain is a very subjective sensation that is an emotional response to the process of nociception: the sum of four separate components beginning with tissue damage, which results in the first component, transduction to a nerve impulse. The next component is transmission to the spinal cord, where the third component occurs: modulation. This modulated signal is then perceived in the cerebral cortex (perception). Pain perception depends on culture, ethnicity, and gender. It is nonlinear, in that a stimulus two times higher does not necessarily result in twice the pain. Pain perception is also based on patient expectations. Studies show that preoperative patient education can reduce patients' pain after major (eg, total knee arthroplasty [TKA]) orthopedic surgery.

Traditional postoperative pain management included the administration of intravenous (IV) or intramuscular narcotic analgesics until oral narcotics were able to control the pain. The patient-controlled analgesia (PCA) is now a mainstay. In this system, morphine is used as the analgesic and typically administered IV at a rate of 1 mg/hour with a patient-controlled dose of 1 mg, which can be administered as often as every 10 minutes. Doses can be increased or decreased to tailor the dose to the patient. Dosing at this level can result in depressed respiration in some patients. However, more cautious dosing can result in insufficient pain relief that can stress the heart, leading to myocardial ischemia in some patients. Other problems can result from traditional pain management with narcotics. Patient rehabilitation can be delayed; nausea, vomiting, constipation, hallucinations, and disorientation can result in lengthened hospital stay and patient dissatisfaction.

Alternative postoperative analgesic methods are proposed. These include epidural and intrathecal administration of local anesthetics and analgesics on a continuous and one-shot basis. These methods have the potential of providing significant pain relief but must be balanced against the alternatives available and the drawbacks that each presents. The one-shot method of adding morphine to the spinal or epidural anesthetic provides pain relief for a limited time, usually on the order of 12 hours, although longer acting forms of morphine (DepoDur) are coming on the market for epidural use, providing pain relief for up to 48 hours. It has the additional problem of limiting additional narcotic analgesia by other routes because overdosing may be possible. Long-term use of continuous epidural or intrathecal analgesia poses the problem of inhibiting rehabilitation. Nurses and physical therapists tend not to mobilize patients with catheters into the spinal canal, and in some hospitals these patients are mandated to go to the intensive care unit. Nerve blocks and injections into joint cavities are limited by the length of action of the local anesthetic agent. Nerve blocks must address all nerves to an area to control postoperative pain. Hence, studies show best results with a longer term effect achieved by the use of pumps that provide a continuous anesthetic flow into the joint or body cavity, with some designs allowing an intermittent bolus for more pain relief. These pumps typically use a long-acting agent such as bupivacaine (0.25% or 0.5%) and infuse at the rate of 2–4 mL/hour. Ropivacaine is reported to have vasoconstrictive properties and less cardiotoxicity than bupivacaine, although at a higher cost.

In the past, non-narcotic pharmacologic treatment of acute postoperative pain was largely restricted to ketorolac, which can be administered by the IV or intramuscular (IM) route in the patient who is restricted in oral intake. Although ketorolac is an effective analgesic through the reduction in the need for morphine, it also increases the perioperative blood loss. After oral intake is permitted, other NSAIDs can be used for analgesics. Neither ketorolac nor other NSAIDs play a routine role in the acute pain management for most orthopedic surgical patients because of the effect these drugs have on the platelets and subsequent blood loss. The availability of COX-2 selective NSAIDs has opened up the possibility of using these drugs as major analgesics for postoperative pain control, without fear of bleeding problems. These drugs act to reduce the need for narcotics with improved pain relief and decreased narcotic side effects. On the horizon are new COX-2 drugs that can be administered parenterally, and these drugs may be of major assistance in the management of early postoperative pain. Such a drug is parecoxib, which is undergoing trials for approval by the Food and Drug Administration (FDA). The use of highly specific COX-2 inhibitors or analgesics came into question with the withdrawal of rofecoxib and valdecoxib from the market because of concern over increased cardiovascular events with long-term use. At this time, other less specific NSAIDs may be considered as alternatives (celecoxib, diclofenac, meloxicam, etodolac) because their effect on platelet function is minimal.

Other analgesics and techniques do not get sufficient recognition for their role in pain control. Acetaminophen is thought to be a central prostaglandin synthase inhibitor and thereby achieves significant relief of pain. It can be tolerated in doses up to 4 g/day, and because it does not act in the same pathway as narcotics, its effect is additive to that of morphine or other narcotics and can reduce the requirement for narcotics. Another analgesic that should be used more often for analgesia is tramadol. This analgesic has very low abuse potential but provides significant analgesia, acting through inhibition of norepinephrine reuptake as well as a weak μ-agonist (similar to morphine) action. Again this mechanism of action is additive to that of traditional opioids and acetaminophen in its analgesic effect. Glucocorticoids are naturally increased in periods of stress such as surgery and are provided exogenously for those patients with suppressed adrenal function. One study showed an increase in cortisol production of 17-fold after TKA, but no such increase after knee arthroscopy. Divided doses of approximately 200 mg of hydrocortisone (8 days normal production) are typically prescribed for such patients. High doses (20 mg) of dexamethasone (equivalent to 400 mg of hydrocortisone) reduce the early postoperative pain in tonsillectomy patients. Although such doses may reduce postoperative nausea, swelling, and pain, as well as create a feeling of well-being, an increased susceptibility to infection may result from longer term dosing. Short courses of relatively high doses of glucocorticoids may be beneficial in reducing postoperative pain. Other methods of pain control may be indirect, such as controlling swelling and pain through hemostasis and cold therapy. Hemostasis may be achieved through the use of bone wax on cancellous bone or through the use of fibrin glue. Vasoconstriction from cold therapy can reduce swelling and also have a direct effect on nociceptive transduction.

A comprehensive approach to pain management can lead to beneficial effects. Multimodal analgesic regimens are suggested using several analgesics that address different points in the nociception process. Combinations of medications can include narcotics, acetaminophen, tramadol, COX-2 inhibitors, and local anesthetics administered through the use of pain pumps. Consideration should be given to administering these medications in the preanesthesia room to preempt the pain of surgery. This can also assist in diminishing peripheral sensitization that occurs with tissue damage. In addition to pharmacological interventions, patient education can reduce preoperative anxiety, reducing pain and increasing satisfaction.

Bianconi M et al: Pharmacokinetics and efficacy of ropivacaine continuous wound instillation after joint replacement surgery. Br J Anaesth 2003;91:830. [PMID: 14633754]

Cook P, Stevens J, Gaudron C: Comparing the effects of femoral nerve block versus femoral and sciatic nerve block on pain and opiate consumption after total knee arthroplasty. J Arthroplasty 2003;18:583. [PMID: 12934209]

Leopold SS et al: Endogenous cortisol production in response to knee arthroscopy and total knee arthroplasty. J Bone Joint Surg Am 2003;85:2163. [PMID: 14630847]

Mallory TH et al: Pain management for joint arthroplasty: Preemptive analgesia. J Arthroplasty 2002;17:129. [PMID: 12068423]

Rasmussen S et al: Increased flexion and reduced hospital stay with continuous intraarticular morphine and ropivacaine after primary total knee replacement: Open intervention study of efficacy and safety in 154 patients. Acta Orthop Scand 2004; 75:606-9. [PMID: 15513495]

Reuben SS et al: Evaluation of the safety and efficacy of the perioperative administration of rofecoxib for total knee arthroplasty. J Arthroplasty 2002;17:26. [PMID: 11805921]

Reuben SS, Sklar J: Pain management in patients who undergo outpatient arthroscopic surgery of the knee. J Bone Joint Surg Am 2000;82:1754. [PMID:11130650]

Sinatra RS, Torres J, Bustos AM: Pain management after major orthopedic surgery: Current strategies and new concepts. J Am Acad Ortho Surg 2002;10:117. [PMID: 11929206]

Sjoling M et al: The impact of preoperative information on state anxiety, postoperative pain and satisfaction with pain management. Patient Educ Couns 2003;51:169. [PMID: 14572947]

B. Deep Venous Thrombosis/Pulmonary Embolus

DVT, a potentially life-threatening disorder, frequently accompanies orthopedic surgery. It is much more of a problem for total joint replacements, spine surgery, and lower extremities immobilized after surgery. This is one of the expected risks after surgery. Venous thromboembolic phenomenon can result in three problems: postphlebitic syndrome, nonfatal PE, and fatal PE. It is necessary to put the risks of PE into appropriate perspective because, contrary to prevailing assumptions in the public and among orthopedic surgeons, PE can occur without surgery (Table 2–2). The risk of having a PE depends on a number of risk factors, including age, weight, the presence of varicose veins, immobility, smoking, previous DVT joint replacement, the season of the year, estrogen therapy, and the location. There is an uncertain relationship between DVT and the probability of having a PE. Obviously one cannot have a PE without having a clot, but which clots are likely to break off and become emboli, and which ones will cause problems are still unresolved issues. It is thought that thigh clots are more important than calf clots because of their size and the potential damage they can do. It is generally conceded, however, that DVT is a marker for PE, and that is the surrogate variable used to determine the effectiveness of treatment of PE. A nonfatal PE can cause cor pulmonale, but this is thought to be an unlikely circumstance, and it is speculated that nonfatal PE would result in a residual effect in the range of 0.1–0.01% of cases. Deep venous thrombosis itself is thought to be a significant problem that results in incompetence of the valves in the deep veins of the calf and thigh. This results in persistent edema, which can progress to brawny edema and ulceration over time. However, many things are thought to cause these changes in addition to DVT. There is a uneven geographic distribution of fatal PE without surgery in the United States, with the West Coast census region having the lowest fatal PE rate. The rate of fatal PE increases with age, although age may simply be a marker for health and activity level. The rate of fatal PE in the general population older than 65 years is in the range of 0.03%, whereas approximate total joint PE rates are typically approximately 0.3%. Thus, there is a 10-fold increase in risk of having a fatal PE with a total hip or knee replacement.

Table 2–2. Rates of complications associated with total hip replacement at the Mayo Clinic.

Complication	Percentage
Death (overall)	0.5
Myocardial infarction	0.5
Pulmonary embolism	0.4
Deep venous thrombosis	1.1

Reproduced, with permission, from Mantilla et al: Poster presented at the Am Acad of Orthopedic Surgeons Annual Mtg; 2001.

Three classes of drugs can be used for chemoprophylaxis of DVT: warfarin (the vitamin K inhibitor), the low-molecular-weight heparins (dalteparin, enoxaparin, and similar drug fondaparinux), and the platelet aggregation inhibitors (aspirin, naproxen, other NSAIDs). Each approach has its advantages and disadvantages. Sodium warfarin has a slow onset of action, sometimes taking several days to reach therapeutic levels, but its oral route of administration is convenient. However, monitoring of the prothrombin time is necessary to ensure appropriate therapeutic levels. The low-molecular-weight heparins do not affect the prothrombin time or the partial thromboplastin time but do affect factor IIa and Xa levels. These do not have to be monitored because the medications are given in standard doses. These medications are provided parenterally. Both warfarin and the low-molecular-weight heparins are associated with bleeding problems. Aspirin and naproxen and other NSAIDs, although causing problems with bleeding at the time of surgery, are really not effective in prevention of DVT. Mechanical means of preventing DVT include compression hose and intermittent pneumatic compression. These are efficacious as adjunctive therapies.

The American College of Chest Physicians regularly performs and publishes metaanalyses of the data available on DVT with updated recommendations. Generally for orthopedic indications after high-risk surgery, either warfarin with an international normalized ratio (INR) of 2–3, a low-molecular-weight heparin starting 12–24 h after surgery, and elastic stockings and intermittent pneumatic compression are useful as supplemental protection against DVT. The recommended period is a minimum of 7 days. Occasionally, use of heparin or vena cava filters is recommended in high-risk situations. Table 2–3 lists the current recommendations.

The community standard in orthopedic surgery probably differs somewhat from that recommended by the American College of Chest Physicians. Newer orthopedic literature seems to suggest that warfarin is the drug of choice but with lower INR values. However, the choice of prophylactic agent is made by the doctor and the patient and is influenced by their interpretation of the risk of thromboembolism and bleeding problems.

Both warfarin and heparin, either low-molecular-weight or regular, have problems that can cause catastrophic side effects in rare cases. Warfarin can cause skin necrosis and venous limb gangrene syndromes unrelated to the operative site. Heparin can induce thrombocytopenia. This is apparently an IgG antibody formation that occurs 5–10 days after starting the drug and can result in a hypercoagulable state that can result in serious problems of coagulation in unintended areas. Some new agents are becoming available, some of which are on the market at the time of this writing but are not indicated for DVT prophylaxis. These drugs are related to the antithrombin drug produced by leeches. Two of these are desirudin and bivalirudin, and they are indicated for anticoagulation in the presence of heparin-induced thrombocytopenia.

In addition, ximelagatran is an antithrombin drug that may soon be available for DVT prophylaxis as an oral prescription. A pentasaccharide (fondaparinux) is approved for DVT prophylaxis and acts in a manner similar to heparin.

Table 2–3. Recommendations for management of DVT prophylaxis for high-risk orthopedic patients

Procedure	Grade	Recommendation
THA/TKA	1A	LMWH started 12–24 h after surgery
		Or
	1A	Fondaparinux 2.5 mg started 6–8 h after surgery
		Or
	1A	Warfarin started immediately after surgery (Target INR 2.5, range 2.0–3.0)
Hip Fractures	1A	Fondaparinux
	1B	LDUH
	1C+	LMWH (As above when safe to use)
	2B	Warfarin (As above)
Trauma	1A	LMWH (As above when safe to use)
	1B	Elastic stockings (ES) and intermittent pneumatic compression (IPC) until LMWH is safe
Acute SCI	1B	LMWH
	1C	ES and IPC

THA = total hip arthroplasty; TKA = total knee arthroplasty; LMWH = low-molecular-weight heparin; LDUH = low dose unfractionated heparin; SCI = spinal cord injury; 1A Grade = clear risk/benefit ratio based on randomized trials without important limitations; 1B Grade = same as 1A but with inconsistent results or methodologic flaws; 1C Grade = clear risk/benefit ratio based on observation studies; 1C+ Grade = same as 1C but based on indirect evidence.

Derived from Geerts WH et al: Prevention of Venous Thromboembolism Seventh ACCP Consensus Conference. Chest (Suppl) 2004;126:338S.

1. Diagnosis—DVT is diagnosed with ultrasound in the postsurgical patient with calf swelling or with Homan's sign in the appropriate clinical setting. Several risk factors can be elicited from the history to increase the suspicion of DVT. These include immobilization, lower extremity or pelvic surgery (in the previous 4 weeks), previous history of DVT, and history of cancer. Ultrasound is a reliable screen for DVT of the thigh veins but less reliable for calf veins. The gold standard for DVT is the venogram, but this method should be used sparingly because it can be quite uncomfortable for patients. Testing for PE has evolved. In nonsurgical patients, *d*-dimer can be helpful in the diagnosis of PE, but the risk of PE continues for weeks after surgery so there may be a role for it in the late postoperative period. Previously, ventilation/perfusion scans were the standard method, followed by pulmonary angiography, if the probability was intermediate. Now spiral CT is quite reliable but is still only reported to be 70% sensitive and 91% specific. In outpatients with a normal ultrasound and a normal lung scan, spiral CT has only a 7% false-positive rate and 5% false-negative rate. Furthermore, evidence from a preliminary study suggests that fibrin monomer discriminates between total hip arthroplasty patients with PE and those without PE. The *d*-dimer was also higher in PE patients but not significantly until 7 days postoperatively.

Ananthasubramaniam K, Shuafra M, Prasad A: Heparin-induced thrombocytopenia and thrombosis. Prog Cardiovasc Dis 2000;42:247. [PMID: 10661778]

Ballard JO: Anticoagulant-induced thrombosis. JAMA 1999;282: 310. [PMID: 10432014]

Brookenthal KR et al: A meta-analysis of thromboembolic prophylaxis in total knee arthroplasty. J Arthroplasty 2001;16:293. [PMID: 11307125]

Freedman KB et al: A meta-analysis of thromboembolic prophylaxis following elective total hip arthroplasty. J Bone Joint Surg Am 2000;82:929. [PMID: 10901307]

Geerts WH et al: Prevention of venous thromboembolism: The Seventh ACCP Conference on Antithrombotic and Thrombolytic Therapy. Chest 2004;126;338S. [PMID: 15383478]

Johnson BF et al: Relationship between changes in the deep venous system and the development of post thrombotic syndrome after an acute episode of lower limb deep vein thrombosis: A one- to six-year follow-up. J Vasc Surg 1995;21:307. [PMID: 7853603]

Kane RE: Neurodeficits following epidural or spinal anesthesia. Anesth Analg 1981;60:150. [PMID: 7011100]

Kubo T et al: Fibrin monomer could be a useful predictor of pulmonary embolism after total hip arthroplasty: Preliminary report. J Orthop Sci 2001;6:119. [PMID: 11484095]

Lilienfeld DE: Decreasing mortality from pulmonary embolism in the United States, 1979–1996. Int J Epidemiol 2000;29:465. [PMID: 10869318]

Lilienfeld DE, Godbold JH: Geographic distribution of pulmonary embolism with mortality rates in the United States, 1980–1984. Am Heart J 1992;124:1068. [PMID: 1529881]

Perrier A et al: Performance of helical computed tomography in unselected outpatients with suspected pulmonary embolism. Ann Intern Med 2001;135:88. [PMID: 11453707]

Salvati E et al: Recent advances in venous thromboembolic prophylaxis during and after total hip replacement. J Bone Joint Surg Am 2000;82;252. [PMID: 10682733]

Turpie AG et al: A synthetic pentasaccharide for the prevention of deep-vein thrombosis after total hip replacement. N Engl J Med 2001;344:(9)619. [PMID: 11228275]

Weitz JI, Hirsh J: New anticoagulant drugs. Chest 2001;119;95S. [PMID: 11157644]

Wells PS et al: Excluding pulmonary embolism at the bedside without diagnostic imaging: Management of patients with suspected pulmonary embolism presenting to the emergency department by using a simple clinical model and D-dimer. Ann Intern Med 2001;135:98. [PMID: 11453709]

Outpatient Care

Economic realities today mandate earlier discharge from the hospital after some procedures and after outpatient surgery in procedures previously done on an inpatient basis. This trend suggests that patients must take more responsibility for their care, and surgeons must provide outpatient access for patients previously treated as inpatients. The indications for discharge have broadened just as the reasons for admission have narrowed. The reasons for keeping a postoperative patient in the acute-care setting are few. The main indications for hospitalization are pain control requiring parenteral narcotics, presence of hemodynamic instability, a need for traction, or a need for frequent physician observation (drains, infection, etc.). Even extended administration of IV antibiotic therapy is not an adequate reason for an acute-care stay. Thus timing of follow-up visits is important, to ensure that the patient is not only unnecessarily inconvenienced but also does not suffer delayed recognition of a complication. In most cases, the first visit should be for suture removal (10–14 days). Again, economic realities mandate a 90-day follow-up as part of the global surgical fee. Follow-up for a total hip replacement patient might be at 2 weeks, 6 weeks, and 12 weeks after surgery. Longer or shorter intervals may be necessary, depending on how the patient is progressing and how much external support the patient is receiving (physical therapy, home nurse visits, home caregivers, and home environment). Joint-replacement patients should be followed up at least yearly on a permanent basis. The American Academy of Orthopedic Surgeons recommends prophylactic antibiotics for joint-replacement patients for procedures such as dental cleaning in which bacteremia may occur, for 2 years after joint replacement, although some surgeons recommend prophylaxis for life, especially when immune compromise is likely (eg, diabetes or renal transplant).

Long-term follow-up for patients with plates, screws, pins, rods, or other fracture devices is not typically necessary after healing of the fracture and rehabilitation of the affected muscles and joints. Antibiotic prophylaxis is not necessary for these patients. In cases of painful hardware, removal may be indicated after healing. Removal of hardware in older (more than 75 years) patients is generally not indicated. In younger (less than 50 years), active patients, hardware removal may be justified to reduce the stress concentration or stress shielding effects of the metal devices to prevent fracture prophylactically. An adequate period (12 weeks or more, depending on activity) of stress protection, especially in torsion, is indicated to reduce the risk of fracture through defects induced in the bone during removal of hardware. For a detailed discussion of rehabilitation, see Chapter 13.

Harrington P et al: Acute compartment syndrome masked by intravenous morphine from a patient-controlled analgesia pump. Injury 2000;31:387. [PMID: 10775698]

Pacheco RJ et al: Gluteal compartment syndrome after total knee arthroplasty with epidural postoperative analgesia. J Bone Joint Surg Br 2001;83:739. [PMID: 11476317]

Richards H et al: Does patient controlled analgesia delay the diagnosis of compartment syndrome following intramedullary nailing of the tibia? Injury 2004;35:296. [PMID: 15124799]

Blood Loss & Replacement

Because blood replacement is now a complicated issue, it is fortunate that not all orthopedic procedures require blood replacement. In California, the surgeon is obligated to give the patient a brochure from the state that describes the blood management options available to the surgeon and the patient when blood transfusion is likely after surgery. Many California hospitals instituted a form for the patient to sign, verifying receipt of this information. Patient involvement in the decision on how to manage blood loss is certainly a good idea. The data on when to transfuse are conflicting, however, and generally the decision is based on the physician's clinical assessment to determine the need for transfusion. Blood volume is approximately 7–8% of body weight, or approximately 5 L in a 70-kg individual. Normal individuals can be resuscitated from acute blood losses of up to 25% with crystalloid/colloid. Greater blood losses can be tolerated if the euvolemic state is maintained, but transfusion should be considered. The status of the clotting system must be monitored in the acute blood loss phase to prevent accelerated blood loss. Blood loss in the postoperative subacute phase can be managed with volume replacement and evaluation of symptomatology to determine the need for transfusion of red cell mass. Patients at risk of stroke, myocardial infarction, or those with decreased cardiac output may need transfusion at higher hemoglobin levels. Younger (less than 50 years), healthier patients may tolerate lower hemoglobin levels unless they have postural hypotension, tachycardia, dizziness, or fainting.

A. Criteria for Blood Transfusion

The decision to transfuse in the immediate postoperative period is predicated on numerous factors, including age, medical condition and cardiac status, estimated blood loss, projected blood loss, availability of blood (autologous, designated donor, or bank), and the patient's perception of risk. Consideration of all factors argues against transfusion in the younger (less than 50 years) or healthier patient until the patient has a hematocrit level of 20–22% or has symptoms that include tachycardia, early and postural hypotension, and dizziness or fainting. Older (more than 60 years) patients at risk of stroke or myocardial infarction would be candidates for transfusion at higher hematocrit levels or with a lower threshold of symptoms.

B. Strategies for Minimizing the Risks Associated with Blood Transfusion

Blood loss is an inevitable part of surgery. With the realization that the banked blood supply is at low risk, but still at risk, of containing infectious agents, strategies to minimize the risk of transmission were developed.

An obvious method of accomplishing this goal is to reduce blood loss. Anesthetic techniques to reduce mean arterial blood pressure can reduce blood loss by reducing the time of surgery as well as the actual blood loss. The patient has to be counseled to avoid antiplatelet drugs in the period prior to surgery. These medications include baby aspirin but also all of the ubiquitous NSAIDs that are in over-the-counter analgesics, cough and cold remedies, and arthritis medications. In the operative period, topical agents such as bone wax, Gelfoam and similar collagen products, thrombin, tranexamic acid and aminocaproic acid (antifibrinolytic), and fibrin glue should be considered. Tranexamic acid can be administered IV or locally to help control bleeding. Surgical technique should be efficient and meticulous to reduce time and therefore blood loss. The patient should be positioned to minimize venous pressure and blood loss, such as positioning a postoperative total knee in flexion to reduce blood loss.

Presurgical banking of autologous blood by the patient (with or without hematopoietic growth factors), immediate preoperative autodonation by hemodilution, and salvage of the patient's intraoperative and postoperatively lost blood with infusion of either washed or unwashed red cells can reduce the patient's exposure to the risks of designated donor blood or homologous banked blood. The problems with autologous blood begin with the cost, but there are other issues. Older (more than 70 years) patients sometimes do not tolerate the anemia from donation. Perhaps the greatest risks are bacterial contamination and clerical error, in which someone gets a potentially fatal ABO-incompatible unit instead of his or her own. Autologous blood that is not used is discarded and not put into the general blood bank pool.

Preoperative hemodilution has the cost associated with the operating room time to draw off the blood and that of the anesthesiologist in supervising the process. Preoperative hematocrit can be boosted through parenteral erythropoietin, which can minimize the effect of surgical blood loss. Erythropoietin is estimated to cost $900 per unit of blood saved, which is more than the cost of autologous blood at $300–400/unit. Furthermore, there may be risks with abnormally high hematocrits. Thus it is only considered when there is little other choice, such as for surgery on Jehovah's Witnesses who refuse transfusions.

Despite initial resistance and continued questions about cost effectiveness by blood bank officials, autologous blood donation has achieved considerable acceptability from patients, physicians, and blood bank administrators. There are disadvantages of autologous donation that counterbalance the obvious advantages of eliminating transfusion-related disease and incompatibility. These are possible bacterial contamination of the blood, perioperative anemia with increased risk of transfusion, administrative error resulting in blood incompatibility from receiving the wrong blood, cost, and wastage of autologous blood that is not used. Blood can be stored for 35 days or can be frozen as a red cell mass for up to 1 year, but loss in viability of the red cells occurs with both storage methods. Use of autologous blood can eliminate the need for banked blood for many but not all orthopedic patients. Some patients, for example, have marginal laboratory test results (eg, Hgb level of 10 g/dL and hematocrit level of 30%) that preclude their predonation of blood. The ability of patients to predonate blood and the amount of blood donated can sometimes be increased through the use of recombinant human erythropoietin therapy. Injections can be given twice weekly and may result in a higher red cell mass collected and a higher hematocrit level at the time of hospital admission. Although expensive, this therapy can be of benefit to patients, especially those who have blood types that are difficult to match or have religious beliefs that conflict with the practice of receiving blood from others.

Red blood cells can be salvaged by suction in the operating room or collected via surgical drains in the recovery room. Adequate loss of blood must be present to make these procedures cost effective. The salvaged blood is generally washed to remove cell debris, fat, and bone fragments. Newer filtration techniques permit the transfusion of blood collected from drains without the washing process.

Bezwada HP et al: Preoperative use of recombinant human erythropoietin before total joint arthroplasty. J Bone Joint Surg Am 2003;85:1795. [PMID: 12954840]

Goodnough LT: Autologous blood donation. Crit Care 2004;8 (Suppl 2):S49. [PMID: 15196325]

Keating EM, Ritter MA: Transfusion options in total joint arthroplasty. J Arthroplasty 2002;17:125. [PMID: 12068422]

Sparling EA et al: The use of erythropoietin in the management of Jehovah's witnesses who have revision total hip arthroplasty. J Bone Joint Surg Am 1996;78:1548. [PMID: 8876583]

Strumper D et al: Clinical efficacy of postoperative autologous transfusion of filtered shed blood in hip and knee arthroplasty. Transfusion 2004;44:1567. [PMID: 15504161]

Zohar E et al: The postoperative blood-sparing efficacy of oral versus intravenous tranexamic acid after total knee replacement. Anesth Analg 2004;99:1679. [PMID: 15562053]

Ethics in Orthopedic Surgery

Ethics in medicine started with Hippocrates and was codified by Thomas Percival in 1803, with the publication of his Code of Medical Ethics. This was extended by the American Medical Association in 1847 and has undergone several revisions over time. Ethics basically define the standards of conduct of honorable or moral behavior by the physician. Many areas of medical ethics, such as abortion or artificial insemination, have little to do with orthopedics. Although many areas of ethics are more restrictive than the law, litigation and legislation have in some cases become the standard by which orthopedists have to abide, with tighter constraints than ethics alone would place. Although ethics as a field is too broad a subject for a text such as this, certain areas that impinge on orthopedics are addressed here.

Clinical Trials

A particularly difficult ethical area is the clinical research study. Although many of these are now more than adequately controlled by institutional review boards (IRBs), the federal government's Office for Human Research Protections, and sponsors of research, the single practitioner in a small orthopedic group is still at risk of performing human, or even animal, research without appropriate ethical controls. The three main areas for concern are the use of ionizing radiation for exams that are not clinically indicated, the use of patient or third-party-payer funds for exams that are not clinically indicated, and the use of patient data in a manner that does not maintain confidentiality. Certainly, ionizing radiation can be used, even for control subjects, if adequate IRB review and patient/subject consent is obtained. This must be done in a formal manner. However, the use of third-party-payer funds for research or revealing patient confidentiality is never ethical. Performing unindicated studies (laboratory, radiographs) at patient expense is certainly unethical. Also, patient confidentiality is fundamental to the doctor–patient relationship. The Health Insurance Portability and Accountability Act changed the way physicians have to look at confidentiality. Verbal, written, and electronic privacy must be maintained in the office and hospital setting. Patient data have to be closely controlled with care taken regarding personal data assistants, scraps of paper with patient identifiers and data, and roentgenographic images. Photos or slides of football injuries in the public domain may be acceptable for presentation, although in some situations this may not be true. Certainly, photos or slides of radiographs with patient identifiers for professional presentations or publications cannot be used without written patient permission. The electronic medical record will produce many potential areas that might violate Health Insurance Portability and Accountability Act (HIPAA) regulations, especially with local area networks that permit laptop access in an entire office or building.

The typical orthopedic clinical research study is a retrospective review of a surgeon's cases. This model of research is considered to be of modest value by researchers doing multicenter, randomized, controlled, double-blind studies, but until the funding is found to do this type of study on something as common as knee replacement, retrospective reviews will have to serve as the database for decision making. This is especially be true for low-volume procedures. These types of studies raise several issues. The main issues are paying for the study (not through patient or third-party funds), maintaining patient confidentiality, and conflict of interest. The first two issues can be resolved by IRB oversight, and private practitioners are advised to obtain that help from their hospital. Conflict of interest has at least two aspects. Physicians may be consultants or designers of the prosthesis or drug and have a financial interest in the success of the product, and they have ego invested in their surgery, that is, they do not want to look like "bad" surgeons and hence may be hesitant to report poor results. Furthermore, they may be professors and need to demonstrate clinical research publications as part of promotion requirements or simply want to "advertise" their abilities through publication. The latter aspects are implied conflicts of interest but are probably as important as a financial conflict. The potential financial conflict should be disclosed to the patient and to other parties such as the hospital and to the journal of publication. Surgeons have an ethical obligation to share medical advances, and presenting surgeons' results with a procedure certainly meets that standard.

Gifts from Industry

The concept that gifts from industry may affect the choice of medication, prosthesis, and so on, is of concern. Generally, the guidelines recommended by the American Medical Association allow gifts, other remuneration, subsidies for meetings, and so on, if the primary purpose is education or of benefit to the patient. Gifts should be of minimal value and related to the physician's work. The pharmaceutical and orthopedic manufacturers are now self-regulated by industry organizations regarding the type of meetings that they can sponsor. Meetings directly sponsored by the company are only allowed to discuss "label" applications of the drug or device, whereas continuing medical education credit courses, which can only be done through an educational institution, can discuss "off-label" uses of products. Payment for travel costs, lodging, and honoraria to attend such meetings is considered inappropriate unless the physician is performing a service, such as faculty duties or consulting. Although it seems unlikely that a physician would change his or her prescribing practice based on a free meal, the appearance of impropriety is important and should be kept in mind.

Cartwright JC et al: Navigating federalwide assurance requirements when conducting research in community-based care settings. J Am Geriatr Soc 2004;52:1567. [PMID: 15341563]

Council on Ethical and Judicial Affairs: *Code of Medical Ethics: Current Opinions with Annotations* (2000–2001 edition). American Medical Association, 2000.

Epps CH: Ethical guidelines for orthopedists and industry. Clin Orthop 2003;412:14. [PMID: 12838046]

Laskin RS, Davis JP: The use of a personal digital assistant in orthopaedic surgical practice. Clin Orthop 2004;421:91. [PMID: 15123932]

Oyama L, Tannas HS, Moulton S: Desktop and mobile software development for surgical practice. J Pediatr Surg 2002;37: 477. [PMID:11877671]

Pancoast PE, Patrick TB, Mitchell JA: Physician PDA and the HIPAA privacy rule. J Am Med Inform Assoc 2003;10:611. [PMID: 14631929]

Musculoskeletal Trauma Surgery 3

Wade R. Smith, MD, Juan F. Agudelo, MD, Anand Parekh, MRCS (Eng), & John R. Shank, MD

The High Cost of Musculoskeletal Trauma

Trauma is the "neglected disease." It is the leading cause of death for people age 1 to 34 years of all races and socioeconomic levels and the third leading cause of death for all age groups. Injuries create a substantial burden on society in terms of medical resources used for treating and rehabilitating injured persons, productivity losses caused by morbidity and premature mortality, and pain and suffering of injured persons and their caregivers. Each year in the United States, one in six residents requires medical treatment for an injury, and one in 10 residents visits a hospital emergency department (ED) for treatment of a nonfatal injury. Data on injury prevalence and costs from the 2000 Medical Expenditure Panel Survey (MEPS) and the National Health Accounts (NHA) reported that injury-attributable medical expenditures cost as much as $117 billion in 2000, approximately 10% of total U.S. medical expenditures. In 2001, there were 157,078 trauma-related deaths, 64% of which were due to unintentional trauma, half of which were caused by motor vehicle crashes. An estimated 29.7 million persons sustained nonfatal injuries during the same period. In 2001, the death rates for motor vehicle-related injuries were 15.3 per 100,000 people, totalling 43,987. Crash injuries result in about 500,000 hospitalizations and four million emergency department visits annually. The economic burden of motor vehicle-related deaths and injuries is also enormous, costing the United States more than $150 billion each year. In 2001, approximately 140,000 Americans sustained gunshot injuries. Twenty-nine thousand of these (21%) died as a result. In the pediatric population, 10,000 deaths associated with trauma are recorded annually in the United States. Trauma accounts for 30% of pediatric emergency room visits and is the most common cause of mortality in the noninfant child.

Musculoskeletal disorders generated 3.5 million admissions to acute-care hospitals in the United States in 1988, more than 40% of which were trauma-related. Musculoskeletal injuries have a tremendous effect on the patient, the family, and the society in general because of the

1. physical and psychologic effects of pain, limitation of daily activities, loss of independence, and reduced quality of life;
2. direct expenditures for diagnosis and treatment; and
3. indirect economic costs associated with lost labor and diminished productivity.

Musculoskeletal injuries occur frequently, result in significant disability, and consume a major portion of health care resources. For example, the cost of hip fracture is estimated at $8.7 billion, or 43% of the total cost of all fractures. Direct costs are about 80% of the total, of which inpatient hospital care amounts to $3.1 billion and nursing home care $1.6 billion. More recent estimates show an increasing effect on the U.S. economy, including over $150 billion per year in direct and indirect cost from lost labor productivity due to trauma.

Mass casualty situations as a result of terrorism are the challenge of the new millennium, requiring a highly organized and effective trauma system. The capability to respond in an organized manner has gained importance after terrorist attacks within United States. In a mass casualty situation, limited resources must be allocated for a great number of victims. The terrorist attacks in Oklahoma City (1995) and at the World Trade Center (1993, 2001) showed the inefficiencies of the civilian disaster response system. The Orthopaedic Trauma Association has developed strategies to educate and optimize the response to mass casualties.

Surveillance for fatal and nonfatal injuries-United States, 2001. Vyrostek SB, Annest JL, Ryan GW. MMWR September 3, 2004/Vol. 53/No. SS-7. CDC.

Medical expenditures attributable to injuries-United States, 2000. MMWR January 16,2004. CDC.

Engelhardt S et al: The 15-year evolution of an urban trauma center: What does the future hold for the trauma surgeon? J Trauma 2001;51:633. [PMID: 11586151]

Praemer A, Furner S, Rice DP: Musculoskeletal conditions in the United States. Am Acad Orthop Surg, Park Ridge IL, 1992.

Soderstrom CA, Cole FJ, Porter JM: Injury in America: The role of alcohol and other drugs—an EAST position paper prepared by the injury control and violence prevention committee. J Trauma 2001;50:1. [PMID: 11253757]

Wynn A et al: Accuracy of administrative and trauma registry database. J Trauma 2001;51:464. [PMID: 11535892]

THE HEALING PROCESS

Bone Healing

Bone is a unique tissue because it heals by the formation of normal bone, as opposed to scar tissue. In fact, it is considered a nonunion when a bone heals by a fibroblastic response instead of by bone formation. Whatever part of the skeleton it comes from, bone has a fine fibroid structure. This is true for cortical and cancellous bone from the diaphysis, epiphysis, or metaphysis. Bone will, therefore, heal by the same mechanism wherever it breaks.

Fracture healing can be divided into primary and secondary healing. In primary healing, the cortex attempts to reestablish itself without the formation of callus (osteonal or haversian healing). This occurs when the fracture is anatomically reduced, the blood supply is preserved, and the fracture is rigidly stabilized by internal fixation. Secondary fracture healing results in the formation of callus and involves the participation of the periosteum and external soft tissues. This fracture healing response is enhanced by motion and is inhibited by rigid fixation.

Fracture healing can be conveniently divided, based on the biologic events taking place, into the following four stages

1. Hematoma formation (inflammation) and angiogenesis.
2. Cartilage formation with subsequent calcification
3. Cartilage removal and bone formation
4. Bone remodeling

A. Hematoma Formation and Angiogenesis

Initially, there is an inflammatory phase characterized by an accumulation of mesenchymal cells around the fracture site. The formed hematoma is a source of growth factors. Transforming growth factor beta (TGF-β) and platelet derived-growth factor (PDGF) are released from platelets at the fracture site. TGF-β induces mesenchymal cells and osteoblasts to produce type II collagen and proteoglycans. PDGF recruits inflammatory cells at the fracture site. Bone morphogenetic proteins (BMPs) are osteoinductive mediators inducing metaplasia of mesenchymal cells into osteoblasts. IL-1 (interleukin-1) and IL-6 recruit inflammatory cells to the fracture site. In fractures where the periosteum is intact, these cells probably come from the cambium. In higher energy fractures where the periosteum has been compromised, the appearance of spindle-shaped cells that are able to differentiate into osteogenic cells has been found to coincide with the appearance of capillary buds. These cells are possibly derived from the pericytes found around capillaries, arterioles, and venules.

Whatever their origin, these cells ensheathe the fracture and differentiate into chondrocytes or osteoblasts. Low-oxygen tension, low pH, and movement favor the differentiation into chondrocytes; high-oxygen tension, high pH, and stability predispose to osteoblasts. Bone morphogenetic proteins (BMPs) and cytokines (IL-1, IL-6) are present during cartilage formation. This initial callus acts as an internal splint against bending and rotational deformation and, less effectively, against shearing and axial deformation. Because the stiffness of this callus in bending and torsion varies with the fourth power of the radius, its distribution around the fracture is important; peripheral distribution adds to rigidity. Clinically, the fracture becomes "sticky," and although some motion is detectable, the fracture is stable.

B. Cartilage Formation with Subsequent Calcification

Radiologic evidence of mineral formation signals the onset of this phase. Cartilage in callus is replaced by woven bone by a process analogous to the endochondral ossification seen in the fetus. The mechanism of mineralization is poorly understood but is thought to involve active transport of minerals and their precipitation from a supersaturated solution. Mineralization causes the chondrocytes themselves to degenerate and die. Capillary buds then invade the mineralized cartilage, bringing osteoblasts, which resorb part of the calcified cartilage and deposit coarse fibroid bone on its residuum. The proliferating cambium layer of the periosteum also lays down new bone on the exposed surface of the bone, if conditions are favorable.

The phase of mineralized callus leads to a state in which the fracture site is enveloped in a polymorphous mass of mineralized tissues consisting of calcified cartilage, woven bone made from cartilage, and woven bone formed directly.

C. Cartilage Removal and Bone Formation

The woven-bone mineralized callus has to be replaced by lamellar bone arranged in osteonal systems to allow the bone to resume its normal function. Before this stage of remodeling can start, it is necessary to consolidate the fracture site. The concept of consolidation is poorly defined but includes filling the gaps left by the previous phase between the ends of the bone; it is also called **gap-healing bone.** This bone has three major characteristics:

1. It forms only under conditions of mechanical stability;
2. It has the ability to replace fibrous or muscle tissue; and
3. It forms within the confines of the bone defect

Gap-healing bone is essentially coarse fibroid bone and, therefore, is not normal lamellar bone.

D. Remodeling

This final phase involves the replacement of woven bone by lamellar bone in various shapes and arrangements and is necessary to restore the bone to optimal function. This process involves the simultaneous meticulously coordinated removal of bone from one site and deposition in another.

Two lines of cells, osteoclasts and osteoblasts, are responsible for this process. Osteoclasts are derived from monocytes and are large multinucleated cells that remove bone. They are located on the resorption surfaces of the bone. Osteoblasts are mononuclear and are responsible for the accretion of bone.

Cartilage Healing

Articular cartilage consists of extracellular matrix (ECM) and chondrocytes. The ECM is formed by water (65% to 80%), collagen (95% type II) and proteoglycans (chondroitin sulfate and keratan sulfate). Collagen in the ECM provides form and tensile strength. Proteoglycans and water give the cartilage stiffness, resilience and endurance.

Chondrocytes are sparse in the adult cartilage, which is not a vascularized tissue. Their nutrition comes from the synovial fluid and depends on the health of the synovial membrane and adequate circulation of the fluid through the spongelike cartilage matrix. Motion of the joint is responsible for most of this circulation. A good part of the rationale behind rigid internal fixation of fractures is to allow early motion of the joints. The same argument can be made for early weight bearing of immobilized joints, which allows cyclical compression of the cartilage and circulation of the synovial fluid.

Rapidly applied forces to the articular cartilage prevent adequate fluid movement and load distribution leading to rupture of the ECM macromolecular framework and cell damage. Articular cartilage lesions are classified according to the type of damage and reparative response:

1. Injuries to the cartilage matrix and cells.
   Caused by acute or repetitive blunt trauma. Evidence of alterations in ECM (decrease in proteoglycans concentration, disruptions of the collagen fibril framework), without macroscopic evidence of damage. It has potential for repair.
2. Chondral fissures, flap tears, or chondral defects.
   Limited, short chondrocytic reparative response. Loss of segmental cartilage.
3. Osteochondral injuries.
   Hemorrhage, fibrin clot formation and inflammatory response. Fibrocartilage formation. Inferior mechanical properties.

Articular cartilage has limited reparative capacities because chondrocytes have a low baseline metabolic rate, a small cell-to-matrix ratio, and a restricted mode of nutrition. If the defect in the cartilage does not go through the calcified plate, the body attempts repair with hyaline cartilage. It will be, however, incomplete, except for the smallest defects. If the calcified plate is violated, the subchondral capillaries bring an inflammatory reaction, which fills the defect with granulation tissue and, eventually, fibrocartilage. The quality of this fibrocartilage can be improved by passive or active motion of the joint. Basic and clinical research has shown the potential of artificial matrices, growth factors, perichondrium, periosteum and transplanted chondrocytes and mesenchymal stem cells to stimulate the formation of cartilage in articular defects.

Tendon Healing

Tendons are specialized structures that allow muscles to concentrate or extend their action. The Achilles tendon, for example, concentrates the action of the bulky muscles of the calf over a small area where a large force needs to be applied for pushoff. Tendons consist of long bundles of collagen scattered with relatively inactive fibrocytes. These cells are nourished by the synovial fluid secreted by the one-cell-thick synovial membrane that covers the tendon (endotenon) and the parietal surface of the sheath (epitenon). The flexor tendons are covered by a richly vascularized adventitia (paratenon).

Muscle Healing

Human skeletal muscle is divided into fiber types depending on their metabolic activity and mechanical function. Type 1 fiber, known as **slow twitch, slow oxidative,** or **red,** muscle, has a slow speed of contraction and the greatest strength of contraction. It functions aerobically and, therefore, is fatigue-resistant. Type 2 fiber, known as **fast twitch** or **white** muscle, is subdivided into two types, according to metabolic activity level: fiber that functions by oxidative and glycolytic metabolism (type 2A) and fiber that is largely glycolytic (type 2B). Both subtypes of white fast-twitch muscles are fatigable but have high strength of contraction and high speed of contraction. Fiber type interconversion can occur, but this is generally believed to happen only under extreme conditions. It is generally conceded that the relative proportions of type 1 and type 2 fibers are defined genetically, with little capacity for change. Thus, sprinters are unlikely to become cross-country runners, and vice versa. Interconversion between type 2A and 2B fibers is much more likely, depending on the type of athletic training.

Traumatic injury to muscle can occur from a variety of mechanisms, including blunt trauma, laceration, or ischemia. Recovery occurs through a process of degeneration and regeneration, with new muscle cells arising from undifferentiated cells. Traumatic injuries include muscle laceration, muscle contusion (blunt injury), and strains resulting from excessive stretching. In addition to muscle regeneration, laceration repair requires reinnervation of denervated muscle areas. Muscle contusion frequently results in hematoma. The normal repair process includes an inflammatory reaction, formation of connective tissue, and muscle regeneration. Blunt trauma may result in myositis ossificans and may cause decreased function. Muscle strains go by a variety of names, including **muscle pull** and **muscle tear.** The failure frequently occurs at the myotendinous junction in experimental animals but may also be within the muscle itself rather than at the bone-tendon junction.

Of particular concern to the traumatologist is the effect of immobilization on muscle tissue. As with all tissues, immobilization and lack of activity result in atrophy. Loss of muscle weight initially occurs rapidly and then tends to stabilize, and loss of strength occurs simultaneously. Resistance to fatigue diminishes rapidly. These changes are minimized if immobilization occurs with some stretching of the muscle. Prevention of "fracture disease" after trauma requires an understanding of muscle physiologic principles.

Nerve Healing

Peripheral nerves have a distinct anatomic structure, with multiple nerve fibers combined to form a fascicle surrounded by perineurium. Multiple fascicles are surrounded by epineurium. Nerves fall into patterns of monofascicular, oligofascicular, and polyfascicular structures. The size and distribution of fascicles change as a function of length, reflecting greater or lesser nerve fibers in each fascicle. Around joints, fascicles typically tend to be multiple and small, perhaps to reduce injury from mechanical trauma. In addition, these nerves tend to have thicker epineurium near joints, with many small fascicles, and this may tend to protect the nerve from flexion and extension cycles. Nerve damage may occur through direct compression or stretching injuries. Ischemic damage from stretching may occur at elongation of 15%. Nerve injuries are now rated from 1 to 5 degrees. First-degree injury is the least severe and is equivalent to neurapraxia. The nerve (axon) is in continuity, and loss of function is reversible. Second-degree injury is equivalent to axonotmesis, with degeneration of the axon. The endoneurial sheath remains in continuity, however, and regeneration occurs by growth of the axon down its original endoneurial tube. Third-degree injury is the same as second-degree injury with the addition of loss of continuity of the endoneurial tube. The perineurium is preserved, however. Because of damage to the fascicle, some misdirection of regenerating axons may occur, and the extent of functional return depends on the extent of misdirection. Fourth-degree injuries preserve only the continuity of the nerve trunk but involve much more extensive degeneration of the fascicles. Despite the continuity of the nerve trunk, this injury may require excision of the damaged segment, with reapproximation of the nerve ends to achieve a functional outcome. Fifth-degree injury involves complete loss of continuity of the nerve trunk. Surgical repair, obviously, is required to achieve restoration of function.

Functional recovery after nerve injury depends on a number of variables. The outcome is much more optimistic for children than adults, and the prognosis diminishes with age. Increasing distance from the nerve injury to the distal point of innervation reduces the likelihood of recovery. Other factors include the length of the damage to the nerve, the technical ability of the surgeon, and the length of time prior to repair.

Buckwalter JA. Articular cartilage injuries. Clin Orthop 2002; 402:21-37. [PMID: 14620787]

Jackson DW, Scheer MJ, Simon TM: Cartilage substitutes: Overview of basic science and treatment options. J Am Acad Orthop Surg 2001;9:37. [PMID: 11174162]

Browne JE, Branch TP: Surgical alternatives for treatment of articular cartilage lesions. J Am Acad Orthop Surg 2000;8:180. [PMID: 10874225]

Lee SK, Wolfe SW: Peripheral nerve injury and repair. J Am Acad Orthop Surg 2000;8:243. [PMID: 10951113]

Robinson LR: Role of neurophysiologic Evaluation in diagnosis. J Am Acad Orthop Surg 2000;8:190. [PMID: 10874226]

ORTHOPEDIC ASSESSMENT & MANAGEMENT OF POLYTRAUMA PATIENTS

A thorough understanding of the pathophysiology of trauma is essential for prompt diagnosis and timely treatment of musculoskeletal injuries. Sound therapeutic principles improve the overall outcome for the patient and optimize the utilization of limited health care resources.

Life-Threatening Conditions: The ABCs of Trauma Care

A systematic approach is required in all cases. The patient is assessed and treatment priorities are established according to the type of injury, stability of vital signs, and mechanism of injury. In a severely injured patient, treatment priorities are dictated by the patient's overall condition, with the first goal being to save life and preserve the major functions of the body. Assessment consists of four overlapping phases:

1. Primary survey (ABCDE)
2. Resuscitation
3. Secondary survey (head-to-toe evaluation and history) and
4. Definitive care

This process, identifies and treats life-threatening conditions, and can be remembered as follows:

*A*irway maintenance (with cervical spine protection);
*B*reathing and ventilation;
*C*irculation (with hemorrhage control);
*D*isability (neurologic status);
*E*xposure and environmental control (undress the patient but prevent hypothermia).

A brief overview of the treatment of polytrauma patients, with special emphasis on the orthopedic aspects, follows:

A. Airway

Great care should be taken while assessing the airway. The cervical spine should be carefully protected at all times and not be hyperextended, hyperflexed, or rotated to obtain a patent airway. The airway should be rapidly assessed for signs of obstruction, foreign bodies and facial, mandibular, or tracheal/laryngeal fractures. A chin lift or jaw thrust maneuver should be used to establish an airway. A Glasgow Coma Scale of 8 or less is an indication for the placement of a definitive airway. The history of the trauma incident is essential because it provides immediate clues to associated injuries. A normal neurologic examination or cross-table lateral radiograph of the cervical spine, including the C7-T1 disk space, does not rule out cervical spine injuries; it only makes them less likely. Any patient with a blunt injury above the clavicle should be considered at risk for cervical spine injury).

B. Breathing

The trauma surgeon should evaluate the patient's chest. Adequate ventilation requires not only airway patency but also adequate oxygenation and carbon dioxide elimination. Remember that the following four conditions, if present, must be addressed emergently:

1. Tension pneumothorax
2. Flail chest with pulmonary contusion
3. Open pneumothorax and
4. Massive hemothorax

C. Circulation

Hemorrhage is the principal cause of postinjury deaths that are preventable. Postinjury hypotension is considered hypovolemic in origin until proved otherwise. Level of consciousness, skin color and pulses are simple to assess and reliably mirror the hemodynamic status of the patient, especially if recorded serially. Fractures of the femur or the pelvis can cause major blood loss, which can severely compromise the ultimate survival of the patient. (See sections on pelvic and femoral fracture.)The orthopaedic surgeon as a member of the trauma team should be alert to the possibility of extremity blood loss and communicate its estimate to the trauma team leader.

D. Disability (Neurologic Status)

The Glasgow Coma Scale (see Chapter 13) should be used to assess neurologic status; it is quick, simple, and predictive of patient outcome. An even simpler way to monitor central neurologic status is to remember the mnemonic AVPU and check if the patient is

*A*lert and oriented,
or responds to *V*ocal stimuli,
or responds only to *P*ainful stimuli,
or is *U*nresponsive.

E. Exposure and Environmental Control

Recognition of lacerations, contusions, abrasions, swelling and deformity can only be accomplished in the completely disrobed patient. The safest way to achieve this is to cut off all clothing. This permits complete examination of the patient, prevents further displacement of fractures and minimizes the risk of overlooking significant problems. Hypothermia must be avoided, as cardiac function may be affected, especially when there is decreased blood volume. Sterile dressings should be applied to any wounds and wound exploration in the emergency department should be avoided to prevent further contamination.

F. Care of Patient before Hospitalization

The diagnosis and treatment of musculoskeletal injuries in polytrauma patients should be initiated in the field by the paramedics. Recognition and appropriate splinting of major fractures, adequate immobilization of the cervical spine, and proper handling of the injured patient are essential to prevent further damage to the neurovascular elements and limit hemorrhage. In many cases, proper care at this stage will prevent or limit shock as well as avoid catastrophic damage to the spinal cord.

The old saying "splint them where they lie" remains especially true when the exact nature and extent of the fractures remain obscure. As a general rule, the following measures should be taken:

1. The joints above and below the fracture should be immobilized.
2. Splints can be improvised with pillows, blankets, or clothing.
3. Immobilization does not need to be absolutely rigid.
4. Apply gentle in-line traction to realign the extremity in severe angulation.
5. Overt bleeding should be tamponaded with available dressings and firm pressure.
6. Tourniquets should be avoided, unless it is obvious that the patient's life is in danger.

Orthopedic Examination

A. History

Injury mechanism: an adequate assessment of the conditions in which the injury was sustained is crucial. Information from paramedics, patient relatives and bystanders should be recorded. Obtain the following information according to injury mechanism:

1. MVA: speed; direction (T bone, rollover etc.); patient location in the vehicle, impact location, postimpact location of the patient (if ejection, determine distance); internal and external damage to the vehicle; restraint use and type.
2. Falls: distance of the fall; landing position.
3. Crush: weight of the object, site of the injury, duration of weight application.
4. Explosion: blast magnitude; patient distance from the blast: primary blast injury (force of the blast wave); secondary blast injury (projectiles).
5. Vehicle-pedestrian: type of vehicle, site of collision, speed.

Environmental exposure, comorbidity, pre-hospital care and observations at the accident scene should be determined. Estimated bleeding, open wounds, deformity, motor and sensory function and delays in extrication or transport are recorded.

B. General Examination

The clinical orthopedic examination requires assessment of the axial skeleton, pelvis, and extremities. The extent of this examination depends on the patient's overall central neurologic status. Swelling, hematomas, and open wounds are assessed visually in the undressed patient. It is obligatory to palpate the entire spine, pelvis, and each joint. Examination soon after trauma may precede telltale swelling in joint or long bone injuries. In the unresponsive patient, only crepitation and false motion may be discerned. Patients with a better mental status, however, can provide feedback regarding pain resulting from palpation. The pelvis is examined by gentle compression of the iliac wings in a mediolateral, anterior-posterior direction and palpation of the pubis. However, if the patient is hemodynamically unstable, manipulation of the pelvis should be avoided in order to prevent increased bleeding. The AP pelvis x-ray must then be used to assess the pelvis as a potential source of shock.

C. Neurologic Examination

The neurologic examination of the extremities should be documented to the fullest extent possible, in light of the patient's mental status, as it is central to subsequent decision making. This examination includes delineation of sensory function in the major nerves and dermatomes in the upper and lower extremities. Perianal sensation is also important. Thus, in the upper extremity, dermatomes from C5–T1 and radial, ulnar, and median nerve function must be assessed.

D. Muscle Examination

Motor examination can be difficult because of pain or impaired mental status, but even in such cases, useful and relatively complete information can be obtained. In the upper extremity, the function of the deltoid, biceps, brachioradialis, extensor pollicis longus, flexor carpi radialis, and intrinsic muscles (first dorsal interosseus and opponens pollicis muscles) must be examined. A more complete examination is indicated if there is obvious trauma to this area. In the lower extremity, the motor supply to the extensor hallucis longus, tibialis anterior, peroneal muscles, gastrocnemius, and quadriceps muscles must be tested and graded. Muscle strength grading is desirable, but demonstration of a minimum of volitional control (even if withdrawal to painful stimuli) is important in verifying the presence of intact central sensory-motor integration.

Particularly important in the face of spinal cord injury or suspected injury are the reflexes of the anal "wink" and bulbocavernosus muscle. Other spinal reflexes (ie, of the biceps and triceps muscles, of the knee and ankle, and the Babinski reflex) are important in "fine-tuning" the neurologic examination. (These are discussed more fully in Chapter 5, "Disorders, Disease, & Injuries of the Spine.")

Imaging Studies

Radiologic assessment follows the same general hierarchy as the clinical assessment. The severely injured polytrauma patient requires plain films of the chest, abdomen, *and* pelvis to indicate sources of respiratory and circulatory compromise. The second level of examination requires the cervical spine cross-table lateral view. The information obtained from this film dictates treatment and the need for any further evaluation of the cervical spine. In the hemodynamically unstable patient, the AP pelvis film is sufficient to make immediate treatment decisions. Complementary pelvis films can be obtained later on.

Subsequent evaluation is dependent on clinical findings. Any long bone or joint with a laceration, hematoma, angulation, or swelling must undergo roentgenographic evaluation. Any long bone fracture requires complete evaluation of the joints proximal and distal to the fracture. At the minimum, two views of the extremities are needed, usually the anteroposterior and lateral views. Coordination of more sophisticated studies with other trauma specialties (eg, neurosurgery or urology) is necessary to allow cardiorespiratory monitoring of the patient while efficiently performing these studies. For example, magnetic resonance imaging (MRI) and computed tomographic (CT) scanning should be performed with the fewest changes of position possible that will also provide the necessary information for all surgical subspecialists.

"Clearing" the Cervical Spine

In the evaluation of the trauma patient, an important consideration is the status of the cervical spine. The cervical spine is easily injured because of the large mass of the head relative to the neck, especially in motor vehicle accidents involving rapid acceleration or deceleration. Consequently, the cervical spine can receive significant force and suffer injury. In the conscious and responsive patient, swelling or tenderness on physical examination of the cervical spine is readily apparent. In the unconscious patient, cervical spine injuries can go undetected, and a careful physical examination must be performed with heavy reliance upon radiographic evaluation.

The essential radiographs for evaluation of the cervical spine include anterior-posterior views, lateral views, and an open-mouth odontoid view. It is essential to be able to see to the top of T1. If this level is not visualized through these conventional views, then a "swimmer's view," which is a lateral cervical spine radiograph with the arm abducted and elevated, should be obtained.

After the cervical spine x-ray films have been reviewed, the ligamentous stability of the cervical spine can be further evaluated. Lateral cervical spine flexion and extension views can be analyzed to see if the lateral alignment of the anterior cervical spinal segments is correct. These can only be obtained in the alert and cooperative patient who can safely sit upright. These films are often delayed for a several-week period.

In the obtunded patient, CT and/or MRI scan is necessary to delineate further soft tissue injury. On the open-mouth view, the lateral masses of C1 should line up with the body of C2. The amount of total overhang of C1 over C2 should be less than 7 mm. On the lateral view, the anterior border of the bodies of the cervical segments should describe an arc. The distance from the basion to the posterior arch of C1 divided by the distance from the opisthion to the anterior arch of C1 should be less than 1 (Powers ratio) (Figure 3–1). A basion to odontoid tip distance above 10mm in children and 5 mm in adults indicates craniocervical dislocation, a potentially fatal injury. The posterior border of the anterior arc of C1 should be within 2–3 mm of the anterior border of C2. There should be no diastasis of the spinous processes, and the joints and facet joints should all be visible. If there is a change in orientation from one cervical spine level to another, then cervical fracture, jumped facets, or dislocation should be suspected. Suspected cervical spine fracture should be investigated with appropriate imaging, such as CT scan, to further delineate the injury pattern. Suspected cervical spine injuries should be treated with provisional stabilization using a cervical collar. Rotational subluxation should be managed with evaluation of soft tissues and reduction maneuvers. In the case of neurologic deficit, careful evaluation of the neurologic status is important, and immediate decompression-stabilization must be considered.

IMMEDIATE MANAGEMENT OF MUSCULOSKELETAL TRAUMA

The orthopedic injuries in the polytrauma patient are seldom truly emergency situations, except for those involving neural or vascular compromise.

For example, fracture-dislocation of the ankle or knee resulting in distal ischemia justifies immediate attempts at reduction to minimize the sequelae of ischemia. A more subtle situation requiring emergent treatment would be dislocation of the hip in which vascular com-

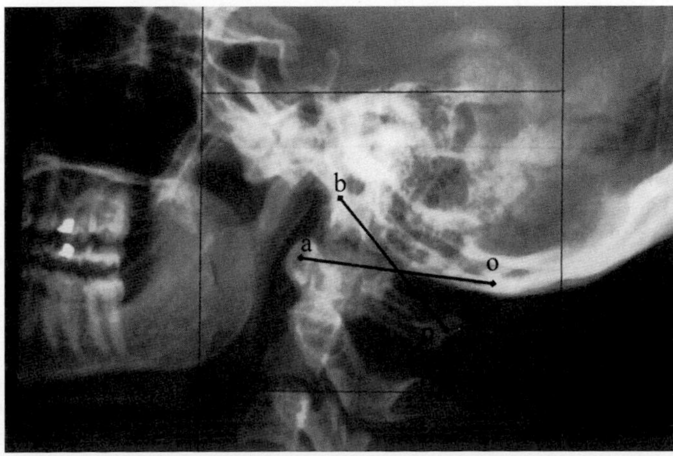

Figure 3–1. Powers ratio: a – anterior arch of atlas, b – basion, p – posterior arch of atlas, o – opisthion. The ratio of bp:oa should be approximately 0.77 in the normal population. Anterior occipito-atlantal dislocation is present when the Powers ratio is greater than 1.15.

promise of the femoral head may result. Arterial bleeding from an open fracture should be treated immediately with pressure to minimize blood loss. Other bone and joint injuries, although urgent, may be approached in a more deliberate manner.

Orthopedic management of traumatic injuries requires consideration of the entire individual as well as the entire extremity. It is short-sighted to treat only the area of injury revealed on radiograph, as the soft-tissue envelope around the bone is essential to fracture healing and the ultimate function of the patient. Repair of soft-tissue damage is clearly important in achieving satisfactory function after healing has occurred. A break in the skin is important, but the damage done to the entire extremity is more important than the extent of laceration.

Complications

From the orthopedist's viewpoint, the major complications associated with trauma are acute respiratory distress syndrome (ARDS), systemic inflammatory response syndrome (SIRS), fat embolism syndrome (FES), multisystem organ failure (MOF), thromboembolic disease, atelectasis, compartment syndrome, sepsis, and ectopic bone formation. The first five disorders involve pulmonary complications and must constantly be kept in mind in managing the polytrauma patient. The institution of early fixation of fractures with concomitant mobilization of the patient has helped to reduce the incidence of these four conditions significantly. They continue to be problems, however, and constant vigilance is necessary to prevent serious consequences. New research has begun to identify subsets of highly injured patients in whom some forms of early definitive fixation may accelerate the development of ARDS, SIRS, and MOF.

A. Acute Respiratory Distress Syndrome

Acute respiratory distress syndrome (ARDS) can be a sequela of trauma with subsequent shock. Massive tissue injury activates the immunological system and releases inflammatory mediators, with subsequent disruption of the microvasculature of the pulmonary system. Some acute orthopaedic procedures have been shown to similarly activate the immune system. Pulmonary endothelial damage results, with decreased partial pressures of oxygen and arterial oxygen saturation and increased carbon dioxide levels. The onset is frequently within 24 hours after trauma and is revealed by hypoxemia, inflammatory reaction, and progressive decrease in arterial oxygen saturation if appropriate treatment is not instituted.

Fat embolism syndrome is a unique orthopedic manifestation of ARDS caused by the release of marrow fat into the circulation following fractures, particularly of the long bones. Pathologic examination of the lungs shows fat droplets, usually diffusely distributed throughout the pulmonary vasculature. This syndrome may also occur in nonfracture situations, as when the medullary canal of a long bone is pressurized during total knee replacement. Fat embolism syndrome occurs frequently as a subclinical occurrence that is insufficient to compromise the patient's pulmonary reserve, but in some cases it can result in severe pulmonary compromise and death.

The clinical diagnosis of ARDS is confirmed by a decrease in arterial P_{O2}, an increase in systemic P_{CO2}, infiltrates on chest radiograph, presence of petechiae, and mental confusion in a patient at risk. Relatively minor injuries can result in this syndrome in patients with limited pulmonary reserve. Treatment is directed toward minimizing hypoxemia with ventilatory support as needed. Prevention is enhanced by early mobilization of the patient, which often implies early fracture fixation.

B. Atelectasis

Atelectasis, or localized collapse of alveoli, is a frequent postoperative complication in elective patients and can be prominent in trauma patients because of the required immobilization. Significant hypoxemia can result, and the onset may be relatively rapid. This may be the source of postoperative fevers in the early recovery phase. Occasionally, radiograph examination, showing platelike collapse of areas of the lung, will confirm the diagnosis. By encouraging coughing and deep breathing, using incentive spirometry, and, in resistant cases, using respiratory therapy, rapid resolution can be expected.

C. Pulmonary Embolism and Deep Venous Thrombosis

Although ARDS and atelectasis are seen in the early postoperative period, pulmonary embolism (PE) is uncommon sooner than 5 days after the onset of immobilization or bed rest. The trauma patient is at risk for PE, and the patient with spinal cord injury even more so. Population based studies have demonstrated recent trauma to be associated with a 13-fold increased risk of venous thromboembolism. Young multiple-trauma patients without prophylaxis have been shown to have a 1–2% incidence of fatal PE, which appears to decrease with a variety of prophylactic measures. Other groups of patients at risk include the elderly (>70 years), the obese, those with a history of prior venous thromboembolism, major surgery of the abdomen, pelvis or extremities, and fractures of the pelvis, hip or leg, and those with malignancy. Although it is uncommon, even a young (<30 years) healthy person can develop deep venous thrombosis (DVT) and be at risk for PE after a long car or airplane trip in which the legs are dependent. Oral contraceptive and smoking use may also increase the risk for a young healthy patient.

Geerts and colleagues examined the incidence of DVT and PE in trauma patients in a prospective series with venography. They found patients to be at significantly increased risk if they had suffered a pelvis or long bone fracture with greater than 5 days immobilization in bed, were obese, had a preexisting coagulopathy or an Injury Severity Score (ISS) greater than 8. Overall, they reported an incidence of 58% with 18% proximal DVT in patients without prophylaxis. The authors noted that fatal PE was the most common yet preventable form of death in the hospitalized trauma patient.

Patients at high risk for PE are those with DVT in the lower extremities, and pelvic veins. Clinically significant PE usually arise from the large veins proximal to the knee. Prevention of DVT in the venous system in this area reduces the risk of PE. Various strategies used to accomplish this include drug therapy with low-dose heparin, low-molecular-weight heparin, pentasaccharide, or sodium warfarin; and mechanical prophylaxis with intermittent pneumatic compression devices or inferior vena cava filters in the high risk patients with contraindications for pharmacologic prophylaxis.

Clinical diagnosis of DVT is unreliable. Definitive diagnosis is made with venography, duplex ultrasound scanning, impedance plethysmography, or CT or MRI venography. Prevention appears to be the best strategy as even routine surveillance screening in a trauma populations is cost-ineffective and does not appear to lower the overall rate of PE.

Pulmonary embolism is suspected in the orthopedic patient suffering an onset of tachypnea and dyspnea usually more than 5 days after an inciting event. The patient frequently reports chest pain and can often point to the painful area. Hemoptysis may also be present. On physical examination, tachycardia, cyanosis, and pleural friction rub can be noted.

Arterial blood gas studies demonstrate hypoxemia, although this is a nonspecific finding. Use of the d-dimer is unreliable in the early trauma patient but may be useful later in the recovery period. Definitive diagnosis is best made with pulmonary angiogram. Perfusion ventilation scanning is less invasive and may help determine whether there is a high or low probability of pulmonary embolus. Spiral CT is becoming useful in diagnosis of PE.

Treatment involves pulmonary support and heparin therapy. The natural history of treated PE is gradual lysis of the emboli, with the return of flow through the pulmonary arterial tree. The natural history of proximal DVT involves recanalization and arborization to bypass the clot. Patients may suffer from postphlebitic syndrome characterized by chronically painful swelling in the extremity.

D. COMPARTMENT SYNDROME

The term **compartment syndrome** refers to pathologic developments in a closed space in the body caused by buildup of pressure. Most commonly, such compartments are circumscribed by fascia and incorporate one or more bones. Pressure rises from edema or bleeding within the compartment, compromising circulation to the contents of the compartment over a period, and can result in necrosis of muscle and damage to nerves.

Compartment syndrome may result from a fracture; a soft-tissue injury; a vascular injury causing ischemia, necrosis, and edema; or from a burn. In an alcohol or drug user, it may be caused by external compression from immobilization that prevents normal postural changes. Failure to redistribute pressure through postural changes results in ischemia of the area under pressure because of collapse of capillaries.

The diagnosis of compartment syndrome must be considered in the postoperative or posttrauma patient who has pain out of proportion to that expected from the inciting injury. As the pain worsens, it can become totally unresponsive to narcotic medication. Epidural narcotics may mask the onset of compartment syndrome in the lower extremity.

The five P's (pulselessness, paresthesia, paresis, pain, and pressure) characteristic of compartment syndrome are helpful, but not diagnostic, for the experienced clinician. Pulses are poor indicators of compartment syndrome as they generally remain intact until late. Paresthesias occur only when the syndrome is significantly advanced. This points to the importance of careful documentation of sensory examination prior to the potential onset of compartment syndrome. Paresis, if present, is an unreliable finding. Subsequent to fracture or injury, pain is likely to induce guarding and thereby is also an unreliable finding. If normal muscle function is present, however, compartment syndrome is unlikely unless it is early. Pain with passive stretching of involved muscles is also a subjective finding and must be differentiated from pain arising from the original injury. To the experienced clinician, pain with passive stretching is a reliable clinical sign. Pressure is a key component of compartment syndrome, but palpation of a soft compartment does not rule out the diagnosis of compartment syndrome. Patients with equivocal clinical findings or those at high risk but without a reliable clinical examination (eg, those who are comatose, have psychiatric problems, or are under the influence of narcotics) should have compartmental pressure measurements. Intracompartmental pressure readings within 30 mm Hg or less of the diastolic blood pressure are indications for fasciotomy. Prior to fasciotomy, circular dressings including casts should be removed, and the patient should be observed for a short period for signs of improvement. Positive clinical findings may justify fasciotomy even despite normal pressures. Late fasciotomy may result in muscle damage or possible necrosis, with resulting risk of infection.

Although compartment syndrome can occur in almost any portion of the body, the two most common locations are the forearm and calf. In the forearm, an extensile volar incision to permit complete release, including the carpal tunnel distally and the lacertus fibrosus proximally, is necessary. Dorsally, a longitudinal incision is used. In the calf, two incisions are used to release the four compartments of the leg. The anterior and lateral compartments are decompressed using a longitudinal incision approximately over the anterior intermuscular septum. Posteromedially, a second incision is used to approach the superficial and deep posterior compartments. While single and limited incision approaches have been described, these may be unreliable and have a higher incidence of iatrogenic nerve injury in the trauma patients.

E. Heterotopic Bone Formation

Clinically significant heterotopic ossification occurs as a consequence of trauma in perhaps 10% of cases and may cause pain or joint motion restriction even to the point of ankylosis. Trauma patients without head injuries frequently manifest heterotopic ossification on radiograph 1–2 months following trauma; if the ossification is clinically significant, resection may be indicated when the bone has matured as indicated by radiographs and bone scan. This can take up to 18 months to achieve.

Resection is accomplished by removing the entire piece of heterotopic bone. Selected patients may benefit from low-dose radiation (7 Gy) and oral indomethacin for 3–6 weeks. Further discussion of this topic can be found in Chapter 13, "Rehabilitation." Heterotopic bone is a much more common occurrence in patients with head injuries. This is believed to result from release of humeral modulators that have not yet been characterized.

Classification of Open Fractures

A. Gustilo and Anderson Classification

Gustilo and Anderson made a significant contribution to trauma care of long bones by introducing their classification of open fractures, which includes the degree of open or closed soft-tissue injury. Their system was initially designed for open tibial fractures; however, it has gone on to include all types of long bone fractures. This system uses three grades and divides the third most severe grade into three subtypes.

Grade I fracture is a low-energy injury with a wound less than 1 cm in length, often from an inside-out injury rather than an outside-in injury. These are generally simple transverse or short oblique fractures.

Grade II fracture involves a wound more than 1 cm long and significantly more injury, caused by more energy absorption during the production of the fracture. Grade II fractures usually display some comminution and have a minimal to moderate crushing component.

Grade III open fracture has extensive wounds more than 10 cm in length, significant fracture fragment comminution, and a great deal of soft-tissue damage. It is usually a high-energy injury. This type of injury results typically from high-velocity gunshots, close range shotgun blasts, motorcycle accidents, or injuries with contamination from outdoor sites such as with tornado disasters or farming accidents. Indeed, any open fracture resulting from a natural disaster, highly contaminated or comminuted, independent of wound size, is automatically classified as a grade III open fracture.

Grade III injuries are divided into subtypes A, B, and C. Grade IIIA fractures have extensive soft-tissue laceration with minimal periosteal stripping and have adequate bone coverage. These injuries include some gunshot injuries and segmental fractures and do not require major reconstructive surgery to provide skin coverage. Grade IIIB fractures, in contrast, have extensive soft-tissue injury with periosteal stripping and require a flap for coverage. Grade IIIC injuries involve vascular compromise requiring surgical repair or reconstruction to allow for reperfusion of the limb. The presence of an intact skin envelope may imply somewhat reduced severity of trauma. The soft-tissue and bony damage may be as severe for closed fractures, however, except for the lower risk of infection.

Severe soft-tissue and bony injuries, especially when open, raise the question of immediate amputation. This problem most frequently arises in the lower extremity between the knee and the ankle. The advent of microvascular surgery has reduced the absolute indication for amputation resulting from ischemia. Two years of reconstruction may be necessary to achieve a united tibia fracture without infection, and even then, function may be compromised by muscle or nerve damage. The patient may have also endured multiple operations, loss of work time, and the emotional trauma accompanying an injury of this magnitude. Prosthetic replacements, particularly in the trauma patient at the below-knee level, may well be a viable alternative to a poorly functioning, insensate lower extremity.

Early Total Care

The desirability of early total and appropriate orthopedic care in multiply injured patients has become well established. Benefits of timely and aggressive treatment include decreased rates of mortality, primarily due to reductions in ARDS and multisystem organ failure (MOF). In a classic study by Bone et al., 178 patients with femoral fractures were entered into an early fixation group (treatment within 24 hours) or a delayed fixation group (treatment after 48 hours). The incidence of pulmonary complications, such as ARDS, fat embolism, or pneumonia, was higher, the hospital stay was longer, and the intensive care unit requirements increased when the femoral fixation was delayed. Bone and collaborators did a follow-up retrospective, multicenter study of 676 patients who had an ISS (Injury Severity Score) greater than 18 and who had major pelvic or long-bone injuries treated under an early fixation protocol within 48 hours at one of six major US trauma centers. These results were compared with historical records of 906 patients from the American College of Surgeons Multiple Trauma Outcomes Study Database. The study, despite shortcomings in methodology, revealed a lower mortality rate for patients whose fractures were stabilized early.

In a study by Reynolds, Richards, and Spain, records of 424 consecutive trauma patients were reviewed. Of these, 105 had an ISS of 18 or greater. These patients did not receive definitive early long bone fixation. In general, femur fractures were stabilized on the day of admission if the patients were hemodynamically stable. These authors noticed that progressive surgical delays caused by decline in the patient's condition resulted in a significant increase in pulmonary complications for patients having an ISS less than 18. However, there was no relation between pulmonary complications and timing of femoral fixation when patients had an ISS of 18 or more. The authors concluded that the severity of injuries, not the timing of fracture fixation, tended to determine patient pulmonary outcome.

Damage Control Orthopaedics

Controversy exists, however, regarding the appropriate timing of orthopedic intervention for specific subsets of severely injured patients, particularly those with head injury or systemic hypotension. Long bone fracture fixation with reamed intramedullary rods, in particular, may cause intraoperative hypotension or an increased release of inflammatory mediators with deleterious results in specific patients.

The multiply injured patient's immunological system is stimulated or primed after trauma (first event). Subsequent resuscitation, hemorrhage, blood products, hypotension and surgery (second event), may produce an exaggerated systemic inflammatory response syndrome (SIRS), potentially leading to ARDS or MOF. Activated neutrophils are the principal effector of the inflammatory response, releasing active oxygen species, which damage the vascular endothelium. Bone marrow contents pushed to the systemic circulation during reaming and nailing can activate neutrophils leading to SIRS in polytrauma patients, particularly during the first 96 hours after trauma. Damage control Orthopaedics aims to decrease the additional surgical trauma through external fixation, and secondary definitive surgery. One study demonstrated that conversion of an external fixator to a reamed intramedullary nail is safe and effective if performed within 2 weeks.

Alternatives to modify the inflammatory response are currently under investigation. The potential advantage is to allow early total fracture care avoiding secondary surgeries.

Soft-Tissue Injuries & Traumatic Arthrotomies

Lacerations of the extremities can result in neural or vascular compromise to an extremity and may also cause traumatic arthrotomies. Compromise of the sterility of any joint requires surgical debridement of that joint. For many joints, arthroscopic irrigation and debridement will minimize trauma and improve the return to function. Other soft-tissue lacerations may require neural or vascular repair. Laceration of a tendon or muscle belly is often involved. Tendon repairs are frequently performed in the foot and the hand. All tendon lacerations of the hand, except for those of the palmaris longus, should be repaired. In the foot, extrinsic tendons are repaired to prevent late imbalance or loss of function. Muscle belly injuries generally require surgical debridement because their subfascial location makes simple irrigation difficult. Laceration involving only the muscle belly requires no surgical repair. Frequently, however, muscle belly laceration involves the continuation of the origin or the insertion tendon of the muscle. In this case, optimal function is obtained by reattaching the lacerated ends. Generally, they can be located by poking into the muscle with a forceps at the site of the blood clot on the surface of the cut end. The tendon portion has retracted and the muscle has expanded because of swelling, leaving a track with a blood clot inside.

In most cases, immediate treatment of open fractures and lacerations consists of surgical debridement. Prior to formal debridement, it is appropriate to splint fractures and cover open wounds with sterile dressings soaked in povidone-iodine. Antibiotic therapy is begun immediately, usually with a cephalosporin bactericidal antibiotic. Tetanus prophylaxis is administered if needed. Antibiotic therapy is continued based on the clinical course.

Irrigation and debridement are intended to convert a clean contaminated wound into a sterile wound. Copious irrigation, using an irrigating solution containing antibiotics, is effective in cleaning the wound. Debridement removes nonviable tissue. Generally, care should be taken to remove only tissue that is necrotic. Skin edges should be debrided, as should dead muscle, and the surface of any contaminated fat or fascia.

After debridement, bone surfaces and exposed tendons should be covered as well as possible with tissue to maintain moistness. Maintain soft tissue attachments to bone whenever possible. Fragments of bone, particularly cortical bone, without attachments, should be removed from the wound. Although the axiom "open fractures should be left open, closed fractures should be left closed" was suitable many years ago, experience has demonstrated that in certain cases minimal risk is assumed in closing the wound. It is acceptable practice, however, to leave any wound open. Grade I wounds may in some cases be closed completely, or the part that was opened to permit debridement may be closed, leaving the original débrided laceration open. This may close spontaneously. Grade II wounds may be treated in a similar fashion, with somewhat more risk. The possibility of gas gangrene must be entertained whenever such a wound is closed. Primary closure of Grade III wounds is rarely if ever done. Adequate closure to cover bone and other structures that may be damaged by desiccation, with-

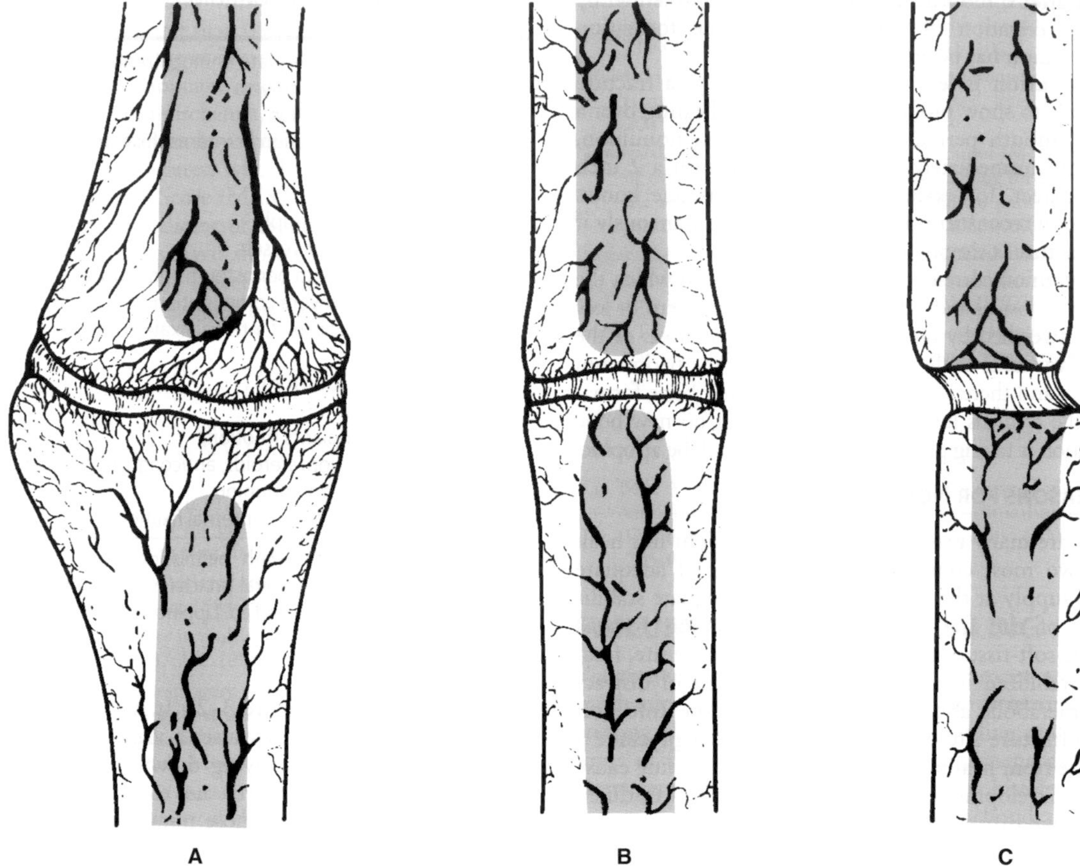

Figure 3–2. Weber and Cech's subclassification of hypertrophic nonunions: elephant's foot (**A**); horse's foot (**B**); oligotrophic (**C**). (This can often resemble atrophic nonunion and is hard to distinguish.) (Reprinted, with permission, from Browner BD et al, eds: *Skeletal Trauma,* 2nd ed. WB Saunders, 1998.)

sick or elderly (>70 years), treatment must also be tailored, as these patients may not be able to safely tolerate surgical intervention.

1. Stimulation of osteogenesis by external forces— It is now known that several pathways exist to stimulate healing of nonunion. The pathways can be divided into the type of force required to stimulate osteogenesis. These inductive forces can be categorized as mechanical, electrical, and chemical and can be applied with varying success both operatively and nonoperatively.

a. Mechanical forces—Application of mechanical forces to achieve bony union has remained the most time-honored, well-tested method to date. Sarmiento has shown that the use of functional bracing incorporated with weight bearing can lead to union of documented tibial nonunions. His results for treating femoral nonunions were less successful using this method. Cyclic mechanical force of ambulation while the fracture reduction is maintained with an external support is the presumed mechanism with which fracture healing is achieved without surgical intervention.

Mechanical forces can also be generated by surgical means. Mechanical stabilization of a long bone nonunion can be achieved either by placement of an intramedullary rod or compression plating. The rod works by providing mechanical stabilization of the fracture, hence allowing for cyclic axial loading of the limb without shearing forces caused by weight bearing. The compression plate provides stability as well as immediate rigid compression across the fracture fragments. These forms of treatment are often all that is necessary in elephant's foot type nonunions.

b. Electrical stimulation—Electrical fields have also been shown to stimulate the dormant chondrocytes and mesenchymal cells in the nonunion cleft to "turn on" and produce bone that results in healing. The mechanism of why this occurs has been postulated but to date is not well understood. Currently, most electrical bone growth stimu-

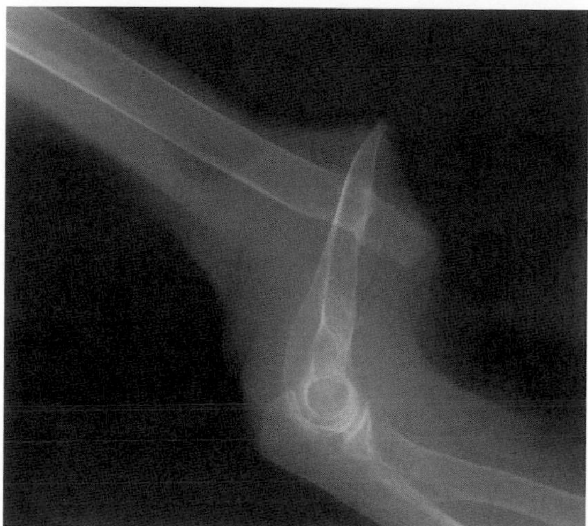

Figure 3–3. Fourteen-year-old distal humeral pseudarthrosis left untreated in an 89-year-old woman. All motion about the elbow is occurring through the pseudarthrosis, as the elbow ankylosed.

lators used are external devices that are incorporated in a cast or functional brace around the site of nonunion. Surgically implanted devices with internal coils wrapped into the nonunion site have also been used with somewhat equivocal success. Sharrard showed in a controlled double-blind study that application of an external pulsed electromagnetic field led to a statistically significant increase in healing of documented delayed tibial unions as compared with a control group. New interest in this field is now focusing on the use of nonpulsed electromagnetic fields and ultrasound. Nonunions being treated with adjuvant electrical fields are in fact being treated with mechanical forces as well, as these fractures are usually immobilized and weight bearing is often allowed on the affected limb.

c. Biological enhancement—Chemical modulators also play an important role in promoting nonunion healing. Application of autogenous cancellous bone graft (most frequently obtained from the iliac crest) is a potent stimulator of fracture healing. As a rigid nonunion will heal with autogenous bone grafting alone and no internal fixation, it is apparent that chemical modulators from the grafted cancellous bone are responsible for stimulating the healing response. There has been recent intense interest in determining the growth factors present in this cancellous bone responsible for "turning on" the healing process. Some surgeons have even reported success by obtaining bone marrow via a large-bore needle from the iliac crest and injecting this into the nonunion site. In the future, it is likely that the humoral modulator responsible will be isolated, synthesized in sufficient quantities by genetic engineering techniques, and simply injected into nonunion clefts to attain union.

d. Pathways of simulation—It is interesting to note that although three separate forces exist that can stimulate healing, it is unknown whether they act via a common pathway. As often happens in the body, these forces could actually work by different pathways so as to allow for some duplicity to help ensure that most fractures will heal.

2. Atrophic nonunions—Atrophic nonunions are not as easily treated as hypertrophic nonunions, and fewer treatment options are available. Electrical stimulation and nonoperative treatment methods have not been effective. The treatment most commonly utilized, and most successfully, is "freshening up" of the avascular bone ends, combined with rigid internal fixation and autogenous bone grafting. This same procedure is used in treating pseudarthroses.

The Ilizarov method has also shown great success in the treatment of complex hypertrophic and atrophic nonunions, sometimes in combination with autogenous bone grafting. This method allows not only for achievement of bony union but also for treatment of any accompanying deformity, segmental bone loss, or shortening that may be present.

Malunion of Fracture

A fracture that has healed with an unacceptable amount of angulation, rotation, or overriding that has resulted in shortening of the limb is defined as malunion. Shortening is better tolerated in the upper than the lower extremity, and angulatory deformities are better tolerated in bones such as the humerus than in the femur or tibia. Hence, no absolute guidelines can be given as to an acceptable versus an unacceptable malunion. Generally, shortening greater than 1 inch is poorly tolerated in the lower extremity. Smaller discrepancies, however, are well treated with just a shoe lift in most situations. When the degree of deformity is sufficient to cause pain (eg. caused by walking on the side of the foot secondary to varus malunion of the distal tibia) or impair normal function, then surgical correction of the malunion is indicated.

When correction of malunion is undertaken, proper preoperative planning is imperative. One must determine the true mechanical axis of the limb to determine the actual site of deformity. If an osteotomy is performed, the surgeon must decide whether to use a closing wedge (where a wedge of bone is removed) or an opening wedge (where a wedge of autogenous or allograft bone is added). This is important, as it will alter the limb length. If the limb is already short, the surgery should also include a limb-lengthening procedure. Proper fixation and often autogenous cancellous bone grafting should be incorporated to ensure that the osteotomy heals, for converting a malunion to a nonunion is only worsening an already bad situation. Special care must be paid to treatment of the soft tissues to prevent wound breakdown and infection.

Determination of the true plane of deformity is essential in planning for the surgical correction. Green and associates have shown in tibial malunions and nonunions that it is rare for the plane of deformity to be in the true sagittal or coronal plane. The true degree of deformity is therefore not fully appreciated on anterior to posterior and lateral radiographs, as the axis is usually in a plane somewhere between these. Thus, treatment of malunions can be appreciated as a difficult task that requires careful planning and execution to achieve anatomic results.

Ilizarov Method

The Ilizarov apparatus and the concepts of distraction osteogenesis have dramatically revolutionized the application of the principles of external fixation in the management of bony defects, nonunions, malunions, pseudarthroses, and osteomyelitis. Since its introduction in Kurgan, Siberia, in 1951 by Gavril A. Ilizarov, surgeons throughout the world have employed this method to pioneer modern limb salvaging and lengthening procedures. This method has numerous advantages, including immediate loading of the limb postoperatively and the use of healthy viable bone to replace devascularized bone in situ by corticotomy, localized transport, and osteogenesis. Accordingly, leg length discrepancy, deformity, nonunions, and infections may all be treated effectively.

The basic premise of the Ilizarov technique is that osteogenesis can occur at a specially controlled osteotomy site (referred to as a **corticotomy**), given the appropriate degree of retained vascularity, fixation, and quantified distraction. Ilizarov realized that healing and neogenesis both required a dynamic state, which could occur in either controlled distraction or compression. This dogma is a function of many principles that Ilizarov classified into three categories: biologic, clinical, and technical. Important biologic concepts include preservation of endosteal and periosteal blood supply via corticotomy and stable fixation. Ilizarov fixation prevents shearing forces but permits axial micromotion with postoperative weight bearing, which enhances bone formation. Distraction osteogenesis occurs at a rate of approximately 1 mm/day. Division of distraction into four equal increments appears to be more physiologically sound than one distraction per day, as used previously in lengthening procedures. At the termination of distraction, neutral fixation is required to allow maturation, calcification, and strengthening of the new bone. In essence, the technique fools the body into believing it is a child again, with the corticotomy site acting as a physis.

Clinical principles such as the geometry of the apparatus once it is constructed, adjustment of the rate of transport, and wound care directly affect the outcome of the procedure. The initial operation for the application of the apparatus is only one small part in the whole treatment scheme. The construct should be as safe and comfortable as possible because for an extended period of time. Pin tract infections are common and must be addressed aggressively with oral antibiotics and local pin care.

From a technical viewpoint, Ilizarov methodology relies on the use of an extremely rigid (in all planes except the axial loading plane), extremely versatile external fixator, employing K-wire fixation under tension. It is this "tension stress" phenomenon of gradually controlled distraction of bone ends at the corticotomy site that makes possible the limb lengthening or osteogenesis required in bone transport. Neogenesis of the accompanying soft tissues, including vessels, nerves, muscle, and skin, also occurs. Likewise, because of the dynamic nature of the apparatus, constant high loads of compression can be maintained across fracture sites to help stimulate fracture healing.

During distraction osteogenesis, the new tissues are aligned parallel to the distraction force vector. Accordingly, the surgeon has fine control over the direction of the regenerating bone. Ilizarov noted that tension stress neogenesis was similar to the natural conditions present in musculoskeletal growth. Mesenchymal cells fill the early distraction gap and soon differentiate into osteoblasts. A hyperemic state exists during distraction osteogenesis, with abundant neovascularization in the distraction gap. The overall blood flow to the affected limb is also increased up to 40%.

As noted earlier, the circular external fixator is attached to the limb using wires under tension. Two diameters of wires are used: 1.5 mm in small children and in upper extremities in adults, and 1.8 mm (twice as stiff in bending) in lower extremities in adults and adolescents. Beaded wires (olive wires) are utilized for bony transport, as well as to provide for rigidity of fixation, to prevent unwanted translation of the bone on the frame. An appropriately applied frame on the lower extremity should allow full weight bearing on the limb, irrespective of the extent of the bony defect present. In fact, Ilizarov felt that ambulation and the restoration of function to the limb were essential to achieve good bone regeneration and union. This cyclic axial loading of the affected limb is a crucial element of the Ilizarov method.

With the incorporation of hinges, plates, rods, and other elements, correction of a deformity can be accomplished in any plane. Hence, the apparatus has become an increasingly useful tool in the treatment of congenital, acquired, and posttraumatic limb deformities, as well as nonunion and malunion. What makes this treatment method unique is that all problems affecting a limb can be managed with the application of one apparatus. For instance, nonunion of the tibia with angulatory deformity and 5 cm of shortening can often be successfully treated with one operation. The surgery would entail application of the Ilizarov apparatus with either acute correction of the angulatory deformity or gradual correction via application of hinges. A corticotomy of the tibia is also performed at the time of surgery to proceed with distraction osteogenesis to restore the 5 cm of limb length. The nonunion is then compressed (once properly aligned) to achieve bony union. The lengthening of the limb is occurring at the same time that the nonunion is being compressed. Ilizarov also found that certain more rigid nonunions could actually heal in distraction. Therefore another treatment approach in the previous example would be primary gradual controlled distraction across the nonunion site for the purpose both of achieving bony union and restoring some of the limb length at the nonunion site. In essence, Ilizarov found that with few exceptions, healing could occur as long as a dynamic force, be it compression or distraction, was properly applied across a nonunion site. This dynamic force, when properly applied, causes the dormant mesenchymal cells in the nonunion gap to differentiate into functioning osteoblasts and allow for bone synthesis and resultant healing.

The Ilizarov method has revolutionized thinking about fracture healing and osteogenesis. It has greatly broadened the scope and indications for limb lengthening and has incorporated limb lengthening as a tool in both fracture and nonunion management. Ilizarov's introduction of the concept of distraction osteogenesis and the tension stress effect have changed Western thinking regarding limb lengthening and fracture healing. Close adherence to Ilizarov's principles makes it now possible to successfully treat a host of orthopedic conditions that previously were fraught with high morbidity rates and poor results. As experience broadens, application of the Ilizarov method will continue to grow.

Bhandari M et al: Reamed versus nonreamed intramedullary nailing of lower extremity long bone fractures: A systematic overview and meta-analysis. J Orthop Trauma 2000;14:2. [PMID: 10630795]

Einhorn TA, Lee CA: Bone regeneration: new findings and potential clinical applications. J Am Acad Orthop Surg 2001; 9:157. [PMID: 11421573]

Hak DJ, Lee SS, Goulet JA: Success of exchange reamed intramedullary nailing for femoral shaft nonunion or delayed union. J Orthop Trauma 2000;14:178. [PMID: 10791668]

Hupel TM et al: Effect of unreamed, limited reamed, and standard reamed intramedullary nailing on cortical bone porosity and new bone formation. J Orthop Trauma 2001;15:18. [PMID:11147683]

Ilizarov GA: The significance of the combination of optimal mechanical and biological factors in the regenerate process of transosseous synthesis. In: Abstracts of First International Symposium on Experimental, Theoretical, and Clinical Aspects of Transosseous Osteosynthesis Method Developed in Kniekot, Kurgan, USSR, September 20–23, 1983.

Ilizarov GA: Transosseous Osteosynthesis. Springer-Verlag, 1992.

Katsenis D et al: Treatment of malunion and nonunion at the site of an ankle fusion with the Ilizarov apparatus. J Bone Joint Surg Am 2005;87:302. [PMID: 15687151]

Lowenberg DW, Randall RL: The Ilizarov method. In: Braverman MH, Tawes RL (eds): Surgical Technology International II, 1993.

Marsh D. Concepts of fracture union, delayed union, and nonunion. Clin Orthop 1998;355S:S22. [PMID: 9917623]

Paley D, Maar DC: Ilizarov bone transport treatment for tibial defects. J Orthop Trauma 2000;14:76. [PMID: 10716377]

Weresh MJ et al: Failure of exchange reamed intramedullary nails for ununited femoral shaft fractures. J Orthop Trauma 2000; 14:335. [PMID: 11029556]

PRINCIPLES OF OPERATIVE FRACTURE FIXATION

Fractures occur when one or more types of stress, in excess of failure strength, are applied to bones. Fractures may occur from axial loading (tension, compression), bending, torsion (a twisting force), or shearing. All of these are observed at one time or another. It is frequently (but not always) helpful to recognize the type of failure in order to treat the fracture. Examples of these mechanisms are shown in Figure 3–4.

Biomaterials Used in Fracture Fixation

Operative fracture fixation requires strength and flexibility of the fixation materials. Two materials found to be useful in these regards are titanium alloy and stainless

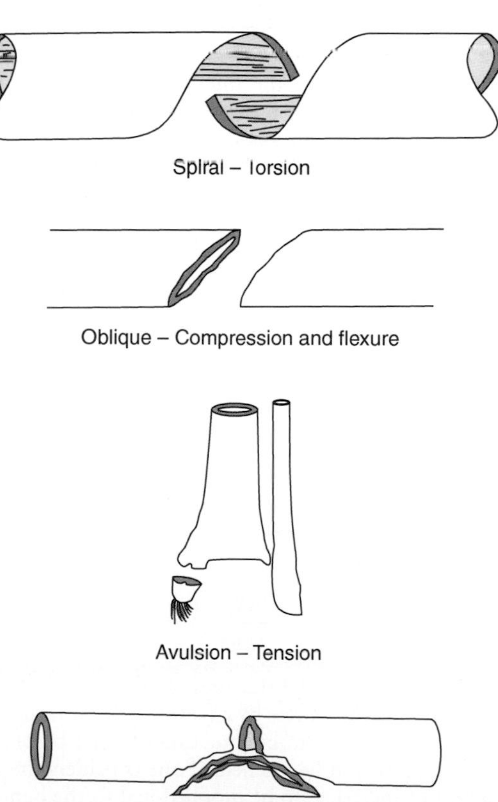

Figure 3–4. Mechanisms of failure of bones.

steel, both of which may be contoured to fit irregularities in bone surfaces at the time of surgery. They provide adequate strength and fatigue resistance to allow fracture healing to occur. The elastic modulus of titanium is half that of stainless steel, resulting in half the flexural rigidity in plates of equal size. Although it is recognized that more flexible devices decrease the disuse osteopenia underneath the plates, the clinical advantage of this difference has not been demonstrated. Other potential materials, including composites, cannot be contoured in the operative suite for particular applications.

Biomechanical Principles of Fracture Fixation

The principles of operative fracture fixation are demonstrated by several examples described here. These examples illustrate the importance of the location of a bone plate on a bone in relation to the loading applied to the bone and plate composite. They will demonstrate the bending stiffness of bone plates as a function of thickness and the load sharing that goes on between bone plates in bone. In addition, the effect of bending on the composite of an intramedullary rod and bone will be examined.

A. Bone Plate Thickness

One approach to solving the problem of bone plate fractures is to increase the thickness of the plate. If a bone plate is subjected to bending stress, the stress in the plate, assuming no loading is carried by the bone, can be calculated from the flexure formula: $s_{max} = Mc/I$, where M is the bending moment applied to the plate, c is one-half the thickness of the plate, and the area moment of inertia, I, is expressed by

$$\frac{bh^3}{12}$$

where h is the thickness of plate and b is the width of the plate. The maximum stress would then be equal to

$$s_{max} = \frac{6M}{bh^2}$$

because c is equal to one-half of h. Doubling the thickness decreases the stress to

$$\frac{6M}{4bh^2}$$

Thus, increasing the thickness of the plate by a factor of 2 reduces the stress by a factor of 4, meaning that the load would have to be four times higher before the failure stress would be reached. If one considers the area moment of inertia, I, to be proportional to the bending stiffness, then doubling the size of the plate would double h, which would mean that the plate is eight times stiffer (but only four times stronger). Because the endurance limit of steel is approximately one-half the ultimate strength, four times higher cyclic loads can be tolerated without fear of failure caused by fatigue.

B. Titanium and Stainless Steel Rods

The second consideration is the difference in the stress carried by an intramedullary rod made of titanium alloy as compared with one constructed of stainless steel. Assume a tibia is a round bone with a hollow, round intramedullary canal 10 mm in diameter. The flexural rigidity is defined as the area moment of inertia times the elastic modulus. A higher flexural rigidity indicates a greater resistance to bending. The area moment of inertia of a thin tube is

$$p^3 r_{ave}^3 t$$

where r is the average radius and t is thickness. Assuming this equation holds for bone also, the ratio of the flexural rigidity of the intramedullary rod to the bone is expressed by the equation

$$\frac{E_m I_m}{E_b I_b} = \frac{r_m^3 t_m E_m}{r_b^3 t_b E_b}$$

The r_{ave} for the metal is 5 mm and for the bone 7.5 mm; t_m is 1 mm and t_b is 5 mm. The ratio E_m/E_b is approximately 10 for stainless steel and 5 for titanium alloy. Thus, the flexural rigidity ratio is

$$\frac{E_m I_m}{E_b I_b} \begin{array}{l} = 0.60 \text{ for stainless steel} \\ = 0.30 \text{ for titanium alloy} \end{array}$$

This indicates that the geometric contribution to stiffness of the construct is greater for bone than for metal. Thus, for a stainless steel rod, the bone and metal rod share the bending stress after healing in a 60:40 ratio, respectively, (75:25 for titanium alloy). It can be seen that the bone is much stiffer than titanium alloy or stainless steel alloy rods. The difference between the two metals is probably not significant for bone remodeling, but maximum strength of the bone would be attained by removal in either case.

C. Bone Plate

The placement of a plate on a bone has a significant bearing on its function. For example, on a curved bone such as the femur, which bows anteriorly, placement of the plate anteriorly tends to place the plate in tension and the posterior cortex of the femur in compression, owing to muscle action of the hamstrings and quadriceps. Conversely, placement of a plate posteriorly tends to cause the fracture to gap open anteriorly because of muscle action. This means that the bone in posterior placement is bearing none of the bending stress resulting from muscle forces and the bone plate has to resist all of this loading. When the bone plate is placed laterally, the axis of bending bisects the broad aspect of the plate, and thus the bone plate is much more able to tolerate the stress caused by muscle load. The plate, however, is susceptible to high stresses if abduction forces are applied to the femur or lower extremity. Thus, optimal placement of a bone plate is on the tension side of the bone, so that the bone will be placed in compressive loading as a result of muscle action. This stimulates healing and minimizes the stresses on the bone plate.

The conventional plate and screw system requires substantial bone exposure for access for open reduction and internal fixation. The surgeon-contoured plate is compressed onto the bone with screws resulting in anatomical reduction and absolute stability. The compressive forces acting on the bone-plate interface can compromise the blood supply and hence the healing process. The Low Contact Dynamic Compression (LCDC) plate was developed to reduce the bone-plate contact surface area.

The recently developed locking plates or internal fixators use a system where the screw head threads into the plate hole, thereby locking the plate just above the bone to minimize contact surface area and the resulting compressive forces. The locked screws in the plate also act as a second bone cortex and therefore self-tapping unicortical screws can be used. This achieves relative stability and therefore promotes callus formation at the fracture site. During fixation, the working length of the plate and screws should be kept in mind with the aim of increasing the working length of the plate and reducing the number of screws used.

D. External Fixation

External fixation is an important treatment modality for musculoskeletal injuries. The basic principles are that pins are placed within the musculoskeletal system proximal and distal to the zone of injury. These pins are then placed on an external frame, a frame outside the confines of the bone and soft-tissue envelope to stabilize fractures. These devices can be useful as temporary treatment for musculoskeletal injuries, or as definitive treatment, depending on their location and the type of bone and soft-tissue trauma. In the upper extremity, they play a significant role in treating comminuted distal radius fractures by providing both provisional and definitive stabilization for healing as well as provisional treatment for grade III open fractures with segmental bone loss and large soft-tissue injuries in the forearm, elbow, and humerus.

For the pelvis, rapidly applied external fixation with compression for pelvic injuries can stabilize the pelvis, reduce blood loss, be of assistance in initial resuscitation, and provide definitive treatment of such injuries. In the lower extremity, external fixators are important in the treatment of tibia fractures, particularly open or comminuted fractures, and in the treatment of open forefoot injuries and femur injuries with segmental defects. For femur and tibia fractures, external fixation may provide excellent initial or provisional stabilization, which can then be followed by intramedullary fixation for definitive care.

These specific uses of external fixation will be discussed in the individual sections on specific fractures.

Bone Substitutes Used in Fracture Fixation

A. Autogenous Bone Grafting

The gold standard for bone grafting material to stimulate bone growth is cancellous bone from the iliac crest. Obtaining bone graft is a process with potential morbidity, blood loss, infection, and, acute and/or chronic pain. Because of these possible problems, alternatives to autogenous bone grafting have been investigated.

B. Osteoconductive Graft Substitutes

Hydroxyapatite and tricalcium phosphate, are inorganic structural bone graft substitutes that are primarily osteoconductive and do not stimulate bone formation. These materials can be injected into fracture sites to provide stabilization from compressive loads. A plethora of materials have come to market with variable degrees of clinical testing. The common denominator is that these are osteoconductive: They provide a scaffold for new bony ingrowth. They have been shown to be effective in well-vascularized areas such as the tibial plateau, distal radius and calcaneus.

C. Donor Bone Allografts

The third alternative bone substitute is allograft derived from living or cadaveric donors. Femoral heads obtained at the time of hip replacement provide a source of living donor bone. Bone collected in the same fashion as transplant organs can also be made available for transplantation. It should be noted that all allograft bone is not the same. Immunogenicity, sterility, mechanical properties, and bone stimulation potential are all dependent on the treatment the bone receives from the time of collection until the time of implantation. The highest risk bone, because of occult viral and bacterial contamination, is that collected in a sterile manner from cadaveric donors and delivered in a sterile manner without further sterilization or processing. This bone also has the highest potential for containing bone growth factors and, therefore, the ability to stimulate new bone formation. Sterilization treatments, such as irradiation and ethylene oxide, are known to compromise these qualities to some extent, with ethylene oxide perhaps being worse than irradiation. Freeze-dried bone is convenient for storage at room temperature but must be sterilized secondarily with ethylene oxide. Because ethylene oxide is unable to penetrate to the depths of large

additional advantage of not devascularizing bony fragments and not creating a surgical wound. In cases of open fractures an external fixator can facilitate wound care. External fixation is effective in preventing loss of reduction and length in situations where there is comminution of bone. In intraarticular fractures, external fixation can be used but reductions are difficult to maintain without percutaneous pins or internal fixation. Complications are common however with external fixation including, pin tract infection, superficial radial nerve neuropathy, pin loosening, and stiffness.

B. Open Reduction and Internal Fixation

1. Plate and screws—Plate and screws can be extremely effective in achieving and maintaining reduction. If bone fragments are large, it is also an effective way to maintain reduction. This technique has a tendency to fail, however, if there are multiple fragments and if there is sufficient comminution so that rigid internal fixation is difficult, or impossible, to achieve. Other drawbacks to this technique include creation of an incision, with potential subsequent scarring, and also the possibility of future hardware removal. Additionally, the operative technique involves soft-tissue stripping and potential devascularization of small fragments during the process of open reduction and internal fixation.

Recently, distal radius plates with fixed-angle screws have been devised specifically for comminuted distal radius fractures. These feature multiple small locking holes in a T configuration, allowing multiple screws for small fragment fixation. This highly stable construct allows early functional treatment. Recent studies indicate that locked plates and early postoperative range of motion may provide improved long-term results.

2. Arthroscopically assisted reduction—Arthroscopically assisted reduction can address the associated ligament injuries improving the final result, with limited scarring. A recent study reported that patients undergoing arthroscopically assisted procedures had a greater degree of supination, flexion, and extension than patients undergoing fluoroscopy-assisted fixation of intraarticular distal radius fractures.

C. Treatment Decisions

Besides fracture type and comminution, additional factors that modify treatment decisions include patient comorbidities, available resources for treatment and surgeon expertise. For a non-comminuted, non-displaced, methaphyseal distal radius fracture, nonoperative treatment with initial splint until the edema subsides and subsequent cast application is the appropriate treatment. In contrast, intraarticular comminuted fractures are difficult if not impossible to reduce and maintain without the addition of hardware. In presence of osteoporosis and intraarticular displacement, ORIF using a fixed angle device is probably the best option. When facing severe comminution, pinning and external fixator can be the most suitable treatment.

1. Extraarticular nondisplaced fractures—Extraarticular nondisplaced fractures can be treated with cast immobilization for 4-6 weeks, until fracture healing occurs, following by mobilization with an off the shelf brace.

2. Extraarticular displaced fractures—Closed reduction should be attempted on extraarticular displaced fractures. If radial length and volar tilt are restored, then a sugar tong splint or long arm cast can be effective in holding the reduction. If the reduction is not adequate by closed means then an external fixator (for ligamentotaxis) and percutaneous pins (to manipulate the fracture) may be necessary. Current trends toward plating via a volar approach with specialized locking plates may improve wrist motion and long-term outcomes even in extraarticular fractures.

3. Intraarticular fractures—The treatment of intraarticular fractures aims to restore the congruity of the articular surface and the anatomic axis of the distal radius in order to improve the outcome. Open reduction and internal fixation is the treatment of choice. For volar Barton's fractures, the treatment of choice is the volar buttress plate. The only contraindications to this treatment are cases with excessive comminution such that open reduction and internal fixation will fail to achieve a stable bony construct. In these situations, use of an external fixator as a distractor and neutralization device is generally indicated. Using a fluoroscopy unit to visualize the fracture will help ascertain that both articular alignment and overall radial length have been adequately restored with external fixation. Minor adjustments as necessary can be effectively done with adjunct percutaneous pins. These maneuvers may fail to achieve the appropriate articular alignment, particularly if some healing has already occurred or if the displacement is severe. In this case, open reduction and internal fixation should be performed. Justification for aggressive treatment of distal radius fractures in young patients (<60 years) comes from several studies. The goal should be articular step-off <2 mm, radial shortening <4 mm, dorsal tilt <15 degrees, volar tilt <20 degrees and loss of radial inclination <10 degrees. Arthroscopically assisted repair of distal radius fractures has been advocated. Intraarticular step-off and associated injuries such as triangular fibrocartilage, scapholunate, and lunotriquetral tears as well as osteochondral lesions can be accurately assessed. Some authors advocate bone grafting in the acute treatment of comminuted fractures.

2. Distal Radioulnar Joint Dislocation

The distal ulna transmits significant loads to the forearm through the distal ulna via the triangular fibrocartilage complex. Even minor disruptions of the precise anatomic relationships between the distal radius and ulna and ulnar carpus results in pain syndromes. The distal radioulnar joint (DRUJ) can be dislocated by a variety of mechanisms, including low- and high-energy trauma. These are associated with disruption of the ulnar soft-tissue triangular fibrocartilage complex, including the articular disk and associated ligaments. There should be a high index of suspicion in order to diagnose this lesion because radiographs that are not taken in the perfect lateral orientation will tend to look relatively normal. A displaced fracture at the ulnar styloid base indicates a high risk of distal radioulnar instability. In the presence of forearm and elbow fracture-dislocations, further evaluation of the radioulnar joint is mandatory.

Clinical Findings

The clinical examination is key, with identification of the distal radioulnar joint surface anatomy and clinical evaluation of the joint. The amount of stability should be carefully assessed and compared with that of the opposite wrist. The patient should position the wrist to reproduce the pain. With the hand pronated, the examiner tries to displace the ulnar head applying a dorsal to volar load 4 cm proximal to the DRUJ (piano key test). Little resistance to ballottement and volar movement of the ulna head corresponds to a positive "piano key test." Subluxation is much more common than anterior or posterior dislocation. Limitation of pronation and supination, or pain associated with such motion, would be expected in such a situation. Palpation of the sixth extensor compart ment during resisted pronation is useful to identify any subluxation. The other common cause of distal radioulnar joint problems is rheumatoid arthritis.

Treatment

Dorsal dislocation, or subluxation, should be treated by reduction of the ulnar head into the sigmoid fossa and placement of the forearm in full supination. The arm should be immobilized in supination, which requires a long-arm cast or splint. Volar dislocation is relatively rare and is usually stable after reduction. If dorsal or volar dislocation or subluxation of the distal ulna cannot be reduced with manipulation in the outpatient setting, closed treatment can be attempted under anesthesia. If this fails, open reduction and soft-tissue reconstruction may be necessary. If this is performed, a retinacular flap may be used to transpose the extensor carpi ulnaris to a more dorsal position to stabilize the distal ulna, as has been described for Darrach reconstruction of the joint.

3. Malunion of Distal Radius

Malunion of the distal radius can have a variety of negative consequences. Alteration of the biomechanical function of the wrist may lead to weakness, limitation of motion, and midcarpal instability. Associated distal radioulnar joint arthrosis may be present, as well as ulnocarpal abutment. Also, rotational deformity is common with angulated malunions. CT of both wrists can be used to identify and measure malrotation preoperatively.

Treatment

The treatment of choice in such a situation, if conservative treatment fails, is reconstructive surgery. Fernandez has elegantly described the strategy. An osteotomy of the radius with iliac crest bone grafting and plate fixation is performed (Figure 3–11). The distal radioulnar joint

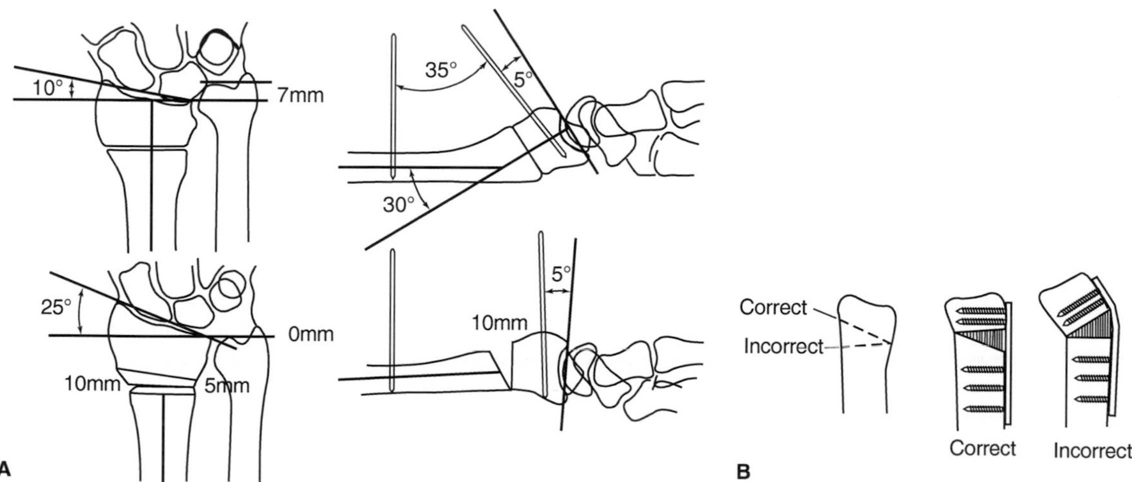

Figure 3–11. Wedge osteotomy of the distal radius with iliac crest bone graft and plate fixation. (Reproduced, with permission, from Green DP, Hotchkiss RN, Pederson WC, eds: *Operative Hand Surgery*, 4th ed. WB Saunders, 1999.)

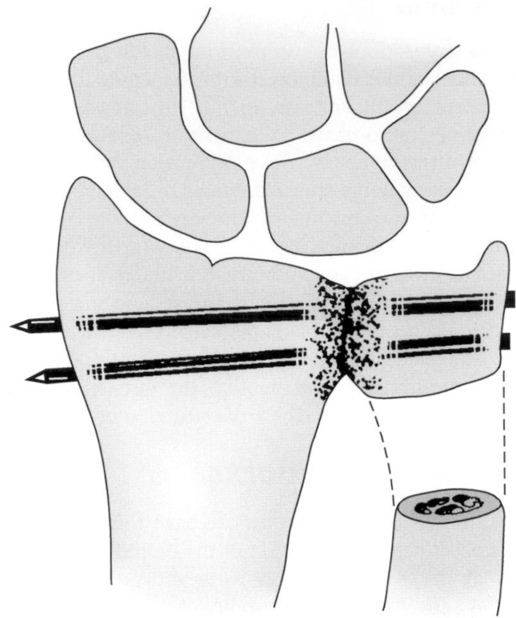

Figure 3–12. Suave-Kapandji reconstruction of the distal radioulnar joint. (Reproduced, with permission, from Green DP, Hotchkiss RN, Pederson WC, eds: *Operative Hand Surgery*, 4th ed. WB Saunders, 1999.)

must be addressed and, depending upon the degree of subluxation or arthrosis, may require closed reduction, open reduction, or reconstruction using the Darrach or Sauve-Kapandji procedures (Figure 3–12). In this procedure, instead of distal ulnar resection as in the Darrach procedure, transverse segmental resection of the ulnar metaphysis is followed by creation of an arthrodesis of the distal ulna to the radius, using the resected bone as grafting material. Forearm rotation occurs through the ulnar metaphyseal pseudoarthrosis. Additionally, restoration of the radial length may be difficult with manipulation alone. Useful adjuncts to achieve restoration of appropriate length and orientation in severe malunion include use of laminar spreaders to distract the proximal and distal fragments of the radius after osteotomy. Alternatively, an external fixator may prove useful in helping to achieve appropriate length after osteotomy.

If the distal radius has settled into a position of shortening and significant angulatory deformity but the fracture is not yet fully healed, osteotomy for early or "nascent" malunion is justified. The advantage of taking down a nascent malunion is that the operation is technically simpler to perform, shortens the time of disability, and leads to better long-term results. Additionally, the distal radioulnar joint can be restored more reliably in these early reconstructions than when osteotomy is required for established malunion. The latter often requires adjunctive distal radioulnar joint reconstruction with Darrach resection, Sauve-Kapandji, hemiresection, or matched resection arthroplasty.

Abboudi J, Culp RW: Treating fractures of the distal radius with arthroscopic assistance. Orthop Clin North Am 2001;32:307. [PMID: 11331543]

Carter PB, Stuart PR: The Sauve-Kapandji procedure for post-traumatic disorders of the distal radio-ulnar joint. J Bone Joint Surg Br 2000;82:1013. [PMID: 11041592]

Chhabra A et al: Biomechanical efficacy of an internal fixator for treatment of distal radius fractures. Clin Orthop 2001;393:318. [PMID: 11764365]

Jakob M, Rikli A, Regazzoni P: Fractures of the distal radius treated by internal fixation and early function. J Bone Joint Surg Br 2000;82-B:341. [PMID: 10813166]

Katz MA et al: Computed tomography scanning of intraarticular distal radius fractures: Does it influence treatment. J Hand Surg Am 2001;26:415. [PMID: 11418901]

Ladd AL, Pliam NB: The role of bone graft and alternatives in unstable distal radius fracture treatment. Orthop Clin North Am 2001;32:337. [PMID: 11331546]

Margaliot Z et al: A meta-analysis of outcomes of external fixation versus plate osteosynthesis for unstable distal radius fractures. J Hand Surg 2005;30:1185. [PMID: 16344176]

May MM, Lawton JN, Blazar PE. Ulnar styloid fractures associated with distal radius fractures: incidence and implications for distal radioulnar joint instability. J Hand Surg (Am). 2002; 27(6):965-71. [PMID: 12457345]

Mehta JA, Bain GI, Heptinstall RJ: Anatomical reduction of intraarticular fractures of the distal radius. J Bone Joint Surg Br 2000;82-B:79. [PMID: 10697319]

Orbay JL, Fernandez DL. Volar fixed-angle plate fixation for unstable distal radius fractures in the elderly patient. J Hand Surg [Am]. 2004 Jan;29(1):96-102. [PMID: 14751111]

Rogachefsky RA et al: Treatment of severely comminuted intraarticular fractures of the distal end of the radius by open reduction and combined internal and external fixation. J Bone Joint Surg Am 2001;83-A:509. [PMID: 11315779]

Schneeberger AG et al: Open reduction and plate fixation of displaced AO type C3 fractures of the distal radius: Restoration of articular congruity in eighteen cases. J Orthop Trauma 2001;15:350. [PMID: 11433140]

Viso R, Wegener EE, Freeland AE: Use of a closing wedge osteotomy to correct malunion of dorsally displaced extraarticular distal radius fractures. Orthopedics 2000;23:721. [PMID: 10917249]

DISLOCATION OF THE RADIOCARPAL JOINT

Dislocation of the radiocarpal joint is usually accompanied by significant carpal-ligamentous injury or fracture. Treatment of these injuries involves restoration of the bony architecture through immediate closed reduction, if possible, elective closed reduction, open reduction and internal fixation, or a combination of these procedures. Associated fractures, such as transscaphoid perilunate or distal radius fracture associated with carpal dislocation, should be treated with open reduction and internal fixation. Ligamentous repair should be performed at this time (see Chapter 10, Hand Surgery). Median nerve evaluation is mandatory, and surgical exploration indicated, if a dense neuropathy is present.

FOREARM SHAFT FRACTURES

In general, any fracture requires evaluation both clinically and radiographically of a joint above and joint below the fracture. It is not uncommon for fractures of the midshaft of the forearm to have significant consequences to either the wrist or elbow.

1. Isolated Fracture of the Ulna (Nightstick Fracture)

Nondisplaced or minimally displaced fractures of the ulnar shaft are fairly common and usually result from a direct blow.

Treatment

A variety of treatment options are possible for managing minimally displaced ulnar diaphyseal injuries. The time to union is about 3 months, with union achieved with cast immobilization and early mobilization of the wrist and elbow. Less stringent immobilization protocols have also resulted in satisfactory results. Sarmiento and Latta achieved excellent results using a functional brace for isolated ulnar fractures. After initial long arm cast fixation for immobilization until acute symptoms and swelling have subsided, cast removal is followed by Orthoplast sleeve or cast bracing with Velcro straps, with no limitation of pronation and supination. Some investigators report excellent results with minimal or no immobilization. In general, some sort of immobilization until pain subsides is preferable. With displaced fractures with angulation greater than 10 degrees or displacement greater than 50%, one must be extremely suspicious of an associated injury at the elbow or wrist. In isolated fractures of the ulna in the adult with displacement >50% or angulation >10 degrees (or both), open reduction and internal fixation is the treatment of choice. Current recommendations include fixation with a 3.5 mm dynamic or limited contact compression plate with six to eight cortices of fixation proximal and distal to the fracture. Intramedullary pinning seems to provide comparable results to plate fixation, but further studies are needed at this point.

2. Isolated Radial Shaft Fractures

A fracture anywhere along the length of the radius with or without associated ulnar fracture with injury to the distal radioulnar joint (DRUJ) is defined as a Galeazzi fracture. Injuries associated with the DRUJ include ulnar styloid fractures, radial shortening >5 mm, and DRUJ dislocation.

Treatment

Open reduction and internal fixation with plate fixation is recommended in adult patients to ensure a reasonable chance of restoration of the distal radioulnar joint. Hughston's series in 1957 had a 92% incidence of poor results with closed treatment. After open reduction and internal fixation of the radial shaft through a volar Henry approach using compression plating, the distal radioulnar joint should be carefully inspected. If it is unstable, pinning in a position of stability (usually full supination) is required. If it is frankly dislocated and cannot be reduced closed, and maintained by closed or percutaneous means, then open stabilization with repair of associated ligaments or removal of interposed soft tissue is mandatory.

3. Monteggia Fracture

Classification of Fractures

In 1814, Monteggia of Milan described an injury involving fracture of the proximal third of the ulna, with anterior dislocation of the radial head. This definition was extended by Bado to include the entire spectrum of these fractures with associated radial head dislocations, regardless of the direction of dislocation. They are classified in the following ways:

Type 1: Fracture of the ulnar diaphysis with anterior angulation and anterior dislocation of the radial head (60% of cases)

Type 2: Fracture of the ulnar diaphysis with posterior angulation or posterior or posterolateral dislocation of the radial head (15% of cases)

Type 3: Fracture of the ulnar metaphysis, with lateral or anterolateral dislocation of the radial head (20% of cases)

Type 4: Fracture of the ulna and radius at the proximal third, with anterior dislocation of the radial head (5% of cases).

Other authors have noted that type 3 fractures may be more common than type 2 fractures, but all agree that type 1 lesions are the most common.

Associated lesions include injury to the radial nerve; palsies of both the deep branch of the radial nerve and the posterior interosseous nerve have been described with Monteggia fractures. It is important to perform an adequate neurovascular examination at the time of evaluation. The index of suspicion must be high because radial head dislocation may be missed if appropriate radiographs are not obtained and scrutinized.

Treatment

Closed treatment is usually satisfactory for children, but open reduction and internal fixation is the treatment of

infraspinatus, and teres minor muscles. The teres major is not a rotator cuff muscle. The cuff muscles serve as depressors of the humeral head to allow the deltoid to efficiently abduct the humerus. The infraspinatus and teres minor are external rotators, while the subscapularis is an internal rotator of the humerus. Two other important muscles in this region are the deltoid and the pectoralis major muscles. These muscles, along with the rotator cuff, cause predictable displacement of fractures around the proximal humerus. Additionally, injury to the rotator cuff, independent of injuries to the insertion of the tuberosities, may be encountered and need to be considered when evaluating the shoulder.

B. Nerve Supply

Injuries to the nerves around the shoulders occur with fractures and dislocations. The brachial plexus and axillary artery can also be injured with anterior shoulder dislocations.

The most important evaluation consists of a neurovascular examination after injury around the arm and shoulder girdle. The radial nerve is commonly injured in humeral shaft fractures, particularly at the junction of the middle and distal third (Holstein-Lewis fracture). Careful evaluation of radial nerve sensory and motor function is critical. Evaluation should include sensation of the dorsal web space between the thumb and index finger, independent digital extension, and wrist extension.

Around the shoulder girdle, fractures of the proximal humerus and fracture-dislocations can on occasion result in axillary nerve and artery injuries. An axillary nerve injury from proximal humeral fracture or fracture-dislocation would result in paralysis of the deltoid muscle and anesthesia over the 'badge' region at the lateral proximal arm. Axillary artery injuries, although uncommon, generally result from fractures or fracture-dislocations in which a medial bone spike injures or penetrates the axillary artery. The index of suspicion is high if the arm, upon evaluation, shows significant color differences compared with the uninjured arm or has a bluish or cadaveric appearance. Pulses should be palpated and evaluated by Doppler studies; even if the pulse is present, if it is significantly different from the uninjured side, arterial injury should be suspected. Appropriate arterial studies should be obtained on an emergent basis or in the operating room. In late diagnosis, the outcome is determined by the neurological morbidity, even though the results of vascular reconstruction are good.

More subtle associated injuries involve the rotator cuff. This can generally be expected with fractures of the tuberosities, but it can also result from strictly soft-tissue injuries such as shoulder dislocations. Generally, rotator cuff avulsion is suspected when radiographs reveal no evidence of fracture but the patient is unable to actively externally rotate the shoulder against resistance. Evaluation of the integrity of the rotator cuff may be difficult in the acute setting, and special studies such as ultrasound, MRI, arthrogram or arthroscopy may be valuable in making this diagnosis.

HUMERAL SHAFT FRACTURE

Fractures of the shaft of the humerus usually result from a direct blow, a fall, an automobile injury, or a crushing injury. Missiles from firearms or shell fragments may pierce the arm and cause an open fracture. Other indirect means of injury, such as a fall on an outstretched upper extremity or violent muscle contracture, can cause midshaft fractures.

Classification

Fractures are classified according to whether they are open or closed and according to the level of the fracture in relation to the insertions of the pectoralis major and deltoid muscles. Characteristics of fracture and associated injury are also factors.

Clinical Findings

Clinical signs and symptoms include a shortened extremity with crepitus and pain at the diaphysis of the humerus. Confirmation should be obtained by radiographs in two planes. Both the shoulder and elbow joints should be thoroughly evaluated, clinically and radiographically, as should the neurovascular status.

Treatment

A. Closed Treatment

The recommended treatment in isolated diaphyseal humeral fractures involves closed methods. Nonoperative methods lead to good results with high union rates. Nonoperative methods include traction by hanging casts, coaptation splints, shoulder spica casts, Velcro bracing, cast humeral bracing, and skeletal traction. Cast bracing appears to be the most effective closed treatment.

1. Hanging cast—Treatment with a hanging cast involves placement of the arm in a Velcro cast with the elbow flexed to 90 degrees, with a sling fashioned over a loop placed on the radial aspect of the wrist. To correct angulation, loops may be placed on the dorsum or volar aspect of the wrist, and anterior or posterior angulation can be adjusted by the length of the sling or suspension apparatus. This treatment requires weekly radiographic evaluations; exercises both for shoulder and digital motion are helpful.

Patients with a large body habitus may develop more significant angulation at the time of healing with this technique, compared with slimmer patients. The vertical position must be maintained even at night. Spiral, comminuted, and oblique fractures have additional advantages of large fracture surfaces for ready healing. Transverse fractures may have more difficulty in healing. The musculature of the upper arm will accommodate 20 degrees of anterior angulation, 30 degrees of varus angulation and 3 cm of shortening without apparent deformity. One risk of this treatment is distraction of the fracture site and eventual nonunion.

2. Coaptation splint—A TU-shaped coaptation splint with cuff and collar is another method for treating humerus fractures. The more modern version of this is functional bracing, as popularized by Sarmiento. The sleeve is ready-made or custom-made from thermoplastic splinting materials and fixed with Velcro straps that can be adjusted to achieve the appropriate level of compression. Stand-alone slings or cuffs are used. Alternatively, a cast brace may be used with a hinge brace at the elbow with upper arm and forearm components. This can control flexion and protect against varus and valgus stresses as well as translational forces; it may be most useful for healing the more distal diaphyseal fractures.

3. Abduction humeral splinting and shoulder casting—Spica casting may be useful in certain unstable fractures, though it is a complex method of immobilization and requires close follow-up.

4. Skeletal traction—In special circumstances, skeletal traction has been used for humeral fractures. When treating other injuries, massive swelling, or open fractures requiring patient recumbency, skeletal traction may be indicated. Increasingly, however, multiple trauma patients are treated with aggressive internal fixation to allow early mobilization. The traction pin is inserted through the olecranon, going from a medial to lateral directions to avoid injury to the ulnar nerve. Differential traction on one side of a Steinmann pin bow or Kirschner wire bow can be used to achieve varus and valgus alignment; traction of the humerus longitudinally and flexion of the forearm and hand suspended overhead help to correct angulation. Positioning is checked with portable radiographs.

5. Sling and swathe—Elderly patients may be best treated by reducing fracture motion in a sling and stockinette body swathe for comfort. Aggressive maintenance of anatomic reduction is not a critical goal in this patient population; shoulder exercises should be initiated as early as possible to avoid shoulder contractures and adhesive capsulitis.

6. External fixation—External fixation is applicable to the humerus in the case of burns, gunshot wounds or severe comminuted open injuries with defects of skin, bone, or soft tissue. Other indications may include osteitis and infected non-union. Because of the soft-tissue envelope around the humerus, one uses external fixation only when other means of management are not applicable or appropriate. Half pins are generally inserted above and below the fracture with access to the soft-tissue defect between the pins.

B. Open Treatment

Special circumstances may merit open reduction and internal fixation. Selected segmental fractures, inadequate closed reduction, "floating" elbow, bilateral humeral fractures, open fractures, multiple trauma, pathologic fractures, and trauma with associated vascular injuries requiring exploration may benefit from internal fixation. There are two general forms of internal fixation: (1) Compression plate and screw fixation using the AO techniques, with posterior, modified lateral and anterolateral surgical approaches. (2) Intramedullary nailing is especially useful in osteopenic bone, segmental and pathological fractures. In multiply injured patients, humeral stabilization, permitting mobilization, pulmonary toilet, and pain control, may be beneficial. The incidence of radial nerve palsy with acute fracture is about 16%; however, current literature does not recommend operative fixation and nerve exploration in these injuries.

FRACTURES & DISLOCATIONS AROUND THE SHOULDER

Classification

The classification of shoulder fractures and dislocations developed by Neer in 1970 is based on the work of Codman in 1934 and before that of Kocher in 1896. This comprehensive system considers the anatomy and biomechanical forces resulting in displacement of fracture fragments as they relate to diagnosis and treatment. Although useful, this system has been demonstrated to have significant interobserver variability. Fractures are classified by the number of parts that are displaced more than 1 cm or angulated more than 45 degrees. Displaced parts can include the anatomical neck, surgical neck, or tuberosities; other categories include fracture-dislocations and head-splitting injuries. The relationship of the humeral head to the displaced parts in the glenoid, as well as the blood supply, is also taken into consideration. The incidence of proximal humerus fractures has been estimated at 4–5% of all fractures. The likelihood of proximal humerus fractures increases in the older age groups (>65 years), especially with concomitant osteoporosis. The incidence of proximal humerus fractures was reported to be 105 per 100,000 people per year in 2002, while the mean patient age has increased from 73 in 1973 to 78 in 2002.

Clinical Findings

Clinical presentation is usually with pain, swelling, and ecchymosis.

Radiographic evaluation is a cornerstone for diagnosis and planning of treatment. The recommended series of radiographs is the so-called Neer trauma series, which consists of an (1) anterior-posterior view, (2) lateral view in the scapular plane, and (3) Velpeau modified axillary view. The lateral radiograph in the scapular plane is the tangential Y-view of the scapula. The combination of three of these views allows evaluation of the shoulder joint in three separate perpendicular planes. The axillary view is important for evaluating the glenoid articular surface and the relationship of the humeral head anteriorly and posteriorly. It can be obtained even in the traumatized patient, with gentle abduction of the arm, with the x-ray beam aimed toward the axilla and the plate placed above the patient's shoulder. On occasion, other studies, including CT scanning for detailing bony anatomy and MRI for detailing soft tissues such as the rotator cuff, may prove helpful.

Treatment

A. Closed Treatment

Approximately 85% of proximal humerus fractures are minimally displaced or nondisplaced and can be treated non-operatively with a sling for comfort and early motion exercises. The remaining 15% require supplemental techniques. The mainstay of closed treatment is initial immobilization and then early motion. Physical therapy or physician-directed exercises are essential and should be started at 7–10 days if possible. Monitoring of the exercises is important to prevent a program that is either too conservative (thus causing unnecessary contractures) or too aggressive (leading to displacement, with excessive pain and swelling).

B. Surgical Treatment

Techniques useful for the smaller percentage of fractures include closed reduction and percutaneous pinning, skeletal traction, and ORIF using a variety of techniques and implants. Good bone quality and simple fracture patterns are essential to make use of the minimal soft tissue dissection in the closed reduction and percutaneous pinning method. For severe fractures, especially four-part fractures or fracture-dislocations in elderly patients, primary prosthetic replacement of the injured humeral head is generally the treatment of choice due to the high risk of avascular necrosis of the humeral head. In younger patients ORIF may be possible even in comminuted fractures.

C. Two-Part Anatomic Neck Fractures

Two-part anatomic neck fractures are rare. No single optimal method of management has been established. Closed reduction is difficult because controlling the articular fragment, which is usually rotated and angulated within the joint capsule, is difficult. The fragment can be preserved in a young (<40 years) patient with ORIF with pins or interfragmentary screws. It may be difficult to obtain adequate screw purchase without violating the articular surface. Additionally, the prognosis for head survival is poor because the blood supply is usually completely disrupted. In general, prosthetic hemiarthroplasty provides the most predictable result in the elderly (>75 years).

D. Two-Part Greater Tuberosity Fractures

Greater tuberosity fractures generally displace posteriorly and superiorly because of traction by the supraspinatus muscle. This is often associated with anterior glenohumeral dislocation. It is appropriate to attempt closed reduction, which may result in an acceptable position for the greater tuberosity. Neer has reported that displacement of the fragment by more than 1 cm is pathognomonic of a rotator cuff defect. The result of fracture healing in this position is subacromial impingement, with limitation of forward elevation and external rotation. In one series, patients with fractures that healed with more than 1 cm of displacement suffered permanent disability, whereas those with less than 0.5 cm of displacement did well. The group of patients in the midrange, 0.5–1 cm of displacement, had a 20% incidence of revision surgery for persistent pain. Open reduction and internal fixation is recommended if displacement is >5 mm with some references recommending ORIF with >3 mm displacement in the high-performance athlete as impingement symptoms may develop in these individuals. A variety of methods, including screws, pins, wires, and suture, can be used to repair the greater tuberosity. Nonabsorbable sutures can be used successfully; the rotator cuff defect can be repaired in a similar fashion. Treatment of this condition should be directed at rotator cuff repair as well as bony reconstruction. Percutaneous pinning tends to be inadequate for preventing re-displacement of greater tuberosity fractures. Despite these injuries being well recognized, there is a need for more studies to specifically evaluate the long-term outcome.

E. Two-Part Lesser Tuberosity Fractures

If the displaced fragment (usually medially by subscapularis) is small, closed reduction of this rare injury is satisfactory. This fracture may be associated with posterior dislocation and may be treated by closed reduction in the acute setting. The position of immobilization in this case would be either neutral or slight external rotation. Larger fragments may require internal fixation.

F. Two-Part Surgical Neck Fractures

In these conditions, both tuberosities remain attached to the head, and the rotator cuff in general remains intact. The diaphysis is often displaced anteromedially by the pull of the pectoralis major muscle. Reduction may be blocked by interposition of the periosteum, biceps tendon, or deltoid muscle, or by buttonholing of the shaft in the deltoid, pectoralis major, or fascial elements. One attempt at closed reduction is advisable; if this fails, operative intervention is recommended. If, on the other hand, the reduction is successful, percutaneous pinning under fluoroscopic control may be an excellent choice for the reducible but unstable fracture (Figure 3–17). If open reduction is required to remove displaced soft tissues, internal fixation can be accomplished by means of percutaneous pinning or intramedullary fixation in conjunction with a tension band wiring technique. In the past, an AO buttress plate has been used; however, complications including screw loosening (particularly in osteoporotic patients), retention of the plate, persistent varus, and interference with the blood supply have been reported. In the osteoporotic patient, wire or suture material for tension banding can be passed through the soft tissues and the rotator cuff, which may be superior to bone for fixation.

Another technique for internal fixation utilizes intramedullary devices such as Enders nails or Rush rods, which can be inserted through a limited deltoid-splitting incision. This may serve well to prevent displacement of the head in relation to the shaft; however, the control of rotational alignment is poor. For elderly (>75 years) or debilitated patients, this may be the best solution to achieve overall alignment with minimal surgical morbidity. Hardware removal is often necessary to treat resultant subacromial impingement. For complicated fractures, patients with osteoporotic bone, or other special circumstances, olecranon traction may be incorporated.

G. Three-Part Fractures

Avascular necrosis in three-part fractures has been reported to be as high as 27%. Open reduction and internal fixation is the treatment of choice with the aim of achieving anatomic reduction and enough stability to allow early rehabilitation. The AO buttress plate has had significant complications, including a high rate of avascular necrosis related in part to extension of soft-tissue displacement and dissection, superior placement of the plate with secondary impingement, loss of plate and screw fixation, malunion, and infections. Recent studies indicate that blade-plate devices tend to have stronger fixation than standard buttress plates. Other studies indicate that Ender nails combined with tension banding are good alternatives in osteoporotic bone. However, the properties of the locking compression plate (low stiffness and elasticity) have been shown to minimize peak stresses at the bone-implant interface. Screws, which lock into the plate, may decrease pullout in osteoporotic fractures. Finally, hemiarthroplasty should be considered in the elderly.

H. Four-Part Fractures

Open reduction and internal fixation of four-part fractures (as with three-part fractures) has generally produced unsatisfactorily high rates of complications such as avascular necrosis and malunion. Some authors recommend gentle open reduction and limited internal fixation in the active patient. In the less active or elderly (>75 years) patient, the accepted method of treatment is hemiarthroplasty, particularly because the avascular necrosis rate may be as high as 90% and the bone is usually osteoporotic. Appropriate prosthesis level and humeral retroversion, as well as the attachment of greater and lesser tuberosities, are critical in achieving a good result. Repair of any rotator cuff defects is necessary to prevent proximal migration of the humeral component as well as loss of rotator cuff power. With rehabilitation post-operatively, generally good pain relief can be expected, however function is usually limited.

I. Fracture-Dislocations

Fracture-dislocations require reduction of the humeral head, and their management is generally based on the fracture pattern. These injuries usually produce impression defects or head-splitting fractures, with concomi-

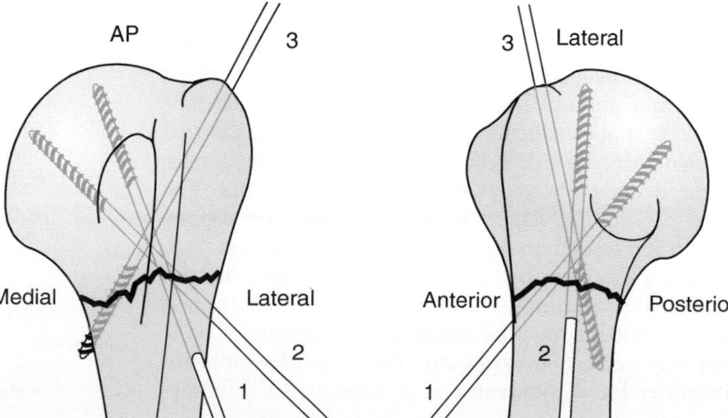

Figure 3–17. **Pinning of the unstable surgical neck fracture.** (Reproduced, with permission, from Fu FH, Smith WR, eds: Percutaneous pinning of proximal humerus fractures. Oper Tech Orthop 2001;11:235.)

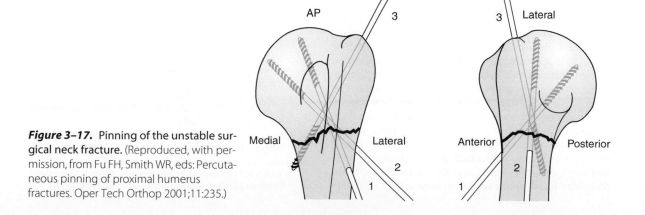

tant posterior dislocation. Management is determined by the size of the impression defect and the time of persistent locked dislocation. Fractures of less than 20% will generally be stable with closed reduction and can be treated with immobilization in external rotation for 6 weeks to restore long-term stability. If the defect is 20–50%, however, transfer of the lesser tuberosity with the subscapularis tendon into the defect by open means is indicated. With impression fractures of greater than 50% or chronic dislocations, hemiarthroplasty may be the best treatment. If concomitant glenoid destruction is present, total shoulder arthroplasty may be required.

Complex Regional Pain Syndrome (CRPS)

This is defined as an abnormal reaction to injury characterized by pain, stiffness, vasomotor changes, swelling and osteoporosis of the affected limb. It is classified into 2 types: Type 1 (formerly reflex sympathetic dystrophy), and Type 2 (formerly causalgia). Type 1 is associated with pain out of proportion to the initial injury, hyperesthesia, restricted mobility and movement disorder, skin changes (color, texture and temperature), edema, patchy osteoporosis and spreading symptoms to become more diffuse. Type 2 includes the features of Type 1 with an identified nerve lesion. CRPS can be precipitated by trauma, infection, myocardial infarction, stroke, surgery, spinal cord disorders, and sometimes, without obvious cause. The pathophysiology is not fully understood but damage to the nervous control of the affected part has been speculated. There is an increased incidence in people aged 40–60. Early diagnosis is key to try to prevent chronic changes (muscle wasting and contractures) and can be made based on history and examination. Investigations include x-rays, bone scans, nerve conduction studies, and thermography. Primarily the cause, if identified, should be treated. Physical and occupational therapy, medications (tricyclic antidepressants, vasodilators and steroids) and sympathetic blockade (chemical or surgical) can be useful.

Clinically, reflex sympathetic dystrophy has three stages, which are not completely distinct from one another. During the first, or early, stage, a burning or aching pain may be present and may be increased by external stimuli; the pain is out of proportion to the severity of the injury and physical findings. The second stage generally develops at approximately 3 months and is characterized by significant edema, cold glossy skin, and joint limitations. Radiographs may reveal diffuse osteopenia. The third, or atrophic, stage is marked by progressive atrophy of skin and muscle and significant joint contractures.

Sudeck's atrophy is a radiographic term that is extended to a clinical condition. Spotty rarefication is distinguished from generalized diffuse atrophy of bone and may occur 6–8 weeks after the onset of symptoms. **Shoulder-hand syndrome** is a variation of this phenomenon that often occurs with upper extremity disorders. Stiffness is characteristic, both at the shoulder and at the wrist and hand level.

Because the cause is unclear, the recommended treatment is an aggressive program of physical therapy modalities to help with soft-tissue sensitivity as well as prevention or treatment of joint contractures. Sympathetic blocks may be important. More recently, multidisciplinary pain management services that incorporate counseling, evaluation of orthopedic musculoskeletal neurologic problems, and sympathetic blocks administered typically by anesthesiologists, have proved successful in helping to limit the time and extent of disability associated with these conditions. Progressive loading of the extremity and progressive resistance-type exercises can also be of benefit in the appropriate setting.

Blum J et al: Clinical performance of a new medullary humeral nail: Antegrade versus retrograde insertion. J Orthop Trauma 2001;15:342. [PMID:11433139]

Chapman JR et al: Randomized prospective study of humeral shaft fracture fixation: Intramedullary nails versus plates. J Orthop Trauma 2000;14:162. [PMID: 10791665]

Cox MA et al: Closed interlocking nailing of humeral shaft fractures with the Russell-Taylor nail. J Orthop Trauma 2000; 14:349. [PMID: 10926243]

Eberson CP et al: Contralateral intrathoracic displacement of the humeral head. J Bone Joint Surg Am 2000;82-A:105. [PMID: 10653090]

Helmy N, Hintermann B: New trends in the treatment of proximal humerus fractures. Clin Orthop 2006;442:100. [PMID: 16394747]

Hintermann B, Trouillier HH, Schafer D: Rigid internal fixation of fractures of the proximal humerus in older patients. J Bone Joint Surg Br 2000;82-B:1107. [PMID: 11132267]

McCormack RG et al: Fixation of fractures of the shaft of the humerus by dynamic compression plate or intramedullary nail. J Bone Joint Surg Br 2000;82-B:336. [PMID: 10813165]

Naranja RJ, Iannotti JP: Displaced three- and four-part proximal humerus fractures: Evaluation and management 2000;8:373. [PMID: 11104401]

Orthoteers: http//www.orthoteers.co.uk/Nrujp-ij33lm/Orthcrps.htm

Palvanen M, et al: Update on the epidemiology of proximal humerus fractures. Clin Orthop 2006;442:87. [PMID: 16394745]

Pickering RM, Crenshaw AH Jr, Zinar DM: Intramedullary nailing of humeral shaft fractures. Instr Course Lect 2002; 51:271–8. [PMID 12064112]

Ruch DS et al: Fixation of three-part proximal humeral fractures: A biomechanical evaluation. J Orthop Trauma 2000;14:36. [PMID: 10630801]

Sarmiento A et al: Functional bracing for the treatment of fractures of the humeral diaphysis. J Bone Joint Surg Am 2000;82: 478. [PMID: 10761938]

Steinmann SP, Moran EA: Axillary nerve injury: Diagnosis and treatment. J Am Acad Orthop Surg 2001;9:328. [PMID: 11575912]

Strothman D et al: Retrograde nailing of humeral shaft fractures: A biomechanical study of its effects on the strength of the distal humerus. J Orthop Trauma 2000;14:101. [PMID: 10716380]

II. TRAUMA TO THE LOWER EXTREMITY

FOOT & ANKLE INJURIES

The appropriate investigation of any foot injury requires obtaining, initially, a precise history of the mechanism of injury. A thorough physical examination will compare the injured extremity to the uninjured contralateral side (looking for ecchymosis, swelling, or deformity), palpating carefully all points of tenderness, stressing the different joints when indicated, and assessing the neurovascular status. Associated injuries and certain systemic disorders (particularly diabetes and peripheral vascular disease) should be identified. An appropriate radiographic evaluation is mandatory. Anteroposterior and lateral views are standard. Oblique and special views are requested according to clinical suspicion. Although some fracture patterns are still best delineated by conventional tomography, CT scanning with 3D rendering has recently proved to be valuable, especially for ankle and calcaneal fractures. Volume rendering helps demonstrate structures surrounding the fracture and shaded surface display is useful for obtaining disarticulated views in intraarticular fractures. Radionuclide imaging is helpful to identify occult injuries. MRI is gaining popularity and is particularly helpful in diagnosing soft-tissue damage to the tibialis posterior tendon or gastrocnemius muscle, osteochondral fractures, and avascular necrosis.

Anatomy & Biomechanical Principles

The foot is a complex, highly specialized structure that permits weight bearing in a smooth, energy-conserving pattern. The delicate balance between bones and soft tissues is necessary for optimal function. When planning treatment of an injured foot, both need to be addressed with equal rigor. High-energy injuries, such as crush injuries, generally have a poorer prognosis, even if the bones are anatomically reduced. Scarring of soft tissues, particularly specialized tissues like the heel fat pad or the plantar fascia, prevents normal function and is often painful.

Embryologically, the foot develops from proximal to distal into three functional segments: the tarsus, metatarsus, and phalanges. Anatomically, it is divided into the hindfoot (talus and calcaneus), the midfoot (navicular, cuboid, and three cuneiforms), and the forefoot (five metatarsals and 14 phalanges). Besides skin, vessels, and nerves, the soft tissues include extrinsic tendons, intrinsic musculotendinous units, a complex network of capsuloligamentous structures, and some uniquely specialized tissues such as fat pads.

The bones, ligaments and muscles of the foot actively maintain the integrity of the 3 arches of the foot. The 2 longitudinal arches aid in weight bearing and absorbing the forces during motion. The transverse arch helps with the movements of the foot.

Classically, the plantar aspect of the foot is divided into four layers, from superficial to deep. The first layer consists of the abductor hallucis, flexor digitorum brevis, and abductor digiti minimi. The second layer is made up of the tendons of the flexor hallucis longus and flexor digitorum longus, flexor digitorum accessorius, the quadratus plantae and lumbricales muscles. In the third layer are the flexor hallucis brevis, adductor hallucis, and flexor digiti minimi muscles. The peroneus longus and tibialis posterior tendons, as well as the unipennate plantar and bipennate dorsal interossei muscles, comprise the fourth and deepest layer.

These 28 bones, 57 articulations, and extrinsic and intrinsic soft tissues work harmoniously as a unit resembling functionally a ball and socket to allow walking, running, jumping, and accommodation of irregular surfaces with a minimal expense of energy.

Energy-effective gait requires optimal integration of all segments involved in locomotion, and proper coordination involves extremely complex pathways. Fluid motion minimizes energy expenditure, and a lot of the fine-tuning to attain this goal occurs in the foot. For example, the subtalar joint everts at heel strike, unlocking the midtarsal joint. Increasing the flexibility of the foot allows for better energy absorption and foot-to-ground accommodation. Conversely, the subtalar joint inverts at push-off, locking the midtarsal joint. This creates a rigid lever more mechanically advantageous for forward propulsion.

This superficial overview of the anatomy and biomechanical principles of the foot serves only to stress the complex relationship between bone and soft-tissue structures. Restoration of this relationship is often challenging, but is the goal of treatment of foot injuries.

FRACTURES COMMON TO ALL PARTS OF THE FOOT

1. Fatigue Fractures

Also known as **stress, march,** or **insufficiency** fractures, fatigue fractures occur when damage from cyclical loading of a bone overwhelms its physiologic repair capacity. Repetitive stress stimulates an attempt to strengthen areas of bone that are experiencing excessive stress. This process begins with resorption of bone to make room for the deposition of new stronger bone. Continued loading can lead to gross failure of the bone weakened by resorption.

This disorder is commonly seen in young active adults involved in vigorous and excessive exercise. A history of a single significant injury is usually lacking. Sites of fracture are most frequently the metatarsals and the calcaneus, but fatigue fractures can be found anywhere.

Clinical Findings

Incipient pain of varying intensity at rest is then accentuated by walking. Swelling and point tenderness are likely to be present. Depending on the stage of progress, radiographs may be normal or may show an incomplete or complete fracture line or only extracortical callus formation that can be mistaken for osteogenic sarcoma. Radionuclide imaging, CT and MRI can be helpful for occult fractures. Persistent unprotected weight bearing may cause arrest of bone healing and even displacement of the fracture fragment.

Treatment

Treatment is by protection in either a short leg cast, walking boot or a heavy stiff-soled shoe. Weight bearing is restricted until pain has subsided and restoration of bone continuity is confirmed radiographically, usually within 3–4 weeks.

2. Multiple High-Energy Injuries

Violent forces applied to the foot may cause more extensive damage than initially appreciated. Certain mechanisms of injury tend to produce specific patterns of lesions, and a high index of suspicion is necessary so as not to overlook some of the associated bony or ligamentous injuries.

Treatment

High-energy fractures are often open, and the basic principles of open fracture management should be applied. The objectives are to preserve circulation and sensation (particularly of the plantar region), maintain a plantigrade position of the foot, prevent or control infection, preserve plantar skin and fat pads, preserve gross motion of the different joints (both actively and passively), achieve bone union, and, ultimately, preserve fine motion. Fasciotomies of the severely injured foot may be necessary to avoid compartment syndromes and their serious sequelae.

Early stabilization of multiple fractures and dislocations will simplify wound management. This can be accomplished through external fixation or internal fixation with K-wires, plates, or screws. Early soft tissue coverage with local or free flaps is also beneficial.

3. Neuropathic Joint Injuries & Fractures

Fractures and other foot disorders often present in the patient with Charcot arthropathy. Neuropathic fractures are frequently seen with diabetes, tabes dorsalis, syringomyelia, peripheral nerve injury or degeneration, leprosy, and other rare neurologic syndromes.

The potential for bone healing is normal if no other comorbidities exist. It has been found, however, that healing of fractures is often delayed in this patient group. Protection, rest, and elevation can result in union without deformity. Open reduction and internal fixation is sometimes necessary. Rarely, arthrodesis is indicated; however, the rate of nonunion is higher than for normal joints.

FOREFOOT FRACTURES & DISLOCATIONS

1. Metatarsal Fractures & Dislocations

Fracture of the metatarsals and dislocation of the tarsometatarsals are frequently caused by a direct crushing or indirect twisting injury to the forefoot. Besides osseous and articular injury, complicating soft tissue lesions are often present. With severe trauma, circulation may be compromised from injury to the dorsalis pedis artery, which passes between the first and second metatarsals.

Metatarsal Shaft Fractures

Undisplaced fractures of the metatarsal shafts cause only temporary disability, unless failure of bone healing occurs. Displacement is rarely significant when the first and fifth metatarsals are not involved because they act as internal splints.

These fractures can be treated with a hard-soled shoe with partial weight bearing, or, if pain is marked, a short leg walking cast.

For displaced fractures of the shaft, it is of paramount importance to correct angulation in the longitudinal axis of the shaft. Residual dorsal angulation causes prominence of the metatarsal head on the plantar surface. The concentrated local pressure may produce a painful skin callus. Residual plantar angulation of the first metatarsal will transfer weight to the heads of the second and third metatarsals. After reduction of angular deformity, a cast should be well molded to the plantar surface to minimize recurrence of deformity and support the transverse and longitudinal arches. If significant angulation or intraarticular displacement persists, open or closed reduction and internal fixation should be considered.

Metatarsal Neck & Head Fractures

Fractures of the metatarsal "neck" are close to the head but remain extraarticular. Dorsal angulation is common and should be reduced to avoid reactive skin callus formation from pressure on the plantar skin. Intraarticular fractures of the metatarsal heads are rare. Even when they heal in a displaced position, some remodeling occurs and the functional outcome is surprisingly good.

The indications for open reduction with or without internal fixation remain controversial.

Closed reduction of metatarsal fractures is best achieved by applying traction (Chinese finger traps) to the involved toes. Reduction is evaluated with intraoperative radiographs, and if judged unacceptable, ORIF with K-wires or plates and screws is indicated. Unstable reductions should also undergo percutaneous pinning under fluoroscopic imaging.

Tarsometatarsal (Lisfranc) Dislocations

The stability of the tarsometatarsal joint complex relies in part on strong ligamentous structures and in part on the bony architecture itself. The base of the second metatarsal is recessed proximally to the base of the other metatarsals in a cleft between the first and third cuneiforms, thus "locking" the joint. Injuries to this structure should alert the clinician to the possibility of other injuries along the entire tarsometatarsal complex.

The original injury, described by Napoleon's field surgeon Lisfranc, was attributed to a soldier falling from his horse with his foot trapped in the stirrup. The mechanism of the injury was an axial load acting on a hyper-plantarflexed foot. Three commonly occurring patterns of this injury are identified: total incongruity, partial incongruity, and divergent (Figure 3–18). The medial border of the second and fourth metatarsals should align with the medial borders of the middle cuneiform and the cuboid, respectively. Associated soft-tissue damage is almost always significant, with open wounds, vascular impairment, swelling, and blistering.

An attempt at closed reduction should be made as soon as possible; however, open reduction is often required. Gentle manipulation can be successful; however, residual instability is common. Postreduction radiographs are obtained, and if anatomic reduction is not obtained, then ORIF with K-wires on the lateral side of the foot to preserve mobility and screws on the medial side of the foot is indicated. The foot is then immobilized and elevated. Timing of hardware removal is controversial with some authors recommending 3 months and others recommending 6 months. Prognosis depends on maintenance of anatomical reduction. However, one study has reported that even in cases where anatomic reduction, normal walking patterns and excellent radiographic results were accomplished post tarsometatarsal fracture dislocation, subjective patient outcomes were less than satisfactory.

Some tarsometatarsal injuries present late (>3–4 weeks), when the healing process will prevent successful closed treatment. If displacement and deformity are significant, open reduction is indicated, but the patient should be advised to expect some residual joint stiffness. If displacement is minimal, it may be better to defer surgery and direct treatment toward functional

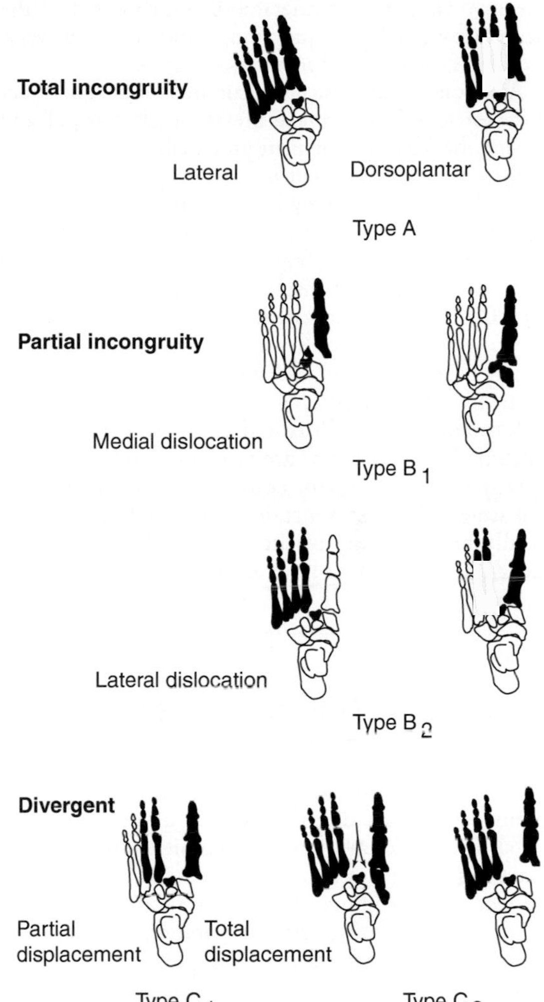

Figure 3–18. Classification of Lisfranc injuries. (Reproduced, with permission, from Coughlin MJ, Mann RA, eds: *Surgery of the Foot and Ankle,* 7th ed. WB Saunders, 1999.)

recovery. Reconstructive operations can be planned more suitably once residual disability is established.

Complications of this injury include chronic foot swelling, residual deformity making shoe fitting difficult, painful degenerative joint disease, and reflex sympathetic dystrophy. Arthrodesis should be considered for symptomatic post-traumatic arthritis.

Fracture of the Base of the Fifth Metatarsal

Three distinct patterns occur: (1) avulsion fracture of a variably sized portion of the tuberosity (styloid process) that may, on rare occasions, involve the joint between the cuboid and the fifth metatarsal; (2) acute Jones fracture involving the intermetatarsal joint(located at the metaphysial-diaphysial junction), and (3) transverse fracture of the proximal metatarsal diaphysis.

Avulsion fractures usually occur after adduction injury to the forefoot. The peroneus brevis muscle may pull and displace the fractured fragment proximally.

Symptomatic treatment is most often successful in a hard-soled shoe, and bony healing rarely fails to occur. Nonunions are rarely symptomatic but can be treated by internal fixation or fragment excision. In the rare event of a significant displaced intraarticular component, ORIF may be indicated.

Acute Jones fractures are best treated in a non-weight bearing cast for 6-8 weeks. Some authors recommend acute ORIF of Jones fractures in the high-performance athlete. Proximal diaphyseal fractures or "chronic Jones fractures" are most probably secondary to fatigue failure. Again, conservative treatment in a non-weight–bearing short leg cast for 6 weeks will usually bring healing of the fracture. Nonunions do occur (due to the poor inherent blood supply) and are often symptomatic. If there is no evidence of bone healing at 12 weeks, internal fixation and bone grafting are recommended.

2. Fractures & Dislocations of the Phalanges of the Toes

Fractures of the phalanges of the toes are most commonly caused by a direct force such as a crush injury. Spiral or oblique fractures of the shaft of the proximal phalanges of the lesser toes may occur as a result of an indirect twisting injury. The injury should be assessed in terms of deformity, soft tissue injury, neurovascular status and radiographically.

Treatment

Comminuted fracture of the proximal phalanx of the great toe, alone or in combination with fracture of the distal phalanx, is a disabling injury. Because wide displacement of fragments is not likely, correction of angulation and support by a splint usually suffices. A weight-bearing removable cast boot may be useful for relief of symptoms arising from associated soft-tissue injury. Spiral or oblique fracture of the proximal or middle phalanges of the lesser toes can be treated adequately by binding the involved toe to the adjacent uninjured toe (buddy taping). Comminuted fractures of the distal phalanx are treated as soft-tissue injuries.

Dislocation of the metatarsophalangeal joints and dislocation of the proximal interphalangeal joints usually can be reduced by closed manipulation. These dislocations are rarely isolated and usually occur in combination with other injuries to the forefoot.

3. Fracture of the Sesamoids of the Great Toe

Fractures of the sesamoid bones of the great toe are rare but may occur as a result of a crushing injury. These injuries must be differentiated from a bipartite sesamoid by comparing radiographs of the contralateral uninvolved foot.

Treatment

Undisplaced fractures require no treatment other than a hard-soled shoe or metatarsal bar. Displaced fractures may require immobilization in a walking boot or cast, with the toe strapped in flexion. Persistent delay of bone healing may cause disabling pain arising from arthritis of the articulation between the sesamoid and the head of the first metatarsal. If conservative modalities have been exhausted excision of the sesamoid may be necessary; however, this should be a last resort treatment.

Calder JD, Whitehouse SL, Saxby TS: Results of isolated LisFranc injuries and the effect of compensation claims. J Bone Joint Surg Br 2004;86:527. [PMID: 15174547]

Haapamaki V, Kiuru M, Koskinen S: Lisfranc fracture-dislocation in patients with multiple trauma: diagnosis with multidetector computed tomography. Foot Ankle Int 2004;25:614. [PMID: 15563381]

Kelly IP et al: Intramedullary screw fixation of Jones fractures. Foot Ankle Int 2001;22:585. [PMID: 11503985]

Kuo RS et al: Outcome after open reduction and internal fixation of Lisfranc joint injuries. J Bone Joint Surg Am 2000;82-A:1609. [PMID: 11097452]

Kura H et al: Mechanical behavior of the Lisfranc and dorsal cuneometatarsal ligaments: In vitro biomechanical study. J Orthop Trauma 2001;15:107. [PMID: 11232648]

Larson CM et al: Intramedullary screw fixation of Jones fractures: Analysis of failure. Am J Sports Med 2002;30:55. [PMID: 11798997]

Nunley JA: Fractures of the base of the fifth metatarsal: The Jones fracture. Orthop Clin North Am 2001;32:171. [PMID: 11465126]

Richter M et al: Fractures and fracture dislocations of the midfoot: Occurrence, causes and long-term results. Foot Ankle Int 2001;22:392. [PMID: 11428757]

Rosenberg GA, Sferra JJ: Treatment strategies for acute fractures and nonunions of the proximal fifth metatarsal. J Am Acad Orthop Surg 2000;8:332. [PMID: 11029561]

MIDFOOT FRACTURES & DISLOCATIONS

1. Navicular Fractures

Avulsion Fractures

Avulsion fractures of the tarsal navicular may occur as a result of severe midtarsal sprain and require neither reduction nor elaborate treatment. Avulsion fracture of the tuberosity near the insertion of the posterior tibialis tendon is uncommon and must be differentiated from a persistent ununited apophysis (accessory navicular) from the supernumerary sesamoid bone, or os tibiale externum. Dorsal lip avulsions also occur.

Body Fractures

Body fractures occur either centrally in a horizontal plane or, more rarely, in a vertical plane. They are occasionally characterized by impaction. Non-comminuted fractures with displacement of the dorsal fragment can be reduced. Closed manipulation by strong traction on the forefoot and simultaneous digital pressure over the displaced fragment can restore normal position. If a tendency to re-displace is apparent, this can be counteracted by temporary fixation with a percutaneously inserted Kirschner wire. Non-weight–bearing immobilization in a cast or splint is required for a minimum of 6 weeks. Comminuted and impacted fractures cannot be anatomically reduced in a closed manner. Where fragments involve >25% of the bone, ORIF may be required to prevent dorsal subluxation of the navicular fragment. Bone graft may be used for depressed areas. Some authorities offer a pessimistic prognosis for comminuted or impacted fractures. It is their contention that even though partial reduction has been achieved, posttraumatic arthritis supervenes, and that arthrodesis of the talonavicular and naviculocuneiform joints will be ultimately necessary to relieve painful symptoms.

Stress Fractures

The navicular is also a frequent site of fatigue fracture in runners. CT or radionuclide imaging is often necessary to make the diagnosis. Six weeks in a non-weight–bearing short leg cast is usually required for fracture healing.

2. Cuneiform & Cuboid Bone Fractures

Because of their relatively protected position in the midtarsus, isolated fractures of the cuboid and cuneiform bones are rarely encountered. Avulsion fractures occur as a component of severe midtarsal sprains. Extensive fractures usually occur in association with other injuries of the foot and often are caused by severe crushing. A "nutcracker" fracture is a compression fracture of the cuboid and, when associated with lateral column shortening, can be treated by lateral column lengthening, ORIF, and bone grafting.

1. Midtarsal Dislocations

Midtarsal dislocation through the naviculocuneiform and calcaneocuboid joints, or more proximally through the talonavicular and calcaneocuboid joints (Chopart's joint), may occur as a result of a twisting injury to the forefoot. Fractures of varying extent of adjacent bones are frequently associated.

When acute treatment is administered, closed reduction by traction on the forefoot and manipulation is generally effective. If reduction is unstable and displacement tends to recur upon release of traction, stabilization for 4 weeks by percutaneously inserted Kirschner wires is recommended.

HINDFOOT FRACTURES & DISLOCATIONS

1. Talus Fractures

Three fifths of the talus is covered with articular cartilage. The blood supply enters the neck area and is tenuous. Fractures and dislocations may disrupt this vascularization, causing delayed healing or avascular necrosis.

Major fractures of the talus commonly occur either through the body or the neck. Head fractures involve essentially a portion of the neck with extension into the head. Indirect injury is usually the cause of most fractures of the talus. Compression fracture or impaction of the tibial articular surface may be caused by the initial injury or may occur later in association with complicating avascular necrosis.

Fractures of the Neck of the Talus

The most common mechanism of talar neck fracture is hyperdorsiflexion with an axial load causing impingement between the talar neck and tibia. The most widely used classification is that of Hawkins:

Type 1: Nondisplaced vertical fracture

Type 2: Displaced fracture of the talar neck with subluxation or dislocation of the subtalar joint

Type 3: Displaced fracture of the talar neck with dislocation of the body of the talus from both the tibiotalar and subtalar joints

Type 4: Later, a type 4 fracture was described by Canale and Kelly to include rare variants which are essentially type 3 injuries with talonavicular subluxation or dislocation (Figure 3–19).

This classification is of prognostic value for avascular necrosis of the body: 0–13% for type 1 fractures, 25–50% for type 2 fractures, 80–100% for type 3 fractures, and 100% for type 4.

Less frequent complications of talar neck fractures include infection, delayed union or nonunion, malunion, and osteoarthritis of the tibiotalar and subtalar joints.

Treatment is aimed at minimizing the occurrence of these complications. Type 1 fractures are best treated with a non-weight–bearing below-knee cast for 2–3 months until clinical and radiologic signs of healing are present. Closed reduction is first attempted for type 2 fractures and, if this is successful in attaining anatomic

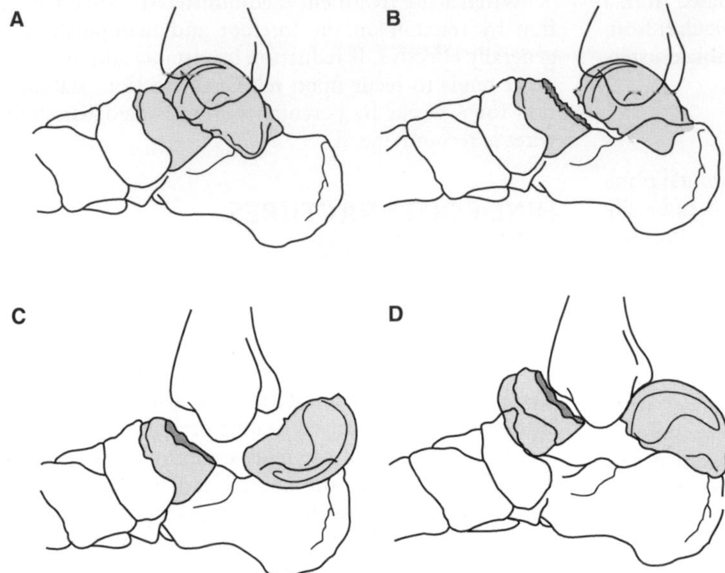

Figure 3–19. **Hawkins classification of talar neck fractures.** (Reproduced, with permission, from Coughlin MJ, Mann RA, eds: *Surgery of the Foot and Ankle,* 7th ed. WB Saunders, 1999.)

alignment, treatment is as for a type 1 fracture. In about 50% of cases, closed reduction is unsuccessful and open reduction and internal fixation with K-wires, pins, or screws is indicated. Closed reduction of types 3 and 4 fractures is almost never successful; ORIF is the rule. The postoperative regimen is the same as above. Progressive weight bearing will be allowed after fracture union if there is no avascular necrosis of the body. This can be determined on the anteroposterior radiograph of the ankle, taken out of the cast by the eighth week, if there is a subchondral lucency in the dome of the talus. This "Hawkins' sign" is possible only if the talar body is vascularized. The most sensitive method, however, appears to be MRI, which can, as early as 3 weeks, clearly define the extent of osteonecrosis in the body of the talus. When avascular necrosis is evident, revascularization can take up to 3 years. To avoid collapse of the talar dome during this process, partial weight bearing is recommended. One should also remember that there is not a direct correlation between avascular necrosis and permanently disabling symptoms.

Fractures of the Body of the Talus

Talus body fractures occur mainly due to shear and axial compression forces. The Hawkins classification describes 5 types of fracture:

Type 1: Osteochondral fracture
Type 2: Coronal, sagittal or horizontal fracture
Type 3: Posterior process fracture
Type 4: Lateral process fracture
Type 5: Crush fracture of the body

Minimally displaced fractures of the talar body are not likely to cause disability if immobilization is continued until union is restored. If significant displacement occurs, the proximal fragment is apt to be dislocated from the subtalar and ankle joints. Associated fractures of the malleoli, talar neck and calcaneus occur frequently. Anterior-posterior, mortise, lateral and Broden (45 degrees internal oblique) views aid radiographic assessment of the injury and enable the quantification of articular surface involvement and displacement. CT is also used to assess comminution and associated fractures.

Reduction by closed manipulation is often difficult but is best achieved by traction and forced plantar flexion of the foot. Immobilization in a short leg cast, with the foot in plantar flexion for about 8 weeks, should be followed by further casting with the foot out of equinus until the fracture line has been obliterated and new bone is present on serial radiographs. Even though prompt adequate reduction is obtained by either closed manipulation or open reduction, extensive displacement of the proximal body fragments may be followed by avascular necrosis. If reduction is not anatomic, delayed healing of the fracture may follow, and posttraumatic arthritis is a likely sequela. If this occurs, arthrodesis of the ankle or subtalar joints may be necessary to relieve painful symptoms.

Osteochondral Fractures of the Talar Dome

These can occur with any type of injury to the ankle area, including sprains. A history of trauma is usual, but not always, present. Classically, lesions of the medial aspect of the talar dome are thicker, more extensive, and less likely to displace, whereas the lateral lesions are shallower, more wafer-like, and more prone to be displaced and symptomatic.

Initial radiograph evaluation often does not demonstrate these lesions. Presently, MRI is the best imaging modality for osteochondral talar lesions.

The Berndt and Harty classification is generally used:

Stage 1: Localized compression

Stage 2: Incomplete separation of the fragment

Stage 3: Completely detached but nondisplaced fragment

Stage 4: Completely detached, displaced fracture

A modified version of this classification to include MRI findings can help radiologists better classify these fractures.

Symptomatic stage 1, 2, and 3 lesions are usually initially treated conservatively with immobilization and restricted weight bearing. Healing is monitored radiographically with anterior-posterior and mortise views. Lesions that fail conservative treatment and all stage 4 lesions require surgical treatment. Reduction and pinning or fixation with screws and excision with or without drilling have been recommended. Arthroscopic management seems to give as good a result as arthrotomy, with fewer complications. Degenerative disease of the tibiotalar joint is a frequent long-term complication.

Compression fractures of the talar dome are rare injuries. They cannot be reduced by closed methods. If open reduction, with or without bone grafting, is elected, prolonged protection from weight bearing is the best means of preventing collapse of the healing area.

Other Talar Fractures

Other rare fractures include those of the lateral (snowboarders' fracture) or posterior process (Shepherd's fracture) or its lateral or medial tubercles. These fractures may be difficult to demonstrate. Special radiographs and radionuclide imaging can be very helpful.

Conservative treatment usually gives excellent results; however, consideration should be given to open reduction and fixation or fragment excision of displaced fractures and those involving the articular surface.

Subtalar Dislocation

Subtalar dislocation, also called **peritalar** dislocation, is the simultaneous dislocation of the talocalcaneal and talonavicular joints. Inversion injuries result in medial dislocations (85%), whereas eversion injuries result in lateral dislocations (15%). Anterior and posterior dislocations are rare.

Prompt gentle closed reduction is usually successful. Immobilization in a non-weight–bearing short leg cast for 6 weeks is usually satisfactory. Soft-tissue interposition, particularly of the posterior tibial tendon, may prevent closed reduction. Open reduction, with or without internal fixation, is then indicated.

Total Dislocation of the Talus

This injury usually results from high-energy trauma, and most are open dislocations. Despite adequate prompt reduction and thorough wound debridement, the complication rate is extremely high, including persistent infection and avascular necrosis. Talectomy and tibiocalcaneal fusion is a frequent final outcome.

2. Calcaneus Fractures

The calcaneus (os calcis) functions to provide support for body weight, maintains the lateral column of the foot and acts as a lever arm for the calf muscles. A fracture causing an impairment of any of the above functions will result in significant gait abnormalities. The most common mechanism of fracture is high-energy axial loading driving the talus downwards (e.g. a fall from a height). Ten percent of calcaneal fractures are associated with compression fractures of the thoracic or lumbar spine, and 5% are bilateral. Comminution and impaction are common features.

Clinical Findings

A. Symptoms and Signs

Pain is usually significant but may be masked by associated injuries. Swelling, deformity, and blistering of the skin occur frequently during the first 36 hours as a result of the severe damage to surrounding soft tissues. The heel pad in particular is a highly specialized fatty structure that acts as a hydraulic cushion. Major disruptions of the heel pad lead to persistent pain and deformity and can produce poor functional results in spite of adequate bony healing.

B. Imaging Studies

Initial radiographs include three views: anteroposterior, lateral, and axial projection (Harris view). Disruption of Böhler's angle and the angle of Gissane can be determined from initial radiographs (Figure 3–20). Oblique

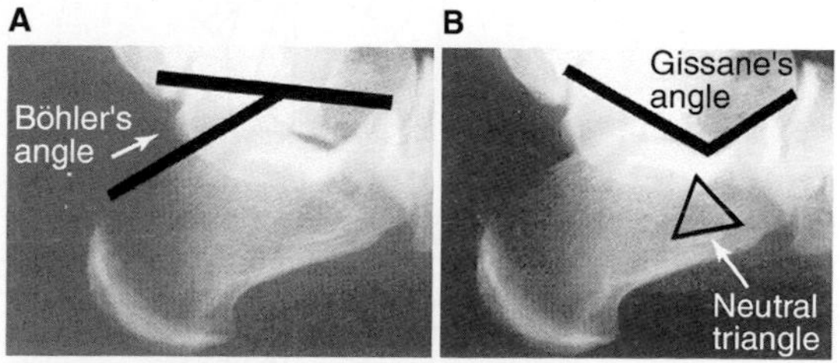

Figure 3–20. Böhler's angle (**A**) and Gissane's angle (**B**), indicating normal anatomic landmarks. (Reproduced, with permission, from Coughlin MJ, Mann RA, eds: *Surgery of the Foot and Ankle,* 7th ed. WB Saunders, 1999.)

or Broden's views are useful to demonstrate subtalar joint incongruity. CT scanning is the diagnostic tool of choice and will further delineate fracture patterns and occult injuries. Bone scanning may be useful to diagnose a stress fracture.

C. Classification

Various classifications have been advocated. Sanders has developed a classification system based upon coronal CT images (Figure 3–21). This classification has been found to be useful in both treatment and prognosis. Type I fractures are nondisplaced articular fractures. Type II fractures are two-part fractures of the posterior facet and are divided into A, B, and C based upon the location of the fracture line. Type III fractures are three-part fractures with a centrally depressed fragment, also divided into A, B, and C. Type IV fractures are four-part articular fractures with extensive comminution. To simplify classification, calcaneus fractures can be divided into intraarticular and extraarticular fractures. Intraarticular fractures occur frequently (75%), have a poorer prognosis, and are further subdivided into nondisplaced, tongue-type, joint depression and comminuted. Extraarticular fractures are rare (25%) and generally have a better prognosis.

Intraarticular Fractures

The subtalar joint is almost always involved, and occasionally the fracture line extends into the calcaneocuboid joint. Isolated fractures of the calcaneocuboid joint are rare.

A. Types of Fractures

1. Nondisplaced fractures—These fractures are successfully treated by protection from weight bearing, for 4–8 weeks, until clinical and radiographic signs of healing are present.

2. Tongue-type fractures—This fracture pattern (Figure 3–22) involves the subtalar joint with a posterior extension in the transverse plane, creating a dorsal fragment.

3. Joint depression—This fracture pattern (Figure 3–23) creates a separate fragment of the posterior facet with joint incongruity.

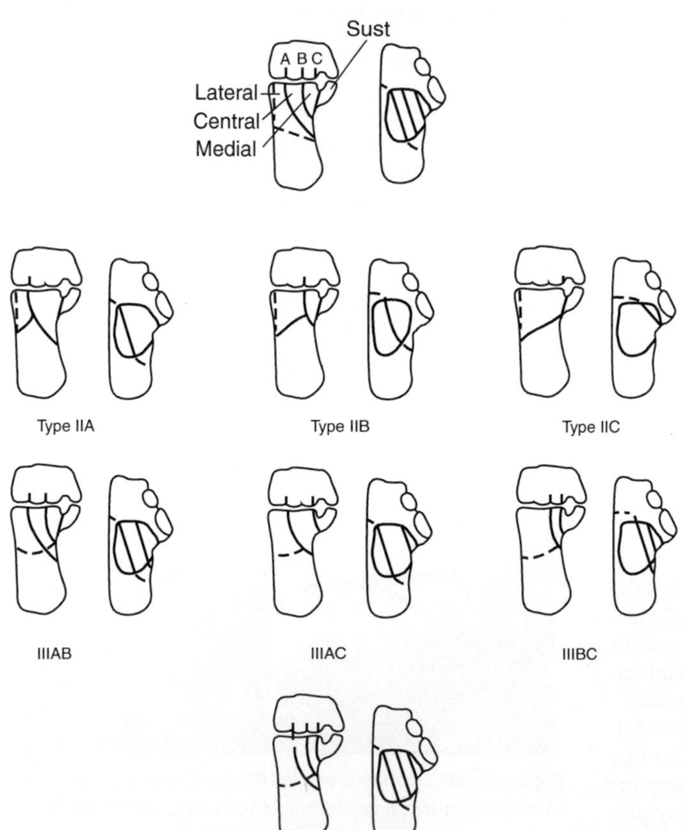

Figure 3–21. **Sanders CT classification of calcaneus fractures.** (Reproduced, with permission, from Coughlin MJ, Mann RA, eds: *Surgery of the Foot and Ankle,* 7th ed. WB Saunders, 1999.)

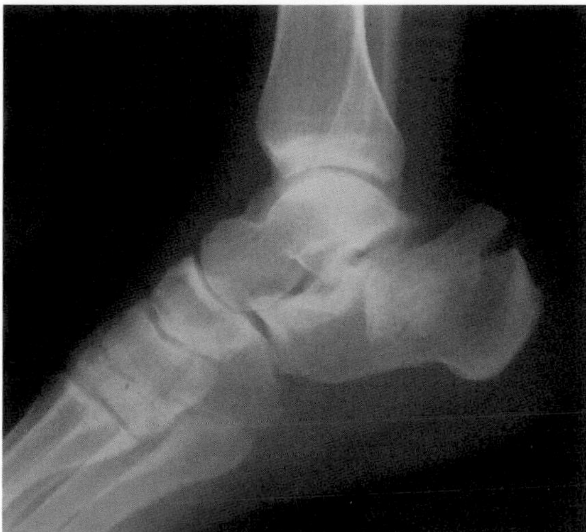

Figure 3–22. Tongue-type fracture of the calcaneus showing involvement of the subtalar joint.

4. Comminuted fractures—Some fracture patterns create such comminution and impaction that they defy classification. They all have in common significant soft tissue injury and subtalar joint incongruity.

B. Treatment

Treatment of displaced intraarticular fractures remains controversial. As already stated, the final outcome is much dependent on soft-tissue as well as bony healing. For the severely displaced fracture, the bursting nature of the injury may defy anatomic restoration.

Some surgeons still advise conservative treatment.

Other surgeons advocate early closed manipulation of displaced intraarticular fractures, to at least partially restore the external anatomic configuration of the heel region. Internal fixation with percutaneous pins may be performed. This is particularly successful for non-comminuted tongue-type fracture patterns. An axial pin is inserted in the tongue fragment, which is then disimpacted and reduced. The pin is then pushed further to stabilize the fracture (Essex-Lopresti technique). Open reduction and internal fixation with pins, screws, or plates, with or without bone grafting, has gained acceptance. The aim of ORIF is to restore Böhler's angle and improve heel alignment through stable fixation. A recent study has demonstrated a correlation between restoration of Böhlers angle and clinical outcome. Some authors advocate primary subtalar arthrodesis for severely comminuted fractures.

C. Complications

The most significant complication is posttraumatic degenerative arthritis. When only the subtalar joint is involved, talocalcaneal fusion is recommended. When the calcaneocuboid joint is also involved, triple arthrodesis should be performed. The rate of wound complications after ORIF has been reported to range from 0 to 12%. Other complications include compartment syndrome, neurovascular and tendon injury, heel pad pain and exostosis and, malunion. Compartment syndrome features in 10% of patients and should be excluded during the examination.

Extraarticular Fractures

Because posttraumatic joint disease is usually not a complication of these fractures, the final outcome is usually much better than that for intraarticular fractures. Fractures can affect any part of the bone.

A. Types of Fractures

1. Fracture of the tuberosity—Isolated fractures of the calcaneal tuberosity are rare.

2. Horizontal fracture—These fractures may be limited to the superior portion of the region of the former apophysis (avulsion type) or extend toward the subtalar joint in the substance of the tuberosity (beak type). A pull from the Achilles tendon may displace the fragment proximally, and reduction may be indicated. If the fragment is big enough, the application of skeletal traction can reduce it to the plantar-flexed foot, and the pin is incorporated in a long leg cast with the knee flexed at 30 degrees. For smaller fragments or when closed reduction is unsuccessful, ORIF with screws, wires, or pullout sutures is indicated.

3. Vertical fracture—Vertical fracture occurs in the sagittal plane somewhat medially through the tuberosity. Because the minor medial fragment normally is not widely displaced, plaster immobilization is not required but may reduce pain. Limitation of weight bearing with crutches will also be helpful.

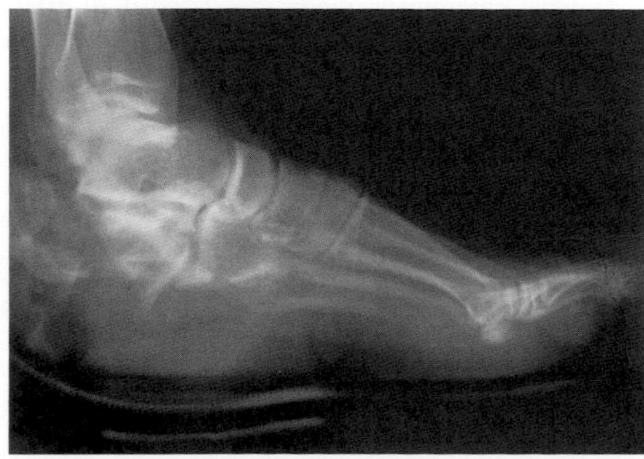

Figure 3–23. Joint depression-type fracture of the calcaneus. The posterior facet is separate fragment.

4. Non-articular fracture of the body—Comminuted fractures of the entire tuberosity, sparing the subtalar joint, are rare. Proximal displacement of the fragments may decrease the subtalar joint angle, but symptomatic degenerative arthritis is not an important sequela, even though some joint stiffness may persist permanently. Marked displacement may benefit from closed reduction to improve heel contour.

5. Fracture of the sustentaculum—A rare injury, fracture of the sustentaculum tali should be suspected in the patient with a history of eversion injury and pain below the medial malleolus, which is often accentuated by passive hyperextension of the great toe. Interposition of the flexor hallucis longus tendon may even prevent reduction. Conservative treatment is usually successful. In the rare instance of symptomatic nonunion, careful excision is indicated.

6. Fracture of the anterior process—Usually caused by forced inversion of the foot, it must be differentiated from midtarsal and ankle sprains. The firmly attached bifurcate ligament avulses a bony flake from the anterior process. Maximal tenderness and swelling occurs midway between the tip of the lateral malleolus and the base of the fifth metatarsal. A lateral oblique radiograph will demonstrate the fracture line.

Treatment is by a non-weight–bearing short leg cast in neutral position for 4 weeks.

7. Fracture of the medial process—This process gives origin to the abductor hallucis and part of the flexor digitorum brevis muscle and can be avulsed in eversion-abduction injuries. Conservative treatment with a well-molded short leg walking cast is usually successful.

B. Complications

Posttraumatic arthritis of the subtalar joint has already been mentioned as the most frequent complication of calcaneal fractures. Other complications include peroneal tendinitis, bone spurs, calcaneocuboid arthritis, and nerve entrapment syndromes (medial or lateral plantar branches and sural nerve, either from posttraumatic or postsurgical scarring).

Beals TC: Applications of ring fixators to complex foot and ankle trauma. Orthop Clin North Am 2001;32:205. [PMID: 11465130]

Berlet GC, Lee TH, Massa EG: Talar neck fractures. Orthop Clin North Am 2001;32:53. [PMID: 11465133]

Boon AJ et al: Snowboarder's talus fracture. Mechanism of injury. Am J Sports Med 2001;29:333. [PMID: 11394605]

Brunet JA: Calcaneal fractures in children. J Bone Joint Surgery Br 2000;82-B:211. [PMID: 10755428]

Fortin PT, Balazsy JE: Talus fractures: Evaluation and treatment. J Am Acad Orthop Surg 2001;9:114. [PMID: 11281635]

Harvey EJ et al: Morbidity associated with ORIF of intraarticular calcaneus fractures using a lateral approach. Foot Ankle Int 2001;22:868. [PMID: 11722137]

Juliano P, Nguyen HV: Fractures of the calcaneus. Orthop Clin North Am 2001;32:35. [PMID: 11465132]

Lim EV, Leung JP: Complications of intraarticular calcaneal fractures. Clin Orthop 2001;391:7. [PMID: 11603691]

Longino D, Buckley RE: Bone graft in the operative treatment of displaced intraarticular calcaneal fractures: Is it helpful? J Orthop Trauma 2001;15:280. [PMID: 11371794]

Rammelt S, Zwipp H: Calcaneus fractures: facts, controversies and recent developments. Injury 2004;35:443. [PMID 15081321]

ANKLE FRACTURES & DISLOCATIONS

Fractures and dislocations of the ankle are among the most common injuries treated by orthopedic surgeons. This injury is seen in all age groups, with a slightly different fracture pattern in children and adolescents than with adults. The ankle joint itself is limited to one plane of motion: plantarflexion and dorsiflexion in the sagittal plane. With incorporation of the motion of the subtalar joint (which allows for inversion and eversion in the coronal plane), the foot is able to move in a complex and varied arc in relationship to the leg.

Anatomy & Biomechanical Principles

The distal tibia and fibula are structures easily palpable because of their minimal soft-tissue coverage. The muscles, tendons, and neurovascular structures in the leg are generally grouped into anterior, lateral, and posterior compartments. In the distal leg, the compartments are predominantly tendinous, with little muscle being present. The tibia has a tubular diaphysis with wide flaring metaphyses both proximally and distally. The shape and size of the bone are markedly different in the proximal versus distal metaphysis. A cross-section of the midshaft tibia is approximately triangular, whereas a cross-section of the distal metaphysis is rounder and smaller in diameter. The inner and distal articular surfaces of the distal tibia and fibula form the ankle mortise (a uniplanar hinge joint). The ankle mortise serves as the "roof" over the talus. The articular portions of the lateral and medial malleoli serve as constraining buttresses to allow for controlled plantarflexion and dorsiflexion in the ankle mortise. This geometric configuration resists rotation of the talus in the ankle mortise. Further constraint and stability are provided by the interosseous membrane, the ankle capsule, the deltoid ligament medially and the lateral ligamentous complex (composed of the anterior talofibular, calcaneofibular, and posterior talofibular ligaments). The syndesmotic ligament connects the tibia to the fibula at the level of the tibial plafond. It allows for 1–2 mm of mortise widening, with ankle plantarflexion and dorsiflexion, accommodating the geometry of the talar dome. The bony architecture of the mortise also provides some constraint to posterior subluxation of the talus. This is provided by the cup-shaped tibial plafond and the slightly increased width of the talar dome anteriorly as compared with posteriorly.

The distal tibia also serves to absorb the compressive loads and stress placed on the ankle. The internal trabecular pattern of the bone helps transmit, diffuse, and resorb the compressive forces. Cross-sectional studies have shown that reduced activity and old age lead to resorption of cancellous bone, thereby decreasing the compressive resistance of the distal tibia.

Fracture-dislocations of the ankle are frequently referred to as **bimalleolar** (fractures of the medial and lateral malleoli) or **trimalleolar** (fractures of the medial, lateral, and posterior malleoli). Fracture of the lateral malleolus with complete rupture of the deltoid ligament (Dupuytren's fracture) or fracture of the medial malleolus with complete disruption of the syndesmosis and a proximal fibular shaft fracture (Maisonneuve's fracture) are also considered bimalleolar fractures on a functional basis.

Classification

The purpose of any classification scheme is to provide a means to better understand the extent of injury, describe an injury, and determine a treatment plan. Presently, the two most widely used classification schemes for describing ankle fractures are the Lauge-Hansen and Weber classifications.

In 1950, Lauge-Hansen described a classification system based on mechanism of injury that described over 95% of all ankle fractures (Figure 3–24). By stressing freshly amputated limbs in combinations of supination, pronation, adduction, abduction, and external rotation, he was able to describe nearly all fracture patterns. Pronation and supination refer to the position of the patient's foot at the instance of injury, while adduction, abduction, and external rotation refer to the vector of the force that is applied. Thus, four mechanisms of injury were described for ankle fractures: (1) supination adduction, (2) supination-external rotation, (3) pronation abduction, and (4) pronation-external rotation. Lauge-Hansen later added a fifth type of injury, the pronation dorsiflexion injury, in order to include a mechanism for tibial plafond fractures. This fifth type is caused by a compression-type injury.

The Weber classification is much simpler, and is based on the level at which the fibular fracture occurs.

Type A: Fracture in which the fibula is avulsed distal to the joint line. The syndesmotic ligament is

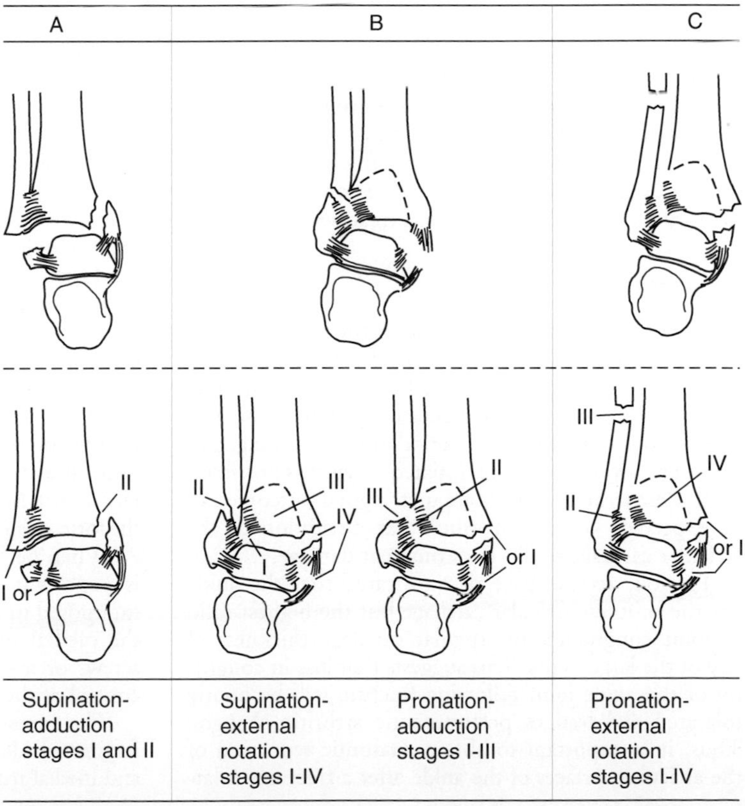

Figure 3–24. Comparison of Lauge-Hansen and Danis-Weber ankle classifications. (Reproduced, with permission, from Browner BD et al, eds: *Skeletal Trauma,* 2nd ed. WB Saunders, 1998.)

left intact, and the medial malleolus is either undamaged or is fractured in a shear-type pattern, with the fracture line angulating in a proximal-medial direction from the corner of the mortise.

Type B: Spiral fracture of the fibula beginning at the level of the joint line and extending in a proximal-posterior direction up the shaft of the fibula. Parts of the syndesmotic ligament complex can be torn, but the large interosseous ligament is usually left intact so that no widening of the distal tibiofibular articulation occurs. Complete syndesmotic disruptions, however can result from this fracture pattern.

The medial malleolus can either be left intact or sustain a transverse avulsion fracture. If the medial malleolus is left intact there can be a tear of the deltoid ligament. Avulsion fracture of the posterior lip of the tibia (posterior malleolus) can also occur.

Type C: Fracture of the fibula proximal to the syndesmotic ligament complex, with consequent disruption of the syndesmosis. Medial malleolar avulsion fracture or deltoid ligament rupture is also present. Posterior malleolar avulsion fracture can also occur. Figure 3–23 shows a comparison of the Weber and Lauge-Hansen schemes.

Many studies have stated that the above classification systems have failed to encompass all possible types of fracture. Furthermore, reproducibility is moderate and the fracture configuration is not predictive of prognosis. In fact, initial talar displacement and number of malleoli injured seem to be important for determining prognosis.

The AO classification system has better reproducibility as it is based on radiographic findings. However, it too cannot clearly separate fracture configurations to identify those that require surgical treatment.

Treatment

Four criteria should be met for the optimal treatment of ankle fractures: (1) dislocations and fractures should be reduced as soon as possible; (2) all joint surfaces must be precisely restored; (3) the fracture must be held in a reduced position during the period of bony healing, and (4) joint motion should be initiated as early as possible.

If these treatment goals are met, a good outcome can be expected, keeping in mind that disruption of the articular cartilage results in permanent damage.

Previous studies have demonstrated that the ankle has the thinnest articular cartilage but the highest ratio of joint congruence to articular cartilage thickness of any of the large joints. This suggests that loss in congruity of the ankle joint following fracture will be poorly tolerated and lead to posttraumatic arthritic changes. Thus, it is important to obtain anatomic reduction of the articular surfaces of the ankle after a fracture. A lateral talar shift of as little as 1 mm will decrease surface contact at the tibiotalar joint by 40%.

Initial treatment of ankle fractures should include immediate closed reduction and splinting, with the joint held in the most normal position possible to prevent neurovascular compromise of the foot. An ankle joint should never be left in a dislocated position. If the fracture is open, the patient should be given appropriate intravenous antibiotics and taken to the operating room on an urgent basis for irrigation and debridement of the wound, fracture site, and ankle joint. The fracture should also be appropriately stabilized at this time.

With the advent of excellent results obtained from the techniques of open reduction and rigid internal fixation as developed by the AO group, the standard of care for displaced ankle fractures has become operative intervention. Exceptions to this rule are nondisplaced, isolated Weber type B lateral malleolar fractures (supination eversion stage 2), distal fibular avulsion fractures, fractures in nonambulatory (ie, paraplegic) patients, and fractures in patients for whom the surgical risks are greater than the consequences of non-anatomic reduction of the fracture. The isolated previously described lateral or medial malleolar fractures may be treated in a well-molded short leg walking cast for 6 weeks. Unstable ankle fractures treated by immobilization should be placed in a long leg cast with the knee flexed to prevent weight bearing on the involved limb. Most non-displaced medial malleolar fractures should be treated with internal fixation because of the risk of nonunion, when these fractures are treated non-operatively.

When performing ORIF of ankle fractures, several principles must be followed. It is important to gently handle the soft tissues about the ankle so as to minimize the risks of infection and wound-healing problems. In the treatment of bimalleolar and trimalleolar fractures, the lateral malleolus should usually be reduced and internally fixed first. This has two benefits: (1) it helps to correctly restore the original limb length, and (2) because of the strong ligamentous connections between the lateral malleolus and talus (anterior and posterior talofibular ligaments), initial fixation of the lateral malleolus will correctly position the talus in the mortise. If a long oblique fracture of the lateral malleolus is present, fixation can sometimes be adequately obtained with two interfragmentary screws. More commonly, however, further fixation, in the form of a neutralization plate and screws, is required.

When performing ORIF of the medial malleolus, it is important to remove any soft tissue or periosteum interposed in the fracture site. It is also preferable to fix the medial malleolus with either two cancellous-type screws or a screw and a K-wire to provide rotational control of the medial malleolar fragment.

The necessity for fixation of the posterior malleolar fragment is dependent on several factors. After the lateral and medial malleolar fractures have been internally fixed, ligamentotaxis often will anatomically reduce the posterior malleolar fragment. If this fragment represents less than 25% of the articular surface of the tibial plafond and there is less than 2 mm of displacement, internal fixation is not always required. If the fragment does not reduce on the intraoperative radiograph with ligamentotaxis, or if the fragment represents more than 25% of the articular surface, most authors agree that it should be internally fixed. Several methods have been described for this, utilizing either direct fixation posteriorly via the lateral or medial incisions, or a lag screw from anterior to posterior.

Following surgery, the limb is placed in a bulky sterile dressing with plaster splints from the ball of the foot to the proximal calf to allow for wound healing. The ankle is kept in neutral position to prevent equinus deformity. After the sutures are removed at 1–2 weeks, the surgeon must decide whether to begin early mobilization of the ankle joint. If the patient is reliable and stable fixation was achieved at the time of surgery, then early range of motion may be initiated, keeping the patient on crutches and not allowing weight bearing. If there is a question about patient reliability or stability of fixation, the limb can be placed in a short leg cast for added protection. Usually at 6 weeks all immobilization is discontinued and weight bearing is slowly advanced. Physical therapy often helps promote ankle motion, strengthening, and regained ankle proprioception.

Barrie J et al: Ankle fractures-Pathomechanics and classification. Blackburn foot and ankle hyperbook: http://www.blackburnfeet.org.uk/hyperbook/trauma/ankle_fractures/pathomechanics_and_classification.htm

Egol KA, Dolan R, Koval KJ: Functional outcome of surgery for fractures of the ankle. J Bone Joint Surg Br 2000;82-B:246. [PMID: 10755435]

Gehrmann RM et al: Athlete's ankle injuries: diagnosis and management. Am J Orthop 2005;34:551. [PMID: 16375063]

Hintermann B et al: Arthroscopic findings in acute fractures of the ankle. J Bone Joint Surg Br 2000;82-B:345. [PMID: 10813167]

Kay RM, Matthys GA: Pediatric ankle fractures: Evaluation and treatment. J Am Acad Orthop Surg 2001;9:268. [PMID: 11476537]

Obremskey WT et al: Change over time of SF-36 functional outcomes for operatively treated unstable ankle fractures. J Orthop Trauma 2002;15:30. [PMID: 11782630]

Pankovich AM: Acute indirect ankle injuries in the adult. J Orthop Trauma 2002;15:58. [PMID: 11782638]

Saltzman R, French BG, Mizel MS: Ankle fracture with syndesmotic injury: case controversies. J Orthop Trauma 2000; 14: 113. [PMID: 10716383]

Tabrizi P et al: Limited dorsiflexion predisposes to injuries of the ankle in children. J Bone Joint Surg Br 2000;82-B:1103. [PMID: 11132266]

Tornetta P: Competence of the deltoid ligament in bimalleolar ankle fractures after medial malleolar fixation. J Bone Joint Surg;82-A:843. [PMID: 10859104]

Tornetta P, Creevy W: Lag screw only fixation of the lateral malleolus. J Orthop Trauma 2001;15:119. [PMID: 11232650]

TIBIA & FIBULA INJURIES

Anatomy

The tibial diaphysis is straight and triangular in cross-section. Its anteromedial border and anterior crest are palpable throughout the entire length of the bone, and are useful landmarks for closed reduction techniques and cast molding with pressure relief, as are the palpable fibular head, distal third of the fibula, medial malleolus and patellar tendon. The distal half of the leg has more tendons and less muscle than the proximal half, and thus soft tissue coverage and blood supply of the distal tibia is more precarious than its proximal portion. The fibula transmits approximately one sixth of the axial load from the knee to the foot and the tibia five sixths.

From a surgical standpoint, the leg has been divided into four compartments. A compartment is defined by the unyielding boundaries, such as bone and fascia, enclosing a given content. The anterior compartment is limited medially by the tibia, posteriorly by the interosseous membrane, laterally by the fibula, and anteriorly by the crural fascia. It contains the tibialis anterior, extensor hallucis longus, extensor digitorum longus, and peroneus tertius muscles, as well as the anterior tibial artery and the deep branch of the peroneal nerve. It is responsible for ankle and toe extension. The lateral compartment contains the peroneus brevis and longus muscles responsible for ankle flexion and foot eversion and the superficial branch of the peroneal nerve. The superficial posterior compartment contains the gastrocnemius, soleus, plantaris, and popliteus muscles and the sural nerve. It is responsible for plantar flexion of the foot and ankle. The deep posterior compartment is enclosed by the tibia, the interosseous membrane, and the deep transverse fascia. It contains the tibialis posterior, flexor hallucis longus, and flexor digitorum longus muscles, and also the posterior tibial and peroneal arteries and the tibial nerve.

1. Tib-Fib Fractures

Fractures of the tibial or fibular diaphysis are the result of direct or indirect trauma, with some of these injuries being open fractures. A thorough assessment of the surrounding soft tissues is mandatory. One must remember that the size of the skin wound does not necessarily correlate with the amount of underlying soft tissue damage. A 1 cm skin laceration can be associated with an extensive muscle and periosteal injury, making the fracture a Gustilo grade 3 instead of 1, with a much poorer prognosis. Also, closed tibia fractures can be associated with significant soft tissue injury. Tscherne and Oestern in 1982 classified the soft tissue injury in ascending order of severity (grades 0 to 3):

Grade 0: soft-tissue damage is absent or negligible.

Grade 1: there is a superficial abrasion or contusion caused by fragment pressure from within.

Grade 2: a deep contaminated abrasion is present associated with localized skin or muscle contusion from direct trauma. Impending compartment syndrome is included in this category.

Grade 3: the skin is extensively contused or crushed and muscular damage may be severe. Also, subcutaneous avulsions, compartment syndrome and rupture of a major blood vessel associated with a closed fracture are additional criteria.

When the fracture is displaced, the clinical diagnosis is usually evident. All compartments should be palpated, and a thorough distal neurovascular examination should be recorded.

Radiographs in the anteroposterior and lateral projections are taken of the entire leg, including the knee and ankle joints. Oblique views are sometimes necessary. Fractures of the distal end of the tibia (pilon or plafond fractures) can be better visualized with CT scanning.

Fibula Diaphysis Fractures

Isolated fibula fractures can be associated with other injuries of the leg, such as fracture of the tibia or fracture-dislocation of the ankle joint. One should pay particular attention to the medial malleolus to rule out deltoid ligament rupture or medial malleolus fracture. Isolated fibula fracture can be the result of a direct or "tapping" mechanism; however, it can also coincide with syndesmosis disruption. If reduction of the mortise is congruent, radiographic follow-up needs to be careful to ensure maintenance of reduction.

Tibia Diaphyseal Fractures

Isolated fractures of the tibial diaphysis are usually the result of torsional stress. There is a tendency for the tibia to displace into varus angulation because of an intact fibula.

Fractures of both the tibia and fibula are more unstable, and displacement can recur after reduction. The fibular fracture usually heals independently of the reduction achieved. The same does not apply to the tibia. There is some controversy as to what is an acceptable reduction of a tibial shaft fracture in the adult. The following criteria are generally accepted: apposition of 50% or more of the diameter of the bone in both anteroposterior and lateral projections, no more than 5 degrees of varus or valgus angulation, 5 degrees of angulation in the anteroposterior plane, 10 degrees of rotation, and 1 cm of shortening. It is assumed that fracture healing in an unacceptable position (ie, malunion) will affect the mechanics of the knee or ankle joint and possibly lead to premature degenerative joint disease.

Acceptable reduction can be obtained in one of many ways, and this is another area of ongoing controversy: closed versus open treatment. The goal of any treatment is to allow the fracture to heal in an acceptable position with minimal negative effect on the surrounding tissues or joints. Closed reduction is obtained under general anesthesia if necessary, and the patient is immobilized in a long leg non-weight–bearing cast. Weekly radiographs for the first 4 weeks will help ensure that displacement does not occur. If it does, angulation can be corrected by "wedging" the cast. This involves dividing the plaster circumferentially and inserting wedges in the appropriate direction after corrective manipulation. At 6 weeks, some shaft fractures are stable enough to be put in a short leg weight-bearing cast, usually a patellar tendon-bearing cast or brace as recommended by Sarmiento. Protected weight bearing should be continued until clinical and radiologic healing is evident.

If acceptable and stable reduction cannot be obtained by closed means, other methods are required. Skeletal traction via a calcaneal transfixing pin is rarely used, although it is an acceptable short-term option in the polytraumatized patient. An external fixator with an outer frame is extremely useful for open fractures, as it provides rigid fixation and still allows access for wound care. This is still the initial treatment for some Gustilo type 3 injuries and in the hemodynamically unstable patient. A reamed intramedullary nail is the recommended treatment for most displaced closed and possibly Gustilo type 1-3a fractures. Intramedullary nails are introduced from a proximal starting point anterior to the tibial tubercle and across the fracture site under fluoroscopic control without opening the fracture site. Dynamic or static interlocking can be achieved with transfixing screws on both ends of the nail, and this maintains length and provides rotational control.

Open reduction and internal fixation with plates and screws using minimally invasive percutaneous plate osteosynthesis (MIPPO) techniques, avoids direct exposure of the fracture site and decreases soft-tissue dissection, devascularization of the bone, risk of infection, and delayed union. This technique is useful in periarticular fractures with diaphyseal extension.

Recent studies comparing tibia fractures treated with cast immobilization with those treated with intramedullary nailing indicate that the intramedullary nail group has a shorter time to healing, a better rate of healing, and an improved functional score. Disadvantages of operative treatment include infection, wound problems, and possible contractures. The advantages of closed treatment are early mobilization with or without weight bearing and a short hospital stay, with less risk of infection from the operative approach. Closed treatment does not preclude further surgical treatment. Disadvantages include residual deformity, knee or ankle joint stiffness, and more difficult wound care. Sound clinical judgment is needed in the decision-making process. An isolated closed tibial fracture in a compliant patient is a much different problem than the same tibial injury in a polytraumatized comatose patient.

Fracture of the Distal End of the Tibia

Also referred to as **pilon** or **plafond** fractures, these fractures involve the distal articular surface of the tibia at the tibiotalar joint. Ruedi and Allgower classified these injuries into I, II, and III based upon the amount of articular displacement and comminution, which represents a wide spectrum of injury (Figure 3–25).

As for any intraarticular fracture, the goal of treatment is to restore an anatomic articular surface. This can be difficult and sometimes impossible. Closed reduction of displaced fractures is almost never successful and external fixation spanning the injury, with or without ORIF of the fibula can be initially performed. Once soft-tissue swelling subsides, minimally invasive open reduction and percutaneous techniques should be attempted. Bone graft can be added to metaphyseal defects to support the articular surface. When the fracture is so comminuted that internal fixation is impossible, an attempt at indirect reduction by ligamentotaxis should be done: ORIF of the fibular fracture to restore length, and closed reduction and external fixation of the tibia. This can usually restore normal contours and alignment of the distal leg and make an eventual tibiotalar fusion easier should disabling posttraumatic arthritisoccur.

These fractures are notorious for associated soft-tissue damage. Swelling can be impressive, and prolonged

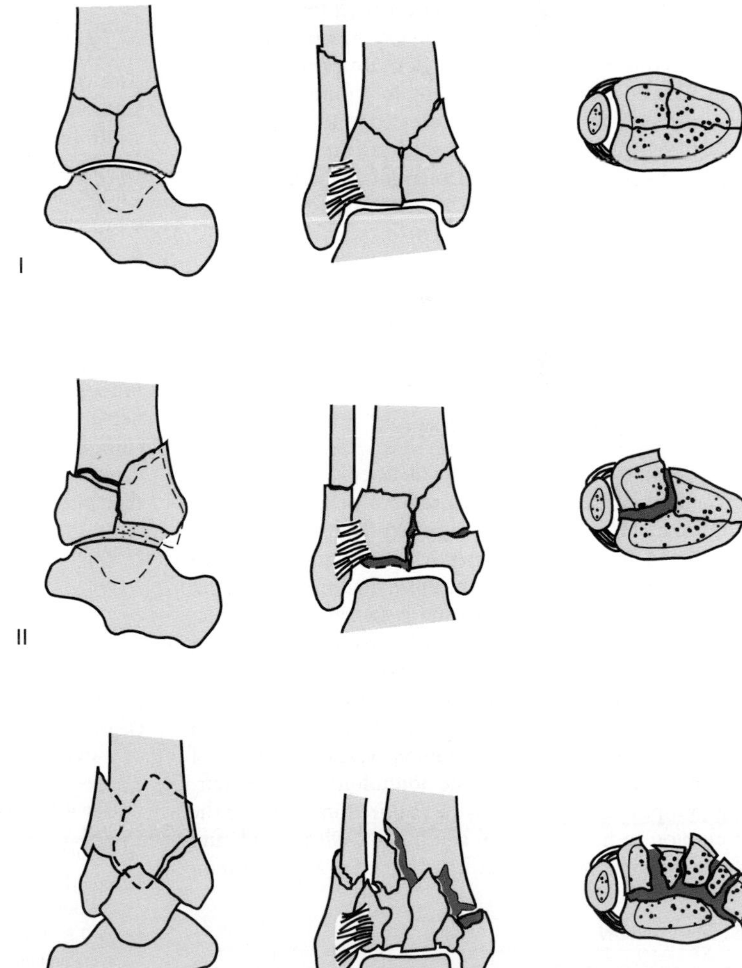

Figure 3–25. Ruedi and Allgower classification of Pilon fractures. (Reproduced, with permission, from Browner BD et al, eds: *Skeletal Trauma,* 2nd ed. WB Saunders, 1998.)

leg elevation is often necessary, especially to prevent surgical wound problems after open reduction. If open surgical treatment of the tibial pilon is planned, the surgery should be deferred until the soft tissue condition improves, usually 7 to 14 days, once the "wrinkle" sign appears. Surgical incisions through hemorrhagic blisters should be avoided. Healing is likely to be slow, and weight bearing should be carefully started only when radiologic evidence of bone healing is present.

Compartment Syndrome

Compartment syndrome is a frequent concern in tibia fractures and is caused by increased pressure in any of the four closed osteofascial spaces, compromising circulation and perfusion of the tissues within the involved compartment. Nerves and muscle tissue are particularly susceptible.

Fasciotomies are performed through a lateral and a medial incision in the skin and fascia of all four compartments. Compartment pressure measurements are taken after decompression to ensure adequate pressure reduction. Tissue debridement is kept to a minimum. The wounds are left open, sterilely dressed, and then treated by delayed primary closure or split-thickness skin grafting 5 days later. Delaying treatment of any compartment syndrome by more than 6–8 hours can lead to irreversible nerve and muscle damage.

Complications

Complications are common after tibia and fibula fractures and may be related to the nature of the injury itself or to its management.

A. Delayed Union or Nonunion

Because of its relatively poor soft-tissue coverage, the tibia, particularly its distal third, is prone to delayed union or nonunion. This occurs more frequently in high-energy, open, and segmental fractures. Pain and motion at the fracture are noted to be present more than 6 months after the injury. Radiographs show the persistence of the fracture line without bridging callus. Sclerosis and flaring of the bone ends characterize the hypertrophic nonunion, whereas osteopenia and thinning of the fragments are seen in atrophic nonunions. Early weight bearing is thought to stimulate bone healing. If nonunion develops in spite of this, rigid fixation (hypertrophic nonunion) or bone grafting (atrophic nonunion) may be required in order for the nonunion to heal. Electrical stimulation, ultrasound, and shock waves have limited efficacy but may achieve union in selected cases.

B. Malunion

Malunion may lead to premature degenerative joint disease. Corrective osteotomies may be required. When associated with shortening, multiple-plane correction and lengthening can be obtained after corticotomy and external fixation with Ilizarov-type devices, which allow progressive correction of the deformity.

C. Infection

Infection of the tibia following open fracture or surgical treatment remains the most severe complication, especially when associated with nonunion. Perioperative prophylactic antibiotic therapy and adequate debridement and irrigation of open fractures are not always successful in preventing this dreaded complication. Recently, the generous utilization of free muscle flaps to increase the local blood supply has significantly improved the overall results of treatment, although amputation is still occasionally required.

D. Complex Regional Pain Syndrome (Reflex Sympathetic Dystrophy)

Complex regional pain syndrome is a fortunately rare complication of unknown cause. It is characterized by pain out of proportion to the original injury. Swelling, pain, and vasomotor disturbances are the hallmarks of this syndrome. Gradual increase in weight bearing and early joint mobilization will minimize the occurrence of this complication. Chemical or surgical sympathetic blockade may be helpful for the more severe forms of this disease.

E. Other Complications

Posttraumatic arthritis is a frequent occurrence after pilon fractures or as a complication of tibial shaft malunion. Joint stiffness and ankylosis may occur after prolonged immobilization. Soft-tissue injuries, including those of nerve, vessels, or muscles, have been discussed in the compartment syndrome section. Sequelae may include dropfoot and claw toe deformities and may require further soft-tissue or bone procedures.

Blauth M et al: Surgical options for the treatment of severe tibial pilon fractures: A study of three techniques. J Orthop Trauma 2001;15:153. [PMID: 11265004]

Finkemeier CG et al: A prospective, randomized study of intramedullary nails inserted with and without reaming for the treatment of open and closed fractures of the tibial shaft. J Orthop Trauma 2000;14:187. [PMID: 10791670]

Gopal S et al: Fix and flap: The radical orthopaedic and plastic treatment of severe open fractures of the tibia. J Bone Joint Surg Br 2000;82-B:959. [PMID: 11041582]

Hernigou P, Cohen D: Proximal entry for intramedullary nailing of the tibia. J Bone Joint Surg Br 2000;82-B:33. [PMID: 10697311]

Keating JF et al: Reamed nailing of Gustilo grade-IIIB tibial fractures. J Bone Joint Surg Br 2000;82-B:1113. [PMID: 11132268]

Larsen LB, Madsen JE, Hoiness PR, Ovre S. Should insertion of intramedullary nails for tibial fractures be with or without reaming? A prospective, randomized study with 3.8 years' follow-up. J Orthop Trauma 2004;18(3):144-9. [PMID:15091267]

Lin J, Hou SM: Unreamed locked tight-fitting nailing for acute tibial fractures. J Orthop Trauma 2001;15:40. [PMID: 11132268]

Nassif JM et al: Effect of acute reamed versus unreamed intramedullary nailing on compartment pressure when treating closed tibial shaft fractures: A randomized prospective study. J Orthop Trauma 2000;14:554. [PMID: 11149501]

Tscherne H, Lobenhoffer P. A new classification of soft-tissue damage in open and closed fractures. Unfallheilkunde. 1982 Mar; 85(3):111–5.

Samuelson MA, McPherson EJ, Norris L: Anatomic assessment of the proper insertion site for a tibial intramedullary nail. J Orthop Trauma 2002;16:23. [PMID: 11782628]

Sarmiento A, Latta LL. 450 closed fractures of the distal third of the tibia treated with a functional brace. Clin Orthop. 2004 Nov;(428):261-71Thordarson DB: Complications after treatment of tibial pilon fractures: Prevention and management strategies. J Am Acad Orthop Surg 2000;8:253. [PMID: 10951114]

Vives MJ et al: Soft tissue injuries with the use of safe corridors for transfixion wire placement during external fixation of distal tibia fractures: An anatomic study. J Orthop Trauma 2001; 15:555. [PMID: 11733671]

Zelle BA et al: Treatment of distal tibia fractures without articular involvement: a systematic review of 1125 fractures. J Orthop Trauma 2006;20:76. [PMID: 16424818]

Ziran BH, Darowish M, Klatt BA, Agudelo JF, Smith WR. Intramedullary nailing in open tibia fractures: a comparison of two techniques. Int Orthop 2004;28(4):235-8. [PMID: 15160254]

INJURIES AROUND THE KNEE

Anatomy & Biomechanical Principles

The knee is a modified synovial hinge joint formed by three bones: the distal femur, the proximal tibia, and the patella. It is often divided into three compartments: medial, lateral, and patellofemoral.

The distal femoral diaphysis broadens into two curved condyles at the metaphyseal junction. Each condyle is convex and articulates distally with its corresponding tibial plateau. Their articular surfaces join anteriorly to articulate with the patella. Posteriorly, they remain separate to form the intercondylar notch. The lateral condyle is wider in the sagittal plane (preventing lateral patella displacement) and extends further proximally. The medial condyle is narrower but extends further distally. This difference in length of both condyles allows for the distance between both knees, when weight bearing, to be smaller than the distance between both hips. Both condylar surfaces form a horizontal plane parallel to the ground and create an anatomic angle (physiologic valgus position) of 5–7 degrees with the femoral shaft. Normally, the centers of the hip, knee, and ankle joints are all aligned to form a mechanical angle of 0 degrees. The supracondylar area of the femur is defined as the distal 9 cm. Fractures proximal to this are considered femoral shaft fractures and carry a different prognosis.

As for the distal femur, the proximal tibia widens proximally at the diaphyseal-metaphyseal junction to form the medial and lateral tibial plateaus (condyles). There is a 7–10 degrees slope from anterior to posterior of the tibial plateaus. The tibial eminence, with its medial and lateral spines, separates both compartments and is the attachment for the cruciate ligaments and the menisci. Distal to the joint itself, the tibia has two prominences: the tibial tubercle anteriorly, where the patellar tendon attaches, and Gerdy's tubercle anterolaterally, where the iliotibial band inserts. Posterolaterally, the under surface of the tibial condyle articulates with the fibular head to form the proximal tibiofibular joint.

The patella is the biggest sesamoid bone in the body. It lies within the substance of the quadriceps tendon. The distal third of the under surface is nonarticular and provides attachment for the patellar tendon. The proximal two thirds articulates with the anterior surface of the femoral condyles and is divided into medial and lateral facets by a longitudinal ridge. The area of contact at the patellofemoral joint varies according to the degree of knee flexion. On each side of the patella are the medial and lateral retinacular expansions formed by fibers of the vastus medialis and vastus lateralis muscles. These expansions bypass the patella to insert directly on the tibia. When intact, they can allow active knee extension even in the presence of a fractured patella. The blood supply to the patella is derived from anastomosis of the genicular vessels from the distal pole proximally. Avascular necrosis of a proximal fracture fragment is not uncommon.

The main plane of motion of the knee is flexion and extension, but physiologically, internal and external rotation, abduction and adduction (varus and valgus), and anterior and posterior translations also occur. The intrinsic bony configuration of the joint affords little stability. A complex soft-tissue network provides joint stability under physiologic loading. It includes passive stabilizers such as medial and lateral collateral ligaments, medial and lateral menisci, anterior and posterior cruciate ligaments, joint capsule, and active stabilizers such as the extensor mechanism, the popliteus muscle, and the hamstrings with their capsular expansions. All these soft tissue components work together in an extremely complex and finely tuned way to prevent excessive displacement of the joint surfaces throughout the full arc of motion under physiologic loading. When abnormal stresses that exceed the soft tissues' ability to resist them are transmitted across the joint, an infinite range of injuries can occur. These may be isolated or combined, partial or complete, and may or may not be associated with bony injuries. An accurate diagnosis, although sometimes difficult, is essential before the appropriate treatment can be decided upon.

LIGAMENTOUS INJURIES

As already stated, a wide spectrum of ligamentous injuries, from partial sprain of an isolated ligament to major soft-tissue disruption are seen in knee dislocations. Associated injuries to bone, cartilage, and menisci are common.

Knowledge of the mechanism of injury is of paramount importance, as certain injury patterns may be anticipated. Dashboard injuries may cause posterior translation of the tibia under the femur with posterior cruciate ligament damage. Hyperextension injuries, as seen in skiers, volleyball players, or basketball players, often involve the anterior cruciate ligament. Tackles at knee level in football often create a valgus flexion external rotation injury with damage to the medial collateral ligament, medial meniscus, and anterior cruciate ligament (The Terrible Triad). A good clinical examination is sometimes difficult, particularly in a young muscular athlete with a large lower extremity, but it is essential and will usually provide key diagnostic information.

Plain radiographs are of limited benefit. They will show fractures, bony avulsions at ligament attachment sites, or capsular avulsion signs such as the lateral capsular sign (Segond fracture), which is diagnostic of anterior cruciate ligament disruption (Figure 3–26).

Tomograms and contrast arthrograms have only limited indications because MRI has become so widely accepted. MRI is now by far the imaging tool of choice for ligamentous injuries of the knee, with an accuracy rate above 95%. Diagnostic arthroscopy is now reserved for cases when MRI is inconclusive or the surgeon is fairly sure that surgical treatment of a lesion will be necessary.

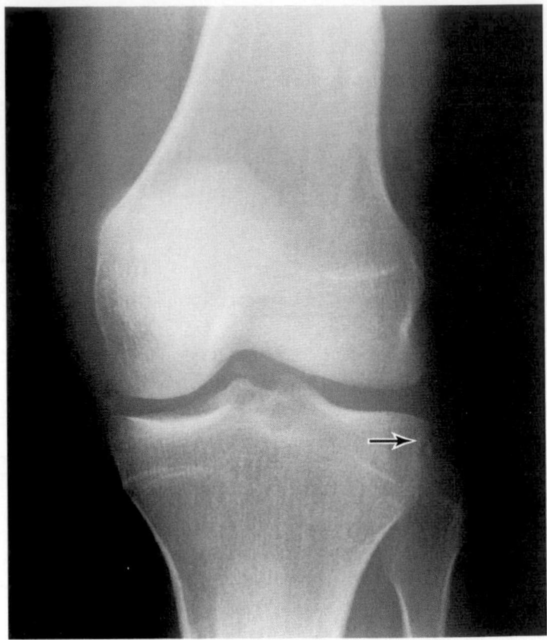

A

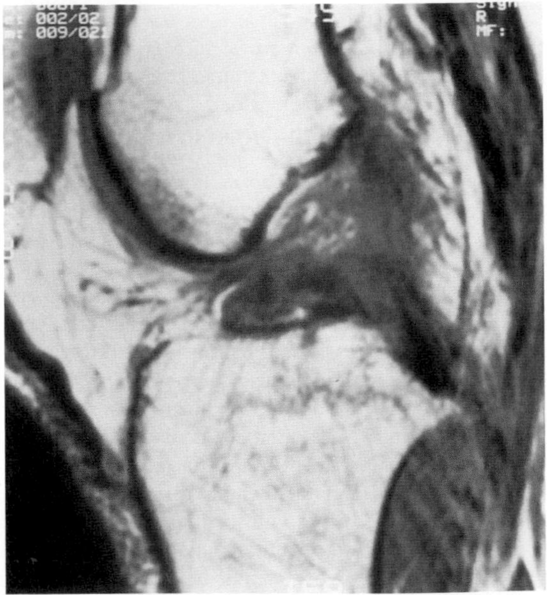

B

Figure 3–26. Lateral capsular sign, diagnostic of anterior cruciate ligament injury, as demonstrated by radiograph (**A**) and MRI studies (**B**).

1. Medial (Tibial) Collateral Ligament Injury

This ligament normally resists valgus angulation at the knee joint. A history of abduction injury, often with a torsional component, is usually obtained. Examination reveals tenderness over the site of the lesion and often some knee effusion. When compared with the contralateral knee, valgus stressing with the knee flexed at 20–30 degrees will show exaggerated laxity at the joint line, signaling a complete tear. Stress radiographs can, on rare occasions, be useful in confirming the diagnosis.

Grade 1 and 2 sprains (incomplete) are treated with protective weight bearing in a hinged brace or cast to prevent further injury while healing progresses. Grade 3 sprains (complete) are rarely isolated. Known associated injuries, such as medial meniscus damage, anterior cruciate ligament tear, or lateral tibial plateau fractures, should be systematically ruled out. Most surgeons now favor conservative treatment of isolated grade 3 medial collateral ligament tears in a long leg hinged-knee brace for 4–6 weeks because surgical repair has not proved to provide any long-term benefit.

2. Lateral (Fibular) Collateral Ligament Injury

This ligament originates from the lateral femoral condyle and inserts on the fibular head. It resists varus angulation at the knee joint. Isolated injuries are extremely rare. Most often, there is a combination of varying degrees of injury to the posterolateral corner, which includes the biceps tendon, posterolateral capsule, popliteus tendon, and iliotibial band. Injury to the peroneal nerve is not uncommon. Pain and tenderness are present over the lateral aspect of the knee, usually with some intraarticular effusion. In severe injuries, there is abnormal laxity on varus stressing compared with the other knee.

Radiographs often show avulsion of the fibular head. When this fragment is of sufficient size, internal fixation with a screw gives excellent results. Conservative management involves protected weight bearing in a long leg hinged-knee brace for 4–6 weeks. Most injuries require operative treatment, although conservative treatment may be indicated for the low-demand patient with mild laxity.

3. Anterior Cruciate Ligament Injury

This ligament originates at the posteromedial aspect of the lateral femoral condyle and inserts near the medial tibial spine. Because it is composed of at least two distinct fiber bundles, part of it remains taut throughout the normal flexion-extension arc of motion. It prevents anterior translation (gliding) of the tibia under the femoral condyles. Isolated injuries are frequent, especially with hyperextension mechanism, but associated medial collateral ligament, medial meniscus, posteromedial capsule, and even posterior cruciate ligament injuries are more common. When the tear is complete, it most often occurs within the substance of its fibers. Rarely, bony avulsion at the femoral or tibial attachment will be seen on plain radiograms.

Clinical Findings

The patient usually recalls the mechanism of injury, and classically feels a popping or snapping sensation in the knee. A moderate effusion usually accumulates during the first few hours is usually the rule. The only clinical finding in acute anterior cruciate ligament deficiency may be a positive Lachman's test, which is the anterior drawer test performed with 20–30 degrees of knee flexion. The classic drawer test, done with the knee flexed at 90 degrees and the foot resting on the table, is not as reliable. The injured knee should always be compared with the uninjured contralateral knee. In chronic anterior cruciate ligament deficiency, secondary restraints have stretched out and other clinical signs, such as the pivot shift and the active drawer sign, become more apparent.

Treatment

Treatment remains controversial despite the abundance of literature on this topic over the last 20 years. Most surgeons feel that surgical reconstruction affords the best long-term results. Non-operative treatment may have a role in the stable knee without signs of quadriceps wasting. When bony avulsions from the femur or tibia are present, surgical repair is indicated as bone-to-bone healing and good long-term results have been demonstrated.

Primary repair of the ligament stumps without reconstruction is likely to fail. The trend presently seems to reserve surgical reconstruction for young high-demand athletes. For others, conservative management with rehabilitation therapy and bracing can give satisfactory results. Those patients who remain unacceptably unstable after conservative treatment can still benefit from delayed reconstructive surgery. Favored techniques at the present include the arthroscopically assisted use of the middle third of the patellar tendon or harvest of an autogenous hamstrings graft.

4. Posterior Cruciate Ligament Injury

The posterior cruciate ligament is a broad thick ligament that extends from the lateral aspect of the medial femoral condyle posteriorly and inserts extraarticularly over the back of the tibial plateau approximately 1 cm below the joint line. It resists posterior translation (gliding) of the tibia under the femoral condyle. It usually ruptures after a posteriorly directed force on the proximal tibia as is sometimes seen in dashboard injuries. Posterior cruciate ligament ruptures can also occur as the end stage of severe hyperextension injuries.

Clinical Findings

The posterior drawer test will be positive, as will the sag test, showing posterior sagging of the tibia with the knee flexed to 90 degrees compared with the opposite side. As for the anterior cruciate ligament, the rupture may be at the bone-ligament junction or more often in the middle substance of the ligament.

Treatment

Reattachment of bony avulsions should restore functional competency of the ligament. Repair of the middle substance tear alone is of no value. Complex reconstructions have been described but remain of unproved value for non-athletic patients. Conservative treatment with rehabilitation (particularly of the extensor mechanism), and even bracing, of isolated posterior cruciate ligament injuries is currently recommended.

5. Meniscal Injury

The meniscus is a fibrocartilage that allows a more congruous fit between the convex femoral condyle and the flat tibial plateau. Both medial and lateral menisci are attached peripherally and have a central free border. They are wedge-shaped and thicker at the periphery. The medial meniscus is C-shaped and the lateral meniscus is O-shaped, with both anterior and posterior horns almost touching medially. They are vascularized only at their peripheral third. Tears involving that vascularized portion have a better repair potential. The menisci spread the load more uniformly on the underlying cartilage, thus minimizing point contact and wear. They are secondary knee stabilizers but are more important in the ligament-deficient knee.

Clinical Findings

Tears can be secondary to trauma or attrition. The medial meniscus is more often involved. Symptoms include pain, swelling, a popping sensation, and occasionally locking and giving way. Examination usually reveals nonspecific medial or lateral joint-line pain, and occasionally grinding or snapping can be felt with tibial torsion and the knee flexed to 90 degrees (McMurray's sign). Radiographs are of minimal value but may rule out other disorders; MRI has replaced contrast arthrography as the diagnostic tool of choice.

Treatment

Initial conservative management with immobilization, bracing, protective weight bearing, and exercises can give good results. Arthroscopic evaluation and treatment is recommended for recurrent or persistent locking, recurrent effusion, or disabling pain. If the tear is large enough and in the vascularized portion, repair should be attempted. For other tears, the affected area should be removed, leaving as much as possible of the healthy meniscus. Routine total meniscectomy has been abandoned because of the high incidence of subsequent arthritis.

6. Chondral & Osteochondral Injuries

The hyaline articular cartilage is avascular and has no intrinsic capability to repair superficial lacerations. Deep injuries involve the bone in the subchondral plate, and extrinsic repair occurs first with a fibrin clot replaced by granulation tissue, which is then transformed to fibrocartilage. Repetitive injury can cause abnormal motion with shearing stresses that can loosen chondral or osteochondral fragments. Compression injuries to the cartilage can lead to posttraumatic chondromalacia.

Clinical Findings

Chondral injuries usually give nonspecific symptoms that mimic meniscal injury. Plain radiographs will often reveal a loose body if the osteochondral fragment is big enough. Tunnel views and patellar tangential views can be helpful in visualizing fragments. Pure chondral fragments will only be seen with contrast arthrograms or MRI, both of which can easily miss the smaller fragments. Arthroscopy remains the most accurate diagnostic procedure.

Treatment

Treatment is controversial. The age of the patient, skeletal maturity and the presence of adequate subchondral bone all play an important part in guiding treatment.

Removal of the free fragment, debridement of the donor site, and drilling of the underlying subchondral bone to promote fibrin clot formation is the most accepted treatment. Rarely, an osteochondral fragment involving weight-bearing cartilage is large enough to warrant reduction and internal fixation.

7. Knee Dislocation

Traumatic dislocation of the knee is a rare injury that often results from high-energy trauma, but may occur from low energy injuries in the elderly. It is classified according to the direction of displacement of the tibia: anterior, posterior, lateral, medial, or rotatory. Complete dislocation can occur only after extensive tearing of the supporting ligaments and soft tissues. Injury to the neighboring neurovascular bundle is common and should be looked for systematically.

Treatment

Knee dislocations require prompt reduction. This is most easily accomplished in the emergency room by applying axial traction on the leg. Rarely, reduction can only be obtained under general anesthesia. The role of angiography is controversial. If pulses and ankle-brachial pressure index are normal, the limb is closely observed. Studies have shown that the isolated presence of abnormal foot pulses is not sensitive enough to detect a surgical vascular injury. Furthermore, one study demonstrated no vascular injury in any of their traumatic knee dislocations with initial normal vascular examination. Angiograms can be useful in the limb with obvious vascular injury, but should not delay treatment. Any vascular injury should be repaired as soon as possible. Ischemia of more than 4 hours implies a poor prognosis for salvage of a functional limb. Prophylactic fasciotomies should be performed at the time of vascular repair to prevent compartment syndrome caused by postrevascularization edema.

The timing of the treatment of the ligamentous damage is also controversial. Most authors now agree that surgical repair of all ligaments is indicated in relatively young (<50 years) active patients. Others still prefer closed management in a cast or braces. Whatever method is used, close follow-up is essential, especially at the beginning, to prevent subluxation, usually posteriorly. If subluxation occurs, the knee should be maintained in a reduced position using a femorotibial external fixator. After 6–8 weeks of immobilization, the knee is protected in a long leg brace and motion is started. Intensive quadriceps and hamstring rehabilitation is necessary to minimize functional loss. The need for a brace for strenuous activities may be permanent.

PROXIMAL TIBIA FRACTURES

1. Tibial Plateau Fractures

Proximal tibia fractures account for 1% of all fractures. There is a wide spectrum of fracture patterns that involve the medial tibial plateau (10–23%), the lateral tibial plateau (55–70%), or both (11–31%). These fractures occur through metaphyseal bone. Like all metaphyseal fractures, the spongiosa is impacted and once reduced, there can be a void with functional bone loss. These fractures usually result from axial loading, as seen in falls from a high place, combined most often with some varus and valgus forces. It is reported that at least 20% of unilateral tibial plateau fractures are associated with ligament rupture of the opposite compartment. The bone fails in compression and shear, with the ligament in tension. This is not easy to determine clinically, because of pain and motion at the fracture site. A thorough neurovascular evaluation should be recorded.

Classification

Many different classification systems have been proposed, none with universal acceptance. The system most widely used today is the Schatzker classification; type I: split fracture of the lateral plateau, type II: split-depression of the lateral plateau, type III: depression of the lateral plateau, type IV: medial plateau fracture, type V: bicondylar fracture, and type VI: a fracture with metaphyseal-diaphyseal dissociation (Figure 3–27). Proper classification is based on quality radiographs, including oblique views if necessary. If fat is present in the knee aspirate and plain films fail to show any obvious fractures, occult injury needs to be ruled out. CT and more recently, MRI have all been used successfully for this purpose. MRI has also been useful to reduce inter-observer disparities in fracture classification, which in turn can affect management.

Treatment

The goal of treatment is to restore anatomic contours to the articular surface, to prevent posttraumatic degenerative joint disease, allow soft-tissue healing in optimal position, and prevent knee stiffness. Both closed and open treatment can achieve these goals. The choice will depend on multiple factors, including the patient's age and general medical condition, the degree of displacement and comminution of the fracture, associated local soft-tissue and bony injuries, local skin condition, residual knee stability, and fracture configuration.

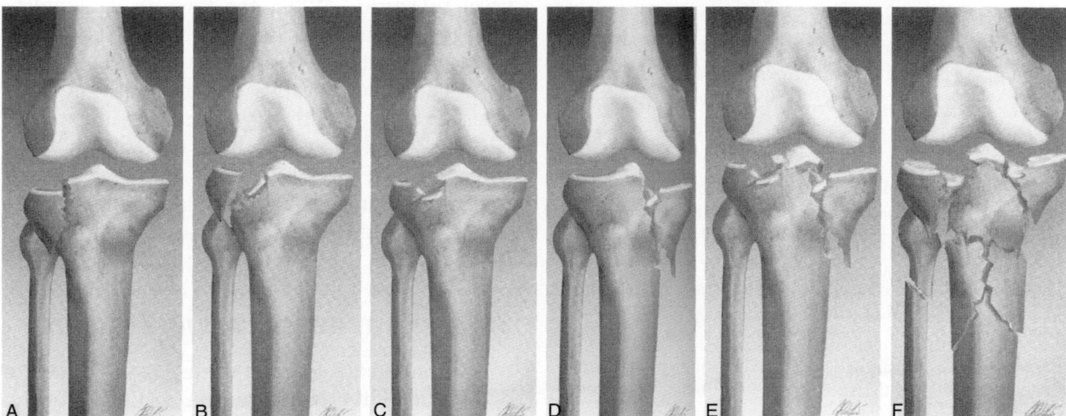

Figure 3–27. Schatzker classification of tibial plateau fractures: **A** (type I: lateral split), **B** (type II: lateral split depression), **C** (type III: lateral depression), **D** (type IV: medial plateau), **E** (type V: bicondylar), **F** (type VI: bicondylar with separation of metaphysis from diaphysis). (Reproduced, with permission, from Rockwood CA et al, eds: *Fractures in Adults,* 4th ed. Lippincott, 1996.)

Closed treatment with a cast or fracture brace is appropriate for minimally displaced fractures with no ligament instability. Definite varus and valgus laxity at full extension is a poor prognostic sign for closed treatment. Articular step-off of 3 mm or less and condylar widening of 5 mm or less can be treated conservatively. Lateral or valgus tilt up to 5 degrees is well tolerated. Medial plateau fractures with any significant displacement should be surgically stabilized. Articular step-off >3 mm should be anatomically fixed. Bicondylar fractures with any medial displacement, valgus tilt >5 degrees or with significant articular step-off should be surgically stabilized. Range of motion is usually allowed after 6 weeks and weight bearing after 3 months. Noncomminuted fractures can undergo closed reduction with fluoroscopic imaging and percutaneous pinning with cannulated screws.

Recently, reduction of the articular fragment under arthroscopic visualization has become more popular, particularly for Schatzker type I, II, III, and IV injuries. The depressed fragment is elevated and bone graft packed underneath to prevent loss of reduction.

Open reduction and internal fixation with plates and screws remains the traditional approach of operative treatment. Reduction should be as anatomically precise as possible, and fixation should be solid enough to allow early mobilization. More recently, Minimally Invasive Plate Osteosynthesis (MIPO) and the Less Invasive Stabilization Systems (LISS) are being used in the treatment of these injuries. Bone defects should be grafted with either autograft, allograft or structural graft substitutes. Early range of motion is allowed according to the stability of the construct. Weight bearing is occasionally allowed at 6–8 weeks but more frequently after 12 weeks.

An external monolateral or ring fixator can be used for provisional and definitive treatment depending upon the clinical situation and experience of the surgical team.

Hybrid and ring external fixators have been found to be useful for bicondylar injuries with severe soft tissue trauma.

Bai B et al: Effect of articular step-off and meniscectomy on joint alignment and contact pressures for fractures of the lateral tibial plateau. J Orthop Trauma 2001;15:101. [PMID: 11232647]

Cain EL, Clancy WG: Treatment algorithm for osteochondral injuries of the knee. Clin Sports Med. 2001 Apr;20(2):321-42. [PMID 11398361]

Chen FS, Rokito AS, Pitman MI: Acute and chronic posterolateral rotatory instability of the knee. J Am Acad Orthop Surg 2000; 8:97. [PMID: 1075373]

Collinge CA, Sanders RW: Percutaneous plating in the lower extremity. J Am Acad Orthop Surg 2000;8:211. [PMID: 10951109]

Geller J et al: Tension wire position for hybrid external fixation of the proximal tibia. J Orthop Trauma 2000;14:502. [PMID: 11083613]

Griffin LY et al: Noncontact anterior cruciate ligament injuries: Risk factors and prevention strategies. J Am Acad Orthop Surg 2000;8:141. [PMID: 10874221]

Kumar A, Whittle AP: Treatment of complex (Schatzker type VI) fractures of the tibial plateau with circular wire external fixation: A retrospective case review. J Orthop Trauma 2000; 14:339. [PMID: 10926241]

Larsson S, Bauer TW: Use of injectable calcium phosphate cement for fracture fixation: a review. Clin Orthop 2002 Feb;(395): 23-32. [PMID 11937863]

Lonner JH, Dupuy DE, Siliski JM: Comparison of magnetic resonance imaging with operative findings in acute traumatic dislocations of the adult knee. J Orthop Trauma 2000;14:183. [PMID: 10791669]

Lundy DW, Johnson KD: "Floating knee" injuries: Ipsilateral fractures of the femur and tibia. J Am Acad Orthop Surg 2001; 9:238. [PMID: 11476533]

Stevens DG et al: The long-term functional outcome of operatively treated tibial plateau fractures. J Orthop Trauma 2001;15: 312. [PMID: 11433134]

Yacoubian SV et al: Impact of MRI on treatment plan and fracture classification of tibial plateau fractures. J Orthop Trauma 2002 Oct;16(9):632-7. [PMID 12368643]

Complications

Early complications include infection, deep vein thrombosis, compartment syndrome, loss of reduction, and hardware failure. Late complications include residual instability and posttraumatic degenerative joint disease that may require total knee replacement arthroplasty or arthrodesis.

2. Tibial Tuberosity Fracture

Tibial tuberosity fractures can occur with a violent quadriceps muscle contraction causing avulsion of the tibial tuberosity. When the fracture is complete, the extensor mechanism is disrupted and active knee extension is impossible.

Although conservative treatment of a nondisplaced avulsion fracture with a cylinder cast in extension for 6–8 weeks will allow it to heal, rigid fixation with percutaneous screws allows much earlier knee mobilization. Closed or open reduction and solid internal fixation is recommended for all fractures displaced by 5 mm or more.

3. Tibial Eminence (Spine) Fracture

A tibial eminence fracture occurs as an isolated injury or as part of the comminution of tibial plateau fractures. The isolated type of injury occurs mostly in the pediatric age group before physeal closure and is believed to be an avulsion fracture at the tibial attachment of the anterior cruciate ligament.

Myers has classified this lesion into three stages and has recommended open reduction for the displaced type 3 fractures. Type 1 and 2 fractures should be treated with a cylinder cast with the knee in extension for 4–6 weeks. When associated with other fractures of the tibial plateau, the tibial eminence fragment usually keeps its attachment to the anterior cruciate ligament, and anatomic reduction with rigid fixation should be obtained.

DISTAL FEMUR FRACTURES

These fractures involve the distal metaphysis and epiphysis of the femur. The incidence of distal femoral fractures has been estimated between 4 and 7% of all femoral fractures. It is important to distinguish between extraarticular (supracondylar) and intraarticular (condylar or intercondylar) fractures, and low energy fractures (usually in the elderly) and high energy fractures (young patient). The distal fragment is usually rotated into extension from traction by the gastrocnemius muscle. The distal end of the proximal fragment is apt to perforate the overlying quadriceps and may penetrate the suprapatellar pouch, causing hemarthrosis. The distal fragment may impinge on the popliteal neurovascular bundle, and an immediate thorough neurovascular examination is mandatory. Absence or marked decrease of pedal pulsations is an indication for immediate reduction. If this fails to restore adequate circulation, an arteriogram should be obtained immediately and the vascular lesion repaired as indicated. Injuries to the tibial or peroneal nerves are less frequent. Treatment should be aimed at restoring the mechanical axis, anatomic reduction of the articular surface and early knee range of motion.

A temporary spanning external fixation can be used to stabilize the fracture in polytrauma patients. Two pins can be rapidly allocated in the femoral shaft and two additional pins in the Tibial shaft. ORIF can be safely done in the first 2 weeks when the patient has been hemodynamically stabilized without increasing the risk of infection, provided that no infection at the pin sites has occurred. Complex Trauma of the Knee encompasses a distal supra or intercondylar femoral fracture combined with a proximal tibial fracture (floating knee); a supra or intercondylar femoral fracture with a second or third degree closed or open injury; or a complete knee dislocation and possible associated neurovascular injuries. Because of the complexity of injury and multidisciplinary team approach, this subset of patients is better treated in level 1 trauma centers.

1. Extraarticular Fractures

Most of these fractures, are best treated with internal fixation, which allows early mobilization of the patient and of the neighboring joints. Most fractures are best treated with fixed-angle plates, locking plates using MIPPO techniques, or retrograde intramedullary nailing. Skeletal traction treatment is reserved for patients for whom surgery is contraindicated and is fraught with all the previously mentioned complications that can accompany prolonged recumbency.

2. Intraarticular Fractures

As for any intraarticular fracture, maximal functional recovery of the knee joint requires anatomic reduction of the articular components and restitution of the mechanical axis. Closed reduction of displaced fragments is almost never successful. Displaced intraarticular fractures usually require open reduction and internal fixation with a variety of methods including Dynamic Compression Screws (DCS), AO buttress plating, LISS, with or without a percutaneous or minimally invasive plate osteosynthesis (MIPPO). For combined intercondylar and supracondylar fractures, or condylar fractures, the transarticular approach and retrograde plate osteosynthesis (TARPO) facilitates anatomic articular reconstruction and percutaneous plate insertion (Krettek et al., 1997).

3. Intercondylar Fracture

A comminuted fracture of the distal femoral epiphysis is classically described as a T or Y fracture, according to the configuration of the articular fragments. Displaced fractures are best treated by open reduction, to restore anatomic alignment of the articular surface, and by internal fixation using screws and condylar plates or screws. Even if the fracture heals in anatomic position, joint stiffness, pain, and posttraumatic arthritis are not uncommon outcomes.

4. Condylar Fracture

Isolated fractures of the lateral or medial femoral condyles are rare. They usually result from varus or valgus stress to the knee joint, and associated ligament injuries should be looked for systematically. Fractures of the posterior portion of one or the other condyle in the frontal plane can also be seen (Hoffa fracture).

Closed reduction of displaced fragments is rarely successful. Open reduction and internal fixation is usually indicated and requires anteroposterior lag screws. Associated ligamentous ruptures are repaired as needed. If fixation is solid, postoperative immobilization is kept at a minimum, and the patient can start moving the knee joint early. Weight bearing is usually allowed at 3 months when clinical and radiologic evidence of bone healing is present.

PATELLAR INJURIES

1. Transverse Patellar Fracture

Transverse fractures of the patella (Figure 3–28) are the result of an indirect force, usually with the knee in flexion. Fracture may be caused by sudden voluntary contraction of the quadriceps muscle or sudden forced flexion of the leg with the quadriceps contracted. The level of fracture is commonly in the middle. Associated tearing of the patellar retinacula depends upon the force of the initiating injury. The activity of the quadriceps muscle causes upward displacement of the proximal fragment, the magnitude of which depends on the extent of the retinacular tear.

Clinical Findings

Swelling of the anterior knee region is caused by hemarthrosis and hemorrhage into the soft tissues overlying the joint. If displacement is present, the defect in the patella can be palpated, and active extension of the knee is lost. A straight leg raise may be preserved if the retinacula is intact.

Treatment

Nondisplaced fractures can be treated with a walking cylinder cast or brace for 6–8 weeks followed by knee rehabilitation. Open reduction is indicated if the fragments are displaced >3 mm or if articular step-off is >2 mm. The fragments must be accurately repositioned to prevent early posttraumatic arthritis of the patellofemoral joint. If the minor fragment is small (no more than 1 cm in length) or severely comminuted, it may be excised and the quadriceps or patellar tendon (depending upon which pole of the patella is involved) sutured directly to the major fragment. Whenever possible, internal fixation of anatomically reduced fragments should be done, allowing early motion of the knee joint. This is best achieved by figure-of-eight tension banding over two longitudinal parallel K-wires.

Accurate reduction of the articular surface must be confirmed by lateral radiographs taken intraoperatively.

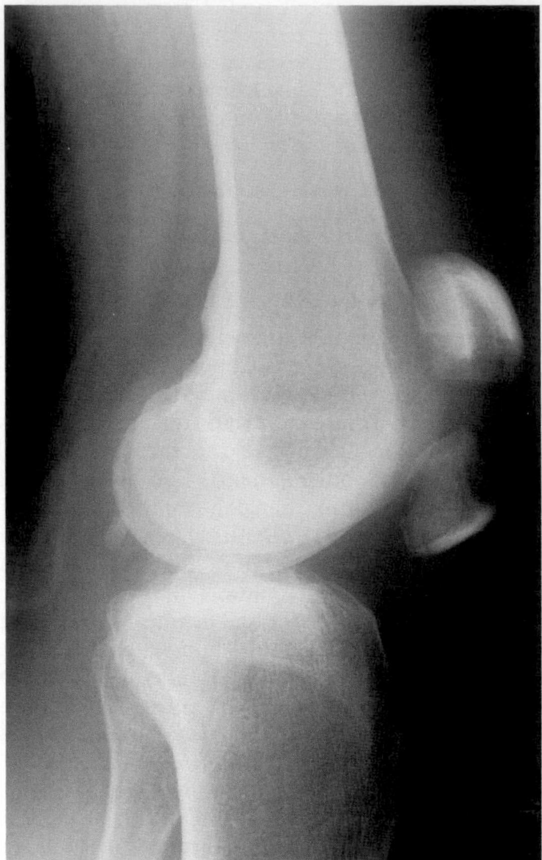

Figure 3–28. Transverse fracture of the patella. (Reprinted from Campbells Operative Orthopaedics, 9/e, Vol. 3, Canale ST [ed], Copyright 1998, Mosby, with permission from Elsevier.)

2. Comminuted Patellar Fracture

Comminuted fractures of the patella are usually caused by a direct force. Most often, little or no separation of the fragments occurs because the quadriceps retinaculum is not extensively torn. Severe injury may cause extensive destruction of the articular surface of both the patella and the opposing femur.

If comminution is not severe and displacement is insignificant, immobilization for 8 weeks in a cylinder extending from the groin to the supramalleolar region is sufficient.

Severe comminution can often be treated with ORIF with addition of a cerclage wire, but on rare occasions excision of the patella and repair of the defect by imbrication of the quadriceps expansion is the only viable alternative. Excision of the patella can result in decreased strength, pain in the knee, and general restriction of activity. No matter what the treatment, high-energy injuries are frequently complicated by chondromalacia patella and patellofemoral arthritis.

3. Patellar Dislocation

Acute traumatic dislocation of the patella should be differentiated from episodic recurrent dislocation, as the latter condition is likely to be associated with occult organic lesions. When dislocation of the patella occurs alone, it may be caused by a direct force or activity of the quadriceps, and the direction of dislocation of the patella is almost always lateral. Spontaneous reduction is apt to occur if the knee joint is extended. If so, the clinical findings may consist merely of hemarthrosis and localized tenderness over the medial patellar retinaculum. Gross instability of the patella, which can be demonstrated by physical examination, indicates that injury to the soft tissues of the medial aspect of the knee has been extensive.

Reduction is maintained in a brace or cylinder cast with the knee in extension for 2–3 weeks. Isometric quadriceps exercises are encouraged. Physical therapy should be initiated to maximize the strength of the vastus medialis. Dynamic bracing may be helpful. Recurrent episodes require operative repair for effective treatment.

4. Tear of the Quadriceps Tendon

Tear of the quadriceps tendon occurs most often in patients over the age of 40. Apparent tears that represent avulsions from the patella occur in patients with renal osteodystrophy or hyperparathyroidism. Preexisting attritional disease of the tendon is apt to be present, and the causative injury may be minor. The tear commonly results from sudden deceleration, such as stumbling or slipping on a wet surface. A small flake of bone may be avulsed from the superior pole of the patella, or the tear may occur entirely through tendinous and muscular tissue.

Pain may be noted in the anterior knee region. Swelling is caused by hemarthrosis and extravasation of blood into the soft tissues. The patient is unable to extend the knee completely. Radiographs may show a bony avulsion from the superior pole of the patella.

Operative repair is recommended for complete tear. Postoperative immobilization should be encouraged in a walking cylinder cast or brace for 6 weeks, at which time knee mobilization is started.

5. Tear of the Patellar Tendon

The same mechanism that causes tears of the quadriceps tendon, transverse fracture of the patella, or avulsion of the tibial tuberosity may also cause the patellar ligament to tear. The characteristic finding is proximal displacement of the patella. A bony avulsion may be present adjacent to the lower pole of the patella if the tear takes place in the proximal patellar tendon.

Operative treatment is necessary for a complete tear. The ligament is resutured to the patella, and any tear in the quadriceps mechanism is repaired. The extremity should be immobilized for 6–8 weeks in a cylinder cast extending from the groin to the supramalleolar region. Guarded exercises may then be started.

Jutson JJ, Zych GA: Treatment of comminuted intraarticular distal femur fractures with limited internal and external tensioned wire fixation. J Orthop Trauma 2000;14:405. [PMID: 1100141])

Meyer RW et al: Mechanical comparison of a distal femoral side plate and a retrograde intramedullary nail. J Orthop Trauma 2000 14;398. [PMID: 11001413]

Stahelin T, Hardegger F, Ward JC: Supracondylar osteotomy of the femur with use of compression. J Bone Joint Surg 2000; 82-A;712. [PMID: 10819282]

Woo SL et al: Healing and repair of ligament injuries in the knee. J Am Acad Orthop Surg 2000;8:364. [PMID: 11104400]

FEMORAL SHAFT FRACTURES

DIAPHYSEAL FRACTURES

Fracture of the shaft of the femur usually occurs as a result of severe trauma. Indirect force, especially torsional stress, is likely to cause spiral fractures that extend proximally or, more commonly, distally into the metaphyseal regions. Most are closed fractures; open fracture is often the result of compounding from within.

Clinical Findings

Extensive soft-tissue injury, bleeding, and shock are commonly present with diaphyseal fractures. The most significant features are severe pain in the thigh and deformity of the lower extremity. Hemorrhagic shock may be present, as multiple units of blood may be lost into the thigh, though only moderate swelling may be apparent. Careful radiographic examination in at least two planes is necessary to determine the exact site and configuration of the fracture pattern. The hip and knee should be examined and radiographs obtained to rule out associated injury. A femoral neck fracture may occur in association with a femur fracture and if overlooked can increase patient morbidity.

Injuries to the sciatic nerve and the superficial femoral artery and vein are uncommon but must be recognized promptly. Hemorrhagic shock and secondary anemia are the most important early complications. Later complications include those of prolonged recumbency, joint stiffness, malunion, nonunion, leg-length discrepancy, and infection.

Classification

No classification is universally accepted for fractures of the femoral diaphysis. Classically, the fracture is described according to its location, pattern, and comminution. Winquist has proposed a comminution classification that is now widely used.

Type 1: Fracture that involves no, or minimal, comminution at the fracture site, and does not affect stability after intramedullary nailing

Type 2: Fracture with comminution leaving at least 50% of the circumference of the two major fragments intact

Type 3: Fracture with comminution of 50–100% of the circumference of the major fragments. Nonlocked intramedullary nails do not afford stable fixation.

Type 4: Fracture with completely comminuted segmental pattern with no intrinsic stability

Treatment

Treatment depends upon the age and medical status of the patient as well as the site and configuration of the fracture.

A. Closed Treatment

This remains a treatment option for some skeletally immature patients. Depending on the age of the pediatric patient and the amount of initial displacement at the fracture site, treatment may consist of immediate immobilization in a hip spica cast, or skin or skeletal traction for 3–6 weeks, until the fracture is "sticky," and then spica casting.

Closed treatment of femoral shaft fractures in the adult is rarely indicated. Acceptable alignment may be difficult to maintain, and joint stiffness is frequent. Other rarer complications of prolonged recumbency, like pressure sores and deep vein thrombosis, can have disastrous consequences.

B. Operative Treatment

Most fractures in the middle third of the femur can be internally fixed by an intramedullary rod. Intramedullary fixation of femoral shaft fractures allows early mobilization of the patient (within 24–48 hour if the fracture fixation is stable), which is of particular benefit to the polytraumatized patient; more anatomic alignment; improved knee and hip function by decreasing the time spent in traction; and a marked decrease in the cost of hospitalization.

Although open nailing procedures have been described, intramedullary fixation is routinely performed closed.

In closed nailing, the fracture is reduced by closed manipulation on a fracture table under fluoroscopic control. An small incision is made proximal to the greater trochanter, and the nail is inserted through the piriformis fossa down into the intramedullary canal, after reaming to the appropriate size. The fracture site is not opened. Closed nailing decreases the chance of infection by decreasing the amount of soft-tissue dissection necessary and by limiting access to the fracture site to the medullary canal. It also does not disturb the periosteal circulation. Some authors feel that bone reamings at the fracture site further promote bone healing. Interlocking nails are the standard of treatment. Screws are inserted percutaneously through holes in both ends of the nail. Dynamic interlocking using screws at only one end of the nail, relies on interference friction of fracture fragments and muscle action to prevent rotation of the unlocked fragment. It allows axial compression at the fracture site. However, up to 10% of dynamic interlocking may undergo secondary rotation or shortening due to unseen fracture lines. Static interlocking (screws at both ends of the nail) provides rotational control and prevents shortening of the bone at the fracture site; this is the recommended technique. Reamed interlocked nailing is recommended for most grade 1, 2, and 3a open fractures. When associated with extensive soft-tissue loss, as in grade 3b and 3c open fractures, temporary bony stability may be achieved with external fixation devices.

Complications of this procedure can arise from technical problems at the time of surgery (eg, choice of a rod that is too short or too narrow) and result in malalignment or shortening. Comminution of the fracture can occur during placement of the rod. Late bone fracture (weeks or months) can occur through interlocking screws, and severely comminuted fractures with weight bearing can suffer rod or screw breakage. Infection can occur after any open procedure but is uncommon with closed nailing. Occasionally, a painful bursa or heterotopic calcification may develop over the proximal end of the nail, causing discomfort when the patient sits or walks. The rod may be removed after healing is complete, usually at 12–16 months. The healing rate of femoral shaft fractures in general is high and approaches 100% after closed nailing techniques.

Other fixation devices are seldom used. Flexible intramedullary rods of the Ender type do not provide sufficient stability in the adult; however, they are routinely used in the pediatric population. Plates and screws require significant soft-tissue dissection and opening of the fracture hematoma and are usually reserved for special cases such as ipsilateral femoral neck and diaphyseal fractures. External fixation remains indicated in some open fractures. In polytrauma patients, initial external fixation may be indicated when early intramedullary nailing (first 24 hours after trauma), can be potentially hazardous due to hemodynamic instability, head or chest trauma. It has also recently gained acceptance as treatment for closed femoral shaft fractures in children to allow earlier mobilization and decreased hospital stays. The distal fragment pins should always be inserted with the knee in flexion to avoid quadriceps tenodesis that will prevent knee flexion. Superficial pin tract infection is common but rarely involves the bone. A course of oral antibiotics, proper pin care, and eventual pin removal, when the fracture is sufficiently healed, are usually all that are needed to control this problem.

SUBTROCHANTERIC FRACTURES

Subtrochanteric fractures occur below the level of the lesser trochanter and are usually the result of high-energy trauma in young to middle-aged adults. They are often comminuted, with distal or proximal extension toward the greater trochanter. Associated soft-tissue damage can be extensive.

The Russell and Taylor classification (Figure 3–29) is a treatment based classification system that incorpo-

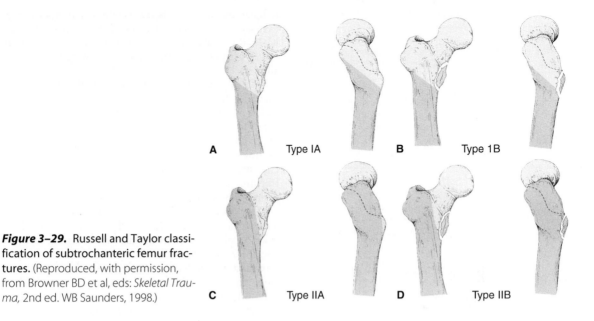

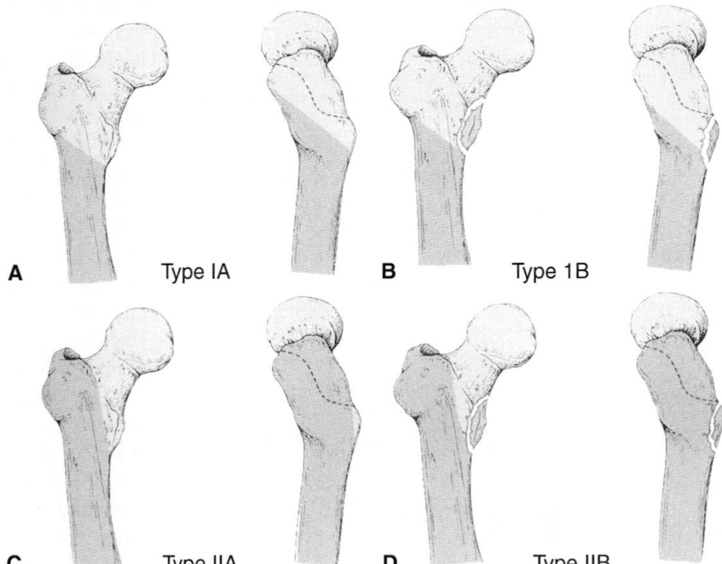

Figure 3–29. **Russell and Taylor classification of subtrochanteric femur fractures.** (Reproduced, with permission, from Browner BD et al, eds: *Skeletal Trauma,* 2nd ed. WB Saunders, 1998.)

rates involvement of the piriformis fossa. Type Ia Russell-Taylor fractures do not involve the piriformis fossa, with the lesser trochanter attached to the proximal fragment. These fractures may be treated with a first-generation intramedullary nail. Type Ib fractures do not involve the piriformis fossa; however, the lesser trochanter is detached from the proximal fragment. These fractures require a second-generation nail, with screw fixation into the head and neck. Type II fractures have fracture extension into the piriformis fossa and are best treated with a sliding hip screw or fixed angle plate. The patient usually presents with a swollen painful proximal thigh with or without shortening or malrotation. If the lesser trochanter is intact, the proximal fragment will tend to displace in flexion, external rotation, and abduction because of the unopposed pull of the iliopsoas and abductor muscles.

In the vast majority of cases, internal fixation (by closed or open methods) is now widely favored. Temporary skeletal traction will maintain femoral length until the definitive surgical procedure can be performed. A variety of devices are available.

Closed intramedullary interlocking nails have gained more popularity recently. Devices with cephalic proximal interlocking are available for those cases where conventional intertrochanteric proximal interlocking is contraindicated. Fixation can be obtained with first-generation intramedullary nails, "gamma nails," intramedullary hip screws, or with a variety of cephalomedullary nails or blades and long sideplates based upon the fracture pattern.

Postoperative activity depends on the adequacy of internal fixation. If fixation is solid, an agile cooperative patient can be out of bed within a few days after surgery and ambulating on crutches with toe-touch weight bearing on the affected side. The fracture is usually healed at 3–4 months, but delayed union and nonunion are not uncommon. Hardware failure in these cases are frequent. Repeat internal fixation with autogenous bone grafting is then the treatment of choice.

Brumback RJ, Virkus WW: Intramedullary nailing of the femur: Reamed versus nonreamed. J Am Acad Orthop Surg 2000; 8:83. [PMID: 10799093]

Dora C et al: Entry point soft tissue damage in antegrade femoral nailing: A cadaver study. J Orthop Trauma 2001;15:488. [PMID: 11602831]

Giannoudis PV et al: Nonunion of the femoral diaphysis. J Bone Joint Surg Br 2000;82-B:655. [PMID: 10963160]

Herscovici D et al: Treatment of femoral shaft fracture using unreamed interlocked nails. J Orthop Trauma 2000;14:10. [PMID: 10630796]

Nowotarski PJ et al: Conversion of external fixation to intramedullary nailing for fractures of the shaft of the femur in multiply injured patients. J Bone Joint Surg Am 2000;82-A:2000. [PMID: 1085909]

Ostrum RF et al: Prospective comparison of retrograde and antegrade femoral intramedullary nailing. J Orthop Trauma 2000; 14:496. [PMID: 11083612]

Patton JT et al: Late fracture of the hip after reamed intramedullary nailing of the femur. J Bone Joint Surg Br 2000;82-B:967. [PMID: 11041583]

Ricci WM et al: Angular malalignment after intramedullary nailing of femoral shaft fractures. J Orthop Trauma 2001;15:90. [PMID: 11232660]

Ricci WM et al: Retrograde versus antegrade nailing of femoral shaft fractures. J Orthop Trauma 2001;15:161. [PMID: 11265005]

Scalea TM, Boswell SA, Scott JD, Mitchell KA, Kramer ME, Pollak AN. External fixation as a bridge to intramedullary nailing for patients with multiple injuries and with femur fractures: damage control orthopedics. J Orthop Trauma. 2004 Sep;18(8 Suppl):S2-10; discussion S10-2. [PMID: 15472561]

Shepherd LE et al: Prospective randomized study of reamed versus undreamed femoral intramedullary nailing: An assessment of procedures. J Orthop Trauma 2001;15:28. [PMID: 11147684]

Tornetta P, Tiburzi D: Antegrade or retrograde reamed femoral nailing. J Bone Joint Surg Br 2000;82-B:652. [PMID: 10963159]

Tornetta P, Tiburzi D: Reamed versus nonreamed anterograde femoral nailing. J Orthop Trauma 2000;14:15. [PMID: 10630797]

HIP FRACTURES & DISLOCATIONS

Epidemiology & Social Costs

Hip fractures include intertrochanteric fractures and femoral neck fractures and constitute a major problem in the United States because of the disabling nature of these injuries. Ambulation is almost impossible in all fractures except femoral neck fractures until they have been treated surgically. These fractures primarily occur in older patients (>55 years), unable in many cases to care for themselves. The incidence of hip fractures sharply rises after menopause in women and the age of 70 in men. Fourteen billion dollars are spent yearly to take care of one million affected Americans. Of these, approximately a quarter regain pre-fracture function. Further, prompt and effective care is necessary to avoid the all too frequent occurrence of death in the elderly (>70 years) patient with a hip fracture (20–30% of patients in the first year after fracture). Thus, this injury justifies state-of-the-art care to minimize not only the societal cost but also the human suffering.

Anatomy & Biomechanical Principles

The hip joint is the articulation between the acetabulum and the femoral head. The trabecular pattern of the femoral head and neck, and that of the acetabulum, is oriented to optimally accept the forces crossing the joint. The total force across the joint is the vector sum of body weight and active muscle force. When the concept of lever arm is factored in, surprising forces across the hip joint are attained: 2.5 times body weight when standing on one leg, five times body weight when running, and 1.5 times body weight when lifting the leg from the supine position with the knee in extension. Using a cane in the opposite hand reduces the force to body weight when standing on that leg. For the same reasons, forces across the joint when the ipsilateral leg is kept in the air are significantly greater than when toe-touch weight bearing is allowed.

The hip capsule is a strong thick fibrous structure that attaches on the intertrochanteric line anteriorly and somewhat more proximally posteriorly. The intracapsular portion of the neck is not covered with periosteum, and fractures of the intracapsular part of the neck cannot heal with periosteal callus formation, only with endosteal union. Interposition of synovial fluid between fracture fragments, as in any joint, can delay or altogether prevent bony union.

The vascular supply of the femoral head is also of paramount importance. There are three main sources of vascular supply: (1) the retinacular vessels arising from the lateral femoral circumflex artery and the inferior metaphyseal artery and then running beneath the synovium along the neck, which they penetrate proximally both anteriorly and posteriorly; (2) the interosseous circulation crossing the marrow spaces from distal to proximal; and (3) unreliably, the ligamentum teres artery. Fractures of the femoral neck always disrupt the interosseous circulation; the femoral head then relies only on the retinacular arteries, which may also be disrupted or thrombosed. Secondary avascular necrosis of part or all of the femoral head can result. Union of a fracture can occur in the presence of an avascular fragment, but the incidence of nonunion is higher. Revascularization of the necrotic fragment occurs through the process of creeping substitution. Part of this process involves replacement of necrotic bony substrate with a "softer" granulation tissue and sets the stage for delayed segmental collapse.

Intertrochanteric fractures usually do not suffer this same fate. The capsule (and vessels) are still attached to the proximal fragment after fracture, and thus the blood supply remains patent.

1. Femoral Neck Fractures

Femoral neck fractures are intracapsular fractures. Because of the already mentioned unusual vascularization of the femoral head and neck, these fractures are at high risk of nonunion or avascular necrosis of the femoral head. The incidence of avascular necrosis increases with the amount of fracture displacement and the amount of time before the fracture is reduced.

Fractures of the femoral neck occur most commonly in patients over age 50. The involved extremity may be slightly shortened and externally rotated. Hip motion is painful, except in the rare cases of nondisplaced or impacted fractures, where pain may be evident only at the extremes of motion. Good quality anteroposterior and lateral radiographs are mandatory.

Classification

The Garden classification for acute fractures is the most widely used system:

Type 1: Valgus impaction of the femoral head

Type 2: Complete but nondisplaced

Type 3: Complete fracture, displaced less than 50%

Type 4: Complete fracture displaced greater than 50%

This classification is of prognostic value for the incidence of avascular necrosis: The higher the Garden number, the higher the incidence. The benefits of either skeletal or skin traction are unclear prior to definitive treatment. Traction may offer comfort in some patients but do not improve overall outcome.

Stable Femoral Neck Fractures

These include stress fractures and Garden type 1 fractures. Stress fractures may be difficult to diagnose. Physical examination, as well as the initial radiographs, may be normal. Repeat radiographs, radionuclide imaging, and MRI may be necessary to confirm the diagnosis. Reviews have shown that age, walking ability, and degree of impaction on the radiographs are important factors influencing fracture healing, and may guide the choice of treatment (conservative management versus internal fixation).

Toe-touch weight bearing (with crutches) until radiologic evidence of healing is usually successful for the compliant patient. Healing is usually complete in 3–6 months. Prophylactic internal fixation may be necessary and is indicated by failure of pain resolution with toe-touch weight bearing or by displacement.

The Garden type 1 fracture is impacted in valgus position and is usually stable. Impaction must be demonstrated on both anteroposterior and lateral views. The risk of displacement is nevertheless significant; most surgeons recommend internal fixation to maintain reduction and allow earlier ambulation and weight bearing. If surgery is contraindicated, closed treatment with toe-touch crutch ambulation and frequent radiographic follow-up until healing can be successful.

Unstable Femoral Neck Fractures

Although undisplaced, a Garden type 2 femoral neck fracture is unstable because displacement is probable under physiologic loading. Garden type 3 and 4 fractures are displaced and often comminuted. They can be life-threatening injuries, especially in elderly patients.

Treatment is directed toward preservation of life and restoration of hip function, with early mobilization. This is best attained by rigid internal fixation or primary arthroplasty as soon as the patient is medically prepared for surgery. Closed treatment in a spica cast is almost always bound to fail. Definitive treatment using skeletal traction requires prolonged recumbency with constant nursing care and is associated with numerous complications, including malunion, nonunion, pressure sores, deep vein thrombosis and pulmonary embolus, osteoporosis, and hypercalcemia, to name a few. If for some reason surgery is not possible, it is better to mobilize the patient as soon as pain permits. Subsequent nonunion can be treated at a later stage, electively. Surgical options are internal fixation or primary arthroplasty. In general, the younger the patient, the greater the effort is justified to save the femoral head.

Treatment

A. Internal Fixation

The goal of internal fixation is to preserve a viable femoral head fragment and provide the optimal setting for bony healing of the fracture while allowing the patient to be as mobile as possible. Because persistent displacement and motion at the fracture site may further jeopardize the femoral head blood supply, surgery should be performed as soon as possible. General or spinal anesthesia is used. The fracture is reduced under fluoroscopic imaging as anatomically accurately as possible. Gentle manipulation is usually sufficient. Rarely, open reduction may be necessary before fixation. Open reduction, if performed, should be approached anteriorly as this results in less disruption of blood supply than a posterior approach. Rigid internal fixation is obtained using multiple parallel partially threaded screws, a dynamic hip screw and plate, or a combination of both. The patient can usually be mobilized the following day, and weight bearing is allowed according to the stability of the construct.

B. Primary Arthroplasty

This procedure is indicated in the elderly patient for Garden type 4 fractures, in which avascular necrosis is highly probable, and for Garden type 3 fractures that cannot be satisfactorily reduced or for femoral heads with preexisting disease. The femoral head is sacrificed, but a definitive procedure is performed, whereas internal fixation of Garden type 4 fractures frequently fails and repeat surgery is required. When the acetabulum is undamaged, the most commonly accepted technique is hemiarthroplasty, using a femoral stem stabilized with methyl methacrylate or a surface that allows biologic fixation with bony ingrowth. If the hip joint itself is already damaged by preexisting disease, total hip replacement may be indicated. Primary head and neck resection (Girdlestone arthroplasty) may be rarely indicated in the presence of infection or local malignant growth.

Complications

The most common sequelae of femoral neck fractures are loss of reduction with or without hardware failure, nonunions or malunions, and avascular necrosis of the femoral head. This latter complication can appear as late as 2 years after injury. According to different series, the incidence of avascular necrosis for Garden type 1 fractures varies from 0 to 15%, for type 2 fractures 10–25%, for type 3 fractures 25–50%, and for type 4 fractures 50–100%. Secondary degenerative joint disease appears somewhat later. The most disabling complication, infection, is fortunately rare.

2. Trochanteric Fractures

Lesser Trochanter Fracture

Isolated fracture of the lesser trochanter is rare. When it occurs, it is the result of the avulsion force of the iliopsoas muscle. Rarely, a symptomatic nonunion may require fragment fixation or excision.

Greater Trochanter Fracture

Isolated fracture of the greater trochanter may be caused by direct injury or may occur indirectly as a result of the activity of the gluteus medius and gluteus minimus muscles. It occurs most commonly as a component of intertrochanteric fracture.

If displacement of the isolated fracture fragment is less than 1 cm and there is no tendency to further displacement (as determined by repeated radiographic examinations), treatment may be bed rest until acute pain subsides. As rapidly as symptoms permit, activity can increase gradually to protected weight bearing with crutches. Full weight bearing is permitted as soon as healing is apparent, usually in 6–8 weeks. If displacement is greater than 1 cm and increases on adduction of the thigh, extensive tearing of surrounding soft tissues may be assumed, and ORIF is indicated.

Intertrochanteric Fractures

By definition, these fractures usually occur along a line between the greater and the lesser trochanter. They typically occur at a later age than do femoral neck fractures. They are most often extracapsular and occur through cancellous bone. Bone healing within 8–12 weeks is the usual outcome, regardless of the treatment. Nonunion and avascular necrosis of the femoral head are not significant problems.

Clinically, the involved extremity is usually shortened and can be internally or externally rotated. The degree of displacement and comminution will determine the instability of the fracture. A wide spectrum of fracture patterns is possible, from the nondisplaced fissure fracture to the highly comminuted fracture with four major fragments (head and neck, greater trochanter, lesser trochanter, and femoral shaft). The Muller/AO system is useful in classifying intertrochanteric femur fractures and has gained more popularity in recent years (Figure 3–30).

The selection of definitive treatment depends upon the general condition of the patient and the fracture pattern. Rates of illness and death are lower when the fracture is internally fixed, allowing early mobilization. Operative treatment is indicated as soon as the patient is medically able to tolerate surgery. Overall mortality decreases if surgery can be performed within 48 hours. Initial treatment in the hospital should be by gentle skin traction to minimize pain and further displacement. Skeletal traction as the definitive treatment is rarely indicated and is fraught with complications such as pressure sores, deep vein thrombosis and pulmonary embolus, deterioration of mental status, and varus malunion. When surgery is contraindicated, it may be preferable to mobilize the patient as soon as pain permits and accept the eventual malunion or nonunion.

The great majority of these fractures are amenable to surgery. The goal is to obtain a fixation secure enough to allow early mobilization and provide an environment for sound fracture healing in a good position. Reduction of the fracture is usually accomplished by closed methods, using traction on the fracture table, and monitored using fluoroscopic imaging. Some surgeons do not attempt to anatomically reduce comminuted fractures but instead prefer to keep the distal fragment medially displaced, to enhance mechanical stability. Internal fixation is most widely obtained with a dynamic screw and sideplate. The screw can slide in the barrel of the sideplate, allowing the fracture to impact in a stable position. The patient can be taken out of bed the next day, and weight bearing with crutches or a walker is begun as soon as pain allows. The fracture usually heals in 6–12 weeks. Other devices used to treat intertrochanteric fractures include second-generation interlocked nails and prosthetic replacement. Recent results of series have shown more complications of fracture fixation with intramedullary techniques compared to the dynamic hip screw.

General complications include infection, hardware failure, loss of reduction, and irritation bursitis over the tip of the sliding screw.

3. Traumatic Dislocation of the Hip Joint

Traumatic dislocation of the hip joint may occur with or without fracture of the acetabulum or the proximal end of the femur. It is most common during the active years of life and is usually the result of high-energy trauma, unless there is preexisting disease of the femoral

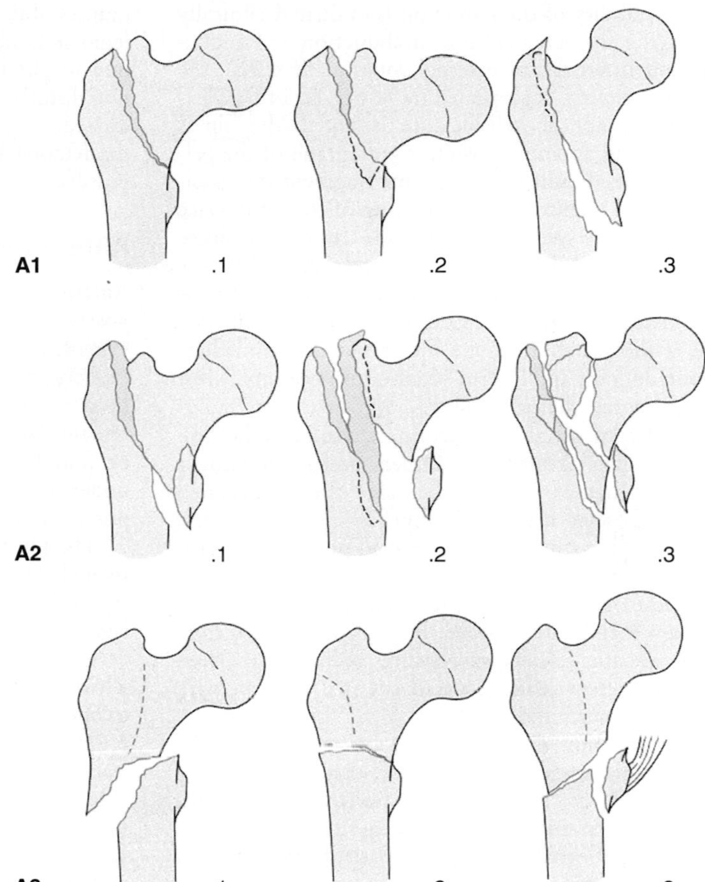

Figure 3–30. **Muller/AO system for intertrochanteric femur fracture classification.** (Reproduced, with permission, from Browner BD et al, eds: *Skeletal Trauma,* 2nd ed. WB Saunders, 1998.)

head, acetabulum, or neuromuscular system. The head of the femur cannot be completely displaced from the normal acetabulum, unless the ligamentum teres is ruptured or deficient because of some unrelated cause. Traumatic dislocations are classified according to the direction of displacement of the femoral head from the acetabulum.

Posterior Hip Dislocation

Usually, the head of the femur is dislocated posterior to the acetabulum when the thigh is flexed, for example, as may occur in a head-on automobile collision when the knee is driven violently against the dashboard. Posterior dislocation is also a complication of hip arthroplasty.

The significant clinical findings are shortening, adduction, and internal rotation of the extremity. Anteroposterior, lateral and, if fracture of the acetabulum is demonstrated, oblique radiographic projections (Judet views) are required. Common associated injuries include fractures of the acetabulum or the femoral head or shaft and sciatic nerve injury. The head of the femur may be displaced through a tear in the posterior hip joint capsule. The short external rotator muscles of the femur are commonly lacerated. Fracture of the posterior margin of the acetabulum can create instability.

If the acetabulum is not fractured or if the fragment is small, reduction by closed manipulation is indicated. General anesthesia provides maximum muscle relaxation and allows gentle reduction. Reduction should be achieved as soon as possible, preferably within the first few hours after injury, as the incidence of avascular necrosis of the femoral head increases with time until reduction. The main feature of reduction is traction in the line of deformity followed by gentle flexion of the hip to 90 degrees with stabilization of the pelvis by an assistant. While manual traction is continued, the hip is gently rotated into internal and then external rotation to obtain reduction.

The stability of the reduction is evaluated clinically by ranging the extended hip in abduction and adduction and internal and external rotation. If stable, the same movements are repeated in 90 degrees of hip flexion. The point of redislocation is noted, the hip is reduced, and an anteroposterior radiograph of the pelvis is obtained. Soft tissue or bone fragment interposition will be manifested by widening of the joint space as compared to the contralateral side. Irreducible dislocations, open dislocations, and those that re-dislocate after reduction despite hip extension and external rotation (usually because of associated posterior wall fracture of the acetabulum) are indications for immediate open reduction and internal fixation if necessary. Most authors agree that a widened joint space on radiograph, despite a stable reduction, is also an indication for immediate arthrotomy. Others prefer obtaining a CT scan first, to further delineate the incarcerated fragments and associated injuries before surgery. Recently, hip arthroscopy has gained popularity, but it remains controversial.

Minor fragments of the posterior margin of the acetabulum may be disregarded, but larger displaced fragments are not usually successfully reduced by closed methods. Open reduction and internal fixation with screws or plates is indicated.

Postreduction treatment will vary according to the type of initial surgery. A strictly soft-tissue injury with a stable concentric reduction may be treated with light skin or skeletal traction for a few days to a week before exercises are begun. A motivated patient can then start crutch ambulation, progressing to full weight bearing at 6 weeks. An unstable reduction can be immobilized in a spica cast or abduction brace for 4–6 weeks. Securely fixed fractures are treated as soft-tissue injuries, but weight bearing is allowed when radiologic signs of bone healing are present. When fixation is tenuous, skeletal traction for 4–6 weeks or hip spica immobilization may be necessary.

Complications include infection, avascular necrosis of the femoral head, malunion, posttraumatic degenerative joint disease, recurrent dislocation, and sciatic nerve injury. Avascular necrosis occurs because of the disruption of the retinacular arteries providing blood to the femoral head. Its incidence increases with the duration of the dislocation. It can occur as late as 2 years after the injury. MRI studies enabling early diagnosis and protected weight bearing until revascularization has occurred are recommended. Sciatic nerve injury is present in 10–20% of patients with posterior hip dislocation. Although usually of the neurapraxia type, these lesions leave permanent sequelae in about 20% of cases. The rare patient who is neurologically intact before reduction but has a deficit after reduction should be explored surgically to see if the nerve has been entrapped in the joint. Associated injuries also, on rare occasions, include fracture of the femoral head. Small fragments or those involving the non-weight–bearing surface should be ignored if they do not disturb hip mechanics; otherwise they should be excised. Large fragments of the weight-bearing portion of the femoral head should be reduced and fixed if at all possible.

Anterior Hip Dislocation

Anterior dislocation of the hip is rare compared to its posterior counterpart. It usually occurs when the hip is extended and externally rotated at the time of impact. Associated fractures of the acetabulum and the femoral head or neck occur rarely. Usually, the femoral head remains lateral to the obturator externus muscle but can be found rarely beneath it (obturator dislocation) or under the iliopsoas muscle in contact with the superior pubic ramus (pubic dislocation).

The hip is classically flexed, abducted, and externally rotated. The femoral head is palpable anteriorly below the inguinal flexion crease. Anteroposterior and transpelvic lateral radiographic projections are usually diagnostic.

Closed reduction under general anesthesia is generally successful. Here also the surgeon must make sure of a concentric reduction comparing both hip joints on the postreduction anteroposterior radiograph. The patient starts mobilization within a few days when pain is tolerable. Active and passive hip motion, excluding external rotation, is encouraged, and the patient is usually fully weight bearing by 4–6 weeks. Skeletal traction or spica casting may rarely be useful for uncooperative patients.

4. Rehabilitation of Hip Fracture Patients

There has been an increased interest in the psychosocial outcome issues of patients with hip fractures. The goal of rehabilitation after hip injuries is to return the patient as rapidly as possible to the pre-injury functional level. Factors influencing rehabilitation potential include age, mental status, associated injuries, previous medical status, myocardial function, upper extremity strength, balance, and motivation.

For the rare patient treated conservatively, rehabilitation focuses early at preventing stiffness and weakness of the other extremities, and at eventually mobilizing the patient out of bed when pain is tolerable. Because the great majority of these injuries are now treated with internal fixation or prosthetic replacement, rehabilitation efforts are focused toward early range of motion, muscle strengthening, and weight bearing. Early full weight bearing as tolerated is encouraged for patients with prosthetic replacements, cemented or not, and for patients with stable fixation of an intertrochanteric fracture to allow compression of the fracture fragments.

Most authors now agree that the same applies for femoral neck fractures with stable internal fixation, although some still prefer partial weight bearing until radiologic evidence of bone healing is present to prevent hardware failure. When internal fixation does not provide stable fixation of the fracture fragments, supplemental protection may be added with a spica cast or brace However, it is highly undesirable in elderly patients. Otherwise, restricted range of motion or weight bearing may be allowed according to the surgeon's specifications.

Conn KS, Parker MJ: Undisplaced intracapsular hip fractures: results of internal fixation in 375 patients. Clin Orthop 2004 Apr;(421):249-54. [PMID 15123955]

Gotfried Y: Percutaneous compression plating of intertrochanteric hip fractures. J Orthop Trauma 2000;14:490. [PMID: 11083611]

Gruson et al: The relationship between admission hemoglobin level and outcome after hip fracture. J Orthop Trauma 2002; 15:39. [PMID: 11782632]

Jaglal S, Lakhani Z, Schatzker J: Reliability, validity and responsiveness of the lower extremity measure for patients with a hip fracture 2000; J Bone Joint Surg Am;82-A:955. [PMID: 10901310]

Kenny AM et al: Osteoporosis in older men and women. Conn Med 2003 Sep;67(8):481–6. [PMID: 14587128]

Parker MJ, Handoll HH, Bhargara A: Conservative versus operative treatment for hip fractures. Cochrane Database Syst Rev. 2000;(4):CD000337. [PMID 11034683]

Parker MJ, Handoll HH: Pre-operative traction for fractures of the proximal femur. Cochrane Database Syst Rev 2001;(3): CD000168. [PMID 11686954]

Parker MJ, Handoll HH: Gamma and other cephalocondylic intramedullary nails versus extramedullary implants for extracapsular hip fractures. Cochrane Database Syst Rev 2004;(1): CD000093. [PMID 14973946]

Rosen JE et al: Efficacy of preoperative skin traction in hip fracture patients: a prospective randomized study. J Orthop Trauma 2001;15:81. [PMID: 11232658]

Shah MR et al: Outcome after hip fracture in individuals ninety years of age and older. J Orthop Trauma 2001;15:34. [PMID: 11147685]

Tidermark J et al: Quality of life related to fracture displacement among elderly patients with femoral neck fractures treated with internal fixation. J Orthop Trauma 2002;15:34. [PMID: 11782631]

PELVIC FRACTURES & DISLOCATIONS

The innominate bones articulate with the sacrum through the sacroiliac joints and between themselves through the symphysis pubis. Upper body weight is transmitted across the hip joint to the lower limbs via the sciatic buttress and the acetabulum. The mechanism and severity of trauma will determine the pattern of injury. Osteoarticular structures and adjacent soft tissues will be involved to varying degrees depending upon the direction and magnitude of applied forces. Pelvic fractures are potentially life threatening with high mortality. A multidisciplinary team approach is necessary to reduce the likelihood of death and disability.

Mechanism of Injury

Four patterns of injury are responsible for pelvic fractures. Anteroposterior compression results in external rotation of the hemipelvis and rupture of the pelvic floor and anterior sacroiliac ligaments. Lateral compression creates compression fractures of the sacrum and disruption of the posterior sacroiliac ligament complex. The sacrospinous and sacrotuberous ligaments remain intact limiting the instability. In high energy lateral compression injuries, the contralateral hemipelvis can be pushed in external rotation, as seen in rollover or crush injuries. Combined external rotation-abduction is common in motorcycle accidents and the deforming forces are transmitted through the femur. The fourth pattern is a shear force vector resulting from fall from heights, where the grade of translational instability is variable.

Clinical Findings

Knowledge of the injury mechanism is of prime importance and should be assessed either by patient history or discussion with the prehospital provider. The physical examination includes inspection of the skin, perineum and rectum. Closed degloving injuries (Morel-Lavallée) should be properly identified. Palpation of the pelvic bony landmarks, including posterior palpation of the sacrum and sacroiliac joint, should be done. Rectovaginal examination is mandatory in all cases to identify open fractures. Bony spikes protruding through the mucosa contaminates the fracture hematoma. Anteroposterior and lateral iliac wing compression maneuvers to assess stability should be performed only once or avoided in hemodynamically unstable patients as excessive manipulation can increase bleeding. Associated injuries should also be systematically sought: lower urinary tract injuries, distal vascular status, and a thorough recorded neurologic examination.

An initial anteroposterior pelvic radiograph as per ATLS protocol is examined to evaluate the pelvic ring as a possible cause of shock. Following successful resuscitation, inlet and outlet views should be obtained. CT scan is essential to further define the fracture pattern Vascular and urologic imaging may also be required.

Open Pelvic Fractures

Open pelvic fractures account for 2–4% of all pelvic fractures. Because a higher energy is required to fracture the immature pelvic ring, the incidence of open pelvic fractures is increased among children. Motorcycle accidents are in part responsible for the increase in open pelvic fractures. Mortality has decreased from 50% in the 80s to 10–25%, probably because of the application of multidisciplinary protocols, including aggressive fracture management, selective fecal diversion and advances in critical care.

Treatment

Significant forces, either directly or indirectly through the lower extremities, are required to destabilize the pelvic ring. A systematic search for associated injuries is mandatory. Hemorrhage and shock are the primary causes of death due to pelvic fracture. The cornerstones of successful treatment include: identification of a significant pelvic injury; rapid resuscitation; hemorrhage control (using angiography or pelvic packing); assessment and treatment of associated injuries, and mechanical stabilization and in selected cases. In the hemodynamically unstable patient the ATLS® protocol should be followed. A pelvic binder or sheet can be used to stabilize the unstable pelvis temporarily. Antiseptic pressure dressings should be applied to bleeding sites. If there is continued hemodynamic instability after initial resuscitation (2 liters of IV fluids), a decision needs to be made in consultation with the trauma surgeon to perform pelvic packing with or without external fixation. If the patient's hemodynamic status stabilizes, the need for definitive versus temporizing mechanical fixation of the pelvis should be determined. This may involve anterior plating of the pubic symphysis, or the application of an external fixation device (pelvic clamp and /or anterior external fixator). Posterior fixation (either surgical or computed tomography guided percutaneous fixation) is usually deferred until a later time. When used to control pelvic fracture motion, the pelvic external fixator is a useful tool to manage volume depletion. It does not provide stable enough fixation to treat complex fractures or most unstable pelvic fractures. It usually resists stresses imposed by sitting but not those from weight bearing, and further internal fixation is often required at a later stage.

In open pelvic fractures, early surgical intervention using a multidisciplinary approach should be undertaken. Seventy-two percent of the open pelvic fractures are grade III open wounds, and should be appropriately treated. Swabs for microbiological examination followed by extensive irrigation and debridement are performed and repeated daily in an attempt to reduce the incidence of pelvic sepsis. Early selective faecal diversion in patients with perineal wounds can reduce sepsis and related mortality. The definitive method of stabilization of open pelvic fractures remains controversial. Internal fixation can be done when no gross contamination is present. Otherwise, external fixation is preferred when faecal or environmental contamination is present.

A. Associated Injuries

1. Hemorrhage—Bleeding associated with pelvic ring fractures usually comes from the small to medium-sized arteries and veins in the surrounding soft tissues and from the bone itself. After blunt trauma, the most common pelvic arteries injured are the superior gluteal artery, internal pudendal, obturator, and lateral sacral arteries. Occasionally, large vessels such as the femoral artery or the common iliac artery or vein are lacerated or torn. An arteriogram is diagnostic. Alternatively, contrast enhanced CT allows the early diagnosis of arterial bleeding. Arterial injuries causing significant bleeding occur only in about 10% of pelvic fractures, and surgery for repair or bypass is urgently required if there is distal ischemia.

2. Thrombosis—It is now well recognized that patients with pelvic fractures have a high incidence of thrombosis of the pelvic veins and, less frequently, of the femoral vein. Those treated with bed rest compound the risk of deep vein thrombosis and secondary pulmonary embolus. More trauma centers now use intermittent pneumatic compression after trauma and pharmacologic anticoagulation once the acute hemorrhagic phase has passed (24–48 hours). Severely traumatized patients with contraindications for pharmacological anticoagulation may benefit from temporary vena cava filters.

3. Neurologic injury—Neurologic injuries are common, with an overall incidence between 10% and 15% in pelvic fractures and are a common cause of disability following pelvic fracture. After unstable vertical shear sacral fractures the incidence rises to 50%. They involve either the roots (L5, S1) as they travel in or around the sacral foramen, or the peripheral nerve itself (sciatic, femoral, obturator, pudendal, or superior gluteal). Neurologic injury following closed or open reduction is not uncommon. Thus it is of paramount importance that a thorough neurologic examination be performed and recorded as soon as possible, searching for sensory or motor deficits in the distribution of all previously mentioned nerves. Peripheral nerve injuries have, overall, a better prognosis than root injuries. Partial nerve injuries also have a better outcome than complete ones. Most of the lesions are of the neurapraxia type, with favorable outcome. It is still accepted that nearly 10% have clinically significant permanent neurologic sequelae.

4. Urogenital injuries—Urogenital injuries are also common, especially in men. The incidence of bladder rupture and urethral disruption is estimated at 5–10% for each. These injuries should be suspected in the conscious patient who is unable to void or who has gross hematuria. Other signs include bloody urethral discharge, swelling or ecchymosis of the penis or perineum, or a high-riding or "floating" prostate on rectal examination. A retrograde urethrogram should be obtained before attempting to introduce a Foley catheter. If unremarkable, catheterization can be safely undertaken and a cystogram obtained later. When a partial or complete urethral disruption is diagnosed, a suprapubic cystostomy should be performed. Late sequelae are common and include urethral strictures, sexual dysfunction, and impotence.

1. Injuries to the Pelvic Ring

Pelvic ring fractures account for 3% of all fractures. There is an extremely wide spectrum between the innocuous avulsion fracture and the life-threatening severely unstable pelvic ring disruption. The choice between different treatment modalities revolves around one key issue: Is the fracture pattern stable or unstable?

From the anatomic standpoint, the posterior sacroiliac ligamentous complex is the single most important structure for pelvic stability. Injuries involving the pelvic ring in two or more sites create an unstable segment. The integrity of the posterior sacroiliac ligamentous complex will determine the degree of instability. Inlet and outlet views and CT scanning are necessary imaging techniques to make this determination. When intact, the hemipelvis will be rotationally unstable but vertically stable. When disrupted, the hemipelvis will be both rotationally and vertically unstable.

Classification & Treatment

Tile devised a dynamic classification system based on the mechanism of injury and residual instability (Table 3–4).

Type A: Fractures that involve the pelvic ring in only one place and are stable.

Type A1: Avulsion fractures of the pelvis, which usually occurs at muscle origins such as the anterosuperior iliac spine for the sartorius, anteroinferior iliac spine for the direct head of the rectus femoris, and ischial apophysis for the hamstring muscles. These fractures occur most often in the adolescent, and conservative treatment is usually sufficient. On rare occasions, symptomatic nonunion occurs, and this is best dealt with surgically.

Type A2: Stable fractures with minimal displacement. Isolated fractures of the iliac wing without intraarticular extension usually result from direct trauma. Even with significant displacement, bony healing is to be expected, and treatment is, therefore, symptomatic. On rare occasions, the soft tissue injury and accompanying hematoma may heal with significant heterotopic ossification.

Type A3: Obturator fractures. Isolated fractures of the pubic or ischial rami are usually minimally displaced. The posterior sacroiliac complex is intact, and the pelvis is stable. Treatment is symptomatic, with bed rest and analgesia, early ambulation, and weight bearing as tolerated.

Type B: Fractures that involve the pelvic ring in two or more sites. They create a segment that is rotationally unstable but vertically stable.

Type B1: Open-book fractures occur from anteroposterior compression. Unless the anterior separation of the pubic symphysis is severe (>6 cm), the posterior sacroiliac complex is usually intact and the pelvis relatively stable. Significant injury to perineal and urogenital structures is often present and should always be looked for. One should remember

Table 3–4. The Tile classification of pelvic ring disruptions.

Type A: Stable, posterior arch intact
A1: Posterior arch intact, fracture of innominate bone (avulsion)
- A1.1 Iliac spine
- A1.2 Iliac crest
- A1.3 Ischial tuberosity

A2: Posterior arch intact, fracture of innominate bone (direct blow)
- A2.1 Iliac wing fractures
- A2.2 Unilateral fracture of anterior arch
- A2.3 Bifocal fracture of anterior arch

A3: Posterior arch intact, transverse fracture of sacrum caudal to S2
- A3.1 Sacrococcygeal dislocation
- A3.2 Sacrum undisplaced
- A3.3 Sacrum displaced

Type B: Incomplete disruption of posterior arch, partially stable, rotation
B1: External rotation instability, open-book injury, unilateral
- B1.1 Sacroiliac joint, anterior disruption
- B1.2 Sacral fracture

B2: Incomplete disruption of posterior arch, unilateral, internal rotation (lateral compression)
- B2.1 Anterior compression fracture, sacrum
- B2.2 Partial sacroiliac joint fracture, subluxation
- B2.3 Incomplete posterior iliac fracture

B3: Incomplete disruption of posterior arch, bilateral
- B3.1 Bilateral open-book
- B3.2 Open-book, lateral compression
- B3.3 Bilateral lateral compression

Type C: Complete disruption of posterior arch, unstable
C1: Complete disruption of posterior arch, unilateral
- C1.1 Fracture through ilium
- C1.2 Sacroiliac dislocation and/or fracture dislocation
- C1.3 Sacral fracture

C2: Bilateral injury, one side rotationally unstable, one side vertically unstable
C3: Bilateral injury, both sides completely unstable

Reproduced, with permission, from Browner BD et al, eds: *Skeletal Trauma,* 2nd ed. WB Saunders, 1998.

that fragment displacement at the time of injury might have been significantly more than what is apparent on radiograph. For minimally displaced symphysis injuries, only symptomatic treatment is needed. The same applies for the so-called straddle (four rami) fracture. For more displaced fracture-dislocations, reduction is done by lateral compression using the intact posterior sacroiliac complex as the hinge on which "the book is closed." Reduction can be maintained by external or internal fixation. "Closing the book" decreases the space available for hemorrhage. It also increases patient comfort, facilitates nursing care, and allows earlier mobilization, which is beneficial to the polytrauma patient.

Type B2 and B3: Lateral compression fractures. A lateral force applied to the pelvis causes inward displacement of the hemipelvis through the sacroiliac complex and the ipsilateral (B2) or, more often, contralateral pubic rami (B3, bucket-handle type). The degree of involvement of the posterior sacroiliac ligaments will determine the degree of instability. The posterior lesion may be impacted in its displaced portion, affording some relative stability. The hemipelvis is infolded, with overlapping of the symphysis. Major displacement requires manipulation under general anesthesia. This should be done soon after injury because disimpaction becomes difficult and hazardous after the first few days. Reduction can be maintained with external or internal fixation, or both. External fixation alone decreases pain and makes nursing care easier but is not strong enough for ambulation if the fracture is unstable posteriorly.

Type C: Fractures that are both rotationally and vertically unstable. They often result from a vertical shear mechanism, like a fall from a height. Anteriorly, the injury may fracture the pubic rami or disrupt the symphysis pubis. Posteriorly, the sacroiliac joint may be dislocated or there may be a fracture in the sacrum or in the ilium immediately adjacent to the sacroiliac joint, but there is always loss of the functional integrity of the posterior sacroiliac ligamentous complex. The hemipelvis is completely unstable. Three-dimensional displacement is possible, particularly proximal migration. Massive hemorrhage and injury to the lumbosacral nerve plexus are common. Indirect radiologic clues of pelvic instability should be looked for such as avulsion of the sciatic spine or fracture of the ipsilateral L5 transverse process. Reduction is relatively easy, with longitudinal skeletal traction through the distal femur or the proximal tibia. If chosen as definitive treatment, traction should be maintained for 8–12 weeks. Bony injuries heal quicker than ligamentous injuries. External fixation alone is insufficient to maintain reduction in highly unstable fractures, but it may help control bleeding and eases nursing care. Open reduction and internal fixation is often required. The surgical technique is demanding, and there is a significant risk of complications. It is best left to experienced pelvic surgeons.

Complications

Long-term complications of unstable pelvic ring disruptions are more frequent and disabling than once thought. Of those patients with residual displacement of more than 1 cm, fewer than 30% are pain free at 5 years. Chronic low back pain and posterior sacroiliac pain is the most frequent long-term complaint, approaching 50% in some series. Nearly 5% of type C injuries are left with a leg length discrepancy of more than 2–5 cm. Residual gait abnormalities are present in 12–32% of cases. The overall nonunion rate is around 3%.

Clinically significant neurologic deficit is present in 6–10% of patients, but abnormal electromyographic findings are present in up to 46%. Long-term urologic complications include urethral strictures in 5–20% of cases and impotence in 5–30% of cases.

2. Fractures of the Acetabulum

The acetabulum results from the closure of the Y or triradiate cartilage and is covered with hyaline cartilage.

Fractures of the acetabulum occur through direct trauma on the trochanteric region or indirect axial loading through the lower limb. The position of the limb at the time of impact (rotation, flexion, abduction, or adduction) will determine the pattern of injury. Comminution is common.

Anatomy

The acetabulum appears to be contained within an arch. It is supported by the confluence of two columns and enhanced by two walls. The posterior column is the strongest one and where more space is available for fixation. It begins at the dense bone of the greater sciatic notch and extends distally through the center of the acetabulum to include the ischial spine and ischial tuberosity. The inner surface forms the posterior wall, and the anterior surface forms the posterior articular surface of the acetabulum. The anterior column extends from the iliac crest to the symphysis pubis. The anterior column rotates 90° just above the acetabulum as it descends. The medial part of the anterior column is the true pelvic brim. The quadrilateral plate is the medial structure preventing medial displacement of the hip, and is an independent structure between the two columns. The acetabular dome or weight-bearing area extends from the bone posterior to the anterior inferior iliac spine to the posterior column.

Classification

Letournel has classified acetabular fractures based on the involved column. Fractures may involve one or both columns in a simple or complex pattern.

Proper fracture classification requires good-quality radiographs. Two oblique views (Judet views) taken 45 degrees toward and away from the involved side complement the standard anteroposterior view of the pelvis. The obturator oblique view is obtained by elevating the fractured hip 45 degrees from the horizontal. This view shows the anterior column and the posterior lip of the acetabulum, and the iliac wing is perpendicular to its broad surface. In this view, the spur sign can be identified in 95% of cases of both-column fractures (Type C), and it corresponds to the area of the iliac wing above the acetabular roof. The Iliac oblique view is obtained by elevating the non-fractured hip 45°. This view best shows the posterior column, including the ischial spine, the anterior wall of the acetabulum, and the full expanse of the iliac wing. In addition, inlet and outlet pelvic views can be complimentary used if any doubt about pelvic ring compromise is present.

CT scanning gives further information on the fracture pattern, the presence of free intraarticular fragments, and the status of the femoral head and the rest of the pelvic ring.

Letournel has classified acetabular fractures into 10 different types: 5 simple patterns (one fracture line) and 5 complex patterns (the association of two or more simple patterns) (Figure 3–31). This is the most widely used classification system, as it allows the surgeon to choose the appropriate surgical approach.

Treatment

The goal of treatment is to attain a spherical congruency between the femoral head and the weight-bearing acetabular dome, and to maintain it until bones are healed. As with other pelvic fractures, acetabular fractures are frequently associated with abdominal, urogenital, and neurologic injuries, which should be systematically sought and treated. Significant bleeding can be present and should be addressed as soon as possible. Examination of the knee ligaments and vascular status of the extremities is mandatory. A careful neurologic

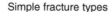

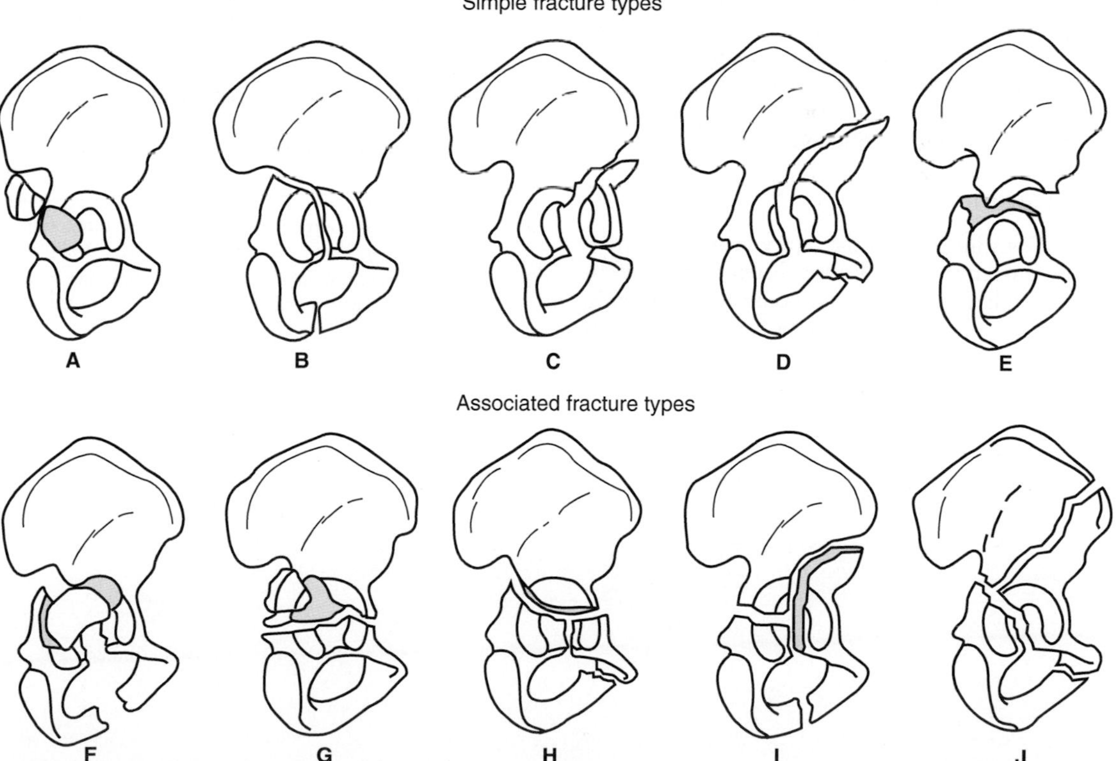

Figure 3–31. Letournel classification of acetabular fractures. (Reproduced, with permission, from Canale ST, ed: *Campbell's Operative Orthopaedics*, 9th ed. Lippincott, 1998.)

examination is necessary. Sciatic nerve compromise occurs in 20% of cases. The peroneal branch is often involved. Also, the tibial branch of the sciatic nerve, the femoral nerve, and the lateral femoral cutaneous nerve can be involved depending upon the fracture pattern and mechanism. Prophylaxis and surveillance for deep vein thrombosis (DVT) should be started soon after trauma. The reported incidence of DVT in patients with pelvic fractures has been as high as 60%.

The stabilized patient should be put in longitudinal skeletal traction through a distal femoral or proximal tibial pin pulling axially in neutral position. A trochanteric screw for lateral traction is contraindicated, as it will create a contaminated pin tract and thus preclude possible further surgical treatment. Postreduction radiographs are obtained. In general, a displaced acetabular fracture is rarely reduced adequately by closed methods. If the reduction is judged acceptable, traction is maintained for 6–8 weeks until bone healing is evident. Another 6–8 weeks is necessary before full weight bearing can be attempted. Surgical indications include intraarticular displacement of 2 mm or more, an incongruous hip reduction, marginal impaction >2 mm, or intraarticular debris. The choice of approach is of primary importance, and sometimes more than one approach will prove necessary. Acetabular surgery uses extensile approaches and sophisticated reduction and fixation techniques and is best performed by trained pelvic surgeons. Other surgical indications include free osteochondral fragments, femoral head fractures, irreducible dislocations, or unstable reductions.

Complications

Complications inherent to the injury include posttraumatic degenerative joint disease, heterotopic ossification, femoral head osteonecrosis, deep vein thrombosis, and other complications related to conservative treatment. Surgery is performed to prevent or delay osteoarthritis, but increases the possibility of complications such as infection, iatrogenic neurovascular injury, and increased heterotopic ossification. When the reduction is stable and fixation is solid, the patient can be mobilized after a few days with non-weight–bearing ambulation, and weight bearing may begin as early as 6 weeks. Most pelvic surgeons now routinely use postoperative prophylactic anticoagulation and heterotopic bone formation prophylaxis with irradiation or indomethacin, or both.

Bellabarba C, Ricci WM, Bolhofner BR: Distraction external fixation in lateral compression pelvic fractures. J Orthop Trauma 2000;14:475. [PMID: 11083609]

Carlson DA et al: Safe placement of S1 and S2 iliosacral screws: the vestibule concept. J Orthop Trauma 2000;14:264. [PMID: 10898199]

Ertel W et al: Control of Severe hemorrhage using C-clamp and pelvic packing in multiply injured patients with pelvic ring disruption. J Orthop Trauma 2001;15:468. [PMID: 11602828]

Grotz MRW, Allami MK, Harwood P, Pape HC, Kretekk C, Giannoudis PV. Open Pelvic Fractures: epidemiology, current concepts of management and outcome. Injury. 2005;1:1–13. [PMID: 15589906]

McCormick JP, Morgan SJ, Smith WR. Clinical effectiveness of the physical examination in diagnosis of posterior pelvic ring injuries. J Orthop Trauma. 2003 APR;17(4):257–61. [PMID: 12679685]

Routt ML, et al. Circumferential pelvic antishock sheeting: A temporary resuscitation aid. J Orthop Trauma 2002;15:45. [PMID: 11782633]

Saterbak AM et al: Clinical failure after posterior wall acetabular fractures: The influence of initial fracture patterns. J Orthop Trauma 2000;14:230. [PMID: 10898194]

Switzer JA, Nork SE, Routt ML: Comminuted fractures of the iliac wing. J Orthop Trauma 2000;14:270. [PMID: 10898200]

Tornetta P: Displaced acetabular fractures: Indications for operative and nonoperative management. J Am Acad Orthop Surg 2001;9:18. [PMID: 11174160]

Sports Medicine

4

Patrick J. McMahon, MD, & Lee D. Kaplan, MD

Introduction

Sports medicine developed in the 1970s as an orthopedic specialty focusing on competitive athletes. Today, sports medicine includes the overall care of athletes from many skill levels. Increasingly, care of recreational athletes has risen to that common for professional athletes. The initial focus of sports medicine on knee injuries now also includes other musculoskeletal injuries, including the shoulder, elbow, and ankle. In addition to the musculoskeletal system, emphasis is placed on the cardiovascular and pulmonary systems, and on training techniques, nutrition, and women's athletics. This wide range of care requires a multidisciplinary team of medical personnel, including athletic trainers, physical therapists, cardiologists, pulmonologists, orthopedic surgeons, and general practitioners.

KNEE INJURIES

Anatomy

The bones of the knee are the distal femur, the proximal tibia, and the patella. These bones depend on supporting ligaments, the joint capsule, and the menisci to provide stability for the joint.

A. Menisci and Joint Capsule

The menisci, or semilunar cartilages, are C-shaped fibrocartilaginous disks in the knee that provide shock absorption, allow for increased congruency between joint surfaces, enhance joint stability, and aid in distribution of synovial fluid.

The medial and lateral menisci provide a concave surface with which the convex femoral condyles can articulate. If the menisci are not present, the convex femoral condyles articulate with the relatively flat tibial plateaus, and the joint surfaces are not congruent. This situation decreases the surface area of contact and increases the pressure on the articular cartilage of the tibia and femur, which may lead to rapid deterioration of the joint surface. The medial meniscus is firmly attached to the joint capsule along its entire peripheral edge. The lateral meniscus is attached to the anterior and posterior capsule, but there is a region posterolaterally where it is not firmly attached (Figure 4–1). Therefore, the medial meniscus has less mobility than the lateral meniscus and is more susceptible to tearing when trapped between the femoral condyle and tibial plateau. The lateral meniscus is larger than the medial meniscus, and carries a greater share of the lateral compartment pressure than the medial meniscus carries for the medial compartment.

B. Ligaments

Within the knee, the anterior cruciate ligament (ACL) travels from the medial border of the lateral femoral condyle to its insertion site anterolateral to the medial tibial spine. This ligament prevents anterior translation and rotation of the tibia on the femur (Figure 4–2). The posterior cruciate ligament (PCL) prevents posterior subluxation of the tibia on the femur. It runs from the lateral aspect of the medial femoral condyle to the posterior aspect of the tibia, just below the joint line (Figure 4–3). On the medial side, the medial collateral ligament has superficial and deep portions (Figure 4–4), which stabilize the knee to valgus stresses. The lateral collateral or fibular collateral ligament runs from the lateral femoral condyle to the head of the fibula. It is the main stabilizer against varus stress (Figure 4–5). The lateral collateral ligament is part of the posterolateral "complex" or "corner" of the knee that also resists external rotation. An important component is the popliteofibular ligament, present in 90% of knees, that runs from the tendon of the popliteus muscle to the styloid on the posterior fibular head.

History & Physical Examination

A. General Approach

The history of knee injury may be obtained by asking the patient the questions listed in Table 4–1. The physical examination begins with observation of the patient's gait. The uninjured knee is then examined as a

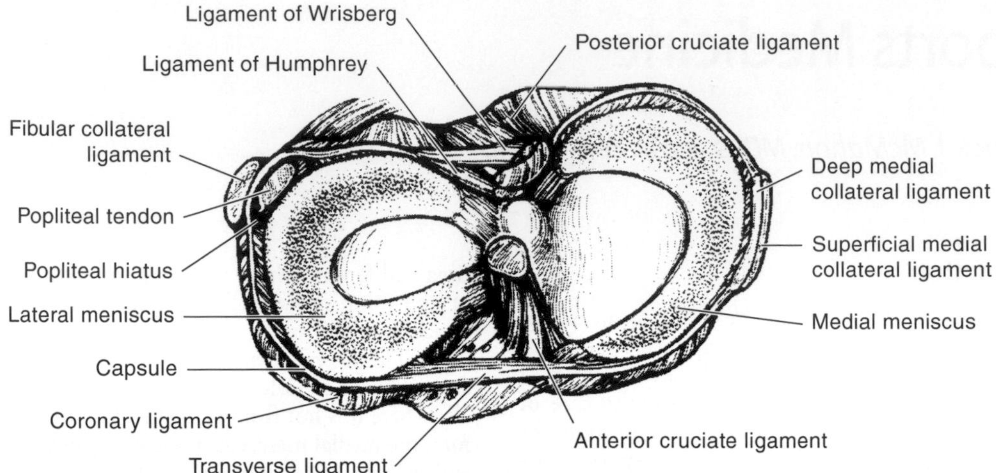

Figure 4–1. **The medial and lateral menisci with their associated intermeniscal ligaments.** ***Note*****: The lateral meniscus is not attached in the region of the popliteus tendon.** (Reproduced, with permission, from Scott WN: *Ligament and Extensor Mechanism Injuries of the Knee: Diagnosis and Treatment.* Mosby-Year Book, 1991.)

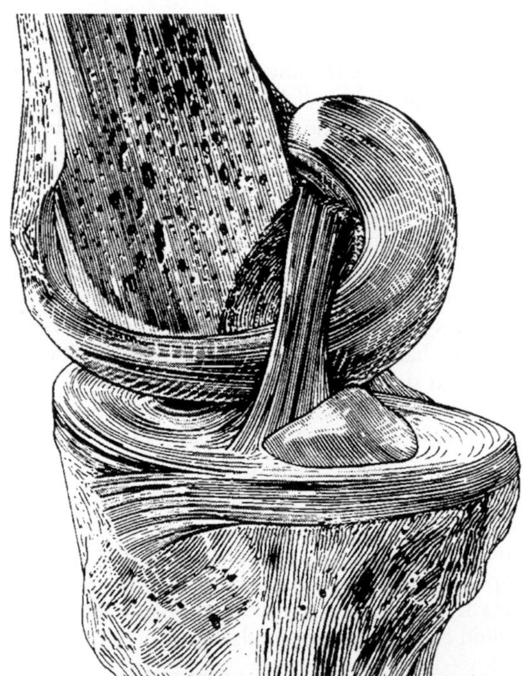

Figure 4–2. **Drawing of the anterior cruciate ligament with the knee in extension, showing the course of the ligament as it passes from the medial aspect of the lateral femoral condyle to the lateral portion of the medial tibial spine.** (Reproduced, with permission, from Girgis FG et al: The cruciate ligaments of the knee joint: Anatomical, functional, and experimental analysis. Clin Orthop 1975;106:216.)

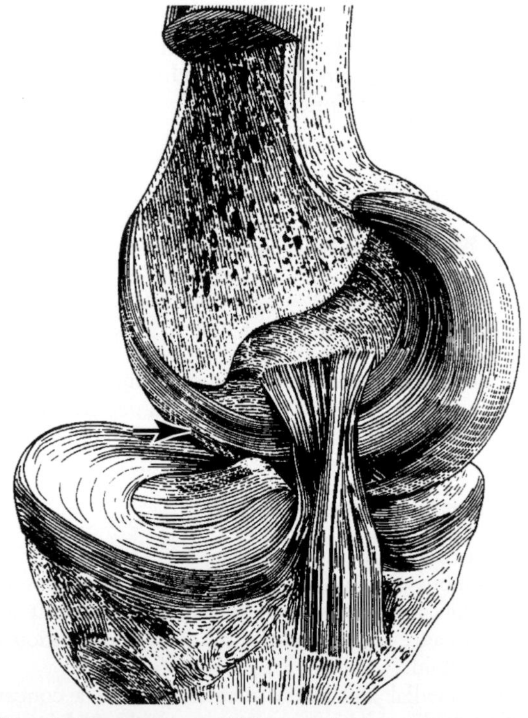

Figure 4–3. **Drawing of the posterior cruciate ligament, showing the course of the ligament as it passes from the lateral aspect of the medial femoral condyle to the posterior surface of the tibia.** (Adapted, with permission, from Girgis FG et al: The cruciate ligaments of the knee joint: Anatomical, functional, and experimental analysis. Clin Orthop 1975;106:216.)

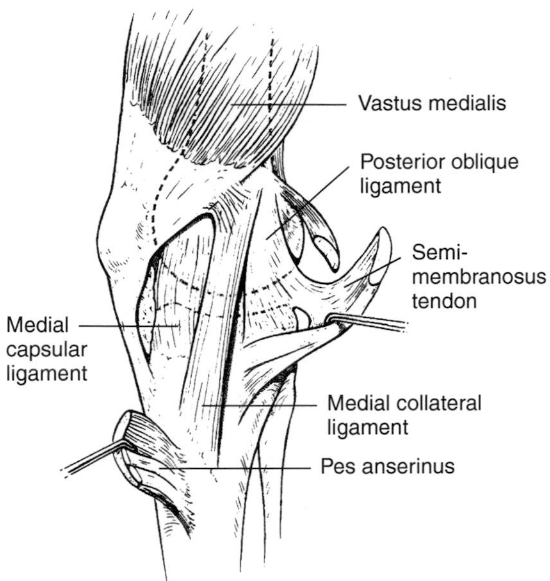

Figure 4–4. Medial capsuloligamentous complex. (Reproduced, with permission, from Feagin JA Jr: *The Crucial Ligaments*. Churchill Livingstone, 1988.)

basis of comparison with the injured knee. Any swelling or effusion should be noted. A small effusion causes obliteration of the recesses on the medial and lateral aspects of the patellar tendon; with a larger effusion, diffuse swelling is present in the region of the suprapatellar pouch. Then, a fluid wave can be palpated on the sides of the patella. Active and then passive range of motion is tested carefully. The knee is palpated to define areas of localized tenderness. The joint lines are located at the level of the inferior pole of the patella when the knee is flexed to 90 degrees.

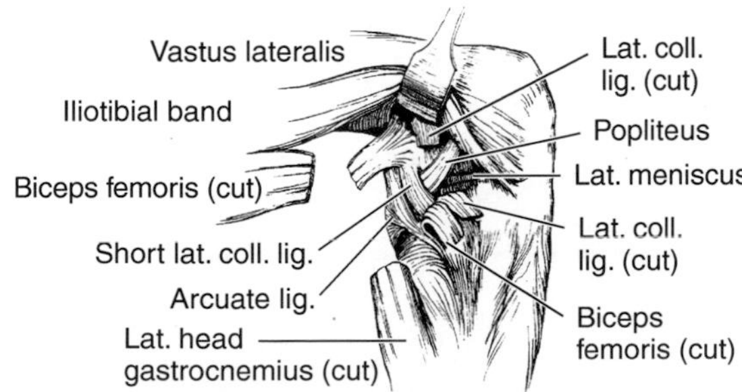

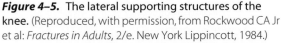

Figure 4–5. The lateral supporting structures of the knee. (Reproduced, with permission, from Rockwood CA Jr et al: *Fractures in Adults*, 2/e. New York Lippincott, 1984.)

Table 4–1. History of a knee injury.

Did an injury occur?	Yes: possible ligament tear or meniscus tear. No: overuse problem or degenerative condition.
Was it a noncontact injury?	Yes: often the ACL is the only ligament torn.
Was it a contact injury?	Yes: possible multiple ligament injuries, including ACL and MCL, ACL and LCL, ACL, PCL, and a collateral ligament.
Did the patient hear or feel a pop?	Yes: a pop often occurs with ACL tears.
How long did it take to swell up?	Within hours: often an ACL tear. Overnight: often a meniscus tear.
Does the knee lock?	Yes: often a meniscus tear flipping into and out of the joint.
Does it buckle (trick knee)?	Yes: not specific; may arise from quadriceps weakness, trapped meniscus, ligament instability, or patella dislocating.
Is climbing or descending stairs difficult?	Often patellofemoral problems.
Are cutting maneuvers difficult?	ACL tear.
Is squatting (deep knee bends) difficult?	Meniscus tear.
Is jumping difficult?	Patellar tendinitis.
Where does it hurt?	Medial joint line: medial meniscus tear or medial compartment arthritis. MCL: MCL sprain. Lateral joint line: lateral meniscus tear, injury, iliotibial band tendinitis, popliteus tendinitis.

ACL = anterior cruciate ligament; MCL = medial collateral ligament; LCL = lateral collateral ligament; PCL = posterior cruciate ligament.

B. Ligament Laxity Evaluation

To determine varus and valgus stability (Table 4–2), the patient's foot is held between the examiner's elbow and hip, with both hands free to palpate the joint (Figure 4–6). Stability should be determined at both full extension and 30 degrees of knee flexion. Grading of laxity is based on the amount of opening of the joint (grade 1, 0–5 mm; grade 2, 5–10 mm; and grade 3, 10–15 mm). Laxity in full extension to varus or valgus angulation is

Table 4–2. Anatomic correlation of clinical ligament instability examination of the knee.

Direction of Force	Position	Ligament Instability
Varus or valgus	Full extension	Posterior cruciate, posterior capsule
Varus	Flexion at 30 degrees	Lateral collateral ligament/complex
Valgus	Flexion at 30 degrees	Medial collateral ligament
Anterior	Flexion at 30 degrees neutral position (AP)	Anterior cruciate ligament
Anterior	Flexion at 90 degrees neutral internal or external rotation	Anterior cruciate ligament
Posterior	90 degrees (sag test)	Posterior cruciate ligament

AP = anteroposterior.

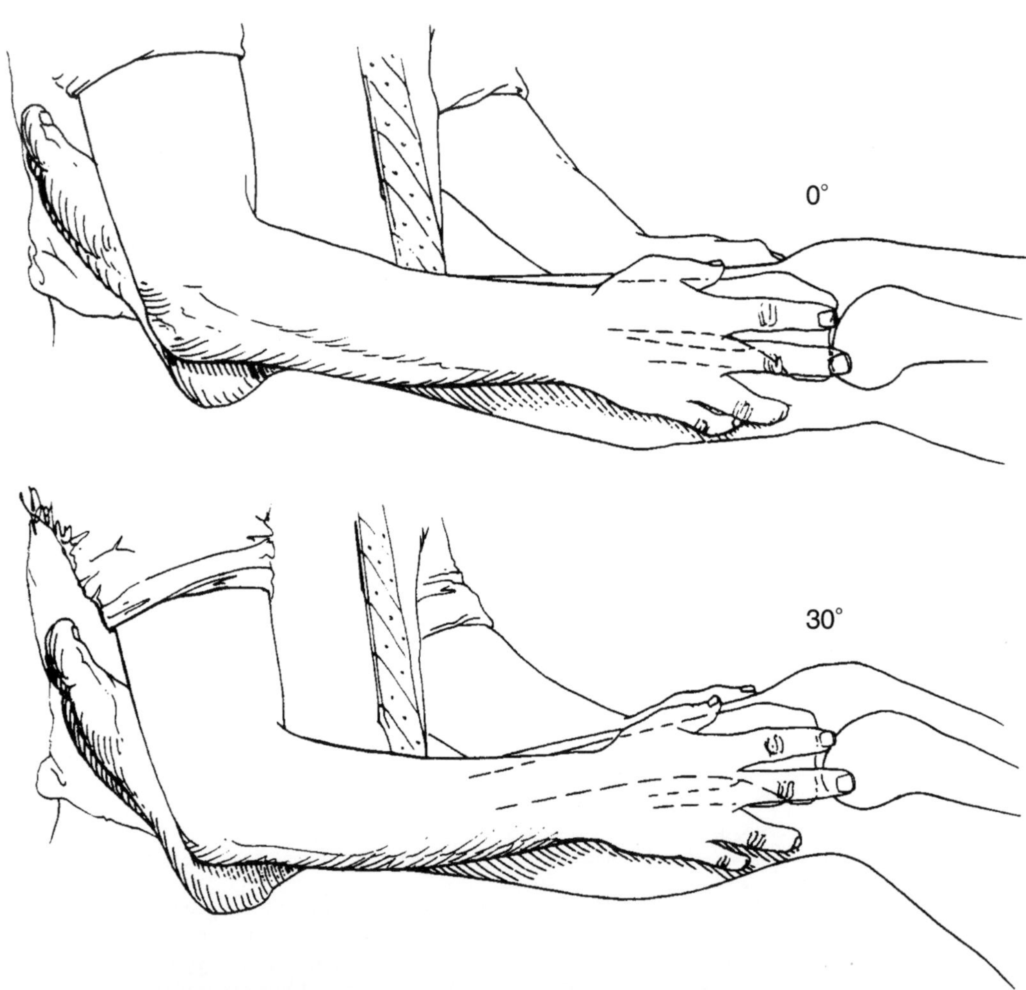

Figure 4–6. **The collateral ligaments being tested in extension and 30 degrees of flexion with the foot held between the examiner's elbow and hip.** (Reproduced, with permission, from Feagin JA Jr: *The Crucial Ligaments.* Churchill Livingstone, 1988.)

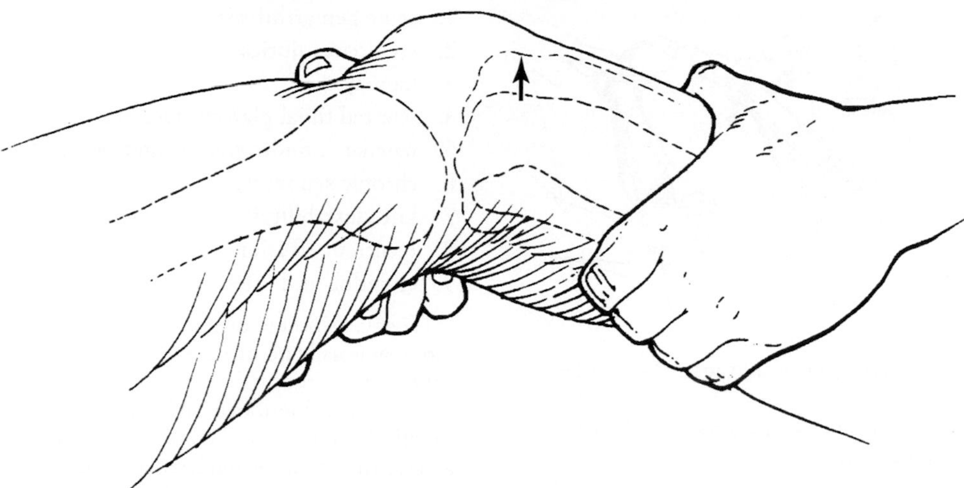

Figure 4–7. **Lachman test.** (Reproduced, with permission, from Feagin JA Jr: *The Crucial Ligaments.* Churchill Livingstone, 1988.)

an ominous sign that indicates disruption of key ligamentous structures. If significant valgus laxity is present in full extension, the posteromedial capsule and medial collateral ligament are torn. With varus laxity in full extension, the posterolateral capsular complex is torn, in addition to the lateral collateral ligament. With either varus or valgus laxity at full extension, anterior and posterior cruciate ligament tears are likely. At 30 degrees of flexion, the posterior capsule and cruciate ligaments are relaxed, and the medial and lateral collateral ligaments can best be isolated. Pain with varus or valgus stress is more suggestive of ligament damage than a meniscus tear.

1. The Lachman test—The Lachman test is the most sensitive test for ACL tears. It is done with the knee flexed at 20 degrees, stabilizing the distal femur with one hand and pulling forward on the proximal tibia with the other hand. (Figure 4–7). With an intact ligament, minimal translation of the tibia occurs and a firm end point is felt. With a torn ACL, more translation is noted, and the end point is soft or mushy. The hamstring muscles must be relaxed during this maneuver to prevent false-negative findings. Comparison of the injured and uninjured knees is essential.

2. Anterior drawer test—The anterior drawer test is done with the knee at 90 degrees of flexion and is not as sensitive as the Lachman test but serves as an adjunct in the evaluation of ACL instability (Figure 4–8). With the patient supine and the knee flexed to 90 degrees (hip flexed to approximately 45 degrees), the foot is restrained by sitting on it, and the examiner's hands are placed around the proximal tibia. Then while the hamstrings are felt to relax and the tibia is pulled forward, the displacement and the endpoint are evaluated.

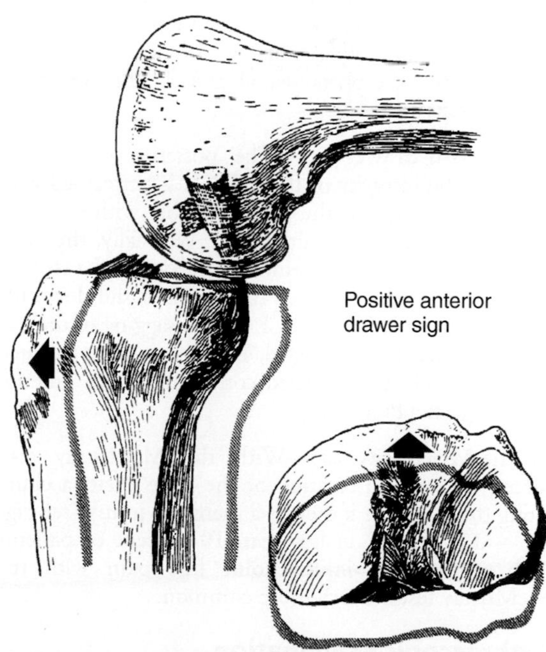

Figure 4–8. **A positive anterior drawer test signifying a tear of the anterior cruciate ligament.** (Reproduced, with permission, from Insall JN: *Surgery of the Knee.* Churchill Livingstone, 1984.)

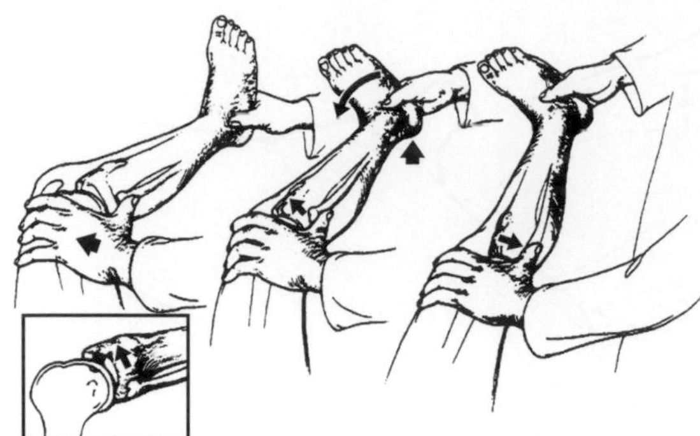

Figure 4–9. The Losee pivot shift test. (Reproduced, with permission, from Scott WN: *Ligament and Extensor Mechanism Injuries of the Knee: Diagnosis and Treatment.* Mosby-Year Book, 1991.)

3. The Losee test—The pivot shift phenomenon demonstrates the instability associated with an ACL tear. Once demonstrated, it is often difficult to repeat because the patient may find this maneuver uncomfortable and will guard against having it done again. As described by Losee, a valgus and internal rotation force is applied to the tibia (Figure 4–9). Starting at 45 degrees of flexion, the lateral tibial plateau is reduced. Extending the knee causes the lateral plateau to subluxate anteriorly with a thud at approximately 20 degrees of flexion. It reduces quietly at full extension. Many other ways of doing this test are described, but the phenomenon and significance of the different tests are similar.

4. Posterior drawer test—The posterior drawer test evaluates the integrity of the PCL. It is performed with posterior pressure on the proximal tibia with the knee flexed at 90 degrees (Figure 4–10). Normally, the tibial plateau is anterior to the femoral condyles, and a step-off to the tibia is palpated when the thumb is slid down the femoral condyles. With a PCL injury, sagging of the tibial plateau may be appreciated, and no step-off is palpated (Figure 4–11). An associated contusion on the anterior tibia suggests a PCL injury.

5. The McMurray test—With the McMurray test, forced flexion and rotation of the knee elicits a clunk along the joint line if there is a meniscus injury (see Figure 4–12). Found in less than 10 percent of patients with a meniscus injury, joint line pain with the McMurray test is much more common.

Arthroscopic Examination

A. Indications for Knee Injuries

Indications for arthroscopic examination in the knee include the following:

1. acute hemarthrosis;
2. meniscus injuries;
3. loose bodies;
4. selected tibial plateau fractures;
5. patellar chondromalacia and/or malalignment;
6. chronic synovitis;
7. knee instability;
8. recurrent effusions; and
9. chondral and osteochondral fractures.

Today, a specific diagnosis of the type of knee injury can now usually be made with a history, physical examination, and appropriate imaging studies. With an examination under anesthesia and arthroscopic evaluation, a specific diagnosis can be confirmed, expanded, or revised, and treatment can be rendered as needed.

B. Technique

Examination under anesthesia is very helpful in diagnosing ligament injuries and instability. It should be performed before the beginning of the procedure, before preparing and draping the extremity. For diagnostic arthroscopy, the knee joint is distended with irrigating fluid (usually saline or lactated Ringer's solution), which washes away blood and debris from the joint. A lateral portal, for the arthroscope, is placed approximately a thumb's breadth above the joint line and just lateral to the patellar tendon. The medial portal is placed at approximately the same level, but just medial to the patellar tendon for introducing arthroscopic tools such as a probe. One approach to the general inspection of the joint is to start in the suprapatellar pouch. Loose bodies and plicas are sought. The patellofemoral joint is then inspected and observed for tracking problems and cartilage damage. The lateral gutter and the popliteus tendon are examined by flexion and

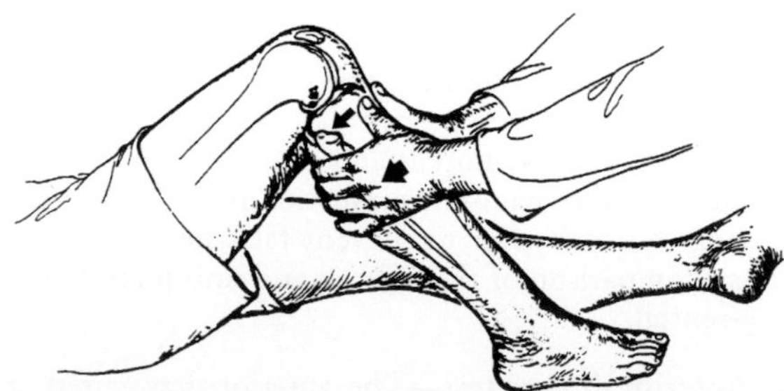

Figure 4–10. The posterior drawer test is done in the same fashion as the anterior drawer test, except that the examiner exerts a posterior force. (Reproduced, with permission, from Scott WN: *Ligament and Extensor Mechanism Injuries of the Knee: Diagnosis and Treatment.* Mosby-Year Book, 1991.)

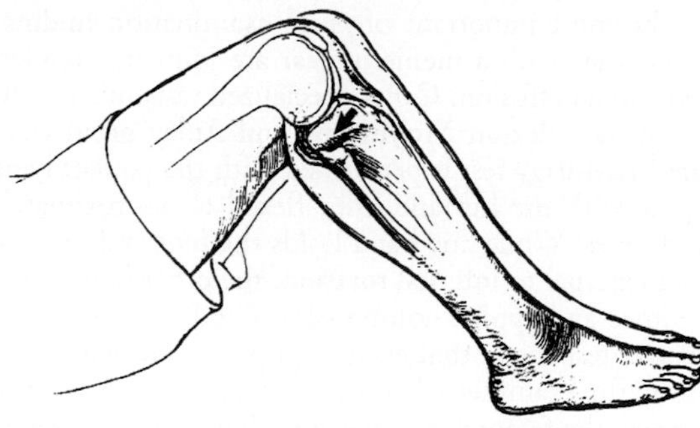

Figure 4–11. **The posterior sag seen in posterior cruciate disruption.** (Reproduced, with permission, from Scott WN: *Ligament and Extensor Mechanism Injuries of the Knee: Diagnosis and Treatment.* Mosby-Year Book, 1991.)

valgus stress to the leg, prior to entering the medial compartment. The medial meniscus is probed using a nerve hook through the medial portal. The intercondylar notch, including the ACL, is inspected. The lateral compartment is then examined in a similar manner. Documentation of findings and procedures performed is important and may be done by videotape, photographs, and diagrammatic sketches. With assessment of the pathologic changes, treatment can be initiated, such as debridement and repair of meniscus tears, removal of loose bodies, or ACL reconstruction.

Imaging & Other Studies

A. Magnetic Resonance Imaging

MRI is a powerful technique for evaluation of the knee joint. Although the diagnosis is usually evident from the history and physical examination, MRI can be used to confirm the suspected injury. Other times, when a physical examination is not possible because of pain or the diagnosis remains elusive, MRI can aid in proper diagnosis. The specificity, sensitivity, and accuracy of MRI are greater than 90% for the medial and lateral menisci and the ACL and PCL. Therefore, MRI is often appropriate for ruling out the need for diagnostic arthroscopic examination. It is less helpful for the diagnosis of problems in knees with previous surgery.

B. Imaging Studies

Roentgenographic examination of the knee is indicated in the evaluation of traumatic injury. In cases of minimal trauma, radiographs may not be needed if the

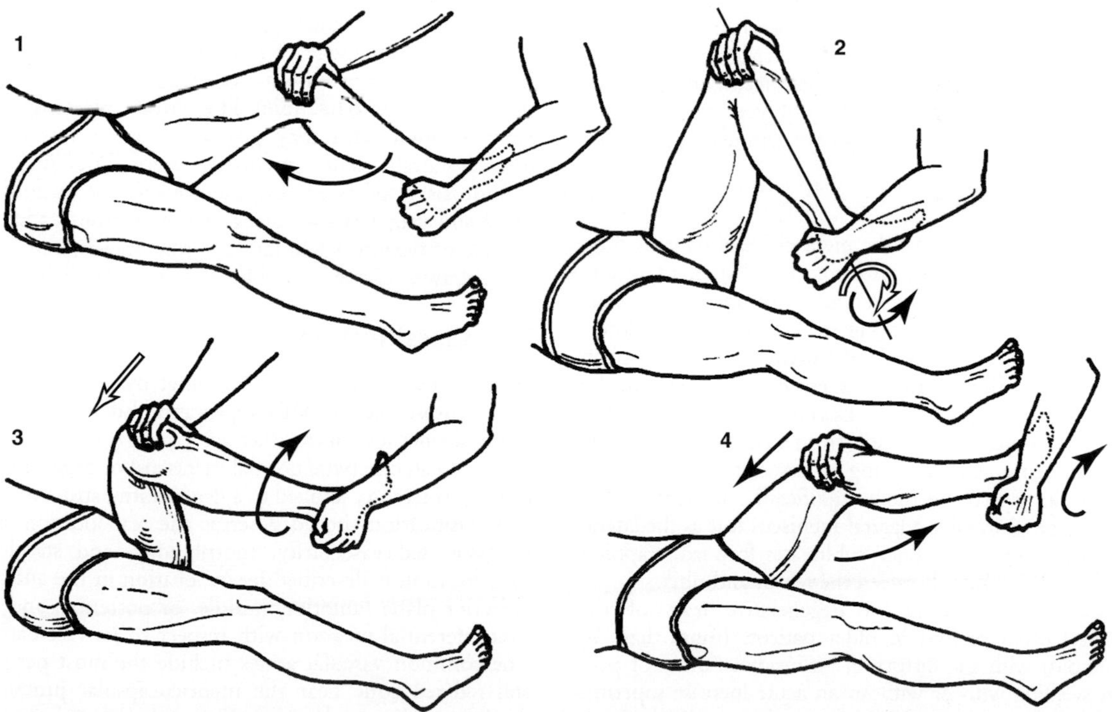

Figure 4–12. **The McMurray test to produce click.** (Reproduced, with permission, from American Academy of Orthopaedic Surgeons: *Athletic Training and Sports Medicine,* 2nd ed., 1991.)

injury proves to be self-limited. Arthrographic examination can be helpful in patients who are unable to undergo MRI because of claustrophobia, metal in the body that may be dislodged, or other contraindications.

C. Laboratory Tests

Laboratory tests may be helpful in ruling out nonmechanical disorders such as inflammatory arthritis as described in Chapter 7.

Chang CY et al: Imaging evaluation of meniscal injury of the knee joint: A comparative MR imaging and arthroscopic study. Clin Imaging 2004;28:372. [PMID: 15471672]

Luhmann SJ et al: Magnetic resonance imaging of the knee in children and adolescents. Its role in clinical decision-making. J Bone Joint Surg Am 2005;87-A:497. [PMID: 15741613]

Sanders TG, Miller MD: A systematic approach to magnetic resonance imaging interpretation of sports medicine injuries of the knee. Am J Sports Med 2005;33(1):131. [PMID: 15611010]

Scholten RJ et al. The accuracy of physical examination diagnostic tests for assessing meniscus lesions of the knee: A meta-analysis. J Fam Pract 2001,50:938. [PMID: 11711009]

MENISCUS INJURY

Meniscal injuries are the most common reason for arthroscopy of the knee. The medial meniscus is more frequently torn than the lateral meniscus because the medial meniscus is securely attached around the entire periphery of the joint capsule, whereas the lateral meniscus has a mobile area where it is not attached. Meniscus injury is rare in childhood, occurs in the late teens, and peaks in the third and fourth decades. After 50 years of age, meniscus tears are more often the result of arthritis than trauma.

Clinical Findings

Acute traumatic tears of the menisci are often caused by axial loading combined with rotation. Patients typically report pain and swelling. Patients with smaller tears may have a sensation of clicking or catching in the knee. Patients with larger tears in the meniscus may complain of locking of the knee as the meniscus displaces into the joint and/or femoral notch. Loss of knee motion with a block to extension may result from a large bucket-handle tear. In acute tears involving an associated ACL injury, the swelling may be more significant and acute. ACL injuries often involve a lateral meniscus tear as the lateral compartment of the knee subluxates forward, trapping the lateral meniscus between the femur and tibia.

Conversely, chronic or degenerative tears of the menisci often present in older patients (more than 40 years old) with the history of an insidious onset of pain and swelling with or without an acute increase superimposed. Often no identifiable history of trauma is obtained, or the inciting event may be quite minor, such as a bending or squatting motion.

The most important physical examination findings in the knee with a meniscus tear are joint line tenderness and an effusion. Other specialized tests include the McMurray, flexion McMurray, and Apley grind tests. The McMurray test is performed with the patient lying supine with the hip and knee flexed to approximately 90 degrees. While one hand holds the foot and twists it from external to internal rotation, the other hand holds the knee and applies compression (see Figure 4–12). A positive test is one that elicits a pop or click that can be felt by the examiner when the torn meniscus is trapped between the femoral condyle and tibial plateau. A variation of this test is the flexion McMurray, in which the knee is held as for the McMurray test. To test the medial meniscus, the foot is externally rotated and the knee maximally flexed. A positive test occurs when the patient experiences pain over the posteromedial joint line as the knee is gradually extended. The Apley grind test requires placing the patient prone with the knee flexed to 90 degrees. The examiner applies downward pressure to the sole of the foot while twisting the lower leg in external and internal rotation. A positive tests results in pain at either joint line.

In addition to the procedure just described, physical examination of the entire leg is essential. Assessing hip range of motion and irritability is useful, especially in children, because referred pain from the hip to the knee area is common. Examining for quadriceps atrophy and the presence of a knee effusion should also be done. Measurement of range of motion may reveal a loss of the normal knee extension. Assessing for tenderness of the femoral condyles, joint lines, tibial plateaus, and patellofemoral joint may give clues as to a possible osteochondral lesion, meniscus lesion, fracture, or chondrosis, respectively. Ligamentous testing, including varus and valgus stress testing at full extension and 30 degrees of flexion; Lachman; anterior drawer; and posterior drawer testing should be done to assess stability.

Tear Classification

Meniscal tears can be classified either by etiology or by their arthroscopic and MRI appearance. Etiologic classification divides tears into either acute tears (excessive force applied to an otherwise normal meniscus) or degenerative tears (normal force applied to a degenerative structure).

Classification should describe the tear location and its associated vascularity, morphology, and stability. Tear location is described by its location in the anteroposterior plane (anterior, middle, or posterior) and its circumferential location with respect to its vascularity. The common vascular zones include the most peripheral red/red zone near the meniscocapsular junction, the intermediate red/white zone, and the most central white/white zone. As tears occur more centrally, the vascularity decreases, as do the associated healing rates.

Tear morphology describes the orientation of the tear within the meniscus and includes vertical or horizontal longitudinal, radial (transverse), oblique, and complex (including degenerative) tears (Figure 4–13). Most acute tears in patients less than 40 years old involve vertical longitudinal or oblique tears, whereas complex and degenerative tears occur more commonly in patients more than 50 years old. Vertical longitudinal, or bucket-handle tears, can be complete or incomplete and usually start in the posterior horn and continue anteriorly a variable distance. Long tears can cause significant mobility of the torn meniscal fragment, allowing it to displace into the femoral notch and cause a locked knee (Figure 4–14). This more commonly occurs in the medial meniscus, possibly owing to its decreased mobility, which leads to increased sheer stresses. Oblique tears commonly occur at the junction of the middle and posterior thirds. They are often smaller tears, but the free edge of the tear can catch in the joint and cause symptoms of catching. Complex or degenerative tears occur in multiple planes, are often located in or near the posterior horns, and are more common in patients more than 50 years old with degenerative menisci. Horizontal longitudinal tears are often associated with meniscal cysts. They usually start at the inner margin of the meniscus and extend toward the meniscocapsular junction. They are thought to result from shear stresses and, when associated with meniscal cysts, they occur in the medial meniscus and cause localized swelling at the joint line.

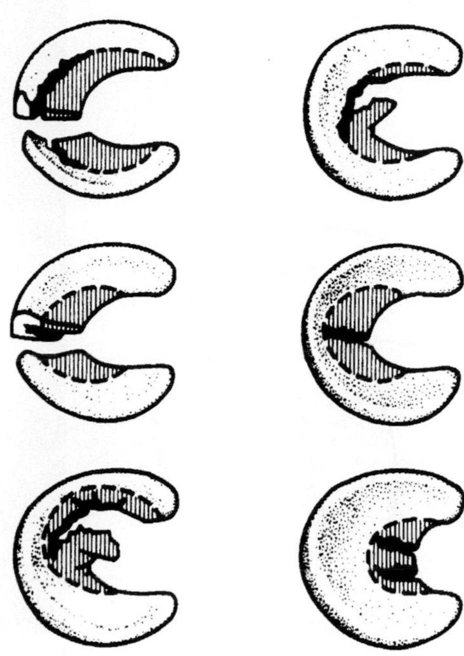

Figure 4–13. Patterns of meniscal tears: bucket-handle, flap, horizontal cleavage, radial, degenerative, and double radial tear of a discoid meniscus. (Reproduced, with permission, from Scott WN: *Arthroscopy of the Knee.* WB Saunders, 1990.)

Treatment & Prognosis

Small stable asymptomatic meniscus tears do not need to be treated surgically. Those causing persistent symptoms should be assessed with the arthroscope. Before the importance of the meniscus was understood and arthroscopy became available, the meniscus was often removed, even when normal. We now attempt to remove only the torn portion of the meniscus or repair the meniscus, if possible.

During arthroscopy, the meniscus should be visualized and palpated with a hooked probe. The inner two thirds of the meniscus is avascular and often requires resection when torn. A biting instrument is used to complete the resection of the torn portion of the meniscus, and the meniscus fragment is removed with a grasping instrument. Power shavers are used to smooth and contour the remaining meniscus to prevent further tearing from a jagged edge. Return to full function may be expected in 6–8 weeks.

Tears in the peripheral third of the meniscus, if small (less than 15 mm), may heal spontaneously because there is a blood supply in this portion of the adult meniscus. Larger tears need to be repaired. Patients who undergo meniscectomy at less than 40 years old are at risk of early osteoarthritis. These changes were first described by Fairbanks and include flattening of the femoral condyle, joint space narrowing, and osteophyte formation. Therefore, if a meniscus can be saved, it should be.

A. Partial Meniscal Resection

Partial meniscectomy has 90% good or excellent results in patients with normal knee stability and no degenerative changes. A major advantage over meniscus repair is a short recovery period, but results after partial meniscectomy are not as satisfactory when degenerative changes or knee ligament injuries are present. Also, results diminish over time; degenerative changes occur with follow-up beyond 10 years. Medial meniscus tears generally do better than lateral tears after partial resection, and an intact meniscal rim and normal articular cartilage surfaces are associated with a better prognosis.

B. Meniscus Repair

Most surgeons attempt a meniscus repair rather than a partial meniscectomy in individuals less than 40 years old. Other commonly accepted criteria for meniscus repair include a complete vertical longitudinal tear greater than

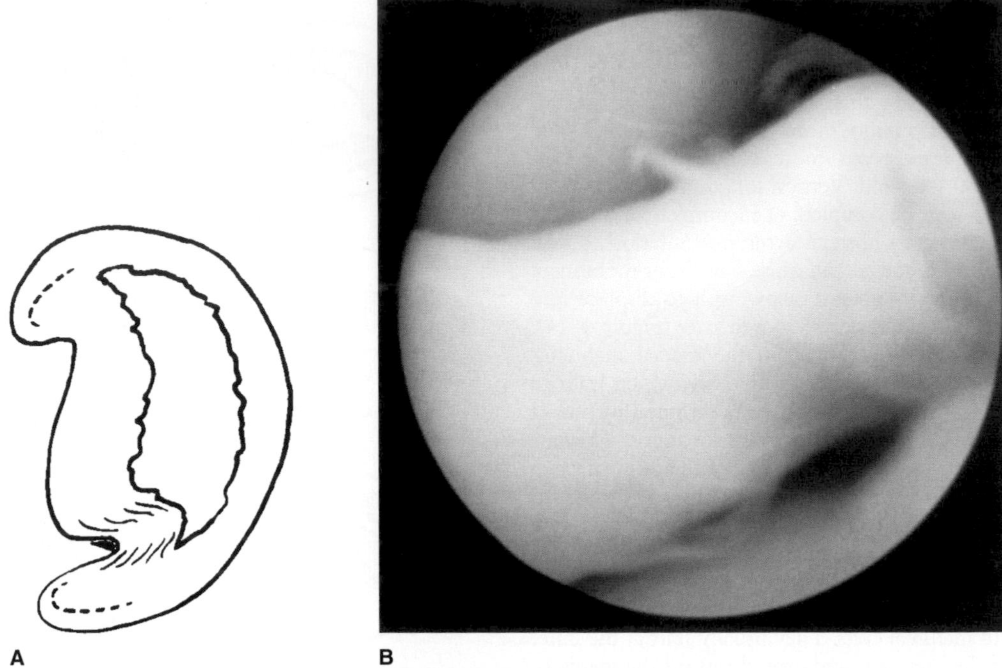

Figure 4–14. **A:** Diagram of a typical bucket-handle tear of the medial meniscus. **B:** Arthroscopic view of a bucket-handle fragment displaced into the intercondylar notch. (Reproduced, with permission, from McGinty JB: *Operative Arthroscopy.* Raven Press, 1991.)

15 mm in length, a tear within the peripheral 10–30% of the meniscus (ie, within 3–4 mm of the meniscocapsular junction), a peripheral tear that can be displaced toward the center of the plateau with a probe, the absence of secondary meniscus degeneration, and a tear in a patient undergoing concurrent ligament or articular cartilage repair.

Multiple factors affect the success of meniscus repair. Although no absolute age limit exists, patients younger than 40 years are thought to have a better chance for healing. Knees with associated ligamentous instability, particularly ACL instability, have inferior rates of meniscus healing because of abnormal meniscus stresses from tibiofemoral instability. The location of the tear and the time lapsed from injury to treatment are also important. Acute tears located in the peripheral red/red or red/white zone have better healing capability than chronic tears located in the red/white or white/white zones. Tears 5 mm or more from the periphery are considered avascular (white zone); those between 3 and 5 mm are variable in vascularity (red/white), and tears in the peripheral 3 mm are considered vascular (red). In areas with marginal vascularization, abrasion of the meniscocapsular junction or use of a fibrin clot may be used. It is thought that a vascular pannus forms from the abraded tissue, which aids in meniscus healing. Finally, the stability of the meniscus repair is a factor, with vertical mattress sutures generally considered the gold standard in meniscus repair.

Meniscus repair is successful in up to 90% of meniscus tears when done in conjunction with ACL reconstructions, as compared to approximately 50% in patients with stable ACLs who had meniscus repairs.

Types of repairs include the traditional open repair and arthroscopic repairs that can be dome with inside-out, outside-in, or all-inside techniques. Inside-out and outside-in repairs require a mini-incision and securing of the meniscus to the capsule with sutures. The all-inside technique has many device options, including both absorbable and nonabsorbable arrows, tacks, darts, and fasteners. Regardless of the type of repair chosen, adequate preparation of the tear site is required. The tear edges should be debrided or abraded with a shaver or rasp to stimulate bleeding. Restoration of biomechanical function is encouraged by anatomic apposition of the tear's edges to ensure good healing potential.

C. Open Meniscal Repair

Open repair of meniscus tears has successful long-term results. The technique involves making a small incision through the subcutaneous tissue, capsule, and synovium to visualize the tear directly. Open repair is most useful in peripheral or meniscocapsular tears, often occurring in conjunction with open repair of a collateral ligament injury or a tibial plateau fracture. Follow-up studies of 10 years or longer show survival rates of repaired menisci of 80–90%, in part influenced by the peripheral nature of the tear and the associated hemarthrosis present in ligament tears or fracture repair cases.

D. Arthroscopic Meniscal Repair

1. Inside-out meniscal repair—Arthroscopic inside-out meniscus repairs are performed using long needles introduced through cannula systems with attached absorbable or nonabsorbable sutures passed perpendicularly across the tear from inside the knee to a protected area outside the joint capsule. These sutures are able to obtain consistent perpendicular placement across the meniscus tear, which gives this method an advantage over other repair techniques. Improved suture placement is gained at the expense of possible neurovascular injury from passing the needle from inside the knee to outside the joint. This technique requires a posteromedial or posterolateral incision to protect the neurovascular structures and safely retrieve the exiting needles. Secondary to its ability to gain vertical mattress suture fixation, this technique remains the gold standard for many surgeons. Numerous retrospective and prospective studies using second-look arthroscopy or arthrography to evaluate healing of the meniscus repairs consistently show rates of 70–90% in isolated repairs and greater than 90% when done in conjunction with an ACL reconstruction. This technique is ideal for posterior and midposterior horn tears. There is difficulty in passing needles in mid- to anterior horn meniscus tears.

2. Outside-in meniscal repair—The arthroscopic outside-in repair was developed in part to decrease the neurovascular risk associated with the inside-out technique. The outside-in technique involves passing a needle from outside the joint, across the tear, and into the joint. Two options then exist for repair of the meniscus tear. One option is to retrieve the suture through an anterior portal, tie a knot outside the knee joint, and then bring the knot back in through the anterior portal placing the knot against the reduced meniscus body fragment. A second option is to use parallel needles and retrieve the suture through the second needle. This can be done using a suture relay. A knot is then tied outside the joint over the capsule. This method is useful for tears in the anterior horn or body of the menisci, but it does not work for tears in or near the posterior horn. Results of the outside-in technique using MRI, arthrography, or second-look arthroscopy to assess healing show complete or partial healing in between 74% and 87% of meniscus repairs that were successful. As expected, more posterior horn tears and tears in unstable knees did worse.

3. All-inside meniscal repair—The popularity of the all-inside repairs has increased as numerous devices and techniques have been introduced in the last few years. Their popularity is due in part to the fact that they do not require accessory incisions thereby saving operative time, and they avoid more technical arthroscopic techniques required in other types of repairs. However, because of the speed of their introduction, their documented clinical effectiveness compared to more traditional techniques has lagged behind their use.

The initial devices introduced in the early 1990s included biodegradable meniscus arrows, meniscus darts, and simple suture devices such as the T-Fix (Acufex, Mansfield, MA). There was a good initial experience with these devices, particularly the meniscus arrows, which were the first to be introduced. Early studies showed success rates of 80% or higher at 1–2 year follow-ups. However, complications with these first-generation devices began to be reported and included retained fragments, foreign body reactions, inflammation, chronic effusions, and articular cartilage injuries. Additionally, mechanical testing of these first-generation devices showed pull-to-failure strengths closer to those of horizontal, not vertical, sutures.

Updated first-generation and second-generation devices were developed in response to these biomechanical strength concerns and to address the early complication rates. Implant design modifications included a change to smaller or rounded heads on the meniscus arrow and darts, polymer composition changes to decrease their resorption times, and the introduction of suture-based implants that did not require arthroscopic knot tying. Examples included contoured and headless arrow designs and suture based implants such as the FasT-Fix (Smith & Nephew, Endoscopy Div., Andover, MA) and RapidLoc (Mitek, Westwood, MA) devices.

It is difficult to compare studies for these updated first-generation devices or second-generation devices, but in general, studies can be classified into two groups: follow-up clinical studies on human implanted devices, and biomechanical cadaveric or animal studies. Secondary to their earlier introduction into clinical use, long-term follow-up studies are most prevalent for updated first-generation meniscus arrow devices. First reported in 1993, multiple studies show 60–90% clinical success rates using either second-look arthroscopy or clinical exam evaluations. Some were even comparable to traditional open suture techniques. Complications, including inflammatory reactions and articular cartilage damage, remain a concern for sutureless devices that may migrate from their original implanted meniscus tear position.

Biomechanical studies on second-generation devices are also published. A follow-up to the initial T-Fix device, the second-generation FasT-Fix suture device, shows superior results. Its biomechanical performance in load-to-failure, stiffness, and cyclic displacement tests has been equivalent to the gold standard of vertical mattress sutures. Other devices including other suture devices and the various meniscus arrows or screws have equivalent biomechanical performance to that of horizontal mattress sutures. It is generally believed that the superiority of vertical mattress over horizontal mattress sutures is derived from the ability of vertical mattress sutures to capture the strong circumferential fibers of the meniscus. Additionally, suture devices in general have a lower risk of loose body reactions because their fixation device is extracapsular. However, there is a learning curve associated with placement of suture devices that may cause their fixation strength to be suboptimal until the technique is mastered.

Caution should be exercised in interpreting biomechanical studies of meniscus repair devices. Virtually all larger studies involve porcine, bovine, or canine models secondary to increased cost and availability issues in obtaining human cadaveric menisci. Studies involving human menisci should also be evaluated for the source of their menisci because as older samples taken from arthritic total joint patients may not accurately reflect in vivo conditions. It is also not known if in vitro load to failure or cyclic loading testing is applicable to the in vivo stress environment.

In general, however, multidevice studies show that (1) vertical mattress sutures are superior to horizontal, (2) arrows and other nonsuture devices have 40–70% of the pull-to-failure strength and cyclic load displacement of vertical mattress sutures, and (3) sutures devices like the FasT-Fix have biomechanical profiles similar to vertical mattress sutures. What remains to be known, however, is the minimal strength that meniscus repair devices need to provide for meniscus healing to occur in vivo.

Repairable meniscus tears often occur with an ACL tear. Stabilizing the knee with ACL reconstruction protects the repaired meniscus from abnormal knee motion, which has a higher rate of success than if the knee is left unstable.

E. Meniscal Transplantation

An alternative to leaving the patient with a meniscus-deficient knee, and almost certain early osteoarthrosis, is meniscus transplantation. This technique yields satisfactory results in approximately two thirds of patients after a short-term follow-up. In the future, biologic scaffolds may enable menisci to be regenerated after meniscectomy.

Ahn JH, Wang JH, Yoo JC: Arthroscopic all-inside suture repair of medial meniscus lesion in anterior cruciate ligament—deficient knees: results of second-look arthroscopies in 39 cases. Arthroscopy 2004;20:936. [PMID: 15525926]

Englund M et al: Patient-relevant outcomes fourteen years after meniscectomy: Influence of the type of meniscus tear and size of resection. Rheumatology (Oxford) 2001,40:631. [PMID: 11426019]

McNicholas MJ et al: Total meniscectomy in adolescence: A thirty-year follow-up. J Bone Joint Surg 2000,82B:217. [PMID: 10755429]

Metcalf MH, Barrett GR: Prospective evaluation of 1485 meniscal tear patterns in patients with stable knees. Am J Sports Med 2004;32:675. [PMID: 15090384]

Rijk PC. Meniscal allograft transplantation—part I: Background, results, graft selection and preservation, and surgical considerations. Arthroscopy 2004;20:728. [PMID: 15483548]

Shelbourne KD, Dersam MD: Comparison of partial meniscectomy versus meniscus repair for bucket-handle lateral meniscus tears in anterior cruciate ligament reconstructed knees. Arthroscopy 2004;20:581. [PMID: 15241307]

Steenbrugge F, Verstraete K, Verdonk R. Magnetic resonance imaging of the surgically repaired meniscus: A 13-year follow-up study of 13 knees. Acta Orthop Scand 2004;75:323. [PMID: 15260425]

KNEE FRACTURE

Articular cartilage injuries of the knee are infrequent, and the examiner must have a high index of suspicion to detect them. Arthroscopy is very helpful with these injuries, especially pure articular cartilage injuries, where radiographs will be normal.

1. Osteochondral Lesions

Osteochondral Fracture

There is much confusion about the nomenclature and etiology of juvenile and adult osteochondral lesions (OCLs) of the knee. Initially, an inflammatory etiology for the condition was suggested. Further inquiry attributed the condition to an ossification abnormality. Still others thought that avascular necrosis might be responsible for the lesions. However, work in basic science, histopathology, and vascular studies did not support any of these etiologies as the cause of OCLs. The term *osteochondral injuries* was used to describe injuries ranging from acute osteochondral fractures to pure chondral injuries. Currently, OCLs are defined as potentially reversible idiopathic lesions of subchondral bone resulting in possible delamination or fragmentation with or without destruction of the overlying articular cartilage. OCLs are subdivided into juvenile and adult forms depending on the presence of an open distal femoral physes. In children, a combination of etiologies is now thought to be responsible for OCL lesions. For example, a stress fracture may develop in the subchondral bone of the distal femoral condyle. Such an injury may provoke further vascular compromise, which results in injury to the subchondral bone that was initially covered with normal articular cartilage. Loss of support from the subchondral bone may result in damage to the overlying articular cartilage. The vast majority of adult OCLs lesions are thought to have arisen from a persistent juvenile OCL lesion, although new lesions in adults are possible as well.

Both adult and juvenile lesions that do not heal have the potential for further sequelae including degenerative osteoarthritis. Juvenile lesions, defined as knees with an open physes, generally have a better prognosis than adult lesions. The classic location of an OCL is the posterolateral aspect of the medial femoral condyle, which accounts for 70–80% of all OCLs. Lateral condyle lesions are seen in 15–20% of patients, and patellar involvement ranges from 5% to 10%. The increased use of MRI and arthroscopy over the past decade may have resulted in greater recognition of OCL lesions.

Clinical Findings

A common presentation of a patient with an OCL is aching and activity-related anterior knee pain that is poorly localized. Pain may worsen with stair climbing or running. Patients with early or stable lesions usually do not complain of mechanical symptoms or knee instability. Mechanical symptoms are more common in patients with unstable or loose OCLs. Parents may note a limp in their child, and patients may complain of knee swelling with possible crepitus.

An antalgic gait may be observed as the patient. An effusion may be variably present, but generally crepitus or pain with range of motion is absent in patients with stable lesions. Tenderness with palpation of the femoral condyle may be observed with various degrees of knee flexion. Loss of range of motion or quadriceps atrophy may be noted in more long-standing cases.

Patients with unstable lesions may have crepitus and pain with range of motion, and an effusion is typically present in these patients. Involvement is bilateral in up to 25% of cases, so both knees should be evaluated regardless of symptoms. Initial evaluation should include anteroposterior, lateral, and tunnel views of both knees. The goal of plain radiographs is to exclude any bony pathology, evaluate the physes, and localize the lesion. Lesion location and an estimation of size can be determined as described by Cahill. MRI is frequently obtained once the diagnosis is confirmed on plain radiographs. MRI can give an estimation of the size of the lesion, the condition of the overlying cartilage and underlying subchondral bone, the extent of bony edema, the presence of a high signal zone beneath the fragment, and the presence of any loose bodies. There are four MRI criteria on T_2-weighted images: a line of high signal intensity at least 5 mm in length between the OCL and underlying bone, an area of increased homogeneous signal at least 5 mm in diameter beneath the lesion, a focal defect of 5 mm or more in the articular surface, and a high signal line traversing the subchondral plate into the lesion. A high signal line is the most common sign in patients found to have unstable lesions that are most likely to fail nonoperative treatment. Patient maturity and lesion size are also important predictors of failure of nonoperative treatment.

Equivocal prognostic value was found in the use of intravenous gadolinium in OCLs. Technetium bone scans were initially proposed to monitor the presence of healing. However, with MRI, that eliminates ionizing radiation and increased time required in bone scanning, it is not widely used.

Treatment & Prognosis

There is general agreement that initial nonoperative management should be pursued in the case of a child with open physes who presents with a stable OCL. The goal of nonoperative treatment is to obtain a healed lesion before physis closure so as to prevent early-onset osteoarthritis. Even if patients are within 6–12 months of physeal closure, a trial of nonoperative treatment is warranted.

As failure of the subchondral bone precedes failure of the overlying articular cartilage, most orthopedists recommend some sort of activity modification. Debate exists whether activity modification should include the use of cast or brace immobilization. The tenet of nonoperative treatment is to reduce the activity level where pain-free activities of daily living are possible. However, there is no optimal immobilization protocol available in the literature.

A general consensus is that patients should at least be non– or partial weight bearing with crutches for 3–6 weeks or until they are pain free. Repeat radiographs are obtained at approximately 6-week intervals. Physical therapy with full weight bearing may be initiated once patients are pain free. Physical therapy should focus on low-impact quadriceps and hamstring strengthening. If patients remain asymptomatic during this phase up to at least 3 months postdiagnosis, activity may be slowly advanced to higher impact activities such as running or jumping. Any recurrence of symptoms or pain or any progression of the OCL on plain radiographs should prompt repeat non–weight bearing and possible immobilization for a longer period. Obvious patient frustration and lack of compliance, especially in adolescents, is common, and a full discussion on the risks and benefits of nonoperative or operative treatment is required.

Operative treatment should be considered in the following instances: (1) detachment or instability of the fragment while the patient is under treatment, (2) persistence of symptoms despite nonoperative treatment in a compliant patient, (3) persistently elevated or worsening radiographic appearance (plain radiographs or MRI), (4) approaching or complete epiphyseal closure. Goals of operative treatment should include achievement of a stable osteochondral fragment that maintains joint congruity and allows early range of motion.

For stable lesions with an intact articular surface, arthroscopic drilling of the lesions is preferred. This creates channels for potential revascularization through the subchondral bone plate. Options include transarticular drilling versus transepiphyseal drilling. Multiple studies show radiographic healing and relief of symptoms in 80–90% of patients with open physes. This decreases to 50–75% in patients with closed physes.

Patients with flap lesions or partially unstable lesions should be managed depending on the status of the subchondral bone. Fibrous tissue between the lesion and subchondral bone should be debrided. If significant subchondral bone loss occurs, packing of autogenous bone graft in the crater prior to fragment reduction and fixation is advised. If significant subchondral bone remains attached to the fragment such that an anatomic fit into its donor site is possible, fixation should be attempted. Various fixation methods are described, including Herbert or cannulated screws and bioabsorbable screws or pins. Complication, however, is associated with these treatments.

Simple excision of the larger fragments shows poor results with more rapid progression of radiographic osteoarthritic changes. For lesions greater than 2 cm^2, drilling or microfracture methods that depend on replacement of the defect with fibrocartilage also show inferior results. These results tend to deteriorate with time with worsening radiographic changes. For these larger lesions, transplantation of autologous osteochondral plugs or autologous chondrocyte implantation was tried. Disadvantages of autologous osteochondral plugs or mosaicplasty include donor site morbidity and incongruent articular fit. Advantages include biologic fixation of autogenous material. Longer term results are now being published in patients less than 40 years old showing successful clinical results in up to 90% of patients. However, additional larger and longer term follow-up studies are needed.

Cepero S, Ullot R, Sastre S: Osteochondritis of the femoral condyles in children and adolescents: Our experience over the last 28 years. J Pediatr Orthop B 2005;14:24. [PMID: 15577303]

KNEE LIGAMENT INJURY

Knee injuries occur during both contact and noncontact athletic activities. Advances in the diagnosis and treatment of ligament injuries now allow athletes at all levels of ability to return to sports at their preinjury level of activity. The ligaments and menisci of the knee work in concert with one another, and frequently more than one structure is damaged when an acute injury occurs.

Ligament injuries are graded as follows: grade 1, stretching of the ligament with no detectable instability; grade 2, further stretching of the ligament with detectable instability, but with the fibers in continuity; and grade 3, complete disruption of the ligament.

Anatomy

Knee stability requires proper functioning of four ligaments. These ligaments include the ACL, the PCL, the medial collateral ligament (MCL), and the lateral collateral ligament (LCL). There are also several accessory or secondary stabilizers of the knee. Secondary stabilizers of the knee include the menisci, iliotibial band, and biceps femoris. These secondary stabilizers become more important when a primary stabilizer is injured.

The MCL is the primary static stabilizer against valgus stress at the knee. The MCL originates from the central sulcus of the medial epicondyle. The sulcus of the C-shaped medial epicondyle is located anterior and distal to the adductor tubercle. The MCL is made up of three main static medial stabilizers of the knee. This includes the superficial MCL, the posterior oblique ligament, and the deep capsular ligament.

The LCL is the primary static stabilizer against varus stress at the knee. The LCL originates from the lateral epicondyle. This is the most prominent point of the lateral femoral condyle. The LCL insertion is on the styloid process of the fibular head, which projects superiorly from the posterolateral fibular head. The LCL joins with the arcuate ligament, the popliteus muscle, and the lateral head of the gastrocnemius to form a lateral arcuate complex to control statically and dynamically varus angulation and external tibial torsion. The iliotibial band and biceps femoris also contribute to stability on the lateral aspect of the knee.

The ACL is the primary static stabilizer of the knee against anterior translation of the tibia with respect to the femur. The ACL originates from the posteromedial surface of the lateral femoral condyle in the intercondylar notch. The ACL inserts on the tibial plateau just medial to the anterior horn of the lateral meniscus, approximately 15 mm posterior to the anterior edge of the tibial articular surface. The blood supply to the ACL and PCL is the middle geniculate artery. Both the ACL and PCL are covered by a layer of synovium, making these ligaments intra-articular and extrasynovial.

The PCL is the primary static stabilizer of the knee against posterior translation of the tibia with respect to the femur. The PCL originates from the posterior aspect of the lateral surface of the medial femoral condyle in the intercondylar notch. The PCL inserts on the posterior aspect of the tibial plateau in a central depression just posterior to the articular surface. The insertion extends distally along the posterior aspect of the tibia for up to 1 cm in length. The PCL is a complex structure consisting of two major bands: the anterolateral and posteromedial bands. The anterolateral band is tight in flexion and loose in extension. The posteromedial band is loose in flexion and tight in extension. The cross-sectional area of the anterolateral band is twice as large as the posteromedial band. The meniscofemoral ligaments, the ligaments of Wrisberg and Humphrey, are the third component of the PCL. The meniscofemoral ligaments travel from the posterior horn of the lateral meniscus to the posteromedial femoral condyle.

Differential Diagnosis of Knee Instability

The differential diagnosis of acute or chronic knee instability can involve any of the knee ligaments and/or the structures of the posterolateral corner. There are often combinations of ligament injuries in addition to injuries of secondary stabilizing structures such as the menisci. The history and mechanism of injury are valuable information, if available. Similarly, the location of pain can help narrow the diagnosis. Clearly, however, a thorough physical examination helps distinguish which ligaments are injured. Additionally, imaging studies are often obtained to confirm clinical suspicions and to evaluate for occult injuries.

Brown JR, Trojian TH: Anterior and posterior cruciate ligament injuries. Prim Care 2004;31:925. [PMID: 15544828]

1. Medial Collateral Ligament Injuries

Clinical Findings

An MCL tear typically presents with medial knee pain after either a noncontact rotational injury or a direct valgus blow to the lateral knee. Instability may or may not be present, depending on the severity of the injury.

Symptoms (History)

How and when the patient was hurt are important parts of the history. Lower grade MCL injuries typically occur in a noncontact external rotational injury, whereas higher grade injuries generally involve lateral contact to the thigh or upper leg. Other important pieces of historical information include the location and presence of pain, instability, timing of swelling, and sensation of a pop or tear. Surprisingly, grade I and II injuries are often more painful than complete MCL rupture. Immediate swelling should make one suspicious of an associated cruciate ligament injury, fracture, and/or patellar dislocation. A prior history of knee injuries or instability should always be sought when evaluating a new knee injury.

Signs (Physical Examination)

MCL injuries are evaluated with a complete knee examination to evaluate for any other coexisting injuries. This is especially true with ACL and PCL evaluation because an injury to either of these ligaments would significantly change the treatment. Given the frequency of coexisting patellar dislocations in MCL injuries, palpation of the patella and the medial parapatellar stabilizing ligaments should be performed in addition to patellar apprehension testing.

Medial joint line tenderness along the course of the MCL is typical at the location of the tear. Laxity to valgus stresses is assessed by the amount of medial joint space opening that occurs at 30 degrees of flexion. It is important to stress the knee at 30 degrees of flexion because with the knee in full extension, the posterior capsule and PCL stabilizes the knee to valgus stress. This stability to valgus stress in full extension could mislead the examiner to believe that the MCL is intact. Zero opening is considered normal, with 1–4 mm indicating a grade I injury; 5–9 mm indicating a grade II injury; and 10–15 mm indicating a complete or grade III injury. Additionally, grade I and II injuries typically have a firm endpoint, whereas a grade III injury tends to have a soft endpoint to valgus stress.

Imaging Studies

A. Radiographs

A series of knee radiographs should be obtained in any patient with a suspected significant knee injury. Radiographs should be inspected for acute fracture, lateral capsular avulsion (the Segond fracture; see ACL imaging), loose bodies, Pellegrini-Stieda lesion (MCL calcification), and evidence of patellar dislocation. Stress radiographs should be obtained in patients prior to skeletal maturity to rule out an epiphyseal fracture.

B. Magnetic Resonance Imaging

MRI is useful for confirming MCL injury and identifying the site of injury as well as the presence of meniscal and other injuries to the knee. Relative indications for an MRI include an uncertain ACL status despite multiple examinations, evaluation of a suspected meniscal tear, or preoperative evaluation for a planned MCL reconstruction or repair.

C. Special Tests

An examination under anesthesia can be valuable when physical examination is unreliable because of the patient guarding the knee. Diagnostic arthroscopy can also be used to evaluate for coexistent pathology. MRI has largely replaced both of these diagnostic methods, however.

Treatment: Nonsurgical & Surgical

Treatment of an isolated MCL injury is generally nonoperative with protection against valgus stress and early motion. Grade I and grade II injuries can be placed in either a cast or a brace and bear weight as tolerated. Generally, knee motion is started within the first week or two, and full recovery is usually achieved more rapidly with early knee range of motion.

Grade III injuries are a bit more controversial. Several authors show increased instability in grade III tears treated nonsurgically, although most of these did not exclude knees with multiligamentous injuries. Comparison of isolated grade III MCL tears treated with surgical reconstruction versus nonsurgical management showed that the nonsurgical treatment group enjoyed better results in both subjective scoring and earlier return to activity.

The exception to the current trend of nonsurgical treatment of grade III injuries is in the setting of a multiligamentous knee injury. In this setting, particularly with a distal tibial avulsion of the MCL, nonsurgical treatment has not fared nearly as well as in isolated MCL injuries. MCL repair in the acute setting can include a primary repair, with shortening if needed, of the torn ligament. Similarly, avulsion fragments are treated with reduction and fixation in the acute setting. Primary repairs can be reinforced with autograft or allograft tissues if the remaining MCL is insufficient for a stand alone repair. Chronic reconstructions also often include autograft or allograft tissue reconstruction.

Traditionally, casting or operative treatment of MCL injuries significantly limited an early return to range-of-motion exercises. With the addition of functional bracing and early motion to a nonsurgical treatment protocol, motion and strengthening of the knee can occur at an early stage while the ligament is protected from valgus stress. As knee motion improves, isotonic strengthening exercises are introduced. As the strength of the extremity improves, the intensity of functional rehabilitation increases accordingly.

Complications

With nonsurgical treatment becoming the standard of care, complications associated with a MCL injury are decreasing. The main complication of nonsurgical therapy is residual valgus laxity or medial knee pain. Radiographs may show residual calcification of the MCL (Pellegrini-Stieda lesion). Potential surgical complications include arthrofibrosis, infection, damage to the saphenous nerve or vein, or recurrent valgus laxity.

Results/Return to Play

In general, good outcomes can be achieved with nonsurgical treatment and rehabilitation of isolated MCL injuries. Return to professional football after nonsurgical treatment of isolated MCL injuries is 98%.

Robinson JR et al: The posteromedial corner revisited. An anatomical description of the passive restraining structures of the medial aspect of the human knee. J Bone Joint Surg Br 2004; 86:674. [PMID: 15274262]

Woo SL, Vogrin TM, Abramowitch SD: Healing and repair of ligament injuries in the knee. J Am Acad Orthop Surg 2000; 8:364. [PMID: 11104400]

2. Lateral Collateral Ligament Injuries

Symptoms (History)

The most consistent symptom of an acute LCL injury is lateral knee pain. However, the symptoms of lateral and posterolateral instability are quite variable and depend on the severity of injury, patient activity level, overall limb alignment, and other associated knee injuries. For example, a sedentary individual with minimal laxity and overall valgus alignment typically has few if any symptoms. However, if LCL laxity is combined with overall varus alignment, hyperextension, and an increased activity level, symptoms are quite pronounced. These patients may complain of lateral joint line pain and a varus thrust of their leg with everyday activities. This is often described as the knee buckling into hyperextension with normal gait.

Signs (Physical Examination)

Patients with a LCL and/or posterolateral corner injury often also have additional ligamentous injuries to the knee. Therefore, a thorough knee examination should be performed to evaluate for coexistent knee pathology. Additionally, a careful neurovascular examination should be performed because the incidence of neurovascular injury, particularly peroneal nerve injury, is reported in 12–29% of posterolateral knee injuries.

The integrity of the LCL is assessed with a varus stress with the knee in full extension and 30 degrees of flexion. Baseline varus opening is widely variable and should be compared to the contralateral leg. The average baseline for varus opening is 7 degrees. Exam findings with an isolated LCL injury should include varus laxity at 30 degrees of flexion and no instability in full extension. This is because of the stabilizing effect that the intact cruciate ligaments provide in full extension.

Note that a significant posterolateral knee injury can be present without significant varus laxity. The most useful test to evaluate for posterolateral instability is the dial test, which is done by externally rotating each tibia and noting the angle subtended between the thigh and the foot. The dial test is performed at 30 degrees and 90 degrees of flexion with a significant difference being an angle 5 degrees or greater than the contralateral leg.

Imaging Studies

A. Radiographs

A series of knee radiographs should be obtained in any patient with a suspected significant knee injury. Radiographs should be inspected for acute fractures, lateral capsular avulsion (Segond fracture; see ACL imaging), loose bodies, fibular head avulsions, and evidence of patellar dislocation. With chronic posterolateral instability, degenerative changes of the lateral compartment are often noted. Lateral joint space narrowing with osteophytes and subchondral sclerosis can be seen. Stress radiographs can help better quantify the amount of varus angulation present.

B. Magnetic Resonance Imaging

MRI is often a useful adjunct for diagnosing posterolateral corner and LCL injuries in the severely injured knee. As mentioned earlier, this posterolateral injury can often go unnoticed during an initial evaluation, and MRI findings can refocus the examination to the posterolateral structures. Pain and guarding at the time of injury can often obscure posterolateral injury, and MRI can prove to be an extremely valuable adjunct in diagnosis.

C. Special Tests/Examinations

1. Reverse pivot shift test—This test involves starting with the knee flexed to 90 degrees. While the knee is extended, the leg is loaded axially with a valgus stress applied to the knee and the foot held in external rotation. A palpable shift is noted as the tibia reduces from its posteriorly subluxed position as the knee is extended.

2. External rotation recurvatum test—This test is performed with the patient supine and the hip and knee fully extended. The leg is lifted off the bed by the toes. Hyperextension, varus instability, and external rotation of the tibial tubercle occurs with adequate quadriceps relaxation in a patient with posterolateral instability.

3. Posterolateral drawer test—A standard posterior drawer test (see PCL physical examination) is performed with the tibia in internal rotation, neutral, and externally rotated positions. With posterolateral injury, the magnitude of the posterior drawer displacement is greatest with external tibial rotation.

4. Examination under anesthesia—An examination while the patient is relaxed under general anesthetic is extremely useful, particularly in the acute setting. If the patient with a multiligamentous knee injury is taken to the operating room, this is an excellent opportunity to examine the knee without guarding to improve the accuracy of the examination.

Treatment

A. Nonsurgical

Isolated LCL ligament injuries, as noted earlier, are rare injuries. However, in the case of an isolated LCL ligament injury with grade II or less magnitude, a period of immobilization from 2 to 4 weeks followed by a quadriceps strengthening program usually yields good results. Grade III injuries often have better results with surgical treatment. The combination of delayed diagnosis along with an uncertain natural history of posterolateral instability make the treatment of these injuries a challenge.

B. Surgical

LCL and posterolateral ligaments, as already discussed, rarely occur in isolation. Therefore, other injuries must also be considered in the treatment plan of the multiligament knee injury. Ideally, the posterolateral and LCL injury is diagnosed in the acute setting. This allows the preferred surgical treatment of a primary repair of the injured structures with augmentation as needed. Primary repair is generally only feasible in the first few weeks following the knee injury.

The knee with chronic posterolateral instability often requires ligamentous reconstruction or advancement to reconstitute a static restraint to varus stresses. The key biomechanical concept of any lateral ligamentous reconstruction is that the isometric point of the LCL lies between the fibular head and the lateral epicondyle. Therefore, regardless of the graft material used to reconstruct the lateral ligamentous complex, a portion of the graft must pass between the lateral femoral epicondyle and the fibular head.

To improve the success rate of reconstruction of chronic lateral ligamentous instability, a proximal tibial valgus osteotomy may be performed to decrease the stress on the lateral structures of the knee.

Rehabilitation

The rehabilitation of the knee after posterolateral reconstructions or repairs is largely guided by associated injuries to the ACL or PCL. It is generally necessary, however, to limit weight bearing for at least 6 weeks and protect the lateral structures with a brace for at least 3 months.

Complications

The peroneal nerve runs just posterior to the fibular head. It is important to isolate the peroneal nerve prior to any lateral knee exposure to minimize the complication of a peroneal nerve injury.

Results

If injuries to the posterolateral corner of the knee are diagnosed and repaired acutely, the results are good for restoration of varus stability and return to play. Chronic posterolateral corner injury reconstructions also perform well when an isometric lateral reconstruction is achieved.

Jakob RP, Warner JP: Lateral and posterolateral instability of the knee. In *Orthopaedic Sports Medicine: Principles and Practice.* Eds. DeLee J, Drez D, Stanitski CL. Philadelphia: WB Saunders, 1994. [NLMID: 9411843]

Ross G et al: Evaluation and treatment of acute posterolateral corner/anterior cruciate ligament injuries of the knee. J Bone Joint Surg Am 2004;86 (Suppl 2):2. [PMID: 15691102]

Shahane SA, Ibbotson C, Strachan R et al: The popliteofibular ligament. An anatomical study of the posterolateral corner of the knee. J Bone Joint Surg Br 1999;81:636. [PMID: 10463736]

3. Anterior Cruciate Ligament Injuries

Symptoms (History)

The mechanism of injury should be elicited in any knee injury evaluation. This can guide the examination to additional structures that may also be injured. ACL injury can occur in a variety of ways; a few mechanisms predominate, however. The most common noncontact ACL injury mechanism involves a deceleration and rotational injury during running, cutting, or jumping activities. The most common contact injury involves either hyperextension and/or valgus forces to the knee by a direct blow.

ACL injury is often associated with a pop heard by the patient at the time of injury. This piece of history is not ACL specific, however. Upon return to competition, the patient often notices instability of the knee or describes the knee "giving out" with twisting activities. Substantial knee swelling secondary to a hemarthrosis typically occurs within the first 4 to 12 hours following the injury.

Signs (Physical Examination)

With the history obtained and a proper physical examination, an ACL tear should be able to be diagnosed without any additional tests. A complete examination of the knee should be performed to evaluate for any other associated injuries. The uninjured knee is examined first to familiarize the patient with the knee examination.

The Lachman test is the most useful test for anterior laxity of the knee. It is performed with the knee in 20–30 degrees of flexion as an anterior force is applied to the tibia while the other hand stabilizes the distal femur. The degree of anterior translation, as well as the presence and character of an endpoint, is assessed. The laxity is graded based on comparison to the uninjured contralateral knee. Grade 1 laxity is 1–5 mm of increased translation. Grade 2 laxity is 6–10 mm of increased translation. Grade 3 laxity is more than 10 mm of translation as compared to the injured contralateral knee.

The anterior drawer test is another test to evaluate anterior tibial translation. This is performed with the knee in 90 degrees of flexion as an anterior force is applied to the tibia. This test is less sensitive than the Lachman test.

In the acute setting of an ACL tear, there is often a window where an accurate examination can occur before extensive knee swelling and guarding inhibit examination. Aspiration of a hemarthrosis can help decrease pain and improve the quality of the examination in the acute setting as well.

The pivot shift test is performed to test the rotational instability associated with an ACL tear. The test is based on the lateral tibial plateau subluxing anteriorly with extension and reduction of the lateral compartment with flexion. The most effective method of achieving this result is by flexing the knee with an axial load from full extension with valgus stress at the knee and internal rotation of the tibia. The reduction of the subluxation should occur at approximately 30 degrees of flexion. MCL injury and some meniscal tears may produce a false-negative test.

The pivot shift test is considered the most functional test to evaluate knee stability after ACL injury. An examination under anesthesia is also often useful in obtaining a more accurate pivot shift test. This can be useful in a patient with an unclear history of instability and an equivocal examination in the office.

Imaging Studies

Plain radiographs of the knee should be obtained to rule out fractures about the knee. The Segond fracture, as discussed earlier, is an avulsion of the anterolateral capsule of the tibia. Before skeletal maturity, an avulsion of the tibial insertion of the ACL can also be seen radiographically. Following radiographs, an MRI is the most useful examination for an evaluation of associated injuries. Although generally not needed for diagnosis of an ACL tear, MRI can diagnose an ACL tear with 95% or better accuracy. Bone bruises of the lateral femoral condyle and lateral tibial plateau are noted in up to 80% of ACL injuries.

Special Studies

Instrumented laxity evaluations can augment the physical examination and provide an objective baseline for future comparison. The most commonly used arthrometer, the KT-1000 (MEDmetric, San Diego, CA), uses a series of standard forces to measure anterior translation of the tibia with the knee in 20–30 degrees of flexion, similar to the Lachman test.

Treatment

A. Nonsurgical

Rehabilitation following an isolated ACL injury should include an effort to regain knee motion and strengthen the muscles about the knee. Returning to activities that produce episodes of instability is discouraged. Once motion and strength are restored, a gradual return to activities can be attempted to determine the functional level that can be attained without instability.

Nonoperative management with rehabilitation after an ACL injury generally yields poor results in patients who return to competitive activities. Significant episodes of instability resulting in pain, swelling, and disability occur in approximately 80% of individuals that participate in sporting activities such as tennis, football and soccer. These episodes of instability are thought to place the menisci and articular cartilage of the knee at risk for further injury (Figure 4–15).

B. Surgical

The decision to reconstruct an ACL tear surgically is individualized and based on the patient's desire to return to competition, age, accompanying degenerative changes, and objective and subjective knee instability. For example, an active patient less than 40 years old with continued desire to compete in cutting and jumping sports with both objective and subjective knee instability may be best treated with surgical reconstruction. But an older patient with some degenerative arthritis of the knee and minimal desire for continued competitive athletics and no subjective instability would be much more suited to nonsurgical care.

Early in the history of ACL surgery, primary repairs of the ligament were found to do poorly. This gave way to ligament reconstruction using a variety of graft materials. Everything from synthetics to autograft and allograft tissues were used for reconstruction of the ACL. Over time, autograft bone-patellar tendon-bone, semitendinosus/gracilis hamstring autograft, and allograft bone-patellar tendon-bone constructs have proven to be the most commonly used grafts and are successful for ACL reconstructions.

The goal of ACL reconstruction is to reproduce the strength, location, and function of the intact ACL. Therefore, once a graft of adequate strength is selected,

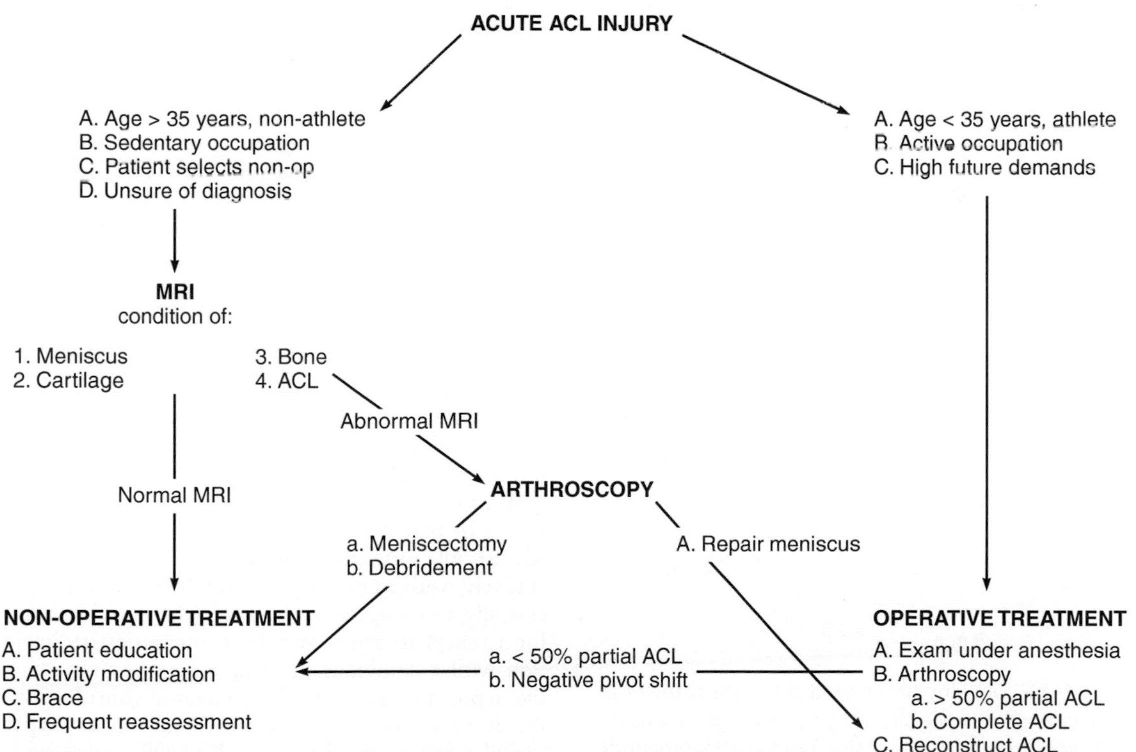

Figure 4–15. Flow chart that summarizes the current management of acute anterior cruciate ligament injuries. (Reproduced, with permission, from Marzo JM, Warren RF: Results of nonoperative treatment of anterior cruciate ligament injury: Changing perspectives. Adv Orthop Surg 1991;15:59.)

the location of the graft is of utmost importance. The graft is generally passed through a bone tunnel in the tibia and a bone tunnel through the femur. The intraarticular placement of the tibial tunnel is generally in the center of the native ACL stump just in front of the PCL origin and just medial to the center of the notch in the coronal plane (Figures 4–16 and 4–17).

Once the graft is in place, the proper tension and fixation of the graft must occur to achieve a successful ACL reconstruction. Establishing proper tension in the graft is important. A lax ACL graft may not restore stability to the knee, and an overtightened graft may cause failure of the graft or limit knee range of motion. Fixation of the graft is achieved through a variety of measures. The most common method involves placing an interference screw up the bone tunnel that captures the graft in the tunnel. The graft can also be fixed via sutures tied over various devices located on the outer cortex of the tunnels.

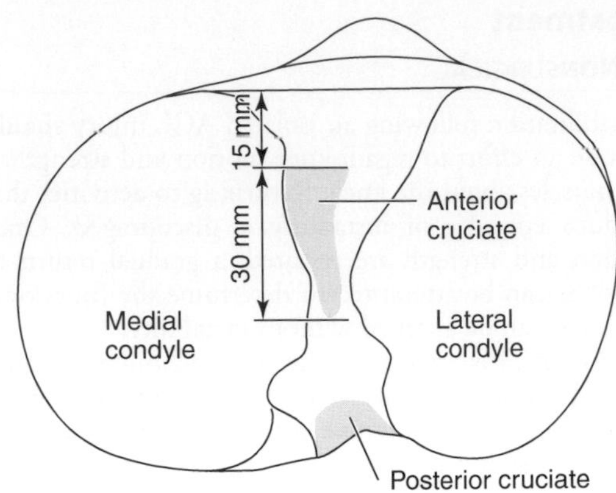

Figure 4–17. The upper surface of the tibial plateau to show average measurements and relations of the tibial attachments of the anterior cruciate ligament. (Reproduced, with permission, from Girgis FC et al: The cruciate ligaments of the knee joint: Anatomical, functional, and experimental analysis. Clin Orthop 1975;106:216.)

Complications

Although ACL reconstruction often results in a successful outcome, several complications can occur. One of the most common is a loss of knee motion, which is minimized by obtaining and maintaining full knee extension immediately following surgery. Knee flexion exercises are begun as soon as possible postoperatively with a goal of 90 degrees by 1 week after surgery. Additionally, patellar mobilization is performed in an attempt to minimize patellofemoral scarring. Another common complication of ACL reconstruction is anterior knee pain. The exact etiology of this pain is unclear; however, it is thought that patellar tendon autograft harvest may increase the incidence of patellofemoral pain. Less common complications (less than 1%) include patellar fracture, patellar tendon rupture, and quadriceps tendon rupture, depending on the graft harvest site.

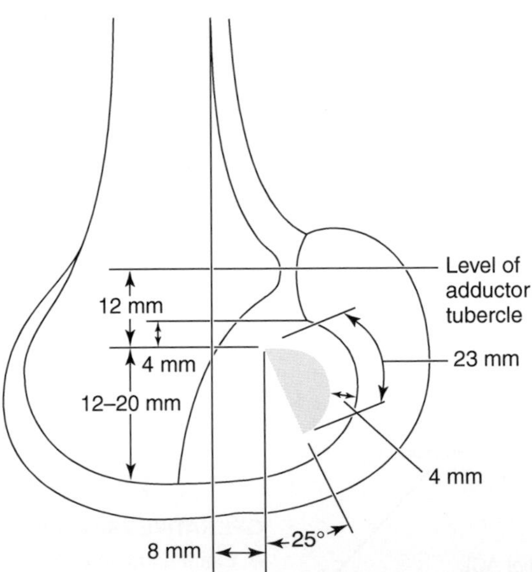

Figure 4–16. Drawing of the medial surface of the right lateral femoral condyle showing the average measurements and body relations of the femoral attachment of the anterior cruciate ligament. (Reproduced, with permission, from Arnoczky SP: Anatomy of the anterior cruciate ligament. Clin Orthop 1983;172:19.)

Results/Return to Play

The goal of any rehabilitation protocol for an ACL reconstruction is to return the patient to the full desired level of activity in a short amount of time as possible while avoiding any complications or setbacks. Through improved surgical techniques and accelerated rehabilitation protocols, most studies show a 90% or better return to play and patient satisfaction. Patients generally are able to return between 4 and 6 months postoperatively, with some professional athletes returning successfully to competition in 3 months. Specific criteria for a return to sports vary from institution to institution with a combination of functional testing, subjective reporting, and clinical examination contributing to the decision. In general, the criteria for return to sports includes full range of motion, KT1000 testing within 2–3 mm of the uninjured knee, 85% or more of quadriceps strength and full hamstring strength, and functional testing within 85% of the contralateral leg.

Herrington L et al: Anterior cruciate ligament reconstruction, hamstring versus bone-patella tendon-bone grafts: A systematic literature review of outcome from surgery. Knee 2005;12:41. [PMID: 15664877]

Hewett TE, Myer GD, Ford KR: Reducing knee and anterior cruciate ligament injuries among female athletes: A systematic review of neuromuscular training interventions. J Knee Surg 2005;18:82. [PMID: 15742602]

Laxdal G et al: A prospective randomized comparison of bone-patellar tendon-bone and hamstring grafts for anterior cruciate ligament reconstruction. Arthroscopy 2005;21:34. [PMID: 15650664]

Marx RG et al: Beliefs and attitudes of members of the American Academy of Orthopaedic Surgeons regarding the treatment of anterior cruciate ligament injury. Arthroscopy 2003;19:762. [PMID: 12966385]

Seitz H et al: Anterior instability of the knee despite an intensive rehabilitation program. Clin Orthop 1996;328:159. [PMID: 8653950]

4. Posterior Cruciate Ligament Injuries

Symptoms (History)

When evaluating a patient for a PCL injury, it is important to obtain the mechanism of injury, the severity of the injury, and any potential associated injuries. In contrast to an ACL tear, it is rare for patients with PCL injuries to report hearing a pop or report any feelings of subjective instability. More commonly, patients complain of knee pain, swelling, and stiffness.

The presentation of a patient with a subacute or chronically injured PCL can range from asymptomatic to significant instability and pain. Patients with significant varus alignment or injury to the lateral structures of the knee often complain of feelings of instability and giving way. There are a few characteristic mechanisms of PCL injury that differ significantly from the mechanism of ACL injuries. One of the most common mechanisms of PCL injury is the so-called dashboard, injury during which the anterior tibia sustains a posteriorly directed force from the dashboard with the knee in 90 degrees of flexion. Sports injuries to the PCL result from an outside force or blow, in contrast to the typical deceleration twisting mechanism of an ACL injury. The most common methods of a sports PCL injury include a direct blow to the anterior tibia or via a fall onto the flexed knee with the foot in plantar flexion. The most common mechanism for isolated PCL injury in the athlete is a partial tear associated with hyperflexion of the knee. Additionally, significant knee multiligamentous injuries with PCL tears can be seen after a varus or valgus stress is applied to the hyperextended knee.

Signs (Physical Examination)

As with other ligamentous injuries, a thorough knee examination is necessary. Specific cues to injury to the PCL on initial inspection include abrasions or ecchymosis around the proximal anterior tibia and ecchymosis in the popliteal fossa. Assessment for meniscal damage and associated ligamentous injury should be performed. Evaluation of ACL laxity in the presence of an acute PCL injury is challenging because of the lack of a stable reference point to perform a Lachman or anterior drawer test.

Examination of the PCL in the acutely injured knee can be challenging. Despite increased awareness of the injury, many PCL injuries go undiagnosed in the acute setting. The most accurate clinical test of PCL integrity is the posterior drawer test. The knee is flexed to 90 degrees with the patient supine, and a posteriorly directed force is applied to the anterior tibia. The amount of posterior translation and the presence and character of the endpoint is noted. The extent of translation is assessed by noting the change in the distance of the step-off between the anteromedial tibial plateau and the medial femoral condyle. The tibial plateau is approximately 1 cm anterior to the medial femoral condyle on average. However, the contralateral knee must be examined to establish a baseline.

Another test for examination of the PCL is the posterior sag or Godfrey test. This test involves flexing the knee and hip and noting the posterior pull of gravity creating posterior "sag" of the tibia on the femur. An adjunct to this test involves watching for a reduction of this subluxation with active quadriceps contraction.

The reverse pivot shift is the analogue to the pivot shift in the evaluation of an ACL injury. This is performed by placing a valgus stress on the knee with the foot externally rotated. The knee is then extended from 90 degrees of flexion and a palpable reduction of the posterolateral tibial plateau is noted between 20 and 30 degrees of flexion.

It is extremely important to evaluate the posterolateral structures of the knee in the setting of a suspected PCL injury. Injury to the posterolateral structures is reported to occur in up to 60% of PCL injuries.

Imaging Studies

A. Radiographs

Given the magnitude of the forces required to injure the PCL, plain radiographs of the knee are essential to evaluate for bony injuries, dislocation, or evidence of other associated injuries. Subtle posterior subluxation on the lateral radiograph may also indicate PCL injury. Stress posterior drawer radiographs and contralateral comparisons may also increase the sensitivity for detecting PCL injuries with plain radiographs. In the chronic setting of PCL injury, radiographs are useful to assess for patellofemoral and medial compartment degenerative changes that can occur over time.

B. Magnetic Resonance Imaging

Although plain films are necessary and useful in the evaluations of these injuries, MRI is the diagnostic study of choice for the knee with a presumed PCL injury. MRI is from 96% to 100% sensitive at diagnosing PCL tears. Equally or more importantly, MRI is extremely valuable in its ability to detect associated injuries. This is particularly important in diagnosing posterolateral corner injuries because these can often be missed on the initial clinical examination. In multiligamentous knee injuries, MRI can also be useful in assessing the ACL because clinical examination of the ACL is challenging in the setting of a complete PCL tear.

C. Special Studies

In the setting of a chronic isolated PCL tear, pain in the medial and patellofemoral compartments are generally evaluated with radiographs. If these are normal, some surgeons proceed with a bone scan to evaluate for increased uptake in these areas. Areas under increased stress demonstrate increased uptake on the bone scan before signs of advanced arthritis occur on radiographs. This subset of patients may benefit from a PCL reconstruction to decrease the stress and delay osteoarthritis.

Treatment

There is significant controversy in the treatment of isolated PCL injuries. Multiple factors must be evaluated in the decision to treat a complete PCL rupture. The patient's age, activity level, expectations, and associated injuries must be taken into account. The literature on operative versus nonsurgical treatment of these injuries can be difficult to interpret, and there is no long-term follow-up studies of randomized patient groups.

A. Nonsurgical

Rehabilitation of the PCL injured knee often largely depends on the associated injuries sustained by the knee. This is particularly true with the commonly associated posterolateral corner injury. Therefore, we focus on the rehabilitation of the isolated PCL injured knee. Regaining motion and strength are the two key objectives of a rehabilitation program. Obtaining full quadriceps strength is essential for achieving the optimal result with nonsurgical treatment. The initial treatment is aimed at keeping the tibia reduced under the femur and minimizing tension on the injured PCL. With partial injuries (grade I and II), the prognosis is quite good, and early motion with weight bearing is the usual course of therapy. In a complete PCL tear, most keep the knee immobilized in extension to protect the posterolateral structures. Early strengthening exercises focus on quadriceps strength with quadriceps sets, straight leg raises, and partial weight bearing in extension.

Overall, most patients benefit from nonsurgical treatment of a PCL tear. Despite objective findings of instability that are often noted on examination, most patients subjectively are satisfied with the function of the knee. Bracing is generally ineffective in controlling PCL laxity clinically.

The main subjective complaint with chronic PCL insufficiency, however, is pain rather than instability. A PCL deficient knee with posterior tibial subluxation places significantly increased stresses on the patellofemoral and medial compartments of the knee. In one series in which patients with PCL injuries were followed with serial radiographs, 60% of patients displayed some degenerative changes of the medial compartment.

B. Surgical

Surgical management of PCL injuries are broken down into avulsion fractures, isolated acute PCL injuries, multiligament injuries, and chronic PCL insufficiency. Avulsion fractures of the PCL are rare fractures. If nondisplaced, these injuries are treated nonsurgically. If significantly displaced, these fractures are generally treated with open reduction and internal fixation.

The majority of surgeons generally still treat isolated PCL injuries with nonsurgical care. However, nonoperative care of these injuries is not without consequences. Although subjective results in these patients are good in the short term, many continue to have objective instability and display degenerative arthritic changes over time. A follow up of PCL deficient knees at an average of 15 years after injury found 89% of patients with persistent pain and half with chronic effusions. All patients in this group showed degenerative changes when followed for 25 years. Therefore, given the risks of continued instability and the potential of an increased chance of arthritic changes, surgical reconstruction of the PCL is a reasonable choice.

Initially, surgical care of complete PCL tears consisted of a primary repair of midsubstance tears. The objective stability of these repairs was generally disappointing. Current reconstruction methods generally involve routing either autograft or allograft tendons through bone tunnels to reconstruct the PCL in an anatomic fashion. Although there are several different methods of reconstructing the PCL, the two main categories of PCL reconstruction consist of single- and double-bundle repairs. Classically, reconstructions of the PCL anatomically replicated the anterolateral bundle of the native PCL with a single-bundle reconstruction. As problems were noted with recurrence of posterior laxity in the postoperative period, a double-bundle technique was derived to reconstruct both the anterolateral and posteromedial bundles of the native PCL. The advantages of the double-bundle technique are thus far theoretical, and there is no long-term clinical follow-up demonstrating the superiority of a double-bundle reconstruction at this time.

The severe instability noted with PCL injuries associated with multiligamentous knee injuries make the argument for ligament reconstruction more compelling in this patient population. Many of the studies involving PCL reconstruction in these complex knee injuries have involved primary repair attempts. Although subjective results were generally good, residual excessive, objective laxity was very common following repairs. More recently ligament reconstructions with allograft and autograft have become the dominant method of PCL reconstruction in this challenging patient population.

Complications

The most common complication following PCL reconstruction is the return of objective posterior laxity on physical examination. This does not present as subjective laxity, however, and patient satisfaction remains high despite objective laxity. Acute PCL reconstructions in the setting of a multiligamentous knee repair/reconstruction can result in arthrofibrosis with extensive postoperative scarring.

Results/Return to Play

Even with nonsurgical management of a PCL injury, the prognosis for a functional recovery and return to competition is very good. A strong quadriceps muscle and extensor mechanism can significantly compensate for PCL laxity. Athletes should spend a minimum of 3 months in rehabilitation before attempting a return to competition. However, there is a subset of patients that experiences significant instability with a grade III PCL injury that does not allow a return to competition. This is a subset of patients that may benefit from PCL reconstruction.

However, the prognosis for a PCL tear associated with a multiligamentous knee injury is guarded with respect to return to play. Although prompt recognition of a multiligamentous injury and appropriately timed treatment, reconstruction, and rehabilitation is essential for optimal recovery, these injuries are such that a significant percentage of patients are not able to return to full competition.

Allen CR, Kaplan LD, Fluhme DJ et al: Posterior cruciate ligament injuries. Curr Opin Rheumatol 2002;14:142. [PMID: 11845019]

Fanelli GC, Edson CJ: Combined posterior cruciate ligament-posterolateral reconstructions with Achilles tendon allograft and biceps femoris tendon tenodesis: 2- to 10-year follow-up. Arthroscopy 2004;20:339. [PMID: 15067271]

5. Patella Dislocation

Dislocation of the patella is a potential cause of acute hemarthrosis and must be considered when evaluating a patient with an acute knee injury. The injury occurs when valgus force and external rotation of the tibia is applied to a flexed leg. It is most common in females in the second decade of life.

Clinical Findings

The patella almost always dislocates laterally. The patient may notice the patella sitting laterally or might say that the rest of the knee has shifted medially. It is unusual to see actual dislocation of the patella except at the time of injury. Reduction occurs when the knee is extended.

Examination demonstrates tenderness over the medial retinaculum and adductor tubercle, which is the origin of the medial patellofemoral ligament. The patient also has pain and apprehension when the patella is pushed laterally with the knee slightly bent. Radiographs, including an axial patellar view, should be obtained to determine whether there are osteochondral fractures. Often, a small fleck of bone is avulsed by the capsule on the medial aspect of the patella. This is not intraarticular and does not require removal. A displaced osteochondral fracture require excisions or internal fixation. Examination of the uninjured knee is recommended to determine whether there are predisposing factors for dislocation, such as patella alta, genu recurvatum, increased Q angle, and patellar hypermobility. Patella alta, or high-riding patella, is identified by measuring the length of the patellar tendon and dividing by the length of the patella. The upper limit of normal is 1.2. The Q angle is formed by a line through the patellar tendon intersecting a line from the anterior superior iliac spine in the center of the patella. A normal Q angle is approximately 10 degrees, with a range of approximately plus or minus 5 degrees. Patients with generalized hypermobility have increased extension of the knee, or genu recurvatum, which in effect gives them patella alta. They also often have hypermobility of all the capsular ligamentous structures, including the static stabilizers of the kneecap, giving them significant patellar hypermobility.

Treatment & Prognosis

A wide variety of treatment options are recommended for patellar dislocations, including immediate mobilization and strengthening exercises, immobilization in a cylinder cast for 6 weeks followed by rehabilitation, arthroscopy with or without retinacular repair, surgical repair of the torn retinaculum, or immediate patellar realignment.

Treatment is based on which predisposing factors are present. Little is lost by functional treatment, similar to the treatment of isolated medial collateral ligament sprains, which is often successful. If dislocation recurs, realignment may be performed. A long-term study showed that patients treated surgically for patellar malalignment problems had a higher incidence of osteoarthritis than those treated nonoperatively.

Atkin DM et al: Characteristics of patients with primary acute lateral patella dislocation and their recovery within the first 6 months of injury. Am J Sports Med 2000;28:472. [PMID: 10921637]

Bensahal H et al: The unstable patella in children. J Pediatr Orthop 2000,9:265. [PMID: 11143470]

Buchner M et al: Acute traumatic primary patellar dislocation: Long-term results comparing conservative and surgical treatment. Clin J Sport Med 2005;15:62. [PMID: 15782048]

KNEE TENDON INJURY

Ruptures of the quadriceps and patellar tendons usually result from a tremendous eccentric contraction of the quadriceps muscle, which may occur when an athlete stumbles and tries not to fall.

1. Rupture of the Quadriceps Tendon

Quadriceps tendon ruptures occur most frequently in patients older than 40 years. Biopsies of fresh rupture sites showed local degenerative changes already present, consistent with the theory that normal tendons do not rupture. Rarely, the injury occurs bilaterally, and it is often associated with gout, diabetes, or steroid use. When it does occur bilaterally with only a small amount of trauma, the diagnosis may be difficult to make because of the small amount of swelling or symptoms of injury.

The cardinal symptom is inability to extend the knee. When extension is attempted, a gap develops in the suprapatellar region. The patella rides at a slightly lower level, and the anterior border of the femoral condyles may be palpated.

Acute complete quadriceps tendon ruptures should be paired surgically. If left untreated, proximal migration and scarring of the quadriceps muscle occurs. Direct-end repair produces excellent results. Neutralizing the forces across the repair is difficult, and immobilization in extension is recommended. Repair of ruptures more than 2 weeks old may be difficult and may require quadriceps lengthening, muscle or tendon transfers, or a combination of these procedures.

Ilan DI et al: Quadriceps tendon rupture. J Am Acad Orthop Surg 2003;11:192. [PMID: 112828449]

Konrath GA et al: Outcomes following repair of quadriceps tendon ruptures. J Orthop Trauma 1998,12:273. [PMID: 9619463]

2. Rupture of the Patellar Tendon

Rupture of the patella tendon occurs more frequently in patients younger than 40 years. The patient cannot actively extend the knee, the patella is high riding, and a defect is palpable beneath the patella. Surgical repair is the treatment of choice. The tendon, along with the medial and lateral retinaculum, should be sewn end to end. A stress-relieving wire may be placed around the patella and through the tibial tubercle. The wire should be removed in 6–8 weeks. Chronic patellar tendon ruptures are very hard to treat. The quadriceps must be freed up from the femur and the patella pulled down to the proper location. The gracilis and semitendinosus tendons can be used to substitute for the patellar tendon.

The extensor mechanism may also be disrupted at the inferior pole of the patella where the patellar tendon originates. This usually occurs in a child between 8 and 12 years of age. The distal pole of the patella plus a large sleeve of articular cartilage is pulled off (Figure 4–18). This may be easily misdiagnosed if the fragment of bone is small. Reestablishment of an intact extensor mechanism is necessary. With displaced fractures, open reduction and internal fixation with tension band wiring are recommended.

KNEE PAIN

Pain in the knee region is a very common complaint of athletes. If there is no history of an acute injury, overuse is commonly the cause. The patient is often able to point to the area of pain. The history of activity must be obtained as well as overall evaluation of the extremities.

1. Anterior Knee Pain

Clinical Findings

A. Symptoms and Signs

Anterior knee pain is a common complaint and frequently bilateral. It is most common in females during the second decade of life. The patellofemoral joint is often the source of pain. Entities such as chondromalacia patella, patellofemoral arthralgia, and lateral patellofemoral compression syndrome are diagnostic considerations.

Patellar pain is often felt when going up or down hills or stairs, and there may be complaints of instability during walking, running, or other sports activities. These activities may create a joint reaction force of several times the body weight on the patella with each step. Swelling is seldom a complaint. If the pain is in one knee only, the patient may alter the way of climbing and descending stairs so that the affected leg is kept straight and each step leads with the same foot. This strategy significantly decreases the joint reaction force on the patellofemoral joint.

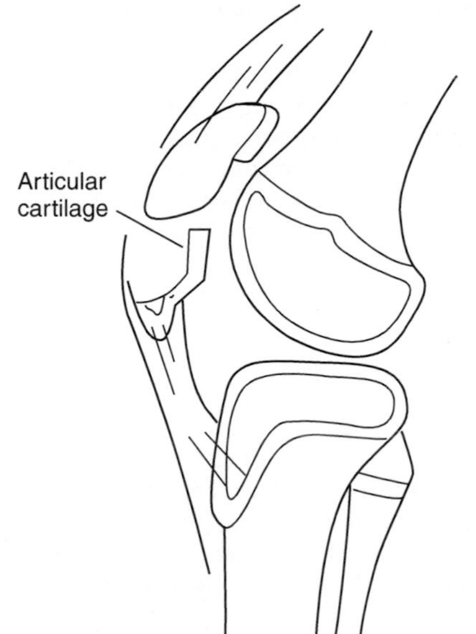

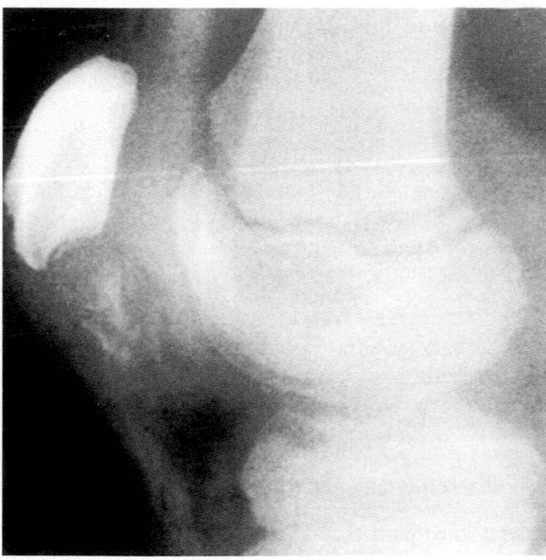

Figure 4–18. Sleeve fracture of the patella. **A:** A small segment of the distal pole of the patella is avulsed with a relatively large portion of the articular surface. **B:** Lateral radiograph of the knee with a displaced sleeve fracture of the patella. Note that the small osseous portion of the displaced fragment is visible, but the cartilaginous portion is not seen. (Reproduced, with permission, from Rockwood CA Jr, ed: *Fractures in Children,* 3rd ed. Lippincott, 1991.)

Many of these problems arise because the patellofemoral joint is semiconstrained, especially in the range of 0–20 degrees of flexion, and the constraint increases as flexion increases. The degree of constraint also depends on a number of other factors, including the angle of the sulcus of the femur, the presence or absence of patella alta, and the generalized ligamentous laxity of the patient. In addition, femoral anteversion and increased Q angle (Figure 4–19) may lead to increased instability of the patellofemoral joint. This lack of constraint may predispose the patella to frank dislocation, although subluxation is a much more common finding. The degree of congruity is anatomically variable and may lead to high-contact stresses caused by anatomic configuration and static and dynamic constraints on the patella. Increased pressure may cause pain and patellofemoral osteoarthritis.

On physical examination of the patient with patellofemoral subluxation, minimal findings in relation to complaints may be present. Occasionally, crepitance, a crackling or clicking sound or feeling, is found with

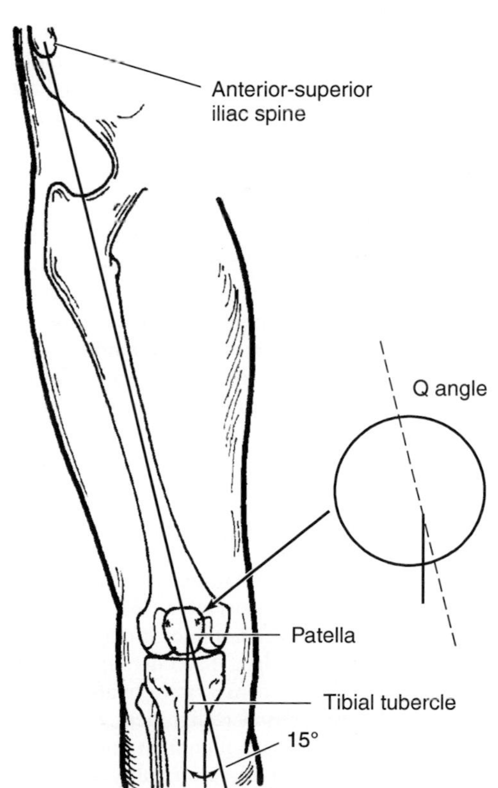

Figure 4–19. Q angle and valgus angulation. (Reproduced, with permission, from American Academy of Orthopaedic Surgeons: *Athletic Training and Sports Medicine,* 2nd ed. AAOS, 1991.)

flexion and extension. Quadriceps strength, tone, and bulk are usually reduced. Pain may be elicited at a particular angle of flexion by putting the knee through its range of motion with resistance. Subluxation may often be diagnosed with the apprehension sign, a rapid contraction of the quadriceps when the patella is passively moved laterally.

B. Imaging Studies

Roentgenographic examination frequently shows a valgus angulation of the knee on anteroposterior views. Occasionally, patella alta may be identified on the lateral view, and tangential views of the patella at various knee flexion angles reveals a lack of contact of the medial facet of the patella with the medial facet of the trochlear groove of the femur. Lateral subluxation of the patellofemoral joint may also be observed.

This syndrome with a normal roentgenographic examination is frequently called chondromalacia patellae; with subluxation identified on radiograph, it is referred to as patellofemoral subluxation. A more accurate term would be patellofemoral arthralgia because patellofemoral subluxation was probably present prior to the onset of pain, and because chondromalacia patellae (softening of the patellar cartilage) is an arthroscopic or pathologic diagnosis. Patellofemoral arthralgia is a clinical diagnosis.

Treatment

A. Chondromalacia Patellae

Initially, treatment is conservative, with the intent of improving quadriceps strength and stamina to stabilize the patellofemoral joint. Weight loss is prescribed to decrease the stress on the patellofemoral joint; reduction in loading the knee in the flexed position also accomplishes pressure reduction. Knee orthotics may be beneficial. When subluxation and fear of dislocation are major concerns, an orthotic that limits extension of the knee may be beneficial because the patella becomes inherently more stable with knee flexion. NSAIDs may be beneficial.

B. Patellofemoral Arthralgia

Only when conservative treatment is exhausted should surgical treatment be considered. Alteration in the alignment of the patellofemoral joint may be beneficial in patellofemoral arthralgia. Lateral retinacular release followed by a period of conservative treatment is beneficial in some cases. Distal realignment may be necessary to achieve appropriate alignment and reduction in pain in those cases with an abnormality such as valgus knee or increased femoral anteversion.

C. Patellofemoral Compression Syndrome

With lateral patellofemoral compression syndrome, there is tenderness along the lateral facet of the patella or along the femoral condyle. Without cartilage damage, an effusion is rarely present. Treatment includes decreasing the activity level, including avoiding hills or step aerobics. Ice-massage, quadriceps and hamstring stretching, and short-arc quadriceps exercises against resistance are recommended to strengthen the vastus medialis obliquus muscle without aggravating the pain. Patellar supports or neoprene sleeves may also be helpful. Most patients respond to this regimen and gradually resume their activities. The role of releasing a contracted lateral patellofemoral retinaculum is controversial.

D. Patellar Tendinitis

Patellar tendinitis, or jumper's knee, is seen in basketball and volleyball players. Tenderness along the tendon, usually at the inferior pole of the patella, is noted. Treatment with ice and avoiding jumping usually suffices. In refractory cases, debridement of mucinous degenerative material from the tendon may be successful.

Prognosis

The prognosis for jumper's knee is quite good. The condition is often persistent but self-limiting. The patient can always alleviate the symptoms by avoiding the activities that cause the problem.

Csintalan R et al: Gender effects on the biomechanical properties of the peripatellar retinaculum. Clin Orthop Rel Res 2002,(402):260. [PMID: 12218492]

Kettunen JA, Visuri T, Harilainen A et al: Primary cartilage lesions and outcome among subjects with patellofemoral pain syndrome. Knee Surg Sports Traumatol Arthrosc 2005;13:131. [PMID: 15756617]

Witvrouw E, Werner S, Mikkelsen C et al: Clinical classification of patellofemoral pain syndrome: Guidelines for non-operative treatment. Knee Surg Sports Traumatol Arthrosc 2005; 13:122. [PMID: 15703965]

2. Lateral Knee Pain

Lateral knee pain that is not located on the joint line may result from iliotibial band friction syndrome. This is a form of bursitis caused by rubbing of the iliotibial band against the lateral epicondyle. Tenderness over the lateral epicondyle at approximately 30 degrees of flexion when the knee is extended is indicative of this diagnosis. Runners and cyclists are commonly afflicted. Crossover gait or running on banked terrain is thought to be a causative factor.

Treatment involves decreasing the athlete's activities, ice-massage, stretching of the iliotibial tract, and use of a lateral wedge orthotic in those patients with heel varus. Running on flat terrain and changing the gait pattern may be helpful. In cyclists, lowering the seat height so the full extension of the knee is not reached and adjusting the pedals so the toes are not internally rotated should help. Steroid injections are infrequently needed, and release of the inflamed portion of the iliotibial band is seldom necessary. As for other overuse syndromes of the knee, the prognosis is good.

Gunter P, Schwellnus MP: Local corticosteroid injection in iliotibial band friction syndrome in runners: A randomised controlled trial. Br J Sports Med 2004;38:269; discussion 272. [PMID: 15155424]

ANKLE OR FOOT PAIN

Evaluation of foot and ankle injuries is described in Chapter 9. Injury specific to athletics includes chronic Achilles tendonitis, heel pain, plantar fasciitis and posterior tibial syndrome.

Clinical Findings

Achilles tendonitis, a frequent complaint in runners, may result from a contracted gastrocsoleus, or hyperpronation may cause overpulling of the medial insertion. Additionally, there may be a bony prominence on the superior-posterior aspect of the calcaneus, causing retrocalcaneal bursitis.

Heel pain is a common problem in runners and difficult to treat because of the uncertainty as to cause. Theories include painful heel spurs, bursitis, fat-pad atrophy, stress fracture, plantar fasciitis, or entrapment of the terminal branches of the posterior tibial nerve.

Many patients have pain localized in the posteromedial surface of the foot just distal to the attachment of the plantar fascia to the calcaneus (plantar fasciitis). This pain is often most severe on initially getting up in the morning and decreases as the day goes on.

Posterior tibial syndrome occurs in runners with hyperpronation. As the longitudinal arch flattens out, the posterior tibial musculotendinous unit elevates the flattened arch and has abnormal strain placed on it.

Treatment

Treatment depends on the cause of the injury, but it includes decreasing running activities, using a heel lift, and performing stretching exercises. If hyperpronation is thought to be the cause, an orthotic may be used. Steroid injections are not recommended because they could lead to weakening and subsequent rupture of the tendon.

Surgical intervention for chronic Achilles tendinitis or retrocalcaneal bursitis is seldom needed. This would be done to remove areas of fibrosis or calcium within the tendon and possibly some bone from the posterior process of the calcaneus. The treatment for plantar fasciitis includes rest, ice-massage, and possibly antiinflammatory medications. A small shock-absorbing type of heel cup often is helpful, and a steroid injection may be given in recalcitrant cases. Acute rupture of the plantar fascia may occur. The pain is usually quite sharp and may cause significant disability for 6–12 weeks.

Hyperpronation may also cause fibular stress fractures. A semirigid orthosis may be recommended to decrease the amount and angular velocity of pronation. Using an orthosis while running actually increases the work of running, but if it decreases abnormal stresses in those who hyperpronate, it may be quite helpful.

Mizel MS et al: Evaluation and treatment of chronic ankle pain. Instr Course Lect 2004;53:311. [PMID: 15116624]

Shalabi A et al: Eccentric training of the gastrocnemius-soleus complex in chronic Achilles tendinopathy results in decreased tendon volume and intratendinous signal as evaluated by MRI. Am J Sports Med 2004;25:149. [PMID: 15244320]

OTHER INJURIES OF THE LOWER BODY

Many disorders seen while caring for athletes may be difficult to diagnose with certainty. The differential diagnosis must be carefully made to rule out more severe injuries. A period of rest followed by gradual return to activities is often the best treatment. During convalescence, application of ice packs, stretching exercises, and gradual strengthening of the injured limb facilitate return to sports activities.

OVERUSE SYNDROMES OF THE LOWER EXTREMITIES

Many athletes, such as runners, cyclists, aerobics enthusiasts, volleyball players, and basketball players, develop painful disorders of the lower extremities without an acute injury. History taking is very important, and the examiner should ask specific questions about the circumstances in which the discomfort occurs. In a runner, for example, the examiner should ask whether there was an increase in the distance run or a change in the running surface, at what point the pain was felt, and what home remedies were tried before the runner sought advice from a physician.

The physical examination should include not only the affected area, but also evaluation of the back, pelvis, leg lengths, genu varum or valgum, femoral and tibial torsion, and cavus or flatfoot deformities. The presence of hamstring and heel cord contracture should be determined, and the gait pattern should be observed. Running shoes should be inspected for wear patterns, which may be quite helpful.

1. Muscle Strains

Muscle strains of the lower extremity are frequent, and disabling muscle injuries, with strain of the distal muscle tendon junction, are the most common. Muscles may stretch to approximately 125% of their resting length before tearing. Strains are graded as mild, moderate, and severe, based on the degree of pain, spasm, and disability that the strain causes. A severe strain would be complete disruption of the muscle, with a palpable defect and balling up of the muscle proximally.

In spite of the frequency of muscle strains and the disability they produce, there is little scientific information on their pathologic basis. Muscles susceptible to more stretching are more susceptible to strains. In the lower extremity, the muscles most frequently injured are the hamstring, quadriceps, and gastrocnemius muscles. These muscles all cross two joints, and they may be unable to resist full stretching across both joints. The most powerful muscles are more likely to be strained, and strains are more common in so-called explosive-type athletics. Eccentric contraction (muscle contraction while the muscle is lengthening) is often thought to be causative in muscle strains.

Clinical Findings

The diagnosis is relatively easy. Often the athlete feels the muscle "grab" while he or she is accelerating. There is localized tenderness over the muscle and pain on stretching of the muscle. Because the two joint muscles are most frequently involved, the muscles should be stretched over both of the joints during examination.

Treatment & Prognosis

The treatment of muscle strains should begin with ice in the immediate postinjury period. Flexibility and strength should be regained prior to return to activity. This may take many months, and if the patient returns to activity too early, there may be a setback to the level of the original injury.

Strengthening of the muscles might make them less susceptible to being torn. It is commonly believed that flexibility helps prevent muscle strains, but there are conflicting reports regarding this idea, and it is still unproved.

Askling C, Karlsson J, Thorstensson A: Hamstring injury occurrence in elite soccer players after preseason strength training with eccentric overload. Scand J Med Sci Sports 2005;15:65. [PMID: 15679576]

Gabbe BJ, Finch CF, Bennell KL et al:. Risk factors for hamstring injuries in community level Australian football. Br J Sports Med 2005;39:106. [PMID: 15665208]

Levine WN et al: Intramuscular corticosteroid injection for hamstring injuries. A 13-year experience in the National Football League. Am J Sports Med 2000;28(3):297. [PMID: 10843118]

2. Shin Pain

Clinical Findings

A. Shin Splints

The term *shin splints* is widely used for shin pain, but it is not a diagnostic term. A more specific diagnosis should be made if possible. Shin splints are usually defined as pain associated with activity in the beginning of training after a relatively inactive period. The pain and tenderness are usually located over the anterior compartment and disappear in 1–2 weeks as the athlete becomes conditioned to the exercise. Care must be taken to differentiate shin splints from stress fractures of the tibia, which cause more localized pain and have many more potential complications if not cared for properly.

B. Medial Tibial Syndrome

Medial tibial syndrome is also seen in runners, occurring along the medial border of the distal tibia. After 3–4 weeks, some hypertrophy of the cortical bone and periosteal new bone formation may be seen on radiograph. It is thought to be either a periostitis or possibly an incomplete stress fracture. The pull of the tibialis posterior muscle from its origin on the tibia and posterior tibial tendinitis are also thought to be possible causes.

Treatment

Treatment for shin splints and medial tibial syndrome is rest and resumption of athletic activities in a graduated fashion.

3. Stress Fractures

Stress fractures may occur in the pelvis, femoral neck, tibia, navicular, and metatarsals. They are usually the result of a significant increase in training and activity. In the female athlete, poor nutrition, low bone density, and a history of menstrual disturbance are associated with a higher prevalence of stress fractures. The history is important in differentiating these injuries from infection or neoplasm, particularly when there is a finding on radiographs. Plain radiographs are normal at first. MRI or technetium bone scans are the best diagnostic tests. If symptoms persist for over a month, radiographs may become positive.

Treatment of stress fractures involves rest and avoidance of high-impact activities until healing occurs. This includes resolution of the tenderness and signs of fracture healing on plain radiographs. Continuous activity with stress fractures may lead to complete fractures. Patients must be made aware of this and all the complications that may develop with a complete fracture.

Armstrong DW III, Rue JP, Wilckens JH et al: Stress fracture injury in young military men and women. Bone 2004;35(3):806. [PMID: 15336620]

Perron AD, Brady WJ, Keats TA: Principles of stress fracture management. The whys and hows of an increasingly common injury. Postgrad Med 2001;110:115.

4. Exertional Compartment Syndromes

Exertional compartment syndromes may result from muscle hypertrophy within the confining osseofascial compartment. As the muscles hypertrophy and the amount of edema within the compartment increases, the blood supply to the nerves and muscles within the involved compartment is diminished, and the pressure continues to increase.

The syndrome presents as recurrent claudication during exertional activity and is relieved by rest. After exercise, the findings of localized pain, pain on passive motion, and hypesthesia are indicative.

Treatment consists activity modification including gradual onset of training. If unsuccessful, compartment pressures may be measured while the patient is exercising on a treadmill, and if the pressures are elevated, surgical fasciotomy is usually effective.

Shah SN, Miller BS, Kuhn JE: Chronic exertional compartment syndrome. Am J Orthop 2004;33:335. [PMID: 15344575]

CONTUSIONS & AVULSIONS OF THE LOWER BODY

1. Contusion to the Quadriceps Muscle

Clinical Findings

A severe contusion to the quadriceps muscle (charley horse) is disabling and results in prolonged inactivity. It frequently occurs in football players. With significant bleeding into the muscle, there is inhibition of movement. Rarely, a compartment syndrome occurs.

Myositis ossificans may occur after these injuries. It may be apparent 2–4 weeks after the injury. Radiographically and histologically, myositis ossificans may be similar to osteogenic sarcoma; therefore, the history of contusion is very important. Radiographs should be obtained after such a contusion to minimize myositis ossificans being confused with cancer.

Treatment & Prognosis

Quadriceps contusions should be treated with elevation of the leg and the hip and knee flexed to tolerance to minimize bleeding. After a few days the knee can be moved with continuous passive motion or so-called drop-and-dangle gravity-assisted exercises. For the latter, the patient is seated on a table high enough to keep the feet off the floor. The patient then hooks the uninjured foot behind the ankle of the injured leg. The uninjured leg extends the knee of the injured leg, and gravity flexes the injured knee. Average length of disability for mild contusions is 2 weeks; for severe contusions, 3 weeks.

If heterotopic ossification is present, no specific treatment is recommended other than treatment for the contusion. Normal function may be obtained, but the recovery period is longer. Because early surgery may cause exacerbation of the heterotopic ossification, it should be avoided.

Cooper DE: Severe quadriceps muscle contusions in athletes. Am J Sports Med 2004;32:820. [PMID: 15090402]

Diaz JA, Fischer DA, Rettig AC et al: Severe quadriceps muscle contusions in athletes. A report of three cases. Am J Sports Med 2003;3:289. [PMID: 12642267]

CONTUSIONS ABOUT THE HIP AND PELVIS

Clinical Findings

Contusions about the pelvis and hip region may be very painful and disabling. Because of the subcutaneous location of the iliac crests and the greater trochanters, these regions are at risk in contact sports.

A contusion over the greater trochanter may cause persistent bursitis, tenderness directly over the greater trochanter, and increased pain with adduction of the leg. Females are more prone to trochanteric bursitis because of their broader pelvis.

A hip pointer is a very painful contusion over the iliac crest that occurs from many contact sports. It must be differentiated from an avulsion fracture in a child and a tear of the muscle aponeurosis in an adult. Profuse bleeding may occur and be very painful.

Treatment & Prognosis

For contusion over the greater trochanter, treatment consists of ice applications and decreased activities. Padding may be helpful to prevent recurrent injuries. The prognosis is good. For hip pointer injuries, initial treatment with ice is helpful. Protective pads are useful in preventing these injuries and returning the athlete to activities sooner.

AVULSION OF THE TIBIAL TUBERCLE

Clinical Findings

Tibial tubercle avulsions occur in adolescent athletes, most often in males between 14 and 16 years of age. They result from a powerful contraction of the quadriceps muscle against a fixed tibia, as in jumping, or with forced passive flexion of the knee against a powerful quadriceps contraction, as in an awkward landing at the end of a jump or fall. Avulsion of the tubercle may occur with either a sudden acceleration or deceleration of the knee extensor mechanism. The patellar tendon must pull hard enough to overcome the strength of the growth plate, the surrounding perichondrium, and the adjacent periosteum.

Swelling and tenderness are located over the proximal anterior tibia. A tense hemarthrosis may be present. A palpable defect in the anterior tibia is associated with a much-displaced avulsion. Proximal migration of the patella occurs, and the patella may seem to float off the anterior aspect of the femur. The knee is held flexed; with displaced fractures, the patient is unable actively to extend the knee.

Watson-Jones defined three types of avulsion fractures, which were subsequently refined as the following three types (Figure 4–20): type 1 fracture, in which the fracture line lies across the secondary center of ossification at the level of the posterior border of the patellar ligament; type 2 fracture, in which a separation breaks out at the primary and secondary ossification centers of epiphysis; and type 3 fracture, in which the separation propagates upward through the main portion of the proximal tibial epiphysis. The degree of displacement depends on the severity of injury to the surrounding soft-tissue moorings. A lateral radiograph with the tibia slightly internally rotated is the best view to see the fracture and the degree of displacement.

Differential Diagnosis

Osgood-Schlatter disease, or osteochondrosis of the tuberosity of the tibia, should not be confused with acute avulsion of the tibial tubercle. In the former, the patient is usually between 11 and 15 years of age and involved in athletics. Pain is located at the tibial tubercle, and it has usually been present intermittently over a period of several months. Walking on a flat surface is not difficult, but ascending or descending stairs causes difficulty. Radiograph examination shows slight separation of the tibial tubercle with new bone formation beneath it (Figure 4–21).

Treatment recommendations vary from decreasing the amount of running and jumping, but continuing participation in athletics, to cylinder cast immobilization for a short period of time. The long-term prognosis is excellent. Although symptoms are often present for 2 years, early short-term cast immobilization may shorten this period of discomfort to 9 months. In most children, casting is not necessary. Explaining the benign nature of the problem to both the patient and the parents, reassuring them that the long-term prognosis is good, and modifying activities usually allows continued

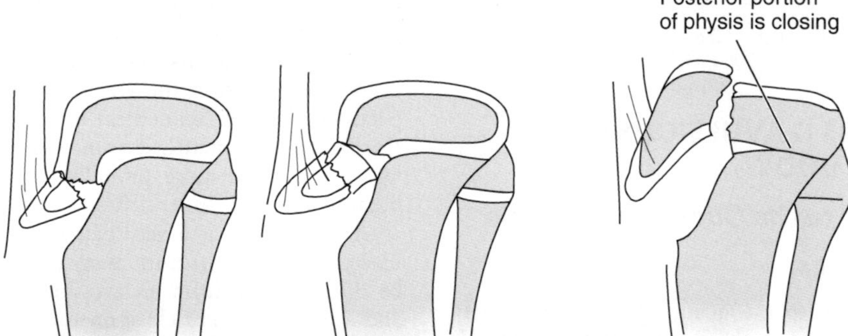

Figure 4–20. Classification of avulsion fractures of the tibial tubercle. Type 1 fracture (**left**) across the secondary ossification center at level with the posterior border of the inserting patellar ligament. Type 2 fracture (**center**) at the junction of the primary and secondary ossification centers of the proximal tibial epiphysis. Type 3 fracture (**right**) propagates upward across the primary ossification center of the proximal tibial epiphysis into the knee joint. This fracture is a variant of the Salter-Harris III separation and is analogous to the fracture of Tillaux at the ankle because the posterior portion of the physis of the proximal tibia is closing. (Reproduced, with permission, from Odgen JA et al: Fractures of the tibial tuberosity in adolescents. J Bone Joint Surg Am 1980;62:205.)

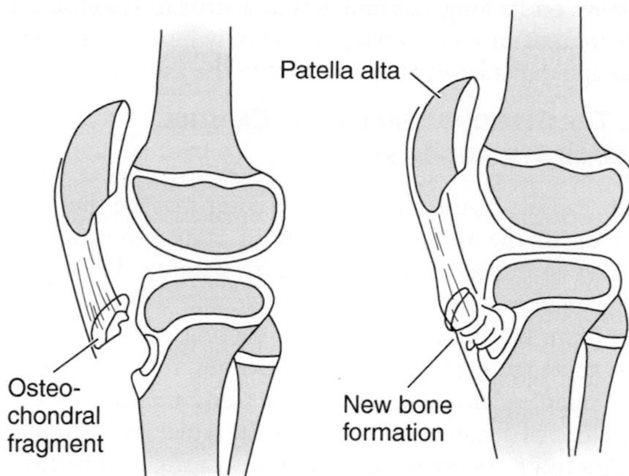

Figure 4–21. Development of Osgood-Schlatter lesion. (**Left**) Avulsion of osteochondral fragment that includes surface cartilage and a portion of the secondary ossification center of the tibial tubercle. (**Right**) New bone fills in the gap between the avulsed osteochondral fragment and the tibial tubercle. (Reproduced, with permission, from Rockwood CA Jr (ed): *Fractures in Children,* 3rd ed. Lippincott, 1991.)

participation in athletics. Hamstring stretching and ice-massage ideally decrease symptoms during the time needed for maturation of the tibial tubercle. The pain goes away when the tubercle unites with the tibia. In a very small number of cases, chronic pain is present if the ossicle fails to unite. Painful ossicles in the adult are treated successfully with simple excision.

Treatment

Full function of the extensor mechanism is necessary, and therefore treatment of tibial tubercle avulsion fractures is aimed at this goal. If the fracture is minimally displaced, and the patient is able to extend the knee fully against gravity, nonoperative treatment is acceptable. A cylinder cast should be applied with the knee extended and worn for 4 weeks. Active range-of-motion and strengthening exercises should then commence. At 6 weeks, quadriceps exercises against resistance are initiated. For displaced fractures, open reduction and internal fixation are recommended, with screws if the piece or pieces are large enough. If rigid fixation of large fragments is obtained, early active flexion and passive extension may be initiated. If a tenuous repair is obtained, protection in a cast is advisable.

Prognosis

Because the injury occurs in children who are close to skeletal maturity, meaningful growth abnormalities at the proximal tibial physis do not occur. Return to activities is allowed after the athlete develops quadriceps mass and strength equal to the contralateral side.

AVULSIONS ABOUT THE PELVIS

Clinical Findings

In the skeletally immature athlete, the apophysis, or growth plate where the muscle attaches to bone, is the weak link in the bone-muscle-tendon unit. Therefore, just as the growth plate is prone to breaking in children's fractures, the bony origin of muscles may be pulled off. This most commonly occurs in athletes between 14 and 25 years of age. Comparison radiographs may be helpful to make sure the avulsion fracture is not just a normal anatomic variant. In the pelvis, this may occur at the iliac crest (abdominal muscles), anterior superior iliac spine (sartorius origin), anterior inferior iliac spine (rectus femoris origin), ischial tuberosity (hamstring origin), and lesser trochanter of the femur (iliopsoas insertion).

Treatment & Prognosis

Symptomatic care with a few days of rest followed by ambulation with crutches for approximately a month is recommended. It is usually 6–10 weeks before athletic activities may be resumed. Long-term athletic activity will probably not be affected. Open reduction and internal fixation do not show superior results, and therefore they are usually not warranted. Abundant calcification may occur in the ischial tuberosity region and may be the cause of chronic bursitis and pain. Excision of the exuberant callous should cure this problem. Another indication for surgery is a painful fibrous nonunion, which also may be cured with excision of the fragment.

Rossi F, Dragoni S: Acute avulsion fractures of the pelvis in adolescent competitive athletes: Prevalence, location and sports distribution of 203 cases collected. Skeletal Radiol 2001;30:127. [PMID: 11357449]

SHOULDER INJURIES

The shoulder is the third most commonly injured joint during athletic activities, after the knee and the ankle. Sports-related injuries of the shoulder may result from a direct traumatic event or repetitive overuse. Any activity that requires arm motion, particularly overhead arm motion such as throwing, may stress the soft tissues surrounding the glenohumeral joint to the point of injury. The shoulder is the most mobile joint in the body, partly as a result of minimal containment of the large humeral head by the shallow and smaller glenoid fossa. The trade-off for this mobility is less structural restraint to undesirable and potentially damaging movements. Thus, a fine balance must be struck to maintain full range of shoulder motion and normal glenohumeral joint stability.

Kim DH et al: Shoulder injuries in golf. Am J Sports Med 200432(5):1324. [PMID: 15262661]

Anatomy

A. The Bony Articulation of the Glenohumeral Joint

The glenohumeral joint is a modified ball-and-socket joint. The glenoid fossa is a shallow inverted, comma-shaped, articular surface one fourth the size of the humeral head. The articular surface of the humeral head is retroverted approximately 30 degrees relative to the transverse axis of the elbow. Because the scapula is oriented anterolaterally approximately 30 degrees on the thorax, relative to the coronal plane of the body, the face of the glenoid fossa matches the humeral head retroversion. The scapula rotates to direct the glenoid superiorly, inferiorly, medially, or laterally to accommodate changing humeral head positions. As a result, the humeral head is centered in the glenoid throughout most shoulder motions. When this centered position is disturbed, instability may result.

B. The Clavicle and Its Articulations

The clavicle articulates medially with the sternum at the sternoclavicular joint and laterally with the acromion of the scapula at the acromioclavicular joint. The clavicle rotates on its long axis and acts as a strut to stabilize the glenohumeral joint, serving as the only bone connecting the appendicular upper extremity to the axial skeleton.

C. The Glenohumeral Joint Capsule, Ligaments, and Labrum

The capsule of the glenohumeral joint may be the most lax of all the major joints, yet in certain positions it makes an important contribution to stability. The capsuloligamentous structures and the glenoid labrum share a common insertion. The anterior capsule is composed of the coracohumeral and superior glenohumeral ligaments, the middle glenohumeral ligament, and the inferior glenohumeral ligament (Figure 4–22). There is a variable relationship between the anterior capsuloligamentous structures and the labrum, such that certain anatomic variations may be associated with joint instability more often than others. For example, an anterosuperior sublabral hole is variably present within the glenohumeral joint, connecting with the subscapularis bursa that lies between the subscapularis tendon and the capsule.

The glenoid labrum not only acts as an attachment site for the capsuloligamentous structures but also as an extension of the articular cavity. Its presence deepens the glenoid socket by nearly 50%, and removal of the labrum decreases joint stability to shear stress. In this way, the triangular cross section of the labrum acts as a chock-block to help prevent subluxation.

D. The Shoulder Musculature

The muscles around the shoulder may be divided into three functional groups: glenohumeral, thoracohumeral, and those that cross both the shoulder and elbow.

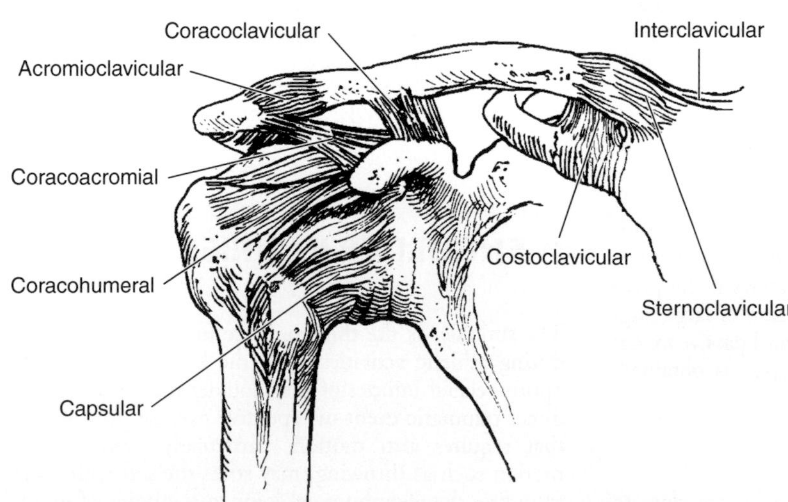

Figure 4–22. Ligaments about the shoulder girdle.

Glenohumeral Muscles

Four muscles compose the rotator cuff: the supraspinatus, subscapularis, infraspinatus, and teres minor. The supraspinatus has its origin on the posterosuperior scapula, superior to the scapular spine. It passes under the acromion, through the supraspinatus fossa, and inserts on the greater tuberosity with an extended attachment of fibrocartilage. The supraspinatus is active during the entire arc of scapular plane abduction; paralysis of the suprascapular nerve results in an approximately 50% loss of abduction torque. The infraspinatus and the teres minor muscles originate on the posterior scapula, inferior to the scapular spine, and insert on the posterior aspect of the greater tuberosity. Despite their origin below the scapular spine, their tendinous insertions are not separate from the supraspinatus tendon. These muscles function together to externally rotate and extend the humerus. Both account for approximately 80% of external rotation strength in the adducted position. The infraspinatus is more active with the arm at the side; the teres minor activates mainly with the shoulder in 90 degrees of elevation. The subscapularis muscle arises from the anterior scapula and is the only muscle to insert on the lesser tuberosity. The subscapularis is the sole anterior component of the rotator cuff and functions to rotate and flex the humerus internally. The tendinous insertion of the subscapularis is continuous with the anterior capsule so that both provide anterior glenohumeral stability.

The deltoid is the largest of the glenohumeral muscles. It covers the proximal humerus on a path from its tripennate origin at the clavicle, acromion, and scapular spine to its insertion midway on the humerus at the deltoid tubercle. Abduction of the joint results from activity of the anterior and middle portions. The anterior portion is also a forward flexor. The posterior portion does not abduct the joint but instead adducts and extends the humerus. The deltoid is active throughout the entire arc of glenohumeral abduction; paralysis of the axillary nerve results in a 50% loss of abduction torque. The deltoid muscle can fully abduct the glenohumeral joint with the supraspinatus muscle inactive.

The teres major muscle originates from the inferior angle of the scapula and inserts on the medial lip of the bicipital groove of the humerus, posterior to the insertion of the latissimus dorsi. The axillary nerve and the posterior humeral circumflex artery pass superior to it through the quadrilateral space also bordered by the teres minor, the triceps, and the humerus. It contracts with the latissimus dorsi muscle, and the two muscles function as a unit in humeral extension, internal rotation, and adduction.

Thoracohumeral Muscles

The pectoralis major and the latissimus dorsi muscles are powerful movers of the shoulder and hence contribute to the joint force that in turn usually stabilizes the glenohumeral joint. The pectoralis major muscle arises as a broad sheet of two distinct heads with the lowermost fibers of the sternal head inserting most proximally on the humerus.

Muscles that have origin on the thorax contribute to glenohumeral stability and may have roles in instability as well. When the shoulder is placed in horizontal abduction, similar to the apprehension position, the lowermost fibers of the sternal head of the pectoralis major muscle are stretched to an extreme. Because anterior instability also occurs from forcible horizontal abduction of the shoulder, the humeral head can be pulled out of the glenoid by passive tension in the pectoralis major and latissimus dorsi muscles.

Biceps Brachii Muscle

Both heads of the biceps brachii muscle have their origin on the scapula. The short head originates from the coracoid and with the coracobrachialis muscle forms the conjoined tendon. The long head of the biceps has its origin just superior to the articular margin of the glenoid from the posterosuperior labrum and the supraglenoid tubercle, and it is inside the synovial sheath of the glenohumeral joint. It traverses the glenohumeral joint, passing over the anterior aspect of the humeral head to the bicipital groove where it exits the joint under the transverse humeral ligament.

Its origin on the scapula and insertion of the radius leaves the long head of the biceps brachii muscle with potential for function at both the shoulder and the elbow. Its function at the elbow is well established to include both flexion and supination. Long considered a depressor of the humeral head, the role of the active biceps was questioned because electromyographic studies showed little or no activity of the biceps when elbow motion was controlled. This does not preclude a passive role or an active role associated with elbow motion because tension in the tendon may then contribute to glenohumeral joint stability.

E. The Neurovascular Supply

The axillary artery traverses the axilla, extending from the outer border of the first rib to the lower border of the teres minor muscle, forming the brachial artery. The axillary artery lies deep to the pectoralis muscle but is crossed in its midregion by the pectoralis minor tendon, just before the tendon inserts on the coracoid process. The axillary vein travels with the axillary artery, and branches of the axillary artery supply most of the shoulder girdle. The brachial plexus consists of the ventral rami of the fifth through eighth cervical nerves and the first thoracic nerve. This network of nerve fibers begins with the joining of the ventral rami proximally in the neck and continues anteriorly and distally, crossing into the axillary region obliquely underneath the clavicle at about the junction area of the distal one third and proximal two thirds. Clavicular fractures in this area have the potential of injuring the brachial plexus. The plexus then lies inferior to the coracoid process, where its cords form the peripheral nerves that continue down the arm. Muscles of the shoulder girdle are supplied by the nerves arising at all levels of the brachial plexus.

Eberly VC, McMahon PJ, Lee TQ: Variation in the glenoid origin of the anteroinferior glenohumeral capsulolabrum. Clin Orthop 2002;400,26. [PMID: 12072742]

Enad JG: Bifurcate origin of the long head of the biceps tendon. Arthroscopy 2004;20:1081. [PMID: 15592239]

Price MR et al: Determining the relationship of the axillary nerve to the shoulder joint capsule from an arthroscopic perspective. J Bone Joint Surg Am 2004;86-A:2135. [PMID: 15466721]

History & Physical Examination

A. General Approach

The history of shoulder complaints must include age, arm dominance, location, intensity, duration, temporal occurrence, aggravating and alleviating factors, radiation of discomfort, physical activity level, occupation, and the mechanism of injury. These responses, combined with the physical findings (Table 4–3) and imaging studies, can lead to accurate diagnosis of shoulder problems. Previous responses to treatment help to characterize their efficacy and establish a pattern of disease or injury progression. The physical examination begins with the patient undressing so both shoulders are fully exposed. Patients should be examined first in the standing position. The surface anatomy should be checked for asymmetry, atrophy, or external lesions. The supraspinatus and infraspinatus fossae are especially important to examine for atrophy. The area of pain should be pointed out by the patient prior to the physician manipulating the shoulder to avoid hurting the patient unnecessarily. A thorough neurovascular examination of the upper extremity should be performed.

B. Shoulder Range of Motion

1. Types of movement—Many terms may be used to describe movements of the shoulder joint (Figure 4–23). Flexion occurs when the arm begins at the side and elevates in the sagittal plane of the body anteriorly. Extension occurs when the arm starts at the side and elevates in the sagittal plane of the body posteriorly. Adduction occurs when the arm moves toward the midline of the body, with abduction occurring as the arm moves away from the midline of the body. Internal rotation occurs when the arm rotates medially, inward toward the body, and external rotation occurs as the arm rotates laterally or outward from the body. Horizontal adduction occurs as the arm starts at 90 degrees of abduction and adducts forward and medially toward the center of the body, and horizontal abduction happens as the arm starts at 90 degrees of abduction and moves outward, away from the body. Elevation is the angle made between the thorax and arm, regardless if it is in the abduction plane, flexion plane, or in between.

2. Evaluation of movement—Range of motion of the injured shoulder should be compared with the opposite shoulder, along with the strength during abduction and rotation. This should be done both passively and actively. The shoulder should be inspected for any changes in synchrony, such as scapular winging, elevation of the scapula, muscle fasciculations indicating abnormal function, and any other irregular or asymmetric movements of the scapula. Information may be gained on loss of flexibility and instability resulting from muscle imbalance, fibrosis, and tendon, capsular, or ligament contractures. Loss of flexibility usually occurs in the capsular tissues of the glenohumeral joint. Sudden pain or clicking may indicate an intraarticular problem. Loss of motion in either internal or external rotation is suggestive of a chronic anterior or posterior dislocation, respectively.

3. Provocative tests—Specific tests are then performed that aid in making the correct diagnosis. The specific tests for instability, impingement syndrome, bicipital tendonitis, and superior capsulolabral/biceps anchor lesions are discussed later.

Imaging & Other Studies

Many varieties of radiologic views and projections are available to examine shoulder injuries. An initial radiographic evaluation of the shoulder should consist of an anteroposterior view of the glenohumeral joint in both internal and external rotation, and an axillary lateral. Additional plain radiographic views depend on the underlying pathology. MRI may be indicated in evaluation of rotator cuff disorders recalcitrant to conservative treatment. An MR arthrogram may be useful in detecting labral pathology. Traditional arthrography is rarely indicated because it is invasive and has little or no advantage over MRI. Ultrasonography is also useful in diagnosis of rotator cuff injury, but it is operator dependent. Electromyographic examination can be useful in identifying shoulder pain of cervical origin.

Arthroscopic Evaluation

A. Indications for Arthroscopic Evaluation of Shoulder Injuries

Indications for arthroscopic examination of the shoulder include the following:

Table 4–3. History and physical examination of the shoulder.

	History	Physical Examination
Cuff tendonitis	Pain over the lateral shoulder with overhead activity Night pain Mild weakness	Neer and Hawkin impingement signs Normal ROM Mild weakness Pain relieved with lidocaine injection into the subacromial space
Cuff tear	Pain over the lateral shoulder with overhead activity Night pain Weakness Loss of ROM	Neer and Hawkin impingement signs Loss of active ROM Weakness Pain relieved with lidocaine injection into the subacromial space
Instability	Joint "slips" out Pain and feelings of instability with shoulder abduction and external rotation (anterior instability only) Asymptomatic with the shoulder at rest	Apprehension of instability with shoulder abduction and external rotation (anterior instability only) Apprehension of instability with shoulder abduction and external rotation relieved by relocation test (if anterior instability only)
AC joint instability (separation)	History of fall onto the "point" of the shoulder Pain on top of the shoulder Pain with cross-body movements Bump at the AC joint	Tenderness at AC joint Deformity at AC joint: acromion displaced inferior to the distal clavicle Pain with cross-body movements Pain relieved with lidocaine injection into the AC joint
AC joint arthritis	Pain on top of the shoulder Pain with cross-body movements	Tenderness at AC joint Pain with cross-body movements Pain relieved with lidocaine injection into the AC joint
Stiffness	Decreased ROM Pain with shoulder at rest but worse at the limits of ROM	Decreased active and passive ROM Pain relieved with lidocaine injection into the glenohumeral joint
Arthritis	Decreased ROM Pain with shoulder at rest but worse with motion Crepitus with motion	Decreased active and passive ROM Crepitus with motion Pain relieved with lidocaine injection into the glenohumeral joint
Biceps tendonitis	Pain over the anterior shoulder with activity	Speed and Yerguson tests Tenderness at the bicipital groove Pain relieved with a lidocaine injection into the bicipital groove

AC = acromioclavicular; ROM = range of motion.

1. impingement syndrome including subacromial bursitis, rotator cuff tendonitis, and rotator cuff tears;
2. acromioclavicular joint osteoarthritis;
3. loose bodies;
4. chronic synovitis;
5. glenohumeral instability;
6. superior capsulolabral/biceps anchor lesions; and
7. adhesive capsulitis (frozen shoulder).

B. Technique

With the patient either in the lateral decubitus or the beach chair position, the arthroscope is inserted into a posterior portal, medial and inferior to the posterolateral

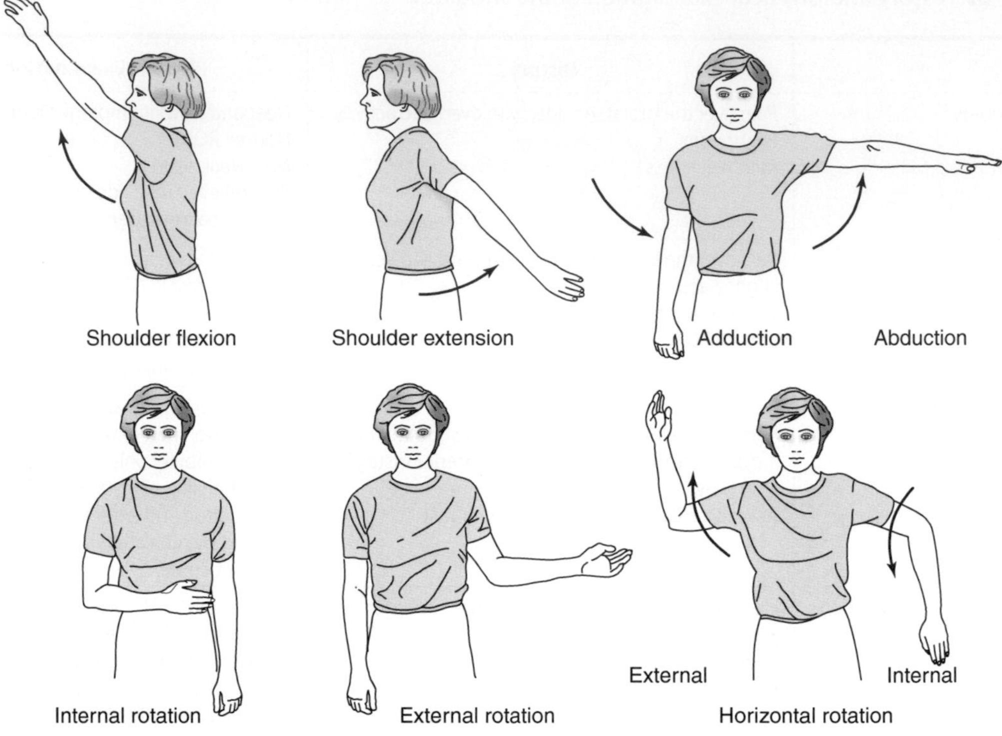

Figure 4–23. Description of shoulder motion.

corner of the acromion. With visualization of the glenohumeral joint, an anterior portal immediately lateral to the coracoid allows additional inflow and entrance of additional instruments. Distal clavicle excision, removal of loose bodies, and capsular release of adhesive capsulitis can be performed. An additional anterior portal inferior to the first is required for instability repair with an arthroscopic technique. The arthroscope is then removed from the joint and placed into the subacromial bursa. Portals lateral to the acromion allow subacromial decompression and rotator cuff repair to be carried out with arthroscopic techniques.

C. Steps in Evaluation

Examination of shoulder range of motion and stability with the patient under anesthesia is helpful in the diagnosis and treatment of shoulder injuries. This should be performed in the operating room prior to arthroscopy. The steps in arthroscopic examination should then include the following:

1. glenohumeral articular surfaces;
2. rotator cuff from inside the joint;
3. labrum including the biceps anchor;
4. anterior capsuloligamentous structures;
5. rotator cuff from the subacromial bursal space;
6. coracoacromial ligament;
7. acromion; and
8. acromioclavicular joint

Applegate GR et al: Chronic labral tears: Value of magnetic resonance arthrography in evaluating the glenoid labrum and labral-bicipital complex. Arthroscopy 2004;20:959. [PMID: 15525929]

Kaplan LD et al: Internal impingement: Findings on magnetic resonance imaging and arthroscopic evaluation. Arthroscopy 2004;20:701. [PMID: 15346111]

Lee DH et al: The double-density sign: A radiographic finding suggestive of an os acromiale. J Bone Joint Surg Am 2004;86-A:2666. [PMID: 15590851]

Lindauer KR et al: MR imaging appearance of 180–360 degrees labral tears of the shoulder. Skeletal Radiol 2005;34:74. [PMID: 15668822]

Magee T, Williams D, Mani N: Shoulder MR arthrography: Which patient group benefits most? AJR Am J Roentgenol 2004;183:969. [PMID: 15385288]

Middleton WD, Teefey SA, Yamaguchi K: Sonography of the rotator cuff: Analysis of interobserver variability. Am J Roentgenol 2004;183:1465. [PMID: 15505321]

Porcellini G et al: Arthroscopic treatment of calcifying tendinitis of the shoulder: Clinical and ultrasonographic follow-up findings at two to five years. J Shoulder Elbow Surg 2004;13:503. [PMID: 15383805]

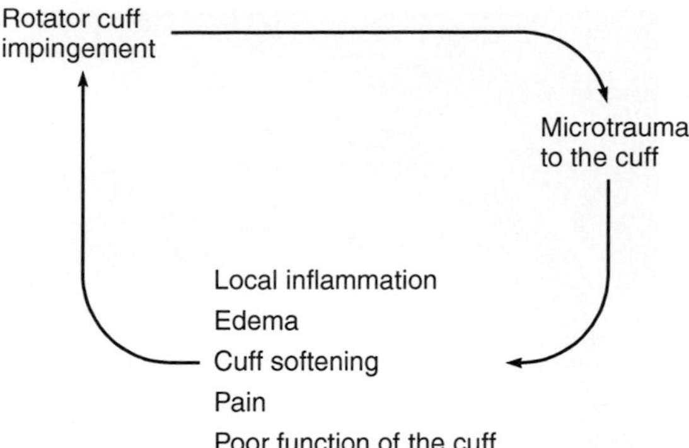

Figure 4–24. The cycle of injury and reinjury resulting from rotator cuff impingement.

SHOULDER TENDON & MUSCLE INJURY

Rotator Cuff Tendon Injuries

Injury to the rotator cuff, a common cause of shoulder pain and disability, has a high prevalence during athletic activities. Injury of the rotator cuff may result in pain, weakness, and decreased range of motion. Symptoms are often worsened by activity, especially when the hand is positioned overhead. Night pain is also common, and many complain of awakening after rolling onto the affected shoulder. Although shoulder weakness and decreased range of motion usually result from a rotator cuff tendon tear, pain alone from subacromial bursitis or rotator cuff tendonitis may also be the cause. Each of these entities most often results from impingement syndrome.

Impingement Syndrome

Any prolonged repetitive overhead activity such as tennis, pitching, golf, or swimming may cause compromise of the space between the humeral head and the coracoacromial arch that includes the acromion, coracoacromial ligament, and the coracoid process. Impingement causes microtrauma to the rotator cuff, resulting in local inflammation, edema, cuff softening, pain, and poor function. These problems may even cause greater impingement, producing a continuous vicious cycle (Figure 4–24). This cycle may be precipitated by acute injury to the rotator cuff tendon itself. Blood supply to this tendon is precarious, thus decreasing its capacity for healing.

1. Subacromial Bursitis

Clinical Findings

Bursitis of the shoulder refers to the inflammation of the subacromial bursa. It has the mildest signs and symptoms of shoulder impingement. Pain is present with overhead activity, and there is usually no or mild pain with the arm at the side.

Active range of shoulder motion is limited by pain. No atrophy of the shoulder muscles is present, and manual muscle testing demonstrates mild weakness. Passively, when the internally rotated shoulder is moved into forward flexion, the patient experiences discomfort. This is called the Neer impingement sign (Figure 4–25). Injection of 10 mL of lidocaine into the subacromial space resolves the pain, and there is a dramatic increase in strength and range of motion with the Neer impingement test.

Radiographic views of the subacromial space, such as the supraspinatus outlet view, may show a spur on the undersurface of the acromion, causing narrowing of the subacromial space. Advances in imaging methods, such as ultrasonography and MRI, now aid in diagnosis of subacromial bursitis, rotator cuff tendonitis, and rotator cuff tendon tear (Figure 4–26).

Treatment & Prognosis

Treatment for impingement syndrome starts with conservative measures such as activity modification, physical therapy, and oral antiinflammatory medications. Activity modification is necessary to minimize overhead arm motion and effect a return to normal overhead throwing biomechanics. Modalities such as heat and cold, iontophoresis or phonophoresis, and microelectric nerve stimulation may also be helpful. Only with normal function of the rotator cuff tendons do glenohumeral mechanics improve and the impingement syndrome cease. If this treatment fails, a subacromial injection of corticosteroids may be helpful.

Surgical intervention is indicated only after failure of a prolonged conservative treatment program (a minimum of 3 months). If the subacromial space is narrow,

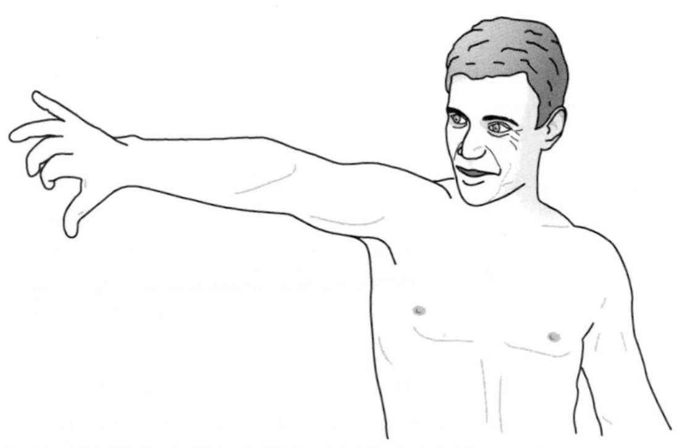

Figure 4–25. Evaluating for impingement of the supraspinatus tendon with the "empty can" test.

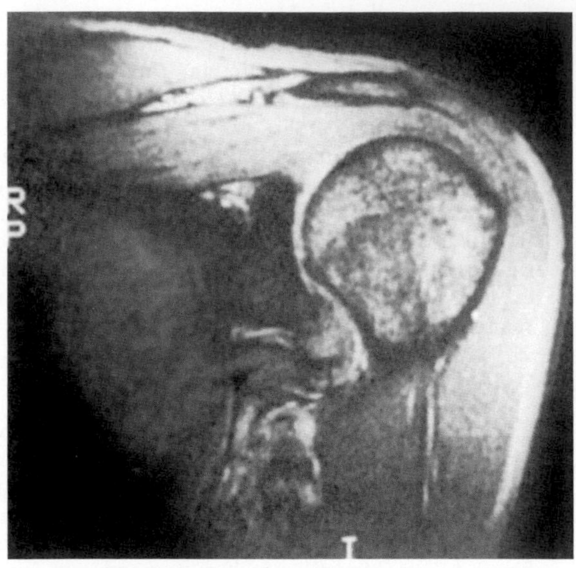
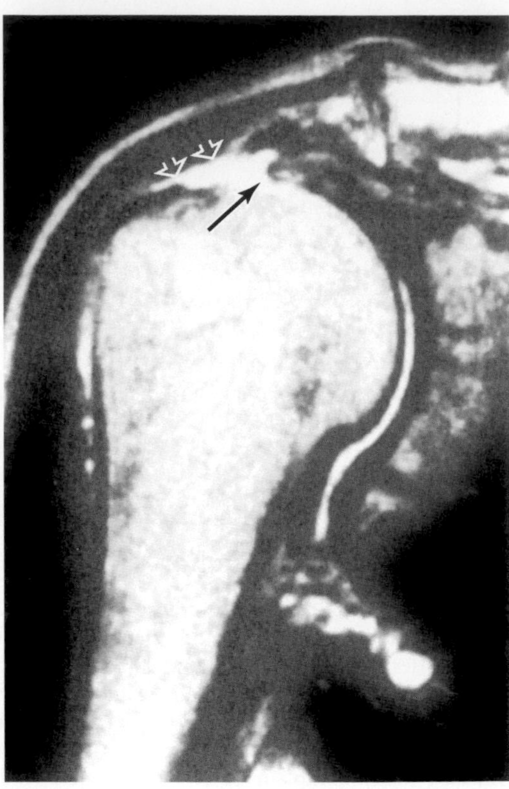

A B

Figure 4–26. MRI demonstrating (**A**) normal shoulder anatomy and (**B**) cystic changes at the greater tuberosity with rotator cuff tear (*arrow*).

release of the coracoacromial ligament combined with shaving the undersurface of the acromion (known as acromioplasty or subacromial decompression) may result in relief of symptoms. This can be done with an arthroscopic technique to decrease postoperative discomfort and minimize the complication of deltoid muscle injuries.

Never has there been more controversy about this surgical procedure. It has been used since the 1930s to diminish symptoms associated with rotator cuff injury. The classic rationale for its efficacy is that any prolonged repetitive overhead activity, such as tennis, pitching, golf, or swimming, may cause compromise of the space between the humeral head and the coracoacromial arch, which includes the acromion, coracoacromial ligament, and the coracoid process. Known as impingement syndrome, microtrauma to the rotator cuff results in local inflammation, edema, cuff softening, pain, and poor function. These problems may even cause greater impingement, producing a continuous vicious cycle. This cycle may also be precipitated by acute injury to the rotator cuff tendon itself. Blood supply to this tendon is precarious, thus decreasing its capacity for healing. Removing subacromial spurs as well as increasing the size of the subacromial space may release pressure on the cuff tendons, ending the vicious cycle and allowing for healing.

Other rationales are proposed for the efficacy of subacromial decompression in treating rotator cuff injuries. The subacromial space, including the subacromial bursa and the subacromial periosteum, is richly innervated, primarily by branches of the suprascapular nerve. Subacromial decompression results in denervation of the subacromial space. Others have found increased inflammatory factors in the subacromial bursa of shoulders with rotator cuff injury that may normalize after subacromial decompression.

Rotator cuff pathology is associated with the shape and geometry of the acromion, especially if there is acromial encroachment onto the supraspinatus tendon. Bigliani and Morrison introduced a commonly used classification to describe the shape of the acromion in 1986. They found a higher incidence of rotator cuff tears in hooked (type III) acromions than in flat (type I) and curved (type

II) acromions. However, several studies show poor to moderate interobserver reliability of this classification, regardless if the clinicians used radiographs, MRI, or cadaveric scapulas to classify the acromions. Routine use of subacromial decompression in the treatment of rotator cuff tears is now questioned. A newer prospective, randomized study of rotator cuff repair found no statistical difference in outcome whether or not a subacromial decompression was done. To confuse matters even more, a study of nearly a hundred patients followed for nearly a decade found subacromial decompression may not prevent progression of impingement syndrome to a tear.

2. Rotator Cuff Tendonitis

Clinical Findings

Of the four rotator cuff muscles, the supraspinatus tendon is most often initially involved. Rotator cuff tendonitis also results from impingement syndrome and is characterized by pain with overhead activity. The patient may occasionally be awakened by pain at night. Active shoulder range of motion is limited by pain. Typically, no atrophy of the shoulder muscles is present and manual muscle testing demonstrates mild weakness. The Neer impingement sign is positive and the pain resolves with subacromial injection of lidocaine.

Treatment & Prognosis

Radiographic evaluation and treatment are similar to subacromial bursitis management. An exception is the athlete less than 40 years old with glenohumeral instability and secondary tendonitis. In this case, the instability should be treated first and the rotator cuff tendonitis then resolves.

3. Rotator Cuff Tendon Tear

Clinical Findings

A rotator cuff tendon tear is characterized by pain with overhead activity. However, the patient is often also awakened at night with pain. The athlete with a chronic rotator cuff tear may describe a gradual loss of strength. Pain may be persistent, occurring even with the arm at the side.

Active range of shoulder motion is limited, and if the tear is severe, there will be atrophy of the shoulder muscles. Manual muscle testing demonstrates weakness. The Neer impingement sign is positive, and the pain resolves with subacromial injection of lidocaine.

Treatment & Prognosis

Radiographic evaluation and treatment are similar to subacromial bursitis management. Unlike acute tears, chronic rotator cuff tears often present insidiously, with slow progression from subacromial bursitis to rotator cuff tendonitis and eventual tendon tear. Differentiating severe rotator cuff tendonitis from partial or small full-thickness chronic rotator cuff tears may be a difficult task.

Tears are most common at the humeral insertion site of the supraspinatus tendon, where stress is greatest with the joint in abduction. Tears may be partial thickness or involve the full thickness of the tendon. The size may be small (less than 1 cm), medium (1–3 cm), large (3–5 cm), or massive (more than 5 cm). Chronic rotator cuff tears may result partly from degeneration within the rotator cuff tendon. Poor vascularity and repetitive activity, especially in the athlete with a restricted subacromial space, may be contributing factors. A minor traumatic event may also cause a full-thickness tear in an athlete with mild or moderate tendon degeneration.

If the tear is small, a prolonged period of rest, lasting 4–9 months, may relieve symptoms. Range-of-motion exercises are also recommended, unless they cause significant discomfort. If this fails to control the symptoms, surgical repair of the tear is recommended. The thin degenerated tissue of a chronic rotator cuff tear makes surgical repair more difficult than repair of an acute tear. Surgical decompression of the subacromial space to remove spurs should also be considered.

Rehabilitation lasts from 6 months to a year with gradual exercise progression needed to restore normal, or near-normal function, and strength. This varies with the tear size repaired and type of surgery performed. Typically, immediately after the procedure, passive motion and isometric strengthening exercises start, along with elbow, hand, and grip strengthening exercises. At 6 weeks, the athlete may be able to begin low-intensity active strengthening exercises against gravity. The goals are to bring the athlete to normal strength with a functional, pain-free range of motion.

Although the lesion location and size are helpful in describing the rotator cuff tear, symptoms do not correlate with these factors alone. Both epidemiologic and imaging studies indicate a high incidence of partial-thickness rotator cuff tears at younger ages and a high incidence of full-thickness rotator cuff tears at older ages. Small full-thickness rotator cuff tears may be asymptomatic as long as the force couple of the anterior and posterior rotator cuff is preserved. Instead, a number of other factors influence the severity of symptoms, including acute/chronic nature of injury, patient age, activity level, humeral head superior migration, shoulder muscle strength, arthritis, pain tolerance, and workers' compensation status.

Partial-Thickness Rotator Cuff Tear

A partial articular sided tendon avulsion is much more common than a bursal side tear of the rotator cuff. As with other rotator cuff injuries, symptoms may resolve with appropriate physical therapy and analgesics. Yet some individuals with a partial-thickness tear have persistent or recurrent symptoms. If a conservative program of exercises and gradual return to activity does not lead to steady improvement, then further diagnostic evaluation with ultrasonography, MRI, or arthroscopy may be helpful. Arthroscopic debridement of the abnormal cuff may promote healing in athletes with partial-thickness posttraumatic tears. Following debridement, immediate resumption of range-of-motion and muscle-strengthening exercises begins. Typically, it requires 6–12 months for a throwing athlete to return to athletics following arthroscopic debridement of a partial-thickness rotator cuff tear.

Gartsman GM, O'Connor DP: Arthroscopic rotator cuff repair with and without arthroscopic subacromial decompression: A prospective, randomized study of one-year outcomes. J Shoulder Elbow Surg 2004;13:424. [PMID: 15220883]

Hyvonen P, Lohi S, Jalovaara P: Open acromioplasty does not prevent the progression of an impingement syndrome to a tear. Nine-year follow-up of 96 cases. J Bone Joint Surg Br 1998;80:813. [PMID: 9768891] See comment as well in J Bone Joint Surg Br 1999;82:743.

Klepps S et al: Prospective evaluation of the effect of rotator cuff integrity on the outcome of open rotator cuff repairs. Am J Sports Med 2004;32:1716. [PMID: 15494338]

Lam F, Mok D: Open repair of massive rotator cuff tears in patients aged sixty-five years or over: is it worthwhile? J Shoulder Elbow Surg 2004;13:517. [PMID: 15383807]

Millstein ES, Snyder SJ: Arthroscopic evaluation and management of rotator cuff tears. Orthop Clin North Am 2003;34:507. [PMID: 14984190]

O'Holleran JD et al: Determinants of patient satisfaction with outcome after rotator cuff surgery. J Bone Joint Surg Am 2005;87-A:121. [PMID: 15634822]

Rebuzzi E et al: Arthroscopic rotator cuff repair in patients older than 60 years. Arthroscopy 2005;21:48. [PMID: 15650666]

Romeo AA et al: Shoulder scoring scales for the evaluation of rotator cuff repair. Clin Orthop 2004;(427):107. [PMID: 15552145]

Sperling JW, Cofield RH, Schleck C: Rotator cuff repair in patients fifty years of age and younger. J Bone Joint Surg Am 2004;86-A:2212. [PMID: 15466730]

BICEPS TENDON INJURIES

1. Bicipital Tendinitis

Clinical Findings

The long head of the biceps muscle is an intraarticular structure deep in the rotator cuff tendon as it passes under the acromion to its insertion at the top of the glenoid. The same mechanism that initiates impingement syndrome symptoms in rotator cuff injuries may inflame the tendon of the biceps in its subacromial position, causing bicipital tendinitis. Tendinitis may also result from subluxation of the tendon out of its groove in the proximal humerus, which occurs with rupture of the transverse ligament. The symptoms of bicipital tendinitis, whether the result of impingement or tendon subluxation, are essentially the same. Pain is localized to the proximal humerus and shoulder joint, with resisted supination of the forearm aggravating the pain. Pain may also occur on manual testing of the elbow flexors and on palpation of the tendon itself. The Yergason test is used to test for instability of the long head of the biceps in its groove.

Treatment & Prognosis

If the tendinitis is associated with shoulder impingement, therapy aimed at treating the impingement syndrome relieves the bicipital tendinitis. If subluxation of the tendon within its groove is the cause of the irritation, conservative therapy includes NSAIDs and restriction of activities, followed by a slow resumption of activities after a period of rest. Strengthening of the muscles that assist the biceps in elbow flexion and forearm supination is also beneficial. Steroid injections into the sheath of the biceps tendon are helpful, but they may be hazardous if placed into the substance of the tendon because they promote tendon degeneration. Persistent symptoms may warrant tenodesis of the biceps tendon directly into the humerus. Recovery from this procedure is difficult, and it is doubtful if a competitive athlete could return to peak performance after such a procedure.

2. Biceps Tendon Rupture

Clinical Findings

The long head of the biceps tendon may rupture proximally, either from the supraglenoid tubercle of the scapula at the entrance of the bicipital groove proximally or at the exit of the tunnel at the musculotendinous junction. The muscle mass moves distally, producing a bulging appearance to the arm. Rupture of the long head of the biceps is predictive of a rotator cuff tear. Rupture of the biceps distally at its insertion involves both heads, and the muscle mass moves proximally. The mechanism is usually a forceful flexion of the arm and is more common in older athletes (greater than 50 years old) or with direct trauma. Microtears probably serve to render the tendon vulnerable to an acute tearing event. The degree of ecchymosis depends on the location of the tear, with avascular areas having less and the musculotendinous junction producing quite a noticeable amount of ecchymosis. Diagnosis is usually easily obvious because the deformity is evident.

Treatment & Prognosis

Surgical treatment of proximal ruptures, if indicated, is usually reserved for patients less than 40 years old. Open surgical repair leaves a long scar and usually does not completely restore the underlying anatomy. The coiled-up distal end of the tendon is usually found beneath the attachment of the pectoralis major. A correlation exists between proximal biceps tendon rupture and rotator cuff tears in middle-age and older athletes (more than 50 years old). Rupture of the distal biceps tendon often warrants surgical repair because of loss of forearm flexion and supination strength. In this case, the tendon is usually found approximately 5–6 cm above the elbow joint, and care must be taken to avoid damage to the lateral antebrachial cutaneous nerve.

Cope MR, Ali A, Bayliss NC: Biceps rupture in body builders: Three case reports of rupture of the long head of the biceps at the tendon-labrum junction. J Shoulder Elbow Surg 2004; 13:580. [PMID: 15383821]

Vidal AF, Drakos MC, Allen AA: Biceps tendon and triceps tendon injuries. Clin Sports Med 2004;23:707. [PMID: 15474231]

PECTORALIS MAJOR RUPTURE

Rupture of the pectoralis major tendon is an uncommon injury, usually occurring during bench press exercises in weight lifting caused by sudden unexpected muscle contraction during pulling or lifting. The athlete usually experiences sudden pain and develops local ecchymosis and swelling. As the swelling subsides, a sulcus and deformity may be visible, and the patient notices weakness of the arm in adduction and internal rotation. The rupture may be partial or complete, and nonoperative treatment usually results in satisfactory function for the activities of daily life. Surgery may be considered if the athlete wishes to return to heavy weight lifting.

Aarimaa V et al: Rupture of the pectoralis major muscle. Am J Sports Med 2004;32:1256. [PMID: 15262651]

GLENOHUMERAL JOINT INSTABILITY

To make the correct diagnosis, the glenohumeral joint must be tested for anterior, posterior, and inferior instability. Different classifications of glenohumeral joint instability are proposed, based on etiology, the direction of the instability, or on various combinations. TUBS is an acronym describing instability caused by a *t*raumatic event, which is *u*nidirectional, associated with a *B*ankart lesion, and often requires *s*urgical treatment. AMBRI refers to *a*traumatic, *m*ultidirectional instability that may be *b*ilateral and is best treated by *r*ehabilitation. In this classification, the etiology of multidirectional instability is thought to be enlargement of the capsule from genetic or microtraumatic origin.

The positive sulcus sign is used as the diagnostic hallmark for multidirectional instability, but we now know that the sulcus sign is sometimes found in asymptomatic shoulders of individuals with increased laxity. Laxity or joint play is a trait of body constitution that differs from one individual to another. Individuals may be loose or tight jointed. A shoulder is hyperlax if the examiner can easily subluxate the humeral head out of the glenoid in the anterior, posterior, and inferior directions without eliciting symptoms. Unfortunately, this makes classification of instability based on etiology, or direction alone, extremely difficult. Instead, classification is best based on the direction of instability that elicits symptoms and the presence or absence of hyperlaxity (Table 4–4).

Gerber C, Nyffeler RW: Classification of glenohumeral instability. Clin Orthop 2002;400:65. [PMID: 12072747]

Glenohumeral Joint Instability Evaluation

A. Anterior Instability

The apprehension test is performed to assess anterior instability. The test applies an anterior directed force to the humeral head from the back with the arm in abduction and external rotation (Figure 4–27). A positive test results from the patient's apprehension that the joint will dislocate. This maneuver mimics the position of subluxation, or dislocation, and causes reflex guarding. Conversely, the relocation test is positive if relief is obtained by applying a posterior directed force to the humeral head (Figure 4–28).

B. Posterior Instability

No single test has high sensitivity and specificity for posterior instability. The posterior apprehension test is performed by applying a posterior directed force to the forward flexed and internally rotated shoulder. To per-

Table 4–4. Classification of glenohumeral instability based on the direction of instability and the presence or absence of hyperlaxity.

Laxity \ Direction	UDI (Unidirectional Instability)	MDI (Multidirectional Instability)
Normal laxity	Very common 60%	Very rare 3%
Increased laxity	Common 30%	Rare 7%

Adapted, with permission, from Gerber C: Observations of the classification of instability. In Warner JJP et al eds: *Complex and Revision Problems in Shoulder Surgery*. Lippincott-Raven, 1997:9–18.

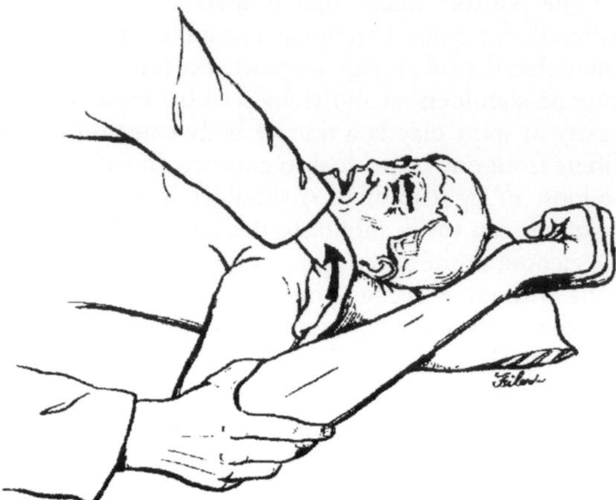

Figure 4–27. The apprehension test for anterior instability.

form the circumduction test, the patient is instructed to move the shoulder actively in a large circle starting from a flexed, internally rotated and cross-body position, then to forward flexion, then to an abducted and externally rotated position, and lastly to the arm at the side. The examiner stands behind the patient and palpates the posterior shoulder. If positive, the joint subluxes in the flexed, internally rotated, and cross-body position, and it reduces as the shoulder is moved. For the Jahnke test, a posteriorly directed force is applied to the forward flexed shoulder. The shoulder is then moved into the coronal plane as an anterior directed force is applied to the humeral head. A clunk occurs as the humeral head reduces from the subluxed position (Figure 4–29).

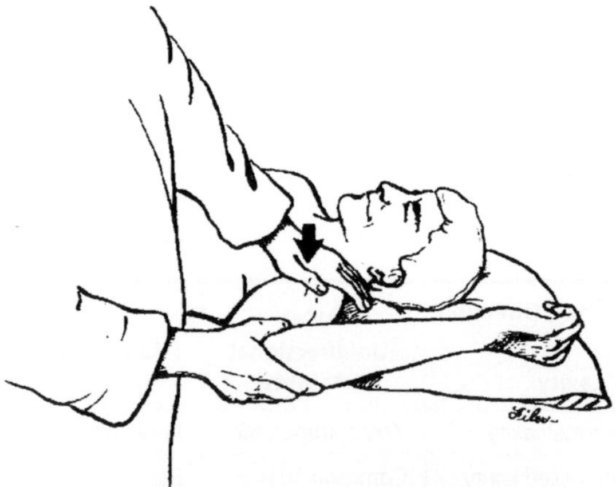

Figure 4–28. The relocation test is positive if relief is obtained by applying a posterior directed force to the humeral head.

C. Inferior Instability

The sulcus sign is used to evaluate laxity and inferior instability. The test is performed with the athlete in a sitting position with the arm at the side. A distraction force is applied longitudinally along the humerus. If positive, discomfort or apprehension of instability are experienced as the skin just distal to the lateral acromion hollows out (Figure 4–30).

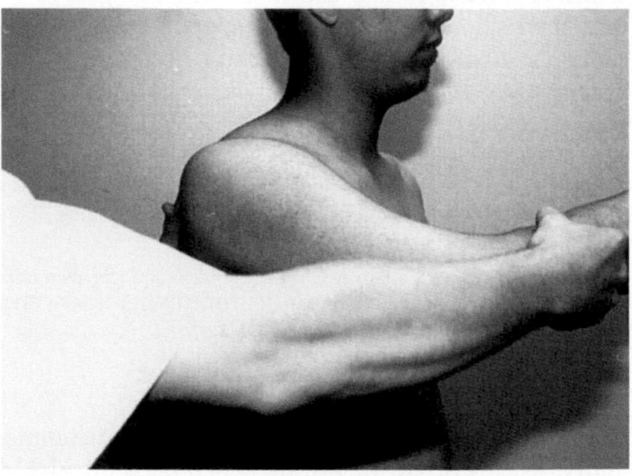

A

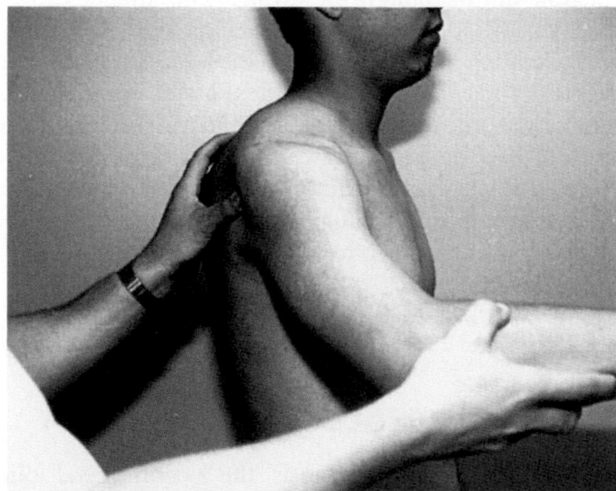

B

Figure 4–29. **The Jahnke test for posterior instability. A: A posterior directed force applied to the forward flexed shoulder (in the upper left column). B: The shoulder is then moved into the coronal plane as an anterior directed force is applied to the humeral head (in the lower left column). A clunk occurs as the humeral head reduces from the subluxed position.** (Reprinted, with permission, from Hawkins RJ, Bokor DJ: Clinical evaluation of shoulder problems. In Rockwood CA et al (eds): *The Shoulder.* WB Saunders, 1998, p. 186.)

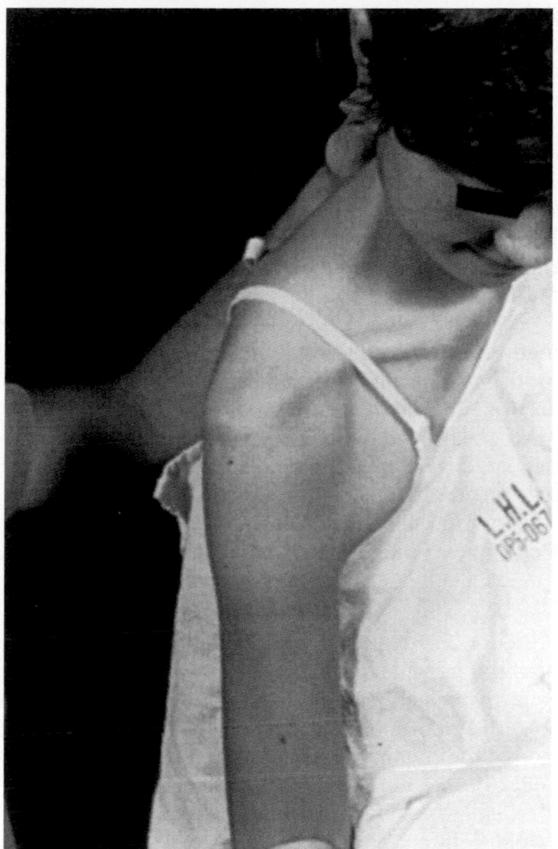

Figure 4–30. The sulcus test for inferior instability. (Reprinted, with permission, from Hawkins RJ, Bokor DJ: Clinical evaluation of shoulder problems. In Rockwood CA et al (eds): *The Shoulder.* WB Saunders, 1998, p. 189.)

1. Glenohumeral Dislocation

When the shoulder is forced beyond the limit of its normal range of motion, the articular surface of the humeral head may displace from the glenoid to varying degrees. The majority of glenohumeral dislocations, or subluxations, are in the anteroinferior direction.

Anterior Dislocation

A. Clinical Findings

Anterior glenohumeral dislocation occurs from either an external rotation or abduction force on the humerus, a direct posterior blow to the proximal humerus, or a posterolateral blow on the shoulder large enough to displace the humeral head. The anterior capsule is either stretched or torn within its attachment to the anterior glenoid. The head may be displaced into a subcoracoid, subglenoid, subclavicular, or intrathoracic position. Two major lesions are typically seen in patients with recurrent anterior dislocations (Figure 4–31). First is the Bankart lesion, an anterior capsular injury associated with a tear of the glenoid labrum off the anterior glenoid rim. The Bankart lesion may occur with fractures of the glenoid rim. Such fractures are often minimally displaced, and treatment is usually dictated by the joint instability. The second major lesion associated with recurrent anterior dislocations is the Hill-Sachs lesion, a compression fracture of the posterolateral articular surface of the humeral head. It is created by the sharp edge of the anterior glenoid as the humeral head dislocates over it. When large, both the Bankart and the Hill-Sachs lesions predispose to recurrent dislocations when the arm is placed in abduction and external rotation. If the glenoid rim fracture involves greater than 20% of the glenoid diameter, the joint becomes prone to instability and treatment with open reduction and internal fixation is indicated. If the fracture is old or the glenoid rim is worn to a similar level, corticocancellous bone grafting of the glenoid rim is indicated.

Other injuries associated with anterior dislocation may occur. These include avulsion of the greater tuberosity from the humerus, caused by traction from the rotator cuff, and injury to the axillary nerve, which may be stretched or torn. Permanent loss of axillary nerve function results in denervation of the deltoid muscle and loss of sensation over the proximal lateral aspect of the arm. Axillary nerve palsy may also occur during

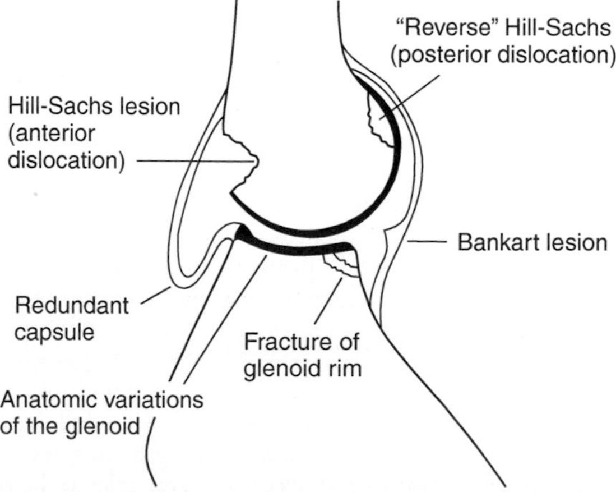

Figure 4–31. Anatomic lesions producing shoulder instability.

reduction of the dislocation, and therefore it should be tested both before and after reduction. The deltoid extension lag sign, described later in the section on axillary nerve injuries, may be the best way to assess function of this nerve. Lastly, the dead arm syndrome may occur after anterior joint instability. For example, a pitcher may report sudden inability to throw, with the arm going numb and becoming extremely weak after the ball release. The symptoms are transient, resolving within a few seconds to minutes.

Athletes who sustain a shoulder dislocation try to hold the injured extremity at the side, gripping the forearm with the opposite hand. Most athletes know their shoulder is dislocated, and they seek help immediately. On physical examination of an anterior dislocation, the examiner notes a space underneath the acromion where the humeral head should lie and a palpable anterior mass representing the humeral head in the anterior axilla.

B. Treatment and Prognosis

One must distinguish between acute and recurrent anterior glenohumeral dislocations because an acute dislocation sustains severe trauma with the increased probability of associated injuries. The recurrent dislocation may occur with minimal trauma, and reduction may be accomplished with much less effort. Anterior dislocations may be reduced by one of several techniques. Longitudinal traction may be exerted on the affected arm with external rotation, followed by internal rotation of the arm. Care must be taken to avoid direct pressure on the neurovascular structures. Another method is to have the patient lie face down on the table and tie or tape a bucket to the injured arm and slowly fill it with water. This allows the musculature around the shoulder to relax from the force of the weight and effects the spontaneous reduction.

Following reduction of an initial dislocation, the shoulder should be immobilized in internal rotation for 2–6 weeks. Healing generally takes at least 6 weeks. Before returning to athletics, the patient should have normal range of motion without pain, and normal strength in the shoulder. Emphasis must be placed on strengthening the rotator cuff muscles to compensate for the laxity of the ligamentous support. When weight training is begun, military press, fly exercises, a narrow grip while bench pressing, and deep shoulder dips must be excluded until considerable time elapses and complete healing is realized.

Recurrent dislocations should be treated with minimal immobilization until the pain subsides, followed by range-of-motion and muscle-strengthening exercises. Many restraining devices are available to help prevent recurrent dislocations during sporting activities, focusing on keeping the arm from going into abduction and external rotation. These orthotics may be effective, but because they limit the athlete's range of shoulder motion, their use is limited for certain competitive activities.

If an athlete has sustained multiple dislocations and is unresponsive to conservative treatment, surgical reconstruction of the shoulder joint may be indicated. There are a wide variety of procedures to correct the instability, with most involving repair of the labral defect and tightening of the anterior capsule and ligamentous structures through an anterior incision (Table 4–5).

For most surgical procedures, aggressive range-of-motion exercises do not start until at least 3 weeks postoperatively. The goal is to have full abduction and 90 degrees of external rotation. By 12 weeks, patients are often progressing well into their initial programs and may begin a variety of weight training exercises, avoiding exercises that strain the anterior capsule.

Posterior Dislocation

A. Clinical Findings

Posterior glenohumeral dislocations result from the posterior capsule being torn, stretched, or disrupted from the posterior glenoid. A reverse Hill-Sachs lesion (Figure 4–31) may appear on the anterior articular surface of the humerus. With a posterior dislocation, the

Table 4–5. Repair of capsule and labrum back to the glenoid rim.

Bankart procedure
duToit procedure
Viek procedure
Eyre-Brook procedure
Moseley procedure
Muscle and capsule plication
Putti-Platt procedure
Symeonides procedure
Muscle and tendon sling procedures
Magnuson-Stack procedure
Bristow-Helfet-Latarjet procedure modifications
Boytchev procedure
Nicola procedure
Gallie-LeMesurier procedure
Boyd transfer of long head of biceps (for posterior dislocation)
Bone block
Eden-Hybbinette procedure
DeAnquin procedure (through a superior approach to the shoulder)
Osteotomies
Weber (humeral neck)
Saha (humeral shaft)

subscapularis, or its insertion on the lesser tuberosity, may be injured. Posterior dislocations are often difficult to diagnose because the patient may have a normal contour to the shoulder or the deltoid of a well-developed athlete may mask signs of a displaced humeral head. The patient holds the injured shoulder in internal rotation and the examiner cannot rotate it externally. Anteroposterior radiographs can be misleading, and axillary views must be obtained to diagnose a posterior dislocation.

B. Treatment and Prognosis

Applying traction in the line of the adducted humerus, with an anterior directed force to the humeral head, reduces a posterior dislocation. Anesthesia often helps decrease the trauma of reduction. Following reduction, the shoulder is immobilized for 2–6 weeks in external rotation and a small amount of abduction. Surgical treatment should be considered if these measures fail to provide the desired results.

Multidirectional Instability

A. Clinical Findings

Some patients have instability in both the anterior and posterior directions, most often subluxation and not dislocation. This situation may result in a painful shoulder, especially if rotator cuff strength decreases. The pain is often primarily a result of rotator cuff inflammation, likely from attempts to stabilize the humeral head during activity.

B. Treatment and Prognosis

A rotator cuff strengthening program is often successful treatment.

Brophy RH, Marx RG: Osteoarthritis following shoulder instability. Clin Sports Med 2005;24:47. [PMID: 15636776]

Good CR, Macgillivray JD: Traumatic shoulder dislocation in the adolescent athlete: Advances in surgical treatment. Curr Opin Pediatr 2005;17:25. [PMID: 15659959]

Kim SH et al: Loss of chondrolabral containment of the glenohumeral joint in atraumatic posteroinferior multidirectional instability. J Bone Joint Surg Am 2005;87-A:92. [PMID: 15634818]

Kim SH et al: Painful jerk test: A predictor of success in nonoperative treatment of posteroinferior instability of the shoulder. Am J Sports Med 2004;32:1849. [PMID: 15572311]

Kirkley A et al: Prospective randomized clinical trial comparing the effectiveness of immediate arthroscopic stabilization versus immobilization and rehabilitation in first traumatic anterior dislocations of the shoulder: Long-term evaluation. Arthroscopy 2005;21:55. [PMID: 15701612]

Krishnan SG et al: A soft tissue attempt to stabilize the multiply operated glenohumeral joint with multidirectional instability. Clin Orthop 2004;(429):256. [PMID: 15577496]

GLENOID LABRUM INJURY

Clinical Findings

The glenoid labrum is a fibrocartilaginous rim around the glenoid fossa that deepens the socket and provides stability for the humeral head. It also is a connection for the surrounding capsuloligamentous structures. Glenoid labrum tears may occur from repetitive shoulder motion or acute trauma. In the athlete with repeated anterior subluxation of the shoulder, tears of the anteroinferior labrum may occur, leading to progressive instability.

Weight lifters may also develop glenoid labrum tears from repetitive bench pressing and overhead pressing. Weakness in the posterior rotator cuff may aggravate this condition. Tears of the glenoid labrum may also occur from acute trauma such as falling on an outstretched arm, but they are also seen in the leading shoulders of golfers and batters when they ground their clubs or bats.

Patients with glenoid labrum injuries may describe their pain as interrupting smooth functioning of the shoulder during their specific activity. On examination, they may have discomfort on forced external rotation at 90 degrees of abduction, with the pain typically not increasing as the arm goes into further abduction. Frequently, a labrum disruption may be felt as a pop or click on forced external rotation. The patient may also experience discomfort on forced horizontal adduction of the shoulder. Manual muscle testing may show associated weakness in the rotator cuff muscles. Diagnostic tests such as a CT scan and MRI following injection of contrast dye into the shoulder joint may allow early detection of glenoid labrum lesions.

Treatment & Prognosis

Range-of-motion exercises and gradual return to activity are often successful in relieving symptoms. However if nonoperative management fails, arthroscopic intervention may be indicated to debride a torn symptomatic labrum. During arthroscopy, care must be taken not to debride the inferior labrum because this may result in increased anterior shoulder instability, escalating the probability of anterior shoulder dislocation. Immediately following surgery, range-of-motion exercises and strengthening training begin. Usually within 2–3 weeks following surgery, the athlete may begin a throwing program. Baseball pitchers may be ready to throw 3 months postoperatively.

SLAP LESIONS

The use of shoulder arthroscopy in the diagnosis and treatment of shoulder disorders has led to increased awareness of superior labrum anterior posterior (SLAP) lesions. SLAP lesions involve the origin of the long head of the biceps brachii (biceps anchor) and the superior capsulolabral structures. A type I lesion has degeneration or fraying of the labrum without instability. Type II lesions are most common, accounting for more than 50% of patients with a SLAP lesion, and they involve detachment of the superior labrum from the glenoid. A type III lesion has a bucket-handle tear of the superior labrum with firm attachment of the remainder of the labrum. Type IV lesions also remain attached to the labrum, but they have an associated bucket-handle tear of the labrum that extends into the biceps tendon (Figure 4–32).

Types V through VII SLAP lesions were later added to this initial four-part classification. A type V lesion is an anterior-inferior Bankhart lesion that continues superiorly to include separation of the biceps tendon. A type VI lesion includes a biceps separation with an unstable flap tear of the labrum. Finally, a type VII is a superior labrum-biceps tendon separation that extends anteriorly beneath the middle glenohumeral ligament.

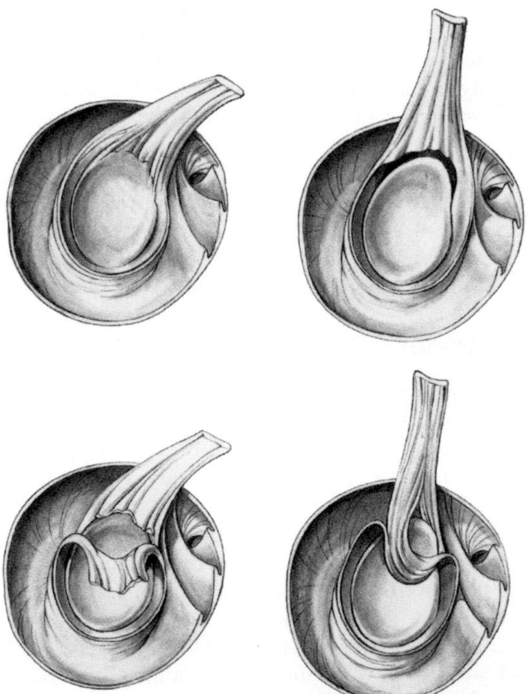

Figure 4–32. The five types of the SLAP lesion include fraying of the superior capsulolabrum (type 1), detachment of the superior capsulolabrum and the biceps anchor (type 2), bucket-handle tearing of the superior capsulolabrum (type 3), detachment of the superior capsulolabrum and tearing into the biceps anchor (type 4), and combinations of these (type 5).

Clinical Findings

Patients present with nonspecific shoulder pain associated with activity. A complicating factor in making the diagnosis is that the majority of SLAP lesions are associated with other shoulder pathology, such as rotator cuff tears, acromioclavicular joint pathology, and instability. Less than 28% of SLAP lesions are isolated.

No single test is both sensitive and specific for diagnosis of SLAP lesions. magnetic resonance arthrography (MRA) can be helpful. However, diagnostic arthroscopy remains the best means to diagnose SLAP lesions definitively. The active compression test may prove to be the most useful single provocative maneuver. The internally rotated shoulder is forward flexed to 90 degrees and then brought across the body in horizontal abduction of approximately 10 degrees. The test is positive if the patient has pain with resisted forward flexion that is relieved by external rotation of the shoulder.

Treatment

Treatment of SLAP lesions can be simplified by noting whether or not the lesion contributes to detachment of either the biceps anchor or the anterosuperior capsulolabrum. Lesions producing meaningful detachment of the anterior capsuloligamentous structures generally require repair of these structures back to the bony glenoid rim. Lesions producing significant defects extending into the biceps tendon may require biceps tenotomy, with or without tenodesis.

Holtby R, Razmjou H: Accuracy of the Speed's and Yergason's tests in detecting biceps pathology and SLAP lesions: comparison with arthroscopic findings. Arthroscopy 2004;20:231. [PMID: 15007311]

Musgrave DS, Rodosky MW: SLAP lesions: Current concepts. Am J Sports Med 2001;30:29. [PMID: 11198828]

Parentis MA, Mohr KJ, El-Attrache NS: Disorders of the superior labrum: Review and treatment guidelines. Clin Orthop 2002;400:77. [PMID: 12072748]

SHOULDER STIFFNESS

Clinical Findings

Often called adhesive capsulitis or frozen shoulder, shoulder stiffness is a painful condition characterized by significant restriction in both active and passive range of motion. The shoulder is characterized as being stiff when the articular surfaces are normal and the joint is stable, yet there is a restriction in range of motion. Stiffness may also result from pathologic connections between the articular surfaces, soft-tissue contracture, bursal adhesions, or a shortened muscle–tendon unit. Often of uncertain etiology, the restrictions of shoulder motion are global. That is, none of the shoulder planes of motion is spared.

Shoulder stiffness may be separated into idiopathic and posttraumatic etiologies. Idiopathic shoulder stiffness is most common in older individuals, especially women between 40 and 60 years of age. Other factors that predispose to idiopathic shoulder stiffness include cervical, cardiac, pulmonary, neoplastic, neurologic, and personality disorders. Patients with diabetes mellitus are also at a high risk of developing shoulder stiffness, with 10–35% of diabetics having restriction of shoulder motion. Diabetics who have been insulin dependent for many years have the greatest incidence and bilateral involvement. The pathophysiology of idiopathic shoulder stiffness remains uncertain, but the pathoanatomy is commonly limited to contracture of the glenohumeral capsule (Figure 4–33). Most prominently involved is the rotator interval that includes the coracohumeral ligament.

Although all patients can recall some traumatic event that preceded their shoulder stiffness, those with distinct trauma such as a prior fracture, rotator cuff tear, or surgical procedure have a posttraumatic etiology. Stiffness after shoulder surgery is typical and usually resolves with time and appropriate rehabilitation. But the shoulder should not be neglected after any surgery about the shoulder girdle. This includes axillary or cervical lymph node dissections, especially when combined with radiation therapy, cardiac catheterization in the axilla, coronary artery bypass grafting with sternotomy, and thoracotomy. All surgeons should be aware that these procedures may result in restricted shoulder motion.

The clinical presentation of idiopathic shoulder stiffness is classically described as having three phases. The first phase is the painful, freezing phase. The pain is typically achy, and sudden jolts or attempts at rapid motion exacerbate the chronic discomfort. The pain may begin at night, and shoulder motion becomes progressively limited. Patients often hold their arm at their side and in internal rotation with the forearm across the belly. They may also be treated for nonspecific shoulder pain with a sling in this position. This inflammatory phase often lasts between 2 and 9 months.

The second phase of progressive stiffness lasts between 3 and 12 months. Stiffness progresses to the point where shoulder motion is restricted in all planes. Essentially, the shoulder has undergone fibrous arthrodesis. Fortunately, pain progressively decreases from the initial inflammatory phase. With time, patients are able to use the shoulder with little or no pain, within the restricted range of motion, but attempts to exceed this range are accompanied by pain. The patient's symptoms then plateau. Unfortunately, this phase may be persistent with symptoms lasting for extended periods. In the resolution, or thawing phase, the shoulder slowly and progressively becomes more supple. It can be as short as a month but typically lasts 1–3 years.

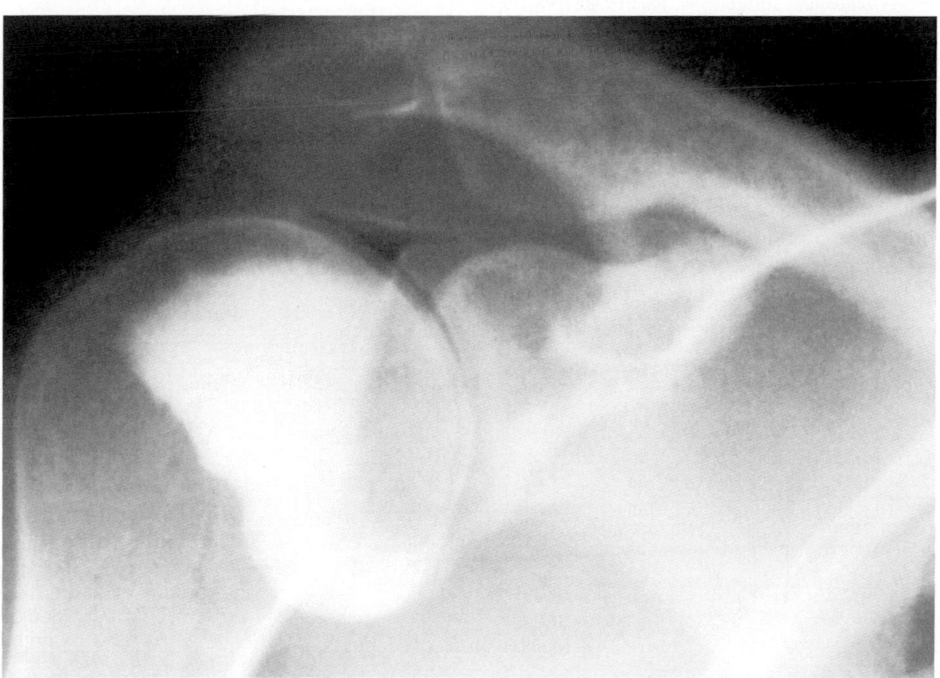

Figure 4–33. Adhesive capsulitis of the shoulder. Note the small irregular joint capsule with addition of contrast material.

On clinical examination, there is loss of both active and passive range of shoulder motion. Often the first motion to be affected is internal rotation demonstrated by an inability to bring the arm up the back to the same level as the normal shoulder. Radiographic confirmation of adhesive capsulitis may be done by arthrography, which demonstrates marked reduction in the capacity of the joint. Often the affected shoulder does not take more than 2–3 mL of dye, although normal capacity is 12 mL.

Treatment & Prognosis

Treatment varies, but conservative modalities and progressive range-of-motion exercises seem effective. Range-of-motion exercises for external rotation and abduction help minimize the length of restriction in motion and dysfunction. Manipulation under anesthesia, long the mainstay of intervention, is being replaced by selective arthroscopic capsular release. Short-term results indicate a quicker return of motion. Whether treated with rehabilitation alone or with capsular release, a return of approximately 80% shoulder range of motion is usual.

Ide J, Takagi K: Early and long-term results of arthroscopic treatment for shoulder stiffness. J Shoulder Elbow Surg 2004; 13: 174. [PMID: 14997095]

Nicholson GP: Arthroscopic capsular release for stiff shoulders: Effect of etiology on outcomes. Arthroscopy 2003;19:40. [PMID: 12522401]

Wolf JM, Green A: Influence of comorbidity on self-assessment instrument scores of patients with idiopathic adhesive capsulitis. J Bone Joint Surg Am 2002;84-A:1167. [PMID: 12107317]

FRACTURES ABOUT THE SHOULDER

CLAVICULAR FRACTURE

The clavicle is one of the most commonly fractured bones in the body, with direct trauma being the usual cause in athletic events (Figure 4–34). Football, wrestling, and ice hockey are the sports most commonly involved in clavicular fractures, which is not surprising because all three are associated with high-speed contact between players.

Clinical Findings

Despite the proximity of vital structures, clavicular fractures that occur during athletic activities are rarely associated with neurovascular damage, and accompanying soft tissue disorders are uncommon. The patient usually gives a history of falling in the area of the shoulder or receiving a blow to the clavicle, experiencing immediate pain and inability to raise the arm. Radiography usually confirms the clinical impression and must show the entire clavicle, including the shoulder girdle, upper third of the humerus, and sternal end of the clavicle. Midclavicular fractures account for 80% of clavicular fractures, with distal fractures at 15% and proximal fractures at 5%. Most fractures of the shaft of the clavicle heal well. The potential for a rare but serious neurovascular complication, such as a tear of the subclavian artery or brachial plexus injury, must be kept in mind when evaluating and treating clavicular fractures, and a neurovascular examination on initial evaluation is very

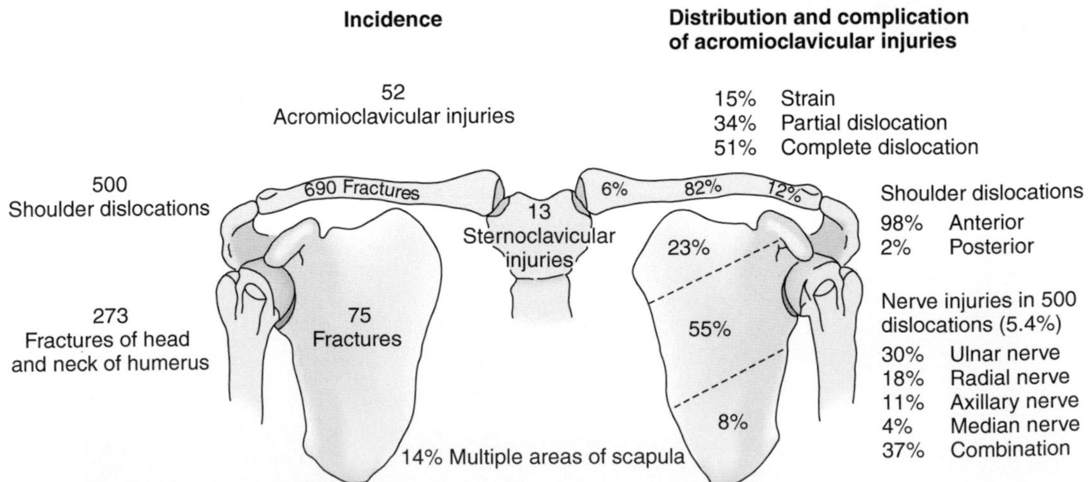

Figure 4–34. Analysis of 1603 shoulder girdle injuries, showing the frequency and location of fractures and dislocations.

important. Pulses in the distal part of the upper extremity, strength, and sensation must be carefully evaluated.

Because the clavicle is the single bone structure that fixes the shoulder girdle to the thorax, a fracture through the clavicle causes the shoulder to sag forward and downward. The pull of the sternocleidomastoid muscle may displace the proximal fragment superiorly. These forces tend to hinder the initial reduction and maintenance of reduction. In addition, distal fractures, which are more common in older age groups (more than 50 years old), may involve tears in the coracoclavicular ligament, which allows the proximal clavicle to ride up superiorly mimicking an acromioclavicular dislocation. Delayed union in this type of fracture is a much greater possibility than with other clavicular fractures.

Treatment & Prognosis

Mid and proximal clavicular fractures are usually treated with a short period of rest, and a sling may be used on the affected side to support the extremity. Immobilization is usually discontinued at 3–4 weeks, and once the clavicular fracture heals, range-of-motion and strengthening exercises should begin. Onset of exercises prior to healing may result in nonunion. Athletes should not be allowed to return to play until achieving their preinjury shoulder strength and range of motion. Generally, no special braces or pads are required when the athlete returns to play.

Grassi FS, Tajana MS, D'Angelo F: Management of midclavicular fractures: Comparison between nonoperative treatment and open intramedullary fixation in 80 patients. J Trauma 2001; 50:1096. [PMID: 11426125]

Robinson CM, Cairns DA: Primary nonoperative treatment of displaced lateral fractures of the clavicle. J Bone Joint Surg Am 2004;86-A:778. [PMID: 15069143]

Robinson CM, Court-Brown CM, McQueen MM et al: Estimating the risk of nonunion following nonoperative treatment of a clavicular fracture. J Bone Joint Surg Am 2004;86-A:1359. [PMID: 15252081]

PROXIMAL HUMERUS FRACTURE

Fractures of the proximal humerus, which represent approximately 4–5% of all fractures, are a relatively uncommon sports injury. They most often present in the early adolescent with open growth plates or in elderly (more than 70 years old) osteoporotic patients. When they do occur in the athlete, they are typically the result of a high-energy impact injury or are secondary to an underlying pathologic bone condition.

Clinical Findings

The proximal humerus consists of four major bony components: the humeral head, the greater tuberosity, the lesser tuberosity and the humeral shaft. Fractures can occur between any or all of these regions, and they are traditionally defined by the location and displacement of the fracture fragments (see Figure 3–15). The patient with a proximal humerus fracture usually is able to report the mechanism of injury and complains of pain, swelling, and inability to use the shoulder. Physical examination often reveals loss of the normal contour of the shoulder, tenderness about the shoulder, ecchymosis that may extend down to the elbow, and crepitus on attempted range of motion. A thorough neurovascular exam is essential because brachial plexus and axillary nerve injuries are reported in association with proximal humerus fractures. Because the axillary nerve is the most commonly injured nerve in these cases, sensation to light touch and pinprick over the lateral aspect of the upper arm and deltoid muscle function must be tested. Accurate radiographic evaluation is necessary to confirm the type and severity of the fracture and is essential in determining the treatment plan. Necessary views include anteroposterior and lateral views in the plane of the scapula as well as an axillary view to rule out an associated glenohumeral dislocation.

Treatment & Prognosis

Most proximal humerus fractures are minimally displaced and can be treated nonoperatively with sling immobilization and early passive range of motion. However, an estimated 20% of these fractures should be treated operatively. Many factors contribute to this decision-making process, including fracture type and degree of displacement, bone quality, activity level, and associated injuries. Surgical options range from closed reduction and percutaneous pinning to open reduction with internal fixation to humeral head replacement.

For minimally displaced fractures, the prognosis is generally good. Loss of motion is the most common complication. It can take 12–18 months to attain the maximal result, so range-of-motion exercises should be continued for an extended period of time.

Fankhauser F et al: A new locking plate for unstable fractures of the proximal humerus. Clin Orthop 2005;430:176.

Iannotti JP, Ramsey ML, Williams GR et al: Nonprosthetic management of proximal humeral fractures. J Bone Joint Surg Am 2003;85:1578. [PMID: 15116630]

Robinson CM, Aderinto J: Posterior shoulder dislocations and fracture-dislocations. J Bone Joint Surg Am 2005;87-A(3):639.

PROXIMAL HUMERAL EPIPHYSEAL FRACTURE

In skeletally immature athletes, epiphyseal fractures of the proximal humerus may occur. The separate growth centers of the articular surface, greater tuberosity, and lesser tuberosity coalesce at approximately 7 years of age, with the remaining growth plates closing at 20–22 years of age. Therefore, fracture separations may occur at any age until the growth plates close. Fortunately, fractures in this area usually do not arrest growth.

Injury can occur to the shoulder of the growing musculoskeletal system from overhead throwing sports. Proximal humerus pain, especially while throwing and associated with widening of the proximal humerus epiphysis, is termed *little league shoulder*. Although widening of the proximal humerus epiphysis can be an adaptive change to throwing, when painful it may represent an overuse fracture.

Dobbs MB et al: Severely displaced proximal humeral epiphyseal fractures. J Pediatr Orthop 2003;23:208. [PMID: 12604953]

Karatosun V et al: Treatment of displaced, proximal, humeral, epiphyseal fractures with a two-prong splint. J Orthop Trauma 2003;17:578. [PMID: 14504580]

ACROMIOCLAVICULAR JOINT INJURY

Clinical Findings

Acromioclavicular dislocations or subluxations, commonly referred to as separations, vary in severity depending on the extent of injury to the stabilizing ligaments and capsule. The typical mechanism of injury is a direct downward blow to the tip of the shoulder. Clinically, pain at the top of the shoulder over the acromioclavicular joint is the predominant symptom, with varying decreases in motion depending on the severity of the injury. The athlete who has sustained this type of injury typically leaves the field holding the arm close to the side.

When checking for instability of the acromioclavicular joint, the examiner should manipulate the midshaft of the clavicle, rather than the acromioclavicular joint, to rule out pain from contusion to the acromioclavicular area. For milder acromioclavicular injuries, the patient should put the hand of the affected arm on the opposite shoulder, and the examiner may then gently apply downward pressure at the patient's affected elbow, noting if this maneuver causes pain at the acromioclavicular joint.

Acromioclavicular joint injuries were initially divided into grades I through III (Figure 4–35). Grade I injuries are typically produced by a mild blow causing a partial tear of the acromioclavicular ligament. When the acromioclavicular ligament is completely torn, but the coracoclavicular ligament remains intact, a grade II injury that involves subluxation or partial displacement results. When the force of injury is severe enough to tear the coracoclavicular and acromioclavicular ligaments in addition to the capsule, a grade III injury occurs.

Three additional injuries were later added to the classification. In grade IV injuries, the clavicle is displaced posteriorly and buttonholed through the fascia of the trapezius muscle. Grade V injuries demonstrate severe inferior displacement of the glenohumeral joint, with the clavicle often 300% superior to the acromion. Lastly, in grade VI injuries, the distal end of the clavicle is locked inferior to the coracoid.

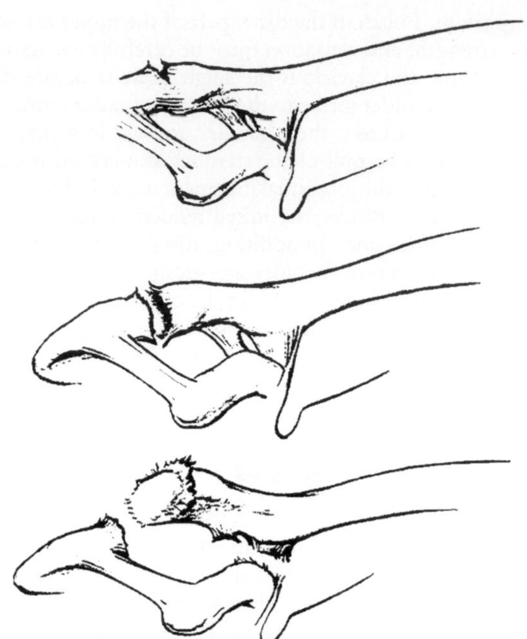

Figure 4–35. Grades of acromioclavicular joint separations.

Acromioclavicular joint displacement is often obvious on physical examination, but it is best classified by radiography. An anteroposterior radiograph that is aimed 10 degrees cephalad allows visualization of the acromioclavicular joint. A radiograph of the entire upper thorax allows the vertical distance between the coracoid and the clavicle on both the involved and uninvolved sides to be compared. Anteroposterior radiographs with weights applied to the upper extremities are usually unnecessary. An axillary lateral radiograph is also essential for proper classification.

Treatment & Prognosis

Management of acromioclavicular joint injuries depends on their severity. Grade I and grade II injuries may be treated with a sling until discomfort dissipates, usually within 2–4 weeks. Next, a rehabilitation program starts, and normal range of motion and strength to the upper extremity begins to be restored. The treatment of grade III injuries or complete dislocations in athletes is controversial. Most feel that grade III injuries are best managed nonoperatively; others advocate operative treatment. Grade IV through VI injuries are best treated with open reduction and internal fixation along with reconstruction of the coracoclavicular ligament.

Nonsurgical treatment may either be a sling for comfort or an acromioclavicular sling to try to achieve reduction. The fit of the device must apply pressure to the distal clavicle sufficient to afford reduction, but not great enough to compromise the skin. Ice and other modalities are used for the acute acromioclavicular injury to reduce soreness and swelling. Pain is the limiting factor in beginning range-of-motion and isometric muscle strengthening exercises. It should be used as a guide for gradual initiation and escalation of these physical therapy regimes. Isotonic exercises may then follow because isometric exercises are more effective earlier when range of motion is limited.

Before resuming athletic activities, the patient must have full range of pain-free motion and no tenderness upon direct palpation of the acromioclavicular joint or pain when manual traction is applied. Athletes who do not require elevation of the arm, such as soccer or football players, tend to return to sports earlier than players who require overhead arm activity, such as tennis, baseball, and swimming athletes.

Fractures of the coracoid process are rare, usually seen in professional riflemen and skeet shooters, although they are also reported in baseball and tennis players. They are identified radiographically, and conservative treatment, including cessation of activity, usually results in uncomplicated healing after 6–8 weeks.

Dumonski M et al: Evaluation and management of acromioclavicular joint injuries. Am J Orthop 2004;33:526. [PMID: 15540856]

Su EP et al: Using suture anchors for coracoclavicular fixation in treatment of complete acromioclavicular separation. Am J Orthop 2004;33:256. [PMID: 15195920]

STERNOCLAVICULAR JOINT INJURY

In the skeletally mature adult athlete, injury to the sternoclavicular joint usually consists of the surrounding soft tissue and capsule tearing, leading to subluxation or dislocation. The mechanism of injury is either a blow to the point of the shoulder, which predisposes to anterior dislocation, or a direct blow to the clavicle or chest with the shoulder in extension, which predisposes to posterior dislocation. The injury may range from a symptomatic sprain to a complete sternoclavicular dislocation with disruption of the capsule and its restraining ligaments.

Anterior Dislocation

The most common type of sternoclavicular dislocation is anterior dislocation, which is recognized clinically by an anterior prominence of the proximal clavicle on the involved side. Radiographic documentation of an anterior sternoclavicular dislocation is difficult because of overlapping of the rib, sternum, and clavicle at the joint, but it may be confirmed by oblique views. A CT scan is usually very sensitive and should be done if radiographic appear normal but the diagnosis is suspected.

Although dislocation of the anterior sternoclavicular joint may cause considerable distress initially, the symptoms usually subside rapidly, with no loss of shoulder function. A variety of surgical and nonsurgical approaches are advocated, but most feel that surgery for anterior dislocations results in significant complications. Closed treatment modalities vary from a sling alone to attempted closed reduction, which may be successful initially but is difficult to maintain.

Posterior Dislocation

Posterior sternoclavicular dislocation is much less common but has more complications because of the potential for injury to the esophagus, great vessels, and trachea. Presenting symptoms range from mild to moderate pain in the sternoclavicular region to hoarseness, dysphagia, severe respiratory distress, and subcutaneous emphysema from tracheal injury.

In most instances, closed reduction of posterior dislocations, if performed early, are successful and stable. To effect reduction, a pillow is placed under the upper back of the supine patient and gentle traction is applied with the shoulder held in 90 degrees of abduction and at maximum extension (Figure 4–36). Rarely, closed reduction under general anesthesia or open reduction is required.

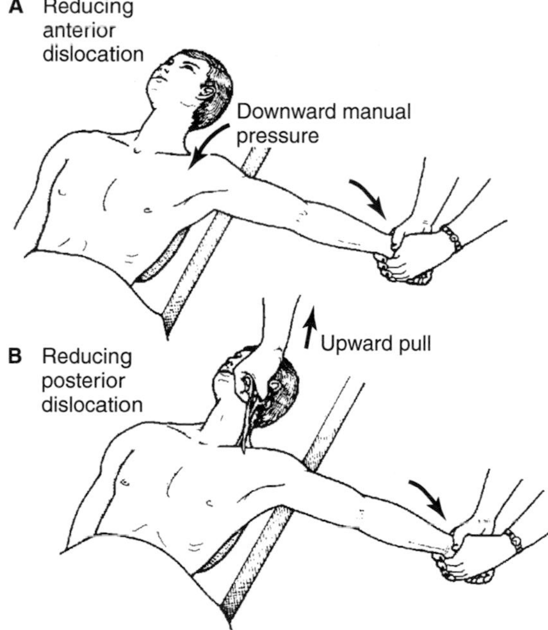

Figure 4–36. Method for reducing (**A**): anterior sternoclavicular dislocation and (**B**): posterior sternoclavicular dislocation.

After reduction, the patient is put in an immobilization splint, instructed to use ice and antiinflammatory agents. Once the joint heals sufficiently, usually within 2–3 weeks, range-of-motion exercises may begin. Elevation of the arm should not be attempted until 3 weeks after injury.

Medial Clavicular Epiphyseal Fracture

In athletes younger than 25 years, sternoclavicular injuries may not result in true dislocations but rather in fractures through the growth plate of the proximal clavicle. These clavicular epiphyseal fractures may appear clinically as dislocations, especially if some displacement is present, and they may be treated conservatively. Typically, these are not associated with growth deformities, and reduction of the fracture is not needed unless there is severe displacement. Symptomatic treatment for pain usually suffices. Sometimes an adolescent presents with an enlarging mass at the sternoclavicular joint and parents are worried about cancer. A careful history reveals trauma several weeks earlier, and the mass represents the callus of a healing clavicular epiphyseal fracture that can be demonstrated radiographically.

Battaglia TC et al: Interposition arthroplasty with bone-tendon allograft: A technique for treatment of the unstable sternoclavicular joint. J Orthop Trauma 2005;19:124. [PMID: 15677929]

SHOULDER NEUROVASCULAR INJURY

Brachial Plexus Injury

Brachial plexus injuries are typically caused by a fall on the shoulder as seen in acromioclavicular joint injuries. Most brachial plexus injuries do not involve motor loss and exhibit paresthesias, which resolve in a period of minutes to weeks, although some cases may persist for months or years. Early in the course of the injury, a transient slowing of conduction across the plexus or a mild prolongation of nerve latency possibly is seen. The "burner" or "stinger" is one of the most common brachial plexus injuries encountered in athletes. The key to diagnosis is short duration of upper extremity paresthesias and shoulder weakness, with pain-free range of motion of the cervical spine. Players may return to competition after shoulder strength and full pain-free range of motion returns.

Rarely, a severe injury occurs (eg, from motorcycle racing). Chronic injuries result in instability of the shoulder that may be treated with trapezius transfer. Arthrodesis is an alternative, initially or after failed muscle transfer.

Peripheral Nerve Injury

A. Long Thoracic Nerve Injury

Traction incidents may cause a long thoracic nerve palsy, with subsequent serratus anterior paralysis and winging of the scapula. Traction and blunt trauma may also cause injury to the spinal accessory nerve, another cause of winging of the scapula. These can be differentiated on physical examination by the position of the scapula. With serratus anterior palsy, the inferior portion of the scapula tends to go medially, whereas the opposite occurs with spinal accessory nerve palsy. Treatment is usually conservative, with return of function in weeks if the nerve is not divided.

Safran MR: Nerve injury about the shoulder in athletes, part 2: Long thoracic nerve, spinal accessory nerve, burners/stingers, thoracic outlet syndrome. Am J Sports Med 2004;32:1063. [PMID: 15150060]

B. Suprascapular Nerve Injury

Entrapment of the suprascapular nerve is often associated with activities such as weight lifting, baseball pitching, volleyball, and backpacking. Traction and repetitive shoulder use are the mechanisms of injury. Compression of the nerve may occur from entrapment at the anterior suprascapular notch of the scapula or at the level of the spinoglenoid notch. The latter occurs in volleyball players and baseball players likely caused by rapid overhead acceleration of the arm. Compression is associated with poorly localized pain and weakness in the posterolateral aspect of the shoulder girdle. This may be followed by atrophy of the supraspinatus or infraspinatus muscles. Eventually, there is weakness of forward flexion and external rotation of the shoulder. The diagnosis is confirmed by electromyography and nerve conduction studies.

Conservative therapy consists of rest, antiinflammatory medication, and physical therapy designed to increase muscular tone and strength. If this is unsuccessful, then surgical exploration is indicated, which may reveal hypertrophy of the transverse scapular ligament, anomalies of the suprascapular notch, and ganglion cysts. Results of surgery vary with the lesion discovered, but many patients return to full function postoperatively.

Safran MR: Nerve injury about the shoulder in athletes, part 1: Suprascapular nerve and axillary nerve. Am J Sports Med 2004; 32:803. [PMID: 15090401]

C. Musculocutaneous Nerve Injury

The musculocutaneous nerve is susceptible to damage from direct frontal blows or surgical procedures. Injury is associated with numbness in the lateral forearm to the base of the thumb and weak to absent biceps muscle function. Most injuries seen in sports are transient and respond to conservative treatment in a matter of days to weeks.

Lo IK, Burkhart SS, Parten PM: Surgery about the coracoid: neurovascular structures at risk. Arthroscopy 2004;20:591. [PMID: 15241309]

D. Axillary Nerve Injury

The usual mechanism of injury is trauma either by direct blow to the posterior aspect of the shoulder or following dislocation of the shoulder or fracture of the proximal humerus. Axillary nerve injury occurs in many sports, such as football, wrestling, gymnastics, mountain climbing, rugby, and baseball. The degree of injury to the nerve varies because the initial presentation may be mild weakness during elevation and abduction of the arm with or without numbness of the lateral arm. The deltoid extension lag sign is indicative of axillary nerve injury. To perform this test, the examiner elevates the arm into a position of near full extension and then releases the arm while asking the patient to hold the arm in this position. If there is complete deltoid paralysis, the arm drops. For partial nerve injuries, the magnitude of the angular drop, or lag, is an indicator of deltoid strength. Approximately 25% of all dislocated shoulder injuries are associated with axillary nerve traction injuries, which respond well to rest, physical therapy, and time. If recovery is not complete within 3–6 months, surgical intervention is recommended with exploration, utilizing neurolysis or grafting, or both, as necessary. Results of surgery are usually favorable, with sensory recovery occurring before motor recovery.

Hertel R et al: The deltoid extension lag sign for diagnosis and grading of axillary nerve palsy. J Shoulder Elbow Surg 1998;7:97. [PMID: 9593085]

THORACIC OUTLET SYNDROME

The symptoms resulting from thoracic outlet compression may be neurologic, venous, or arterial. Obstruction of the subclavian vein may lead to stiffness, edema, and even thrombosis of the limb. Arterial obstruction may be the result of direct compression and manifests with pallor, coolness, and forearm claudication. Doppler examination reveals changes in arterial and venous flow. Electromyography and nerve conduction studies are also helpful in diagnosis.

Nonoperative treatment is recommended for less severe forms of this syndrome, and once the pain subsides, an exercise program to strengthen the pectoral girdle muscles is beneficial. Special exercises to strengthen the upper and lower trapezius, along with the erector spinae and serratus anterior muscles, yields good results. Correcting poor posture and an ongoing maintenance program are mandatory once improvement is reached. Progression of symptoms or failure of nonoperative treatment are indications for surgical exploration and correction of the pathologic factors encountered.

Degeorges R, Reynaud C, Becquemin JP: Thoracic outlet syndrome surgery: Long-term functional results. Ann Vasc Surg 2004;18:558. [PMID: 15534735]

ELBOW INJURIES

EPICONDYLITIS (TENNIS ELBOW)

Tennis elbow is the term given to many painful conditions about the elbow. An anatomic location may usually be found and specific diagnosis made.

Lateral Epicondylitis

Lateral tennis elbow involves the common tendon to the extensor muscles of the wrist and hand. Patients who perform repetitive wrist extension against resistance (such as the backhand stroke in tennis) are at risk. Their pain is usually chronic and more bothersome than disabling. Tenderness is located over the lateral humeral epicondyle, and pain is produced by extending the wrist against resistance. The tendon of the extensor carpi radialis brevis is identified as the most common site of the lesion. Other causes for lateral elbow pain should be considered, including radiocapitellar arthritis and posterior interosseous nerve compression. Radiographs only rarely reveal soft-tissue calcification near the lateral humeral epicondyle, and MRI is of questionable aid in making the diagnosis.

Treatment includes decreasing specific activities and using a tennis elbow band to distribute the tension of the muscular pull over a larger area, thereby decreasing the force per unit area. A lighter racquet, smaller grip on the racquet, and correcting backhand technique are also helpful. Exercises to strengthen the wrist extensor muscles should be included in the treatment plan. If this approach fails, an injection of local anesthetic and cortisone into the most tender region is often curative. Surgical treatment is needed in recalcitrant cases. Multiple procedures are described to take care of this malady. Commonplace in all procedures is release of the common extensor origin. Histologic studies of the afflicted tendon show degenerative changes with angiofibroblastic proliferation. These are thought to be similar to the pathologic changes of the torn rotator cuff, with diminished vascularity, an altered nutritional state, and tearing of the susceptible tendon.

Medial Epicondylitis

Medial epicondylitis involves the common flexor pronator origin. Treatment is similar to the management of lateral tennis elbow. Ulnar nerve compression at the elbow may occur in conjunction with medial tennis elbow. In approximately 60% of the cases treated surgically, ulnar nerve compression was present. The common flexor origin is an important medial stabilizer of the elbow, so if surgical treatment is indicated, the debrided tendon should be reattached rather than released from the medial epicondyle.

Ciccotti MC, Schwartz MA, Ciccotti MG: Diagnosis and treatment of medial epicondylitis of the elbow. Clin Sports Med 2004;23:693 [PMID: 15474230]

Jobe FW, Ciccotti MG: Lateral and medial epicondylitis of the elbow. J Am Acad Orthop Surg 1994;2:1. [PMID: 10708988]

ELBOW INSTABILITY

Rupture of the collateral ligaments of the elbow occurs most commonly from elbow dislocation. This can result from excessive valgus force, and initially the ulnar collateral ligament ruptures. Excessive posterolateral rotatory force may also result in rupture of the lateral ulnar collateral ligament. In either case, the elbow may dislocate, and typically the direction is posterior. Treatment after relocation and brief immobilization consists of active range-of-motion exercises. Recurrent instability is rare, and instead a small loss of elbow extension, usually less than 10 degrees, commonly results.

Valgus Instability

Valgus instability may result from overuse in overhead throwing sports, such as baseball, football, and javelin throwing. With acute medial collateral ligament rupture, a pop may be felt during a throw. Tenderness is present on the medial side of the elbow, usually just distal to the medial epicondyle. Instability can then be appreciated when a valgus force is applied to the elbow. This must be done with the elbow flexed 20 degrees because failure to unlock the olecranon from within the olecranon fossa in full extension creates a false sense of stability. Comparison to the contralateral side aids in making the correct diagnosis. If the ulnar collateral ligament was injured but remains intact, the valgus stress test may elicit pain but no instability. Then the so-called milking maneuver (Figure 4–37) also elicits pain along the medial side of the elbow. Eliciting pain while moving the elbow in flexion and extension with valgus stress during the milking maneuver may be the best test for diagnosing medial collateral ligament injuries in the elbow.

A stress radiograph may aid in making the diagnosis. An anteroposterior radiograph can be taken while the examiner performs the valgus stress test. Alternatively, gravity can be used to apply the valgus stress. For this, an anteroposterior radiograph of the elbow is taken with the shoulder externally rotated at 90 degrees with the elbow flexed at approximately 20 degrees. When instability is present, there will be a wider medial opening than on the contralateral normal side. MRI may also be useful, especially if an arthrogram is performed concurrently, because dye leaking through the ulnar collateral ligament is diagnostic of a rupture.

Surgical repair may be indicated in overhead throwing athletes who suffer an acute rupture of their ulnar collateral ligament and still want to continue to participate in their sport. Soccer players, basketball players, and other athletes participating in nonoverhead throwing may be treated with a program of early active range-of-motion exercises with expectation of full return to their sport. Chronic ulnar collateral ligament injuries resulting from overuse are best treated with rehabilitation, NSAIDs, and avoidance of throwing for as long as 3 months. Only those with residual pain and instability after participation in such a program should undergo reconstruction of the anterior band of the ulnar collateral ligament. In this surgery, pioneered by Dr. Frank

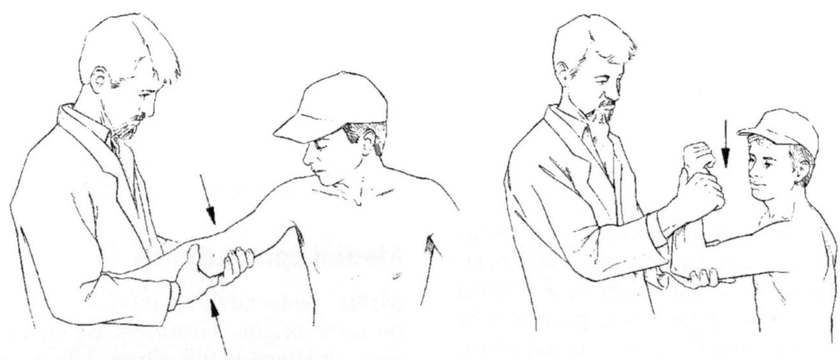

Figure 4–37. **The valgus stress and milking maneuver tests for medial ulnar collateral ligament injury.** (Reprinted, with permission, from Chen FS et al: Medial elbow problems in the overhead-throwing athlete. J Am Acad Orthop Surg 2001;9(2):102.)

Jobe, the palmaris longus tendon is woven through drill holes in the medial humeral epicondyle and olecranon. Nearly 70% of athletes are able to return to highly competitive throwing after such surgery.

Chen FS, Rokito AS, Jobe FW: Medial elbow problems in the overhead-throwing athlete. J Am Acad Orthop Surg 2001; 9(2):99.

O'Driscoll SW, Lawton RL, Smith AM: The "moving valgus stress test" for medial collateral ligament tears of the elbow. Am J Sports Med 2005;33:231. [PMID: 15701609]

Thompson WH et al: Ulnar collateral ligament reconstruction in athletes: Muscle-splitting approach without transposition of the ulnar nerve. J Shoulder Elbow Surg 2001;10:152. [PMID: 11307079]

Posterolateral Rotatory Instability

Posterolateral rotatory instability of the elbow may result from a fall on the outstretched upper extremity, surgery of the lateral side of the elbow, or chronic varus stress as may occur in long-term crutch walkers. The instability covers a spectrum of severity from mild subluxation to recurrent dislocation. Those with mild forms complain of intermittent symptoms on the lateral side of the elbow associated with supination of the forearm, such as pain, snapping, or catching. More severe symptoms include locking or sensations of elbow instability. To perform the posterolateral rotatory instability test, a valgus stress is applied to the supinated elbow with the patient supine and the upper extremity over the head (Figure 4–38). Subluxation of the radial head occurs with the elbow in extension and resolves when the elbow is flexed. This maneuver also reproduces the patient's symptoms. A lateral stress radiograph, done with the elbow in extension as described for the posterolateral rotatory instability test, may also demonstrate the instability (see Figure 4–38). Treatment for acute cases consists of an elbow brace to hold the forearm in pronation and restricted terminal elbow extension for 6 weeks. Chronic cases are best treated with reconstruction of the lateral ulnar collateral ligament. Postoperatively the patient is put in the same brace as used for acute posterolateral rotatory instability for 6–12 weeks.

Olsen BS, Sojbjerg JO: The treatment of recurrent posterolateral instability of the elbow. J Bone Joint Surg Br 2003;85:342 [PMID: 12729105]

Sanchez-Sotelo J, Morrey BF, O'Driscoll SW: Ligamentous repair and reconstruction for posterolateral rotatory instability of the elbow. J Bone Joint Surg Br 2005;87:54. [PMID: 15686238]

OTHER ELBOW OVERUSE INJURIES

Posterior Elbow Impingement

Impingement may result from mechanical abutment of bone and soft tissues in the posterior elbow, which may or may not be associated with injury of the ulnar collateral ligament. Hyperextension injuries with an intact ulnar collateral ligament occur in gymnasts, football linemen, weight lifters, and others. The lesion is usually located in the center of the posterior elbow, and the pain is reproduced by forcible extension of the elbow. If there is insufficiency of the ulnar collateral ligament, as is often the case when there is posterior elbow impingement in overhead athletes, the lesion is posteromedial. In this case, the impingement is between the medial aspect of the olecranon and the lateral side of the medial

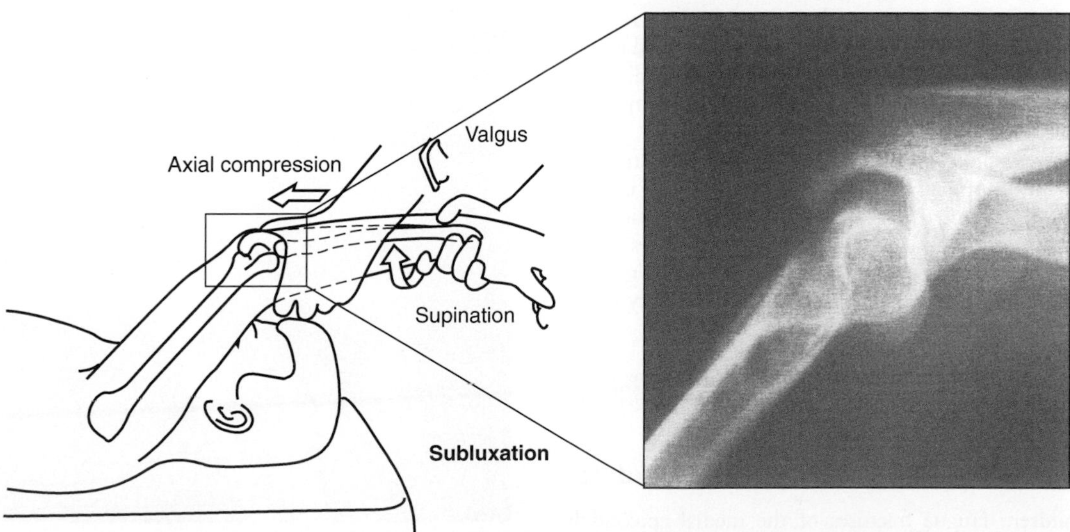

Figure 4–38. The posterolateral rotatory instability test reproduces the patient's symptoms.

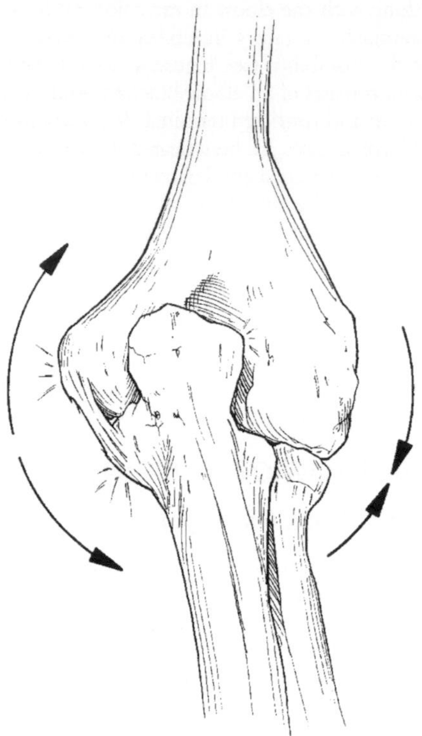

Figure 4–39. Mechanism of posteromedial impingement between the medial aspect of the olecranon and the lateral side of the medial wall of the olecranon fossa. (Reprinted, with permission, from Chen FS et al: Medial elbow problems in the overhead-throwing athlete. J Am Acad Orthop Surg 2001;9(2):105.)

wall of the olecranon fossa (Figure 4–39). Pain may be reproduced with the valgus stress test as described earlier for valgus instability, but the pain is posteromedial and medial. Radiographs may demonstrate osteophytes of the olecranon of the olecranon fossa.

As with most injuries caused by repetitive trauma, treatment begins with prevention. The number of innings pitched is probably the most important factor relating to injury. If symptoms persist, removal of osteophytes is successful treatment, providing no ulnar collateral ligament injury is present. Treatment of the valgus instability is also required for successful outcome.

Moskal MJ, Savoie FH III, Field LD: Arthroscopic treatment of posterior elbow impingement. Instr Course Lect 1999;48:399. [PMID: 10098066]

Fatigue Fracture of the Medial Epicondyle

In children, fatigue fractures of the medial epicondyle cause pain and swelling. This was blamed on throwing curve balls, but some studies show that a properly thrown curve ball causes no more injuries than the traditional fastball. Prevention or minimization of damage involves several steps. First, it is important to maintain proper conditioning by continuing pitching practice in the off-season or beginning the baseball season in a slow progressive fashion. Second, pain and inflammation should be avoided, and if the elbow becomes painful, the athlete should stop throwing immediately. An accurate pitching count should be kept during a game, and a stopping point should be planned in advance. If the pitcher begins having pain or shows loss of control, pitching should be temporarily terminated, and treatment to decrease the swelling and inflammation should begin. No competitive throwing is allowed until full range-of-motion returns and no pain or tenderness is associated with throwing.

Osteochondritis Dissecans of the Capitellum

Osteochondritis dissecans of the capitellum usually affects pitchers older than 10 years (Figure 4–40). Changes in the radiocapitellar joint are very worrisome because of possible permanent loss of function. If fragmentation occurs, loose bodies may require excision.

Stubbs MJ, Field LD, Savoie FH: Osteochondritis dissecans of the elbow. Clin Sports Med 2001;20:1. [PMID: 11227698]

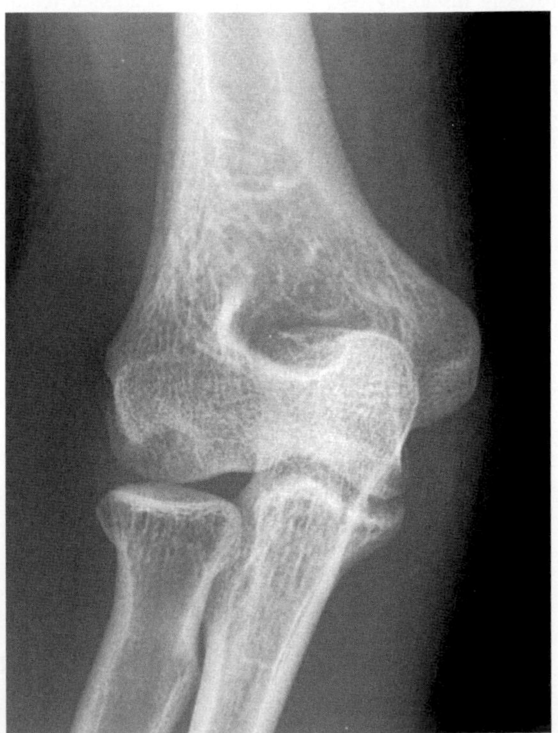

Figure 4–40. AP view of an elbow with osteochondritis dissecans of the capitellum.

SPINE INJURIES

CERVICAL SPINE INJURY

Cervical spine injuries in athletes are relatively infrequent, but the potential for serious injury to the nervous system exists. If spine injury is suspected, it is wise to be extremely cautious until a proper diagnosis can be made. This is the best way to prevent conversion of a repairable injury to a catastrophic outcome. Most often, a spine injury results from a collision, and sometimes it includes associated head injuries. The head and neck must be immobilized right away, and ease of breathing and level of consciousness ascertained immediately.

1. Brachial Plexus Neurapraxia

The most common cervical injury is pinching or stretching neurapraxia of the nerve root and brachial plexus. The injury is of short duration, and the patient has a full pain-free range of motion of the neck. These injuries are commonly called "stinger" or "burner" injuries. They result from lateral impact of the head and neck with simultaneous depression of the shoulder. This may cause stretching and pinching of the nerves of the brachial plexus, with burning pain, numbness, and tingling extending from the shoulder down into the hand and arms. Symptoms frequently involve the C5 and C6 root levels. Recovery is usually spontaneous within a few minutes after the acute episode.

Patients who demonstrate full muscle strength of the intrinsic muscles of the shoulder and upper extremity and have full pain-free range of motion of the cervical spine may return to their activities. If they have residual weakness or numbness, they should not be allowed to re-enter the game. Absence of neck pain should alert one to the possibility of a cervical spine injury, as neck pain is not part of the syndrome.

Persistence of paresthesia or weakness requires further evaluation before returning to play. This includes neurologic, electromyographic, and radiographic evaluation. The athlete should not participate in contact sports until full muscle strength is achieved and a repeat electromyogram shows evidence of axonal regeneration, usually at least 4–6 weeks.

Prevention of so-called stinger injuries is chiefly through correct head and neck techniques and strengthening of the neck musculature. Additionally, the use of cervical rolls may eliminate extremes of motion during impact.

2. Cervical Strain

Acute strains of the muscles of the neck are probably the most frequent cervical injuries in athletes. The word *strain* implies injury to a muscle, whereas a *sprain* is a ligamentous injury. A strain happens when a muscle tendon unit is overloaded or stretched. The clinical picture is common to all musculotendinous injuries. Motion of the neck becomes painful, reaching a peak after several hours or the next day. NSAIDs, heat, massage, and other modalities are beneficial.

3. Cervical Sprain

With cervical sprain, there is damage to the ligamentous and capsular structure connecting the facet joints and vertebra. It is often difficult to differentiate from a strain. There is limited motion and pain in the area of the injury and along the muscle groups overlying the area of the injury. Ligamentous disruption may be extensive enough to result in instability with associated neurologic involvement. Routine cervical spine radiographs are indicated. In those athletes with diminished motion as well as pain, stability of the cervical spine should be documented, which may be done with flexion and extension radiographs.

Treatment of a cervical sprain consists of immobilization, rest, support, and antiinflammatory therapy. Return to participation is permitted when motion and muscle strength normalize.

4. Cervical Spinal Cord Neurapraxia with Transient Tetraplegia

The phenomenon of cervical spinal cord neurapraxia with transient tetraplegia is a distinct clinical entity. Sensory changes include a burning pain, numbness, tingling, or loss of sensation. Motor changes include weakness or complete paralysis, which is usually transient, with complete recovery occurring in 10–15 minutes, although in some cases gradual resolution occurs over 36–48 hours. Complete motor function and full pain-free cervical motion returns. Routine radiographs of the cervical spine are negative for fractures or dislocations. Some radiographic findings include spinal stenosis, congenital fusions, cervical instability, and intervertebral disk disease. To determine whether cervical spinal stenosis is present, the anteroposterior diameter of the spinal canal is measured, and this figure is divided by the anteroposterior diameter of the vertebral body (Figure 4–41). If the ratio is less than 0.80, stenosis is present.

Athletes who have suffered transient tetraplegia are not known to be at any greater risk for permanent tetraplegia. Patients who have this syndrome and associated instability of the cervical spine or cervical disk disease should be precluded from further participation in contact sports. Those who have spinal stenosis alone should be treated on an individual basis.

More severe injuries, including fractures and dislocation of the cervical spine, may occur. Treatment of these

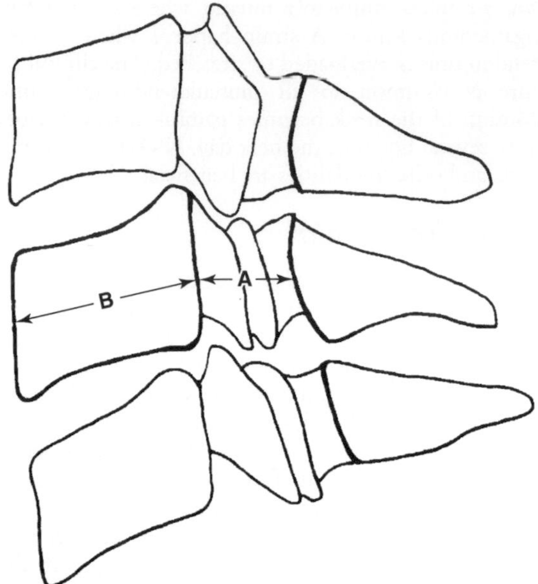

Figure 4–41. The ratio of the spinal canal to the vertebral body is the distance from the midpoint of the posterior aspect of the vertebral body to the nearest point on the corresponding spinolaminar line (**A**) divided by the anteroposterior width of the vertebral body (**B**). (Reproduced, with permission, from Torg JS et al: Neurapraxia of the cervical spinal cord with transient quadriplegia. J Bone Joint Surg Am 1986;68:1354.)

begins on the playing field, with immobilization of the spine. A face mask, if worn, may be cut off with bolt cutters. After thoroughly stabilizing the spine, the patient is moved to a spine board. Sandbags are used to immobilize the head and neck. The patient may then be transported to a local emergency room for further evaluation and treatment. Fractures and dislocations with or without permanent neurologic injury are treated like other spine injuries.

Torg JS et al. Cervical cord neurapraxia: Classification, pathomechanics, morbidity, and management guidelines. J Neurosurg 1997;87:843. [PMID: 9384393]

Torg JS et al: Neurapraxia of the cervical spinal cord with transient quadriplegia. J Bone Joint Surg Am 1986;68:1354. [PMID: 3782207]

LUMBAR SPINE INJURY

Clinical Findings

Spondylolysis is a disruption of the pars interarticularis, whereas spondylolisthesis involves anterior slippage of one vertebral body over the next. Spondylolysis is most often found at L5 and L4 but may occasionally be seen at L3 and L2. It is believed to result from repeated stress around the pars interarticularis during hyperextension of the lumbar spine. If continued hyperextension activity occurs, spondylolysis may become spondylolisthesis. Sports in which spondylolisthesis is commonly found include gymnastics, football, and weight lifting. Female teenage gymnasts, for example, often have back pain but normal early radiographs. Approximately 3–6 weeks later, a stress response may be seen around the pars interarticularis, with increased density developing. At this time, the bone scan is positive, indicating an impending stress fracture that will show up on plain radiographs in 2–4 weeks. A physician who is aware of which sports put stress on the pars interarticularis should consider a bone scan to rule out spondylolisthesis.

Treatment & Prognosis

The treatment of spondylolisthesis involves cessation of all aggravating sports and other actions producing spinal hyperextension. A certain percentage of these fractures heal spontaneously. Healing time for spondylolysis of the lumbar spine is usually approximately 6 months. If after that period of time no significant signs of healing are apparent, it is unlikely that spontaneous healing will take place. At this point, spinal fusion should be considered, or the patient should be willing to confine activities to less stressful pain-free sports.

Many patients with spondylolisthesis engage in high-level sporting activities without significant pain or neurologic deficit. Only a small percentage actually present for evaluation and care. Complete evaluation and treatment recommendations for spondylolisthesis and spondylolysis are found in the section on the spine.

Bono CM: Low-back pain in athletes. J Bone Joint Surg Am 2004;86-A:382. [PMID: 14960688]

Miller SF, Congeni J, Swanson K: Long-term functional and anatomical follow-up of early detected spondylolysis in young athletes. Am J Sports Med 2004;32:928. [PMID: 15150039]

Disorders, Diseases, & Injuries of the Spine

5

Serena S. Hu, MD, Clifford B. Tribus, MD, Bobby K-B Tay, MD, & Nitin N. Bhatia, MD

OSTEOMYELITIS OF THE SPINE

Osteomyelitis of the spine comprises approximately 1% of all cases of pyogenic skeletal infections. Pathogenic organisms can infect the vertebra, the intervertebral disk, or the spinal canal through multiple mechanisms, including local spread from an adjacent infection or as a result of seeding from a noncontiguous source of infection either hematogenously or through the lymphatics. Bacteria can also be introduced directly to compromised tissues as a result of trauma, surgery, diskography, or intravenous or intradural catheterization. Although many organisms are implicated, the most frequently cultured organisms are *Staphylococcus aureus* and *Pseudomonas aeruginosa. Salmonella* should be strongly considered as a potential pathogen in patients with sickle cell disease. Infection with *Mycobacterium tuberculosis* is often seen in less developed countries and in prison populations. Spinal sepsis is most common in adolescents, the elderly (more than 60 years), intravenous drug abusers, patients with diabetes or renal failure, and patients who have undergone spinal surgery. Osteoporosis is also implicated as a predisposing factor secondary to increased blood flow. Eismont and Bohlman reported several risk factors for neurologic deterioration including patients with diabetes, rheumatoid arthritis, steroid use, age greater than 50 years, a cephalad level of infection, and infection with *S. aureus.* For additional information on osteomyelitis, see Chapter 8.

Clinical Findings

A. Symptoms and Signs

Patients with osteomyelitis of the spine may or may not present with symptoms relating to their spine. Pyogenic osteomyelitis is fundamentally different from tubercular osteomyelitis. In the latter, patients generally complain of indolent, chronic back pain. In pyogenic osteomyelitis, the symptoms of acute spontaneous back pain, fever, and weight loss are common but not always present. On physical examination, patients with diskitis or pyogenic osteomyelitis of the spine often exhibit significant percussion tenderness posteriorly over the affected vertebral segments. Paraspinal muscle spasm may be seen in more than 90% of patients. A history of fevers is found in less than 50% of affected patients. Neurologic involvement, fortunately, affects less than 10% of all patients with spinal infections. When the infection involves the cervical spine, patients may develop Horner syndrome, or dysphagia. Pyogenic osteomyelitis should be suspected in any patient who presents with back pain and a recent history of an acute systemic infection (eg, appendicitis, perinephritic abscess, pneumonia, genitourinary tract infection, or meningitis).

B. Laboratory Studies

The results of laboratory tests can be equivocal. The white cell count is elevated in only 42% of patients and often is normal. Both blood and spinal cultures may also be negative. Blood cultures are accurate in only 25% of cases, and closed biopsy techniques are diagnostic in only 70% of cases. The ESR rate is elevated in more than 90% of patients, and the C-reactive protein level (CRP) is also elevated at an earlier point in the infectious process. However, both of these tests are systemic indicators of inflammation and are relatively nonspecific. Thus, there is often a significant delay in diagnosis because many of the signs and symptoms of pyogenic vertebral osteomyelitis are subtle. Clearly, the diagnosis relies on having a high index of suspicion in at-risk patients as well as initiating the appropriate evaluation that will identify the organism and determine the extent of infection.

C. Imaging Studies

Radiographic signs of osteomyelitis typically lag behind symptomatic progression of the disease. MRI with vascular-based contrast enhancement (gadolinium) is the gold standard for early neurodiagnostic imaging. Radiographic findings may appear normal.

In pyogenic osteomyelitis, early radiographic changes may include loss of disk space height, erosion of the vertebral endplates, and vertebral destruction and collapse (Figure 5–1). In advanced cases, the vertebral bodies may become fused because of the inflammation and destruction of the intervertebral disk.

In tubercular osteomyelitis, radiographic studies typically demonstrate anterior vertebral body destruction with sparing of the intervertebral disk. Loss of bone stability in the cervical or thoracic spine may lead to kyphotic deformity and paralysis. Progression to solid fusion may occur but usually later than seen in pyogenic osteomyelitis.

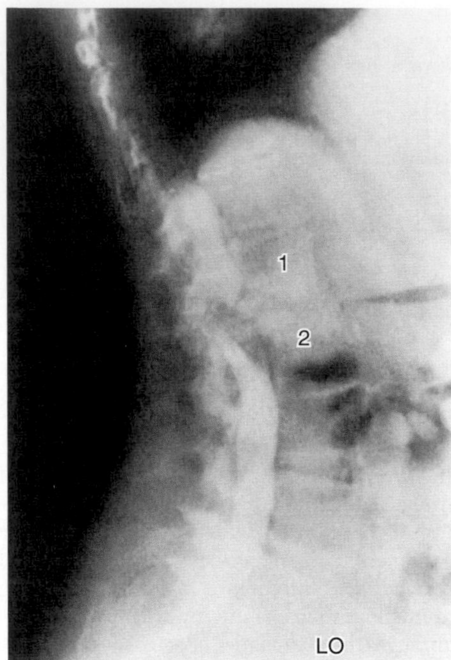

A

B

Figure 5–1. Imaging studies in patients with osteomyelitis of the spine. **A:** Radiograph showing an epidural abscess and advanced collapse between L1 and L2. **B:** CT scan showing destruction of the vertebral body.

Treatment

Early diagnosis and identification of the responsible organism is the cornerstone of treatment. Once the organism is confirmed by biopsy or blood culture, appropriate intravenous antibiotics should be initiated and continued for at least 6 weeks. Short-term bed rest for pain management is appropriate. Spinal column bracing is often necessary for pain relief, immobilization of the affected segments, and minimizing the progression of spinal deformity. Success of nonoperative treatment is linked to patient age younger than 60 years, immunocompetency, infection with *S. aureus,* and a decreasing erythrocyte sedimentation rate (ESR) with appropriate medical treatment. Indications for surgery other than tissue diagnosis include moderate to advanced destruction of the spine with instability, neurologic compromise, sequestrum formation, and failure to respond to intravenous antibiotics. Paraspinal abscesses may be managed conservatively with intravenous antibiotics unless the patient meets one of the surgical criteria just listed.

Pediatric diskitis often responds to spinal column bracing, immobilization, and rest. Although controversial, antibiotic therapy in the pediatric diskitis patient appears to improve nonoperative resolution of symptoms.

The incidence of epidural abscesses may be on the rise, associated with older patients and chronic illness. Epidural abscesses are best treated with early recognition, antibiotic therapy, and immediate surgical decompression. Preoperative paralysis and neurologic deterioration are poor prognostic factors of the disease. MRI is as sensitive as myelography with CT. For diagnostic purposes, MRI offers the advantage of being noninvasive and being able to delineate other disease entities, making it the imaging modality of choice.

For surgical candidates with osteomyelitis or diskitis, the treatment of choice consists of anterior surgical debridement and stabilization with an autogenous structural graft bone graft. Often posterior instrumentation and spinal fusion over the affected segments is necessary to prevent collapse of the anterior graft and to prevent late deformity. Foreign bodies, such as methylmethacrylate, are relatively contraindicated in spinal stabilization, although newer studies suggest that instrumentation can be safely used in an anterior column infection. Antibiotic-impregnated polymethylmethacrylate (PMMA) cement used as a temporary spacer may be useful in grossly contaminated sites. New minimally invasive surgical techniques that use laparoscopy and thoracoscopy appear to be an excellent alternative for operative management of spinal infections. These techniques employ similar surgical principles with expand-

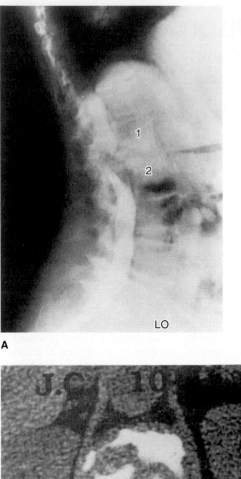

ing surgeon experience, although currently a thorough decompression of the spinal canal is not possible with the minimally invasive technique.

Dimar JR et al: Treatment of pyogenic vertebral osteomyelitis with anterior debridement and fusion followed by delayed posterior spinal fusion. Spine 2004;29:326; discussion 332. [PMID: 14752357]

Eismont FJ et al: Pyogenic and fungal vertebral osteomyelitis with paralysis. J Bone Joint Surg Am 1983;65:19. [PMID: 6849675]

Emery SE, Chan DP, Woodward HR: Treatment of hematogenous pyogenic vertebral osteomyelitis with anterior debridement and primary bone grafting. Spine 1989;14:284. [PMID: 2652335]

Fayazi AH et al: Preliminary results of staged anterior debridement and reconstruction using titanium mesh cages in the treatment of thoracolumbar vertebral osteomyelitis. Spine J 2004;4:388. [PMID: 15246297]

Frazier DD et al: Fungal infections of the spine. Report of eleven patients with long-term follow-up. J Bone Joint Surg Am 2001;83:560. [PMID: 11315785]

Gasbarrini AL, Bertoldi E, Mazzetti M et al: Clinical features, diagnostic and therapeutic approaches to haematogenous vertebral osteomyelitis. Eur Rev Med Pharmacol Sci 2005;9:53. [PMID: 15852519]

Hee HT et al: Better treatment of vertebral osteomyelitis using posterior stabilization and titanium mesh cages. J Spinal Disord Tech 2002;15:149. [PMID: 11927825]

Muckley T et al: The role of thoracoscopic spinal surgery in the management of pyogenic vertebral osteomyelitis. Spine 2004;29:E227. [PMID: 15167673]

Ogden AT, Kaiser MG: Single-stage debridement and instrumentation for pyogenic spinal infections. Neurosurg Focus 2004;17:E5.

Schuster JM et al: Use of structural allografts in spinal osteomyelitis: A review of 47 cases. J Neurosurg 2000;93(1 Suppl):8. [PMID: 10879752]

Tay BK, Deckey J, Hu SS: Spinal infections. J Am Acad Orthop Surg 2002;10:188. [PMID:12041940]

Weinstein MA, Eismont FJ: Infections of the spine in patients with human immunodeficiency virus. J Bone Joint Surg Am 2005; 87:604. [PMID: 15741629]

TUMORS OF THE SPINE

PRIMARY TUMORS OF THE SPINE

Primary tumors of the spine account for 0.04% of all tumors and 10% of all primary tumors of bone. The overwhelming majority of spinal tumors are metastatic. As with tumors elsewhere in the musculoskeletal system, primary lesions in the spine may be osteogenic, chondrogenic, fibrogenic, hematopoietic, neurogenic, or vascular. Generally, benign tumors typically occur in the younger age group (younger than 21 years), whereas up to 70% of malignant tumors are found in patients older than 21 years.

Principles of Diagnosis

A. History and Physical Examination

If the presence of a spinal tumor is suspected, a thorough history and physical examination must be performed. Pain is the common presenting symptom. Persistent pain, especially at night, is the chief complaint in more than 80% of cases. The average time from onset of symptoms until diagnosis in patients with benign lesions is 19 months, whereas that in patients with metastatic disease is 4 months. The age of the patient is important in establishing the differential diagnosis (see Chapter 6). In adults, malignant lesions of bone occur twice as frequently as benign lesions. In children younger than 10 years, however, only 15–20% of tumors are malignant. Location within the spinal column also aids in establishing the diagnosis. Although 75% of tumors located in the vertebral bodies or pedicles are malignant, only 35% of those in the posterior elements are malignant.

On examination, the patient may complain of tenderness over the involved region of the spine. Although rare initially, radiculopathy secondary to nerve root compression may be the only finding. Signs and symptoms may mimic a herniated nucleus pulposus and may progress to localized weakness, sensory loss, and bowel or bladder dysfunction. Up to 70% of patients may develop motor weakness by the time the diagnosis is made. Pathologic fractures may present with acute onset of pain and paraparesis. Examination of the spine may reveal scoliosis, as occurs with osteomas or osteoblastomas, or it may reveal a painful kyphosis.

B. Imaging Studies

The workup begins with high-quality plain radiographs, followed by CT scanning, radioisotope bone scanning, and MRI as necessary. The routine anteroposterior view may reveal the presence of the so-called winking owl sign, which is indicative of early pedicle destruction. As with other bony tumors, the more slowly expanding bony tumors of the spine are well circumscribed with reactive ossification. More aggressive lesions have a moth-eaten or erosive appearance. It is important to realize that radiographic evidence of bony destruction is not apparent until 30–50% of the trabecular bone is lost. Vertebral collapse with preservation of the disk space is a common finding.

Early on it is often difficult on plain radiographs to distinguish a neoplastic process from an infectious one. Technetium bone scans are an accurate and sensitive modality in detecting metastatic disease. False-positive results are acceptably low and usually a result of osteoarthritis. If the osteoblastic response is impaired, as in multiple myeloma or in highly lytic lesions, false-negative results may occur. However, with the advent of MRI, bone scanning is limited in its usefulness in staging of the tumor.

CT scanning with or without myelography is of great benefit in detecting and evaluating osseous lesions and dural impingement. CT scanning also allows an accurate assessment of the extent of bony destruction to help in preoperative planning. Evaluation of soft tissue and marrow has improved immensely with the advent of MRI. Tumor resolution is outstanding (Figure 5–2), and preoperative planning is greatly enhanced.

Arteriography enables the surgeon to evaluate the vascular supply to the tumor and the extent of vascular neogenesis. Highly vascular tumors, such as metastatic renal cell tumors, thyroid carcinoma, hemangiosarcoma, and aneurysmal bone cysts, are well visualized. Partial or complete embolization of highly vascular tumors may make operative resection significantly easier and safer. In addition, identification of feeder vessels in tumors in the lower thoracic spine may help identify possible vascular supply to the tumor from the artery of Adamkewitz. Inappropriate ligation of this major vessel may result in spinal cord ischemia and paralysis.

MRI is the study of choice in the diagnosis and evaluation of primary neoplasms of the spine. Its advantages include superior soft-tissue visualization, the availability of multiplanar images, and the ability to evaluate the extent of neural compression or infiltration.

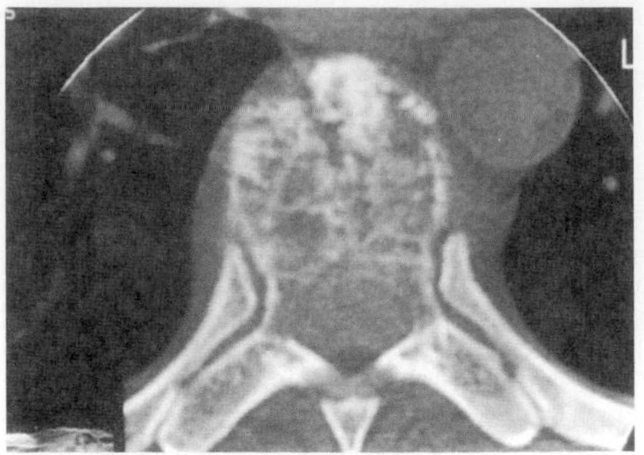

A

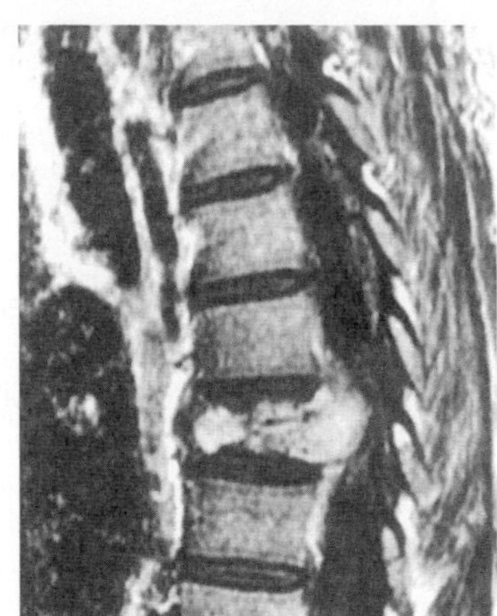

B

Figure 5–2. Imaging studies in a patient with a hemangioendothelioma. **A:** CT scan showing the tumor invading the spinal canal. **B:** MRI of the thoracic spine, demonstrating tumor extension.

C. Biopsy

An open or closed percutaneous biopsy may be necessary for establishing the diagnosis. If the workup is consistent with a benign symptomatic tumor such as an osteoid osteoma, an excisional biopsy may be appropriate. When malignancy is suspected, needle biopsy should be performed prior to resection. Because the accuracy rate for needle biopsy is 75% or less, several specimens should be obtained. Open biopsy is necessary if aspiration is nondiagnostic.

D. Surgical Treatment

The surgical treatment of spinal tumors depends on (1) biologic tumor type, (2) location within spine, (3) percentage of vertebral involvement, (4) neurologic involvement, (5) potential for spine failure and instability, and (6) anticipated life expectancy of the patient.

Bauer HC: Controversies in the surgical management of skeletal metastases. J Bone Joint Surg Br 2005;87:608.

Bilsky MH et al: Operative management of metastatic and malignant primary subaxial cervical tumors. J Neurosurg Spine 2005;2:256. [PMID: 15796349]

Degen JW et al: CyberKnife stereotactic radiosurgical treatment of spinal tumors for pain control and quality of life. J Neurosurg Spine 2005;2:540. [PMID: 15945428]

Fisher CG et al: The surgical management of primary tumors of the spine: Initial results of an ongoing prospective cohort study. Spine 2005;30:1899. [PMID: 16103863]

Flemming DJ et al: Primary tumors of the spine. Semin Musculoskelet Radiol 2000;4:299. Review. [PMID: 11371321]

Saad RS et al: Fine needle aspiration biopsy of vertebral lesions. Acta Cytol 2004;48:39. [PMID: 14969179]

Vialle R et al: Chondroblastoma of the lumbar spine. Report of two cases and review of the literature. J Neurosurg Spine 2005; 2:596. [PMID: 15945435]

Weinstein JN, McLain RF: Primary tumors of the spine. Spine 1987;12:843. [PMID: 3441830]

1. Benign Tumors

Benign primary tumors of the spine include osteoid osteoma, osteoblastoma, osteochondroma, aneurysmal bone cyst, hemangioma, eosinophilic granuloma, and giant cell tumor. For additional discussion of these tumors, see Chapter 6.

Osteoid Osteoma

Osteoid osteoma and osteoblastoma are osteoblastic lesions that are differentiated from each other by size. Lesions smaller than 2 cm are arbitrarily called osteoid osteomas, whereas tumors larger than 2 cm are called osteoblastomas. Osteoid osteoma affects males more frequently than females and is generally seen in patients between 10 and 20 years of age. This benign tumor is usually located in the posterior elements and most frequently involves the lumbar spine, followed by the cervical and then the thoracic spine.

The patient presents with a complaint of a progressive localized ache that may or may not have a radicular component but is usually relieved by the use of salicylates. Tenderness, muscle spasm, neurologic abnormalities, and even scoliosis may be present on examination. Torticollis may be associated with scoliosis of the cervical spine. Pelvic tilt may be seen in conjunction with lumbar spine scoliosis. Minimal correctability is seen with side bending. In the majority of cases, the tumor is located on the concave side of the curve.

Osteoid osteomas appear radiographically as a nidus surrounded by densely sclerotic bone. Tumors that grow close to the periosteum may cause a fusiform thickening of the overlying cortex secondary to hyperemia. Both the nidus and periosteal reaction can sometimes be seen on plain radiographs but are most easily delineated on the axial cuts of a CT scan. Although spontaneous resolution is reported in some cases, treatment of osteoid osteoma generally requires thorough local excision of the lesion because recurrence is likely. Spinal fusion is usually not indicated at the time of excision. In most cases, any scoliosis present preoperatively improves over the following 6–12 months. If the scoliosis is severe (more than 40 degrees) or the spine was rendered unstable by resection of the articular facets and pedicle, fusion should be considered.

Osteoblastoma

When osteoid osteomas grow larger than 2 cm, they are called osteoblastomas. Benign osteoblastomas account for fewer than 1% of all bone tumors. Although cases are rare, more than 40% of them involve the spine, and half of these spinal cases are associated with scoliosis. Osteoblastomas are more common in males than females and seen most frequently in patients younger than 30 years.

Patients generally complain of localized pain or scoliosis. Fifty-three percent of spinal osteoblastomas are found in the lumbar spine, and the rest are equally distributed in the thoracic and cervical spine.

Radiographic examination may reveal an expanded sclerotic cortex, although there are no classic characteristics. Rarely is the lesion lobulated. The posterior elements and pedicles are more frequently involved than the vertebral body. Vertebral involvement almost always occurs because of secondary expansion from the pedicle, and there may be an associated soft-tissue mass.

Curettage can offer a high rate of disease remission when the lesions are well contained within the vertebral bone. Wide excision of the lesion is always curative and may also provide reliable pain relief and resolution of the spinal deformity. However, marginal excision is safer, provides an excellent cure rate, and is the treatment of choice for these tumors. Even partial excision may offer symptom resolution if the nidus is removed. This can be aided by the use of adjuvant radiotherapy. The local recurrence rate can be up to 10% for some osteoblastomas, but malignant degeneration is a rare occurrence.

Osteochondroma

Osteochondromas result when metaplastic cartilage cells in the periosteum undergo progressive endochondral ossification. Multiple osteochondromatosis is the most common of all skeletal dysplasias, and approximately 7% of these patients have vertebral involvement. Spinal cord compression may occur and is the main indication for excision, which is almost always curative.

Aneurysmal Bone Cyst

Aneurysmal bone cysts result from an expansile hyperemic osteolytic process that erodes through bone. Approximately 80% of patients are younger than 20 years. An estimated 12–30% of these neoplasms occur in the spine, especially the lumbar areas. The tumor involves the posterior elements 60% of the time. Symptoms and signs include a rapid evolution of pain in the spine and radiculopathy. Radiographs reveal the presence of an osteolytic tumor with poor demarcation, peripheral ballooning, and cortical erosion with osseous septa within its substance. Like the chordoma but unlike most other tumors, the aneurysmal bone cyst may cross the intervertebral space. Scoliosis or kyphosis may be present.

The differential diagnosis includes giant cell tumors and cavernous hemangioma. Giant cell tumors usually occur in an older patient population and tend to involve the sacrum. A cavernous hemangioma is usually located in the vertebral body.

Appropriate treatment of aneurysmal bone cysts requires recognition that it may arise from or coexist with a preexisting neoplasm. For the isolated lesion, the treatment of choice is aggressive debulking. If the size and location of the tumor preclude complete surgical removal, incomplete curettage can be undertaken and usually eradicates the lesion. Bone grafting is often necessary. Spinal instrumentation, fusion, or both may be necessary, depending on the extent of the lesion.

Profound hemorrhage is a risk with primary surgical resection and may be controlled with preoperative embolization. Although aneurysmal bone cysts are sensitive to radiation, complications of irradiation-induced myelopathy and sarcoma are noted.

Hemangioma

Hemangiomas, common tumors of the vertebral column, arise from embryonic angioblastic tissue. They comprise approximately 7% of all benign tumors. They are much more common in females than in males and have a predilection for the lower thoracic and upper lumbar spine.

Hemangiomas are frequently asymptomatic. In some cases, they are found serendipitously on screening radiographs. In other cases, they are associated with a compression fracture, with the patient presenting with pain and neurologic symptoms. Radiographically, they present with classic vertebral striations resulting from the abnormally thickened bony trabeculae. CT scans easily delineate the lesion, and MRI shows high signal intensity on T_2-weighted images and low signal intensity on T_1-weighted images. If the patient presents with pain without neurologic deficit, low-dose irradiation is extremely effective in ameliorating the symptoms. If the patient shows signs of neurologic dysfunction, treatment should consist of anterior decompression, mass excision, and anterior fusion. Preoperative embolization of the feeding artery may facilitate surgical management.

Eosinophilic Granuloma (Langerhans Cell Histiocytosis)

Eosinophilic granuloma is a proliferative disorder of the Langerhans cells that is commonly seen in children younger than 10 years and rarely in adults. The disease has a male preponderance. Vertebral involvement is seen in 7–15% of cases and typically presents with a sudden onset of neck pain and torticollis.

Patients frequently present with localized pain. Spinal cord compression is a rare but reported event.

Eosinophilic granuloma can present with a spectrum of radiographic manifestations depending on the stage of the tumor. Early on, the tumor presents as a central lytic lesion with poorly defined margins. On plain radiographs, there is permeative bony destruction with a marked periosteal reaction. At this stage, the tumor is difficult to distinguish from a high-grade sarcoma such as Ewing sarcoma. Later in the evolution of the tumor, there is vertebral body collapse leading to a flattening of the vertebral bone between the adjacent intact disks. This phenomenon results in the classic "coin-on-end" appearance and "vertebra plana."

The differential diagnosis includes Ewing sarcoma and infection, and biopsy may be necessary to confirm the diagnosis.

Eosinophilic granuloma usually resolves spontaneously. If the patient suffers from disseminated Langerhans cell histiocytosis, chemotherapy may be appropriate. Local infiltration with corticosteroids is of some benefit. Low-dose irradiation (500–1000 rads) is used in cases associated with neurologic compromise. The use of anterior decompression and anterior fusion is the treatment of choice in patients with neurologic symptoms.

Giant Cell Tumor

Giant cell tumors comprise approximately 10% of all primary bone tumors. These tumors occur in people between 20 and 40 years of age with a slight female predominance (70.8%). Spinal involvement is seen in patients in the third and fourth decades of life. This tumor is locally aggressive and presents most commonly in the anterior vertebral structures. The presenting complaint is typically pain; however, as many as 50% of patients may present with neurologic deficits. Plain radiographs show a lytic lesion with matrix calcification and sclerosis. Aggressive surgical curettage or en bloc excision depending on the location and extent of tumor yield the best results. Because of the risk of sarcomatous transformation, radiation therapy should be reserved for patients with incomplete excision or local recurrence. There is a higher recurrence rate in those patients with soft-tissue extension, anterior and posterior tumor, and spinal canal involvement.

Bertram C, Madert J, Eggers C: Eosinophilic granuloma of the cervical spine. Spine 2002;27:1408. Review. [PMID: 12131737]

Brown CW et al: Treatment and outcome of vertebral Langerhans cell histiocytosis at the Children's Hospital of Eastern Ontario. Can J Surg 2005;48:230. [PMID: 16013628]

Fidler MW: Surgical treatment of giant cell tumours of the thoracic and lumbar spine: Report of nine patients. Eur Spine J 2001;10:69. [PMID: 11276839]

Garg S, Mehta S, Dormans JP: Modern surgical treatment of primary aneurysmal bone cyst of the spine in children and adolescents. J Pediatr Orthop 2005;25:387. [PMID: 15832161]

Kak VK et al: Solitary osteochondroma of the spine causing spinal cord compression. Clin Neurol Neurosurg 1985;87:135. [PMID: 4028590]

Ozaki T et al: Osteoid osteoma and osteoblastoma of the spine: experiences with 22 patients. Clin Orthop 2002;397:394. [PMID: 11953633]

Papagelopoulos PJ et al: Treatment of aneurysmal bone cysts of the pelvis and sacrum. J Bone Joint Surg Am 2001;83:1674. [PMID: 11701790]

Zileli M et al: Osteoid osteomas and osteoblastomas of the spine. Neurosurg Focus 2003;15:E5. Review. [PMID: 15323462]

2. Malignant Tumors

Primary malignant tumors of the spine are rare and carry a poor prognosis. Multiple myeloma is the most common. Osteosarcoma, Ewing sarcoma, chondrosarcoma, and chordoma occur much less frequently. For additional discussion of these tumors, see Chapter 6.

Solitary Plasmacytoma & Multiple Myeloma

Multiple myeloma and solitary plasmacytoma are B-cell lymphoproliferative diseases composed of abnormal aggregates of plasma cells. The neoplasm has a peak occurrence between 50 and 60 years of age with an equal sex distribution. Multiple myeloma is a multifocal plasma cell cancer of the osseous system whose neoplastic cells produce complete or incomplete immunoglobulins. The annual incidence of myeloma is approximately 2–3 per 100,000 among the general population. Genetic analysis of the tumor cells demonstrates abnormalities in band q32 of chromosome 14. The diagnosis is made on serum and urine evaluation for abnormal immunoglobulin levels. Serum protein electrophoresis shows increases in the levels of one of the immunoglobulin classes. The M-component is IgG in 55% of cases, IgA in 25% of cases, and rarely IgE, IgD, or IgM. Urine protein electrophoresis may detect the presence of immunoglobulin light chains called Bence Jones proteins in up to 99% of patients. In 60% of patients afflicted with multiple myeloma, both Bence Jones proteins and abnormal serum immunoglobulin levels are detected.

The initial treatment of myeloma consists of chemotherapy and irradiation. Chemotherapy is an effective means of controlling the advancement of the disease process but may increase the risk of secondary leukemia. The commonly employed agents include melphalan and prednisone. Newer agents such as gallium nitrate may attenuate the rate of skeletal bone loss from the disease and from steroid treatment. Radiation to affected osseous sites may reduce pain and prevent vertebral collapse, deformity, and neural compression. Patients with solitary plasmacytoma have a 5-year survival rate of 60%. In contrast, patients with multiple myeloma have only an 18% 5-year survival rate and a median survival of 24 months.

Osteosarcoma

Primary osteosarcoma is a malignant tumor of mesenchymal cells characterized by the direct formation of osteoid or bone by the tumor cells. It is the second most common primary neoplasm of bone behind myeloma. Most appear in persons younger than 20 years of age before epiphyseal closure. There is a slight male preponderance. In a series of patients with osteosarcoma, Barwick noted that 1–2% arose initially in the spine.

Patients with retinoblastoma (caused by a hereditary mutation in the q14 band of chromosome 13 that codes for a tumor suppressor gene) have a 500-fold greater risk of developing osteosarcoma. The overall consensus is that these tumors have a multifactorial origin involving genetic, constitutional, and environmental influences.

Radiographically, osteosarcomas present as mixed lytic and sclerotic lesions that cause cortical destruction and soft-tissue calcification. In advanced stages, vertebral collapse occurs from replacement of the structural elements of the spine with tumor. Traditional therapy involved limited tumor resection and radiotherapy. A more aggressive approach, as described by Sundaresan and Weinstein, with wide resection, combination chemotherapy, and local radiotherapy demonstrated promising early results. Secondary spinal osteosarcoma caused by malignant transformation of pagetoid or previously irradiated bone is extremely aggressive and associated with early metastasis. A 5-year survival rate of 17% is reported in cases involving pagetoid bone, and the prognosis is even poorer in cases involving irradiated bone.

Ewing Sarcoma

Ewing sarcoma is a malignant round cell tumor with a peak incidence in the second decade of life. The sarcoma was first described in 1921 by James Ewing, who called it an "endothelial myeloma." The neoplasm occurs twice as often in men as in women. Spinal involvement is seen in 3.5% of all Ewing sarcomas, and a large proportion of these arise in the sacrum.

Metastatic involvement of the spine is more common in the late stage of the disease. The vertebral body involvement seen on radiographs in patients with Ewing sarcoma can mimic the vertebra plana seen in patients with eosinophilic granuloma.

When the lesion is localized to the sacrum, the prognosis is worse because these particular lesions tend to be more aggressive and less responsive to chemotherapy and irradiation.

Chondrosarcoma

Chondrosarcoma is the third most common primary bone tumor behind myeloma and osteosarcoma. Although chondrosarcoma rarely affects the spine, it does so more often than osteosarcoma or Ewing sarcoma. The peak incidence of chondrosarcoma is in the fourth to sixth decade, with males affected four times more often than females. An estimated 6–10% of all chondrosarcomas arise in the spine.

Pain in the area of involvement is the first symptom. Fifty percent of patients have a palpable mass before being diagnosed. Approximately 4.5% have some form of neurologic deficit, varying from sensory deficits to frank paraplegia.

Radiographs show typical cortical destruction and paraspinal soft tissue calcification. MRI helps delineate the extent of soft-tissue and bony involvement.

Chondrosarcomas are radio resistant. Thus, the mainstay of treatment is wide excision. Survival is closely related to obtaining a clear surgical margin at the time of surgical excision. In the Mayo clinic series, 15 of 20 (75%) of the patients with chondrosarcoma died of local progression. Their 5-year survival rate was 21–55%, with a median survival of 6 years. High-dose irradiation therapy may have limited benefit for inoperable lesions.

Chordoma

A chordoma is a slow-growing tumor that arises from notochordal cells in the vertebral body. Physaliphorous cells, containing abundant vacuoles filled with glycogen and oxidative enzymes, are the distinctive cells of this neoplasm. Molecular analysis shows that chordoma cells express galectin-3, a carbohydrate binding protein that plays a role in cell differentiation, morphogenesis, and cancer biology. The neoplasm usually occurs in the fifth and sixth decades of life and afflicts men twice as often as women. Chordomas are found in the sacrum and coccyx in 55% of cases, in the basilar skull in 30%, and in the lumbar and cervical spine in 15%. The clinical course is indolent, and detection is often delayed until after metastasis occurs. Symptoms and signs include local pain, radiculopathy, and bowel or bladder dysfunction. Patients with cervicothoracic tumors can present with progressive dyspnea. Rectal examination can reveal a presacral mass.

After wide surgical resection, the local recurrence rate varies from 28–64%. Great care must be taken to prevent tumor spillage during resection because this can increase the local recurrence rate from 28% to 64%. Adjuvant radiation therapy is indicated when complete resection is not possible or when there is tumor spillage at the time of resection. Radiation therapy may allow an increased continuous disease-free survival. The 5-year survival rate in patients treated with irradiation alone is approximately 50%; that in patients treated with irradiation plus surgical resection is 71%. Virtually all patients eventually die from tumor recurrence.

Boriani S et al: Chondrosarcoma of the mobile spine: Report on 22 cases. Spine 2000;25:804. [PMID: 10751291]

Fourney DR, Gokaslan ZL: Current management of sacral chordoma. Neurosurg Focus 2003;15:E9. [PMID: 15350040]

Ilaslan H et al: Primary vertebral osteosarcoma: Imaging findings. Radiology 2004;230:697. Epub accessed January 28, 2004. [PMID: 14749514]

Lane JM et al: Kyphoplasty enhances function and structural alignment in multiple myeloma. Clin Orthop Relat Res 2004;426:49. [PMID: 15346051]

McLain RF, Weinstein JN: Solitary plasmacytomas of the spine: A review of 84 cases. J Spinal Dis 1989;2:69. [PMID: 2520065]

Ozaki T et al: Osteosarcoma of the spine: experience of the Cooperative Osteosarcoma Study Group. Cancer 2002;94:1069. [PMID: 11920477]

Papagelopoulos PJ et al: Chordoma of the spine: Clinicopathological features, diagnosis, and treatment. Orthopedics 2004;27:1256. [PMID: 15633956]

Sell M et al: Chordomas: A histological and immunohistochemical study of cases with and without recurrent tumors. Clin Neuropathol 2004;23:277. [PMID: 15584212]

Venkateswaran L et al: Primary Ewing tumor of the vertebrae: Clinical characteristics, prognostic factors, and outcome. Med Pediatr Oncol 2001;37:30. [PMID: 11466720]

Zeifang F et al: Long-term survival after surgical intervention for bone disease in multiple myeloma. Ann Oncol 2005;16:222. [PMID: 15668274]

METASTATIC DISEASE OF THE SPINE

Although the skeleton is the third most common site for metastatic disease, the spine, especially the thoracic spine, is the most frequently involved region of the skeleton. Approximately 70% of patients who die of cancer have evidence of vertebral metastasis on postmortem examination.

Lung, breast, prostate, renal, thyroid, and gastrointestinal carcinomas are all reported to metastasize to the spine, where lesions can lead to multilevel spinal instability and cord compression. Unfortunately, 30–50% of the bone must be destroyed before the metastatic involvement becomes evident on radiographs.

Many patients with spinal metastasis are asymptomatic. Symptoms, when they do occur, are typically a result of invasion of the tumor into the paravertebral soft tissues, compression of the spinal cord or nerve roots, or pathologic fracture and spinal instability. In these cases, patients frequently complain of severe, unrelenting back pain with or without neurologic sequelae. The pain typically wakes the patient up at night. The course may be rapid, leading to paraplegia or quadriplegia.

Technetium bone scanning reveals multiple sites of radioisotope uptake. MRI is the imaging study of choice to assess the extent of the tumor. Biopsy is necessary when the primary tumor is unknown and typically can be performed under CT guidance.

Most patients who do not develop progressive instability or neurologic compromise can be managed nonoperatively with systemic chemotherapy, local irradiation, and bracing.

Radiation therapy and chemotherapy protocols depend on the primary source of carcinoma. From 80% to 90% of patients suffering from spinal metastatic disease are reported to gain significant relief with radiation therapy. Irradiation can be started as early as 2 weeks after surgical decompression and fusion. Surgical intervention is warranted in patients who have severe pain and have failed to respond to conservative management. It is also indicated in patients who have significant neurologic dysfunction or spinal instability. Factors found to affect survival include preoperative neurologic status, anatomic site of primary

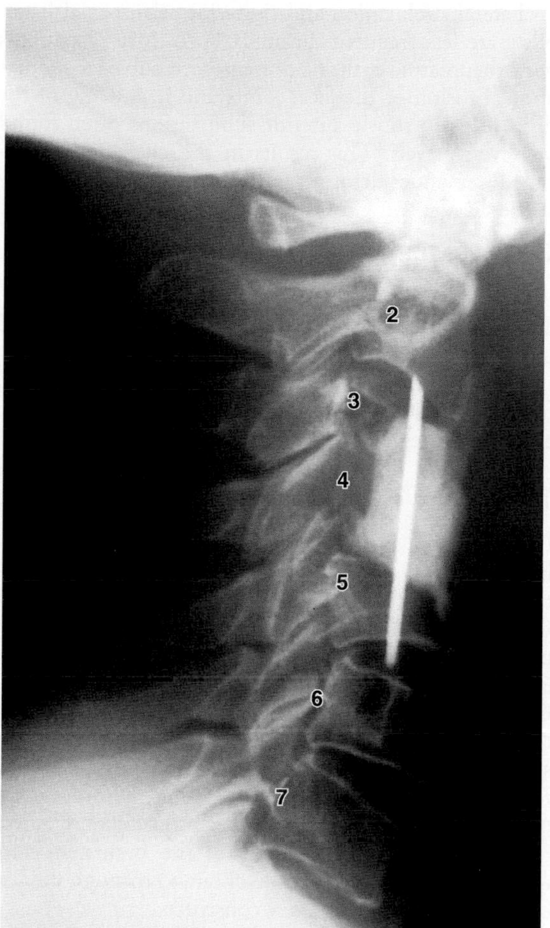

Figure 5–3. Radiograph showing metastasizing adenocarcinoma of C4 and C5, treated with excision, methylmethacrylate, and K-wire.

carcinoma, and number of vertebral bodies involved. Patients with a slower onset of neurologic compromise have a better prognosis for recovery of neurologic function than patients with acute onset of neurologic compromise. Stabilizing constructs can consist of bone, metal, or methylmethacrylate (Figure 5–3).

Alvarez L et al: Vertebroplasty in the treatment of vertebral tumors: Postprocedural outcome and quality of life. Eur Spine J 2003;12:356. Epub accessed March 22, 2003. [PMID: 12687441]

Barr JD et al: Percutaneous vertebroplasty for pain relief and spinal stabilization. Spine 2000;25:923. [PMID: 10767803]

Chataigner H, Onimus M: Surgery in spinal metastasis without spinal cord compression: Indications and strategy related to the risk of recurrence. Eur Spine J 2000;9:523. [PMID: 11189921]

Ghogawala Z, Mansfield FL, Borges LF: Spinal radiation before surgical decompression adversely affects outcomes of surgery for symptomatic metastatic spinal cord compression. Spine 2001;26:818. [PMID: 11295906]

Holman PJ et al: Surgical management of metastatic disease of the lumbar spine: experience with 139 patients. J Neurosurg Spine 2005;2:550.

Jeremic B: Single fraction external beam radiation therapy in the treatment of localized metastatic bone pain. A review. J Pain Symptom Manage 2001;22:1048. [PMID 11738168]

Manabe J et al: Surgical treatment of bone metastasis: Indications and outcomes. Int J Clin Oncol 2005;10:103. [PMID: 15864695]

North RB et al: Surgical management of spinal metastases: Analysis of prognostic factors during a 10-year experience. J Neurosurg Spine 2005;2:564. [PMID: 15945430]

Ryu S et al: Image-guided and intensity-modulated radiosurgery for patients with spinal metastasis. Cancer 2003;97:2013. [PMID: 12673732]

Togao O et al: Percutaneous vertebroplasty in the treatment of pain caused by metastatic tumor. Fukuoka Igaku Zasshi 2005; 96:93. [PMID: 15991606]

EXTRADURAL TUMORS

Extradural tumors include hemangiomas, lipomas, meningiomas, and lymphomas. Surgical management usually involves laminectomy and tumor excision. This is often all that is needed for symptomatic relief in these slow-growing tumors.

Loblaw DA et al: Systematic review of the diagnosis and management of malignant extradural spinal cord compression: The Cancer Care Ontario Practice Guidelines Initiative's Neuro-Oncology Disease Site Group. J Clin Oncol 2005;23:2028. [PMID: 15774794]

INFLAMMATORY DISEASES OF THE SPINE

RHEUMATOID ARTHRITIS

Rheumatoid arthritis is the most common form of inflammatory arthritis. It affects 3% of women and 1% of men. The disease frequently affects the spine. The same inflammatory cells that destroy peripheral joints affect the synovium of apophyseal and uncovertebral joints, causing painful instability and neurologic compromise. Up to 71% of patients with rheumatoid arthritis show involvement of the cervical spine. The most common patterns of involvement are C1-C2 instability, basilar invagination, and subaxial subluxation. Sudden death associated with rheumatoid arthritis, most probably secondary to brain stem compression, is reported.

Clinical Findings

A. Symptoms and Signs

From 7% to 34% of patients present with neurologic problems. Documentation of neurologic function can be difficult because loss of joint mobility leads to general muscle weakness. Although many patients complain of nonspecific neck pain, atlantoaxial subluxation is the most common cause for pain in the upper neck, occiput, and forehead in patients with rheumatoid arthritis. Symptoms are aggravated by motion. Increasing compression of the spinal cord results in severe myelopathy with gait abnormalities, weakness, paresthesias, and loss of dexterity. Findings may also include Lhermitte sign (a tingling or electrical feeling that occurs in the arms, legs, or trunk when the neck is flexed), increased muscle tonus of the upper and lower extremities, and pathologic reflexes.

B. Imaging Studies

Instability of the upper cervical spine is determined on lateral flexion-extension radiographs. An atlantodens interval (ADI) that exceeds 3.5 mm is abnormal. Subluxation with an atlasdens interval of 10–12 mm indicates disruption of all supporting ligaments of the atlantoaxial complex (transverse and alar ligaments). The spinal cord in this position is compressed between the dens and the posterior arch of C1. Although the ADI is an important measurement for traumatic instability of the C1-C2 complex, the posterior atlantodens interval (PADI) is more prognostic to assess neurologic compromise. The PADI is a direct measure of the space available for the spinal cord at the C1-C2 level. The PADI is measured from the posterior aspect of the odontoid process to the nearest posterior structure (the foramen magnum or the posterior ring of the atlas). If the space available for the spinal cord is less than 13 mm, the likelihood that the patient will develop myelopathy is extremely high.

Cranial settling is present in from 5% to 32% of patients. The odontoid process should not project more than 3 mm above the Chamberlain line, which is a line between the hard palate and the posterior rim of the foramen magnum. The tip of the dens should not project more than 4.5 mm above the McGregor line, which is a line connecting the posterior margin of the hard palate to the occiput. The Clark classification divides the axis into thirds in the sagittal plane. In severe cases of cranial settling, the anterior arch of C1 moves from station 1 (the upper third of C2) to station 3 (the lower third of C2). Neurologic compromise occurs as a result of impingement of the dens into the brainstem and the upper cervical spinal cord. The vertebral arteries can also become occluded as they course between the dens and the foramen magnum to enter the skull.

Lateral subluxation and posterior atlantoaxial instability are less frequent. From 10% to 20% of patients with rheumatoid arthritis present with subaxial subluxation. Erosion of the facet joints and narrowing of the disks leads to subtle anterior subluxations often found on several levels. This results in the characteristic so-called stepladder deformity that occurs most commonly at the C2-C3 and C3-C4 levels.

C. Laboratory Studies

Rheumatoid factor is positive in up to 80% of patients. The ESR rate is elevated and the hemoglobin is decreased in the active phase of the disease.

After plain radiographs, which should include lateral flexion-extension views, MRI is the study of choice to evaluate the degree of neural compression and deformity.

Treatment

Indications for surgery are severe neck pain and increasing loss of neurologic function. Most commonly, a posterior arthrodesis between C1 and C2 is performed. A Gallie type or Brooks type of fusion can be done, or posterior transarticular screw fixation can be used. The latter obviates the need for postoperative halo immobilization. In cases of basilar invagination (cranial settling), extension of the fusion to the occiput is necessary. Preoperative halo traction is often required to reduce the subluxation or pull the odontoid process out of the foramen magnum. Often a suboccipital craniectomy is necessary to decompress the brainstem adequately. Good fixation can be obtained through the use of plate-screw and rod-screw constructs.

Alberstone CD, Benzel EC: Cervical spine complications in rheumatoid arthritis patients. Awareness is the key to averting serious consequences. Postgrad Med 2000;107:199. [PMID 10649674]

Boden SD et al: Rheumatoid arthritis of the cervical spine. A long-term analysis with predictors of paralysis and recovery. J Bone Joint Surg Am 1993;75:1282. [PMID: 8408150]

Christensson D, Saveland H, Rydholm U: Cervical spine surgery in rheumatoid arthritis. A Swedish nation-wide registration of 83 patients. Scand J Rheumatol 2000;29:314. [PMID: 11093598]

Clark CR, Goetz DD, Menezes AH: Arthrodesis of the cervical spine in rheumatoid arthritis. J Bone Joint Surg Am 1989; 71:381. [PMID: 2925711]

Faraj AA, Webb JK, Prince H: Surgical treatment for rheumatoid neck arthritis bilateral occipitospinal fusion with plate fixation. Acta Orthop Belg 2001;67:164. [PMID: 11383295]

Graziano GP, Hensinger R, Patel CK: The use of traction methods to correct severe cervical deformity in rheumatoid arthritis patients: A report of five cases. Spine 2001;26:1076. [PMID: 11337628]

Grob D: Posterior occipitocervical fusion in rheumatoid arthritis and other instabilities. J Orthop Sci 2000;5:82. [PMID: 10664444]

Haid RW Jr et al: C1-C2 transarticular screw fixation for atlantoaxial instability: A 6-year experience. Neurosurgery 2001; 49:65. [PMID: 11440461]

Kauppi MJ, Barcelos A, da Silva JA: Cervical complications of rheumatoid arthritis. Ann Rheum Dis 2005;64:355.

Matsunaga S, Ijiri K, Koga H: Results of a longer than 10-year follow-up of patients with rheumatoid arthritis treated by occipitocervical fusion. Spine 2000;25:1749. [PMID: 10888940]

Matsuyama Y et al: Long-term results of occipitothoracic fusion surgery in RA patients with destruction of the cervical spine. J Spinal Disord Tech 2005;18(Suppl):S101. [PMID: 15699794]

van Asselt KM et al: Outcome of cervical spine surgery in patients with rheumatoid arthritis. Ann Rheum Dis 2001;60:448. [PMID: 11302865]

ANKYLOSING SPONDYLITIS

Ankylosing spondylitis is a chronic seronegative inflammatory disease that affects the axial skeleton, especially the sacroiliac joints, hip joints, and spine. Extraskeletal involvement is found in the aorta, lung, and uvea. The incidence of ankylosing spondylitis is 0.5–1 per 1000 people. Although males are affected more frequently than females, mild courses of ankylosing spondylitis are more common in the latter. The disease usually has its onset during early adulthood. However, juvenile ankylosing spondylitis affects adolescents (younger than 16 years) and has a predisposition toward hip involvement. The HLA-B27 surface antigen is found in 88%–96% of patients, and investigators postulate that an endogenic component (ie, HLA-B27) and an exogenic component (eg, *Klebsiella* or *Chlamydia*) are responsible for triggering of the disease process. The ESR is elevated in up to 80% of the cases but does not accurately reflect disease activity. The serum creatine phosphokinase (CPK), however, is a good indicator of the severity of the disease process.

Clinical Findings

A. Symptoms and Signs

The onset is insidious, with early symptoms including pain in the buttocks, heels, and lower back. Patients complain typically of morning stiffness, the improvement of symptoms with activity during the day, and the return of symptoms in the evening. The earliest changes involve the sacroiliac joints and then extend upward into the spine. Spinal disease results in loss of motion and subsequent loss of lordosis in the cervical and lumbar spine. Synovitis in the early stages leads to progressive fibrosis and ankylosis of the joints during the reparative phase. Enthesitis occurs at the insertion of the annulus fibrosus on the vertebral body with eventual calcification that results in the characteristic "bamboo spine." The pain from the inflammatory process subsides after full ankylosis of the affected joints occurs. Approximately 30% of patients develop uveitis, and 30% have chest tightness. Limited chest expansion indicates thoracic involvement. Fewer than 5% of patients have involvement of the aorta, characterized by dilation and possible conduction defects. In addition, patients may suffer from renal amyloidosis and pulmonary fibrosis.

B. Imaging Studies

The earliest radiographic changes are visible in the sacroiliac joints. Symmetric bilateral widening of the joint space is followed by subchondral erosions and ankylosis. Bony changes in the spine affect the vertebral body. Changes include loss of the anterior concavity of the vertebral body, squaring of the vertebra, and marginal syndesmophyte formation, which give the spine the appearance of bamboo. Ankylosis of the apophyseal joints also develops. The disease generally starts in the lumbar spine and migrates cephalad to the cervical spine. Atlantoaxial instability is seen occasionally.

Treatment

The natural history of ankylosing spondylitis, with its slow progression over several decades, has to be considered in planning treatment. Initially, treatment consists of exercises and indomethacin. Approximately 10% of patients develop severe bony changes that eventually require surgical intervention. These changes characteristically include a fixed bony flexion deformity that limits their ambulatory potential. Hip disease should be addressed before correction of spinal deformities because correction of hip flexion deformities may allow significant compensation of the spinal kyphosis to allow adequate horizontal gaze.

Loss of lumbar lordosis can be treated by multilevel V-shaped osteotomies posteriorly (the Smith-Petersen procedure), by a decancellation procedure (the Heinig procedure) of L3 or L4, or by pedicle subtraction osteotomy based at L3 or L4. (Figure 5–4).

The spine is then fused in the corrected position. Utilization of modern fixation systems such as a pedicle screw system allows for early mobilization of the patient. Thorough preoperative assessment of the deformity and measuring of the chin-eyebrow-to-floor angle are helpful for the exact planning of the corrective osteotomy. Relative contraindications to surgery are poor general health and significant scarring of the major vessels, which may be injured when the spine is extended.

The cervical osteotomy is performed between C7 and T1. This approach avoids injury to the vertebral artery that usually enters the transverse foramen of C6. Although the procedure is usually performed under local anesthesia, the evolution of somatosensory and motor evoked potential monitoring of the spinal cord permits the use of general anesthesia. After removal of the poste-

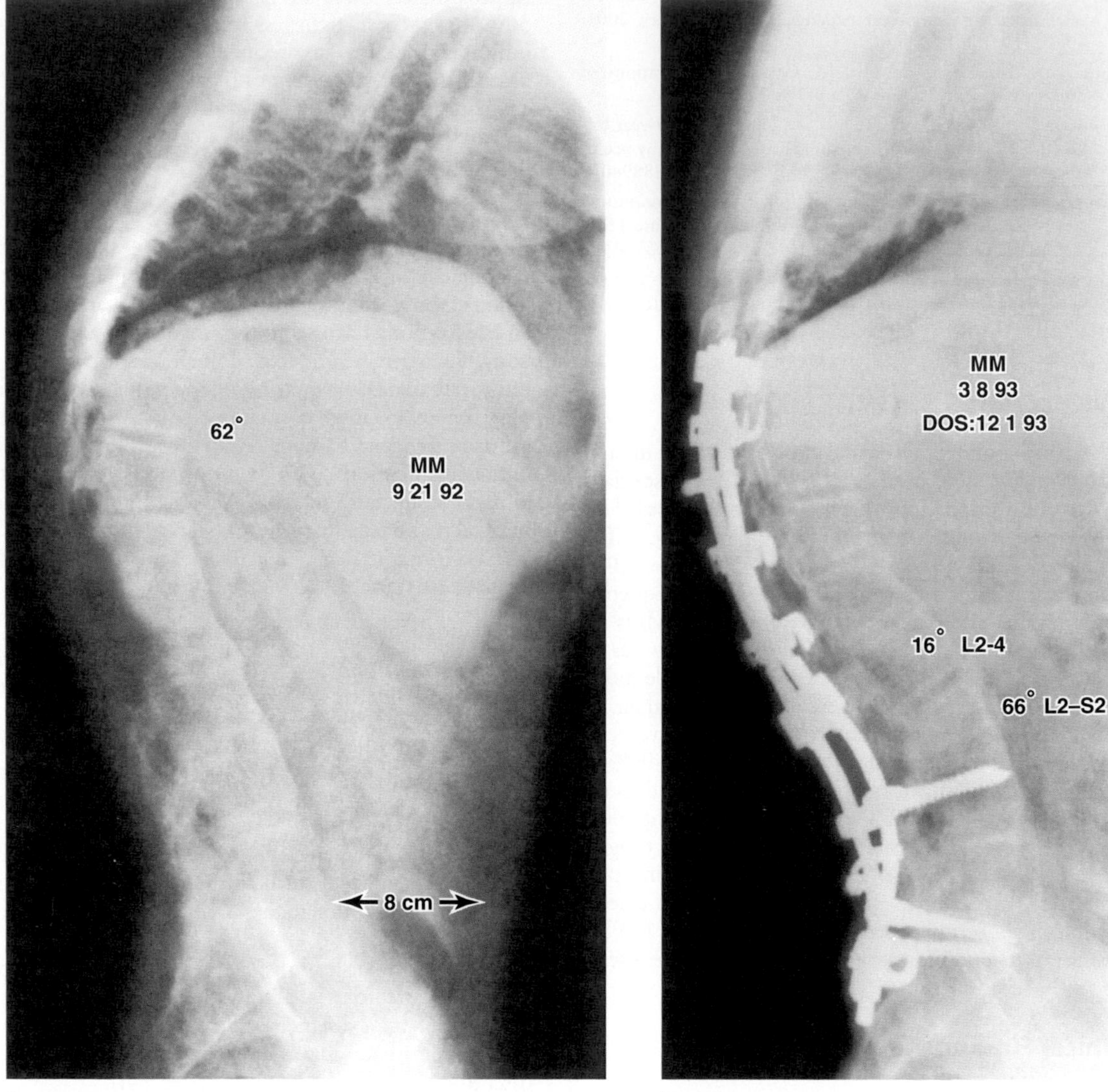

Figure 5–4. Imaging studies in a patient with ankylosing spondylitis. **A:** Radiograph demonstrating flat back deformity, junctional kyphosis, and sagittal decompensation. **B:** Radiograph taken after a decancellation procedure of L3 and posterior fusion were performed to correct the alignment.

rior elements and neural decompression, the kyphotic deformity is corrected with gentle extension of the head. The head is held in the corrected position using internal fixation with plate-screw constructs or plate-rod constructs with adjunctive halo-vest immobilization.

Berven SH et al: Management of fixed sagittal plane deformity: Results of the transpedicular wedge resection osteotomy. Spine 2001;26:2036. [PMID: 11547205]

Braun J et al: Therapy of ankylosing spondylitis. Part II: Biological therapies in the spondyloarthritides. Scand J Rheumatol 2005;34:178. [PMID: 16134723]

Chen IH, Chien JT, Yu TC: Transpedicular wedge osteotomy for correction of thoracolumbar kyphosis in ankylosing spondylitis: Experience with 78 patients. Spine 2001;26:E354. [PMID: 11493864]

Danisa OA, Turner D, Richardson WJ: Surgical correction of lumbar kyphotic deformity: Posterior reduction "eggshell" osteotomy. J Neurosurg 2000;92(Suppl 1):50. [PMID: 10616058]

Kim KT et al: Clinical outcome results of pedicle subtraction osteotomy in ankylosing spondylitis with kyphotic deformity. Spine 2002;27:612. [PMID: 11884909]

Kubiak EN et al: Orthopaedic management of ankylosing spondylitis. J Am Acad Orthop Surg 2005;13:267.

Taggard DA, Traynelis VC: Management of cervical spinal fractures in ankylosing spondylitis with posterior fixation. Spine 2000;25:2035. [PMID: 10954633]

van der Linden S, van der Heijde D: Clinical aspects, outcome assessment, and management of ankylosing spondylitis and postenteric reactive arthritis. Curr Opin Rheumatol 2000; 12:263. Review. [PMID: 10910177]

DISEASES & DISORDERS OF THE CERVICAL SPINE

Principles of Diagnosis

In evaluating the cervical spine, the use of appropriate imaging studies is critical to a timely and precise diagnosis. Available imaging techniques include plain radiography, tomography, myelography, CT, CT with myelography, three-dimensional reconstruction CT, MRI, and scintigraphy. An understanding of the advantages and disadvantages of each technique is necessary for the proper selection of imaging studies and interpretation of results.

A. Plain Radiography

In evaluating the patient with neck pain, cervical spine radiographs are important in the initial search for a possible lesion. In the trauma setting, when a head or neck injury is suspected, radiographic studies must be carried out appropriately or a life-threatening lesion may be overlooked. The trauma series includes anteroposterior (AP), right oblique, left oblique, and open-mouth (odontoid) views in addition to an initial cross-table lateral view. When all five views are taken, sensitivity is 92%. Cervical spine precautions must be implemented throughout the radiographic evaluation (see Injuries of the Cervical Spine later in the chapter). In the absence of a history of trauma, the oblique and odontoid views are not always required.

The lateral view reveals the majority of traumatic lesions if performed correctly. Inadequate views can miss more than 20% of cervical spine injuries, however. All seven vertebrae should be clearly visible. Gentle traction on the upper extremities may be necessary to view C7. If this is unsuccessful, a swimmer's view may be necessary. Careful scrutiny of the prevertebral soft tissue, the anterior border of the vertebral bodies, the vertebral bodies themselves, the posterior border of the bodies, the spinal canal proper, and the posterior elements must be done.

The prevertebral region may reveal swelling consistent with a hematoma, and this may serve as the only clue to a traumatic lesion. The upper limits for the prevertebral space are 10 mm at C1; 5 mm at C2; 7 mm at C3 and C4; and 20 mm at C5, C6, and C7. The contours of the cervical bony structures are regular, and subtle incongruities may indicate significant instability. Variations in normal cervical anatomy do exist, however, and a familiarity with them may prevent an overzealous workup. The ADI normally measures less than 3 mm in adults and less than 4 mm in children.

In reviewing the AP radiograph, careful assessment of the interspinous distance must be undertaken. Vertical widening at a given level greater than 1.5 times the level above and below indicates a hyperflexion injury with posterior instability or interlocking of the posterior facets. Traumatic tilting may also be noted in the AP plane while not appreciated on the lateral view.

Oblique views taken at 45 degrees allow visualization of the articulations of the facet joints. The open-mouth view permits evaluation of the odontoid process, the lateral masses, and the articulations of the lateral masses, and it also permits assessment of the distance between each lateral mass and the odontoid process. In atlantoaxial rotatory subluxation, the lateral mass of the atlas that is rotated forward is closer to the midline (medial offset); the opposite mass is farther away from the midline (lateral offset). Burst fractures of the C1 ring cause overhang of the C1 lateral masses on C2. A combined overhang exceeding 6.9 mm is highly correlated with insufficiency of the transverse ligament and C1-C2 sagittal instability.

This radiographic series is equally important in evaluating infants and children with suspected congenital or developmental defects and adults with insidious neck pain. Arthritic changes may be subtle or readily apparent with osteophytes, disk space narrowing, and facet sclerosis. Bone quality can also be assessed on plain radiographs.

B. Computed Tomography

CT scans allow excellent visualization of the bony architecture and the paravertebral soft tissues of the cervical spine. The pedicles, laminae, spinous processes, and bony spinal canal can be examined with significantly better resolution when CT is used than when conventional radiographs are taken. CT with myelography or intrathecal contrast enhancement permits a visualization of the spinal canal contents.

CT is an appropriate modality for evaluating congenital variations and malformations, including spinal canal stenosis and spina bifida. Pars defects, atlantoaxial joint diseases, inflammatory changes, primary tumors, and metastatic carcinoma are well appreciated with CT. Although cervical disk disease is detectable when thin cuts and contrast enhancement are used with CT, it is better visualized with MRI.

In the trauma patient with questionable findings on plain radiographs, CT is integral in evaluating possible fractures or instability. Atrophy, deformity, and displacement of the spinal cord from acute or chronic injury are all appreciable with the use of intrathecal contrast. With the advent of MRI, however, CT is now reserved for the assessment of the bony architecture, which it does better than MRI.

Three-dimensional reconstruction of CT images gained wide clinical acceptance with the advancement of computer graphics. The reconstructions can be rotated in space to evaluate the anatomy from almost any perspective. This technique is valuable in the understanding of atlantoaxial rotatory subluxations or complex fractures of the spinal column.

C. Magnetic Resonance Imaging

MRI permits axial, sagittal, coronal, or oblique plane analysis of the anatomy. It is routinely noninvasive, requiring contrast material in only selected cases.

MRI is the standard for assessing cervical spinal cord damage. Spinal cord tumors and trauma as well as central disk herniation can be easily visualized. In the preoperative evaluation of patients with spondylosis or disk herniation, MRI is the neuroimaging test of choice.

Intravenous paramagnetic agent gadolinium is commonly used to differentiate tissues receiving higher blood flow. This is helpful in the diagnosis of infection, tumor, and postsurgical scar.

D. Scintigraphy

Bone scans that employ technetium-99m phosphate permit assessment of physiologic processes within the musculoskeletal system. Metabolic, metastatic, and inflammatory abnormalities can be detected. Technetium-99m phosphate is incorporated into the hydroxyapatite in bone and reflects increased bone osteogenesis in a given region of bone. Early-phase imaging with technetium-99m gives blood flow information. Accordingly, subtle fractures, avascular necrosis, and osteomyelitis can be detected. Other radioisotopes used in scintigraphy include gallium-67 citrate, which labels serum proteins, and indium-111, which labels white blood cells. These labeling techniques are helpful in discerning areas of neoplasia or acute infection.

Daffner RH: Controversies in cervical spine imaging in trauma patients. Semin Musculoskelet Radiol 2005;9:105. [PMID: 15278699]

Holmes JF, Akkinepalli R: Computed tomography versus plain radiography to screen for cervical spine injury: a meta-analysis. J Trauma 2005;58:902. Review. [PMID: 15920400]

Larsson EM et al: Comparison of myelography, CT myelography and magnetic resonance imaging in cervical spondylosis and disk herniation. Pre- and postoperative findings. Acta Radiol 1989;30:233. [PMID: 2736175]

Mower WR et al: NEXUS Group. Use of plain radiography to screen for cervical spine injuries. Ann Emerg Med 2001;38:1. [PMID: 11423803]

Sanchez B et al: Cervical spine clearance in blunt trauma: Evaluation of a computed tomography-based protocol. J Trauma 2005;59:179.

Schuster R et al: Magnetic resonance imaging is not needed to clear cervical spines in blunt trauma patients with normal computed tomographic results and no motor deficits. Arch Surg 2005;140:762. [PMID: 16103286]

Taneichi H et al: Traumatically induced vertebral artery occlusion associated with cervical spine injuries: Prospective study using magnetic resonance angiography. Spine 2005;30:1955.

CONGENITAL MALFORMATIONS

The atlantooccipital region is a frequent location for abnormalities. Various combinations involving bone and nervous structures are possible. During embryologic development, 42 somites are formed from the paraxial mesoderm. The somites divide into sclerotomes, which form the vertebral bodies after separation into a caudal and cephalad portion. The middle portion builds the intervertebral disk. The second, third, and fourth somites fuse and become the occiput and posterior part of the foramen magnum. The fate of the first somite is unclear. The development of the neural tube progresses simultaneously with that of the cartilaginous skeleton.

Disturbances of embryologic development can result in incomplete development or absence of a tissue or part, as found in dysraphism, aplasia of the odontoid process, incomplete closure of the atlas, or absence of the atlas facet. Lack of segmentation results in atlantooccipital fusion, block vertebrae, and possible instability at adjacent cervical levels. A disturbance of neurologic development, alone or in combination with bony defects, can lead to basilar impression, Arnold-Chiari malformation, and syringomyelia, all of which manifest in myelopathy.

1. Os Odontoideum

Os odontoideum is an uncommon type of pseudarthrosis between the odontoid process and the body of the axis. It can cause significant atlantoaxial instability and myelopathy and can result in sudden death. The development of cervical myelopathy is thought to be a function of the amount of space available for the spinal cord. Because of the instability between C1 and C2, the spinal cord can become compressed against the anterior portion of the axis or the posterior ring of the atlas. In some cases, extrinsic compression of the vertebral arteries results in ischemic insult to the brain.

Clinical Findings

A. Symptoms and Signs

Patients with os odontoideum may be asymptomatic or may present with symptoms and signs that relate to atlantoaxial instability, such as ill-defined neck complaints or focal or diffuse neurologic deficits. A careful history may be needed to rule out trauma, although congenital os odontoideum may come to the attention of the surgeon secondary to a reported but inconsequential neck injury.

B. Imaging Studies

The radiographic findings may be extremely subtle and difficult to distinguish. In the mature skeleton, os odontoideum appears as a radiographic lucency. In children younger than 5 years, however, an anomalous gap may be confused with a normal neural synchondrosis. Flexion-extension views must therefore be obtained to demonstrate motion between the odontoid process and the body of the axis. The ossicle in os odontoideum is either round or ovoid, with a smooth surface and uniform cortical thickness. It is usually approximately half the size of the normal odontoid process. In traumatic nonunion, the edge is irregular with a narrow gap. The fracture line may involve the body of C2 as well. An additional radiologic finding in os odontoideum is hypertrophy of the anterior ring of the atlas with a corresponding hypoplastic posterior ring. In flexion-extension views, the ossicle travels with the anterior ring of the atlas (Figure 5–5). In cases that are difficult to diagnose, further studies include open-mouth views, tomograms, and CT reconstructions.

Treatment

Patients diagnosed with os odontoideum must be warned of the gravity of the situation because minimal trauma can be fatal. Patients with cervical myelopathy can be treated with traction, immobilization, or both, but they often require subsequent posterior fusion. Sometimes symptoms are reversible with or without intervention. Management of asymptomatic patients with instability is controversial. The benefits of surgical stabilization in an attempt to avoid potentially lethal injury from relatively minor trauma are counterbalanced by the possible complications of surgery.

If fusion is indicated, usually a posterior fusion of C1-C2 is adequate. Different fusion techniques are available. Most surgeons use the Gallie technique or the Brooks technique. The Gallie technique involves the use of a single block-shaped bone graft between the posterior ring of C1 and the spinous process of C2. A single sublaminar wire holds the graft in place. The Brooks technique uses from two to four sublaminar wires, and two bone grafts are wedged between the laminae of C1 and C2. The loss of motion between atlas and axis results in an overall decrease of 50% of cervical rotation. Use of transarticular

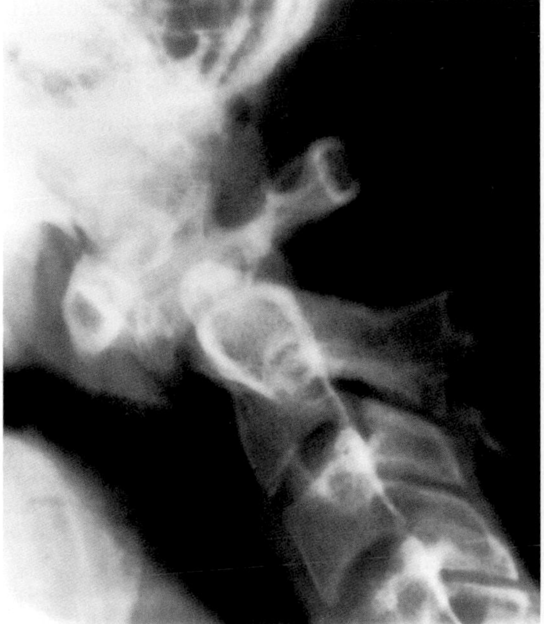

A

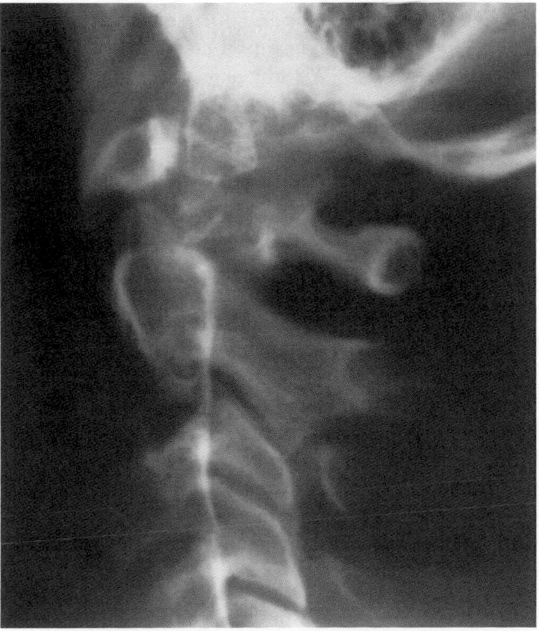

B

Figure 5–5. Imaging studies in a patient with os odontoideum. **A:** Radiograph in flexion. The ossicle moves with the anterior ring of the atlas. **B:** Radiograph in extension.

screws or screw-rod constructs that purchase into the lateral masses of C1 and the pedicle of C2 are rigid enough to allow the patient to mobilize without a halo vest.

Dai L et al: Os odontoideum: Etiology, diagnosis, and management. Surg Neurol 2000;53:106. [PMID: 10713186]

Gluf WM, Brockmeyer DL: Atlantoaxial transarticular screw fixation: A review of surgical indications, fusion rate, complications, and lessons learned in 67 pediatric patients. J Neurosurg Spine 2005;2:164. [PMID: 15739528]

2. Klippel-Feil Syndrome

Klippel-Feil syndrome refers to an array of clinical disorders associated with congenital fusion of one or more cervical vertebrae. The fusion, which may be multilevel, results from a failure of the normal division of the cervical somites during the third through eighth weeks of embryogenesis. The cause of this failure is unknown. The syndrome was first described in 1912 by M. Klippel and A. Feil as a triad of clinical features: a short "web" neck, a low posterior hair line, and limited cervical neck motion. Interestingly, only 50% of patients with the syndrome that now bears the names of Klippel and Feil present with this classic triad.

Various conditions were subsequently seen in association with congenitally fused cervical vertebrae. These include scoliosis (seen in approximately 60% of cases), renal abnormalities (in 35%), deafness (in 30%), Sprengel deformity (in 30%), synkinesis or mirror movement (in 20%), congenital heart defects (in 14%), brainstem anomalies, congenital cervical stenosis, adrenal aplasia, ptosis, Duane contracture, lateral rectus palsy, facial nerve palsy, syndactyly, and upper extremity diffuse or focal hypoplasia.

Clinical Findings

A. Symptoms and Signs

Decreased range of motion is the most frequent finding in patients with cervical spine involvement. Involvement of only the lower cervical spine or fusion of fewer than three vertebrae results in minimal loss of motion, however. Patients may also be able to compensate at other cervical interspaces, masking any loss of motion.

Neck shortening is difficult to detect unless extreme. Webbing of the neck (pterygium colli), facial asymmetry, or torticollis is seen in fewer than 20% of patients. Webbing of the neck can nevertheless be dramatic, with underlying muscle involvement extending from the mastoid to the acromion. Sprengel deformity, which results from a failure of either or both scapulae to descend from their embryologic origin at C4, is seen in approximately 30% of patients. Sometimes an omovertebral bone bridges the cervical spine to the scapulae and limits the neck and shoulder motion.

Cervical spine symptoms in Klippel-Feil syndrome are related to the secondary hypermobility of the unfused vertebrae. Except for atlantoaxial joint involvement, resulting in a significant decrease in occipital rotation, the fused joints at a given level are asymptomatic. Because of the increased mechanical demands placed on the uninvolved joints, secondary osteoarthritis, disk degeneration, spinal stenosis, and instability may result at these levels. Neurologic sequelae, usually confined to the head, neck, and upper extremities, result from impingement of the cervical nerve roots. With progressive cervical instability, the spinal cord may become involved, leading to spasticity, weakness, hyperreflexia, and even quadriplegia or sudden death from minor trauma.

B. Imaging Studies

Radiographic findings (Figure 5–6) of congenital cervical vertebral fusion are diagnostic of Klippel-Feil syndrome. This may present as synostosis of two vertebral bodies or as a multilevel fusion, as originally described in 1912. Other noteworthy findings are flattening of the involved vertebral bodies and the absence of disk spaces. Hypoplastic cervical disks in a child are often hard to appreciate radiographically. If suspected, flexion-extension views can be taken. CT scanning and MRI have improved the assessment of bony and nerve root involvement.

Spinal canal stenosis is not usually seen until adulthood. Although anterior spina bifida is infrequent, the posterior form is not. Enlargement of the foramen magnum with fixed hyperextension often accompanies the cervical spina bifida. Hemivertebrae are also noted.

Involvement of the upper thoracic spine can occur and may be the first sign of an undiagnosed cervical synostosis.

Because of the potential for multiorgan involvement in patients with Klippel-Feil syndrome, an electrocardiogram and renal ultrasound are also recommended.

Treatment

Treatment of the cervical spine abnormalities is limited. Multilevel involvement leads to hypermobility at uninvolved joints, so affected patients should be cautious in their activities. Prophylactic surgical stabilization is not routinely performed in asymptomatic patients because the risk-benefit ratio has not been well defined. In some cases, however, surgical fusion is performed.

Secondary osteoarthritis may be treated in the usual manner, including use of a cervical collar, traction, and antiinflammatory agents. Nerve root impingement requires careful evaluation before surgical decompression because more than one level may be involved and there may also be central abnormalities.

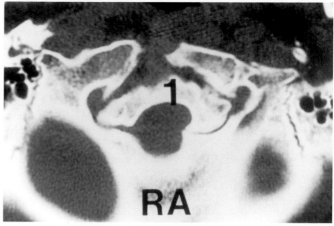

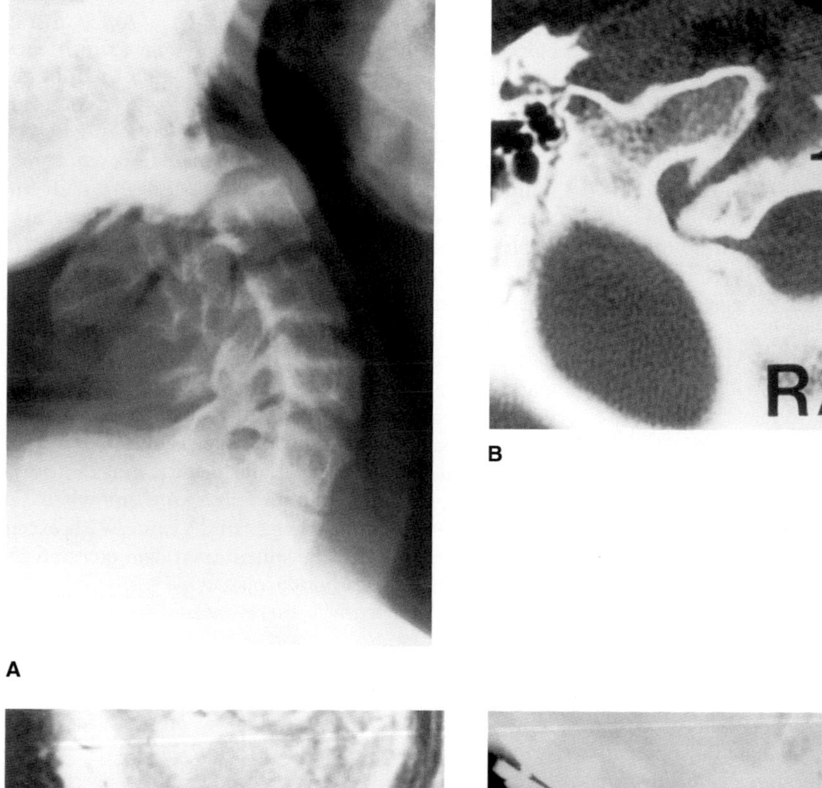

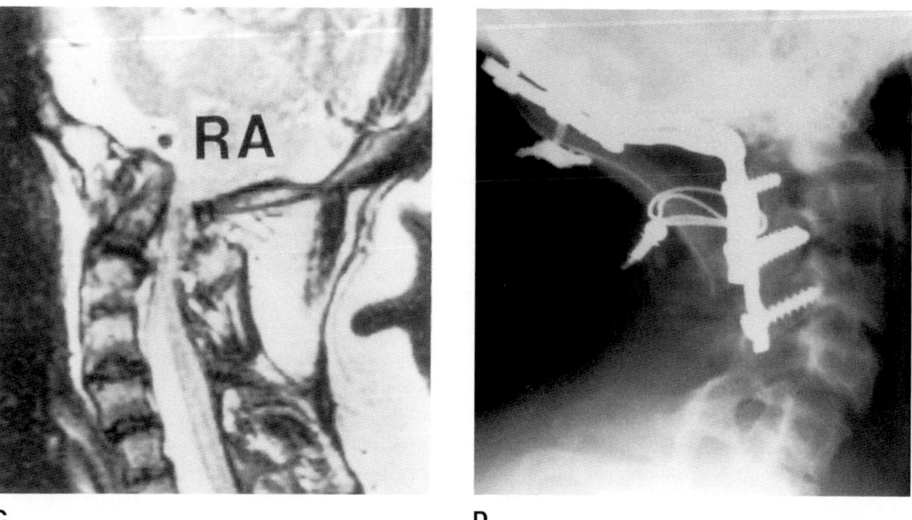

Figure 5–6. Imaging studies in a patient with Klippel-Feil syndrome and cervical myelopathy. **A:** Radiograph showing fusion of the atlas and the occiput and autofusion of the posterior elements of C3 and C4. **B:** CT scan demonstrates this as well. **C:** MRI demonstrating severe stenosis of the spinal canal. The odontoid process is above the level of the foramen magnum. **D:** Radiograph following posterior decompression and fusion between the occiput and C4.

Surgical correction of the aesthetic deformities is only moderately successful. Carefully selected candidates may benefit from soft tissue Z-plasty or tenotomies. This may improve the appearance of the patient but does not affect cervical motion.

Prognosis

Children with mild involvement can be expected to grow up to lead healthy, normal lives. Patients with more severe involvement can do comparably well if the associated conditions are successfully treated at an early age.

Herman MJ, Pizzutillo PD: Cervical spine disorders in children. Orthop Clin North Am 1999;30:457. Review. [PMID: 10393767]

Tracy MR, Dormans JP, Kusumi K: Klippel-Feil syndrome: Clinical features and current understanding of etiology. Clin Orthop 2004;424:183. [PMID: 15241163]

CERVICAL SPONDYLOSIS

Cervical spondylosis is defined as a generalized disease process affecting the entire cervical spine and related to chronic disk degeneration. In approximately 90% of men older than 50 years and 90% of women older than 60 years, degeneration of the cervical spine can be demonstrated by radiographs. Initial disk changes are followed by facet arthropathy, osteophyte formation, and ligamentous instability. Myelopathy, radiculopathy, or both may be seen secondarily. Cervical myelopathy is the most common form of spinal cord dysfunction in people older than 55 years. People older than 60 years are more likely to have multisegmental disease. The incidence of cervical myelopathy is twice as great in men as in women.

Pathophysiology

The relationship between the spinal cord and its bony arcade has been studied extensively. The first publication on the subject was written in the early 1800s and gave the first account of a "spondylotic bar," which was actually a thickened posterior longitudinal ligament protruding into the canal secondary to disk degeneration. Subsequent work revealed that disk degeneration and osteoarthritis could lead to spinal cord and nerve root impingement.

Acute traumatic disk herniation was distinguished from the chronic spondylotic process in the mid-1950s. Concurrently, anterior spinal artery impingement by the disk or osteophyte was proposed as part of the pathogenesis. As indicated in these studies, disk degeneration starts with tears in the posterolateral region of the annulus. The subsequent loss of water content and proteoglycans in the nucleus then leads to a decrease of disk height. The longitudinal ligaments degenerate and form bony spurs at their insertion into the vertebral body. These so-called hard disks have to be distinguished from soft disks, which represent acute herniation of disk material into the spinal canal or into the neural foramen. The most frequently involved levels are the more mobile segments: C5-C6, C6-C7, and C4-C5. The converging of the cervical disk space may result in buckling of the ligamentum flavum, with further narrowing of the spinal canal. Segmental instability results in hypertrophic formation of osteophytes by the uncovertebral joint of Luschka and by the facet joints. These prominent spurs result in compression of both the exiting nerve roots and the spinal cord.

Further work revealed that the sagittal cervical canal diameter was appreciably smaller (3 mm on average) in the myelopathic spondylotic spine than in the normal spine. The anterior-posterior dimensions of the cervical spinal canal measure between 17 and 18 mm in normal individuals. Spinal canal stenosis is present when the canal diameter becomes less than 13 mm. With extension of the neck, both the spinal canal diameter and the neuroforaminal diameter decrease.

Clinical Findings

A. Symptoms and Signs

Headache may be the presenting symptom of cervical spondylosis. Usually, the headache is worse in the morning and improves throughout the day. It is commonly located in the occipital region and radiates toward the frontal area. Infrequently, patients complain of a painful, stiff neck. Signs include decreased range of motion, crepitus, or both. With more advanced cases, radicular or myelopathic symptoms may be present.

1. Cervical spondylotic radiculopathy—Cervical radiculopathy in spondylosis can be quite complex, with nerve root involvement seen at one or more levels and occurring either unilaterally or bilaterally. The onset may be acute, subacute, or chronic, and impingement on the nerve roots may be from either osteophytes or disk herniation. With radiculopathy, sensory involvement in the form of paresthesias or hyperesthesia is more common than motor or reflex changes. Several dermatomal levels may be involved, with radiation into the anterior chest and back. The chief complaint is radiation of pain into the interscapular area and into the arm. Typically, patients have proximal arm pain and distal paresthesias.

2. Cervical spondylotic myelopathy—Cervical myelopathy has a variable clinical presentation, given the complex pathogenic mechanisms involved. These include static or dynamic canal impingement, facet arthropathy, vascular ischemia, and the presence of spondylotic transverse bars. In addition, given its neuronal topography, the cord may be affected in dramatically different ways by relatively minor differences in anatomic regions of compression. The clinical course of myelopathy is usually progressive, leading to complete disability over a period of months to years with stepwise deteriorations in function.

Patients often present with paresthesias, dyskinesias, or weakness of the hand, the entire upper extremity, or the lower extremity. Deep aching pain of the extremity, broad-based gait, loss of balance, loss of hand dexterity, and general muscle wasting are found in patients with advanced myelopathy. Impotence is not uncommon in these patients.

Hyperextension injuries of the spondylotic cervical spine can precipitate a central cord syndrome in which motor and sensory involvement is typically greater in the upper extremities than the lower extremities. Recovery from this injury is usually incomplete. Complete quadriplegia can also occur if the preexisting stenosis is severe. In this setting, the 1-year mortality approaches 80%.

Deep tendon reflexes can be either hyporeflexic or hyperreflexic, with the former seen in anterior horn cell (upper extremity) involvement and the latter seen in corticospinal tract (lower extremity) involvement. Hyporeflexia is found at the level of compression; hyperreflexia occurs on the level below. Long-tract signs, such as the presence of the Hoffmann reflex or Babinski reflex, indicate an upper motor neuron lesion. Clonus is often present though asymmetric. Upper extremity involvement is often unilateral, whereas lower extremities are affected bilaterally. High cervical spondylosis (C3-C5) leads to complaints of numb and clumsy hands; myelopathy of the lower cervical spine (C5-C8) presents with spasticity and loss of proprioception in the legs.

Abdominal reflexes are usually intact, enabling the clinician to differentiate spondylosis from amyotrophic lateral sclerosis, in which reflexes are often absent. Multiple compressions of the spinal cord cause more severe deterioration functionally and electrophysiologically than a single-level compression does.

B. Imaging Studies

Although spondylosis results from cervical spine degeneration, not every patient with radiographic evidence of cervical disk degeneration has symptoms. Furthermore, patients with all the radiographic stigmas of cervical spondylosis may be asymptomatic, and others with clinical evidence of myelopathy may show only modest radiographic changes. This paradox is explainable by canal size differences, with the smaller-diameter canal having less space to buffer the degenerative lesion.

The average AP diameter of the spinal canal measures 17 mm from C3 to C7. The space required by the spinal cord averages 10 mm. The dural diameter increases by 2–3 mm in extension. The smallest sagittal anteroposterior diameter is measured between an osteophyte on the inferior aspect of the vertebral body to the base of the spinous process of the next vertebra below. An absolute spinal canal stenosis exists with a sagittal diameter of less than 10 mm. The stenosis is relative if the diameter measures 10–13 mm.

Plain film findings also vary according to the stage of spondylosis at which they were taken. Radiographs may appear normal in early disk disease. Alternatively, they may show single or multilevel disk space narrowing with or without osteophytes. C5-C6 and C6-C7 are the two most commonly involved segments (Figure 5–7). Vertebral body sclerosis at the adjacent base plates may also be seen. Cortical erosion is uncommon and indicates an inflammatory process such as rheumatoid arthritis.

Oblique views permit evaluation of the facet joints and detection of osteophytosis and sclerosis. The superior facets undergo degeneration more frequently than their inferior counterparts. The superior joints may then subluxate posteriorly and erode into the lamina below. Inferior osteophytes, however, may prevent significant slippage. If instability seen on flexion-extension views is significant (greater than 3.5 mm when measured at the posteroinferior corner of the vertebral body), foraminal stenosis as well as vertebral artery impingement may result.

MRI permits visualization of the entire cervical canal and spinal cord by showing the spinal cord and nerve roots in two planes. The use of a contrast-enhanced CT scan is occasionally required in elderly (more than 60 years) patients with advanced degenerative bony changes of the cervical spine. Accurate identification of the location and extent of pathologic changes is necessary to determine the optimal approach for decompression. Selective nerve root blocks and electromyography may be useful to identify the level of involvement.

Differential Diagnosis

Inflammatory, neoplastic, and infectious conditions can mimic cervical spondylotic radiculopathy and myelopathy.

The cervical spine is affected in most rheumatoid arthritis patients. Atlantoaxial subluxation or subaxial instability can cause symptoms similar to those seen in degenerative cervical myelopathy. A primary tumor or metastatic disease can present with unremitting neck pain, often more intense at night. MRI can distinguish neoplastic conditions from degenerative disorders. Infections of the cervical spine occur in children and in elderly (more than 60 years) or immunocompromised individuals. Multiple sclerosis should be considered in the differential diagnosis. It occurs in younger patients but can present with similar motor signs. Pancoast tumors may invade the brachial plexus, resulting in upper extremity symptoms. Syringomyelia presents with tingling sensations plus motor weakness. A low protein concentration in the cerebrospinal fluid and characteristic changes on MRI are found. Disor-

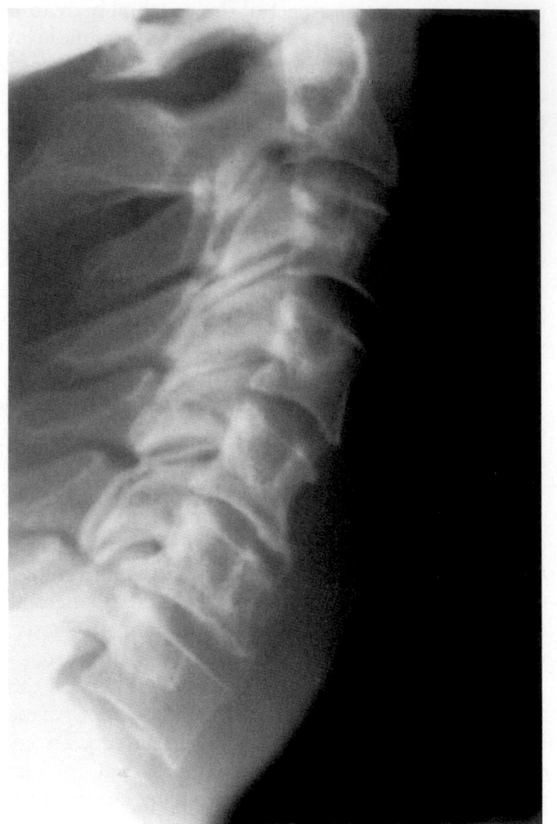

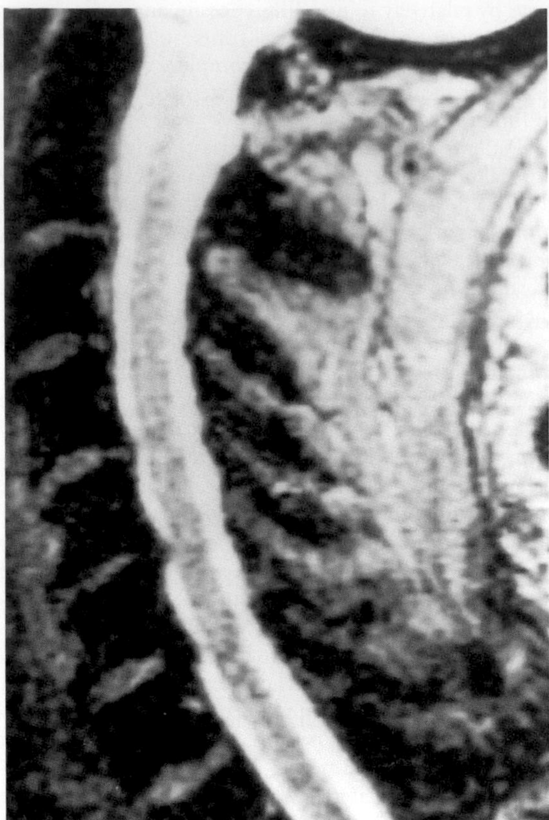

Figure 5–7. Imaging studies in a patient with cervical spondylosis and chronic neck pain. **A:** Radiograph showing collapsed disk space between C5 and C6 and a large posterior osteophyte at the inferior endplate of C6. **B:** MRI showing collapsed disk spaces, a mild stenosis of the spinal canal, and effacement of the spinal cord by an osteophyte at C6.

ders of the shoulder, especially rotator cuff tendinitis, can imitate cervical radiculopathy. Compressive peripheral neuropathies, such as thoracic outlet syndrome, also have to be ruled out.

Treatment

Patients should be divided into three groups, according to the predominance of their symptoms: neck pain alone, radiculopathy, and myelopathy. The duration and progression of symptoms need to be considered in the planning of treatment. Several studies suggest that patients with cervical radiculopathy or myelopathy have better long-term results from surgery if symptoms are of short duration.

A. Conservative Treatment

Initial management of patients with cervical spondylosis may involve a soft collar, antiinflammatory agents, and physical therapy consisting of mild traction and the use of isometric strengthening and range-of-motion exercises. The soft cervical collar should be worn only briefly, until the acute symptoms subside. Analgesics are important in the acute phase, and muscle relaxants are helpful in breaking the cycle of muscle spasm and pain. Diazepam should be avoided because of its side effects as a clinical depressant. Epidural corticosteroid injections may be efficacious in patients with radicular pain. Trigger point injections are an empirical form of therapy that seems to work well in patients with chronic neck pain.

The value of cervical traction remains unclear. It is contraindicated in patients with cord compression, rheumatoid arthritis, infection, or osteoporosis. A careful screening of roentgenograms before treatment is mandatory. No evidence indicates that home traction is more effective than manual traction. Isometric strengthening exercises of the paravertebral musculature should be started after the acute symptoms resolve. The patient should be instructed to start a home exercise program early, to avoid long-term dependency on passive therapy modalities. Although ice, moist heat, ultrasound, and transcutaneous electrical nerve stimulation (TENS) are safe to use, there is no scientific proof of their efficacy.

B. Surgical Treatment

Surgical intervention should be considered if the patient does not respond to a conservative treatment protocol or shows evidence of deteriorating myelopathy or radiculopathy. The spinal cord can be effectively decompressed by either anterior, posterior, or combined approaches.

The anterior approach allows multilevel diskectomy, vertebrectomy, foraminotomy, and fusion with tricortical iliac crest bone grafts or strut grafts. Newer instrumentation techniques, such as cervical plates (Figure 5–8), alleviate the need for halo immobilization. However supplemental posterior fixation and fusion should be added if more than three vertebral levels are decompressed anteriorly. Posterior fixation minimizes the risk of anterior dislodgement of the graft even in the presence of solid anterior fixation. Anterior interbody fusion after decompression for a herniated cervical disk (Figure 5–9) has a high success rate.

Cervical disk replacement prostheses were also developed to provide a motion-sparing alternative to anterior cervical diskectomy and fusion. By maintaining existing motion or restoring motion to a diseased motion segment, these prostheses have the potential to decrease the rate of symptomatic adjacent segment degeneration. Currently, clinical trials approved by the Food and Drug Administration (FDA) are under way to assess the efficacy of these devices against the outcomes that can be obtained with anterior cervical diskectomy and fusion.

The number of involved levels may be important in deciding which of the surgical approaches to use. Patients with cervical myelopathy and involvement of more than three vertebral body levels may be best managed by a posterior approach. Multilevel laminectomy or laminoplasty shows excellent results. If laminectomies are performed, the facet joints and capsules should be preserved to minimize the chance of postlaminectomy deformity. Late swan-neck deformities after laminectomy can be avoided with simultaneous posterior fusion using lateral mass plates. Laminoplasty is advantageous in that the cervical spinal cord can be decompressed without the high risk of developing late deformity. In addition, the morbidity associated with instrumentation and fusion can be avoided.

Operative treatment in cases of cervical spondylotic radiculopathy and myelopathy must be individualized for every patient.

Prognosis

Cervical spondylosis is generally a progressive, chronic disease process. In a study of 205 patients with neck pain, Gore et al. found that many patients had decreased pain at the 10-year follow-up, but those with the most severe involvement did not improve. Conservative measures may retard the disease process in its early stages. If myelopathy or radiculopathy becomes clinically evident, surgical intervention is often necessary. For disease involving less than three vertebral levels, early anterior decompression and fusion improves the clinical outcome, particularly in the elderly (more than 60 years) individual who suffers from cervical myelopathy.

Belanger TA et al: Ossification of the posterior longitudinal ligament. Results of anterior cervical decompression and arthrodesis in sixty-one North American patients. J Bone Joint Surg Am 2005;87:610. [PMID: 15741630]

Chagas H et al: Cervical spondylotic myelopathy: 10 years of prospective outcome analysis of anterior decompression and fusion. Surg Neurol. 2005;64(Suppl 1):S1:30. [PMID: 15967227]

Edwards CC II et al: Cervical myelopathy. current diagnostic and treatment strategies. Spine J 2003;3:68. Review. [PMID: 14589250]

Edwards CC II, Heller JG, Murakami H: Corpectomy versus laminoplasty for multilevel cervical myelopathy: An independent matched cohort analysis. Spine 2002;27:1168. [PMID: 12045513]

Emery SE: Cervical spondylotic myelopathy: Diagnosis and treatment. J Am Acad Orthop Surg 2001;9:376. Review. [PMID: 11767723]

Epstein N: Anterior approaches to cervical spondylosis and ossification of the posterior longitudinal ligament: Review of operative technique and assessment of 65 multilevel circumferential procedures. Surg Neurol 2001;55:313. Review. [PMID: 11483184]

Heller JG et al: Laminoplasty versus laminectomy and fusion for multilevel cervical myelopathy: An independent matched cohort analysis. Spine 2001;26:1330. [PMID: 11426147]

Mehdorn HM, Fritsch MJ, Stiller RU: Treatment options and results in cervical myelopathy. Acta Neurochir Suppl 2005; 93:177. [PMID: 15986751]

Onari K et al: Long-term follow-up results of anterior interbody fusion applied for cervical myelopathy due to ossification of the posterior longitudinal ligament. Spine 2001;26:488. [PMID: 11242375]

Phillips FM, Garfin SR: Cervical disc replacement. Spine 2005; 30(Suppl 17):S27.

Takayama H et al: Proprioceptive recovery of patients with cervical myelopathy after surgical decompression. Spine 2005;30: 1039.

Wada E et al: Subtotal corpectomy versus laminoplasty for multilevel cervical spondylotic myelopathy: A long-term follow-up study over 10 years. Spine 2001;26:1443. [PMID: 11458148]

Wang MY, Shah S, Green BA: Clinical outcomes following cervical laminoplasty for 204 patients with cervical spondylotic myelopathy. Surg Neurol 2004;62:487. [PMID: 15576110]

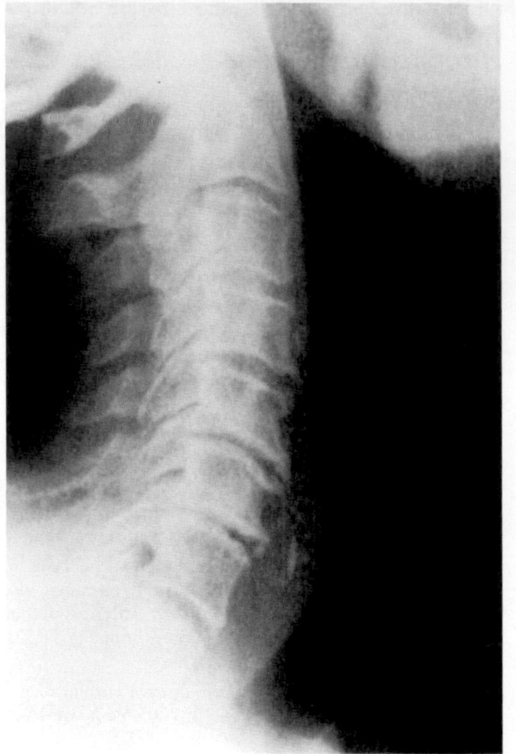

A

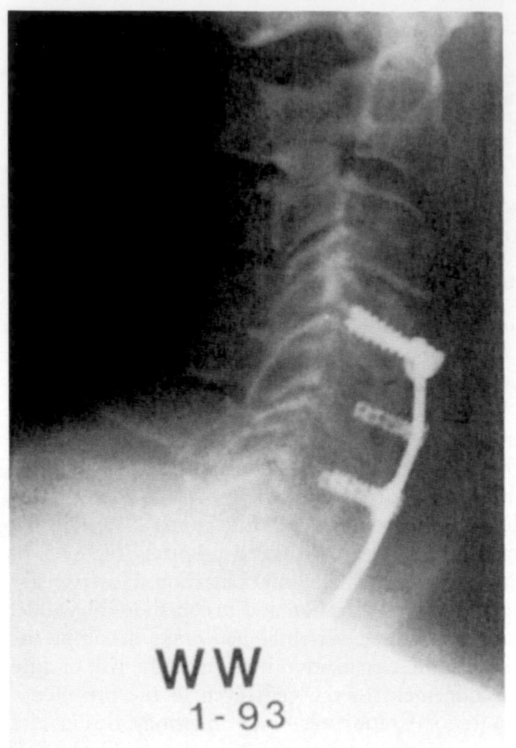

B

WW
1/93

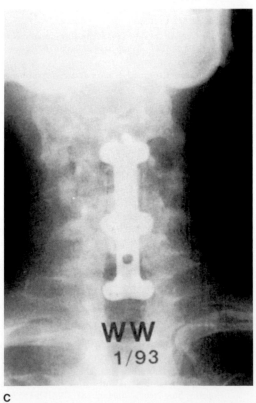

C

Figure 5–8. Imaging studies in a patient with cervical spondylotic myelopathy. **A:** Radiograph showing degenerative changes between C4 and C7. **B** and **C:** Radiographs taken after anterior vertebrectomy of C5 and C6, iliac crest strut graft, and anterior plate fixation.

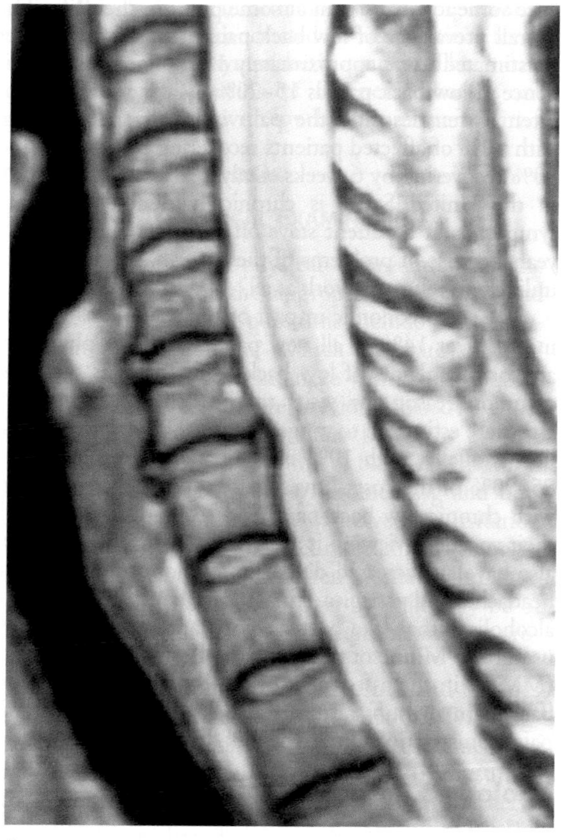

A

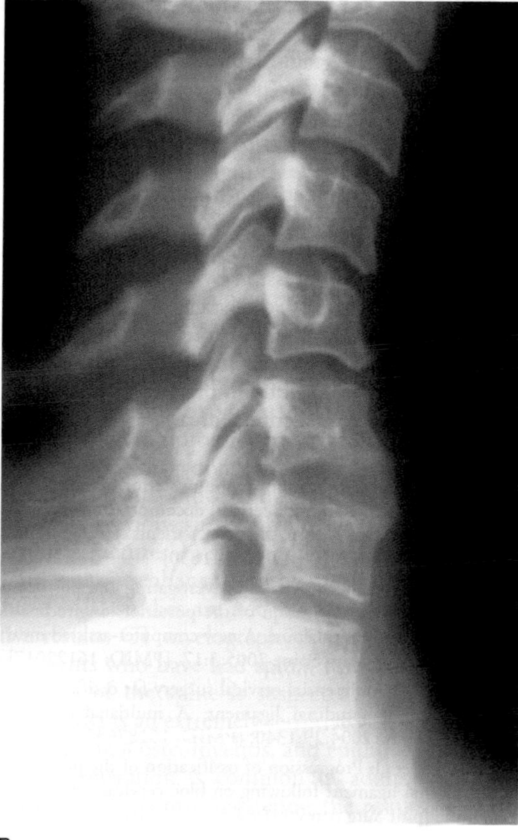

B

Figure 5–9. Imaging studies in a patient with cervical disk herniation. **A:** MRI showing herniation at C6-C7. **B:** Radiograph taken after anterior cervical fusion with a tricortical graft from the pelvis.

OSSIFICATION OF THE POSTERIOR LONGITUDINAL LIGAMENT

Ossification of the posterior longitudinal ligament (OPLL) is a relatively common cause of spinal canal stenosis and myelopathy in the Asian population. Its overall incidence is 2–3% in Japan, compared with 0.6% in Hawaii and 1.7% in Italy. Males are affected more often than females, and the peak age at onset of symptoms is the sixth decade. Although the cause of the disorder is unknown, it may be controlled by autosomal dominant inheritance because it is found in 26% of the parents and 29% of the siblings of affected patients. The disorder is associated with several rheumatic conditions, including diffuse idiopathic skeletal hyperostosis (DISH), spondylosis, and ankylosing spondylitis.

Clinical Findings

Almost all patients have only mild subjective complaints at the onset, although 10–15% of them complain of clumsiness and spastic gait. Nevertheless, minor trauma can lead to acute deterioration of symptoms and can result in quadriplegia. Spastic quadriparesis is the most common neurologic presentation.

Ossification of the posterior longitudinal ligament can easily be diagnosed on plain lateral radiographs. The levels most frequently involved are C4, C5, and C6. A segmental type of disorder is distinguished from the continuous, local, and mixed type on the basis of the distribution of lesions behind the vertebral bodies. CT scanning is helpful in assessing the thickness, lateral extension, and AP diameter of the ossified ligament. More than 95% of the ossification is localized in the cervical spine, although extension into the thoracic spine is reported to be a cause of persistent myelopathy following cervical decompression.

Enchondral ossification is mainly responsible for the formation of the ossified mass, which connects to the upper and lower margins of the vertebral bodies. In many cases, the ossified material is closely adherent to

Pathophysiology

Some physiologic narrowing of the canal occurs with age. There are also normal variations in the cross-sectional areas and shapes of the lumbar spinal canal, with the narrowest area found between L2 and L4. The canal volume increases in flexion and decreases in extension. Narrowing of the spinal canal can further occur by bulging of the disk anteriorly, by buckling of the ligamentum flavum posteriorly, and by encroachment of the articular facets. Degeneration of the intervertebral disk causes increased stress on the facet joint and can lead to arthrosis and hypertrophy of facets and adjacent structures. This ultimately compromises the spinal canal. The decrease in canal volume occurs at such a slow and gradual pace that the neurologic structures in most patients accommodate to it, with the result that there may be surprisingly few neurologic symptoms even in patients with advanced degenerative stenosis.

The cause of pain experienced by patients with stenosis is perplexing and is attributed to mechanical, ischemic, inflammatory, and various other mechanisms. The simplest explanation, of course, is pure mechanical compression of cord and adjacent roots. The hourglass configuration and bulging of the dura as it is decompressed attests to the increased pressures within the stenotic canal. According to the neuroischemic explanation, the nerve fibers are nutritionally deprived by compression of the small nutrient vessels. Inflammatory conditions of the dura and exiting nerve roots are equally suspect. Common surgical findings are an adhesive arachnoiditis of the pia and the presence of friction neuritis, and these may constrict or tether the neural elements. The hypertrophic membranes also have reduced permeability and may obstruct the free flow of cerebrospinal fluid (CSF) from perfusing the root tissues. This can compromise the metabolism of nerve fibers because nearly 50% of their nutrients are derived from CSF.

According to a vascular and nutritional explanation for the onset of pseudoclaudication, the nerve fibers in the resting state diminish metabolic requirements that enable them to conduct sufficient impulses for minimal activity of the muscles. With increases in exertion, however, the metabolic requirements of the compromised nerve rise rapidly. The tension of root fixation and the reduced permeability to CSF hamper the delivery of necessary nutrients and the removal of noxious accumulations. The resulting relative neuroischemia renders the nerve more mechanosensitive, causing ectopic impulses to be conducted and to produce pain, paresthesias, and pseudoclaudication.

Gross morphologic changes include a compressed caudal sac, diffuse ligamentous and facet joint hypertrophy, disk space narrowing with or without concomitant protrusion, encroachment of the lamina, and occasional degenerative olisthesis. Microscopic changes include quantitative losses of neurons with numerous empty axons, various degrees of demyelinization, diffuse interstitial fibrosis with venous congestion, and coiled arterial "pigtails" on either side of the compressed lesion.

Classification

Spinal stenosis is classified as congenital or acquired. The congenital type is caused by developmental spinal anomalies that compromise the neural elements. This type is seen, for example, in patients with achondroplasia (Figure 5–11). The acquired type is more common and further divided into the degenerative, olisthetic-scoliotic, posttraumatic, and postoperative subtypes. Although the original shape of the spinal canal may be round, oval, or trefoil, the trefoil shape is most commonly associated with stenosis and may be a predisposing factor.

The location of stenosis can be central or lateral. In central stenosis, hypertrophied structures cause circumferential pressure of the spinal cord. Lateral stenosis is associated with narrowing of the foraminal canal, which is divided into three separate zones: the entrance zone, the middle zone, and the exit zone.

Clinical Findings

A. Symptoms and Signs

In degenerative spinal stenosis, which occurs primarily in elderly (more than 70 years) individuals and is seen more commonly in men than in women, the lower lumbar segments are affected the most severely. The

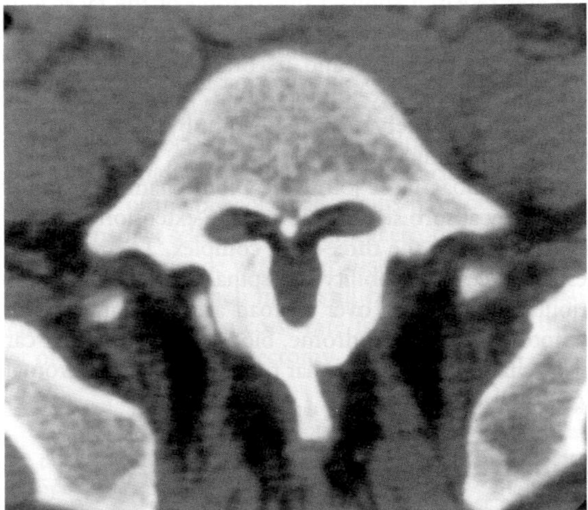

Figure 5–11. CT scan showing severe stenosis and typical trefoil shape of the lumbar spine in a patient with achondroplasia.

pattern of complaints varies among patients. In many cases, there is an insidious onset and slow progression of pain in the lower back, buttock, and thigh. The pain is generally diffuse rather than neurosegmental and is episodic. Nearly all patients report that their lower extremity pain is altered by changes in position. It generally occurs with standing or walking and is relieved by rest, lying, sitting, or adopting a position of flexion at the waist. In addition, patients may find it easier to walk uphill (when their trunk is flexed) than downhill (when their trunk is extended). They may also have greater walking tolerance pushing a shopping cart because they are able to ambulate in a more flexed position. These are the hallmarks of pseudoclaudication. Neurogenic and vascular claudication may be difficult to distinguish from each other. Thus, all patients should have their distal pulses examined as a part of the overall neurologic evaluation. Mistaken diagnoses are not uncommon.

In a study of 172 patients who had symptoms of claudication, were found on myelogram and CT to have lumbar stenosis, and were treated operatively, investigators found that 65% of the patients demonstrated objective weakness and 25% exhibited diminished deep tendon reflexes. Only 10% had positive results in the straight leg–raising test, indicating entrapment of a nerve root. Nine patients had peripheral vascular disease identified by ultrasound and arteriography, and six of these nine required additional vascular bypass surgery for persistent symptoms of lower extremity claudication.

B. Imaging Studies

Findings on plain radiographs include degenerative disk disease, osteoarthritis of the facets, spondylolisthesis, and narrowing of the interpedicular distance as seen on the AP view. Although myelography was commonly used in the past to evaluate spinal cord or root compression, it is an invasive procedure with possible side effects and no longer used routinely. CT scanning is commonly used to evaluate the spinal elements and allows for accurate measurement of the canal dimensions when combined with contrast enhancement. A dural sac with an anteroposterior diameter of less than 10 mm correlates with clinical findings of stenosis.

MRI is comparable to contrast-enhanced CT scanning in its ability to demonstrate spinal stenosis and is now the imaging modality of choice to assess the spinal canal and the neural structures. (Figure 5–12).

Differential Diagnosis

A complete physical examination is essential to exclude other causes of referred pain in the low back, such as retroperitoneal tumors, aortic aneurysms, peptic ulcer disease, renal lesions, and pathologic processes of the hips or pelvis.

Psychologic factors of low back pain often give rise to symptoms independent of spinal canal narrowing and can lead to confusing differential diagnoses. Depression is common in the elderly (more than 70 years), and prompt recognition and treatment of underlying depression as the cause of somatic complaints may result in marked diminution of symptoms.

Treatment

A. Conservative Treatment

Initial management of the patient with symptoms suggestive of spinal stenosis should consist of salicylates or nonsteroidal agents and an exercise program tailored to the patient's goals or lifestyle. Surprisingly, many patients show an appreciable response to this form of treatment. Narcotics may induce dependency and should be avoided. Epidural corticosteroid injections have a short-term success rate of 50% and a long-term success rate of 25%.

B. Surgical Treatment

If conservative methods fail, the patient's quality of life must be a key factor in deciding when to proceed with surgery. Decompressive laminectomy has a short-term success rate between 71% and 85%. Approximately 17% of older patients require reoperation for recurrent stenosis or instability. The disk should be preserved under any circumstances, to avoid postoperative instability. The best surgical results are seen in patients without coexisting morbid conditions (Figure 5–13).

Postoperative instability is reported in approximately 10–15% of patients treated. Preoperative risk factors for developing instability include disk space narrowing, osteoporosis, preexisting spondylolisthesis, and multilevel decompression. Late instability can occur when 50% of bilateral facets were resected, or when 100% of one facet joint was resected. In these cases, a prophylactic instrumented lateral fusion should be performed.

Atlas SJ et al: Long-term outcomes of surgical and nonsurgical management of lumbar spinal stenosis: 8 to 10 year results from the Maine lumbar spine study. Spine 2005;30:936. [PMID: 15834339]

Chang Y et al: The effect of surgical and nonsurgical treatment on longitudinal outcomes of lumbar spinal stenosis over 10 years. J Am Geriatr Soc 2005;53:785. [PMID: 15877553]

Galiano K et al: Long-term outcome of laminectomy for spinal stenosis in octogenarians. Spine 2005;30:332. [PMID: 15682015]

Ghiselli G et al: Adjacent segment degeneration in the lumbar spine. J Bone Joint Surg Am 2004;86:1497. [PMID: 15252099]

Ikuta K et al: Short-term results of microendoscopic posterior decompression for lumbar spinal stenosis. Technical note. J Neurosurg Spine 2005;2:624. [PMID: 15945442]

Knaub MA et al: Lumbar spinal stenosis: Indications for arthrodesis and spinal instrumentation. Instr Course Lect 2005;54: 313. [PMID: 15948459]

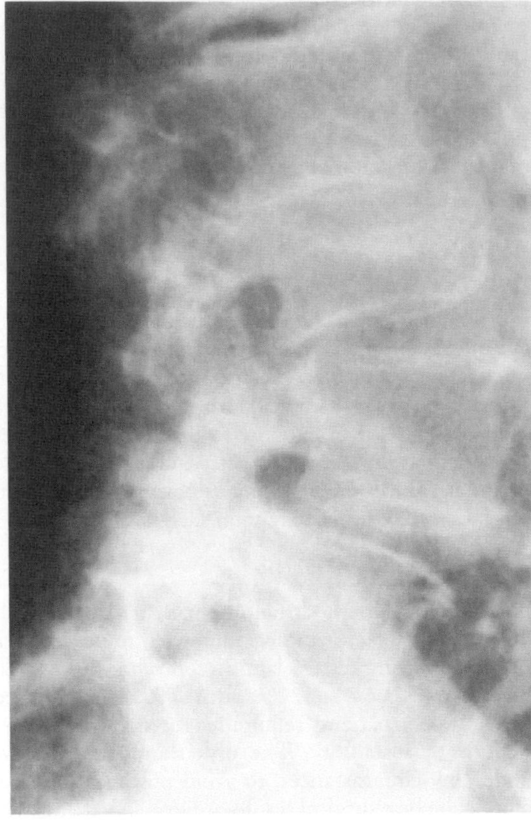

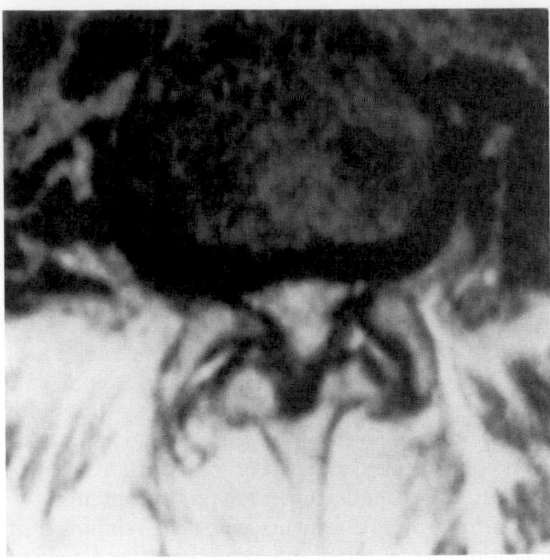

A

B

Figure 5–12. Imaging studies in a patient with degenerative stenosis of the lumbar spine. **A:** Radiograph showing degenerative spondylolisthesis between L4 and L5, as well as an old compression fracture of L3. **B:** MRI showing severe stenosis of the spinal canal at L4-L5, marked facet hypertrophy and ligamentous hypertrophy resulting in central canal stenosis, and lateral recess stenosis.

Kornblum MB et al: Degenerative lumbar spondylolisthesis with spinal stenosis: A prospective long-term study comparing fusion and pseudarthrosis. Spine 2004;29:726. [PMID: 15087793]

Lin SI, Lin RM: Disability and walking capacity in patients with lumbar spinal stenosis: Association with sensorimotor function, balance, and functional performance. J Orthop Sports Phys Ther 2005;35:220. [PMID: 15901123]

Palmer S, Turner R, Palmer R: Bilateral decompressive surgery in lumbar spinal stenosis associated with spondylolisthesis: Unilateral approach and use of a microscope and tubular retractor system. Neurosurg Focus 2002;13:E4. [PMID: 12296681]

Saint-Louis LA: Lumbar spinal stenosis assessment with computed tomography, magnetic resonance imaging, and myelography. Clin Orthop 2001;384:122. [PMID: 11249157]

Sengupta DK, Herkowitz HN: Lumbar spinal stenosis. Treatment strategies and indications for surgery. Orthop Clin North Am 2003;4:281. [PMID: 12914268]

Shapiro GS, Taira G, Boachie-Adjei O: Results of surgical treatment of adult idiopathic scoliosis with low back pain and spinal stenosis: A study of long-term clinical radiographic outcomes. Spine 2003;28:358. [PMID: 12590210]

Simotas AC: Nonoperative treatment for lumbar spinal stenosis. Clin Orthop 2001;384:153. [PMID: 11249160]

Truumees E: Spinal stenosis: Pathophysiology, clinical and radiologic classification. Instr Course Lect 2005;54:287. [PMID: 15948457]

Yuan PS, Booth RE Jr, Albert TJ: Nonsurgical and surgical management of lumbar spinal stenosis. Instr Course Lect 2005;54:303. [PMID: 15948458]

OSTEOPOROSIS AND VERTEBRAL COMPRESSION FRACTURES

Osteoporosis is characterized by a decline in overall bone mass in the axial and appendicular skeleton. The disease affects between 15 and 20 million people in the United States. Peak bone mass, attained between 16 and 25 years of age, slowly declines with age as the rate

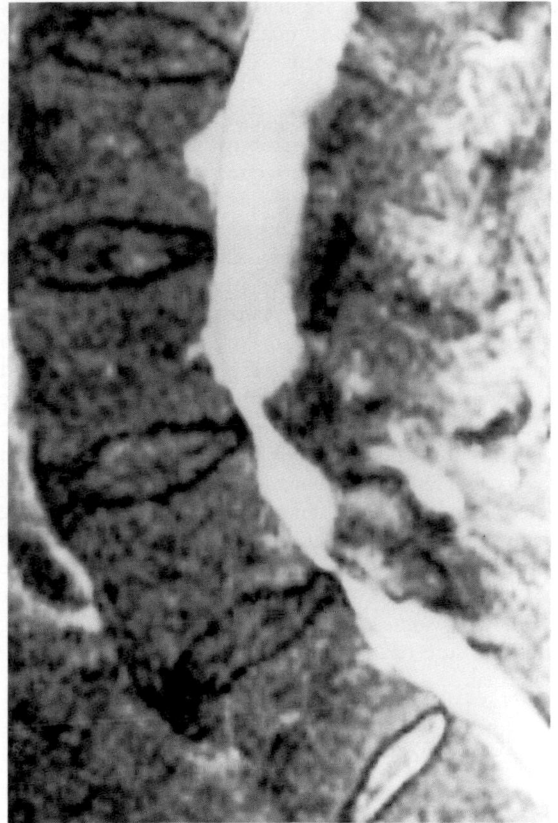

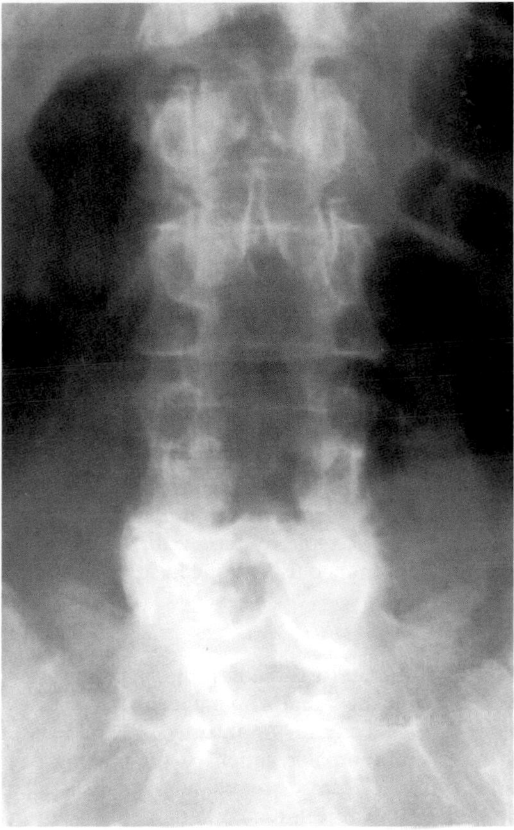

A B

Figure 5–13. Imaging studies in a patient with stenosis of the lumbar spine and leg pain. **A:** MRI showing stenosis at L3-L4. **B:** Radiograph taken after two-level laminectomy, which led to resolution of the preoperative leg pain.

of bone resorption exceeds that of bone formation. This phenomenon occurs in both men and women and is known as senile osteoporosis. Women are also susceptible to postmenopausal osteoporosis that occurs during the 15–20 years after the onset of menopause and is directly linked to estrogen deficiency. Environmental factors also play a role in accelerating the rate of skeletal bone loss. These include chronic calcium deficiency, smoking, excessive alcohol intake, hyperparathyroidism, and inactivity. Genetic influences may also play a role.

Vertebral compression fractures are one of the most frequent manifestations of osteoporosis in the elderly (more than 60 years). Over 700,000 vertebral compression fractures occur each year. Fortunately, the overwhelming majority of patients are asymptomatic.

Clinical Findings

Patients with symptomatic vertebral compression fractures typically complain of axial pain localized to the fractured level. Occasionally, the patient's family notices that the patient's back is becoming increasingly rounded and significant loss of height has occurred. This spinal deformity is known as the dowager's hump. In general, there is no neurologic dysfunction and no radiation of the pain in any dermatomal distribution. There is often no history of significant trauma or an inciting event.

Imaging

Plain radiographs and densitometric scans are the major imaging modalities in the assessment of osteoporotic bone and their pathologic counterparts (insufficiency fractures). Dual-energy x-ray absorptiometry (DXA) is the most useful of the densitometric imaging techniques because it carries a high degree of precision (0.5–2%) and subjects the patient to minimal amounts of radiation. It is also quite accurate for assessment of osteoporosis in both the axial and appendicular skeleton. Other imaging modalities include single-energy x-ray absorptiometry (SXA), quantitative computed tomography (QCT), and radiographic absorptiometry.

Posterior/anterior and lateral radiographs of the affected area of the spine are likely to reveal the location and severity of the osteoporotic fracture(s). In the thoracic spine, wedge compression fractures are most commonly encountered. In the lumbar spine, both compression and burst fractures can occur. Other imaging modalities include technetium bone scans and MRI scans. These studies should be reserved for the evaluation of fractures that remain symptomatic or progress after a course of conservative treatment. MRI is extremely useful in differentiating nonunited fractures from those that have healed and in differentiating osteoporotic fractures from those caused by malignancy.

Bone biopsy is indicated if a metabolic bone disease or a malignancy is suspected as the cause of the osteoporosis. The sample, typically retrieved from the anterior iliac crest, is examined using bone histomorphometry.

Treatment

Prevention still remains the best treatment for osteoporosis. Maximizing bone mineral density prior to the onset of bone loss and minimizing the bone loss that occurs is the optimal regimen to prevent the painful sequelae of the disease. In women, estrogen replacement therapy can be initiated if there is no history of breast cancer, thromboembolic disease, or endometrial disease. Routine gynecological examination is necessary once therapy is initiated. Calcitonin therapy can be used if estrogen therapy is contraindicated. Parathyroid hormone is currently under clinical trials for the treatment of osteoporosis. Early evidence suggests that it may help to increase skeletal bone mass significantly and may be useful as a first-line treatment for severe osteoporosis.

The bisphosphonates, etidronate and alendronate, prevent osteoclastic resorption of bone. They are the only FDA-approved compounds in widespread use that increase bone mineral density. However, the increase is relatively small.

The initial treatment of symptomatic vertebral compression fractures involves a trial of analgesic therapy and bracing for comfort. Evaluation and treatment for osteoporosis can be initiated if not done already. Conservative therapy should be attempted for at least 6–12 weeks or longer if the patient is improving.

Surgical Treatment

Patients who have fractures that cause neurologic deficits or significant spinal cord compression should be treated with anterior decompression and fusion followed by posterior segmental instrumentation and fusion. The poor bone quality makes correction of deformity and maintenance of posterior constructs a challenging task.

Patients who have recalcitrant back pain from a nonunited vertebral compression fracture who have failed a course of conservative management can obtain excellent symptomatic relief from fracture stabilization through injection of PMMA bone cement into the fracture through a percutaneous technique. The two most popular procedures, vertebroplasty and kyphoplasty, are both safe and efficacious. In both techniques, a cannula is inserted intrapedicularly or extrapedicularly (lateral to the pedicle) into the anterior portion of the affected vertebral body, and acrylic cement is instilled into the fractured bone under fluoroscopic control. Once the cement cures, the fracture is immediately stabilized. In the kyphoplasty technique, a balloon is inflated in the vertebral body in an attempt to compress the existing bone, create a void for instillation of more viscous cement under lower pressure, and correct the wedge deformity. This technique has the theoretical advantage of allowing some deformity correction and preventing high-pressure-related extrusion of PMMA into the spinal canal.

The mechanism of pain relief achieved through vertebroplasty and kyphoplasty is unclear. Multiple mechanisms may play a role, including fracture stabilization, denervation of pain fibers by the heat generated during the cement curing process, and neurotoxicity of the PMMA monomer. In addition, longer follow-up has raised concerns over predisposing the adjacent segment to fracture by overstiffening the affected level. These concerns are currently under active investigation.

Coumans JV, Reinhardt MK, Lieberman IH: Kyphoplasty for vertebral compression fractures: 1-year clinical outcomes from a prospective study. J Neurosurg 2003;99(Suppl 1):44. [PMID: 12859058]

Diamond TH, Champion B, Clark WA: Management of acute osteoporotic vertebral fractures: A nonrandomized trial comparing percutaneous vertebroplasty with conservative therapy. Am J Med 2003;114:257. [PMID: 12681451]

Do HM et al: Prospective analysis of clinical outcomes after percutaneous vertebroplasty for painful osteoporotic vertebral body fractures. AJNR Am J Neuroradiol 2005;26:1623. [PMID: 16091504]

Grohs JG et al: Minimal invasive stabilization of osteoporotic vertebral fractures: A prospective nonrandomized comparison of vertebroplasty and balloon kyphoplasty. J Spinal Disord Tech 2005;18:238. [PMID: 15905767]

Guglielmi G et al: Percutaneous vertebroplasty: Indications, contraindications, technique, and complications. Acta Radiol 2000;46:256. [PMID: 15981722]

McGraw JK et al: Prospective evaluation of pain relief in 100 patients undergoing percutaneous vertebroplasty: results and follow-up. J Vasc Interv Radiol 2002;13:883. [PMID: 12354821]

Nussbaum DA, Gailloud P, Murphy K: A review of complications associated with vertebroplasty and kyphoplasty as reported to the Food and Drug Administration medical device related web site. J Vasc Interv Radiol 2004;15:1185. [PMID: 15525736]

Phillips FM et al: Minimally invasive treatments of osteoporotic vertebral compression fractures: Vertebroplasty and kyphoplasty. Instr Course Lect 2003;52:559. Review. [PMID: 12690882]

Steinmann J, Tingey CT, Cruz G et al: Biomechanical comparison of unipedicular versus bipedicular kyphoplasty. Spine 2005; 30:201. [PMID: 15644756]

Uppin AA et al: Occurrence of new vertebral body fracture after percutaneous vertebroplasty in patients with osteoporosis. Radiology 2003;226:119. [PMID: 12511679]

DEFORMITIES OF THE SPINE

SCOLIOSIS

Scoliosis is an abnormal curvature of the spine as viewed in the coronal plane. It is also generally associated with a rotational deformity, and it is the rotational component, manifested as a rib hump, prominent scapula, waist asymmetry, or lumbar fullness, that is most likely to call attention to the spinal curvature.

Etiology, Classification, & Pathophysiology

Scoliosis is classified according to its cause, with the most common causes summarized in Table 5–1. For example, if the curvature is secondary to a structural bony abnormality, it is described as congenital scoliosis. If it is caused by a neurologic disturbance or muscle disease (myopathy), it is described as neuromuscular scoliosis. If no cause can be determined, it is described as idiopathic scoliosis. The idiopathic type is the most common. Proposed etiologies for idiopathic scoliosis include abnormalities in melatonin, growth hormone or other hormones, platelet abnormalities, and posterior column abnormalities (ie, impaired proprioception and vibratory sensibility.

Particularly in idiopathic cases, scoliosis can also be classified according to the patient's age at onset. The age ranges for infantile, juvenile, adolescent, and adult scoliosis are shown in Table 5–1. Many surgeons consider juvenile scoliosis not to be a true separate entity, but rather a mix of late-presenting infantile scoliosis and early-developing adolescent scoliosis.

The curvature is named according to the side of the convexity, as well as the level of the apex, which is the most rotated vertebral body in the curve. For a cervical curve, the apex is at C1 through C6; for a cervicothoracic curve, C7 through T1; for a thoracic curve, T2 through T11; for a thoracolumbar curve, T12 or L1; for a lumbar curve, L2 through L4; and for a lumbosacral curve, L5 or lower.

The most common types of curves in cases of idiopathic scoliosis are the right thoracic curve, followed by the double curve (right thoracic and left lumbar) and the right thoracolumbar curve. The primary curve or curves are considered structural. A secondary curve, known as a compensatory curve, permits the head to be centered over the pelvis. Compensatory curves are of lesser magnitude, more flexible, and less rotated; when

Table 5–1. Classification of scoliosis by cause.

- I. Idiopathic scoliosis
  - A. Infantile (under 3 years of age)
  - B. Juvenile (from 3 to 10 years of age)
  - C. Adolescent (from 10 years of age to skeletal maturity)
  - D. Adult
- II. Neuromuscular scoliosis
  - A. Neuropathic
    - 1. Upper motor neuron
      - a. Cerebral palsy
      - b. Charcot-Marie-Tooth disease
      - c. Syringomyelia
      - d. Spinal cord trauma
    - 2. Lower motor neuron
      - a. Poliomyelitis
      - b. Spinal muscular atrophy
      - c. Myelomeningocele
  - B. Myopathic
    - 1. Arthrogryposis
    - 2. Muscular dystrophy
- III. Congenital scoliosis
  - A. Failure of formation
  - B. Failure of segmentation
  - C. Mixed failure of formation and segmentation
- IV. Neurofibromatosis
- V. Connective tissue scoliosis
  - A. Marfan syndrome
  - B. Ehlers-Danlos syndrome
- VI. Osteochondrodystrophy
  - A. Diastrophic dwarfism
  - B. Mucopolysaccharidosis
  - C. Spondyloepiphyseal dysplasia
  - D. Multiple epiphyseal dysplasia
  - E. Achondrodysplasia
- VII. Metabolic scoliosis
- VIII. Nonstructural scoliosis
  - A. Postural, hysterical
  - B. Secondary to nerve root irritation

Modified and reproduced, with permission, from Winter RB: Classification and terminology of scoliosis. In Lonstein JE et al, eds: *Moe's Textbook of Scoliosis and Other Spinal Deformities,* 3rd ed. WB Saunders, 1994.

they become less flexible and rotation is evident, it may be difficult to determine which curve is the primary one, and indeed they may be considered structural.

The natural history of spinal curvatures is affected by factors such as the magnitude of the curve, the age of the patient, and the underlying cause of the problem. With curve progression, the deformity can become severe, leading in some cases to a so-called razor-back deformity secondary to rib rotation. With thoracic curves measuring more than 60–90 degrees (depending on the chest anterior-posterior dimension), cardiopulmonary function can become compromised, and a secondary restrictive lung disease may result from the chest deformity. Curve progression is most common during continued skeletal growth; however, it is now evident that moderate curves of 40–50 degrees should be observed for progression in adulthood. Although the extent of progression in adulthood varies widely among patients, the average amount is 1 degree per year. Taking radiographs every 2–5 years appears to be satisfactory for adults who have idiopathic scoliosis without other clinical signs of progression. The likelihood of progression is greater in patients whose scoliosis is associated with conditions such as neurofibromatosis or connective tissue diseases, including Marfan syndrome and Ehlers-Danlos syndrome.

Principles of Diagnosis

A. History and Physical Examination

In a patient with a spine deformity, the history should include the age when the deformity was first noted; the manner in which it was noted (by the patient or family member, by the pediatrician or other health professional during examination or school screening, etc.); the perinatal history; developmental milestones; other illnesses; and family history of scoliosis or other diseases that may affect the musculoskeletal system. Although the incidence of scoliosis in the general population is approximately 1%, the incidence is greater in the children of women with scoliosis and particularly in the daughters of these women. For this reason, the children of women with scoliosis should be screened repeatedly throughout their preadolescent and adolescent years. Idiopathic scoliosis of the adolescent type (see Table 5–1) is more common in females, whereas that of the infantile type is more common in males.

In children and adolescents, the curvature is generally not painful. If the patient complains of pain, appropriate diagnostic tests should be performed to determine whether the curvature is secondary to the presence of a bony or spinal tumor, herniated disk, or other abnormality.

The patient's skin, habitus, and back should be carefully inspected. The presence of café au lait spots, skin tags, or axillary freckles is suggestive of neurofibromatosis. The presence of hairy patches or dimples over the spine is suggestive of spinal dysraphism. Numerous clinical syndromes are associated with scoliosis (see Table 5–1), and some of these include unusual facies. Tall, long-limbed patients may have Marfan syndrome and should be examined for high-arched palate, cardiac murmur, and dislocated lenses. Dwarfs have a high incidence of spinal deformity, both kyphosis (see section on kyphosis) and scoliosis, as well as spinal instability.

In patients with scoliosis, the shoulders or pelvis may not be level, or waist asymmetry may be noted. Most commonly, these patients have scapular prominence, with rotational deformity and rib prominence. The rib hump, or the lumbar prominence of a lumbar curve, can be accentuated by having the patient lean forward from the waist, permitting the arms to hang down; the examiner then views the spine from above or below (Figure 5–14). The rib hump can be quantified by direct measurement of its height or by using a scoliometer, which permits measurement of angular deformity. Also important in the patient's examination is measurement of decompensation, if present. This can be deter-

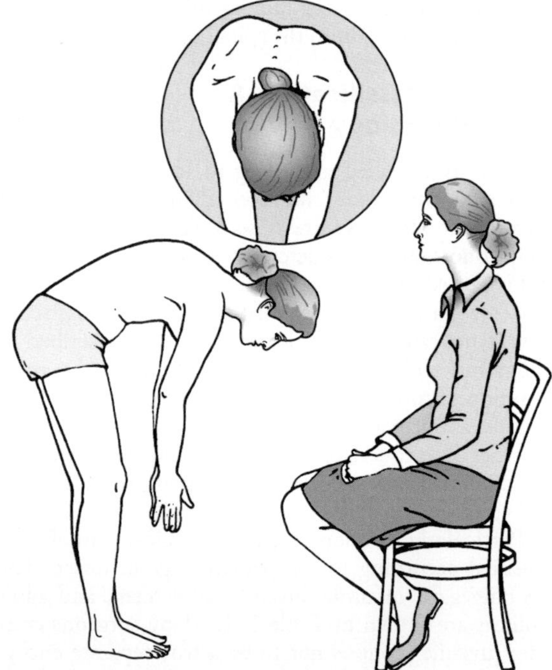

Figure 5–14. **The rotational deformity of scoliosis is manifested by a rib hump, which is accentuated by having the patient bend forward.** (Reproduced, with permission, from Day LJ et al: Orthopedics. In Way LW, ed: *Current Surgical Diagnosis & Treatment*, 9th ed. Stamford: Appleton & Lange, 1991.)

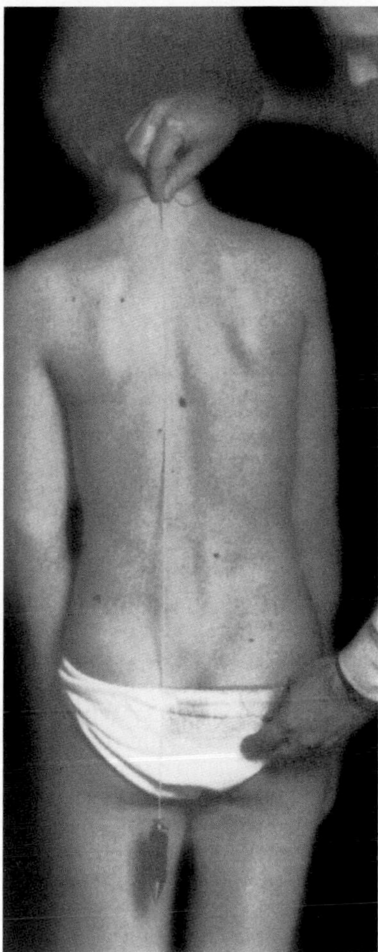

Figure 5–15. Use of a plumb bob to measure coronal decompensation in a patient with scoliosis. (Reproduced, with permission, from McCarthy RE: Evaluation of the patient with deformity. In Weinstein SL, ed: *The Pediatric Spine*. Raven, 1994.)

mined by dropping a plumb bob from the prominence of the C7 spinous process and measuring where it falls with respect to the gluteal line (Figure 5–15).

Flexibility of the curve can be qualitatively assessed by having the patient bend in the direction that effects curve correction. The spinous processes within the curve as well as the rib hump can then be assessed for flexibility of the deformity.

B. Neurologic Tests

Patients should demonstrate a normal gait and be able to walk on their toes and heels, unless other concomitant conditions are present. Motor and sensory testing of the lower extremities should be performed, and testing of the upper extremities should also be done if the curve pattern is atypical or if a neuromuscular condition is suspected. Reflexes should be tested, and the presence of asymmetry or a pathologic reflex (eg, clonus, a positive Babinski sign, or a positive Hoffmann sign) should be noted and suggest a nonidiopathic etiology.

An asymmetric abdominal reflex is the most common neurologic abnormality noted with an intracanal lesion, such as a syrinx, diastematomyelia, or spinal cord tumor. The abdominal reflex is assessed by gently scratching each of the four quadrants of the abdomen, just a few centimeters away from the umbilicus. The response is considered normal if the umbilicus moves slightly toward the direction scratched.

Abnormal neurologic test results are an indication for further workup, such as a spine MRI, particularly if the patient has an atypical curve (eg, a left thoracic curve) or a rapidly progressive spinal deformity.

C. Imaging Studies

AP and lateral radiographs of the entire length of the spine should be taken, and this generally requires the use of an extra-long x-ray cassette. When the radiographs are taken, the patient should be in the standing position. If neuromuscular problems make it impossible for the patient to stand, however, radiographs can be taken with the patient sitting. Curves are measured using the Cobb method, as shown in Figure 5–16.

Views taken with the patient bending away from the concavity may be helpful or necessary, particularly if levels for fusion are being selected. These bend views allow for the assessment of the maximal correction of the curve. For curves measuring greater than 90 degrees or if the patient cannot perform the bending movement, traction films can be obtained by having two assistants exert longitudinal traction on the patient, either by grasping the legs and arms or via application of a head halter.

For severe curves (more than 90 degrees), the rotational deformity of the spine may distort the detail on an AP view. For this reason, a special Stagnara view should be obtained. The x-ray cassette is positioned parallel to the rib hump, and the x-ray beam is directed perpendicular to this to obtain an AP view of the spine, rather than of the patient (Figure 5–17).

For patients with abnormal results in the neurologic examination, atypical curve patterns, rapidly progressive curvatures, or congenital scoliosis, evaluation of the spinal canal is indicated. MRI or myelograms with CT scanning can be used. For young patients, sedation is often required. The radiologist should be advised to look for the following: a syrinx (a fluid-filled cyst within the spinal cord); a tethered cord (a fibrous band that is located distally and can prevent the normal cephalad migration of

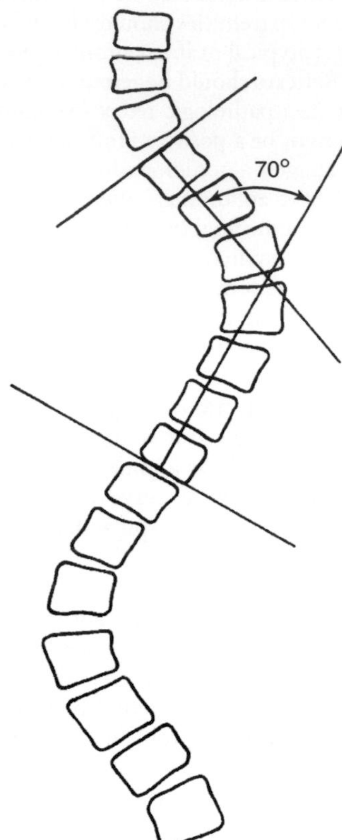

Figure 5–16. Use of the Cobb method to measure the scoliotic curve. First, lines are drawn along the endplates of the upper and lower vertebrae that are maximally tilted into the concavity of the curve. Next, a perpendicular line is drawn to each of the earlier-drawn lines. The angle of intersection is the Cobb angle. (Reproduced, with permission, from Day LJ et al: Orthopedics. In Way LW, ed: *Current Surgical Diagnosis & Treatment,* 9th ed. Stamford: Appleton & Lange, 1991.)

the cord); a diastematomyelia (a bony or fibrous defect that divides the spinal cord and may cause a tether); or a diplomyelia (a reduplication of the spinal cord).

D. Other Studies

If the patient has a finding of intracanal abnormalities, particularly if surgical correction of the deformity is contemplated, neurosurgical evaluation may be indicated. In many cases, the release of a tethered cord or decompression of a syrinx can be performed prior to or at the same time as the scoliosis surgery.

Patients with curves greater than 60 degrees, those with respiratory complaints, and those with scoliosis resulting from a neuromuscular cause should undergo pulmonary function testing, particularly if surgery is being considered. In cases in which pulmonary function test values are less than 30% of predicted values based on the age, sex, and size of the patient, some clinicians recommend an aggressive approach with preoperative tracheostomy placement. We prefer, however, to caution patients about the possibility of tracheostomy placement if postoperative weaning from the respirator is prolonged, and we have rarely found tracheostomy to be necessary.

Principles of Treatment

Although general principles of treatment are discussed here, additional details about treatment of idiopathic scoliosis in adults, neuromuscular scoliosis, neurofibromatosis, and congenital scoliosis are given in subsequent sections of this chapter.

A. Conservative Treatment

Mild curves (less than 20 degrees) can generally be managed conservatively. In most cases, curves less than 10 degrees require observation only, except in very young patients who have neuromuscular scoliosis and a high risk of progression in their collapsing-type curves.

Although some skeletally immature patients with curves greater than 20 degrees require bracing, others do not. If an adolescent has less than 2 years of skeletal growth remaining, has not demonstrated progression,

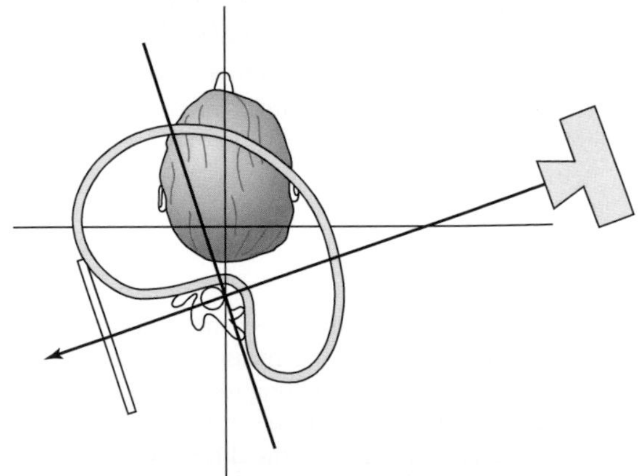

Figure 5–17. In cases of severe curvature, the x-ray beam and cassette are positioned as shown to obtain an anteroposterior view of the curve itself, rather than of the patient. This view is known as the Stagnara view. (Reproduced, with permission, from Lonstein JE: Patient evaluation. In Bradford DS et al, eds: *Moe's Textbook of Scoliosis and Other Spinal Deformities,* 2nd ed. WB Saunders, 1987.)

and has a curve that is still less than 30 degrees, the clinician may consider observation even at this point; however, considerations such as rotational deformity or a positive family history may suggest a more aggressive treatment for certain patients in this group. Any skeletally immature patient with a significant curve who shows progression of the curvature should be referred to an orthopedic surgeon with experience in treating scoliosis for possible brace treatment. Because the error of measurement of the Cobb angle is 3–5 degrees, progression of more than 5 degrees is considered significant.

Several types of braces are available for the treatment of scoliosis. The Milwaukee brace, which is also called the **cervical thoracolumbosacral orthosis,** can be used for nearly all curvatures, but its high profile makes it less desirable, particularly for a self-conscious adolescent. This brace (Figure 5–18) has a pelvic mold to which upright metal struts are attached. The struts are then joined to a neck ring. Corrective pads can be fastened to the metal struts, applying pressure to the rib at the apex of the convexity. If shoulder asymmetry is significant, a shoulder ring can be applied.

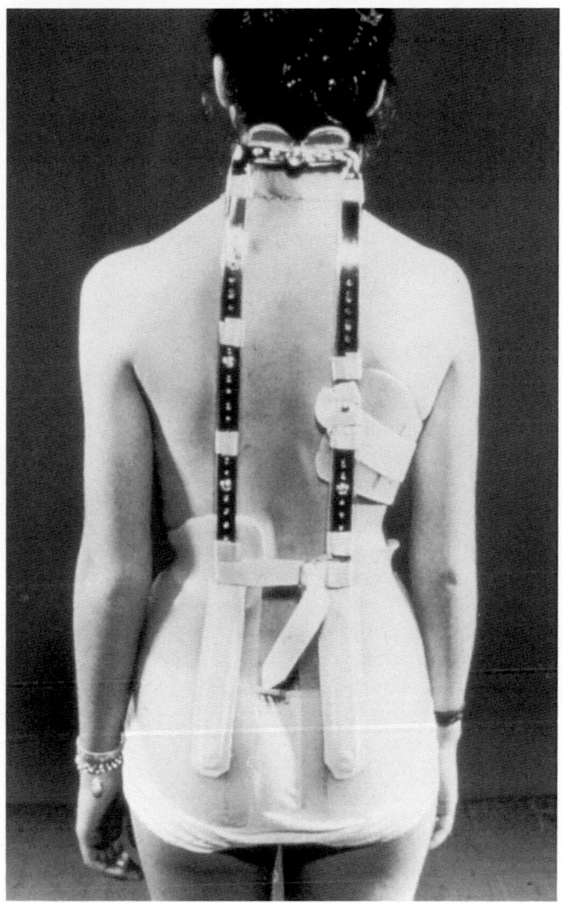

Figure 5–18. The Milwaukee brace, which is also known as the cervical thoracolumbosacral orthosis (CTLSO), can be used to treat scoliosis.

The thoracolumbosacral orthosis is a more cosmetically acceptable brace, but its use is limited to patients whose curves have an apex at T8 or below. The thoracolumbosacral orthosis is an external shell orthosis that is generally constructed of copolymer (largely polypropylene but with a small portion of polyethylene to prevent cracking). The shell is molded to the patient, and corrective pads are placed. One pad applies pressure at the apical rib, at the most prominent area. A second pad can be applied over the lumbar prominence if a double-curve pattern is present. If the patient shows significant decompensation to the left or right, a trochanteric extension can be included on that side to correct this tendency.

Because of the corrective forces being placed posteriorly, bracing may aggravate thoracic lordosis. For this reason, particular care should be made to place pads as laterally as possible. A decrease of normal thoracic kyphosis is common in idiopathic scoliosis and in fact contributes to the cardiovascular problems seen in patients because of the resultant decreased AP diameter of the thoracic cage.

For isolated lumbar curves, a lumbosacral orthosis can be used (Figure 5–19). Although the Boston brace is the most well-known type of lumbosacral orthosis, others are available. The various types of lumbosacral orthosis all use the corrective effect of flattening of lumbar lordosis to facilitate curve correction.

Although braces are designed to apply corrective forces to the spinal curvature and corrective effects are frequently noted on follow-up radiographs taken with the patient in the brace, braces do not afford long-term correction. Success may be achieved in preventing curve progression during the growth period of the patient and improvement may even be noted, but the curvature generally returns to the preorthotic level of severity.

Unlike most braces, the Charleston night bending brace is worn only during the night. When this brace was used in the treatment of idiopathic scoliosis, with patients braced in maximal correction only at night, early results suggested that it was as effective as full-time brace wear; however, most of the patients had not yet achieved skeletal maturity.

Infants may require casting for management of severe curves. When the patients become large enough in size, a Milwaukee brace may be used.

Patients who are wearing braces for the treatment of scoliosis should be reexamined at intervals ranging from 4 to 6 months, depending on how close they are to their growth spurt. Some clinicians prefer that patients

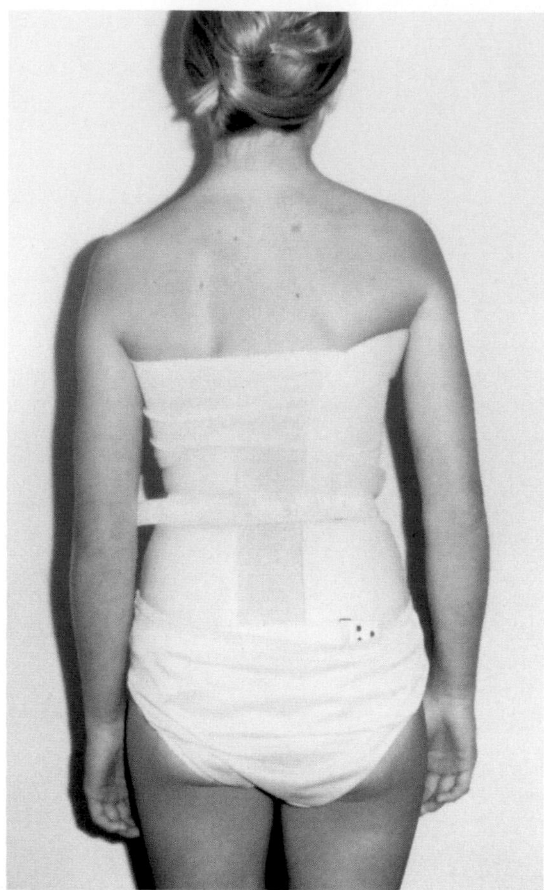

Figure 5–19. The underarm brace, which is also known as the lumbosacral orthosis (LSO), can be used to treat lumbar scoliosis.

wear their braces during follow-up radiographs, but others prefer that the braces be removed on the day of the office visit and while radiographs are taken. Generally, it is felt that full-time brace wear (23 hours a day) is best, and some studies indicate that compliance with brace wear is correlated with the success of braces. Patients may be permitted to remove the brace during athletic activities. As children grow, corrective pads may not be applying force at the appropriate area, which should be checked clinically as well as with confirming radiographs where appropriate.

If an idiopathic curvature can be controlled with bracing, bracing should be continued until the end of skeletal growth. This progress can be assessed clinically by measuring the patient's height during each office visit as well as by following the patient's history (in female patients, for example, growth generally continues for approximately 2 years after menarche). Skeletal growth can be assessed radiographically by evaluating the iliac apophysis (Risser sign, as shown in Figure 5–20) or by taking radiographs of the various physes in the wrist and comparing them with radiographs published in *Gruelich and Pyle's Radiographic Atlas of Skeletal Development of the Hand and Wrist.* Weaning from the brace can be begun as the patient nears the end of skeletal growth. Depending on the severity of the final curvature, follow-up radiographs may be necessary to assess the loss of correction. Some loss of correction should be expected; again, it is important not to anticipate permanent curve correction.

B. Surgical Treatment

Curves greater than 40 degrees are difficult to control with bracing because of the greater pressures that must be exerted to effect correction. Moreover, curves greater than 50 degrees are at risk for progression, even in adulthood. When conservative treatment is not possible, several options are available for surgical intervention.

Posterior fusion and Harrington rod instrumentation was historically used. This involves placing hooks on a ratcheted rod in distraction at the ends of the curve to be fused and then performing a fusion and bone grafting. Sublaminar wiring, because of the passage of each wire around the lamina and therefore into the spinal canal at each level, carries an

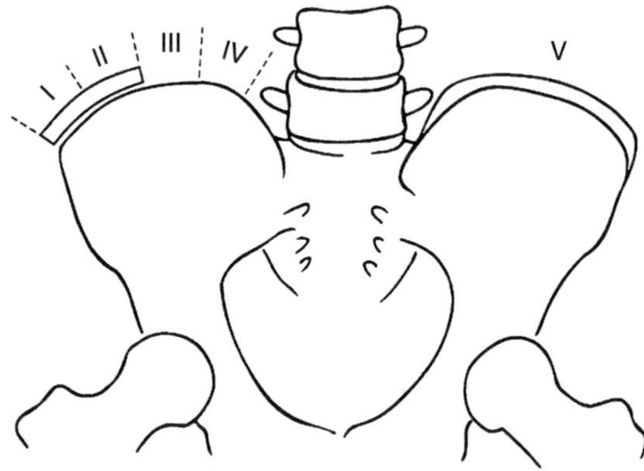

Figure 5–20. The Risser sign for skeletal maturity. The iliac apophysis first appears laterally and grows medially. Risser I is less than 25% ossification; Risser II is 50% ossification; Risser III is 75% ossification; Risser IV is completion of ossification; and Risser V denotes that the apophysis has fused with the iliac crest or complete skeletal maturity has occurred. (Reproduced, with permission, from McCarthy RE: Evaluation of the patient with deformity. In Weinstein SL, ed: *The Pediatric Spine*. Raven, 1994.)

increased risk of neurologic complications but gives better gradual and segmental control. The sublaminar wiring technique is generally reserved for neuromuscular scoliosis patients because of the need for better fixation in the generally osteoporotic bone, as well as for other patients who may have significant osteoporosis, such as older patients (more than 60 years).

Currently, variable hook-rod systems permit placement of hooks or screws at multiple selected sites

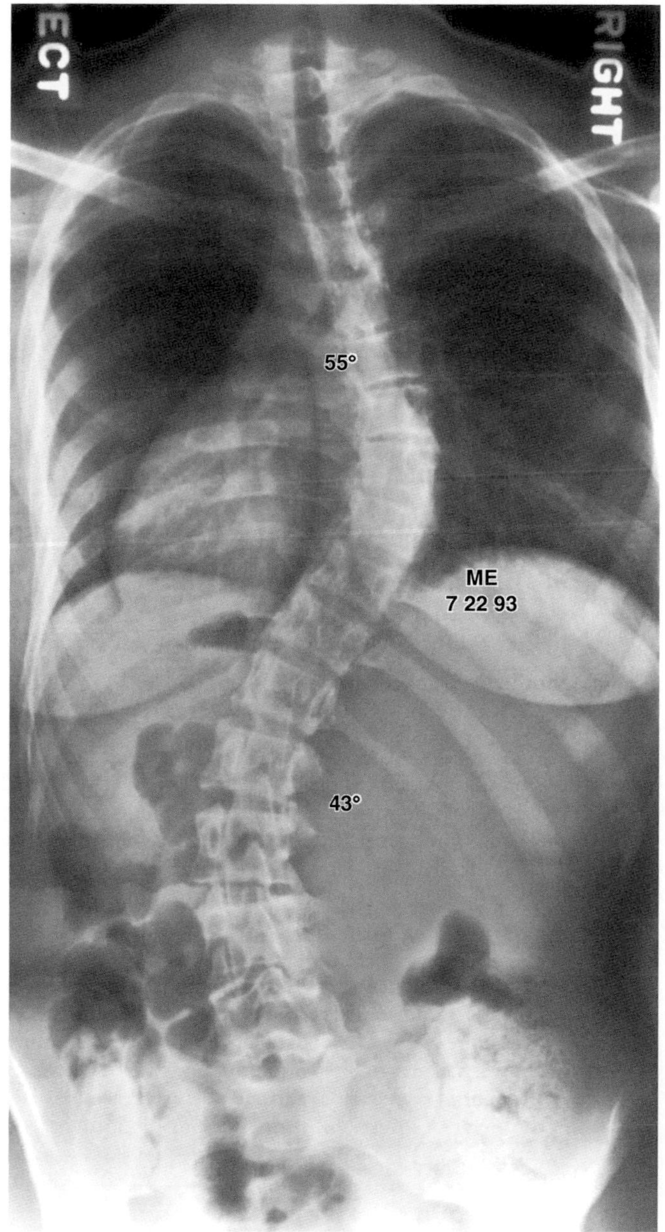

A

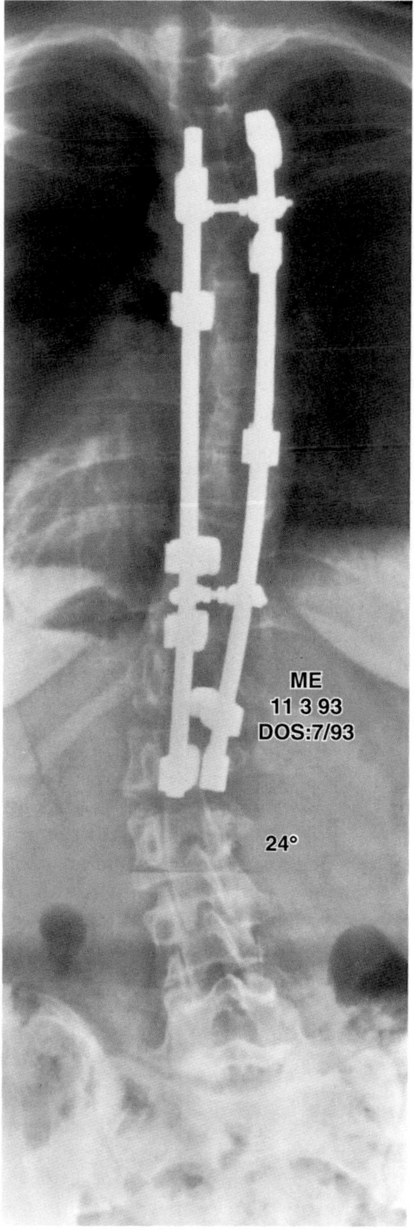

B

Figure 5–21. Imaging studies in a patient with scoliosis. **A:** Radiograph showing preoperative curvature. **B:** Radiograph taken after treatment using Cotrel-Dubousset instrumentation.

along the deformity and the application of distraction or compression, as appropriate, to correct the curve (Figure 5–21). Detailed descriptions of the various instrumentation patterns are beyond the scope of this chapter, but the basic principle is to distract on the concavity of a curve and compress across the convexity. The patient's sagittal contours can also be corrected, if needed, by applying compression to decrease kyphosis or maintain lordosis and by applying distraction to increase kyphosis. The sagittal contours can also be improved by carefully bending the rod prior to insertion so that rotation of the rod converts the coronal curve to the sagittal kyphosis if desired. The systems use a concave and a convex rod. These two rods are usually cross-linked, and they provide rigid fixation so that postoperative brace wear is not needed for most young patients.

For more rigid curves, such as may be found in older patients (over 25 years), it may be necessary to perform an anterior release and fusion as well. With an anterior approach, the disk material can be removed completely, gaining additional mobility and correction and, because an anterior fusion is then performed as well, increasing the fusion rate through this region. Additional factors that may suggest the need for anterior release and fusion include rigid kyphosis, prior failed fusion, and the presence of severe spasticity, as found in some cases of neuromuscular scoliosis. When possible, the two operations are performed at the same surgical sitting, which appears to decrease the perioperative complications. Increasing use of pedicle screws throughout the lumbar and thoracic spine appears to decrease need for anterior release and fusion in many cases.

Some single curves, particularly thoracolumbar and lumbar curves, can be treated with an anterior approach rather than with a posterior approach if desired by the surgeon. In some cases, this can decrease the number of levels fused, which is particularly desirable in the lumbar spine. Screws are placed into the vertebral body on the convex side of the curve during the anterior fusion, connected to a rod, and compression is applied to gain correction (Figure 5–22). They are generally not used lower than the level of L4 because the common iliac vessels would then lie over them and face potential erosion.

Complications & Risks of Surgery

The incidence of complications in adolescent patients is quite low, although the complications outlined here should be discussed with the parent and child during obtaining of informed consent. The risk of major complications in adult scoliosis surgery is reported to be upward of 30%, with increased rates found in association with more complex cases, older patients, and patients with coexisting medical conditions.

A. Neurologic Compromise

Among the risks faced by patients who undergo major spine fusion are paralysis and death. The incidence of paralysis, however, according to reports of the Scoliosis Research Society, is 0.4%, including both temporary and permanent deficits. Some of the neurologic risk appeared to be greater in the earlier days of using the variable hook-rod systems. These systems are powerful, and overcorrection and overdistraction can result. Because this is better understood today, the risk appears to have decreased.

B. Cardiopulmonary Problems

Cardiopulmonary complications are unusual in adolescents, but the incidence increases in older individuals. In patients with severe pulmonary disease or a history of cigarette smoking, prolonged intubation may be required. In older patients with a preexisting disease, the risk of cardiac ischemia is increased, particularly with long surgeries, significant blood loss, and controlled hypotension as might be induced by the anesthesia team. Controlled hypotension is used to minimize blood loss during many procedures but should be tailored to what can be tolerated by a given patient.

The risk of thromboembolic complications after spine surgery ranges from 0.5% to 50%. Many surgeons use antithromboembolic hose, sequential compression boots, or low-molecular-weight heparin during and after surgery. Pharmacologic anticoagulation poses the risk of postoperative bleeding into the surgical site, which can result in an epidural hematoma and compression of the neural elements and thus should be used with caution and only in high-risk patients. Although their efficacy is well documented with hip and knee arthroplasty, benefits are not yet demonstrated for spinal surgery patients.

C. Infection

Although perioperative antibiotics should and usually are given, patients undergoing spinal surgery are at risk for infection. We have found prior infection, smoking history, diabetes, staged anterior and posterior spinal fusion, and increasing age to result in increased risk for postoperative infection.

D. Pseudarthrosis

Rarely occurring in the adolescent but seen occasionally in adults is pseudoarthrosis, or the failure of fusion. This can result in persistent pain or loss of curve correction. Although tomograms or bone scans are difficult to interpret because of the presence of metallic artifacts,

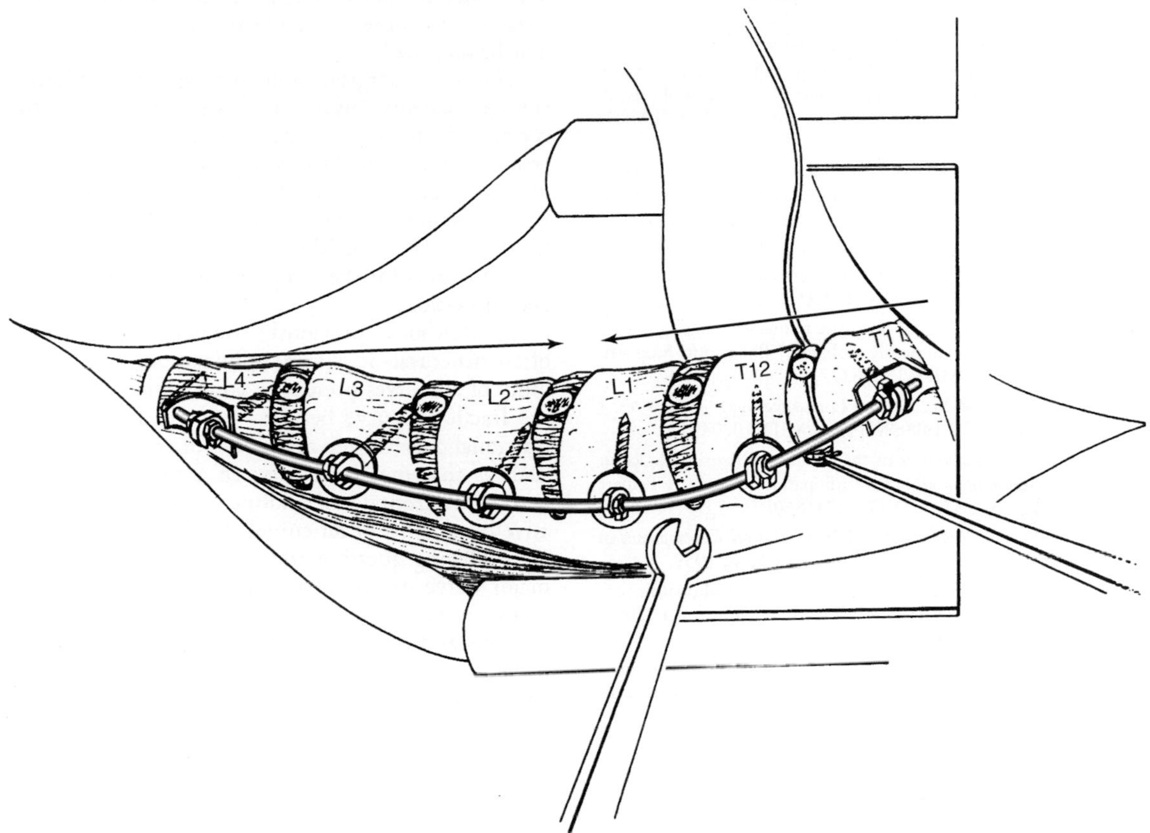

Figure 5–22. Illustration of the use of anterior instrumentation on a Thoracolumbar Scoliosis Curve.

they may help delineate suspicious areas. High suspicion for pseudarthrosis may necessitate reexploration and refusion, sometimes supplemented by anterior fusion. Instrumentation that is painful or broken may be an indication of pseudoarthrosis.

E. Decompensation

In cases of decompensation, the patient leans with the trunk shifted to one side. Decompensation, particularly in the coronal plane, can generally be attributed to overcorrection of the instrumented curves such that the flexibility of the compensatory curves is insufficient to allow righting of the patient.

F. Flat Back Syndrome

Seen less frequently now that contoured rods are used, flat back syndrome can be a debilitating complication and reinforces the need to restore or maintain the normal sagittal contours of the spine. The distraction required to achieve curve correction by Harrington rods, when applied across the lumbar spine, flattens the normal lumbar lordosis. This can also occur if the patient is positioned such that the spine is not adequately extended. Patients may need to hyperextend their hips to stand fully upright, or a hip-flexed, knee-flexed gait may be adopted. This is generally a late complication as patients lose their ability to compensate; affected patients note increasing back fatigue or pain and the inability to stand up straight. Surgical correction of flat back syndrome has a high rate of complications, although patient satisfaction is generally high.

G. Low Back Pain

Lower distal levels of fusion appear to correlate with increasing risk of low back pain. This raises the concern of late degeneration below the spine fusion. If the clinician can attribute a patient's symptoms to a specific unfused level, extension of the fusion may be indicated.

Ascher M et al: Safety and efficacy of Isola instrumentation and arthrodesis for adolescent idiopathic scoliosis: Two- to 12-year follow-up. Spine 2004;29:2013. [PMID: 15371702]

Daneilsonn AJ, Nachemson AL: Back pain and function 22 years after brace treatment for adolescent idiopathic scoliosis: A case-control study—part I. Spine 2003;28:2078 [PMID: 14501917]

Daneilsson AJ, Nachemson AL: Back pain and function 23 years after fusion for adolescent idiopathic scoliosis: A case-control study—part II. Spine 2003;28:E373. [PMID: 14501939]

Danielsson AJ, Nachemson AL: Radiologic findings and curve progression 22 years after treatment for adolescent idiopathic scoliosis. Spine 2001;26:516. [PMID: 11242379]

Davids JR et al: Indications for magnetic resonance imaging in presumed adolescent idiopathic scoliosis. J Bone Joint Surg Am 2004;86:2187. [PMID: 15466727]

Dickson RA, Weinstein SL: Bracing (and screening)—Yes or no? J Bone Joint Surg Br 1999;80:193. [PMID: 10204919]

Gepstein R et al: Effectiveness of the Charleston bending brace in the treatment of single curve idiopathic scoliosis. J Pediatr Orthop 2002;22:84. [PMID: 11744860]

Gruelich W, Pyle S: *Radiographic Atlas of Skeletal Development of the Hand and Wrist.* Stanford University Press, 1959.

Lenke LG: Lenke classification system of adolescent idiopathic scoliosis: Treatment recommendations. Instr Course Lect 2005; 54:551. [PMID: 15948478]

Lenke LG et al: Radiographic results of arthrodesis with Cotrel-Dubousset instrumentation for the treatment of adolescent idiopathic scoliosis: A 5 to 10-year follow-up study. J Bone Joint Surg Am 1998;80:807. [PMID: 9655098]

Nachemson AL, Petersen P-E, and members of the Brace Study Group of the Scoliosis Research Society: Effectiveness of treatment with a brace in girls who have adolescent idiopathic scoliosis. J Bone Joint Surg Am 1995;77:815. [PMID: 7782353]

Parent S et al: Adolescent idiopathic scoliosis: Etiology, anatomy, natural history, and bracing. Instr Course Lect 2005;54:529. [PMID: 15948477]

Petersen L-E, Nachemson AL, and members of the Brace Study Group of the Scoliosis Research Society: Prediction of progression of the curve in girls who have adolescent idiopathic scoliosis of moderate severity. J Bone Joint Surg Am 1995:77:823. [PMID: 7782354]

Rowe DE et al: A meta-analysis of the efficacy of nonoperative treatments for idiopathic scoliosis. J Bone Joint Surg Am 1997;79:664. [PMID: 9160938]

1. Idiopathic Scoliosis in Adults

Indications for intervention in adults with scoliosis are pain and progression. Painful scoliosis can be treated with conservative measures, including antiinflammatory agents and physical therapy, in an approach similar to the treatment of low back pain without a deformity. Bracing of the curvature is rarely indicated because these patients have no skeletal growth remaining; however, a patient who cannot tolerate surgery for medical reasons may be braced as a salvage measure. In an otherwise reasonably healthy patient, if progression greater than 5 degrees can be documented or if symptoms are refractory to conservative measures, surgical correction may be indicated.

The same surgical principles apply to adults as younger patients. Adults are more likely to have rigid curves, which may require a combined anterior and posterior approach. Depending on the deformity and region of pain, fusion to the sacrum may be indicated. Patients with significant leg pain should have preoperative CT scanning or MRI to assess whether spinal stenosis accounts for the symptoms and warrants surgical decompression.

In adulthood, previously compensatory curves are often structural. It is important to consider the flexibility of all curves present in adult patients, including the fractional curve between L4 and the sacrum. (A fractional curve is one that does not cross the midline, such as that measured between a tilted L4 endplate and the horizontal and midline sacrum.) The preoperative bend films of all curves should be reviewed and the following question addressed: If correction of the major curve or curves is achieved as would be predicted by the curve flexibility, will the patient still be able to stand centered head over pelvis? If not, the clinician may need to consider fusing a lesser curve to balance the spine.

Another concern is the need to correct sagittal plane deformity, particularly kyphosis, or maintain normal sagittal contours.

Anterior release and fusion may be indicated prior to posterior instrumentation in some cases to permit the patient to stand upright with the head over the sacrum and the knees and hips straight. Before subjecting a patient to the significantly greater surgical risk of a combined anterior and posterior procedures, however, the surgeon should take into account issues such as spinal stenosis, hip disease, and pain from the patient's condition that may affect the patient's ability to stand fully upright.

For older patients, particularly women, osteoporosis may prevent optimal fixation of the instrumentation to the spine. Sublaminar wires, as previously mentioned, can improve the rigidity of the fixation because the multiple sites of attachment spread the load over more bony attachments. There is, however, a theoretical increase in risk of neurologic damage during surgery when this approach is used.

Use of iliac screws (Figure 5–23) should be considered for long fusions to the sacrum because it appears best at resisting flexion moments that are experienced at the lumbosacral junction. In complex and difficult cases such as the one discussed here, surgery should only be undertaken for relatively healthy patients who have failed to respond to nonoperative intervention and who have a clear under-

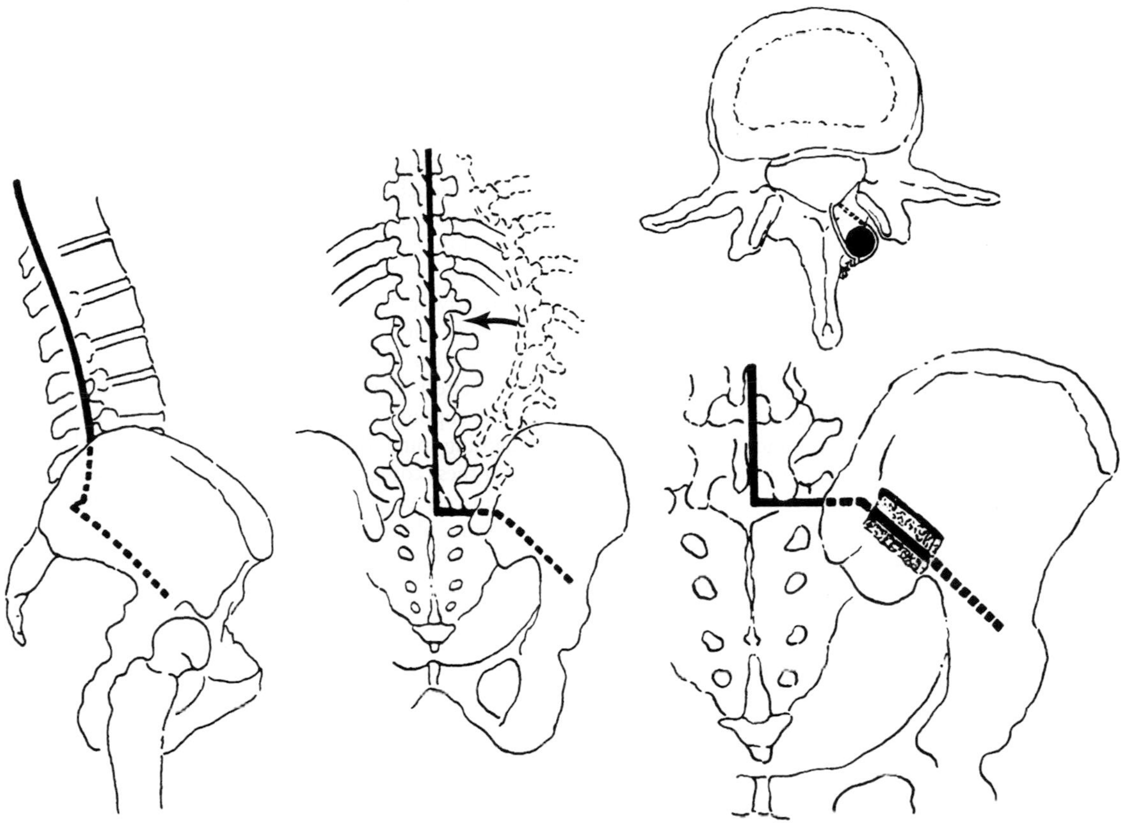

Figure 5–23. **Use of the Galveston technique to obtain pelvic fixation.** (Reproduced, with permission, from Shook JE, Lubicky JP: Paralytic spinal deformity. In Bridwell KH, DeWald RL, eds: *The Textbook of Spinal Surgery*. Lippincott, 1991.)

standing of the goals and the significant perioperative risks of surgery.

Postoperative care in the adult patient undergoing major reconstructive surgery requires detailed attention to the patient's systemic needs, much more so than is generally required by patients undergoing other orthopedic procedures. Those patients who require thoracotomy or thoracoabdominal approaches will have postoperative chest tubes and are at higher risk for pulmonary complications.

Fluid shifts can be significant after lengthy procedures, particularly those with large blood losses. Anterior approaches, although largely retroperitoneal, can lead to prolonged ileus, a problem compounded by the use of postoperative narcotics that all orthopedic patients require.

Bradford DS et al: Adult scoliosis: Surgical indications, operative management, complications, and outcomes. Spine 1999; 24(24):2617. [PMID: 10635525]

Connolly PJ et al: Adolescent idiopathic scoliosis. J Bone Joint Surg Am 1995;77A:1209. [PMID: 7642667]

Dickson JH et al: Results of operative treatment of idiopathic scoliosis in adults. J Bone Joint Surg Am 1995;77A:513. [PMID: 7713967]

Eck KR et al: Complications and results of long adult deformity fusions down to L4, L5 and the sacrum. Spine 2001;26(9): E182. [PMID: 11337635]

Grubb SA et al: Results of surgical treatment of painful adult scoliosis. Spine 1994;19(14):1619. [PMID: 7939999]

Kim YJ et al: Pseudoarthrosis in primary fusions for adult idiopathic scoliosis: Incidence, risk factors, and outcome analysis. Spine 2005;30(4):468. [PMID: 15706346]

Schwab F et al: Adult scoliosis: A health assessment analysis by SF-36. Spine 2003;28(6):603. [PMID: 12342769]

Schwab FJ et al: Adult scoliosis: A quantitative radiographic and clinical analysis. Spine 2002;27(4):387. [PMID: 11840105]

Weinstein SL et al: Health and function of patients with untreated idiopathic scoliosis: A 50 year natural history study. JAMA 2003;289(5):559. [PMID: 12578488]

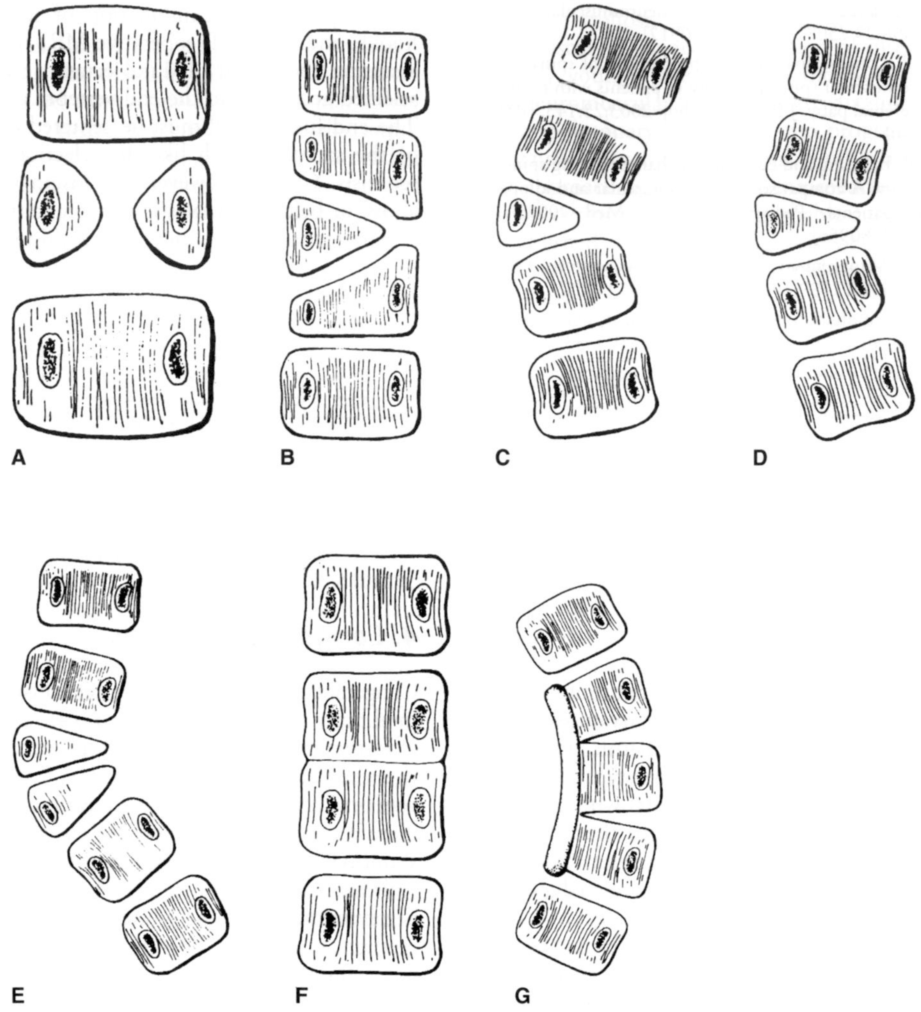

Figure 5–24. The major types of congenital scoliosis are failure of formation, as shown in diagrams A through E, and failure of segmentation, as shown in diagrams F and G. (Reproduced, with permission, from Hall JE: Congenital scoliosis. In Bradford DS, Hensinger RN, eds: *The Pediatric Spine*. Thieme, 1985.)

malities (10–50%). Abdominal ultrasound or other imaging tests should be used to rule out absent or abnormal kidneys. Intracanal abnormalities may include a syrinx (cyst within the cord), diastematomyelia or diplomyelia (division or reduplication of the cord, respectively), and tethered cord (presence of a tight filum terminale that does not permit the conus medullaris to migrate upward normally with growth).

If surgical intervention in patients with congenital scoliosis is indicated, several options are available. Fusion in situ is the simplest procedure. For very young (less than 10 years) patients, however, a posterior fusion alone results in tethering of the posterior elements while the anterior elements continue to grow. This situation may lead to the crankshaft phenomenon, whereby the anterior growth in the spine results in a twisting deformity around the fused posterior elements. For this reason, combined anterior and posterior fusion is usually recommended for very young patients, halting growth circumferentially about the spine. (The crankshaft phenomenon can also occur in very young patients with noncongenital forms of scoliosis who were treated by posterior fusion. Age younger than 10 years, Risser stage 0 or 1, and the presence of an open triradiate cartilage are indicators of skeletal maturity at risk for development of crankshaft.)

In some cases of hemivertebra, hemiepiphysiodesis may be performed, arresting growth on the curve convexity but permitting continued growth on the curve concavity, with resultant gradual curve correction. This procedure has good results in selected patients but can be unpredictable with respect to the amount of actual correction that can be achieved.

In cases in which a hemivertebra is accompanied by significant coronal decompensation and compensatory growth would not be adequate to result in spinal balance, consideration can be given to hemivertebra excision via a combined anterior and posterior approach. Although this procedure is technically more demanding and has greater potential risks, it allows for better overall curve correction and improvement of coronal balance. Hemivertebra excision may be the preferred option in the lumbar spine or lumbosacral junction, where the neurologic risk is to the cauda equina rather than the spinal cord and where oblique takeoff of the vertebra above the hemivertebra can result in significant truncal decompensation.

Bradford DS: Partial epiphyseal arrest and supplemental fixation for progressive correction of congenital spinal deformity. J Bone Joint Surg Am 1982;64:610. [PMID: 7068703]

Bradford DS, Boachie-Adjei O: One-stage anterior and posterior hemivertebral resection and arthrodesis for congenital scoliosis. J Bone Joint Surg Am 1990;72:536. [PMID: 2324140]

Deviren V et al: Excision of hemivertebrae in the management of congenital scoliosis of the thoracic and thoracolumbar spine. J Bone Joint Surg Br 2001;83:496. [PMID: 11380117]

Holte DC et al: Excision of hemivertebrae and wedge resection in treatment of congenital scoliosis. J Bone Joint Surg Am 1995;77A:159. [PMID: 7844121]

Kim YJ, Otsuka NY, Flynn JM et al: Surgical treatment of congenital kyphosis. Spine 2001;26:2251. [PMID: 11598516]

Nakamura H, Matsuda H, Konishi S et al: Single-stage excision of hemivertebrae via the posterior approach alone for congenital spine deformity: Follow-up period longer than ten years. Spine 2002;27:110. [PMID: 11805647]

Prahinski JR, Polly DW Jr, McHale KA et al: Occult intraspinal anomalies in congenital scoliosis. J Pediatr Orthop 2000;20:59. [PMID: 10641690]

Thompson AG et al: Long term results of combined anterior and posterior convex epiphysiodesis for congenital scoliosis due to hemivertebrae. Spine 1995;20:1380. [PMID: 7676336]

KYPHOSIS

The normal sagittal contour of the spine includes cervical lordosis, thoracic kyphosis, and lumbar lordosis (Figure 5–25). Increases or decreases in any of these can be seen. If they are severe enough, they can cause disability, as discussed later in the cases of congenital kyphosis and Scheuermann kyphosis.

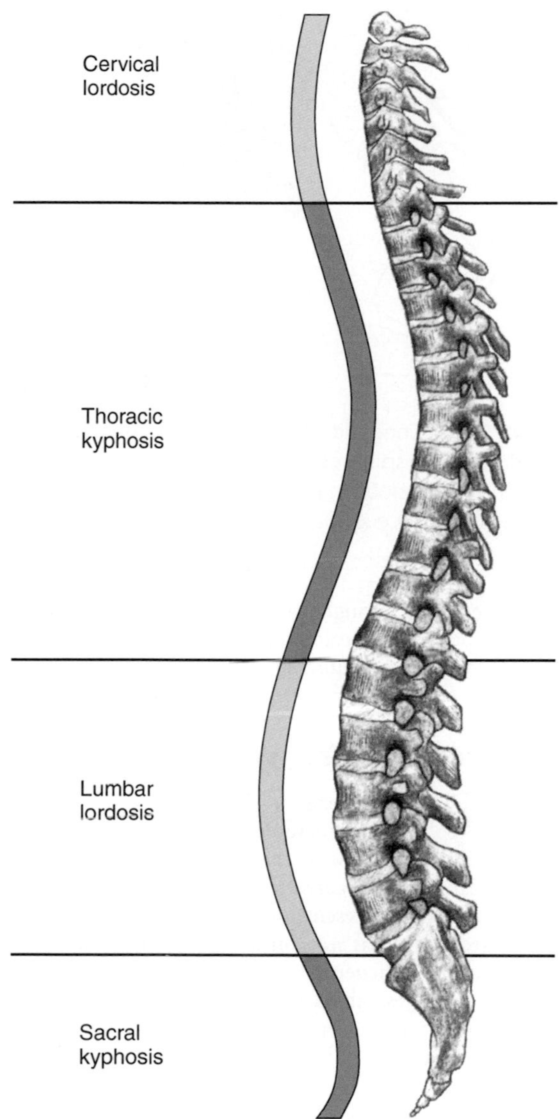

Figure 5–25. The normal sagittal contour of the spine. (Reproduced, with permission, from Bullough PG, Boachie-Adjei O: *Atlas of Spinal Diseases.* Gower, 1988.)

1. Congenital Kyphosis

As in congenital scoliosis (see previous discussion), congenital kyphosis can result from a failure of formation or a failure of segmentation. In congenital kyphosis, however, failures of formation have a much more dangerous clinical prognosis. These can lead to congenital or progressive "dislocation" of the spinal column (Figure 5–26) and paralysis if not treated appropriately. If

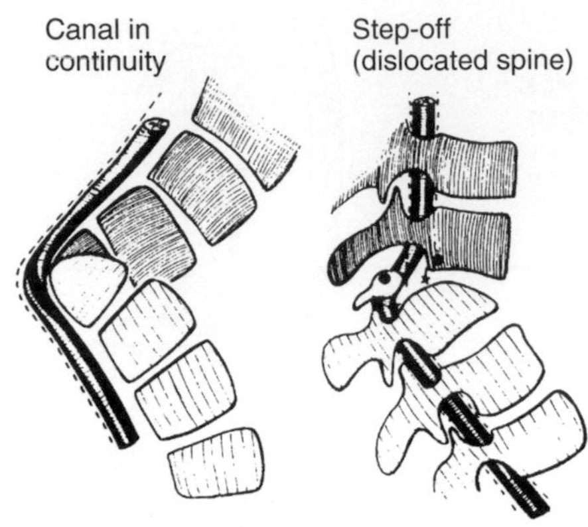

Figure 5–26. Congenital kyphosis and congenital "dislocation" of the spinal column. (Reproduced, with permission, from Dubousset J: Congenital kyphosis. In Bradford DS, Hensinger RN, eds: *The Pediatric Spine.* Thieme, 1985.)

performed early enough, posterior fusion may be sufficient to prevent neurologic problems. Severe deficiencies, however, may require anterior and posterior fusion to achieve stability.

2. Scheuermann's Kyphosis

Normal thoracic kyphosis ranges from 25 to 45 degrees. Postural kyphosis can increase this curvature, but if no abnormalities are present, the curve is flexible and the posture can be easily corrected by the child. If endplate abnormalities are present and three or more vertebral bodies are wedged as seen on the lateral radiograph, the diagnosis of Scheuermann kyphosis can be made. Schmorl nodules, characterized by herniation of the disk material at the vertebral endplates, and increased thoracic kyphosis are also seen. Clinically, patients with this type of kyphosis have a curvature that is more abrupt than that observed in people with postural roundback, and this type is only partly correctable by forced extension. It can be demonstrated either by having the patient hyperextend or by taking a lateral radiograph with the patient lying over a pad at the apex of the kyphosis so the Cobb angle can be measured. Thoracic curves may cause pain and discomfort, although some report that pain is more commonly seen in thoracolumbar curves.

Bracing can be instituted if the kyphosis measures more than 45 or 55 degrees in a skeletally immature patient, particularly if the curvature is progressive or accompanied by pain. If lesser degrees of deformity are symptomatic, they can be treated with physical therapy exercises and observed for progression. Brace treatment requires the use of the Milwaukee brace, with two paraspinal pads placed over the apical ribs posteriorly. Radiographs should be taken with the patient in the brace to confirm that adequate correction is being effected. The brace can be removed for sports and bathing but should otherwise be worn 23 hours a day. Repeat lateral radiographs should be taken at intervals of 4–6 months. If bracing is successful at controlling the curve, it should be continued until the patient nears skeletal maturity. Weaning should be performed slowly, so as to maintain correction. Although some correction may be lost, proper use of the Milwaukee brace can result in long-lasting improvement in many patients with kyphosis (which is not the case with brace treatment of adolescent idiopathic scoliosis).

Surgical treatment of kyphosis may be indicated if the curve magnitude increases despite bracing, if the patient has significant associated symptoms, or if the patient who is nearing skeletal maturity has a severe curvature. Posterior spinal fusion with a variable hook-rod system, such as the Cotrel-Dubousset system, is the treatment of choice in these cases. If the curve flexibility does not permit adequate correction as demonstrated on a hyperextension lateral radiograph, an anterior release and fusion prior to the posterior spinal fusion is indicated.

Reports describe the natural history of Scheuermann kyphosis, suggesting some functional limitations but little actual interference with lifestyle. The deformity can worsen over time. It appears clear, however, that many patients have their symptoms of back pain and deformity improved by surgery. Proper patient education and selection are essential for appropriate treatment of these patients.

Arlet V, Schlenzka D: Scheuermann's kyphosis: Surgical management. Eur Spine J 2005;14:817. [PMID: 15830215]

Lowe TG, Kasten MD: An analysis of sagittal curves and balance after Cotrel-Dubousset instrumentation for kyphosis secondary to Scheuermann's disease. Spine 1994;19:1680. [PMID: 7973960]

Murray PM et al: The natural history and long-term follow-up of Scheuermann's kyphosis. J Bone Joint Surg Am 1993;75:236. [PMID: 8423184]

MYELODYSPLASIA

Neural tube defects can result in complex spinal deformities secondary both to the neuromuscular collapsing nature of the spine and to the vertebral anomalies that can give rise to congenital kyphosis or congenital scoliosis. Myelomeningocele or meningocele is present at birth in a patient whose neural tube failed to close in utero. Sac closure is usually performed shortly after birth. In many cases, the affected infant also requires placement of a ventriculoperitoneal shunt because of hydrocephalus. The level of neurologic function usually corresponds to the level of the defect. For example, a low thoracic myelomeningocele patient has no lumbar nerve roots functioning and therefore no lower extremity function. An L4 myelomeningocele patient has a functioning tibialis anterior but no extensor hallucis and no gastrocnemius and usually no voluntary bowel and bladder control.

Neurologic function in patients with myelodysplasia is static and should not deteriorate with growth. Neurologic changes, especially during growth spurts, require evaluation for tethered cord, a common occurrence in affected children.

Orthopedic management includes maximizing the function of patients through the use of braces, ambulatory aids, wheelchairs, or surgery. The degree of spinal deformity is related to the neurologic level, with spinal collapse more likely in those with a higher neurologic level of involvement than in those with a lower level. The presence of bony abnormalities can affect this prognosis, of course.

As with many neuromuscular spinal deformities, curvatures may present early in life. If the clinician elects to treat a patient with bracing, it is important to remember that bracing in the presence of insensate skin can result in pressure sores if the brace is not adequately padded and the parents are not instructed regarding skin care.

In many cases, the curvature eventually requires surgical stabilization. Because of the magnitude and stiffness of the curvature as well as the absence of posterior elements, the preferred treatment is anterior and posterior fusion. Anterior instrumentation may improve rigidity of the surgical construct. In patients with myelodysplasia, fusion to the sacrum is invariably required because of pelvic obliquity or lack of sitting balance. Luque-Galveston instrumentation to the proximal thoracic spine is preferred, as with many neuromuscular deformities.

The lack of posterior elements in the myelodysplastic spine can lead to congenital kyphosis. Although kyphosis in these patients does not compromise neurologic function, it can lead to pressure sores over the prominent area. The treatment of choice for this problem is posterior kyphectomy and fusion.

Banit DM et al: Posterior spinal fusion in paralytic scoliosis and myelomeningocele. J Pediatr Orthop 2001;21:117. [PMID: 11176365]

Parsch D et al: Surgical management of paralytic scoliosis in myelomeningocele. J Pediatr Orthop 2001;10:10. [PMID: 11269805]

SPONDYLOLISTHESIS & SPONDYLOLYSIS

Spondylolisthesis is the slipping forward of one vertebra upon another. Spondylolysis is characterized by the presence of a bony defect at the pars interarticularis, which can result in spondylolisthesis.

The classification system most commonly used in spondylolisthesis was originated by Wiltse et al. in 1976 and subsequently modified by others. Type I, the dysplastic form of spondylolisthesis, is a congenital deficiency of the superior sacral facet, the inferior fifth lumbar facet, or both. Type II, the isthmic form, is caused by a defect in the pars interarticularis but can also be seen with an elongated pars. Types I and II are most commonly seen in younger (less than 15 years) patients and most likely to occur at the L5-S1 level. Type III, the degenerative form of spondylolisthesis, is seen in older patients and most frequently involves the L4-L5 level. Type IV, the traumatic form, is located other than at the pars. Type V, the pathologic form, is caused by conditions such as a neoplasm. The Wiltse classification of spondylolisthesis is shown in Figure 5–27.

Marchetti and Bartolozzi proposed a classification of spondylolisthesis that separates developmental and acquired types of spondylolisthesis. Developmental spondylolisthesis is divided into high dysplastic and

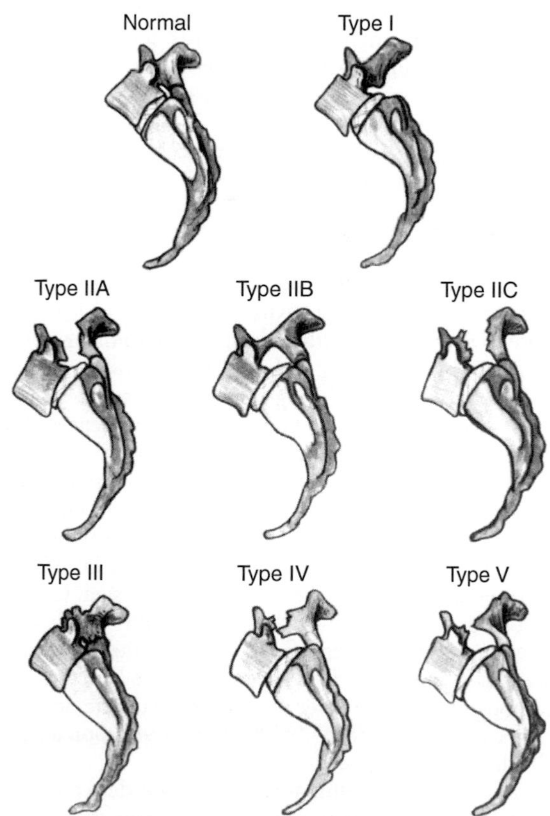

Figure 5–27. Classification of spondylolisthesis. (Reproduced, with permission, from Bradford DS, Hu SS: Spondylolysis and spondylolisthesis. In Weinstein SL, ed: *The Pediatric Spine*. New York: Raven, 1994.)

low dysplastic types, with each of these subdivided into those with lysis of the pars interarticularis or elongation of the pars interarticularis. Acquired types include degenerative, traumatic, postsurgical, and pathologic. A new classification based on clinical presentation and spinal morphology is now suggested for children and adolescents.

Bridwell KH, DeWal RL, eds: *The Textbook of Spinal Surgery*, 2nd ed. Lippincott-Raven, 1997.

Herman MJ, Pizzutillo PD: Spondylolysis and spondylolisthesis in the child and adolescent: A new classification. Clin Orthop 2005;434:46. [PMID: 15864031]

Marchetti PG, Bartolozzi P: Classification of spondylolisthesis as a guideline for treatment. In Wiltse LL et al: Classification of spondylolisthesis and spondylolysis. Clin Orthop 1976;117:23. [PMID: 11277669]

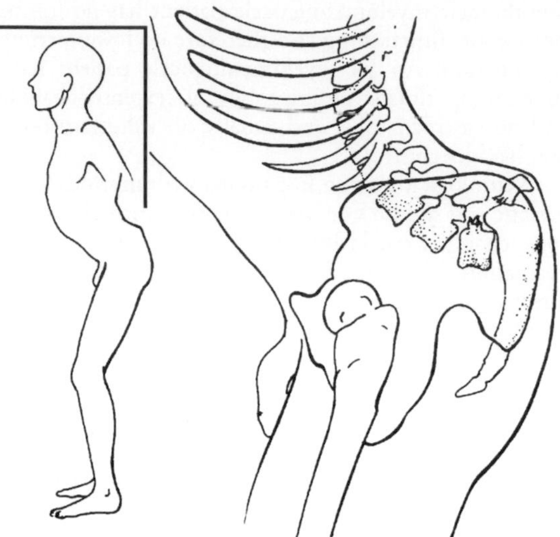

Figure 5–28. **Diagram showing how high-grade spondylolisthesis results in a short trunk, with the rib cage approaching the iliac crests.** (Reproduced, with permission, from Bradford DS, Hu SS: Spondylolysis and spondylolisthesis. In Weinstein SL, ed: *The Pediatric Spine*. Raven, 1994.)

1. Isthmic Spondylolisthesis

The cause of isthmic spondylolisthesis may be developmental, with a congenital defect of dysplasia predisposing some individuals to spondylolysis. The overall incidence of spondylolysis is approximately 6%. The high incidence of spondylolysis in gymnasts, football players, weight lifters, and other athletes who place their lumbar spines in hyperextension suggests that repetitive injury may be a contributing mechanism. Biomechanical studies also suggest that the pars interarticularis is under the greatest stress in extension.

Clinical Findings

Spondylolysis and spondylolisthesis may be asymptomatic, or they may present with back pain and leg pain. Rarely, they present with radicular symptoms or bowel and bladder symptoms. Isthmic spondylolisthesis most commonly presents during the preadolescent growth spurt, between 10 and 15 years of age. The extent of slippage may not be correlated with the severity of pain. The L5 pars interarticularis defect, with resultant slippage of L5 forward on the sacrum, is most commonly seen.

In young patients, regardless of the extent of slippage, there may be tight hamstrings and a knee-bent, hips-flexed gait, the classic Phalen-Dickson sign. Careful palpation of the spine of the patient with spondylolisthesis may reveal a step-off secondary to the prominent spinous process of L5. With more severe slippage, the lumbosacral junction becomes more kyphotic and the trunk appears shortened, with the rib cage approaching the iliac crests (Figure 5–28).

Radiographic examination shows the defect on the lateral view, with the percentage of slippage measurable from this view. The Meyerding classification is most commonly used (Figure 5–29). Oblique radiographs demonstrate the "collar" or "broken neck" on the "Scottie dog" (Figure 5–30). If a unilateral defect is present, the contralateral pars or lamina may show sclerosis. If the history is suggestive of an early stress fracture and radiographic findings are negative, bone scans may be useful. CT scanning shows spondylolysis as an incomplete ring.

The slip angle, a measure of lumbosacral kyphosis, is useful in determining the likelihood of progression to higher grades of slippage in patients. A line is drawn along the posterior cortex of the sacrum, and the angle between its perpendicular and a line drawn along the inferior border of L5 is measured (Figure 5–31). If the slip angle is greater than 50 degrees, the likelihood of progression is high.

In patients with radicular symptoms or bowel or bladder impairment, CT scanning or MRI is essential if surgical intervention is considered.

Treatment

A. Conservative Treatment

Low-grade spondylolisthesis (Meyerding grade I or II) can usually be managed with conservative measures, including restriction of the aggravating activity, bracing to reduce lumbar lordosis, and physical therapy. Patients with grade I slips who respond to conservative therapy may be permitted to resume all activities. For those with grade II slips who are improved with conservative treatment, it is usually recommended that they

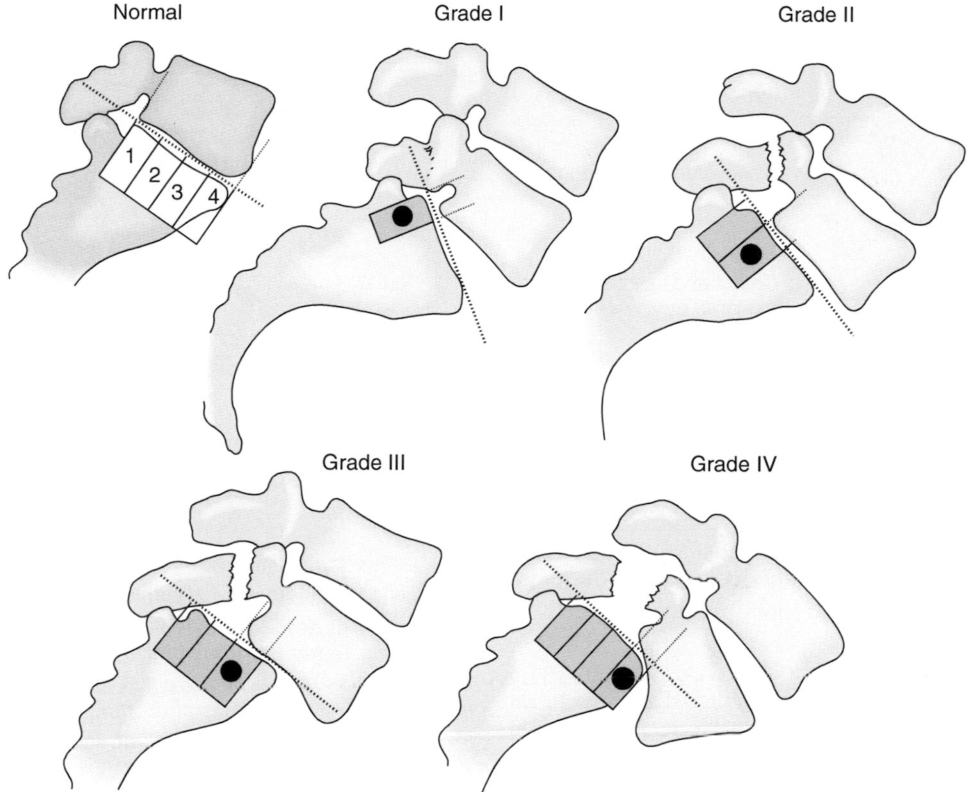

Figure 5–29. Meyerding classification of degree of slippage in spondylolisthesis. Grade I is 1–25% slippage; grade II is 26–50% slippage; grade III is 51–75% slippage; and grade IV is 76–100% slippage. (Reproduced, with permission, from Bradford DS, Hu SS: Spondylolysis and spondylolisthesis. In Weinstein SL, ed: *The Pediatric Spine.* Raven, 1994.)

refrain from activities that hyperextend the spine. Skeletally immature patients with grade III or higher slips are at significant risk for progression, and they are recommended for fusion.

B. Surgical Treatment:

1. Fusion and decompression—Fusion is indicated for patients who fail to respond to conservative measures, demonstrate progression, or have greater than 50% slippage and are skeletally immature. For most patients, fusion in situ is indicated. If slippage is less than 50%, fusion from L5 to S1 is sufficient. If slippage is greater than 50%, it is necessary to fuse from L4 to S1 to achieve a fusion bed that is under compression. Intertransverse fusion can result in fusion rates of 95% and good to excellent clinical outcomes in 75–100% of patients. This technique can be performed through two parallel paraspinal skin incisions. Alternatively, a midline skin incision with paraspinal fascial incisions, approximately two fingerbreadths off the midline, can be employed. The sacrospinalis fibers can be split, and access to the transverse processes is obtained. The transverse processes, pars interarticularis, facet joint, and adjacent lamina are exposed and decorticated. Iliac crest bone graft is harvested and placed in corticocancellous strips over the fusion bed (Figure 5–32).

If neurologic findings such as numbness, leg pain, leg weakness, or bowel and bladder compromise are present, decompression may be needed. Central and foraminal stenosis can be evaluated with a CT scan or MRI. In many cases, fibrocartilaginous scarring at the site of the pars defect accounts for the compressive symptoms. Particularly for young (less than 18 years) patients, an isolated decompression without fusion is likely to result in slip progression, so decompression should be combined with fusion. Some reports indicate that signs of nerve root irritation, including hamstring tightness, resolve when fusion is used without surgical decompression. It may take up to 18 months for these signs to resolve after fusion alone.

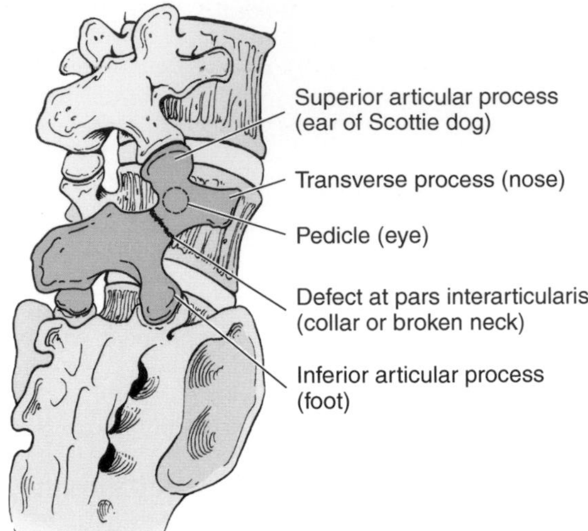

Figure 5–30. Diagram showing the "Scottie dog" (dark shaded area) seen on oblique radiographs of the lumbar spine in patients with spondylolisthesis.

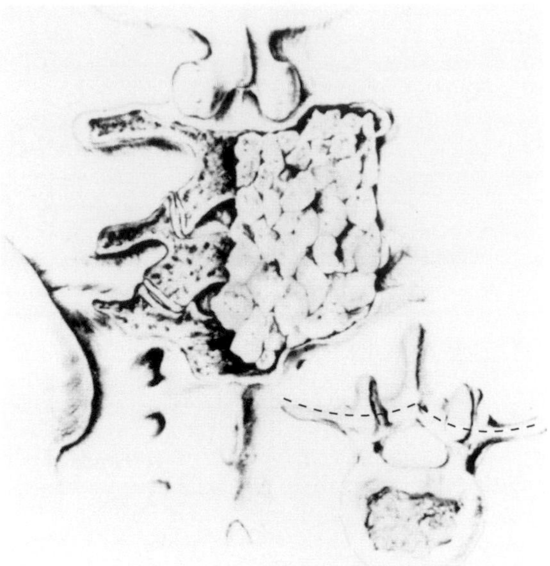

Figure 5–32. Schematic diagram of fusion for spondylolisthesis, as described by Wiltse. (Reproduced, with permission, from Bradford DS, Hu SS: Spondylolysis and spondylolisthesis. In Weinstein SL, ed: *The Pediatric Spine*. Raven, 1994.)

Bracing or casting may be indicated after fusion and may consist of the use of a lumbar corset, a thoracolumbar orthosis, or a thoracolumbosacral orthosis with leg extension or pantaloon spica cast, depending on the preference of the surgeon. Once the patient's fusion is solid, full activities are permitted.

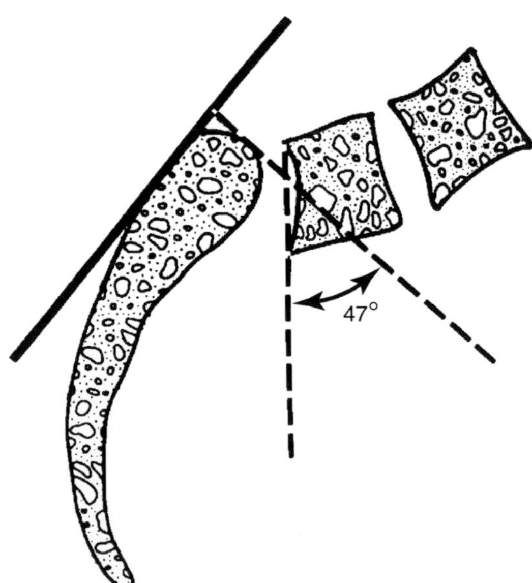

Figure 5–31. Measurement of the slip angle as a predictor of progression in spondylolisthesis. (Reproduced, with permission, from Bradford DS, Hu SS: Spondylolysis and spondylolisthesis. In Weinstein SL, ed: *The Pediatric Spine*. Raven, 1994.)

2. Pars repair—Pars repair may be indicated for young (less than 18 years) patients who have single-level or multiple-level L1-L4 pars defects without evidence of disk damage. Screw fixation or wiring of the transverse process to the spinous process (Figure 5–33) yields good results in appropriately selected patients.

3. Fibular strut graft—Bohlman and Cook described a technique for one-stage posterior decompression and interbody fusion for treatment of grade V spondylolisthesis (spondyloptosis). After wide decompression, a drill hole is prepared between the L5 and S1 nerve roots, passing through the sacrum to the L5 vertebral body that has slipped in front of the sacrum. The configuration is similar to that diagrammed in Figure 5–34 for anterior strut graft fusion. Autograft or allograft fibula is inserted and then countersunk to avoid dural impingement. Posterolateral fusion is also performed at this time.

4. Anterior fusion—Another option for achieving fusion is via an anterior transperitoneal or retroperitoneal approach. The surgeon can either perform disk space grafting with tricortical iliac crest or place a fibular graft through a drill hole from the L5 vertebral body to the sacrum (see Figure 5–34). For high-grade slips, anterior fusion places the graft in compression. Clearly,

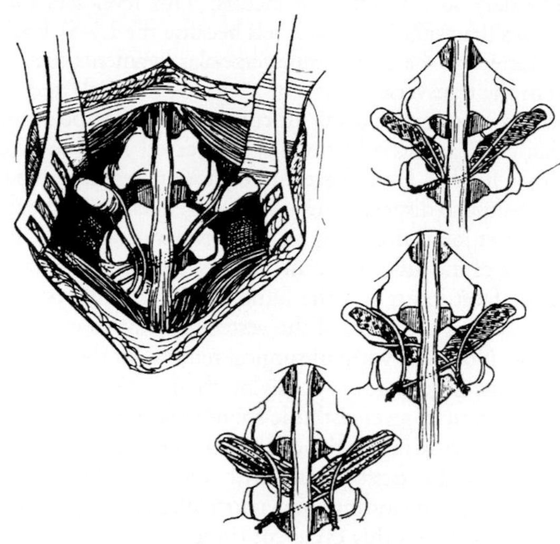

Figure 5–33. Illustration of pars repair, which can be performed in younger patients with minimal slippage, particularly above L5. Wires are placed around the transverse process and wired around the spinous process. The pars defect itself must be cleared of fibrous tissue and then bone grafted. (Reproduced, with permission, from Bradford DS, Hu SS: Spondylolysis and spondylolisthesis. In Weinstein SL, ed: *The Pediatric Spine.* Raven, 1994.)

there are significant risks with the anterior approach, including the risk of vascular damage in male and female patients and the risk of retrograde ejaculation secondary to damage of the sympathetic nervous system in male patients. Because of these risks and because good results can generally be achieved with posterolateral fusion, anterior fusion is best reserved for patients with high-grade slippage or patients who have undergone unsuccessful posterior arthrodesis treatment.

5. Reduction—Reduction of high-grade spondylolisthesis remains controversial but may be considered in patients who have high-grade slippage and are unable to stand balanced with their head over the sacrum while keeping their knees straight. Reduction can improve the patient's overall trunk appearance, which is characterized by a short waist, transverse abdominal skin fold, and heart-shaped pelvis, all of which become more prominent with high-grade spondylolisthesis. Improvement of the slip angle may prevent slip progression.

Although even fusion in situ of high-grade slips can lead to neurologic compromise and cauda equina syndrome, concern is raised over the neurologic risk with reduction techniques. Closed reduction using halo-pelvic or halo-femoral traction allows for gradual reduction while permitting the awake patient to have repeated neurologic assessments. It is less commonly used because of the availability of smaller pedicle screws. A posterolateral fusion can be performed after traction is completed or initially at the time of decompression. Anterior fusion may or may not be indicated,

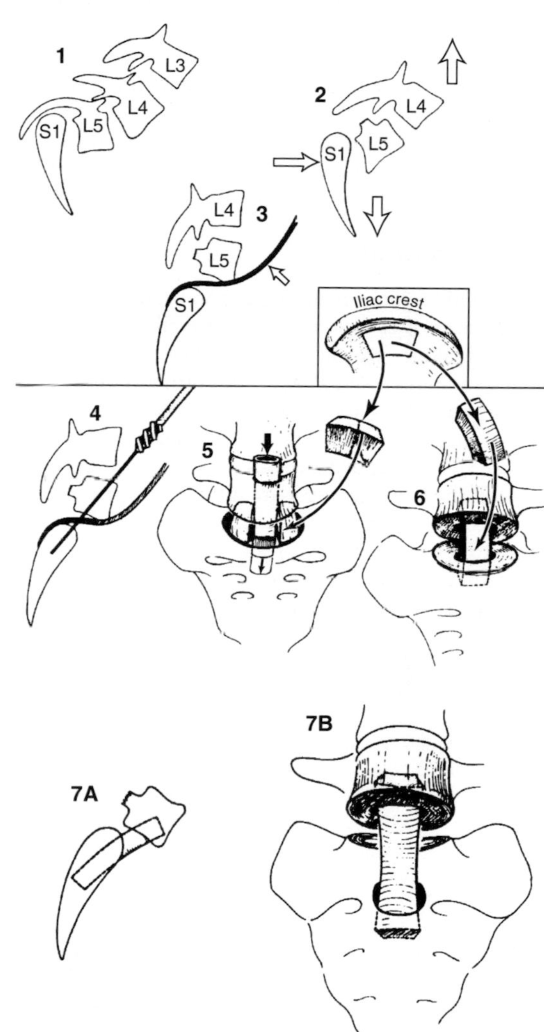

Figure 5–34. Diagram showing the steps involved in an anterior strut grafting procedure for high-grade spondylolisthesis. This approach permits grafting of iliac crest or fibula from the L5 vertebra to the sacrum, with the graft being placed under compression. (Reproduced, with permission, from Bradford DS, Hu SS: Spondylolysis and spondylolisthesis. In Weinstein SL, ed: *The Pediatric Spine.* Raven, 1994.)

depending on the particular patient and on the reduction achieved.

Pedicle screw instrumentation can be used by experienced surgeons to distract and then posteriorly translate the slipped vertebra. Neurologic complications may occur but in most cases are temporary. Supplemental techniques, such as intrasacral rods with iliac buttressing, or iliac screws, appear to improve distal fixation as does performing an interbody fusion.

For severe slips, L5 vertebrectomy with reduction of L4 onto S1 is successfully performed. The technique shortens the spine and therefore theoretically poses less neurologic risk, but surgical manipulation of the nerve roots and posterior translation of L4 can result in neurologic compromise such as footdrop.

Complications

As noted earlier, neurologic compromise sometimes results even after fusion in situ. Particularly with decompression alone (which is rarely indicated) but also with high-grade slips even after fusion, progression of the slip can occur. This happens if there is pseudarthrosis (failure of fusion), but slippage can also occur postsurgically before the fusion becomes solid, or the fusion mass can bend if the forces across it are sufficiently great.

Incomplete pain relief is rare in adolescents but is sometimes a complaint of adults. The reasons for this are not entirely clear, but it is noted that secondary degenerative changes can occur either at the level of the spondylolisthesis or at the level above.

Frennered AK et al: Natural history of symptomatic isthmic low-grade spondylolisthesis in children and adolescents: A seven-year follow-up study. J Pediatr Orthop 1991;11:209. [PMID: 2010523]

Kakiuchi M: Repair of the defect in spondylolysis. J Bone Joint Surg Am 1997;79:818. [PMID: 9199377]

Labelle H et al: Spondylolisthesis, pelvic incidence, and spinopelvic balance: A correlation study. Spine 2004;29:2049. [PMID: 15371707]

Laursen M et al: Functional outcome after partial reduction and 360° fusion in grade III-V spondylolisthesis in adolescent and adult patients. J Spinal Dis 1999;12:300. [PMID: 10451045]

Minamide A et al: Transdiscal L5-S1 screws for the fixation of isthmic spondylolisthesis: A biomedical evaluation. J Spinal Disord Tech 2003;16:114. [PMID: 12679668]

Ogilvie JW: Complications in spondylolisthesis surgery. Spine 2005;30:S97. [PMID: 15767893]

Petraco DM et al: An anatomic evaluation of L5 nerve stretch in spondylolisthesis reduction. Spine 1996;21:1133. [PMID: 8727186]

2. Degenerative Spondylolisthesis

Unlike isthmic spondylolisthesis, degenerative spondylolisthesis is found more commonly at the L4-L5 level, secondary to a number of factors. This level sees more stresses than other lumbar levels because the L5-S1 level is protected by the strong transverse-alar ligaments that run from the transverse process of L5 to the sacral ala and also because the lumbosacral junction usually lies below the iliac crest and is additionally protected from motion. Other lumbar levels have more motion segments above and below to disperse stress. With degeneration at the disk and facet joints occurring at a somewhat greater rate, narrowing of the disk can occur. Because of the configuration of the facet joints and the lumbar lordosis, this results in some slippage forward of the vertebral body upon the one below. Note that without surgical removal of the posterior elements, degenerative spondylolisthesis rarely reaches the severity seen in severe isthmic spondylolisthesis.

The narrowing at the disk level can lead to increased stresses at the facet joints, with resultant degenerative facet disease, including joint narrowing and hypertrophy of the facets. As this cycle continues, the hypertrophied facets and the redundant ligamentum flavum can result in spinal stenosis. The forward displacement of one vertebra upon the other can further narrow the canal.

Most patients with degenerative spondylolisthesis demonstrate symptoms of spinal stenosis with dysesthesias or leg pain. The spinal stenosis pattern of pain when walking beyond a well-defined distance (neurogenic claudication) is often present, relieved only by sitting down or bending over.

If degenerative spondylolisthesis is refractory to conservative measures (described earlier for isthmic spondylolisthesis), surgery may be indicated. Surgical intervention should consist of decompression. Fusion enhances surgical results after decompression for degenerative spondylolisthesis. Instrumentation such as pedicle screws may enhance fusion rates and prevent further slippage during the postdecompression period before the fusion consolidates.

Boden SD et al: Orientation of the lumbar facet joints: Association with degenerative disc disease. J Bone Joint Surg Am 1996; 78:403. [PMID: 8613448]

Fischgrund JS et al: Degenerative lumbar spondylolisthesis with spinal stenosis: A prospective randomized study comparing decompressive laminectomy and arthrodesis with and without spinal instrumentation. Spine 1997; 22:2807. [PMID: 9431616]

Herkowitz HN: Spine update. Degenerative spondylolisthesis. Spine 1995;20:1084. [PMID: 7631240]

Kuntz KM, Snider RK, Weinstein JN et al: Cost-effectiveness of fusion with and without instrumentation for patients with degenerative spondylolisthesis and spinal stenosis. Spine 2000; 25:1132. [PMID: 10788859]

Nork SE et al: Patient outcomes after decompression and instrumented posterior spinal fusion for degenerative spondylolisthesis. Spine 1999;24:561. [PMID: 10101820]

Sengupta DK, Herkowitz HN: Degenerative spondylolisthesis: Review of current trends and controversies. Spine 2005;30:S71. [PMID 15767890]

3. Thoracic Disk Disease

Disk herniation is found much less commonly in the thoracic spine than in the cervical and lumbar spine, presumably because of the decreased mobility seen in this region with the rib cage and sternum. Herniated thoracic disks account for 1–2% of operative disks, although the reported incidence in autopsy series is 7–15%.

Patients with thoracic disk disease may present with radicular symptoms at the level of involvement and complain of back or lower extremity pain, extremity weakness, numbness corresponding to the level of the disk herniation or below, and bowel or bladder dysfunction. They may demonstrate a spastic gait, with long-tract signs, if the disk is more central. Diagnosis is made by myelography, sometimes in conjunction with CT scanning or MRI.

In the absence of long-tract signs and paraparesis, conservative measures may include rest, antiinflammatory medications, and physical therapy, with a 70–80% success rate.

Surgical treatment is recommended for patients with signs of myelopathy, including paraparesis or hyperreflexia. Decompression is most safely performed via an anterior approach. The anterior extrapleural approach is advocated and yields good results.

When an anterior approach is used, 58–86% of patients show neurologic improvement and 72–87% experience pain relief. Neurologic deterioration is reported in up to 7% of patients who undergo surgery via an anterior or anterolateral approach and in 28–100% of patients who undergo posterior decompression. Posterior laminectomies are associated with a high rate of complications, including worsening neurologic function from manipulation of the cord and incomplete decompression of an inadequately visualized disk.

Bohlman H, Zdeblick T: Anterior excision of herniated thoracic discs. J Bone Joint Surg Am 1988;70:1038. [PMID: 3403572]

Brown CW et al: The natural history of thoracic disc herniation. Spine 1992;17:97. [PMID: 1631725]

Levi N, Gjerris F, Dons K: Thoracic disc herniation. Unilateral transpedicular approach in 35 consecutive patients. J Neurosurg Sci 1999;43:37. [PMID: 10494664]

Otani K et al: Thoracic disc herniation. Spine 1988;13:1262. [PMID: 3206285]

Regan JJ et al: A technical report on video-assisted thoracoscopy in thoracic spinal surgery. Spine 1995;20:831. [PMID: 7701398]

Vanichkachorn JS, Vaccaro AR: Thoracic disk disease: Diagnosis and treatment. J Am Acad Orthop Surg 2000;8:159. [PMID: 10874223]

Wood KB et al: Thoracic discography in healthy individuals. A controlled prospective study of magnetic resonance imaging and discography in asymptomatic and symptomatic individuals. Spine 1999;24:1548. [PMID: 10457574]

INJURIES OF THE CERVICAL SPINE

The cervical spine is the most mobile area of the spine, and as such it is prone to the greatest number of injuries. Injuries to the cervical spine and spinal cord are also potentially the most devastating and life altering of all injuries compatible with life. In the United States, approximately 10,000 spinal cord injuries occur each year. An estimated 80% of the victims are younger than 40 years, with the highest proportion of injuries reported in those between 15 and 35 years of age. Approximately 80% of all people who suffer from spinal column injuries are male. Falls account for 60% of injuries to the vertebral column in patients older than 75 years. In younger patients, 45% of injuries result from motor vehicle accidents, 20% from falls, 15% from sports injuries, 15% from acts of violence, and the remainder from other causes.

With the use of seat belts and air bags in motor vehicles and the advent of trauma centers and improved emergency service awareness of potential cervical injuries, fewer patients with cervical spine injuries are dying secondary to respiratory complications. The approach in treating these patients is early recognition of cervical spine injuries with rapid immobilization to prevent neurologic deterioration while the evaluation and treatment of associated injuries are carried out. After the patient is stabilized, the goals are restoration and maintenance of spinal alignment to provide stable weight bearing and facilitate rehabilitation.

Identification & Stabilization of Life-Threatening Injuries

Eighty-five percent of all neck injuries requiring medical evaluation are a result of a motor vehicle accident. Many of the affected patients are multiple-trauma victims and therefore may have more urgent life-threatening conditions. The ABCs of trauma are followed in order of priority, with *a*irway, *b*reathing (ventilation), and *c*irculation secured before further evaluation proceeds. Throughout the evaluation of other body systems, the cervical spine should be presumed injured and thus immobilized. Approximately 20% of patients with cervical trauma are hypotensive upon presentation. The hypotension is neurogenic in origin in approximately 70% of cases and related to hypovolemia in 30%. Concomitant bradycardia is suggestive of a neurogenic component. Another finding suggestive of cervical spine injury is an altered sensorium secondary to head trauma or lacerations and facial fractures. Appropriate diagnosis and fluid management are critical in the early hours of postinjury management. After all life-threatening injuries are identified and stabilized, the secondary evaluation, including an extremity examination and neurologic examination, can be safely carried out.

History & General Physical Examination

Details of the history of the injury should be obtained. If the patient is conscious, much of the information can be obtained directly. If not, family members or witnesses of the injury should be questioned. In the case of a motor vehicle accident, for example, pertinent questions include the following: Which part of the patient's body was the point of impact? Was the patient thrown from the car? Was there head trauma or a loss of consciousness? Were there any transient signs of paresis? Was the patient able to move any of his or her extremities at any time following the accident and before loss of function? What were the speeds of the involved motor vehicles? Was the patient restrained with a seat belt? Did an air bag deploy?

The history taken from the patient or family members should also include information about preexisting conditions such as epilepsy or seizures and about preexisting injuries. If the patient had any previous radiographic examinations, the radiographs might be useful for comparison.

It is helpful to question patients about what they are experiencing at the time of the examination. Are there areas of numbness, paresthesia, or pain? Can they move their extremities? The examiner should then proceed with the physical evaluation, beginning by observing the face and head of the patient for any areas of potential injury and attempting to determine the potential mechanism of injury. For instance, any lacerations or contusions to the forehead might indicate a hyperextension type injury. Observation should next include watching the extremities for any signs of motion. A genital examination should be performed because a sustained penile erection may be indicative of severe spinal cord injury. Then without moving the patient, palpation can be performed. Although palpation can be helpful in identifying potential levels of injury of the spine, it should not be used as the sole screening examination because false-negative results are possible.

Neurologic Evaluation

A meticulous neurologic examination should be performed following the history and general physical examination.

A. Neurologic Tests

The neurologic evaluation should start with documentation of the function of the cranial nerves, working proximally to distally. Observation is particularly important in the unconscious patient. Spontaneous motion in an extremity may be a sole source of information regarding spinal cord function. Respiratory efforts made with intrathoracic musculature versus abdominal musculature are also significant. In the conscious patient who is able to follow commands, a motor examination should be fairly straightforward. Rectal and perirectal sensations should be documented because these may be the sole signs for distal spinal cord function.

An extensive sensory examination should also be performed with careful attention to dermatomal innervation. In the acute setting, it is useful to document sharp and dull sensations as well as proprioception. Sharp and dull sensations are carried via the lateral spinothalamic tract, whereas proprioception is carried through the posterior columns. Sharp and dull sensations are effectively tested with the sharp and blunt ends of a pen, and proprioception is tested by having the patient verify the position of the large toe and other joints as the examiner places them in dorsiflexion and plantarflexion. It proves helpful to make ink markings directly on the patient's skin to show the level of the dermatomal deficit, which decreases the chance for intraobserver or interobserver error over sequential examinations.

Reflexes should be checked bilaterally. In the upper extremity, the biceps reflex at the flexor side of the elbow evaluates the C5 nerve root, and the brachioradialis stretch reflex at the radial aspect of the forearm just proximal to the wrist checks the C6 nerve root. The triceps reflex is innervated by C7. In the lower extremity, the knee jerk reflex is innervated by L4, and the ankle jerk is innervated by S1.

The presence or absence of the four reflexes listed in Table 5–2 should be checked. The Babinski reflex (plan-

Table 5–2. Evaluation of reflexes in patients with injuries of the cervical spine.

Reflex	Root	Positive Response	Significance
Babinski	Upper motor neurons	Extension and spread of toes	Upper motor neuron lesion is present
Bulbocavernosus	S3 and S4	Contraction of anal sphincter	Spinal shock is over
Cremasteric	T12 and L1	Retraction of scrotal sac	Spinal shock is over
Anal wink	S2, S3, and S4	Contraction of anal sphincter	Spinal shock is over

tar reflex) is evaluated by firmly stroking the lateral plantar aspect of the foot distally and then medially over the metatarsal heads and then observing the toes. If the toes flex, the response is considered negative (normal). If the toes extend and spread, the response is considered positive (abnormal) and indicative of an upper motor neuron lesion. The bulbocavernosus reflex has its root in the S3 and S4 nerves and is evaluated by squeezing on the glans in a male patient or applying pressure to the clitoris in a female patient. This action should elicit a contraction of the anal sphincter. If a Foley catheter is in place, simply pulling on the Foley catheter can stimulate the anal sphincter contraction. The cremasteric reflex is evaluated by stroking the inner thigh and observing the scrotal sac, which should retract upward secondary to contraction of the cremasteric muscle. This function is innervated by T12 and L1. Finally, the anal wink, innervated by S2, S3, and S4, is elicited by stimulating the skin about the anal sphincter and eliciting a contraction.

The presence of spinal shock causes the absence of all reflexes and typically lasts up to 24 h after the injury. The bulbocavernosus reflex is the reflex that returns first (see Table 5–2), thus marking the end of spinal shock. This point has prognostic importance because recovery from a complete neurologic deficit that is still present at the end of spinal shock is extremely unlikely. A complete neurologic examination should be repeated over time as the patient is manipulated and treated.

B. Anatomic Considerations

The ability to interpret the results of a patient's neurologic examination appropriately depends on a thorough knowledge of the anatomy of the spinal cord and peripheral nerves.

Peripheral nerves are a combination of afferent fibers, which carry information from the periphery to the central nervous system, and efferent fibers, which carry information away from the central nervous system. As the peripheral nerve approaches the spinal cord, it becomes known as the spinal nerve. Proximal to the spinal cord, the fiber splits, with the afferent fibers becoming the dorsal root or sensory root and the efferent fibers becoming the ventral root. The afferent fibers are often regrouped in various plexuses that are located between the spinal cord and the periphery. This regrouping takes place before the fibers enter the dorsal root, therefore leading to significant overlap between the dorsal root and the respective dermatomes. The implications of this anatomic fact should be kept in mind by the clinician when performing a sensory examination. For example, a sectioned peripheral nerve is demonstrated by a highly specific sensory loss in that particular dermatome, whereas the clinical findings are more variable for a sectioned dorsal root.

The spinal cord is a caudal continuation of the brain, extending in an organized fashion from the foramen magnum at the base of the skull down to the proximal lumbar spine. The spinal cord has three primary functions: It provides a relay point for sensory information; it serves as a conduit for ascending sensory information and descending motor information; and it mediates body and limb movements because it contains both interneurons and motor neurons. Headed from caudal to rostral, the spinal cord is highly organized with a central butterfly-shaped area of gray matter and surrounding white matter.

The overall diameter of the spinal cord varies as a relative percentage of the spinal canal. The cord fills approximately 35% of the canal at the level of the atlas but increases to approximately 50% of the canal in the lower cervical spine. This variation results from the relative increasing and decreasing size of the spinal gray matter and spinal white matter. As the spinal roots become larger, as occurs at the base of the cervical spine, the size of the gray matter increases relative to the white matter, whereas the size of the white matter decreases linearly from cephalad to caudal.

The gray matter, so called because it appears gray on unstained cross sections, is divided into three zones: the dorsal horn, the intermediate zone, and the ventral horn. Made up predominantly of lower motor neurons, it is prominent in the cervical swellings and lumbar swellings, where axons concentrate before exiting to innervate the upper extremities and lower extremities, respectively.

The white matter derives its name from the fact that the axons in this area are myelinated, casting a white hue on unstained sections. White matter is functionally and anatomically divided into three bilaterally paired columns: the ventral columns, the lateral columns, and the dorsal columns.

The two major ascending systems that relay somatic sensory information are the dorsal columns and the anterolateral system. The ascending axon has its cell body located in the dorsal root ganglion before proceeding without synapsing through the dorsal horn at that level and then ascending along the dorsal column before synapsing at the approximate level of the medulla and crossing over to the contralateral side before proceeding to the cerebral cortex. The topography of the dorsal column is such that the sacrum and lower extremities are medial, with the trunk and cervical region being lateral. The anterolateral system carries pain and temperature sensorium. The afferent fibers have a cell body in the dorsal root ganglion and then synapse at that given level in the dorsal horn before crossing directly to the contralateral side and traveling up the spinothalamic tract.

Motor pathways originate in the cerebral cortex and travel distally to the contralateral side approximately at the level of the medulla and travel down the lateral corticospinal tract before synapsing with the lower motor

clinician should inspect the lateral masses. The facet joints are typically angled away from the vertical and therefore not clearly seen on the AP projection. If, however, the facet joint can be seen at a particular level, this is indicative of a fracture through the lateral masses and a rotational malalignment of the facet.

The open-mouth (odontoid) view is the projection most useful for looking at C1-C2 anatomy. It permits visualization of both the dens in the AP plane, and the lateral masses of C1 on C2.

The right and left oblique views can be taken of the cervical spine with the patient in the supine position. These views are useful as confirmatory studies in ruling in or out lateral mass injuries.

3. Stress radiographs—Two techniques are used in obtaining cervical stress radiographs. The first is to apply axial distraction to the cervical spine through a halo or traction device and obtain a lateral radiograph. This technique should be carefully performed in the presence of a physician and only after gross instabilities of the cervical spine are ruled out. Serial lateral radiographs are taken as weight is sequentially added, reaching an amount equivalent to approximately a third of body weight or 30 kg, depending on the level of suspected injury. Occult instability can be inferred by noting an interspace angulation of at least 11 degrees or an interspace separation of at least 1.7 mm (Figure 5–37).

The second technique, which should only be performed in a fully alert and cooperative patient, is used to obtain flexion-extension lateral radiographs that are helpful in the diagnosis of late instability. The technique is to have the patient flex the head forward as far as possible while a lateral radiograph is taken and then to have the patient put the head in full extension while another radiograph is taken. Findings presumptive of instability are facet subluxation, forward subluxation of 3.5 cm of one vertebral body on the next, and interbody angulation of greater than 11 degrees.

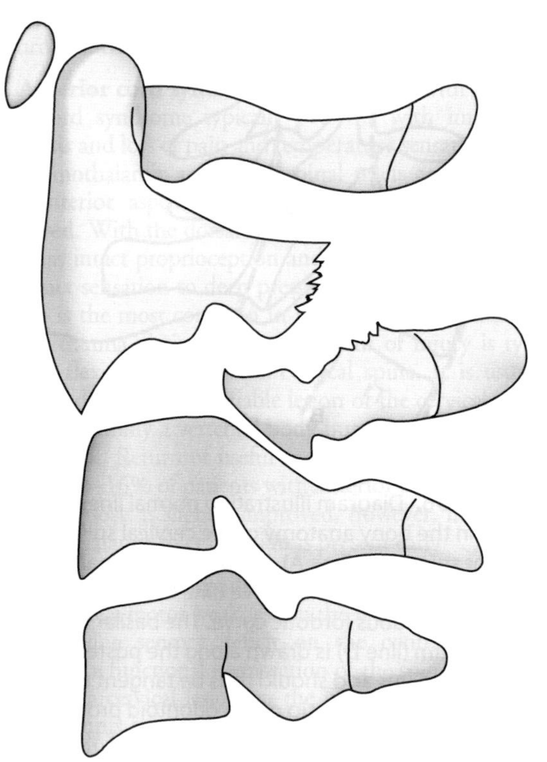

A

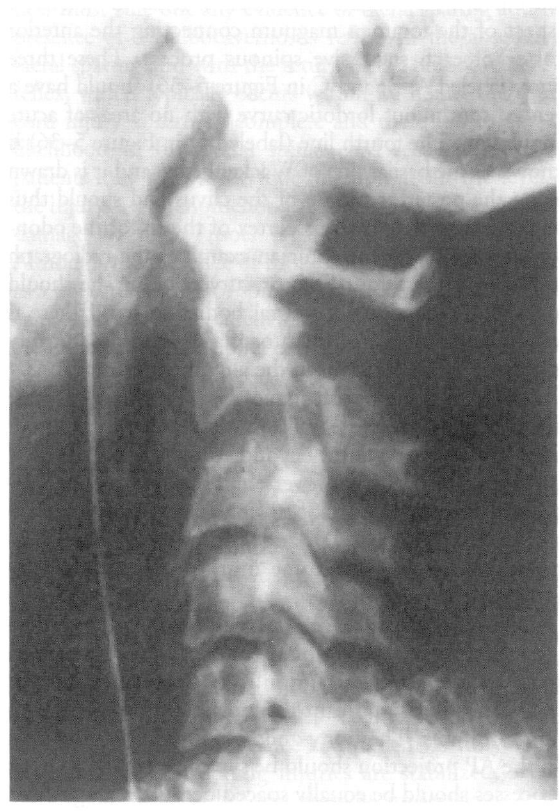

B

Figure 5–37. **A:** Diagram illustrating an increase of the C2-C3 interdisk space in a patient with type IIA traumatic spondylolisthesis. **B:** Radiograph demonstrating an increased space. (Reproduced, with permission, from Levine AM, Rhyne AL: Traumatic spondylolisthesis of the axis. Semin Spine Surg 1991;3:47.)

B. Computed Tomography

CT scanning is the most useful means for definitive delineation of bony fracture anatomy. Its advantages are its ready availability and its ability to be performed with a minimal amount of patient manipulation. CT scans provide excellent axial detail, and if the sections are taken with close enough cuts, the computer can reconstruct images in sagittal, coronal, or oblique planes. CT scans can now even be reformatted into a three-dimensional construct for excellent visualization of the bony anatomy.

C. Magnetic Resonance Imaging

MRI is the most effective way to evaluate the soft-tissue component of cervical trauma. The major advantage of MRI is that it can visualize occult disk herniation, hematoma, or edema about the spinal cord, as well as ligamentous injury. Current disadvantages are that MRI is disrupted by metallic objects, so these should be removed from the area of examination, and it also requires a prolonged amount of time to perform, therefore making close monitoring of the acutely ill patient difficult.

Diagnostic Checklist of Spinal Instability

The concept of spinal stability is central to the understanding and treatment of cervical spine injuries. In a broad sense, patients with injuries that are deemed unstable require surgical intervention, whereas those deemed to have stable injury patterns can be treated nonoperatively. Spinal injuries, however, are not readily divided into unstable and stable injuries, and in actuality they fall along a spectrum of spinal instability.

White and Panjabi's diagnostic checklist of spinal instability (Table 5–3) has nine categories, each of which is assigned a point value. If a total of 5 points is present in a given patient, the injury is deemed unstable.

Holdsworth's two-column theory of spine stability, as well as Denis's three-column theory, proposed for application to the thoracolumbar spine, are also applied to the cervical spine in an attempt to better predict stability in the neck.

General Principles of Managing Acute Injuries of the Cervical Spine

Management of acute cervical spine injury is predicated on two principles: protection of the uninjured spinal cord and prevention of further damage to the injured spinal cord. This is accomplished by following spine precaution principles from the very onset of medical care, starting at the accident scene. The cervical spine should be considered injured until proven otherwise and securely immobilized before the patient is transported to a medical center. The equipment for initial immobilization should not be removed until the definitive means of immobilization can be put in place or the cervical spine is cleared of injury. Use of a spinal board, with the patient's head taped to the board and held between two sandbags, is the most secure form of immobilization readily available in the field. This technique can be supplemented by a Philadelphia collar. When the medical center is reached, if a definitive cervical spine injury is identified and deemed unstable, skeletal traction for immobilization, reduction, or both may be applied. Gardner-Wells traction is easily applied and adequate for axial traction. Halo traction affords the added advantage of four-point fixation and thus controlled traction in three planes. Halo traction can also be easily converted at a later time to halo-vest immobilization.

Table 5–3. White and Panjabi's diagnostic checklist of spinal instability.

Checklist Category	Description	Point Value[a]
1	Disruption of the anterior elements, with greater than 25% loss of height	2
2	Disruption of the posterior elements	2
3	Sagittal plane translation of greater than 3.5 mm or greater than 20% of the anteroposterior diameter of the vertebral body	2
4	Intervertebral sagittal rotation of greater than 11 degrees	2
5	Intervertebral distance of greater than 1.7 mm on a stretch test	2
6	Evidence of cord damage	2
7	Evidence of root damage	1
8	Acute intervertebral disk space narrowing	1
9	Anticipated abnormally large stress	1

[a]If a total of 5 points is present in a given patient, the injury is deemed unstable.

Modified and reproduced, with permission, from White AA III, Panjabi MM: Update on the evaluation of instability of the lower cervical spine. Instr Course Lect 1987;36:513.

Among the various agents that show potential benefits in laboratory studies of models of spinal cord injury are corticosteroids, opiate receptor antagonists (such as naloxone or thyrotropin-releasing hormone), and diuretics (such as mannitol). The National Acute Spinal Cord Injury Studies (NASCIS) II and III reported neurologic improvement with steroid treatment given within 8 hours of injury. Those treated within 3 hours did best; those treated between hours 3 and 8 only did better by extending to 48 hours of treatment. Criticism of the NASCIS studies called to question the validity of the conclusions, and many professional organizations downgraded their enthusiasm for the use of methylprednisolone in the patient with the acutely injured spinal cord. However, many hospitals still use the protocol in blunt trauma cord injuries if the medicine can be administered within 3 hours of the injury. The recommended dosage of methylprednisolone in an acute setting is 30 mg/kg given as a bolus and followed by 5.4 mg/kg/h for 24 hours. However, some thought should be given to its use because, for example, the Congress of Neurological Surgeons stated that steroid therapy "should only be undertaken with the knowledge that the evidence suggesting harmful side effects is more consistent than any suggestion of clinical benefit."

Bracken MB et al: Administration of methylprednisolone for 24 or 48 hours or tirilazad mesylate for 48 hours in the treatment of acute spinal cord injury; Results of the Third National Acute Spinal Cord Injury Randomized Control Trial. JAMA 1997;277:1597.

Denis F: The three-column spine and its significance in the classification of acute thoracolumbar spinal injuries. Spine 1983; 8:817.

Nesathurai S: Steroids and spinal cord injury: revisiting the NASCIS 2 and NASCIS 3 trials. J Trauma 1998;45(6):1088.

White AA III, Panjabi MM: Update on the evaluation of instability of the lower cervical spine. Instr Course Lect 1987;36:513.

INJURIES OF THE UPPER CERVICAL SPINE

With the exception of occipitoatlantal dissociation, traumatic injuries to the upper cervical spine are less frequently associated with significant neurologic injury than are traumatic injuries to the lower cervical spine. This is secondary to the fact that the spinal cord occupies only a third of the upper spinal canal versus a half of the lower spinal canal.

Occipitoatlantal Dissociation

Occipitoatlantal dissociation is a disruption of the cranial vertebral junction, and it implies a subluxation or complete dislocation of the occipitoatlantal facets. This injury is typically fatal, yet the clinician must be aware of it because unrecognized occipitoatlantal dissociation may have catastrophic results. The mechanism of dissociation is poorly understood, but it most likely results from either a severe flexion or distraction type of injury. Anterior translation of the skull on the vertebral column is a common presentation and most likely a hyperflexion injury. Bucholz, however, presented the pathologic anatomic findings of fatal occipitoatlantal dissociation and proposed a mechanism of hyperextension with resultant distractive force applied across the craniovertebral junction.

When the dissociation is a frank dislocation, the findings are clear on a lateral radiograph. When the dissociation is a subluxation, however, findings may be more subtle. In normal individuals, the distance between the tip of the dens and the basion (the anterior aspect of the foramen magnum) should be no greater than 1.0 cm, and the previously described Wackenheim line should run from the base of the basion tangentially to the tip of the dens. If the dens penetrates this line, anterior translation of the cranium is implied. Calculation of the Powers ratio can also be helpful in securing the diagnosis. Powers and his colleagues described a ratio of two lines (Figure 5–38), the first of which runs from the tip of the basion to the midpoint of the posterior lamina of the atlas (line BC) and the second of which runs from the anterior arch of C1 to the opisthion (line AO). When the ratio of BC to AO is greater than 1:1, anterior occipitoatlantal dissocia-

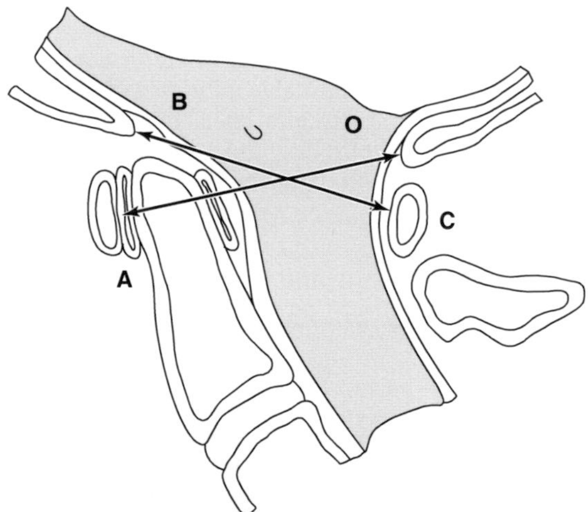

Figure 5–38. Diagram showing lines used in the calculation of the Powers ratio, which is helpful in diagnosing occipitoatlantal dissociation. The distance between the basion (point B) and the posterior arch (point C) is divided by the distance between the anterior arch of C1 (point A) and the opisthion (point O). The normal ratio of BC to AO is 1:1. A ratio of greater than 1 suggests the head is dislocated anteriorly on the spine.

tion is present. Other radiographic signs include marked soft-tissue swelling and the presence of avulsion fractures at the occipitovertebral junction.

Early recognition and surgical stabilization are the mainstays of treatment in cases of occipitoatlantal dissociation.

Fractures of Vertebra C1 (Atlas Fractures)

The mechanism of injury in the fracture of the atlas is most typically axial compression with or without extension force, and the anatomic findings of the fracture are indicative of the specifics of the force and the position of the head at the time of impact. In 1920, Jefferson presented his classic description of the four-part fracture of the atlas following an axial injury. This fracture is a burst type that occurs secondary to the occipital condyles being driven into the interior portions of the ring of the atlas and driving the lateral masses outward, resulting in a two-part fracture of the anterior ring of the atlas as well as a two-part fracture of the posterior ring. More common than the classic four-part atlas fracture, however, are the two-part and three-part fractures. Isolated anterior arch fractures are the least common, and they are typically associated with fractures of the dens, whereas the more common posterior arch fracture is typically the result of a hyperextension injury.

A fracture of the atlas is typically diagnosed on plain radiographs. Findings may be subtle on the lateral cervical spine radiograph. The open-mouth (odontoid) view may show asymmetry of the lateral masses of C1 on C2 with overhang (Figure 5–39). A bilateral overhang totaling more than 6.9 mm is presumptive evidence of a disruption to the transverse ligament and suggests potential late instability. Presumptive evidence for transverse ligament disruption can also be seen on the lateral radiograph if the ADI is greater than 4 mm.

The treatment for fractures of the atlas as isolated injuries is typically nonoperative (Figure 5–40). If there are signs of transverse ligament disruption, halo traction is indicated with later transfer to halo-vest immobilization for a total of 3–4 months. Immediate halo-vest application is indicated in cases involving a moderately displaced fracture with lateral mass overhang up to 5 mm, although collar immobilization is preferred in cases involving a minimally displaced fracture of the atlas. At completion of bony union, flexion-extension views should be obtained to rule out any evidence of late instability. If late instability is present and the bony elements were allowed to heal, a limited C1-C2 fusion can address the instability. If a nonunion is present or if the posterior arch remains disrupted, an occiput to C2 fusion is necessary to control the late instability.

Dislocations & Subluxations of Vertebrae C1 & C2

A. Atlantoaxial Rotatory Subluxation

Atlantoaxial rotatory subluxation is most common in children and may be associated with minimal trauma or even occur spontaneously. Although some patients are asymptomatic, others present with neck pain or torticollis (a position in which the head is tilted toward one side and rotated toward the other). Inasmuch as the mechanism of injury is often unclear, the propensity for the C1-C2 location is based on anatomic factors. In approximately 50% of cases, cervical spine rotation occurs at the C1-C2 junction, where the facet joints are more horizontal and less inherently stable in rotation.

The diagnosis of atlantoaxial rotatory subluxation is typically suspected on the basis of radiographs taken in several views. The odontoid view may show displacement of the lateral masses with respect to the dens; a lateral view may show an increased ADI; and the AP view may show a lateral shift of the spinous process of C1 on C2. CT scanning can be used to confirm the diagnosis, and a dynamic CT scan with full attempted right and left rotation can demonstrate a fixed deformity.

There are four types of atlantoaxial rotatory subluxations. In type I, the ADI is less than 3 mm, which suggests the transverse ligament is still intact. In type II, the interval is 3–5 mm, which suggests the transverse ligament is not structurally intact. In type III, the interval exceeds 5 mm, which is indicative of disruption of the transverse ligament as well as secondary stabilization of the alar ligament. In type IV, there is a complete posterior dislocation of the atlas on the axis, a finding typi-

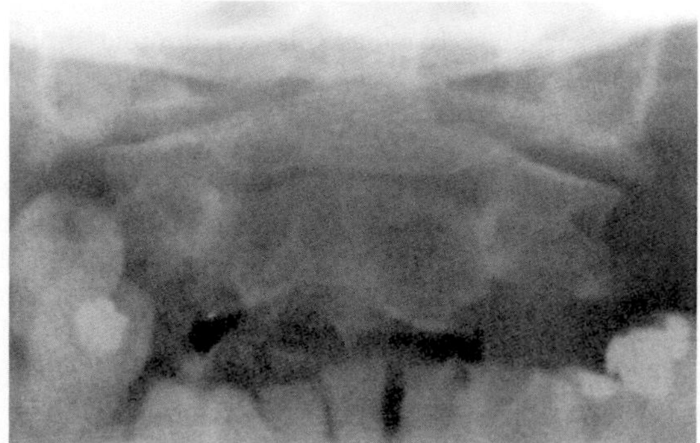

Figure 5–39. **Open-mouth (odontoid) radiographic view demonstrating asymmetry of the lateral masses of C1 on C2 with overhang in a patient with a Jefferson fracture.** (Reproduced, with permission, from El-Khoury GY, Kathol MH: Radiographic evaluation of cervical spine trauma. Semin Spine Surg 1991:3:3.)

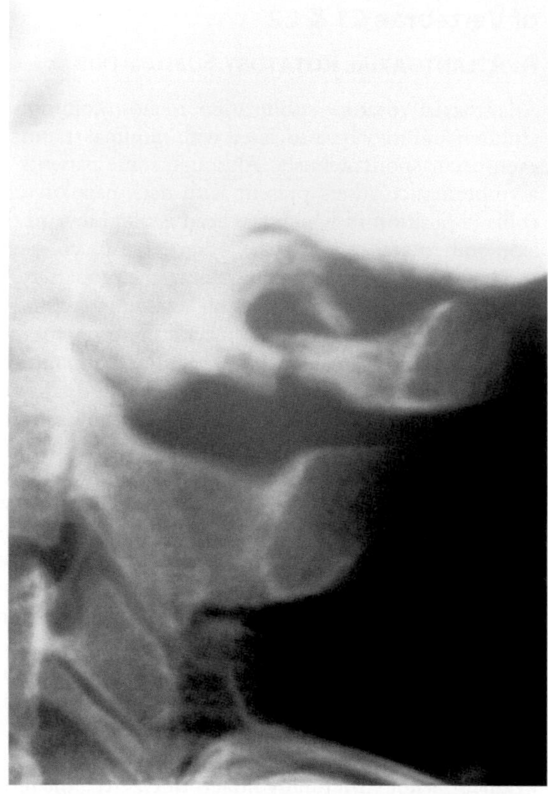

A

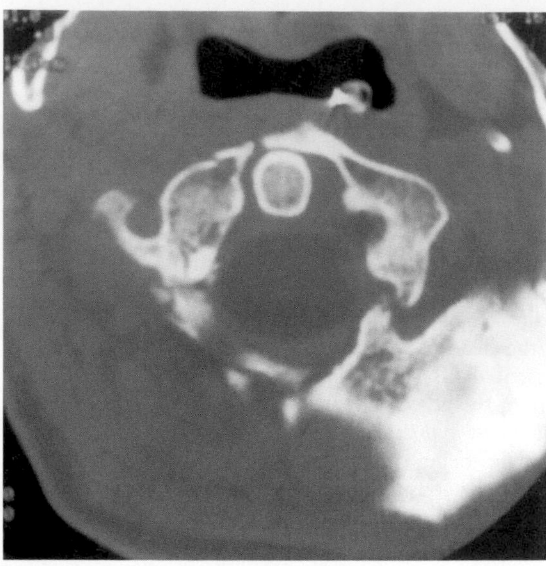

B

Figure 5–40. Imaging studies in a patient who was in a motor vehicle accident and sustained a distractive extension injury to his cervical spine and a three-part fracture of his atlas (a Jefferson fracture). **A:** Lateral radiographic view showing a fracture of the posterior arch. **B:** Axial section of a CT scan further delineating the fracture anatomy. This injury was deemed stable and treated nonoperatively in a halo vest.

cally associated with a hypoplastic odontoid process such as that seen in several forms of mucopolysaccharidosis (eg, the Morquio syndrome).

Treatment of atlantoaxial subluxation is typically conservative, consisting of traction followed by immobilization. Approximately 90% of patients respond to this treatment regimen. There is a high incidence of recurrence, however. For patients who do not respond to conservative measures and for patients with recurrent problems, C1-C2 arthrodesis may be required to control the deformity.

B. Disruption of the Transverse Ligament

The transverse ligament and secondarily the alar ligament are the main constraints to anterior displacement of C1 on C2. It was previously presumed that because anterior subluxation of C1 on C2 typically involves a fracture through the dens, the transverse ligament is in fact stronger than the bony elements of the dens. Fielding and his colleagues, however, showed that experimentally this was not the case, yet clinically the higher association of anterior dislocation of dens fractures still holds true.

The mechanism of disruption is typically a flexion injury, and the diagnosis is made on lateral radiographs. The ADI should not exceed 3 mm in the adult. If the interval is 4 mm or larger and the dens is intact, a rupture of the transverse ligament is presumed.

High-resolution CT scan can be used to categorize this injury into two types. Type 1 is a disruption in the substance of the transverse ligament, whereas type 2 involves an avulsion fracture of the insertion of the transverse ligament on the lateral mass of C1. Type 1 injuries predictably fail conservative treatment and should be managed with a C1-C2 arthrodesis. A trial of nonoperative care in type 2 injuries using a rigid cervical orthosis may be a reasonable alternative. A 74% success rate can be anticipated, with surgery reserved for patients who fail nonoperative care, showing persistent instability after 12 weeks in mobilization.

C. Fracture of the Odontoid Process

Fracture of the odontoid process is typically associated with high-velocity trauma, and the mechanism of injury is flexion in most cases. Depending on the fracture pattern, extension may be the predominant force in a smaller subset of cases. Associated injuries, particularly fractures of the ring of the atlas, should be ruled out. Neurologic involvement is relatively rare with odontoid fractures. In a study of 60 patients with acute fractures of the odontoid process, Anderson and D'Alonzo reported that 15 had some neurologic deficit on presentation, but only 5 of the 15 had major neurologic involvement, and only 2 of this group of 5 remained quadriparetic at follow-up.

Odontoid fractures may be suspected on the basis of clinical presentation and confirmed on plain radiographs, although spasm and overlying shadows can obscure the diagnosis. CT scan with sagittal and coronal reconstruction is the most sensitive study to diagnose these injuries. CT scan with axial sectioning alone may miss the horizontal fracture line typical of these injuries; thus, the reconstructions are necessary.

Both the risk of nonunion with delayed instability and the method of treating odontoid fracture depends on the classification of the fracture. Reported rates of nonunion range from 20% to 63%. According to the classification system proposed in 1974 by Anderson and D'Alonzo, there are three types of fracture of the odontoid process (Figure 5–41).

Type I is a fracture through the tip of the odontoid process. In this configuration, the blood supply is maintained through the base of the odontoid process and through the attachment of the alar transverse ligaments. The mechanical stability of this fracture pattern is left intact. Symptomatic care and immobilization are the treatment of choice.

Type II, the most common type, is a fracture through the base of the odontoid process at its junction with the body of the axis. In this configuration, soft-tissue attachments to the fracture fragment cause distraction at the fracture site. Because the amount of cancellous bone available for opposition is limited, a high nonunion rate is expected, particularly if displacement is significant or the patient is older (more than 60 years). In this case, primary surgical treatment may be indicated. Anterior screw fixation of the odontoid process is now the treatment of choice for most type 2 odontoid fractures. Although it is technically demanding, it does allow for the maintenance of motion at C1-C2 (Figure 5–42).

Type III is a fracture through the body of the axis. The blood supply is maintained through soft-tissue attachments, and abundant cancellous bone opposition at the fracture site facilitates a high rate of union. The treatment, therefore, is conservative, consisting of halo traction or halo-vest immobilization until bony union occurs.

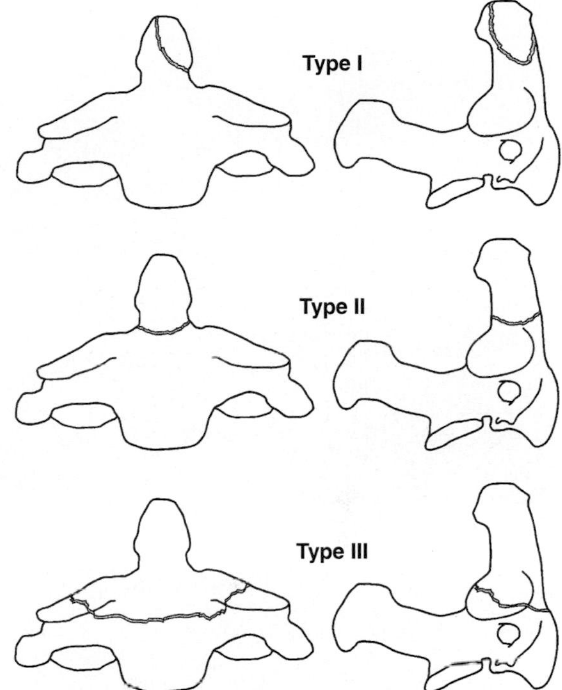

Figure 5–41. Diagram showing the three types of fractures of the odontoid process.

D. Hangman's Fracture (Traumatic Spondylolisthesis of Vertebra C2)

Hangman's fracture occurs when a fracture line passes through the neural arch of the axis. The anatomy of the axis is such that the superior facets are anterior and the inferior facets are posterior, thus concentrating stress through the neural arch. Because of the high ratio of spinal canal size to spinal cord size at this level, neurologic damage associated with hangman's fracture should be unusual. However, in his postmortem studies, Bucholz reported that traumatic spondylolisthesis was second only to occipitoatlantal dislocations in cervical injuries leading to fatalities.

According to the scheme proposed by Levine and Rhyne, hangman's fractures can be classified on the basis of anatomic factors and the presumed mechanism of injury. Treatment depends on the type of fracture. Imaging studies in a patient with hangman's fracture are shown in Figure 5–43.

Type I is typically caused by hyperextension with or without additional axial load. There is no angulation of the deformity, and the fracture fragments are separated by less than 3 mm. Treatment should consist of immobilization in a cervical collar or halo vest until union occurs, which is typically 12 weeks.

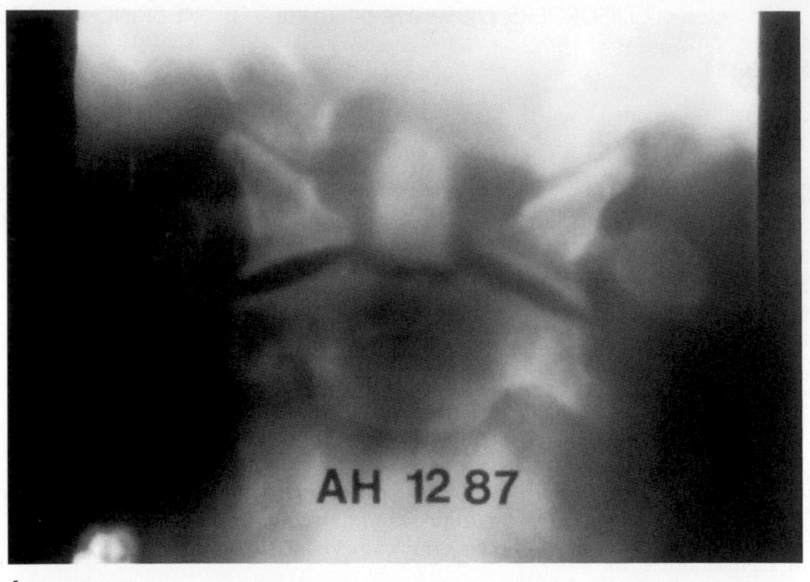

A

B

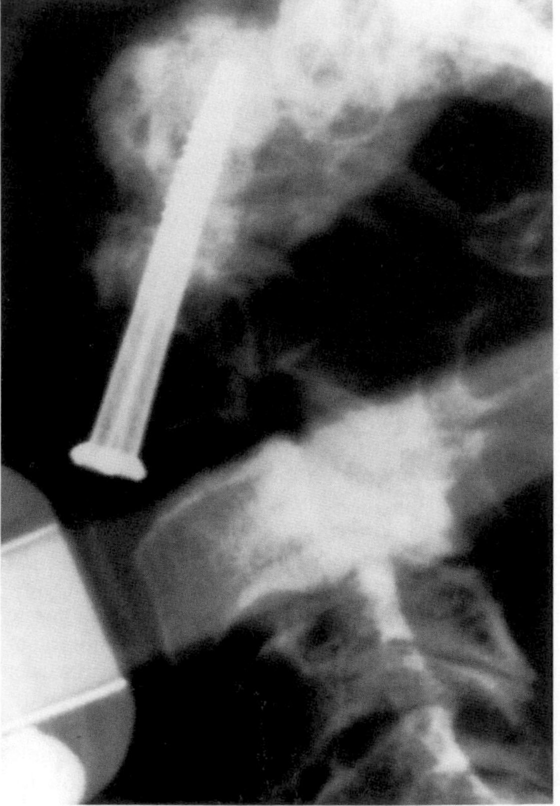

C

Figure 5–42. Imaging studies in a patient with a type II odontoid fracture nonunion. **A:** Open-mouth radiographic view showing the fracture line at the base of the odontoid process. **B:** Sagittal reconstruction using CT scanning to better delineate the fracture anatomy. **C:** Radiograph taken after the patient underwent anterior placement of two odontoid screws under fluoroscopic control using a cannulated screw system.

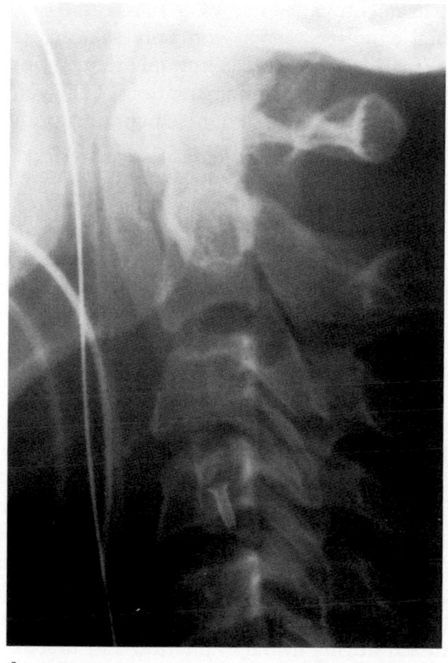

A

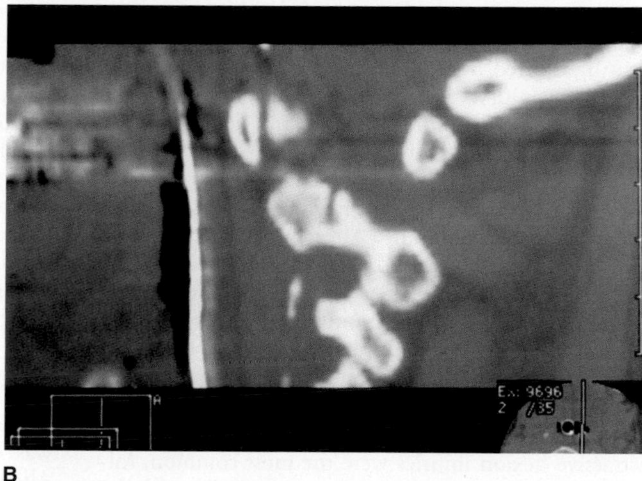

B

Figure 5–43. Imaging studies in a patient who was in a motor vehicle accident and sustained a hangman's fracture, or traumatic spondylolisthesis of C2. **A:** Lateral radiographic view, which is largely unremarkable. **B:** Sagittal reconstruction using CT scanning to better delineate the fracture site at the base of the posterior elements. The patient was treated nonoperatively.

Type II is thought to be caused by hyperextension and axial load with a secondary flexion component leading to displacement of the fracture. Reduction of the anterior angulation in this type of fracture is necessary and typically obtained by traction therapy and then followed by placement of a halo vest until union occurs. An atypical type II hangman's fracture is described. This fracture occurs through the posterior aspect of the vertebral body, potentially resulting in cord compromise as the anterior aspect of the vertebral body flexes forward. A higher likelihood of neurologic injury with this atypical pattern is seen, and halo-vest immobilization is recommended.

Type IIA has the same fracture pattern as type II but with a component of distraction that also occurred at the time of injury and led to disruption of the C2-C3 disk space, rendering this injury inherently unstable. Traction should be avoided in cases of type IIA fracture because it exacerbates the injury. Treatment should consist of immediate halo-vest application, with the patient's head positioned in slight extension to afford a reduction.

Type III includes a fracture through the neural arch, a facet dislocation, and a disruption of the C2-C3 disk space that renders the injury highly unstable. Treatment generally consists of early closed reduction of the facet dislocation and application of a halo vest to maintain the reduction. If the reduction cannot be obtained in a closed fashion or cannot be maintained conservatively, treatment with open reduction of the dislocation and anterior or posterior fusion is indicated.

Anderson LD, D'Alonzo RT: Fractures of the odontoid process of the axis. J Bone Joint Surg Am 1974;56:1663.

Govender S et al: Fractures of the odontoid process. J Bone Joint Surg Br 2000;82(8):1143. [PMID: 11132275]

Powers B et al: Traumatic anterior atlanto-occipital dislocation. Neurosurgery 1979;4:12.

Vieweg U, Schultheiss R: A review of halo vest treatment of upper cervical spine injuries. Arch Orthop Trauma Surg 2001; 121(1–2):50. [PMID: 21034862]

Ziai WC, Hurlbert RJ: A six year review of odontoid fractures: The emerging role of surgical intervention. Can J Neurol Sci 2000;27(4):297. [PMID: 11097519]

INJURIES OF THE LOWER CERVICAL SPINE

As stated earlier, fractures and dislocations of the lower cervical spine have a greater frequency of catastrophic neurologic involvement because of the decreased ratio of spinal canal to spinal cord in the lower levels. Treatment of affected patients again relies on early recognition of the injury, recognition of inherent stability or instability of the injury pattern, and institution of appropriate definitive care.

In 1982, Allen and colleagues developed a classification system for closed indirect fractures and dislocations of the lower cervical spine. After reviewing numerous cases previously described by other authors as well as 165 of their own cases, they grouped the injuries into six categories, based on the position of the cervical spine at the time of impact and on the dominant mode of failure. The six categories were compressive flexion, vertical compression, distractive flexion, compressive extension, distractive extension, and lateral flexion. Of these, the distractive flexion injuries were the most common, followed by the compressive extension injuries and the compressive flexion injuries. Some of the categories were further divided into stages, as described next.

Compressive Flexion Injury

There are five stages of compressive flexion injuries, which are labeled compression flexion stage (CFS) I through V (Figure 5–44). CFS I shows a slight blunting and rounding to the anterior superior vertebral margin, without any evidence of posterior ligamentous damage. CFS II shows some additional loss of height of the anterior vertebral body, again sparing the posterior elements. CFS III has an additional fracture line passing from the anterior surface of the vertebral body through to the inferior subchondral plate, with minimal displacement. CFS IV has less than 3 mm of displacement of the inferior posterior vertebral fragment into the neural canal. CFS V has severe displacement of the inferior posterior fragment into the canal, with widening of the spinous processes posteriorly, indicative of three-column disruption.

Within the compressive flexion category are two types of fractures, more commonly referred to as the **compression fracture** and the **teardrop fracture.** Most compression fractures without disruption of the posterior elements are thought to be stable, so no surgical intervention is required. The more severe compression fracture injuries, however, can result in displacement of bone into the spinal canal, and if a neurologic injury is present, these require anterior decompression and stabilization. All patients should be carefully checked with flexion-extension views at the completion of their treatment to rule out any evidence of late instability.

Vertical Compression Injury

Vertical compression spinal (VCS) injuries occur secondary to axial loading and are divided into three stages. VCS I consists of an endplate central fracture with no evidence of ligamentous failure. VCS II is a fracture of both vertebral endplates, again with only minimal displacement. VCS III is the more commonly termed **burst fracture** with a spectrum of fragmentation of the vertebral body, with or without posterior element disruption.

The treatment for VCS injuries is typically nonoperative. Traction is applied to obtain and maintain alignment, and bony union is generally complete after 3 months of halo-vest immobilization. Flexion-extension views should be obtained at the completion of healing because a posterior ligamentous injury can result in late instability.

Distractive Flexion Injury

The category of distractive flexion spinal (DFS) injury was the most common injury category reported by Allen and colleagues, and it includes both unilateral and bilateral facet subluxation and dislocation. There are four stages of DFS injury. DFS I, termed a **flexion sprain,** is characterized by subluxation of the facet joint, with possible interspinous process widening. This injury has subtle radiographic findings and may easily be missed during initial evaluation and therefore result in late symptomatic instability (Figure 5–45). DFS II is a unilateral facet dislocation, the diagnosis of which can be confirmed on plain radiographs. The lateral radiograph would reveal an anterior subluxation of one vertebra of approximately 25% of vertebral body width at the affected level. The facet itself may be perched or fully dislocated. DFS III is a bilateral facet dislocation with approximately 50% anterior dislocation at the affected level. DFS IV, which is also termed a **floating vertebra,** is a bilateral facet dislocation with displacement of a full vertebral width.

Treatment of DFS injuries depends on the severity of the injury. Achievement of anatomic alignment and spinal stability yields the best results. Patients with unilateral facet dislocation should be treated with closed reduction in the acute phase, followed by immobilization. If closed reduction is not possible, open reduction and fusion are indicated (Figure 5–46). Bilateral facet dislocations are associated with a higher incidence of both neurologic injury and instability. Treatment consisting of closed reduction and immobilization is feasible, but because it results in a high percentage of late instability, which eventually requires posterior fusion, the use of early posterior fusion is indicated.

Another fracture pattern that should be included in the discussion on flexion injuries is the clay shoveler's fracture, which is a fracture of the spinous process, typically at level C6, C7, or T1. This is an avulsion injury that generally occurs in flexion by the counteractive forces of the muscular attachments. As an isolated injury, it is considered stable and usually treated nonoperatively.

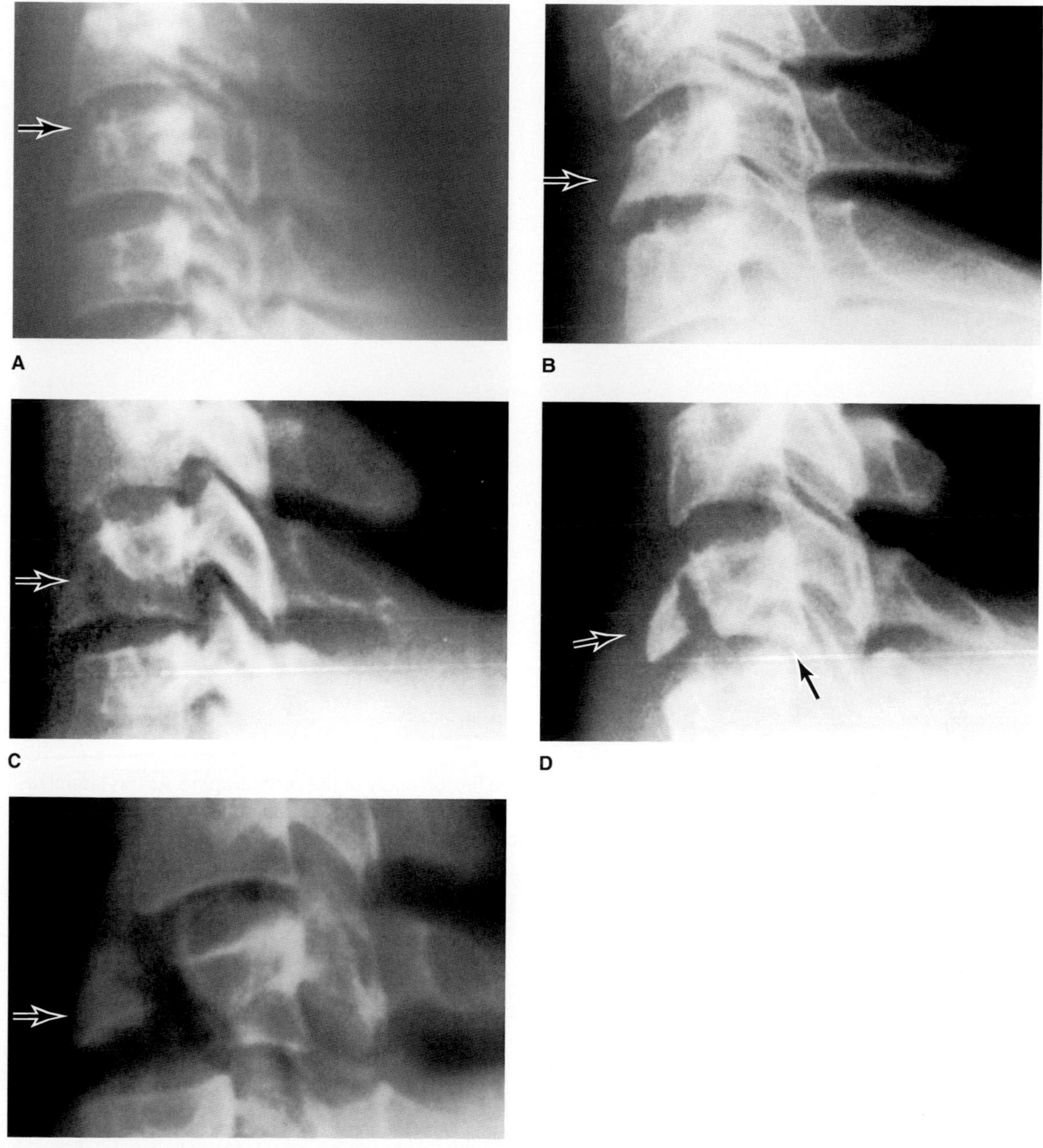

Figure 5–44. Radiographs showing the five stages of compressive flexion injury. **A** shows CFS I. **B** shows CFS II. **C** shows CFS III. **D** shows CFS IV. **E** shows CFS V. (Reproduced, with permission, from Allen BL et al: A mechanistic classification of closed, indirect fractures and dislocations of the lower cervical spine. Spine 1982;7:1.)

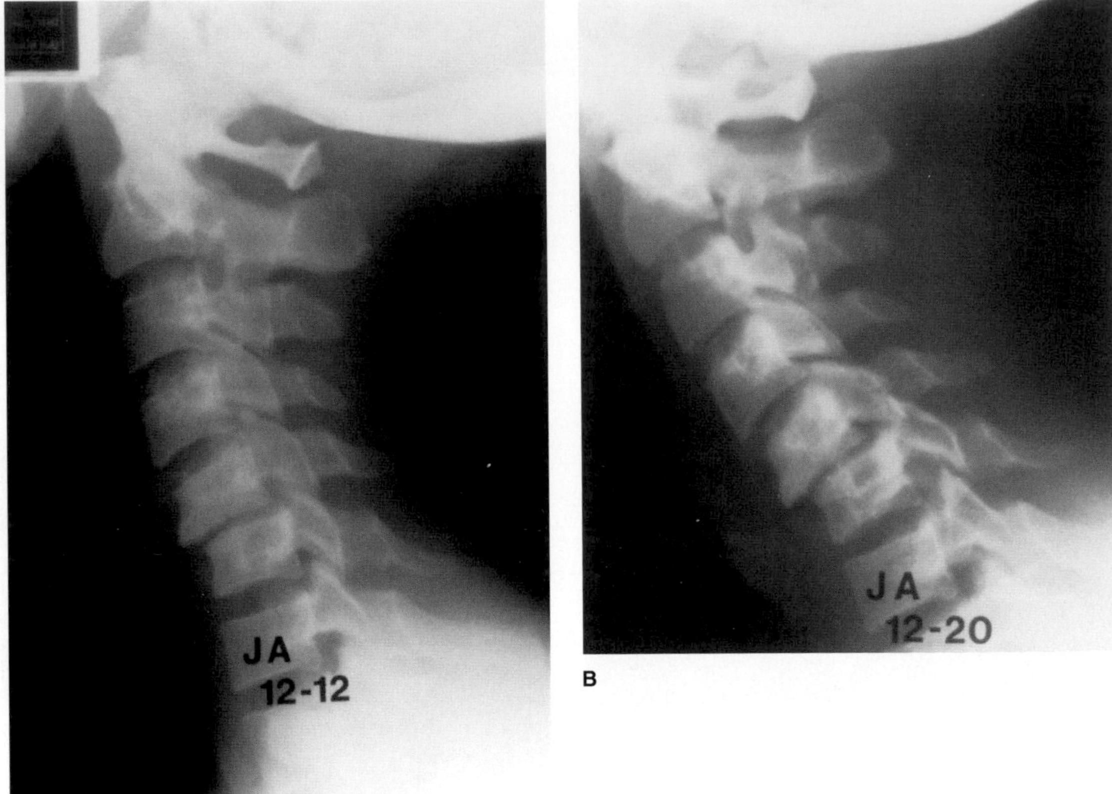

A B

Figure 5–45. Imaging studies in a patient with a distractive flexion injury of the cervical spine. **A:** This lateral radiographic view demonstrates anterior subluxation of C5 on C6. **B:** The follow-up radiograph shows progression of the subluxation. The patient was treated with a posterior spinal fusion of C5-C6.

Compressive Extension Injury

The category of compressive extension (CES) injury was the second most common injury category reported by Allen and colleagues. It is divided into five stages. CES I is a fracture of the vertebral arch unilaterally, with or without displacement, and CES II is a bilateral fracture. CES III and CES IV were not encountered in the series reported by Allen and colleagues but are theoretic interpolations between CES II and CES V. CES III is a bilateral fracture of the vertebral arch articular processes, lamina, or pedicle without vertebral displacement, whereas CES IV is the same fracture pattern but with moderate vertebral body displacement. Three patients in the Allen series had CES V injuries, which were bilateral vertebral arch fractures with 100% anterior displacement.

Treatment of CES injuries is related to the three-column theory. Stabilization with a posterior, anterior, or combined approach is indicated if there is significant disruption of the middle column or of two of the three columns.

Distractive Extension Injury

Distractive extension (DES) injuries are typically soft-tissue lesions and divided into two stages. DES I is a disruption of the anterior ligamentous complex or, rarely, a nondisplaced fracture of the vertebral body. Radiographs may appear entirely normal. One clue to the diagnosis is widening of the disk space, which is sometimes present. DES II is a disruption of the posterior soft-tissue complex, which can allow posterior displacement of the upper vertebral body into the spinal canal. This lesion is often reduced at the time of lateral radiographs and may show only subtle or no changes on routine radiographs. When neurologic involvement is present, it is most commonly a central cord syndrome, and provided that no coexisting compression lesions are present, some neurologic recovery is expected.

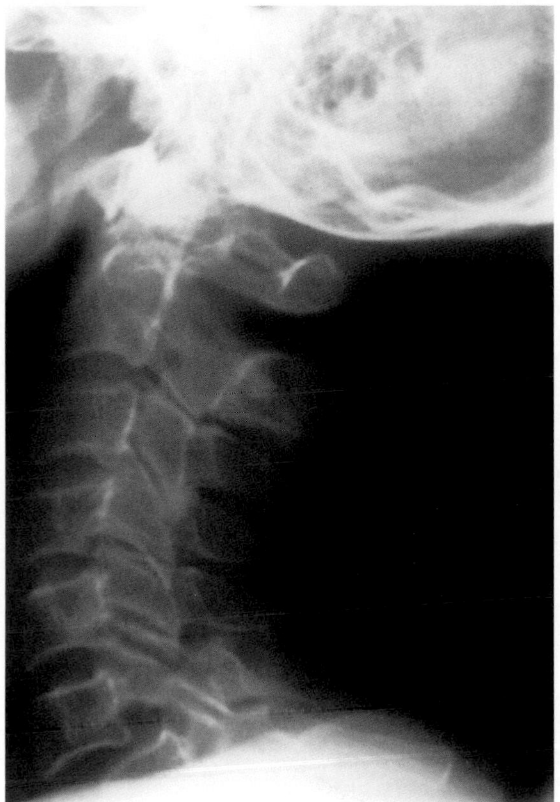

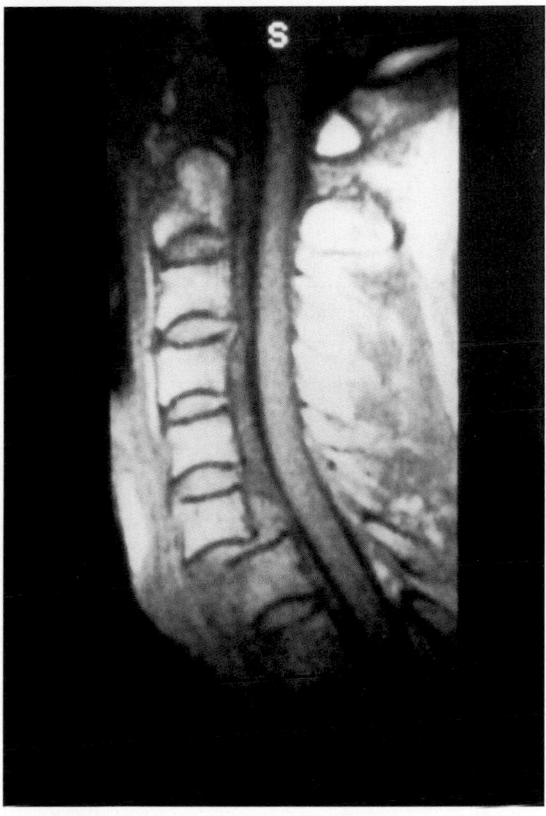

A B

Figure 5–46. Imaging studies in a man who fell from a height and suffered a C6-C7 fracture-dislocation with a perched facet but remained neurologically intact. **A:** Lateral radiographic view demonstrating the fracture-dislocation at C6-C7. **B:** MRI demonstrating the anterior subluxation of C6 on C7, with the intervertebral disk retropulsed behind the C6 vertebral body. The patient was treated with an anterior diskectomy, reduction, and fusion.

The DES injury is usually stable and does not require surgical intervention. Late flexion-extension views, however, are indicated to rule out any evidence of late instability.

Lateral Flexion Injury

Allen and colleagues included the injuries of five patients in the category of lateral flexion (LFS) injury. This category is further divided into two stages. LFS I is an asymmetric compression fracture of the vertebral body and ipsilateral posterior arch, with no displacement in the coronal plane. LFS II has a similar fracture pattern but with displacement in the coronal plane, which suggests ligamentous disruption on the tension side of the injury. This mechanism can lead to brachial plexus injuries of varying degrees on the distracted side.

Because of the rarity of LFS injuries, treatment protocols are not well established. Surgical stabilization should be considered if late instability is expected or if there is a neurologic deficit.

Treatment Decisions

Ultimately the treating physician must decide on a treatment plan. The Allen classification, although quite useful to describe an injury, is a mechanistic system that is challenging to apply to the individual patient to assess operative indications. The decision whether to operate is based on a spectrum of spinal stability and neurologic compromise. A patient with a three-column injury, continued neurologic compression, and neurologic symptoms has a clear operative indication either through an anterior, posterior, or combined approach. A fully neurologically intact patient with a one-column

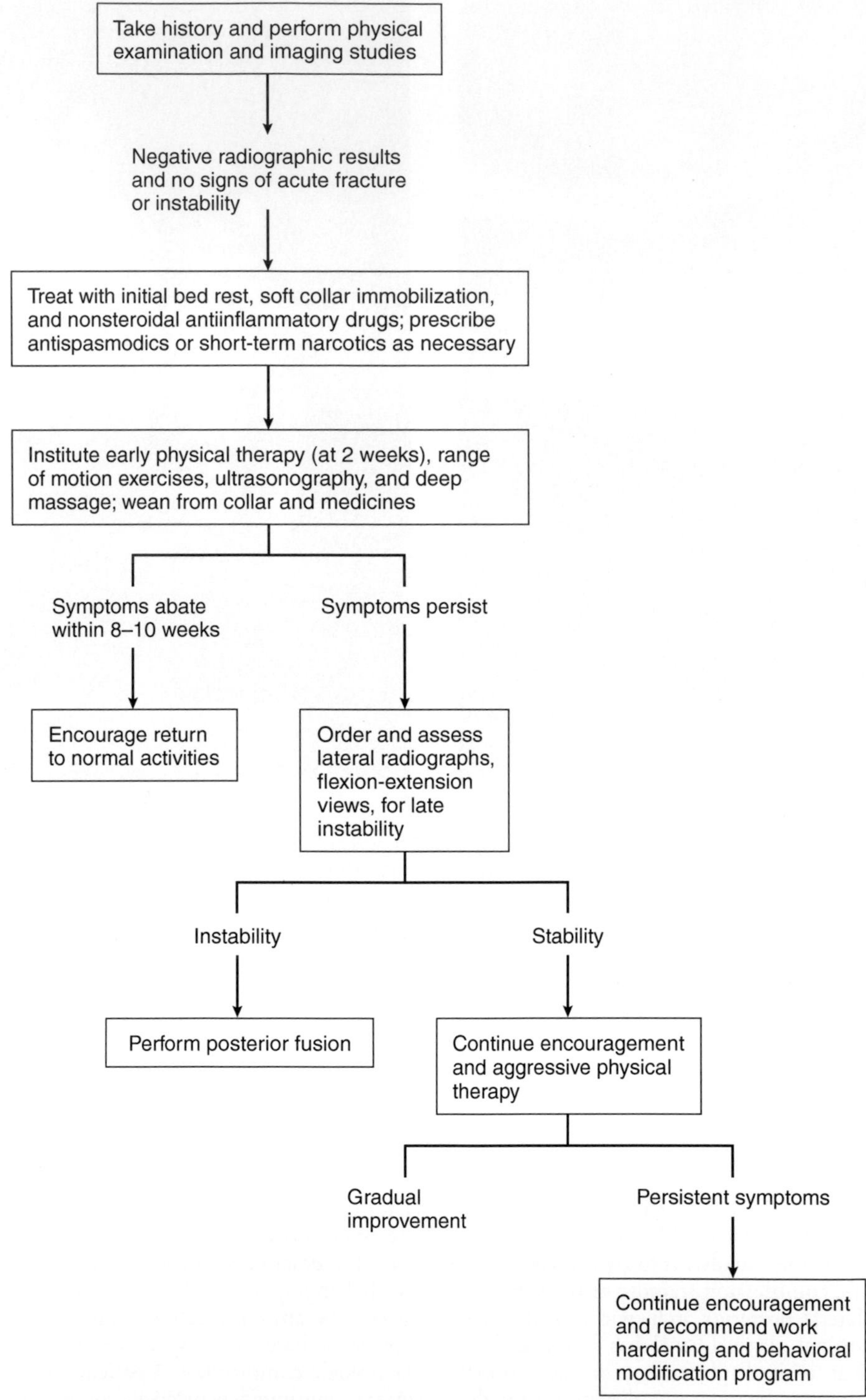

Figure 5–47. Algorithm for management of patients with cervical strain.

injury generally does fine in a brace. Patients with injury patterns in between must be treated on a case-by-case basis.

Cervical Strains & Sprains (Whiplash Injury)

Cervical strains and sprains, which are commonly referred to as a whiplash injury when associated with motor vehicle accidents, can produce a protracted and confusing clinical picture. Pain is typically the one unifying feature, yet there may be numerous other complaints, including local tenderness, decreased range of motion, headaches that are typically occipital, blurred or double vision, dysphagia, hoarseness, jaw pain, difficulty with balance, and even vertigo. It is often difficult for the physician to correlate radiographic findings, diagnostic test results, and other objective findings with the subjective complaints of the patient. The constellation of symptoms is fairly uniform, however, and should certainly not be discounted, and many investigators propose an anatomic basis for the clinical complaints. McNabb proposed that paresthesias in the ulnar distribution may be secondary to spasm of the scalenus muscle, and certainly symptoms such as hoarseness and dysphagia can be related to retropharyngeal hematoma. The cervical zygapophysial joint and facet capsule are implicated as a source for chronic pain after whiplash injury.

Figure 5–47 presents an algorithm for management of cervical strain. Radiographs should be taken because the amount of neck trauma that the patient has sustained may be significant. Radiographic findings, however, may be subtle or entirely negative. Cervical lordosis may be reversed, indicating spasm. Subtle signs of instability may also be present, and these can be further delineated on flexion-extension views if symptoms persist. The prevertebral soft-tissue window should be within normal limits to rule out any prevertebral hematoma.

Once the stability of the spine is ensured, the care of the cervical sprain or whiplash injury should be symptomatic. Initial rest, bed rest if necessary, and soft collar immobilization are indicated, along with the use of antiinflammatory medications. Early mobilization with progressive range of motion and weaning from external supports should be encouraged, however. Frequent reassurance is often necessary because the symptoms may be long lasting.

Approximately 42% of patients have persistent symptoms beyond 1 year, with approximately a third having persistent symptoms beyond 2 years. Most patients who do improve do so within the first 2 months. Factors associated with a poor prognosis include the presence of occipital headaches, interscapular pain, or reversal of cervical lordosis. Women have a worse prognosis than men, and hyperextension injuries are thought to have a worse prognosis than hyperflexion injuries.

Hartling L et al: Prognostic value of the Quebec classification of whiplash associated disorders. Spine 2001;26(1):36. [PMID: 11148643]

McNabb I: The "whiplash syndrome." Orthop Clin North Am 1971;2:389.

Siegmund GP et al: Mechanical evidence of facet capsule injury during whiplash—A cadaveric study using combined shear, compression, and extension loading. Spine 2001;26(19):2095. [PMID: 11698885]

Yoganandan N et al: Whiplash injury determination with conventional spine imaging and cryomicrotomy. Spine 2001;26(22): 2443. [PMID: 11707708]

Musculoskeletal Oncology

6

R. Lor Randall, MD, and Bang H. Hoang, MD

Tumors of the musculoskeletal system are an extremely heterogeneous group of neoplasms consisting of well over 200 benign types of neoplasms and approximately 90 malignant conditions. The relative incidence of benign to malignant disease is 200:1. The tumors uniformly arise from embryonic mesoderm and are categorized according to their differentiated or adult histology. Current classification schemes are essentially descriptive. Each histologic type of tumor expresses individual, distinct behaviors with great variation between tumor types. Benign disease, by definition, behaves in a nonaggressive fashion with little tendency to recur locally or to metastasize. Malignant tumors or sarcomas, such as osteosarcoma and synovial cell sarcoma, are capable of invasive, locally destructive growth with a tendency to recur and to metastasize.

Neoplastic processes arise in tissues of mesenchymal origin far less frequently than those of ectodermal and endodermal origin. In 2004, soft-tissue and bone sarcomas had an annual incidence in the United States of more than 8600 and 2400 new cases, respectively. When compared with the overall cancer mortality of 563,000 cases per year in 2004, sarcomas are a small fraction of the problem. However, although a relatively uncommon form of cancer, these mesenchymal tumors behave in an aggressive fashion with reported current mortality rates in some series greater than 50%. According to the National Cancer Institute's Surveillance, Epidemiology, and End Results (SEER) program, approximately 8600 new soft-tissue sarcomas developed in the United States in 2004 with over 3600 sarcoma-related deaths. The associated morbidity is much higher. These tumors inflict a tremendous emotional and financial toll on individuals and society alike. Furthermore, sarcomas are more common in older patients, with 15% percent affecting patients younger than 15 years and 40% percent affecting persons older than 55 years. Accordingly, as the population ages, as it is doing at a rapid rate, the incidence of these tumors will increase.

ETIOLOGY OF MUSCULOSKELETAL TUMORS

Tumorigenesis is a complex multiple-step process by which healthy tissue progressively transforms from a normal phenotype into an abnormal colony of proliferating cells. During this process, cells acquire genetic abnormalities in oncogenes, tumor suppressor genes, and other genes that directly or indirectly control proliferation. Such a process may progress beyond the controlled state of benign disease to become a dedifferentiated, aggressive, and immortal phenotype by genomic instability. It is this instability that allows the cell to progress to fulminant malignancy. DNA regulation and, correspondingly, integrity is ultimately lost and a cancer is born.

To appreciate how bone or soft-tissue tumors develop, one must have a basic understanding of the cell cycle during which cell division occurs. The cell cycle is divided into four distinct phases: G1 (gap 1), S (DNA synthesis), G2 (gap 2), and M (mitosis). DNA synthesis occurs during the S phase, with chromosomal separation and cell division occurring in the M phase. The majority of cell growth takes place during G1. The mature state for mesenchymal tissues is normally in a resting, nonproliferative phase designated G0. It is the factors that affect the exit of the cell from G0, with entrance into G1, that is the hallmark of neoplastic disease.

Control of the cell cycle is a function of numerous regulatory proteins and checkpoints. The checkpoints allow for the monitoring and correction in the genetic sequence. The proteins are encoded by two basic gene types: oncogenes (stimulatory) and tumor suppressor genes (inhibitory). The retinoblastoma (Rb) protein and its phosphorylation state are critically important in regulating cell cycle progression (from G1 to S phase). Therefore, the activation state of Rb is a highly regulated cellular event. In addition, multiple cyclins and cyclin-dependent kinases are being studied actively to elucidate their role in regulation of the cell cycle.

Oncogenes, encoding a variety of growth factors, promote progression of the cell through G1, effecting a mitogenic signal. Suppressor genes, such as wild-type *TP53,* act to arrest the cell cycle. Specifically, *TP53* acts to stop the cell cycle at the G1/S border as a final attempt to abort proliferation. Other suppressor genes work earlier to keep reproduction at bay. A complex array of molecules can serve as either an induction or suppressor function. When this pathway is not orchestrated properly, a given cell obtains the potential for limited or even immortal proliferation. A normal cell progresses through a preneoplastic state on its way to becoming neoplastic via the accumulation of mutations. A critical step during tumor progression is the loss of suppressor gene function, which occurs by a variety of defects, including deletions, translocations, promoter silencing, loss of heterozygosity, point mutations, microsatellite changes, and telomeric associations. The degree to which the daughter cells dedifferentiate into a malignant phenotype is a function of the amount of genomic instability that arises with each subsequent mitosis. Mutation begets mutation as the checkpoints and regulatory machinery continually fail to repair the genetic code.

Factors that influence these mechanisms include both inheritable genetic conditions (eg, Li-Fraumeni syndrome, retinoblastoma) or environmental factors. It is well established that oncogenic viruses, radiation, and chemical carcinogens can affect these processes, ultimately compromising genomic stability.

The neoplastic process may arrest in the so-called benign state, with further genomic instability curtailed, or it can almost progress to a sarcomatous state. For example, if the cell type of origin is a lipocyte, then a lipoma or liposarcoma may develop. Furthermore, a liposarcoma can progress in its dedifferentiation such that its phenotype, as a high-grade lesion, minimally reflects its lipocytic origin. This possibility does not imply, however, that all benign lesions are necessarily at risk for malignant degeneration. It is not a surgical indication to remove a lipoma because of concern over developing a liposarcoma.

Although a plethora of molecular markers are being studied, understanding the details of genomic instability and subsequent tumor formation is lacking. The initiation of the neoplastic process and subsequent disease progression is a complex multistep process in gene expression and deregulation. There is no single pathway by which all neoplasms arise; instead, multiple genetic targets are altered in a variety of sequences with the common result of cellular proliferation that is tumorigenesis.

EVALUATION & STAGING OF TUMORS

History & Physical Examination

When evaluating a new patient with a possible tumor, the workup must commence with a thorough history and physical examination. Prior to ordering any diagnostic studies, particular questions must be answered, and the physical characteristics of the mass in question must be assessed. This procedure prevents unnecessary tests and better enables the physician to determine which tests will be most helpful in diagnosing the condition as well as facilitating therapeutic interventions if needed.

The clinical history is of paramount importance (Table 6–1). The age of the patient permits the generation of a list of potential diagnoses (Table 6–2), which,

Table 6–1. Questions that must be asked in the workup of a possible tumor.

1. **The patient's age.** Certain tumors are relatively specific to particular age groups.
2. **Duration of complaint.** Benign lesions generally have been present for an extended period (years). Malignant tumors usually have been noticed for only weeks to months.
3. **Rate of growth.** A rapidly growing mass, as in weeks to months, is more likely to be malignant. Growth may be difficult to assess by the patient if it is deep seated, as can be the case with bone. Deep lesions may be much larger than the patient thought ("tip-of-the-iceberg" phenomenon).
4. **Pain associated with the mass.** Benign processes are usually asymptomatic. Osteochondromas (see text) may cause secondary symptoms because of encroachment on surrounding structures. Malignant lesions may cause pain.
5. **History of trauma.** With a history of penetrating trauma, one must rule out osteomyelitis. With a history of blunt trauma, healing fracture must be entertained.
6. **Personal or family history of cancer.** Adults with a history of prostate, renal, lung, breast, or thyroid tumors are at risk for developing metastatic bone disease. Children with neuroblastoma are prone to bony metastases. Patients with retinoblastoma are at an increased risk for osteosarcoma. Secondary osteosarcomas and other malignancies can result from treatment of other childhood cancers. Family history of conditions such as Li-Fraumeni syndrome must raise suspicion of any bone lesion. Furthermore, certain benign bone tumors can run in families (eg, hereditary multiple exostoses; see text).
7. **Systemic signs or symptoms.** Generally there should be no significant findings on the review of systems with benign tumors. Fevers, chills, night sweats, malaise, change in appetite, weight loss, and so on, should alert the physician that an infectious or neoplastic process may be involved.

Table 6–2. Distribution of bone tumors by age (years).

Type of Tumor	0	10	20	30	40	50	60	70	80
Benign bone tumors									
Osteoid osteoma									
Osteoblastoma									
Osteofibrous dysplasia									
Enchondroma									
Periosteal chondroma									
Osteochondroma									
Chondroblastoma									
Chondromyxoid fibroma									
Fibrous cortical defect									
Nonossifying fibroma									
Fibrous dysplasia									
Solitary bone cyst									
Aneurysmal bone cyst									
Epidermoid cyst									
Giant cell tumor									
Hemangioma									
Malignant bone tumors									
Classic osteosarcoma									
Hemorrhagic osteosarcoma									
Parosteal osteosarcoma									
Periosteal osteosarcoma									
Secondary osteosarcoma									
Low-grade intramedullary osteosarcoma									
Irradiation-induced osteosarcoma									
Multicentric osteosarcoma									
Primary chondrosarcoma									
Secondary chondrosarcoma									
Clear cell chondrosarcoma									
Dedifferentiated chondrosarcoma									
Mesenchymal chondrosarcoma									
Ewing sarcoma									
Lymphoma									
Multiple myeloma									
Solitary plasmacytoma									
Fibrosarcoma									
Malignant fibrous histiocytoma									
Adamantinoma									
Vascular sarcoma									
Chordoma									
Metastatic carcinoma									

Table 6–3. Aspects of physical exam that should be documented when evaluating a patient with a mass.[a]

1. **Skin color**
2. **Warmth**
3. **Location**
4. **Swelling.** Swelling, in addition to the primary mass effect, may reflect a more aggressive process.
5. **Neurovascular exam.** Changes may reflect a more aggressive process.
6. **Joint range of motion** of all joints in proximity to the region in question, above and below.
7. **Size.** A mass greater than 5 cm should raise the suspicion of malignancy.
8. **Tenderness.** Tenderness may reflect a more rapidly growing process.
9. **Firmness.** Malignant tumors tend to be firmer on examination than benign processes. This applies more to soft-tissue tumors than osseous ones.
10. **Lymph nodes.** Certain sarcomas (eg, rhabdomyosarcoma, synovial sarcoma, epithelioid, and clear cell sarcomas) all have increased rates of lymph node involvement.

[a]*Note:* These findings assume the absence of trauma.

when combined with the history and a few additional studies, should permit establishing a diagnosis. The duration of symptoms, rate of growth, the presence of pain, and a history of trauma can help elucidate the diagnosis. A careful past medical history, family history, and review of systems must not be overlooked either.

A thorough physical exam is also critical (Table 6–3). The clinician must assess the location and size of the mass, the quality of the overlying skin, the presence of warmth, any associated swelling, the presence of tenderness, and the firmness of the lesion. Range of motion of all joints in proximity to the tumor, above and below, must be recorded as well as a complete neurovascular exam. An assessment of the related lymph node chains as well as an examination for an enlarged liver or spleen should be performed.

The clinician must also consider pseudotumors in addition to true neoplastic conditions. A history of trauma suggests a possible stress fracture or myositis ossificans as a diagnosis. The history of stress-related physical activity and the exact timing of symptom presentation and variations of symptoms with the passage of time are important considerations in establishing a differential diagnosis.

Imaging Studies

A. Radiography

Initial evaluation should begin with plain radiography. In every patient with a suspected tumor, orthogonal anteroposterior (AP) and lateral views of the affected area should be taken. This includes soft-tissue masses as well. In many cases, radiographic examination is diagnostic, and no further imaging studies are indicated. However, in the case of a more aggressive process, the diagnosis may be determined on the plain radiographs but further evaluation with advanced studies is usually indicated to determine the extent of local soft-tissue involvement as well as to assess the extent of disseminated disease (staging).

The initial radiographic images must be scrutinized. For bone lesions, the location within the bone (eg, epiphyseal, metaphyseal, or diaphyseal) facilitates the diagnosis. Epiphyseal tumors are usually benign. The more malignant primary sarcomas, such as osteosarcoma, are typically seen in a metaphyseal location; however, round cell tumors, such as Ewing sarcoma, multiple myeloma, and lymphomas, are usually medullary diaphyseal lesions. A tumor arising from the surface of a long bone may be a benign lesion, such as an osteochondroma, or it may be a low-grade sarcoma, such as a parosteal osteosarcoma.

Terms such as *geographic, well circumscribed, permeative,* and are used to describe the appearance of radiographic abnormalities. Geographic or well circumscribed implies that the lesion has a distinct boundary and is sharply marginated, suggesting a benign tumor (Figure 6–1). A poorly defined, infiltrative process is described as permeative or moth eaten and reflects a more aggressive processsuch as a malignancy (Figure 6–2), although aggressive but benign processes can have this radio-

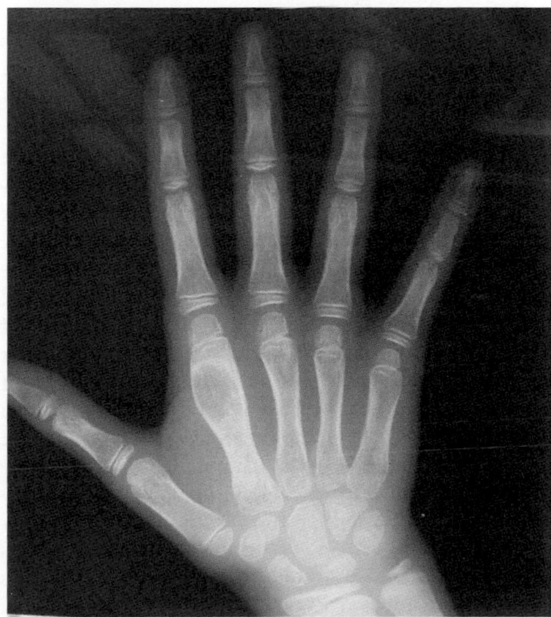

Figure 6–1. Radiograph of an enchondroma of the second metacarpal. Notice its geographic appearance.

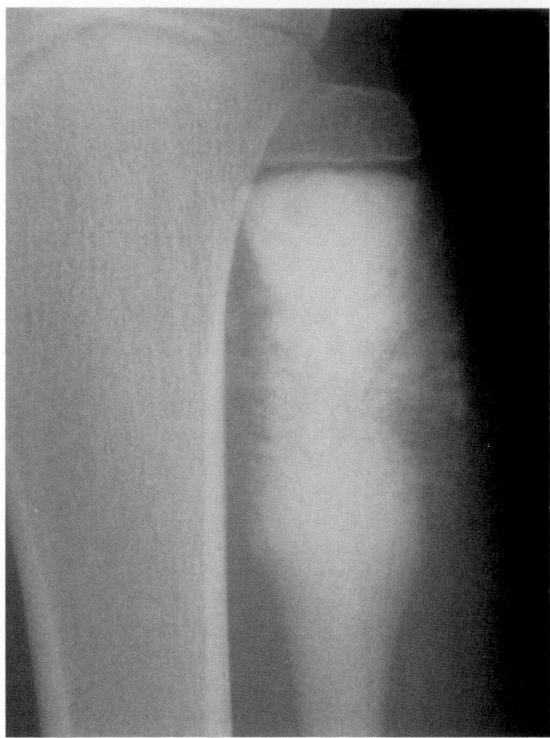

Figure 6–2. Radiograph of a proximal fibular osteosarcoma demonstrating the destructive, permeative nature of malignant bone tumors.

graphic quality as well (Figure 6–3). An exception to this rule is multiple myeloma, which frequently demonstrates a punched-out, well-demarcated appearance but in multiple locations.

With a careful history, physical, and appropriate radiographs, the physician can reach a working diagnosis of the lesion. Although benign and malignant tumors can mimic each other, some tumors can be ruled out on the basis of the history, the age of the patient, the location of the tumor (in which bone and where in the bone), and the radiographic appearance of the tumor, as shown in Tables 6–1 through 6–6. For example, a 20-year-old man with a 3-month history of pain in the knee is found to have an epiphyseal lesion in the distal femur. The lesion has a benign geographic appearance. If the tumor is benign, the criteria of the patient's age (see Table 6–2) eliminates only solitary bone cyst and osteofibrous dysplasia, but all other benign tumors remain possibilities. If the tumor is malignant, it is likely to be an osteosarcoma (various types), Ewing sarcoma, fibrosarcoma, vascular sarcoma, or, possibly, chondrosarcoma, according to the age criterion. The most common site for bone tumors is about the knee, especially the distal femur. The likely benign tumors are giant cell tumor, nonossifying fibroma, chondroma, osteochondroma, and chondroblastoma. The likely malignant tumors in this age group are osteosarcoma, Ewing sarcoma, fibrosarcoma, and, possibly, chondrosarcoma. Most malignant tumors are metaphyseal. Based on location in the bone (Table 6–4), the most likely benign tumors are chondroblastoma and giant cell tumor. Most malignant tumors are metaphyseal. The geographic appearance implies a benign radiographic appearance. Thus, the working diagnosis would be chondroblastoma or, possibly, giant cell tumor if the lesion were benign, whereas it would be osteosarcoma or chondrosarcoma if the lesion were malignant, which is less likely. In this age group, metastatic disease is very unlikely, but low-grade infection may mimic a tumor, particularly if the patient is immunocompromised, as can be determined from the patient's history. Table 6–5 indicates the most useful studies for further workup.

B. Isotope Bone Scanning

Technetium-99 radioisotope scans are used to assess the degree of osteoblastic activity of a given lesion

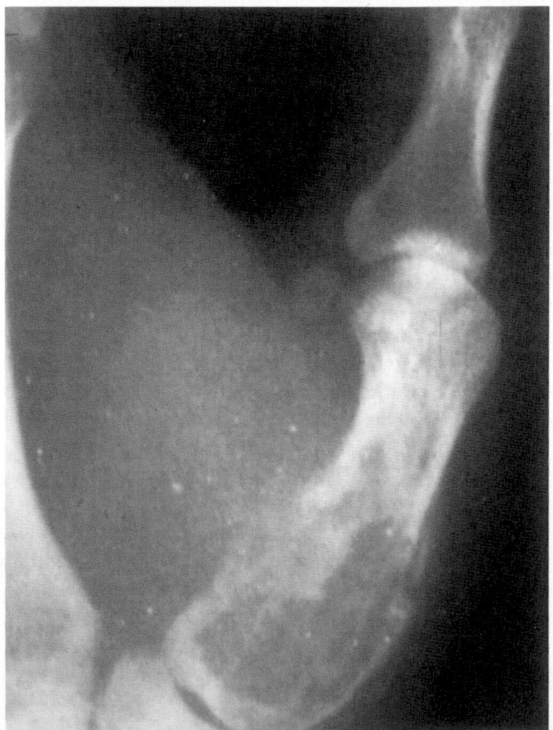

Figure 6–3. Radiograph of a giant cell tumor of the thumb. This is a typical moth-eaten appearance.

(Figure 6–4). In general, they are quite sensitive, with a few exceptions, for active lesions of bone. Accordingly, technetium-99 scans are excellent screening tools for remote lesions (staging). The best indication for a bone scan is suspected multiple bony lesions, such as those commonly seen in metastatic carcinomas and lymphomas of bone. Isotope bone scanning is far simpler to perform, less expensive, and requires less total body irradiation than skeletal surveys. It is common practice to use serial isotope scans to follow patients with suspected metastatic disease and at the same time evaluate the effectiveness of their systemic therapy program.

Isotope scanning is also used in the staging process of a primary sarcoma such as an osteosarcoma to make sure the patient does not have an asymptomatic remote skeletal lesion. Technetium-99 scans are also useful in distinguishing blastic lesions of bone. Given that the study reflects metabolic activity, an enostosis (bone island) would not demonstrate significant increased activity compared with a blastic prostate metastasis. Inflammatory disease and trauma also show increased activity. It is important to note, however, that multiple myeloma and metastatic squamous cell carcinoma may not demonstrate technetium uptake (ie, a false-negative result). Skeletal surveys are preferable for screening for additional sites of involvement in such cases.

C. Computed Tomography and Magnetic Resonance Imaging

Computed tomography (CT) remains a standard imaging procedure for use in well-selected clinical situations. Perhaps the best indication for CT is for smaller lesions that involve cortical structures of bone or spine (Figure 6–5). In such cases, CT is superior to MRI because the resolution of cortical bone using MRI is inferior. CT scan of the lung is the modality of choice for evaluating patients with sarcoma for possible lung metastases. Abdominal CT scan is invaluable in surveying for a primary tumor in patients who present with bone metastases. For tumors involving the pelvis and sacrum, CT can help elucidate the extent of bone involvement (Figure 6–6). In cases involving a soft-tissue lesion, MRI is far superior to CT unless there is a heavily calcified process.

MRI is the imaging modality of choice for evaluating bone marrow involvement as well as noncalcific soft-tissue lesions. The two most commonly used MRI sequences are the T_1-weighted and T_2-weighted spin echo (Figure 6–7). MRI can also demonstrate the normal anatomy of soft structures, including nerves and vessels, thereby nearly eliminating the need for arteriography and myelograms. Dynamic-enhanced MRI, with its ability to estimate tumor blood flow by examining the rate of contrast uptake and clearance, may serve as a predictor of clinical outcome or tumor response to chemotherapy.

Laboratory Studies

A. Biopsy

The biopsy should usually be the final staging procedure. Although the biopsy can distort the imaging studies, such as MRI, pathologic evaluation and interpretation may require information provided by the prior workup. Complications relating to the biopsy are not infrequent. Accordingly, careful preoperative planning is imperative. The imaging studies aid the surgeon in selecting the best site for a tissue diagnosis. In most cases, the best diagnostic tissue is found at the periphery of the tumor, where it interfaces with normal tissue. For example, in the case of a malignant bone tumor, soft-tissue invasion is usually evident outside the bone, and this area can be sampled without violating cortical bone and thus without causing a fracture at the biopsy site. If a medullary specimen is needed, a small round or oval hole should be cut to decrease the chance of fracture. If the medullary specimen is malignant, the cortical hole should be plugged with bone wax or bone cement to reduce soft-tissue contamination following the procedure.

Obtaining an adequate specimen is critical. A frozen section determines if viable and adequate tissue were obtained. A few experienced tumor centers may make a definitive diagnosis based on a frozen section, allowing the surgeon to proceed with definitive operative treatment of the tumor. However, freezing artifact can cause overinterpretation of the material, so an aggressive resection should always be deferred until the permanent analysis is complete. Additional studies beyond conventional light microscopy, such as immunocytochemistries and cytogenetics, may also be necessary.

The placement of the biopsy site is a major consideration. If the surgeon is inexperienced and not familiar with surgical oncologic principles, a serious contamination of a vital structure such as the popliteal artery or sciatic nerve may occur. Such an error might necessitate an amputation instead of a limb-sparing procedure. To avoid this problem in the case of a suspected malignant condition, the surgeon who performs the biopsy should be the same surgeon who will perform the definitive operative procedure.

Transverse incisions should be avoided because removing the entire biopsy site with the widely resected subjacent tumor mass is difficult. Adequate hemostasis is mandatory to avoid formation of a contaminating hematoma. A drain may be helpful but frequently is unnecessary. If a drain is used, it must be placed in line with the incision.

Table 6–6. Distribution of soft-tissue tumors by age (years).

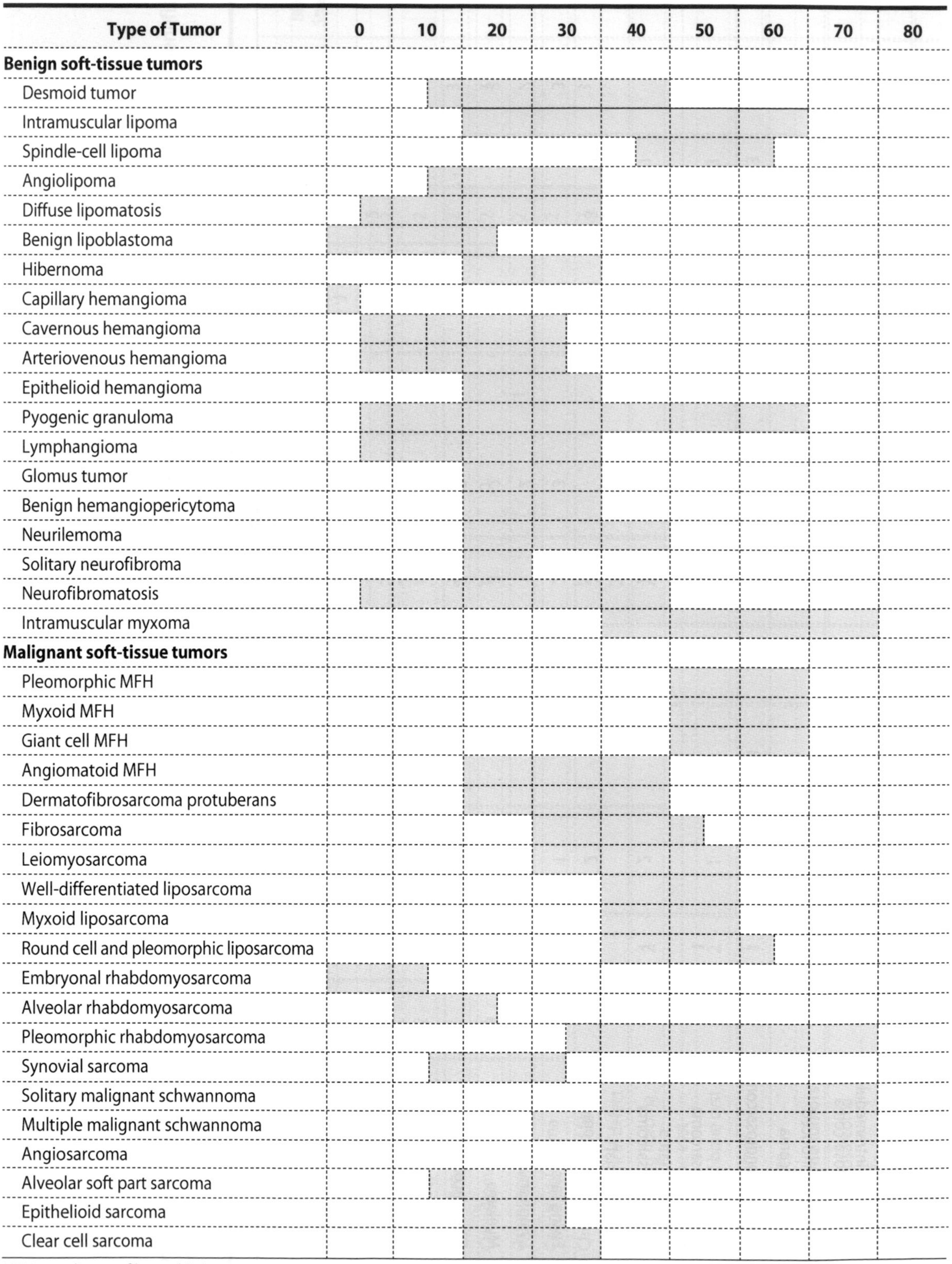

Type of Tumor	0	10	20	30	40	50	60	70	80
Benign soft-tissue tumors									
Desmoid tumor		▐	■	■	■				
Intramuscular lipoma			■	■	■	■	■		
Spindle-cell lipoma					▐	■	▌		
Angiolipoma		▐	■	■					
Diffuse lipomatosis	▐	■	■	■					
Benign lipoblastoma	■	■	▌						
Hibernoma			■	■					
Capillary hemangioma	▌								
Cavernous hemangioma	▐	■	■	▌					
Arteriovenous hemangioma	▐	■	■	▌					
Epithelioid hemangioma			■	■					
Pyogenic granuloma	▐	■	■	■	■	■	■		
Lymphangioma	▐	■	■	■					
Glomus tumor			■	■					
Benign hemangiopericytoma			■	■					
Neurilemoma			■	■	■				
Solitary neurofibroma			■						
Neurofibromatosis	▐	■	■	■	■				
Intramuscular myxoma					■	■	■	■	
Malignant soft-tissue tumors									
Pleomorphic MFH						■	■		
Myxoid MFH						■	■		
Giant cell MFH						■	■		
Angiomatoid MFH			■	■	■				
Dermatofibrosarcoma protuberans			■	■	■				
Fibrosarcoma				■	■	▌			
Leiomyosarcoma				■	■	■			
Well-differentiated liposarcoma					■	■			
Myxoid liposarcoma					■	■			
Round cell and pleomorphic liposarcoma					■	■	▌		
Embryonal rhabdomyosarcoma	■	▌							
Alveolar rhabdomyosarcoma		■	▌						
Pleomorphic rhabdomyosarcoma				▐	■	■	■	■	
Synovial sarcoma		▐	■	▌					
Solitary malignant schwannoma					■	■	■	■	
Multiple malignant schwannoma				■	■	■	■	■	
Angiosarcoma					■	■	■	■	
Alveolar soft part sarcoma		▐	■	▌					
Epithelioid sarcoma			■	▌					
Clear cell sarcoma			■	■					

MFH = malignant fibrous histiocytoma.

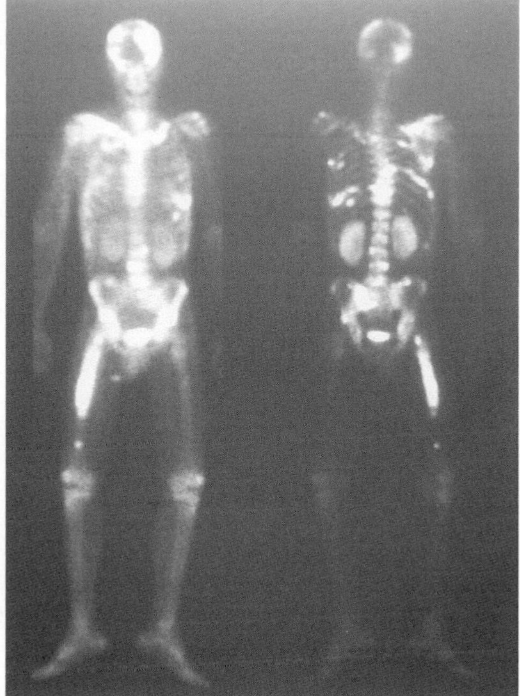

Figure 6–4. Technetium-99 scan demonstrating extensive osteoblastic activity in a patient with metastatic adenocarcinoma.

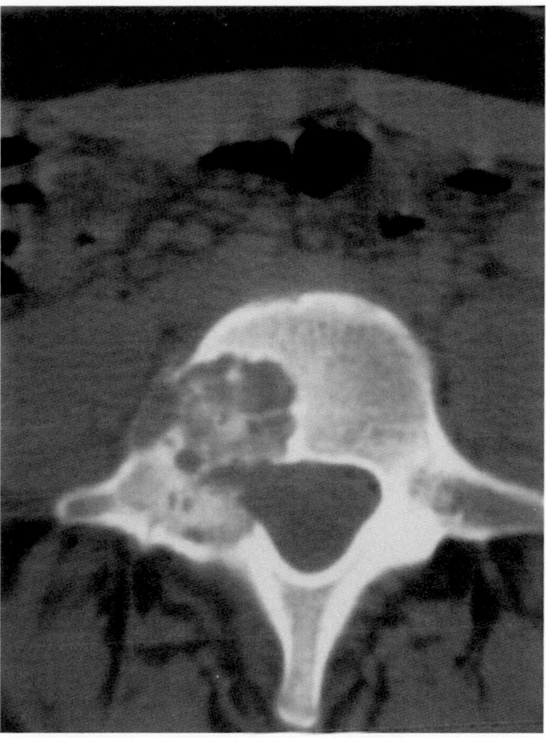

Figure 6–5. CT scan of an osteoblastoma arising from the right pedicle of a lumbar vertebral body.

Needle biopsies, either core or fine needle, can be used by experienced tumor centers, especially for lesions that are easily diagnosed, such as metastatic carcinomas or round cell tumors. Because the subtype of sarcoma is proving to be very important, architecture of the tumor is generally needed, which requires a core biopsy rather than a fine-needle aspirate. Core biopsies also allow the surgeon to sample various areas of the tumor to avoid sampling error in a heterogeneous tumor. In the case of a deep pelvic lesion or a spinal lesion, a CT-guided nee-

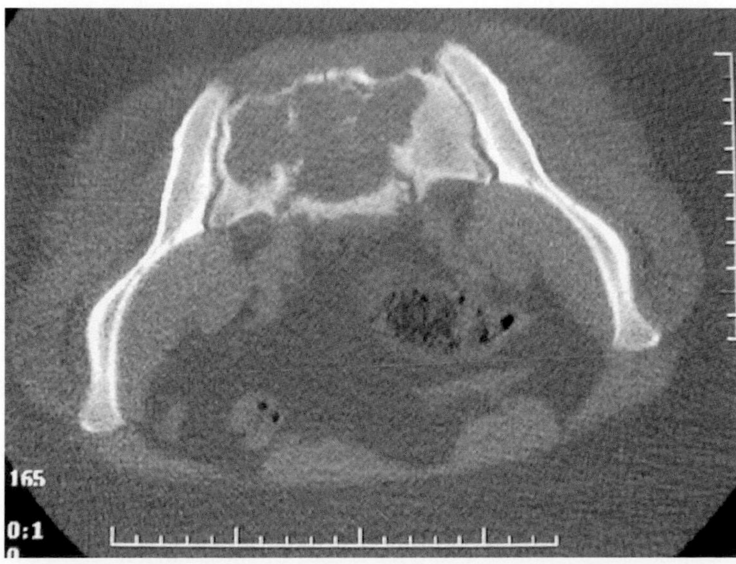

Figure 6–6. Pelvic CT demonstrating the bony destruction of the sacrum caused by a giant cell tumor.

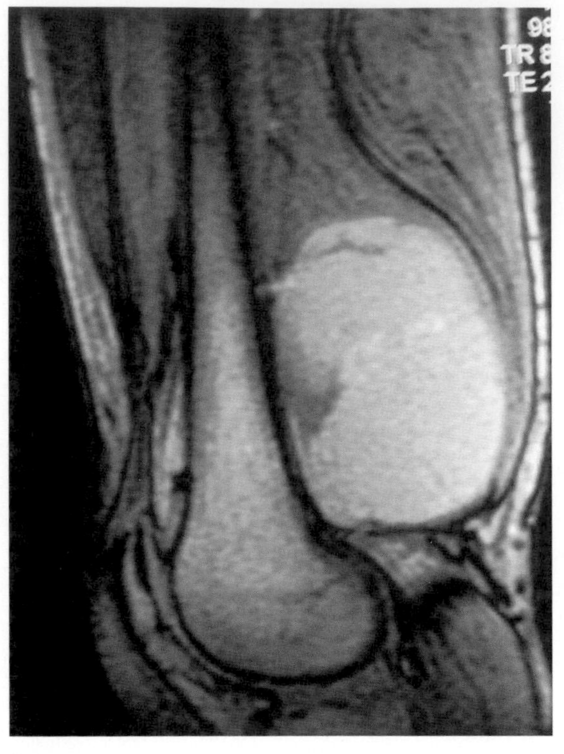

A

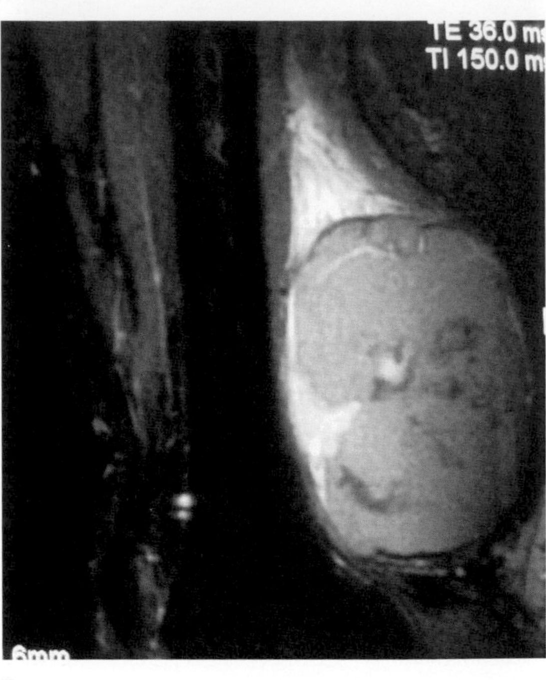

B

Figure 6–7. Synovial sarcoma involving the popliteal fossa. (**A**) T_1 weighted. (**B**) T_2 weighted.

dle biopsy is ideal because it avoids excessive multicompartmental contamination.

In general, excisional biopsies are discouraged unless the lesion is particularly small (less than 2–3 cm) or in an area where a cuff of healthy uninvolved tissue of at least 1 cm can be removed as well. This technique ideally avoids a second procedure to remove the entire biopsy site if the lesion turns out to be malignant.

B. Cultures and Special Studies

The damage of biopsy specimens after retrieval can make it impossible to perform special studies such as immunohistochemistry, cytogenetics, flow cytometry, and electron microscopy. For this reason, the biopsy surgeon should consult with the pathologist before specimens are retrieved and handled. Furthermore, many current studies require fresh tissue (no formalin). It is also a good habit to obtain cultures for bacterial culture (anaerobic and aerobic) as well as fungal and acid-fast bacteria if clinical suspicion warrants.

Molecular diagnostics is on the verge of revolutionizing sarcoma diagnostics. Specific translocations were found in a variety of tumors (Table 6–7). Furthermore, therapeutics are beginning to be designed against specific molecular defects in malignancies. Gastrointestinal stromal tumor (GIST), a malignant mesenchymal tumor arising from the gastrointestinal (GI) tract, omentum, and mesentery, overexpresses a mutant form of c-*kit.* The *KIT* gene encodes a tyrosine kinase receptor for the growth factor named stem cell factor or mast cell growth factor. Therapy directed against c-*kit* is having an early and remarkable effect on the previously difficult treatment of malignancy. Similar pathways are being elicited in other sarcomas.

Staging Systems

After the appropriate studies are completed, staging begins. *Staging* refers to an assessment of the grade of the tumor and the extent to which the disease has spread. There are several staging systems, but all have the purpose of helping the physician plan a logical treatment program and establish a prognosis for the patient. The two major systems are discussed here.

A. System of the American Joint Committee on Cancer

The American Joint Committee on Cancer (AJCC) system (5th edition) is used by most surgical oncologists

Table 6–7. Common translocations seen in sarcomas.

Ewing/primitive neuroectodermal tumor: t(11;22) (q24; q12), (t21; 22) (q22; q12), (t7; 22) (p22; q12)
Myxoid chondrosarcoma: t(9; 22) (q22; q12)
Myxoid & round cell liposarcoma: t(12; 16) (q12; p11)
Synovial sarcoma: t(X; 18) (p11; q11)
Alveolar rhabdomyosarcoma: t(2; 13) (q35; q14), t(1; 13) (p36; q14)
Alveolar soft parts sarcoma: t(X; 17) (p11.2; q25)
Desmoplastic small round cell tumor: t(11; 22) (p13; q12)
Congenital fibrosarcoma: t(12; 15)

when dealing with soft-tissue sarcomas. It classifies sarcomas according to their histologic grade (low or high), depth (superficial or deep), and size (with large tumors more than 5 cm in greatest dimension). Adverse prognostic factors include large tumor size, deep location within the extremity, and high histologic grade.

B. System of the American Musculoskeletal Tumor Society (Enneking System)

Orthopedic oncologists generally prefer the Enneking system, which addresses the unique problems related to sarcomas of the extremities and applies to tumors of the bone as well as those of soft tissue. The Enneking system has a 3-point scale for classifying tumors as stage I, II, or III on the basis of their histologic and biologic appearance and their likelihood of metastasizing to regional lymph nodes or distant sites such as the lung. Stage I refers to low-grade sarcomas with less than 25% chance of metastasis. Stage II refers to high-grade sarcomas with more than 25% chance of metastasis. Stage III is for either low-grade or high-grade tumors that have metastasized to a distant site, such as a lymph node, lung, or other distant organ system.

The Enneking system further classifies tumors on the basis of whether they are intracompartmental (type A) or extracompartmental (type B). Type A tumors are constrained by anatomic boundaries such as muscle fascial planes and stand a better chance for local control of tumor growth with surgical removal than type B tumors do. A lesion contained in a single muscle belly or a bone lesion that has not broken out into the surrounding soft tissue would be classified as a type A tumor. A lesion in the popliteal space, axilla, pelvis, or midportion of the hand or foot would be classified as a type B tumor. Although compartmentalization of a tumor is an important concept, studies show that the size of the tumor rather than whether it is contained within a compartment is more prognostic. Larger tumors, greater than 5 cm, are prognostically unfavorable.

A low-grade fibrosarcoma located inside the fascial plane of the biceps muscle and having no evidence of metastasis would be classified as a stage IA tumor. A typical malignant osteosarcoma of the distal femur with breakthrough into the surrounding muscle as determined by MRI would be classified as a stage IIB lesion. If CT scanning revealed metastatic involvement of the lung, the osteosarcoma would then be classified as a stage IIIB lesion.

Enneking WF: A system of staging musculoskeletal neoplasms. Clin Orthop 1985;204:9.

Mankin HJ et al: The hazards of the biopsy, revisited. J Bone Joint Surg Am 1996;78:656. [PMID 8642021]

Miettinen M et al: Gastrointestinal stromal tumors—Definition, clinical, histological, immunohistochemical, and molecular genetic features and differential diagnosis. Virchows Arch 2001;438(1):1. [PMID: 11688571]

Moley JF et al: Soft-tissue sarcomas. Surg Clin North Am 2000; 80(2):687. [PMID: 10836012]

Oliveira AM et al: Grading in soft tissue tumors: Principles and problems. Skeletal Radiol 2001;30(10):543. [PMID: 11685477]

Reddick WE et al: Dynamic MR imaging (DEMRI) of microcirculation in bone sarcoma. J Magn Reson Imaging 1999;10(3): 277. [PMID: 10508287]

Simon MA et al: Diagnostic strategy for bone & soft tissue tumors. J Bone Joint Surg Am 1993;75:622. [PMID: 8478392]

Skrzynski MC et al: Diagnostic accuracy and charge savings of outpatient care needle biopsy compared with open biopsy of musculoskeletal tumors. J Bone Joint Surg Am 1996;78:644. [PMID: 8642019]

Zahm SH et al: The epidemiology of soft tissue sarcoma. Semin Oncol 1997;24(5):504. [PMID: 9344316]

DIAGNOSIS & TREATMENT OF TUMORS

BENIGN BONE TUMORS

Benign bone tumors have certain characteristics that favor their diagnosis over malignant conditions. If the condition is benign, the patient is frequently asymptomatic, and the radiograph usually shows a well-defined geographic lesion with sclerotic reactive margins that suggest a long-standing process associated with slow growth potential. In contrast, if the condition is malignant, the patient usually complains of pain, and the radiograph commonly shows a more permeative lesion with lytic destruction and poorly defined margins that suggest rapid progression. In many cases, further studies such as MRI or bone isotope studies are not necessary for a typical benign tumor, such as fibrous dysplasia, enchondroma, or nonossifying fibroma. A system of staging exists for benign bone tumors. Stage 1 lesions are considered latent. They generally are asymptomatic but not always. Although they can progress, they usually resolve. Initially, these lesions should be observed. Stage 2 lesions are considered active. They tend not to resolve spontaneously and are less well demarcated than stage 1 lesions. They frequently require surgical intervention with aggressive treatment. Recurrence is not infrequent. Stage 3, or aggressive lesions, demonstrate extensive destruction. Treatment often requires wide en bloc resection.

The more common types of benign bone tumor seen by the practicing orthopedic surgeon are discussed in this section.

Benign Osteoid-Forming Tumors

A. Osteoid Osteoma

The most common benign osteoid-forming tumor is the osteoid osteoma, accounting for 10% of all benign bone tumors. It is more common in males than in females, with a peak incidence in the second decade of life. The proximal femur is the most common site. Dull aching pain is the most frequent symptom. Symptoms are relieved with nonsteroidal antiinflammatory drugs (NSAIDs) secondary to a high concentration of prostaglandins in the nidus. Osteoid osteoma may have a unique pathogenic nerve supply as well, a unique finding among bone tumors.

The characteristic radiographic feature of the osteoid osteoma is the central lytic nidus that measures up to 1 cm in diameter. In the common cortical lesion (Figure 6–8), an extensive reactive sclerosis is evident, creating a fusiform bulge on the bone surface. However, if the nidus is more centrally located in metaphyseal bone, less sclerosis is seen and the radiographic appearance is less diagnostic. If the nidus is close to a joint or actually in the joint, as in the case of a femoral neck lesion, inflammatory synovitis results and suggests the diagnosis of a pyarthrosis or rheumatoid disease. Technetium bone scans are invariably positive. A CT scan is helpful to better anatomically locate the lesion in preoperative planning.

In the spine, the typical location for an osteoid osteoma is in the posterior elements, such as the lamina or pedicle. The lumbar spine is most commonly involved; the dorsal spine is the second most commonly involved. A secondary scoliosis may develop, with the convexity toward the lesion. Furthermore, if the nidus is in proximity to a nerve root, root irritation can develop. In the lumbar spine, this pain can present as sciatica and suggest the diagnosis of a herniated disk.

Previously, some investigators believed that the osteoid osteoma was an inflammatory process such as a Brodie abscess, which has a similar clinical and radiographic appearance. Currently, it is accepted that osteoid osteoma is a true osteoid-forming neoplasm and absent of lymphocytes or plasma cells. Histologically, the nidus shows aggressive but benign woven bone formation, with large numbers of osteoblasts and osteoclasts in a vascular fibrous stroma. No chondroid areas are seen.

Most cases of osteoid osteoma are stage 1 lesions and can be treated symptomatically with aspirin or NSAIDs. If the patient fails such treatment, surgical intervention is warranted. If surgery is undertaken, the entire symptomatic nidus must be eradicated. Removal of a large amount of the surrounding sclerotic bone should be avoided because it can severely weaken the bone and may result in a pathologic fracture. If the lesion is in cortical bone, adequate exposure is required so the surgeon can visualize the bulging cortex. Intralesional resection via the so-called burr-down technique is generally preferred over en bloc resection. The nidus can be identified visually by the hyperemic pink color in the reactive bone adjacent to it. Simple curettage of the nidus followed by high-speed burring to advance the margin another 2–3 mm is all that is necessary. If the lesion is not visible on the surface, as in the case of a medullary lesion, radiographic markers should be placed intraoperatively prior to placing the round cortical window. CT-guided radiofrequency ablation (RFA) is reported as an effective, less invasive method of treating osteoid osteoma. This method employs probes with high-frequency alternating current to induce ionic agitation and frictional heat to cause tumor necrosis. RFA is used extensively as a less invasive treatment modality with similar success rate as surgical excision.

B. Osteoblastoma

Osteoblastoma is a large osteoid osteoma that demonstrates a propensity for the posterior elements of the spine. The tumors are found more commonly in males than in females and occur in the same age group as osteoid osteomas. Osteoblastomas are less common than osteoid osteomas, accounting for 1% of all bone tumors. A few can be found in the metaphyses of long bone (raising suspicion about a possible osteosarcoma), and a few can be seen in the ankle and wrist areas. These lesions are usually stage 1–2 lesions.

Radiographically, the osteoblastoma has a more lytic and destructive appearance than the osteoid osteoma. Its nidus, which is greater than 1–2 cm, has a less sclerotic reactive bone at the periphery and may take on the appearance of an aneurysmal bone cyst. Histologically, the nidus of the osteoblastoma is nearly identical to that

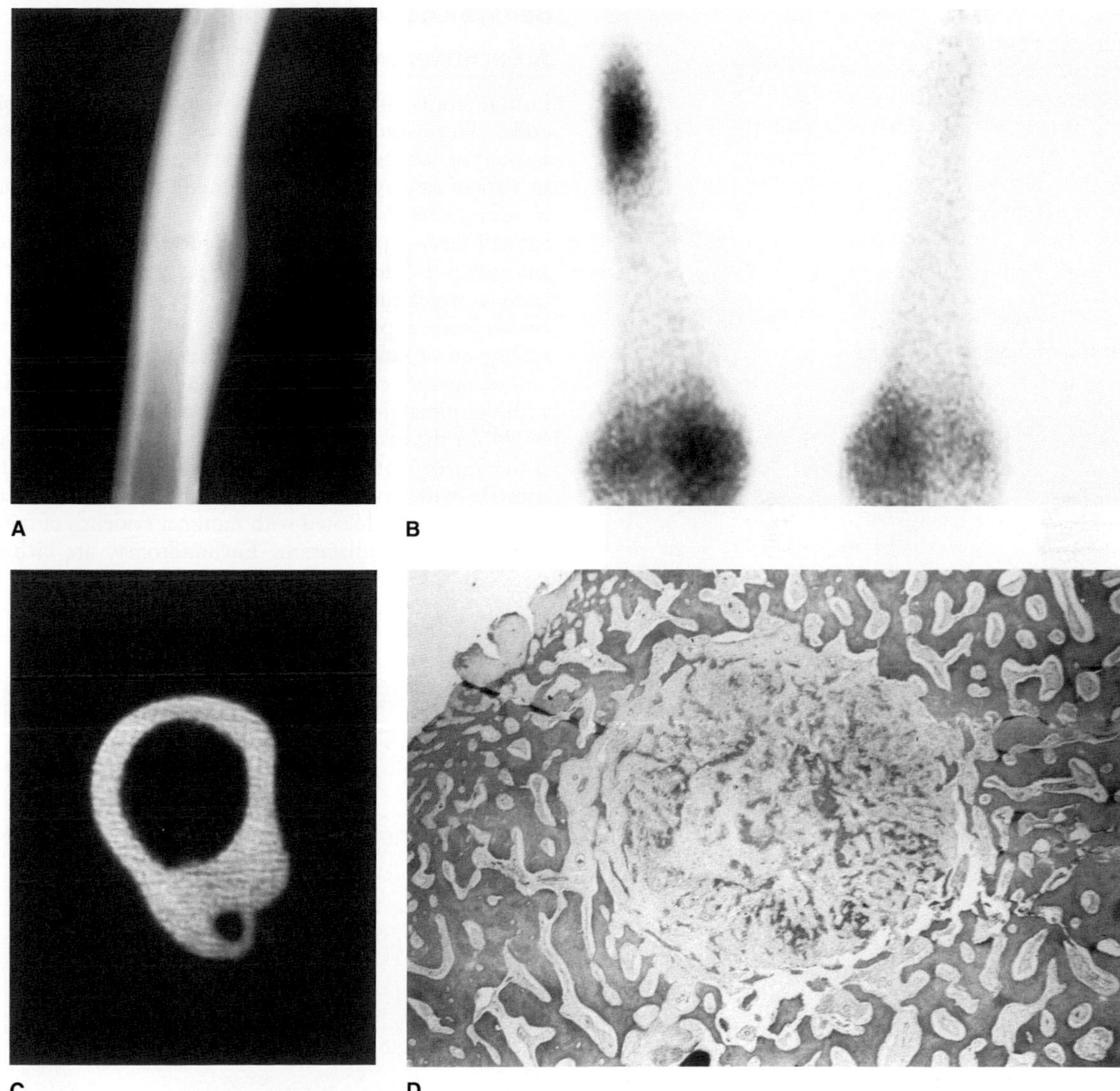

Figure 6–8. Radiograph (**A**), isotope bone scan (**B**), CT scan (**C**), and photomicrograph (**D**) of an osteoid osteoma in the femur of a 19-year-old man.

of the osteoid osteoma and shows excessive osteoblastic activity and osteoid formation with numerous giant cells in a vascular fibrous stroma.

In the spine area, the effects of osteoblastoma are similar to those of osteoid osteoma, with pressure on nerve roots causing pain down the leg or arm (Figure 6–9). In the thoracic area, a large lesion could result in cord compromise.

In patients with osteoblastomas, treatment usually consists of a vigorous curettage of the lesion, which may require a bone graft if instability results. Radiofrequency ablation may also prove useful in the management of this lesion.

C. Osteofibrous Dysplasia

Osteofibrous dysplasia is a rare condition that is seen almost exclusively in the tibia of children younger than 10 years. It is more common in boys than in girls and usually asymptomatic. It commonly affects the diaphysis and results in anterior cortical bowing. Osteofibrous dysplasia can occur in the fibula and even more rarely can be seen bilaterally. It is most likely a hamartoma-

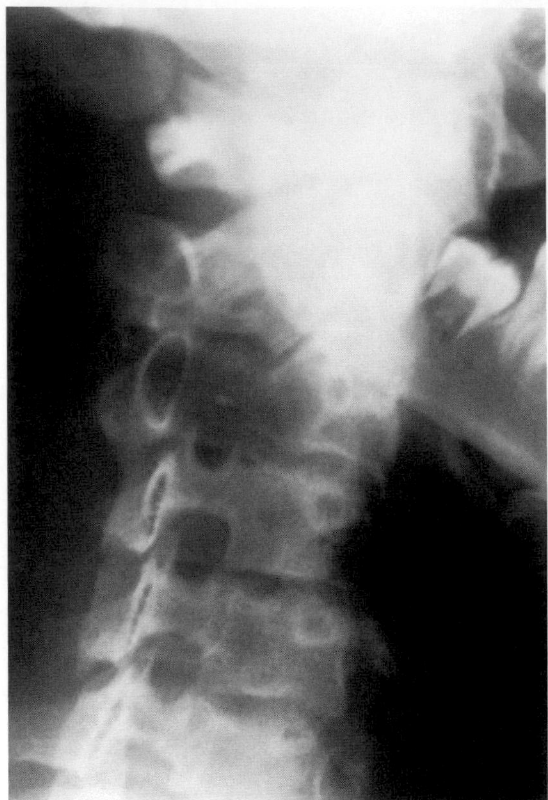

Figure 6–9. Radiograph of osteoblastoma in the pedicle area of the C3 vertebra of a 14-year-old boy.

tous process and tends to involute spontaneously with skeletal maturity.

In osteofibrous dysplasia (Figure 6–10), the lytic changes seen in the anterior tibial cortex surrounded by sclerotic margins, thus creating a soap-bubbly appearance similar to the radiographic picture of both fibrous dysplasia and adamantinoma. Histologically, the lytic lesion shows a benign trabecular alphabet-soup pattern in a fibrous stroma. The histologic findings are similar to those in fibrous dysplasia, although the lesions of fibrous dysplasia lack the prominent surface layer of osteoblasts seen in osteofibrous dysplasia. These lesions are stage 1–2.

In a report of experience with 35 cases of osteofibrous dysplasia, investigators indicated that early attempts at curettage and grafting of the lesions resulted in a high failure rate because of recurrence. For this reason, they suggested waiting until patients reach the age of 15 years and their disease arrests spontaneously before proceeding with a definitive debridement and bone grafting.

Benign Chondroid-Forming Tumors

A. Enchondroma

Enchondroma refers to a centrally located chondroma of bone. These tumors are relatively common lesions, accounting for greater than 10% of benign bone tumors. In 50% of cases, the tumor is found in the small tubular bone of the hands and feet. It arises in growing bones as a hamartomatous process but is frequently asymptomatic and may avoid detection until the patient reaches adulthood, at which time the lesion may be discovered in association with a pathologic fracture or as an incidental finding on a routine radiographic examination.

Radiographs of enchondromas show geographic lysis with sharp margination and central calcification (Figure 6–11). In the case of an enchondroma of the hand, the cortex is frequently thinned out with slight dilation. In contrast, with involvement of the large long bones, the lesion is centrally located with minimal evidence of cortical erosion or dilatation. Enchondromas are either stage 1 or 2 lesions.

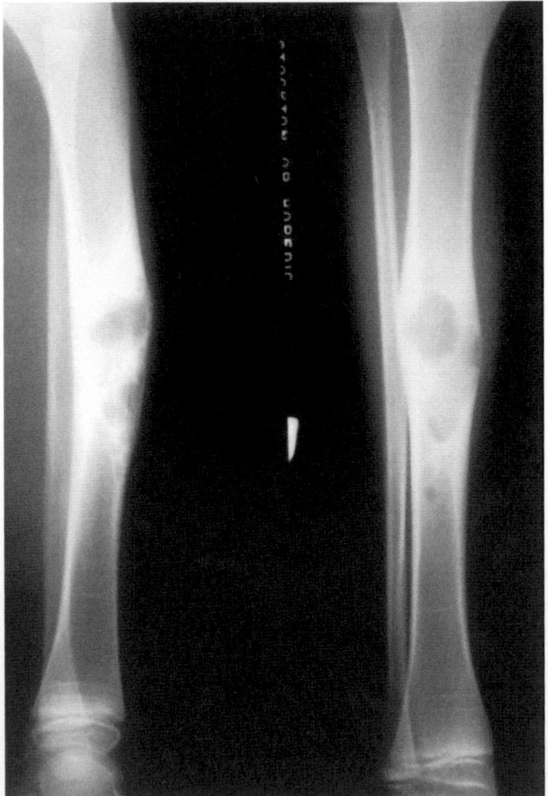

Figure 6–10. Radiograph of osteofibrous dysplasia in the tibia of an 8-year-old boy.

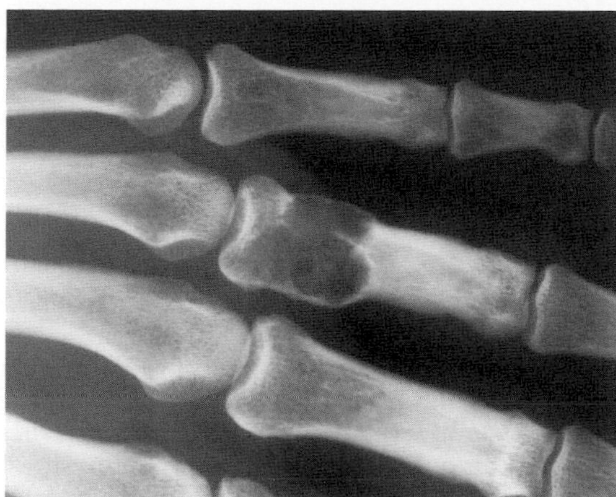

Figure 6–11. Radiograph of an enchondroma of the proximal phalanx of the ring finger.

Multiple enchondromatosis, or Ollier disease (Figure 6–12), is a rare nonfamilial dysplasia typically seen on half of the body and appears similar to fibrous dysplasia. This condition can be quite extensive, with significant involvement of metaphyseal areas resulting in bowing and shortening of the long bones. Such dramatic changes are rarely seen in cases of a solitary enchondroma. In patients with Maffucci syndrome, enchondromatosis is seen in association with multiple soft-tissue hemangiomas.

A large solitary enchondroma in a large bone converts to a low-grade chondrosarcoma in fewer than 5% of cases, and the conversion takes place during adulthood. A solitary enchondroma on the hand rarely converts to a chondrosarcoma. A secondary chondrosarcoma in enchondromatosis can arise in up to 20% of cases and may be related to inactivation of particular tumor suppressor genes.

There is no need to treat an asymptomatic patient with a solitary enchondroma of the hand or foot. If the patient has a pathologic fracture, it is best to allow the fracture to heal and then at a later date to perform a simple curettage and bone grafting procedure, which usually results in good function and a low chance of recurrence. Patients with Ollier or Maffucci disease must be followed carefully because of the increased risk of malignant degeneration.

B. Periosteal Chondroma

A benign chondroma seen on the surface of a bone is called a periosteal chondroma. Patients usually have more than one lesion, and the most common location is on the proximal humeral metaphysis. Radiographically, the lesions appear to lie on the cortical surface and appear to saucerize the underlying cortex (Figure 6–13). These lesions are stage 1–2. Periosteal chondromas can grow to a sizable mass, but anything larger than 4 cm suggests a peripheral primary chondrosarcoma.

Management of periosteal chondromas generally consists of observing the lesion at intervals to make sure it does not continue growing as the patient reaches adulthood. In cases in which simple local resection without bone graft is indicated, the procedure is associated with a low recurrence rate.

C. Osteochondroma

The nonossifying fibroma of bone is the most common benign tumor of bone, and the solitary osteochondroma is the second most common. Like the enchondroma, the osteochondroma is a developmental, or hamartomatous, process that arises from a defect in the outer edge of the growth plate on the metaphyseal side and results in an exostosis that always points away from the joint of origin as the lesion moves away from the growth plate during the growing years.

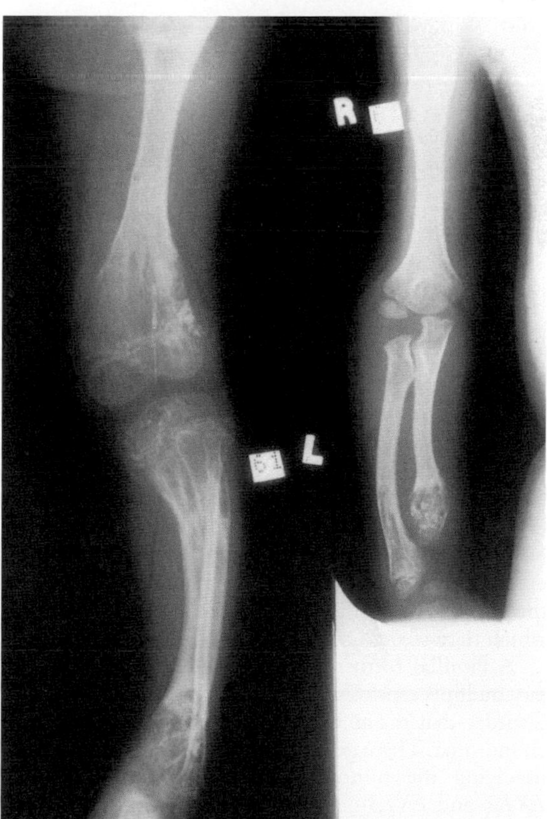

Figure 6–12. Radiograph of Ollier disease of the upper and lower extremities.

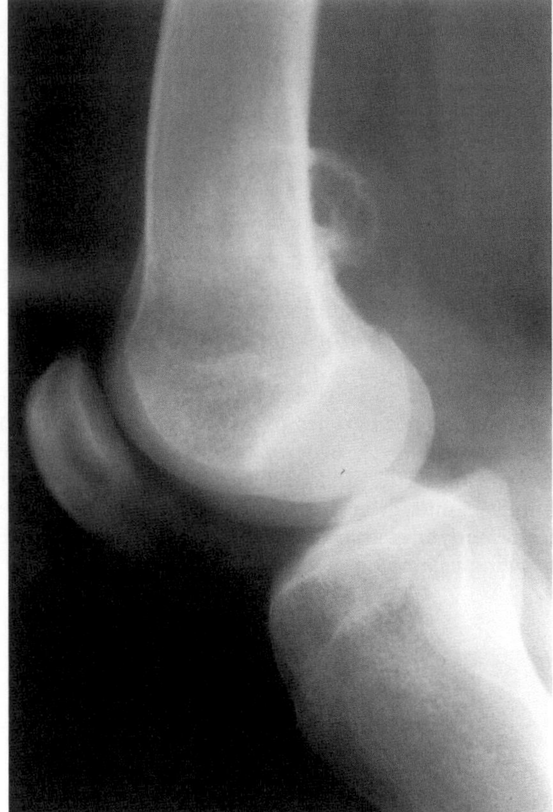

Figure 6–13. Radiograph of a periosteal chondroma of the distal femur.

The bony base of an osteochondroma is in direct communication with the medullary canal of the bone from which it arises. These lesions can be either pedunculated, as is commonly seen around the knee, or sessile, as is typically seen in the proximal humerus. There must be an associated cartilaginous cap on the bony base to make the diagnosis of osteochondroma (Figure 6–14). This cap has the histologic features of a normal growth plate during the growing years. However, osteochondroma growth plate activity subsides at the same time as the activity in the larger plate from which the osteochondroma arose.

A familial form of osteochondroma, called hereditary multiple exostosis (HME), is an autosomal-dominant disorder that is one tenth as common as solitary osteochondroma. Three genetic loci are associated with HME involving the tumor suppressor *EXT* genes (*EXT1, EXT2,* and *EXT3*). This condition can vary from quite mild to extensive involvement with symmetric limb shortening. Forearm involvement can be quite deforming. The metaphyseal portions of long bones are deformed and widened (Figures 6–15 and 6–16). The histologic findings in multiple exostoses are similar to those in solitary osteochondroma.

Conversion of solitary osteochondroma to chondrosarcoma occurs only during adulthood. The overall rate of conversion for all types of solitary lesions is quite rare. In HME, there is approximately a 1% chance of malignant conversion to secondary chondrosarcoma in the cartilaginous cap, especially in the larger, more proximal lesions.

Osteochondromas are stage 1 lesions. Most children and adults with a solitary osteochondroma are asymptomatic and therefore do not require surgical treatment. In some cases, the lesion may be palpable and irritating. Surgical removal is appropriate in these cases to address the symptoms only and not as a prophylaxis for chondrosarcomatous degeneration. In HME, symptomatic lesions are addressed surgically as needed. Corrective osteotomy is occasionally required because of angulatory deformity in the lower extremity. If a previously quiescent lesion begins to enlarge, in adults with either a solitary osteochondroma or with multiple exostoses, it

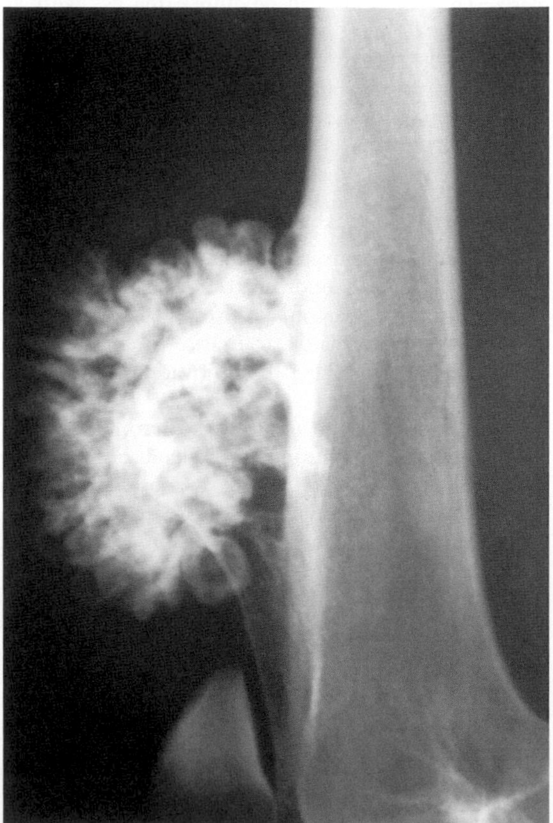

Figure 6–14. Radiograph of an osteochondroma of the distal femur.

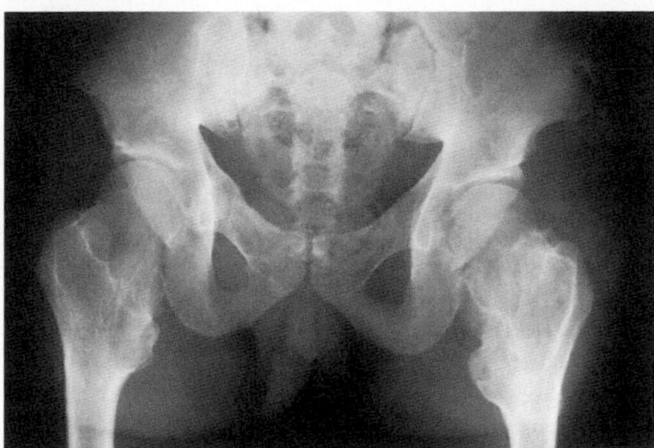

Figure 6–15. Radiograph of multiple exostoses of both hips.

should be removed. The surgical margin should be wide enough to include the entire cartilaginous cap because this is where malignant degeneration can occur.

D. Chondroblastoma

The term *chondroblastoma* suggests a benign cartilage-forming tumor, but in fact this epiphyseal lesion of childhood has a histologic appearance that is more typical of the benign metaphyseal-epiphyseal giant cell tumor of young adulthood. The chondroblastoma is approximately one fifth as common as the giant cell tumor. It differs from other bone tumors in that it is almost always associated with epiphyseal or apophyseal bone. The majority of cases arise in the second decade of life. Males are affected more often than females. The most common location is the outer portion of the proximal humeral epiphysis, but other common locations are the distal femoral and proximal tibial epiphyseal areas. Because of its proximity to a joint, chondroblastoma can present with a symptomatic joint effusion.

In cases of chondroblastoma, the radiograph demonstrates a lytic tumor with a sharp sclerotic margin and central stippled or flocculated calcification occurring in the chondroid portion of the tumor (Figure 6–17). As the growth plate closes, the tumor can expand gradually into the metaphyseal area, and it sometimes becomes quite aneurysmal, as in the case of a giant cell tumor. The chondroblastoma has the histologic appearance of a giant cell tumor, with numerous macrophages seen usually in areas of hemorrhage. The stromal cells of the chondroblastoma are polyhedral, like those of a giant cell tumor, but with associated halos that give the chondroblastoma a so-called chicken-wire appearance. Although chondroid metaplasia in the chondroblastoma is not easy to find, it must be present to firmly establish the diagnosis. Most chondroblastomas are stage 2 lesions, but some can be stage 3.

The spontaneous conversion of chondroblastoma to a malignant tumor is extremely rare. However, as with the case of giant cell tumors, conversion to sarcoma can occur following radiation treatment. Even though the chondroblastoma is considered benign, it is reported to metastasize to the lung on rare occasions. Nevertheless, it carries an excellent prognosis.

Treatment for chondroblastoma consists of aggressive intralesional resection with curettage; bone graft or bone cement (polymethyl methacrylate) may be used to reconstruct the defect. It is our experience that this suffices, with local recurrence less than 10%. Some authors, however, recommend more aggressive marginal or wide resection.

E. Chondromyxoid Fibroma

The chondromyxoid fibroma, a very rare tumor, generally affects males in the second or third decade of life. The most common location of the tumor is the proximal tibial metaphysis, followed by the distal femur and the first ray of the foot. The tumor is slow growing and accompanied by mild pain symptoms.

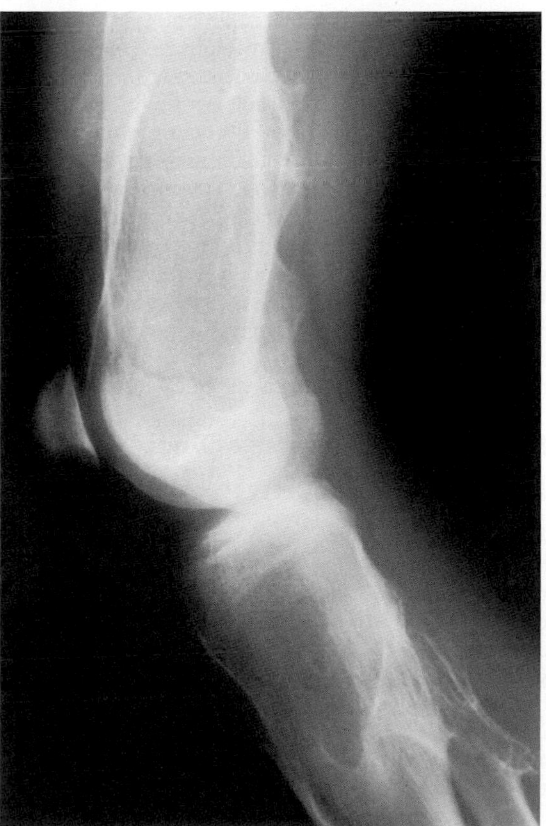

Figure 6–16. Radiograph of multiple exostoses in the knee.

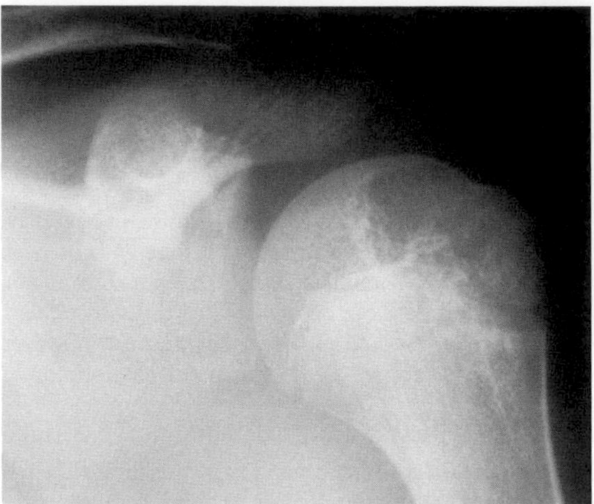

Figure 6–17. Radiograph of a chondroblastoma in the proximal humeral epiphysis of a 15-year-old boy.

Radiographs of chondromyxoid fibroma show a lytic tumor with sharp sclerotic margins and a pseudoloculated pattern resembling that of a bone cyst. The tumor is eccentrically located in metaphyseal bone with a slightly dilated and thinned-out cortex similar to that shown in Figure 6–18. Histologic findings include a strange but specific mixture of fibrous, myxomatous, and chondroid tissues, which could mistakenly suggest the diagnosis of a chondrosarcoma. The findings also commonly include giant cells, which may suggest the diagnosis of a chondroblastoma seen in epiphyseal bone. This stage 2 lesion is quite active locally, especially in children. With simple curettage and bone grafting, the recurrence rate can approach 25%. Aggressive marginal excision should be performed. The conversion of chondromyxoid fibroma to chondrosarcoma is extremely rare.

Benign Fibrous Tumors of Bone

A. Fibrous Cortical Defect

Fibrous cortical defects, or cortical desmoids, are small hamartomatous fibromas seen almost exclusively in the metaphyseal areas of the lower extremities of growing children. They can be multiple, and as many as 25% of normal children demonstrate these asymptomatic lesions at 5 years of age. The lesions tend to disappear as the result of bone remodeling before skeletal maturity. If excessive stress is placed across the lesions, they can become symptomatic and can also cause findings of increased activity on an isotope bone scan.

In the case of fibrous cortical defects, microscopic studies show benign-appearing fibroblasts with an occasional area of histiocytes, foam cells, and benign giant cells. The radiographic appearance is so characteristic of this entity (Figure 6–19) that a biopsy is usually not necessary. These are stage 1 lesions and can generally be observed.

B. Nonossifying Fibroma

Just as the osteoblastoma is considered a larger or more extensive form of osteoid osteoma, the nonossifying fibroma is considered a larger form of the fibrous cortical defect. It is typically seen in the lower extremity of children. Because of its size, it may not entirely resolve by skeletal maturity and can persist into adult life. If the lesion is quite large, approaching 50% of the diameter of the bone, pathologic fracture may ensue. The fracture-healing process may facilitate resolution of the lesions. Careful consideration to fracture prophylaxis should be reserved for large lesions only in children older than 10 years. Nonossifying fibromas are stage 1 lesions, and neither they nor fibrous cortical defects require biopsy because their radiographic appearance is so characteristic.

With nonossifying fibroma, multiple lesions may take on the appearance of fibrous dysplasia and can be associated with café au lait skin defects. Large lesions in the

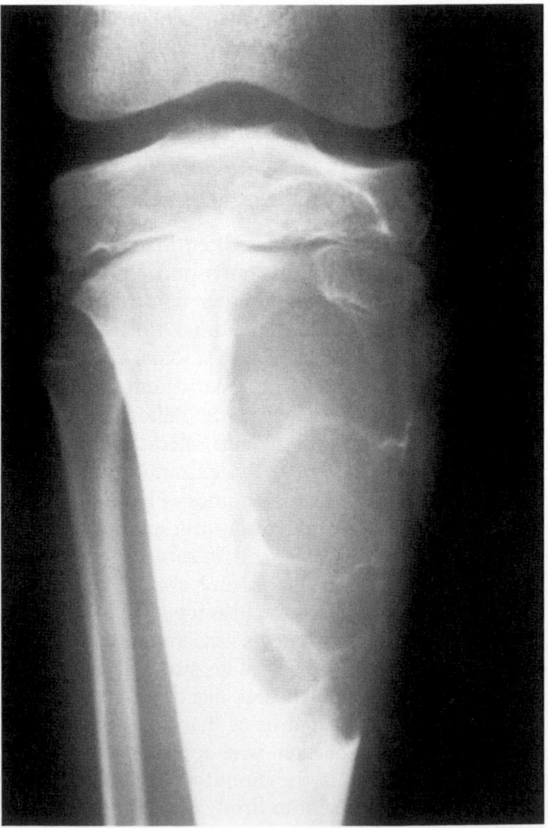

Figure 6–18. Radiograph of a chondromyxoid fibroma in the proximal tibia of an 11-year-old boy.

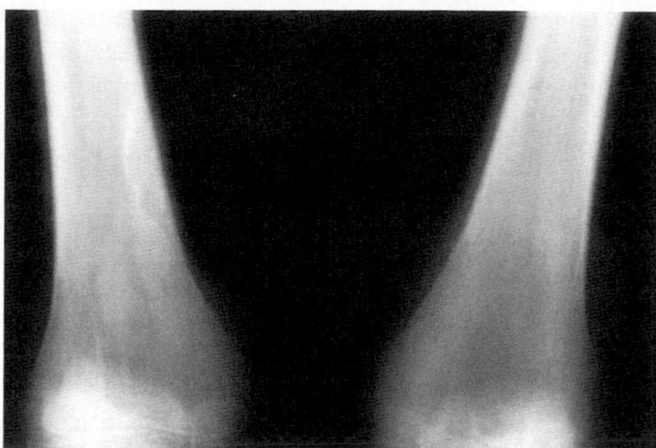

Figure 6–19. Radiograph of a metaphyseal fibrous defect in a 15-year-old boy.

proximal tibia can assume the appearance of a chondromyxoid fibroma (Figure 6–20). The lesions have a well-defined sclerotic margin and a pseudomultiloculated lytic center that gives them a soap-bubbly radiographic appearance. Histologically, they appear identical to fibrous cortical defects and are characterized by benign fibrous tissue speckled with areas of histiocytes, foam cells, and giant cells. As the lesion involutes in adulthood and the number of giant cells and histiocytes diminishes, large areas of cholesterol deposits become evident, which may suggest the diagnosis of a xanthofibroma or xanthoma of bone. Nonossifying fibromas are clearly separated from fibrous dysplasia by the absence of the metaplastic osteoid formation in the fibrous stroma.

C. Fibrous Dysplasia

Fibrous dysplasia can present in a variety of ways: monostotic, polyostotic, and with or without associated syndromes (Figure 6–21). Most cases are diagnosed within the first three decades and have a distinct female predilection. The monostotic presentation is more common than polyostotic. This condition is a dysplastic anomaly of bone-forming mesenchymal tissue with an inability to produce mature lamellar bone. Accordingly, the bone is arrested in the woven state with a resultant proliferation of spindle cell fibroblasts. In the polyostotic form, it tends to involve one side of the body rather than bilaterally. Nevertheless, it can involve any bone of the body. The most common location is the proximal femur, where it results in the so-called shepherd's crook deformity. Other areas frequently involved include the tibia, pelvis, humerus, radius, and ribs.

In addition to bony involvement, patients can demonstrate café au lait skin pigmentation. These patches usually have a rough border, in contrast to the smooth border of those seen in neurofibromatosis. Patients with fibrous dysplasia may have associated endocrine problems. For example, 5% of patients with the polyostotic form of fibrous dysplasia also exhibit precocious puberty (McCune-Albright syndrome). Other associated endocrine abnormalities include hyperthyroidism, acromegaly, Cushing disease, and hypophosphatemic osteomalacia. Polyostotic fibrous dysplasia with soft-tissue myxomas is known as Mazabrand syndrome. Fibrous dysplasia can also involve the skull and jaw bones, mimicking ossifying fibroma of jaw bone.

In fibrous dysplasia, microscopic findings include an alphabet-soup pattern of metaplastic woven bone scattered through a benign fibrous tissue stroma. This woven stroma has an absence of osteoblastic rimming. Foam cells, giant cells, and cholesterol deposits can be seen. Large cystic areas and even areas of cartilage formation are commonly present.

The molecular basis for fibrous dysplasia is associated with mutations affecting the alpha subunit of G protein. These mutations affect cells of the osteoblastic lineage, resulting in decreased differentiation and increased proliferation. These mutations cause constitutive elevation of cAMP in fibrous dysplasia and thus alter cAMP target genes such *c-fos*, *c-jun*, IL-6, and IL-11.

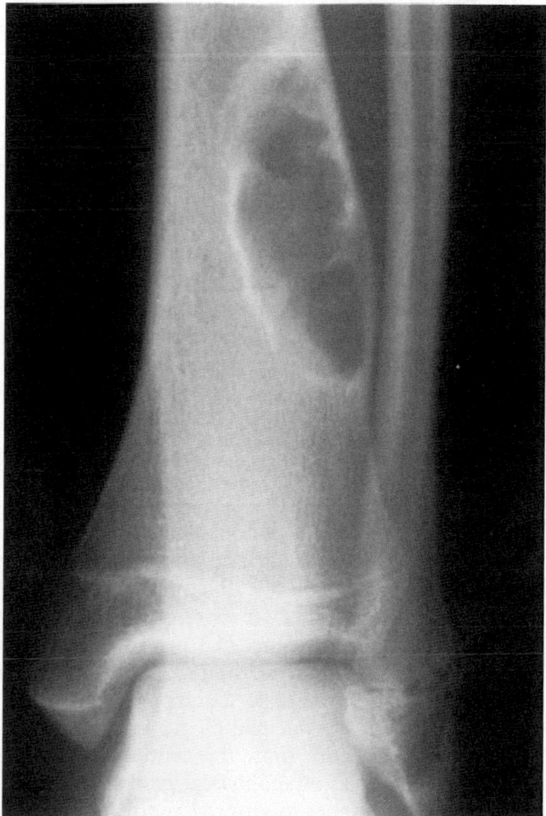

Figure 6–20. Radiograph of a nonossifying fibroma of the distal tibia.

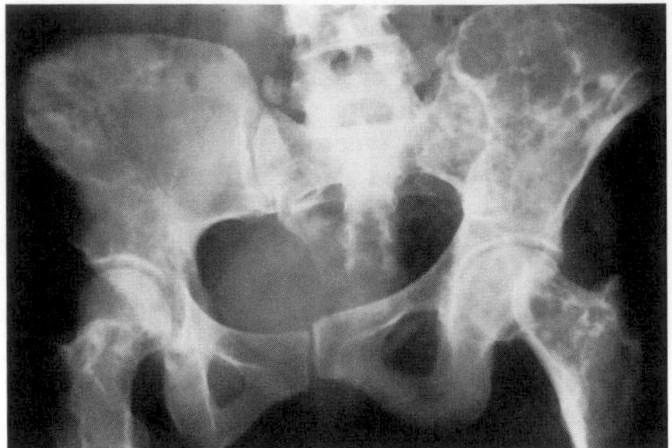

Figure 6–21. Radiograph of polyostotic fibrous dysplasia of the pelvis.

Fibrous dysplasia tends to be active during the growing years and then burns out in adult life. Fewer than 1% of lesions convert to osteosarcoma, fibrosarcoma, or even chondrosarcoma. If conversion does occur, it almost always happens during adulthood. Generally, this disease is either stage 1 or 2.

In pediatric patients with active disease, curettage and grafting should be avoided because of high recurrence rates. The goals in treating pediatric patients should be the prevention and treatment of deformity, especially in the lower extremity. Most cases should become quiescent with skeletal maturity. If not, the best surgical treatment in adults consists of rigid fixation with an intramedullary implant with strut grafting as needed. The best surgical treatment in adults consists of the use of long autogenous fibular struts combined with autogenous cancellous bone graft. This treatment has a higher success rate in the adult group than in the pediatric group. Medical management with bisphosphonates is of benefit in some cases. Irradiation is contraindicated because it may lead to irradiation-induced sarcoma at a later date.

Cystic Lesions of Bone

A. Simple Bone Cyst

Simple bone cysts are a common pseudotumor of bone and the most frequent cause of pathologic fractures in children. Bone cysts typically affect patients between 5 and 15 years of age and occur more often in boys than in girls (2:1) with an incidence of 1 per 10,000 children per year. They are found in the proximal humerus in 50% of cases and in the upper femur in 25%. Patients are asymptomatic until a pathologic fracture occurs. Fractures seem to arise from the central metaphyseal side of an epiphyseal or apophyseal growth plate. The cystic process continues to grow away from the physis. When it remains in contact with the physis it is termed "active." When it separates it is termed "inactive."

Radiographs typically show a solitary cyst that is centrally located in the metaphyseal area and has marked thinning of the adjacent cortical bone and a pseudoloculated appearance (Figure 6–22). The bone cyst is filled with a clear serous fluid, and there is increased pressure during the active phase. The fact that this pressure gradually decreases as the cyst becomes inactive suggests a hydrodynamic mechanism.

The cyst cavity, lined with a fibrinous membrane that contains giant cells, foam cells, and a slight osteoid formation, is similar to the fibrous tissues seen in other fibrous bone lesions, including fibrous dysplasia. The periosteal covering in the area of a cyst is normal, and thus the pathologic fractures heal normally and in most cases do not require surgery. Unfortunately, the cyst usually persists after fracture union and requires further treatment. Bone-resorbing factors, such as matrix metalloproteinases, prostaglandins, IL-1, IL-6, tumor necrosis factor alpha (TNF), and oxygen free radicals, are demonstrated in the cyst fluid. Elevated nitrate and nitrite levels are also noted to be higher in the cyst fluid than in serum.

Before the mid-1970s, the standard treatment for a solitary bone cyst was aggressive curettage or even resection followed by bone grafting. In patients with active disease, the recurrence rate was 30–50%, and repeated grafting was frequently necessary. In patients with inactive disease, particularly those older than 15 years, the surgical results were much better and the recurrence rate was lower. Unicameral bone cysts are generally considered

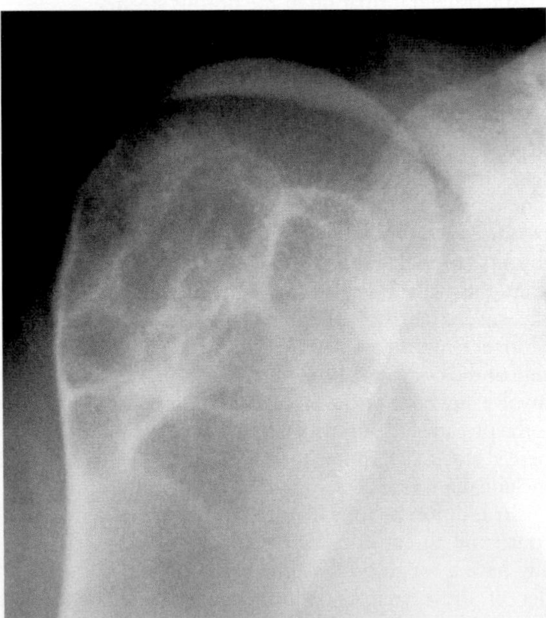

Figure 6–22. Radiograph of a solitary bone cyst on the proximal humerus of a 13-year-old boy.

stage 1 lesions, but occasionally they may be stage 2. Currently, treatment is a function of location. In weight-bearing bones, such as the proximal femur, lesions should be treated aggressively. Initial management usually involves aspiration/injection with either bone marrow or corticosteroid. The injections are carried out with bone biopsy needles and are repeated three to five times at intervals of 2–3 months, depending on the radiographic response. The best results are when the patient is between 5 and 15 years of age, at which time the disease is active and macrophage activity is greatest in the cyst lining. Curettage and bone grafting may also be an effective modality. Demineralized bone matrix injected in combination with autogenous bone marrow shows encouraging results, with an approximately 20% recurrence rate and low morbidity.

Physicians should note that sarcomas can take on the radiographic appearance of a solitary bone cyst. For this reason, if needle aspiration does not reveal cystic fluid or if it is impossible to inject contrast material and obtain radiologic confirmation of the diagnosis, an open biopsy is indicated to rule out a sarcoma.

B. Aneurysmal Bone Cyst

Aneurysmal bone cyst is a hemorrhagic lesion with many characteristics of a giant cell tumor but occurs only half as frequently. Although 75% of the cases of aneurysmal bone cyst occur in patients 10–20 years old, giant cell tumor is rare in patients younger than 20 years of age. Both aneurysmal bone cyst and giant cell tumor are more common in females than in males. The femur is the most frequently affected site, followed by the tibia, pelvis, and spine. In the spine, two thirds of aneurysmal bone cysts arise from posterior elements and one third arise from the vertebral body, whereas most giant cell tumors arise from the vertebral body.

Initially, the aneurysmal bone cyst appears on radiograph as an aggressive osteolytic lesion with extensive permeative cortical destruction that gives the impression of a malignant process such as Ewing sarcoma or hemorrhagic osteosarcoma. Next, a large aneurysmal bulge occurs outside the bone, with a thin reactive shell of bone forming at the outer edge. Less soap-bubbly pseudoseptation is seen in an aneurysmal bone cyst than in a solitary cyst (Figure 6–23).

At the time of biopsy, the aneurysmal bone lesion demonstrates large hemorrhagic cysts, but bleeding is modest. The hemorrhagic cysts are broken up by thick spongy fibrous septa that histologically contain great numbers of large giant cells and have thin osteoid seams. Even if a few mitotic figures are seen, the diagnosis of a benign lesion can remain. A carefully placed biopsy with multiple samples is needed to rule out other well-known skeletal tumors that may demonstrate an aneurysmal component. These include giant cell tumor, chondromyxoid fibroma, and malignant hemorrhagic osteosarcoma. Some authors believe there is no such entity as the aneurysmal bone cyst and that it is merely a morphologic variant of some other underlying neoplastic process. Like the solitary bone cyst, this cyst may have a hydraulic pressure origin that is secondary to hemorrhage and could be traumatically induced. However, abnormal cytogenetic findings were noted in aneurysmal bone cysts, which may suggest a distinct cellular pathogenetic etiology. Specifically, a t(16,17) translocation resulting in a CDH11-USP6 fusion gene product is frequently observed in aneurysmal bone cyst. Aneurysmal bone cyst is either a stage 2 or 3 lesion and frequently symptomatic.

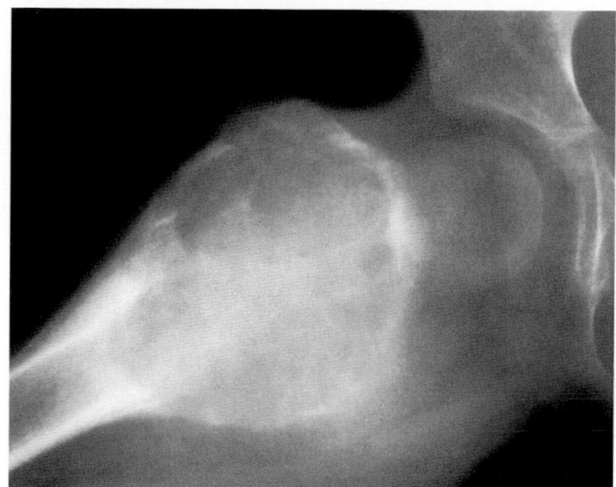

Figure 6–23. Radiograph of an aneurysmal bone cyst on the proximal femur of a 5-year-old boy.

If an aneurysmal cyst is left untreated, it may involute spontaneously, during which time it develops a heavy shell of reactive bone at the periphery. This involutional process can be hastened by surgical curettage and bone grafting. Radiation is no longer recommended. Another option for treating extremely large lesions is repeated embolization to reduce the rate of hemorrhagic expansion.

C. Epidermoid Cyst

The least common bone cyst is the epidermoid bone cyst. This lesion is found either in the distal phalanx or in the skull. No other bone is affected. In the case of the phalanx, the cyst is usually the result of nail bed epithelium being driven into the subjacent distal phalanx by a crushing blow. The ectopic squamous epithelium produces a keratinized cavity that is filled with clear fluid and creates a surface erosion with a sclerotic reactive base (Figure 6–24). The bulbous cyst seen at the fingertip transilluminates with flashlight examination. Other conditions that might have a similar appearance are the glomus tumor and the enchondroma. The epidermoid cyst is treated with a simple curettage and, in some cases, a bone graft.

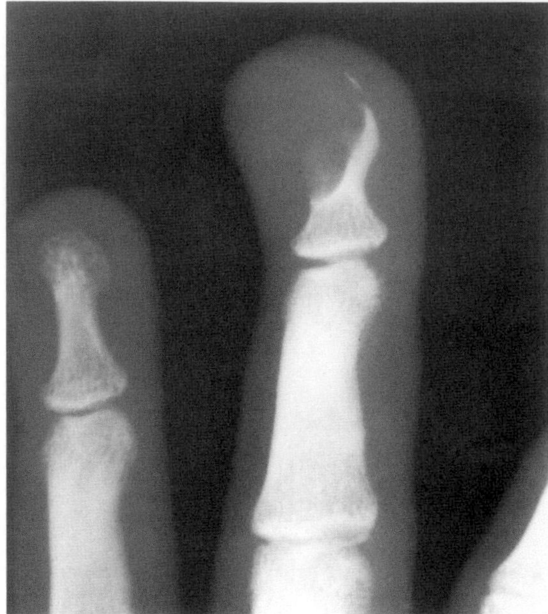

Figure 6–24. Radiograph of an epidermoid cyst in the distal phalanx.

Giant Cell Tumor of Bone

Numerous types of tumors contain giant cells but are not true benign giant cell tumors. Most of the variants are seen in children and include aneurysmal bone cyst, chondroblastoma, simple bone cyst, osteoid osteoma, and osteoblastoma. The giant cell–rich osteosarcoma is the most malignant of the variants, and it is sometimes difficult to distinguish from an aggressive benign giant cell tumor. The giant cell reparative granuloma is a benign variant seen in jaw bones or hand bones and has more spindle cells than a classic giant cell tumor. The brown tumor of hyperparathyroidism is a nonneoplastic variant seen in both primary and secondary hyperparathyroidism. Only after all of the variant conditions are excluded can the diagnosis of benign giant cell tumor be made. Giant cell tumor of bone is now associated with overexpression of osteoprotegerin ligand (OPGL), an important stimulator of osteoclast differentiation, suggesting overactivity of osteoclast in the etiology of this neoplasm.

Between 5% and 10% of all benign bone tumors are true giant cell tumors, occurring most frequently in the third decade of life. They are more frequently found in females than in males. In approximately half of the cases, the tumor is found about the knee. The next most common locations are the distal radius and sacrum. The tumor is usually painful for several months prior to diagnosis and can cause a pathologic fracture. It can also cause a painful effusion because of its juxtaposition to a major joint. Giant cell tumors may present as either stage 2 or stage 3 disease and less frequently as stage 1. On radiograph, the lesion appears lytic in nature and is located in the epiphyseal-metaphyseal end of a long bone (Figure 6–25). The lesion grows toward the joint surface and frequently comes into contact with articular cartilage but rarely breaks into the joint.

Like the chondroblastoma, the benign giant cell tumor has a 1–2% chance of metastasizing to the lung. Recurrent tumors have a 6% chance. Accordingly, pulmonary staging is an importantcomponent in the initial evaluation and follow-up of giant cell tumor of bone. The prognosis for survival with this complication is favorable, and the tumors may resolve spontaneously. The benign giant cell tumor can later convert to a malignant condition such as an osteosarcoma or malignant fibrous histiocytoma. It is generally believed that this is secondary to treatment. A conversion rate of 15–20% is reported in patients who were treated previously with more than 3000 cGy of radiation, with conversion occurring 3 or more years after treatment. The conversion rate in patients who do not receive radiation therapy is less than 5%. This finding has come into question with newer radiation therapy modalities.

Until recent years, the standard treatment for giant cell tumor was curettage and bone grafting. The recurrence

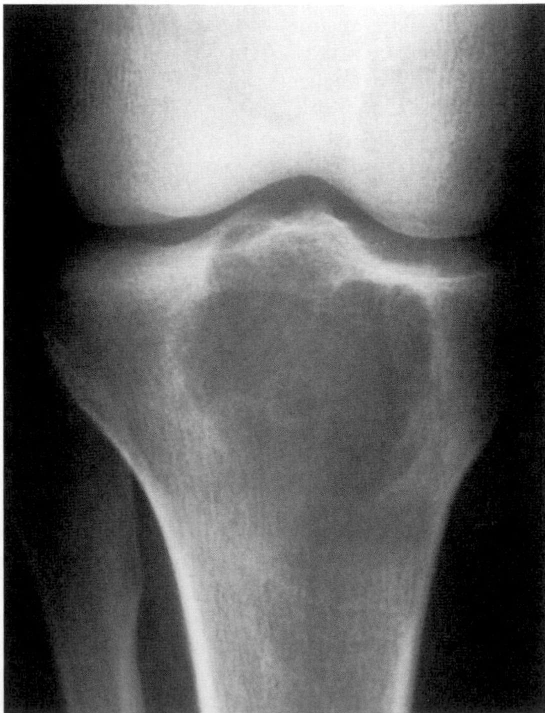

Figure 6–25. Radiograph of a giant cell tumor on the proximal tibia of a 22-year-old woman.

rate with this treatment was reported as up to more than 50%. Follow-up treatment consisted of an aggressive resection of the recurrent lesion and reconstruction with a large osteoarticular allograft, endoprosthesis, or an excisional arthrodesis. Currently, most surgeons elect an aggressive curettage, followed by high-speed burring and adjuvant phenol, hydrogen peroxide, or liquid nitrogen and by the subsequent packing of the defect with bone cement. With this new approach, the recurrence rate is between 10% and 25%. When giant cell tumor infrequently involves an expendable bone such as the proximal fibula or ilium, it should be primarily resected. En bloc resection continues to be used to treat multiple recurrent tumors, intensive soft-tissue involvement, or massively destructive cases. Embolization may also prove palliative or curative in unresectable cases. For advanced, multiply recurrent, or aggressive metastatic cases, investigators are developing experimental medical protocols. Close follow-up for locally recurrent disease and pulmonary involvement is critical. Surveillance should include a plain chest radiograph every 6–12 months for the first 2–3 years at least.

Hemangioma

Hemangioma of bone is a hamartomatous process that occurs more frequently in females than in males. It is most commonly found in vertebral bodies (Figure 6–26). It is found only rarely in the diaphysis of long bone. Hemangiomas of bone can be associated with hemangiomas of soft tissue. The spinal lesion is usually discovered as an incidental radiographic finding and demonstrates a characteristic vertically oriented honeycombed or moth-eaten appearance. On rare occasions, a lesion can cause cord compression that may require surgical resection. In such cases, preoperative angiography is critical in evaluating the vascular blood supply to the spinal cord. Alternatively an attempt at arterial embolization may prove successful and is less aggressive.

Gorham disease, characterized by massive osteolysis in children or young adults, is usually associated with the presence of benign cavernous hemangiomas or lymphangiomas of bone. This strange condition usually affects a particular area (such as the spine or the hip) but can involve multiple bones of that area and tends to resolve spontaneously.

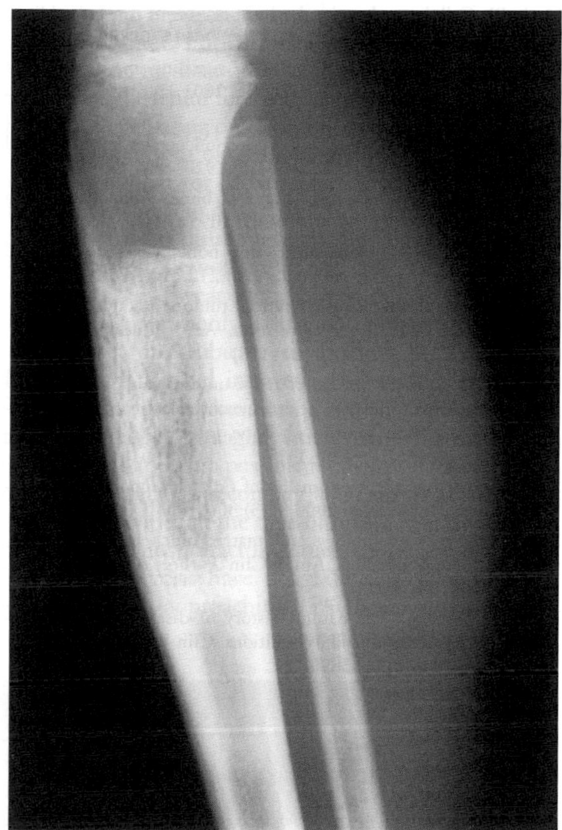

Figure 6–26. Radiograph of a hemangioma of the tibia in a 14-year-old boy.

Baruffi MR et al: Aneurysmal bone cyst with chromosomal changes involving 7q and 16p. Cancer Genet Cytogenet 2001;129(2): 177. [PMID: 11566352]

Bottner F et al: Cyclooxygenase-2 inhibitor for pain management in osteoid osteoma. Clin Orthop 2001;393:258. [PMID: 11764357]

Boutou-Bredaki S et al: Prognosis of giant cell tumor of bone. Histopathological analysis of 15 cases and review of the literature. Adv Clin Path 2001;5(3):71. [PMID: 11753878]

Bovee JV et al: Malignant progression in multiple enchondromatosis (Ollier's disease): An autopsy-based molecular genetic study. Hum Pathol 2000;31(10):1299. [PMID: 11070122]

Cantwell CP et al: Current trends in treatment of osteoid osteoma with an emphasis on radiofrequency ablation. Eur Radiol 2004;14(4):607. [PMID: 14663625]

Cheung P et al: Etiological point mutations in the hereditary multiple exostoses gene EXT1: A functional analysis of heparan sulfate polymerase activity. Am J Hum Genet 2001;69(1):55. [PMID: 11391482]

Flemming DJ et al: Primary tumors of the spine. Semin Musculoskelet Radiol 2000;4(3):299. [PMID: 11371321]

Gallazzi MB et al: Percutaneous radio-frequency ablation of osteoid osteoma: Technique and preliminary results. Radiol Med (Torino) 2001;102(5-6):329. [PMID: 11779979]

Kivioja A et al: Chondrosarcoma in a family with multiple hereditary exostoses. J Bone Joint Surg Br 2000;82(2):261. [PMID: 10755438]

Komiya S et al: Increased concentrations of nitrate and nitrite in the cyst fluid suggesting increased nitric oxide synthesis in solitary bone cysts. J Orthop Res 2000;18(2):281. [PMID: 10815830]

Lindner NJ et al: Percutaneous radiofrequency ablation in osteoid osteoma. J Bone Joint Surg Br 2001;83(3):391. [PMID: 11341426]

Maki M et al: Comparative study of fibrous dysplasia and osteofibrous dysplasia: Histopathological, immunohistochemical, argyrophilic nucleolar organizer region and DNA ploidy analysis. Pathol Int 2001;51(8):603. [PMID: 11564214]

scopic evaluation demonstrating the presence of malignant-appearing stromal cells with giant cells.

Because hemorrhagic osteosarcoma is a high-grade, purely lytic tumor, the incidence of pathologic fracture in the early course of the disease is high. If significant contamination of the adjacent neurovascular structures results, a pathologic fracture may necessitate amputation rather than limb salvage (Figure 6–33). This situation must be carefully evaluated with a preoperative MRI. Accordingly, in cases with significant risk for fracture during the preoperative treatment regiment, it may be appropriate to immobilize the involved extremity or proceed with limb-sparing surgery earlier than usual. Prior to the advent of aggressive multidrug chemotherapy, the prognosis for patients with hemorrhagic osteosarcoma was extremely poor. At present, however, it is the same as the prognosis for patients who have classic osteosarcoma and is treated with similar protocols.

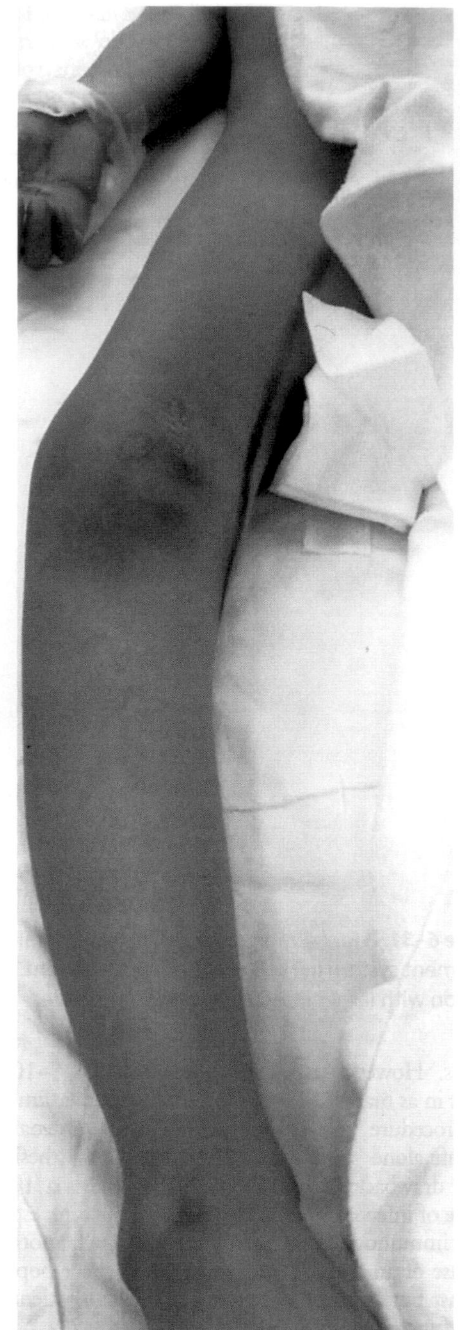

Figure 6–33. Clinical photograph of patient that sustained a pathologic fracture through a distal femur osteosarcoma contaminating the neurovascular structures precluding limb salvage.

C. Parosteal Osteosarcoma

Parosteal osteosarcoma is a low-grade variant arising in an exophytic pattern from the cortical surface of bone. There is no medullary involvement. It is low-grade with a 5-year survival rate in excess of 90% and a 10-year survival rate of 80%. It accounts for 3–4% of all osteosarcomas.

The tumor is composed of a spindle-cell fibroblastic component with well-developed bone trabeculae. There also may be areas of cartilage present. Osteoblasts are well differentiated, and few mitotic figures are present.

Parosteal osteosarcoma is more common in females than in males and affects a slightly older age group than classic osteosarcoma (see Table 6–2). It is a slow-growing tumor with minimal symptoms initially. It is metaphyseal in origin, with the vast majority of cases involving the posterior aspect of the distal femur (Figure 6–34).

Because the parosteal osteosarcoma is low grade, it does not respond well to either chemotherapy or radiation therapy. Therefore, the only treatment is wide surgical resection. This usually requires distal femoral removal, but in smaller cases side resection of the posterior cortex and tumor only may be feasible, sparing the knee joint. Nevertheless, a negative tumor margin is imperative. Otherwise, recurrence is likely. Recurrence may occur as late as 5–10 years because of the tumor's slow growth.

On occasion, low-grade parosteal osteosarcoma can dedifferentiate into a high-grade sarcoma. Such a lesion carries a similar prognosis to classic osteosarcoma.

D. Periosteal Osteosarcoma

Periosteal osteosarcoma is another surface osteosarcoma of low to intermediate grade. This lesion represents less than 2% of all osteosarcomas. It arises beneath the periosteum, elevating it and inducing vigorous neoosteogenesis with a predominant chondroblastic differentiation. It is slightly more common in females, with a peak incidence in the

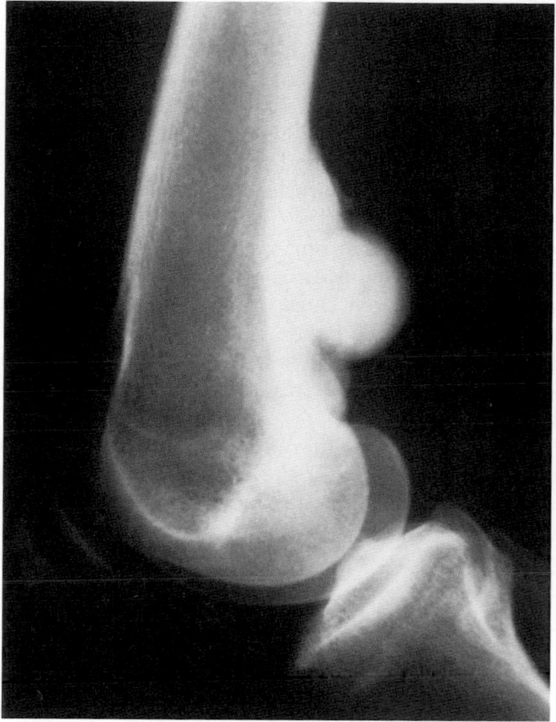

A

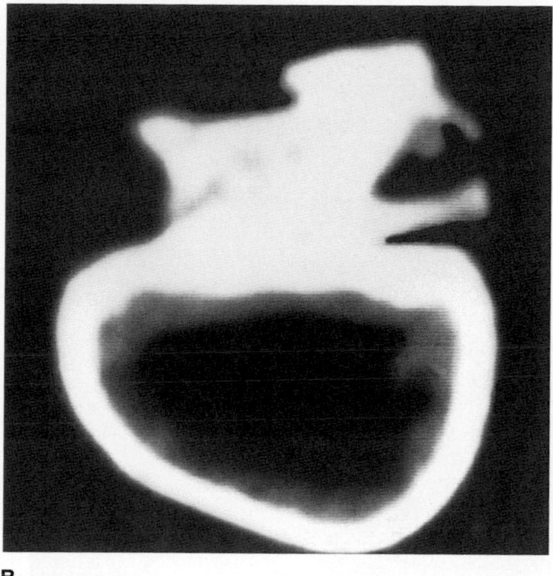

B

Figure 6–34. Radiograph (**A**) and CT scan (**B**) of a parosteal osteosarcoma of the distal femur in a 21-year-old woman.

second decade of life. It almost exclusively arises in the long bone. The lesion can mimic an aneurysmal bone cyst or periosteal chondroma radiographically (Figure 6–35).

Because of its low to intermediate grade, periosteal osteosarcoma is generally not treated with chemotherapy but may be in more advanced cases. Wide surgical resection is the modality of choice. Because periosteal osteosarcoma is a low-grade tumor, it carries a better prognosis than the classic osteosarcoma. Approximately 25% of patients succumb to metastatic disease within 2–3 years. The surgical treatment is usually a limb-sparing procedure, and because the tumor is more diaphyseal in location, the adjacent joints may often be spared.

E. Secondary Osteosarcoma

Osteosarcoma can arise from benign disease through a process that may involve a second mutation and usually occurs at a later age (see Table 6–2). Among the benign conditions that can result in secondary osteosarcoma are Paget disease, osteoblastoma, fibrous dysplasia, benign giant cell tumor, bone infarction, and chronic osteomyelitis.

The classic example of a secondary osteosarcoma is seen in a small percentage of patients with Paget disease. Pagetic osteosarcomas, which represent approximately 3% of all osteosarcomas, are the most common osteosarcomas in the older (more than 65 years) age group. The most frequent location for pagetic osteosarcoma is the humerus, followed next by the pelvis and femur. The typical patient has a long history (15–25 years) of dull, aching pain associated with the inflammation of Paget disease before a new acute pain arises in an area of recent lytic destruction and the diagnosis of pagetic osteosarcoma is established (Figure 6–36). The prognosis for patients with pagetic osteosarcoma is extremely poor (5-year survival rate of approximately 8%). Because of the older age group involved, chemotherapy is usually not an option secondary to intolerance.

F. Low-Grade Intramedullary Osteosarcoma

Another rare and low-grade osseofibrous variant of osteosarcoma is the central or intramedullary form. Although this variant has a microscopic appearance similar to that of the parosteal osteosarcoma, it is usually located in metaphyseal bone about the knee joint in adults between 15 and 65 years of age. Males and females are equally affected. Radiographically, intramedullary osteosarcoma creates a sclerotic density in metaphyseal bone (Figure 6–37). Like the parosteal osteosarcoma, the low-grade intramedullary osteosar-

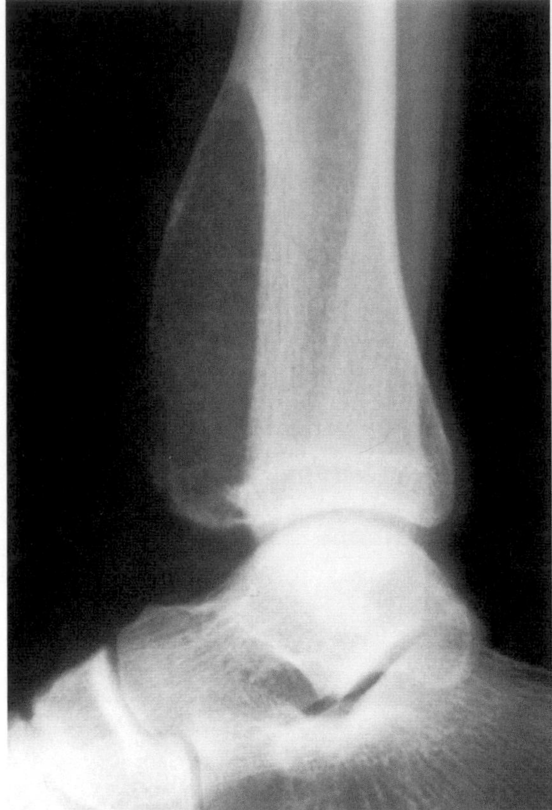

Figure 6–35. Radiograph of a periosteal osteosarcoma of the distal tibia in a 15-year-old boy.

coma carries an excellent prognosis and can be treated with local surgery alone.

G. Irradiation-Induced Osteosarcoma

Radiation-induced osteosarcoma may arise after any form of significant radiation exposure (in excess of 30 Gy) (Figure 6–38). Onset is usually delayed an average of 15 years (range: 3–55). Other irradiation-induced sarcomas, besides the osteosarcoma type, include irradiation-induced fibrosarcoma and malignant fibrohistiocytoma. All of these secondary sarcomas are invariably high grade and carry a poor prognosis for survival, with a very high rate of metastasis.

H. Multicentric Osteosarcoma

Multicentric osteosarcoma has two clinical presentations: (l) synchronous, occurring in childhood and adolescents, and (2) metachronous, occurring in adults. The synchronous type is a high-grade sclerosing intramedullary type, which is lethal. The adult form is less aggressive, with a lower histologic appearance, but prognosis remains grim (Figure 6–39).

I. Soft-Tissue Osteosarcoma

Osteosarcoma can occur in muscle tissue outside bone and accounts for approximately 4% of all osteosarcomas (Figure 6–40). Soft-tissue osteosarcoma is rarely seen in patients younger than 40 years. The number of cases is equal in males and females, and the tumor is usually seen in large muscle groups of the pelvis and thigh areas.

Soft-tissue osteosarcoma must be differentiated from the more common myositis ossificans. Although soft-tissue osteosarcoma shows heavy mineralization in the central area (see Figure 6–40), myositis ossificans has a zonal pattern of ossification, with the mature dense ossification concentrating at the periphery of the lesion.

The treatment of the soft-tissue form of osteosarcoma is the same as for the high-grade osseous form and includes a wide resection and adjuvant chemotherapy. The prognosis is worse with the soft-tissue form of osteosarcoma, with a high rate of chemotherapy resistance.

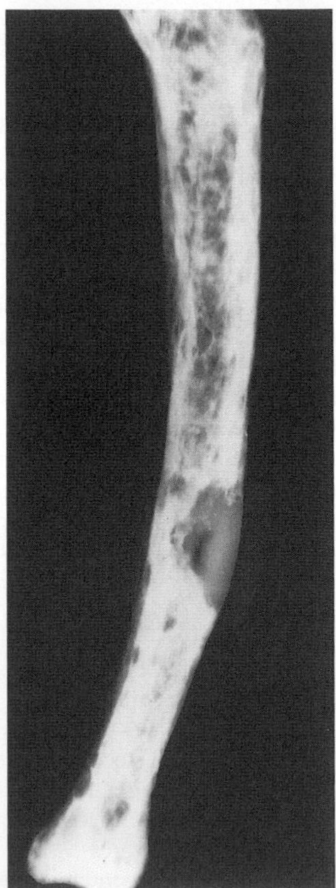

Figure 6–36. Radiograph of a pagetic osteosarcoma of the tibia.

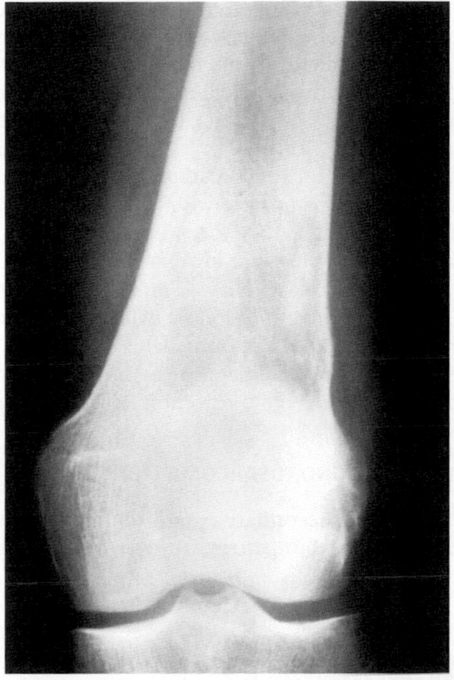

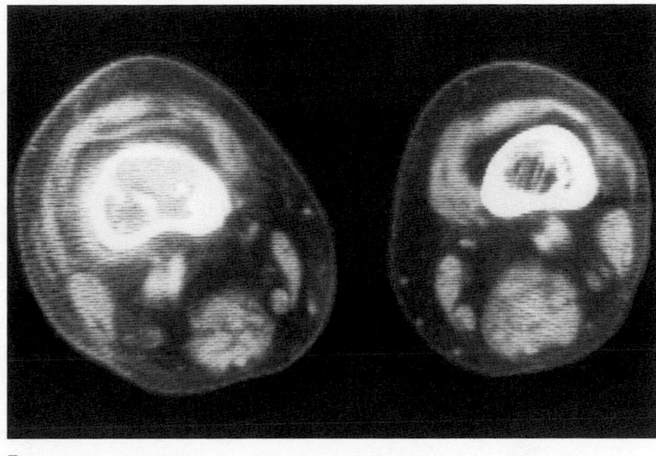

Figure 6–37. Radiograph (**A**) and CT scan (**B**) of a low-grade intramedullary osteosarcoma in the distal femur of a 65-year-old man.

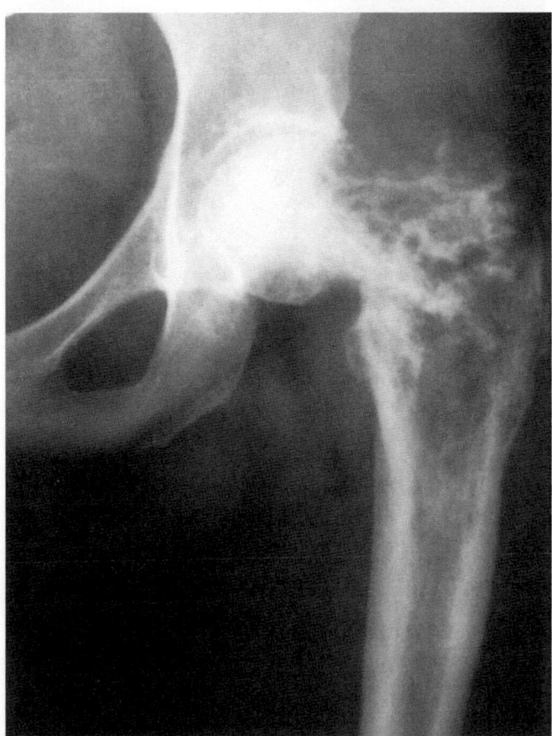

Figure 6–38. Radiograph of irradiation-induced osteosarcoma of the peritrochanteric area in a 35-year-old woman.

Chondroid-Forming Sarcomas

Chondroid-forming sarcomas are a heterogenous group of neoplasms consisting of a cartilage-based histology. A cornerstone to the diagnosis of chondrosarcoma is the absence of osteoid formation. If any osteoid is present with a malignant stroma, the tumor is considered an osteosarcoma with chondroblastic features. It is important to make the distinction because chondrosarcomas behave differently from osteosarcomas. However, this can be a difficult task. The surgeon must consider the age of the patient and carefully assess the radiographic and histologic features to confirm the diagnosis.

A. Primary or Central Conventional Chondrosarcoma

The typical primary chondrosarcoma is a low-grade tumor seen in adults between 30 and 60 years of age. The tumor is found more frequently in men than in women. Minimal symptoms of pain may occur over a period of several years before a radiograph is obtained. The pelvis and femur are the most common locations, followed by the rib cage, proximal humerus, scapula, and upper tibia. Primary chondrosarcoma is extremely rare in small bones, including the hand and foot. The metaphysis is the most common location in a long bone; however, a diaphyseal location is not unusual.

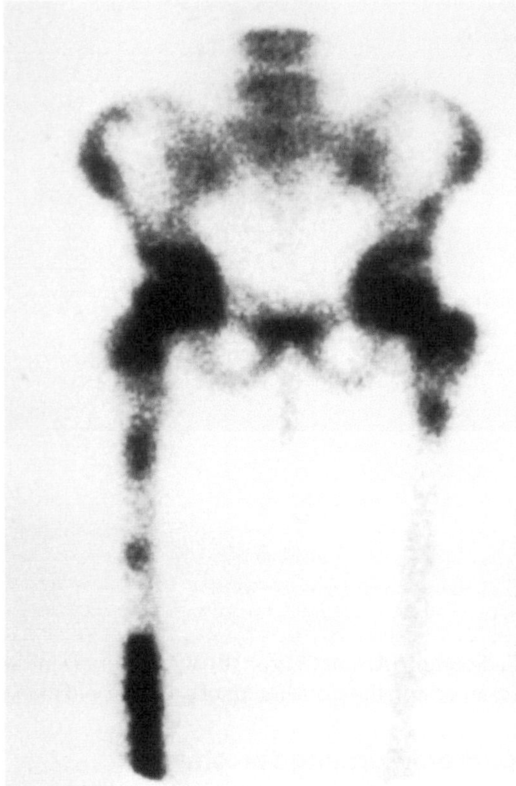

Figure 6–39. Isotope bone scan of multicentric osteosarcoma in an 8-year-old girl.

Approximately 85% of central chondrosarcomas are low-grade lesions with a typical matrix calcification that can be described as flocculated. The high-grade lesions are rare, and radiographically they lose their typical lobulated and calcific pattern and take on the appearance of a more permeative high-grade tumor, such as a malignant fibrous histiocytoma. At the same time, histologically the high-grade chondrosarcomas lose their chondroid matrix pattern, which is replaced with that of a more aggressive spindle-cell tumor.

The radiologic feature that clearly separates this lesion from a benign enchondroma is the permeative lysis seen in the surrounding cortex (Figure 6–41). Because of the weakened cortex, the patient usually complains of local pain not experienced with an enchondroma. Because most chondrosarcomas are low grade, they do not respond well to adjuvant irradiation or chemotherapy. Therefore, aggressive surgical management is imperative. However, optimal surgical management is controversial. Although wide en bloc resection is ideal from a margin standpoint, it can often produce considerable morbidity. On the contrary, aggressive intralesional resection (curettage) and margin expansion with an adjuvant therapy (eg, phenol or liquid nitrogen) can reduce morbidity and may provide equal local control. In fact, some authors found that for grade 1 chondrosarcoma the margin of resection is not significant in terms of local recurrence or disease progression.

In general, the prognosis for low-grade central chondrosarcoma is very good, with a low rate of pulmonary metastasis if the primary lesion is widely resected. Nevertheless, recurrences can occur late, even over 15 years later. For any intermediate- or high-grade chondrosarcoma, wide, en bloc resection is mandatory (Figure 6–42).

B. Secondary Chondrosarcoma

The vast majority of secondary chondrosarcomas arise from osteochondromas in patients afflicted with HME.

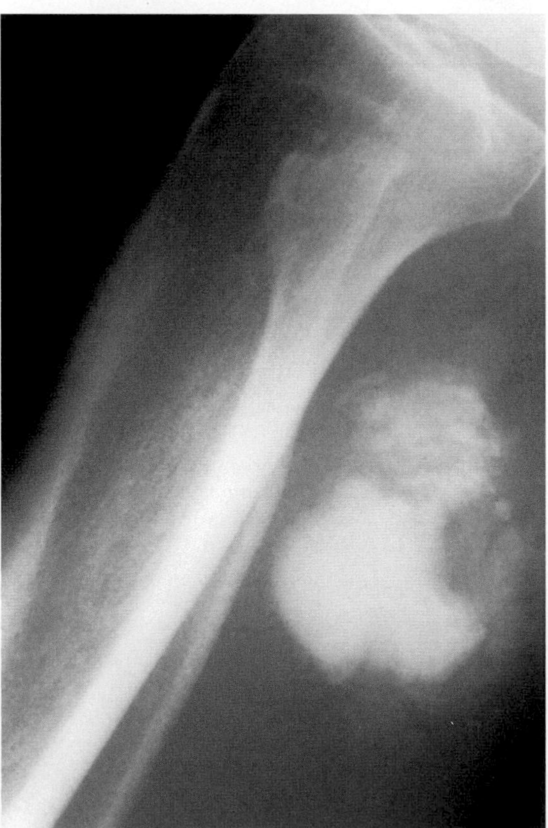

Figure 6–40. Radiograph of a soft-tissue osteosarcoma in the calf area of a 67-year-old man.

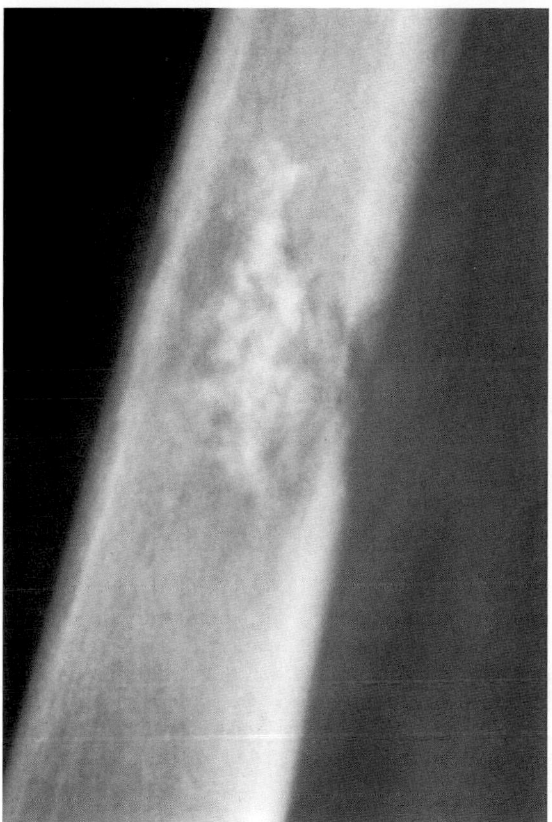

Figure 6–41. Radiograph of a low-grade primary chondrosarcoma in the distal femur of an 83-year-old man.

Patients with solitary osteochondromas do not generally form secondary chondrosarcomas in their lesions, making prophylactic removal unnecessary and unwarranted unless the solitary lesion is otherwise symptomatic. Even in patients with HME, the rate of malignant degeneration is less than 1% and generally does not occur in patients prior to skeletal maturity. However, patients with secondary chondrosarcoma tend to be younger than those with primary chondrosarcomas (see Table 6–2). The lesions tend to be slow growing with minimal to mild symptoms. The most common site is the pelvis, followed by the proximal femur, proximal humerus, and ribs. Plain radiographs demonstrate a flocculated calcific pattern (Figure 6–43). Anything thicker than 1–2 cm should raise suspicion of a secondary chondrosarcoma. The overall prognosis for patients with secondary or peripheral chondrosarcoma is even better than that for patients with primary or central chondrosarcoma. Surgical removal, without violation of the cartilage cap, is the only effective treatment modality.

C. Dedifferentiated Chondrosarcoma

Dedifferentiated chondrosarcoma is the most malignant variant of chondrosarcoma, accounting for between 5% and 10% of all chondrosarcomas. It is heralded by the transformation of areas of conventional chondrosarcoma into malignant fibrous histiocytoma or osteosarcoma. Histologically, it is characterized by two distinct but neighboring areas of low- to intermediate-grade malignant chondroid tumor and heterogenous high-grade sarcoma. Dedifferentiated chondrosarcoma occurs in older patients, usually between 50 and 70 years of age. It is found in the same areas affected by central primary chondrosarcomas, including the pelvis, femur, and proximal humerus (Figure 6–44). Radiographs show areas of rarefication within the tumor with cortical attenuation. Pathologic fracture is not uncommon.

The prognosis in dedifferentiated chondrosarcoma is bleak, with the majority of patients developing and dying of metastatic disease within 1 year (historically, 1-year survival rate approached 10%). Chemotherapy and radiation therapy are less effective than in a malignant fibrous histiocytoma or osteosarcoma that arose de novo. Surgical resection remains the mainstay of treatment, with adjuvant modalities employed in younger patients.

D. Clear Cell Chondrosarcoma

Clear cell chondrosarcoma is a rare low-grade variant of chondrosarcoma. Clear cell lesions occur more often in males than in females and are usually seen in patients between 20 and 50 years of age. The vast majority of lesions are found in the femoral head (Figure 6–45). The radiographic appearance is one of a lytic tumor with sharp margination and a central matrix calcification, creating the appearance of a chondroblastoma. Although microscopic examination reveals the presence of some giant cells, as seen in a chondroblastoma, areas of low-grade chondrosarcoma are also evident in which no giant cells are seen. Even on gross examination, the clear cell chondrosarcoma does not look like a chondrosarcoma, which explains why it is frequently mistaken for a chondroblastoma in younger adult patients. The tumor cells have abundant glycogen, giving them their characteristic clear cell phenotype. Although no significant genetic alteration is found in clear cell chondrosarcoma, newer findings show that alkaline phosphatase activity may correlate with prognosis.

The treatment for clear cell chondrosarcoma is a wide excision and reconstruction. The prognosis with this type of treatment is good. In contrast, when lesions are mistaken for chondroblastomas and treatment consists of a simple curettage and bone grafting, the prognosis is poor and the recurrence rate is high.

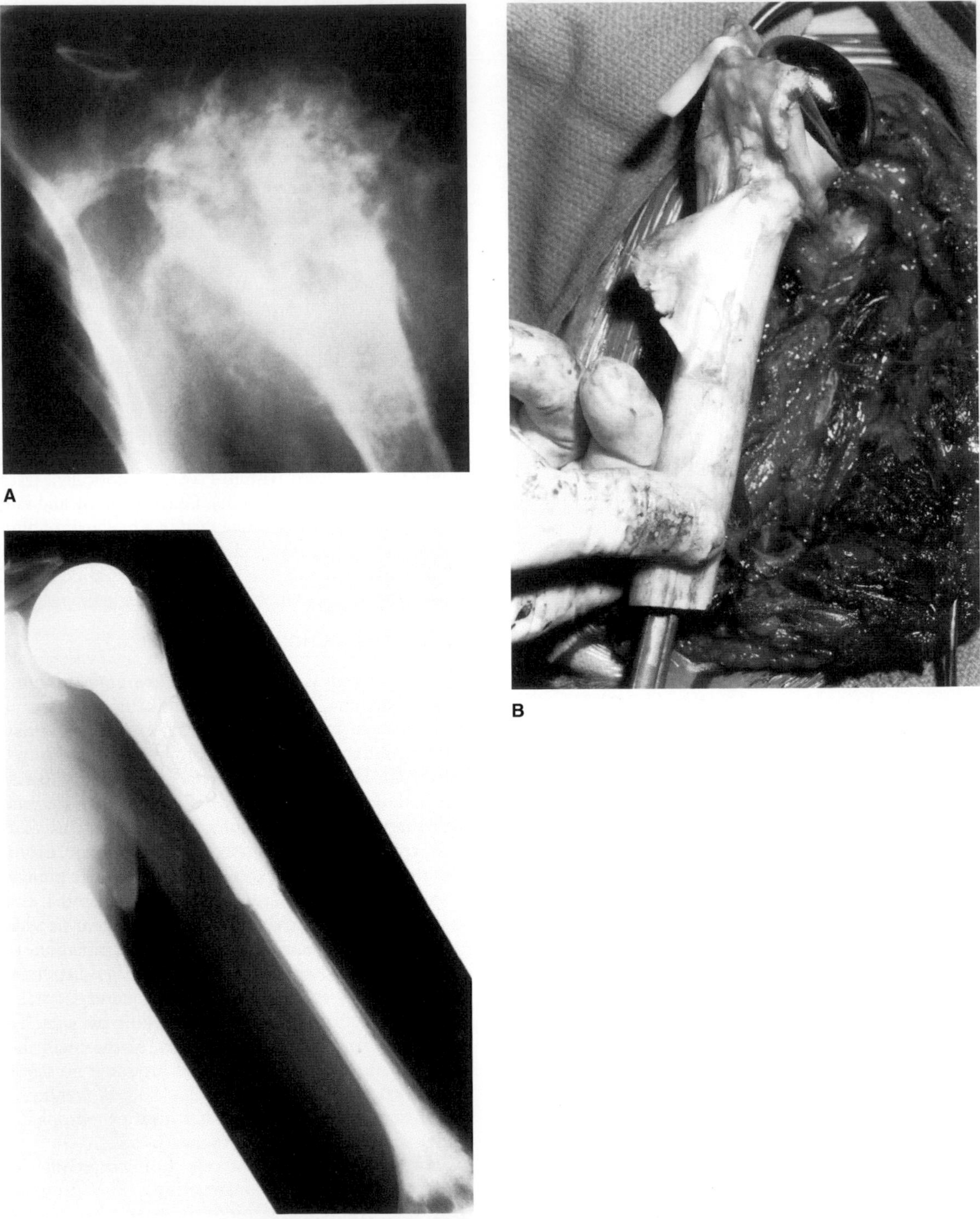

Figure 6–42. Preoperative radiograph of a large central chondrosarcoma in the proximal humerus of a 52-year-old woman (**A**), placement of a Neer prosthesis (**B**), and postoperative radiograph (**C**).

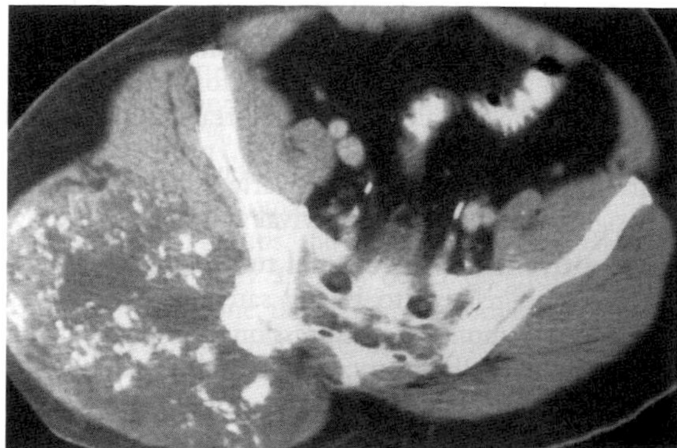

Figure 6–43. CT scan of a secondary peripheral chondrosarcoma in the ilium of a 56-year-old man with multiple exostoses.

E. Mesenchymal Chondrosarcoma

Another rare variant of chondrosarcoma is the mesenchymal chondrosarcoma. It is a highly cellular tumor composed of primitive mesenchymal cells with foci of cartilage differentiation. This tumor involves the soft tissue in a third of cases, occurs more frequently in females than in males, and is seen in young adults (see Table 6–2). The jaw is the most common location, followed by the spine and ribs, with very few cases noted in long bones.

Mesenchymal chondrosarcoma is a high-grade tumor with histologic features of low-grade chondrosarcoma. Heavily calcified areas, mixed with areas of malignant round cells, may give it the appearance of Ewing sarcoma or hemangiopericytoma.

Treatment consists of resection, with a wide margin if possible, and adjuvant chemotherapy and radiation therapy. Despite aggressive treatment, the prognosis is very poor, with a high incidence of pulmonary metastasis.

Round Cell Sarcomas

This so-called group of tumors is composed of distinct tumors that, other than their similar microscopic appearance using hematoxylin-eosin stain, are quite different. They behave and are treated in a variety of ways, given that each arises from a different cell type.

A. The Ewing Family of Tumors

1. Ewing sarcoma—Ewing sarcoma is a well-known clinical entity originally described by James Ewing as a diffuse endothelioma of bone. Since the time of his description, many theories have evolved regarding the tumor's true histogenesis. Based on electron microscopic and immunohistochemical findings, experts currently believe the tumor represents an undifferentiated member of the family of neural tumors distinct from neuroblastoma. Cytogenetic studies identified a chromosomal abnormality with a reciprocal translocation in chromosomes 11 and 22 seen in 90% of cases. This translocation is also seen in primitive neuroectodermal tumor (PNET) and Askin tumors. The breakpoints were cloned, and it is now known that the Ewing sarcoma and *FLI1* genes are involved. The Ewing sarcoma gene encodes a homologous sequence to the RNA binding site in RNA polymerase II. The FLI product is a transcription factor. Accordingly, in the resultant fusion protein, the *FLI1* transcription factor is placed under control of the Ewing sarcoma promoter. Two other translocations are also described in Ewing/PNET: t(21:22) and t(7:22).

In 90% of cases, Ewing sarcoma is found in patients between 5 and 25 years of age. If the patient is younger

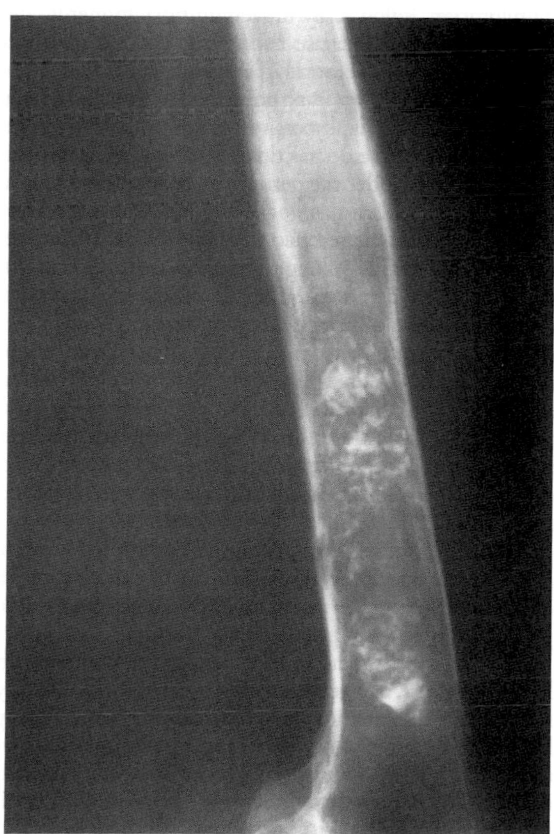

Figure 6–44. Radiograph of dedifferentiated chondrosarcoma in the distal femur of a 73-year-old woman.

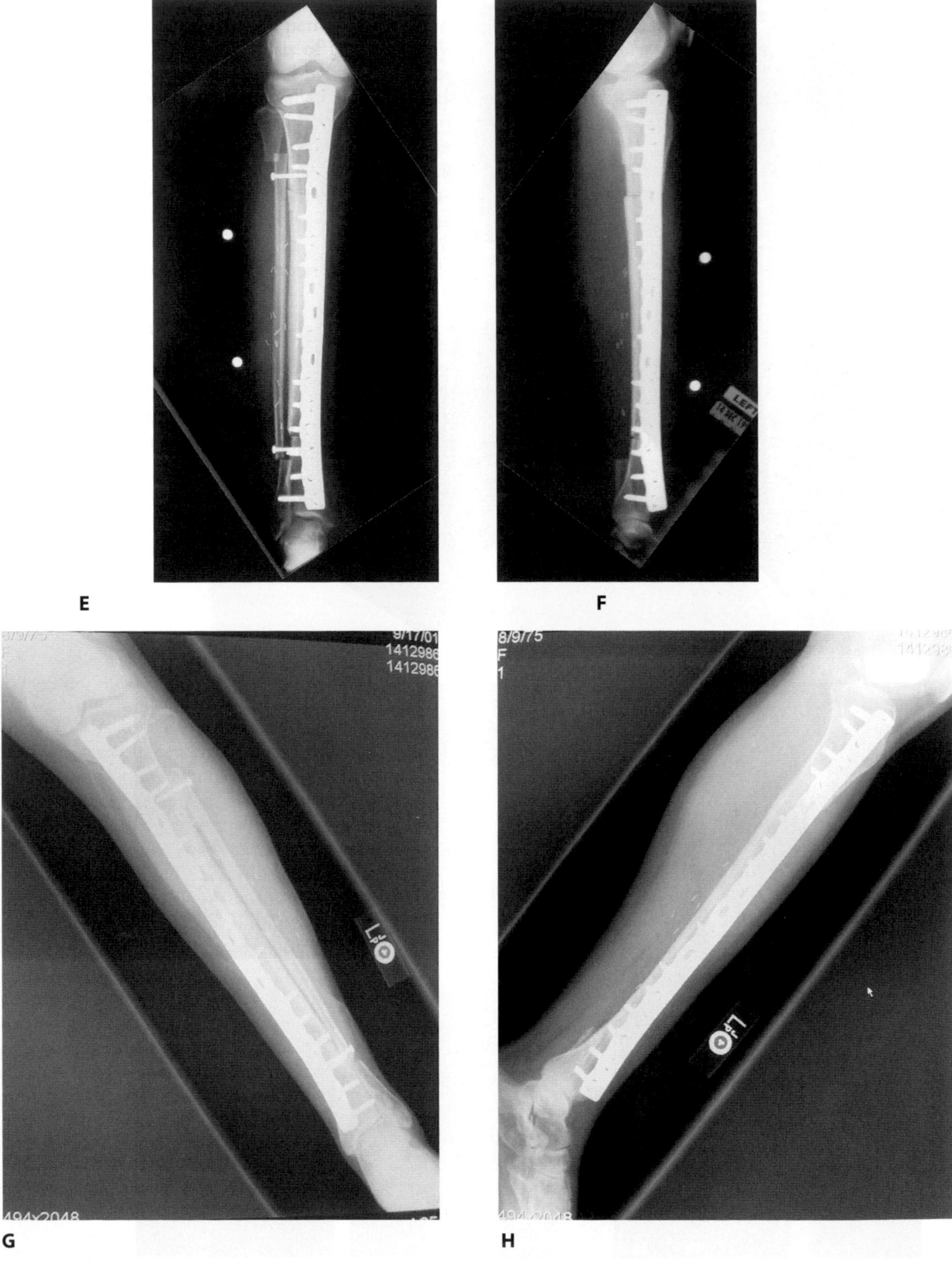

Figure 6–51. (Continued) Immediate postoperative after resection with intercalary allograft reconstruction and vascularized fibula transport anteroposterior radiograph (**E**), lateral radiograph 3 years postoperative (**F**), anteroposterior radiograph (**G**), lateral radiograph (**H**). *Continued.*

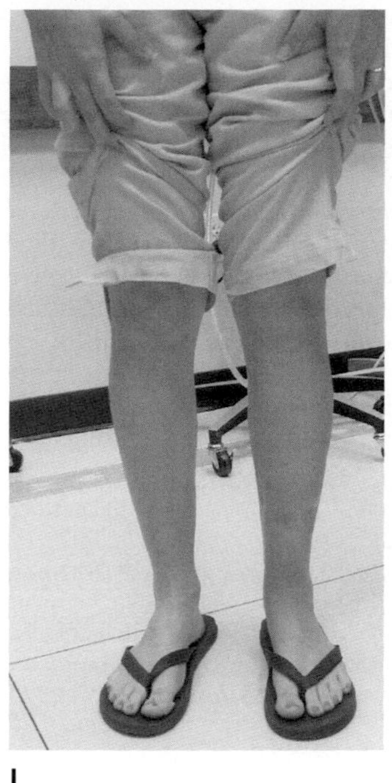
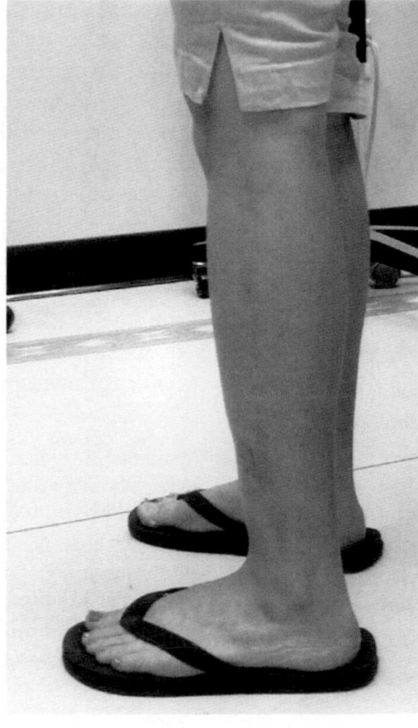
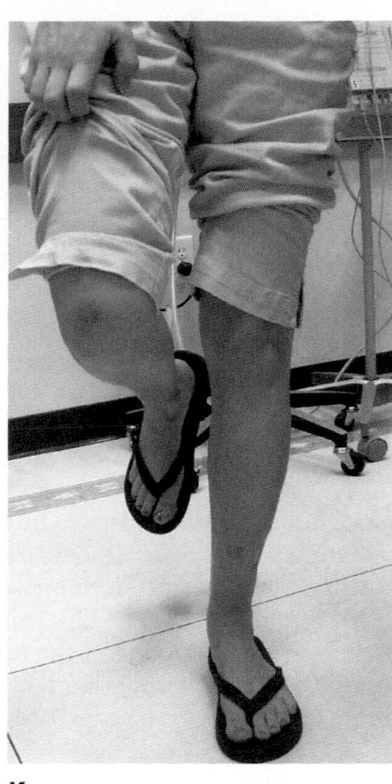

I J K

Figure 6–51. (Continued) **I–K:** Clinical photos 3 years postoperative.

diagnosis is that osteofibrous dysplasia is painless, whereas pain is a frequent symptom in adamantinoma. Another is that fibrous lesions of bone stop growing at bone maturity, whereas the adamantinoma continues on into adult life, at which point a biopsy of the progressive lytic portion of the disease should be performed. There have been cases of osteofibrous dysplasia combined with small areas of adamantinoma scattered in the benign osseofibrous tissue. Adamantinoma is also occasionally found in both the tibia and fibula, so the physician should look for multiple sites.

Microscopic findings include nests or cords of epithelial or angioid tissue growing in a fibrous tissue stroma, which can give adamantinoma the appearance of a low-grade angiosarcoma or a metastatic carcinoma.

Adamantinoma grows extremely slowly, over many years, but on occasion metastasizes to regional lymph nodes and the lung. For this reason, it should be treated by a wide resection, which in most cases is a segmental diaphyseal resection followed by an allograft reconstruction over an intramedullary nail. Because of the low-grade nature of this tumor, adjuvant irradiation or chemotherapy is rarely indicated. Even if pulmonary metastases occur, they can be resected, and there is a fairly good prognosis for survival.

Vascular Sarcomas of Bone

Vascular sarcomas are relatively rare. They include the hemangioendothelioma, angiosarcoma, and hemangiopericytoma of bone. The terms *hemangioendothelioma* and *angiosarcoma* are frequently used synonymously; however, the first term refers to a low-grade tumor, and the second term usually suggests a higher grade lesion with a poorer prognosis. The vascular sarcomas have two different cell-line origins: endothelial cells for the hemangioendotheliomas, in contrast to hemangiopericytes for the hemangiopericytomas.

A. Hemangioendothelioma

The hemangioendothelioma, which is more common in males than in females, is seen in a wide range of ages between the second and seventh decades. The femur, pelvis, spine, and ribs are the usual sites of origin, and the diaphyses and metaphyses of the long bones are also involved. One third of cases are multicentric, usually in the same bone or limb.

Radiographically, the lesion appears lytic, with surrounding sclerotic bone. The more anaplastic the disease process is, the less reactive bone is. The clinical picture varies widely, depending on the histologic grade of the tumor. The low-grade lesions look like benign hemangiomas, are slow growing, and carry an excellent prognosis. The high-grade lesions are fast-growing lytic lesions with a poor prognosis.

Treatment depends on the histologic grade. The low-grade lesions do well with simple curettement and bone graft, but the high-grade lesions require a more aggressive wide resection and reconstruction. Adjuvant chemotherapy and radiation therapy can be considered for high-grade lesions, especially in patients with multifocal disease.

B. Hemangiopericytoma

The hemangiopericytoma is an extremely rare form of vascular sarcoma that also has a wide spectrum of clinical presentations, depending on the histologic grading. This tumor is the malignant counterpart of the glomus tumor, discussed later in the section on soft-tissue tumors. The hemangiopericytoma is a round cell tumor located outside the endothelial membrane of the vascular channel. This can be demonstrated clearly by a silver staining of the reticulum fibers lying between the inner endothelial cells and the outer hemangiopericytes.

Chordomas

Chordoma of bone is rare and accounts for 4% of malignant bone tumors. It takes its origin from the primitive notochord and has the clinical appearance of a chondrosarcoma. Chordomas affect males more frequently than females and are seen in patients between 30 and 80 years of age. Although 50% of the tumors are sacrococcygeal in origin, 37% arise in the sphenoccipital area, and the remainder arise from vertebral bodies of the cervical or lumbar spine. The cranial lesions are seen in a younger age group and carry a poor prognosis because of the dangerous location next to the brain, where surgical removal is difficult.

On radiograph, the chordoma appears as a centrally located lytic process that has minimal sclerotic response at the periphery and may show slight matrix calcification, as in a chondrosarcoma. If the sacrum is involved, the lesion is seen usually in the lower three sacral segments and presents as an extracortical lobulated mass both in front and behind the sacrum. Because of the slow tumor growth, pain may not occur early, but constipation can be an early symptom that results from pressure on the rectum. Because the true anatomic borders are not readily defined by routine radiography, it is best to image this tumor with CT or MRI (Figure 6–52). Microscopically, nests or cords of cells, sprinkled in a sea of mucinous tissue, give an appearance similar to low-grade chondrosarcoma. In most cases, large vacuolated cells appear like a signet ring and are referred to as physaliferous cells.

Treatment for the sacral lesions is an aggressive wide resection, which can be difficult because of excessive bleeding. Significant neurogenic bowel and bladder deficits can result. At the present time, it is common to use adjuvant radiation therapy to help reduce the chance of postoperative recurrence. Newer studies recommend using up to 5000 cGy preoperatively, followed with a boost of 1500 cGy postoperatively. If the surgeon is successful in obtaining clean margins, the local recurrence rate is approximately 30%. With contaminated margins, the recurrence rate climbs to 65%. Recurrence 10–15 years following surgery is common. Because of the low-grade characteristics of the chordoma, it is rare to see a pulmonary metastasis, even after a local recurrence following an inadequate local surgical resection.

Anthouli-Anagnostopoulou FA et al: Juxtacortical osteosarcoma. A distinct malignant bone neoplasm. Adv Clin Path 2004(3):127. [PMID: 11080792]

Bacci G et al: Neoadjuvant chemotherapy for osteosarcoma of the extremity: Long-term results of the Rizzoli's 4th protocol. Eur J Cancer 2001;37(16):2030. [PMID: 11597381]

Bacci G et al: Histologic response of high-grade nonmetastatic osteosarcoma of the extremity to chemotherapy. Clin Orthop 2001;(386):186. [PMID: 11347833]

Bacci G et al: Telangiectatic osteosarcoma of the extremity: Neoadjuvant chemotherapy in 24 cases. Acta Orthop Scand 2001; 72(2):167. [PMID: 11372948]

Barrille-Nion S et al: Advances in biology and therapy of multiple myeloma. Hematology (Am Soc Hematol Educ Program) 2003;248–278. Review. [PMID: 14633785]

Berend KR et al: Adjuvant chemotherapy for osteosarcoma may not increase survival after neoadjuvant chemotherapy and surgical resection. J Surg Oncol 2001;78(3):162. [PMID: 11745799]

Bruns J et al: Chondrosarcoma of bone: An oncological and functional follow-up study. Ann Oncol 2001;12(6):859. [PMID: 11484965]

Crapanzano JP et al: Chordoma: A cytologic study with histologic and radiologic correlation. Cancer 2001;25;93(1):40. [PMID: 11241265]

Ewing J: Diffuse endothelioma of bone. Proc NY Pathol Soc 1921; 21:17.

Gokgoz N et al: Comparison of p53 mutations in patients with localized osteosarcoma and metastatic osteosarcoma. Cancer 2001;92:2181. [PMID: 11596036]

Gorlick R et al: Expression of HER2/erbB-2 correlates with survival in osteosarcoma. J Clin Oncol 1999;17(9):2781. [PMID: 10561353]

Hoang BH et al: Expression of LDL receptor-related protein 5 (LRP5) as a novel marker for disease progression in high-grade osteosarcoma. Int J Cancer 2004;109(1):106. [PMID: 14735475]

Hoang MP et al: Mesenchymal chondrosarcoma: A small cell neoplasm with polyphenotypic differentiation. Int J Surg Pathol 2000;8(4):291. [PMID: 11494006]

Kanamori M et al: Extra copies of chromosomes 7, 8, 12, 19, and 21 are recurrent in adamantinoma. J Mol Diagn 2001;3(1): 16. [PMID: 11227067]

Kaste SC et al: Thallium bone imaging as an indicator of response and outcome in nonmetastatic primary extremity osteosarcoma. Pediatr Radiol 2001;31(4):251. [PMID: 11321742]

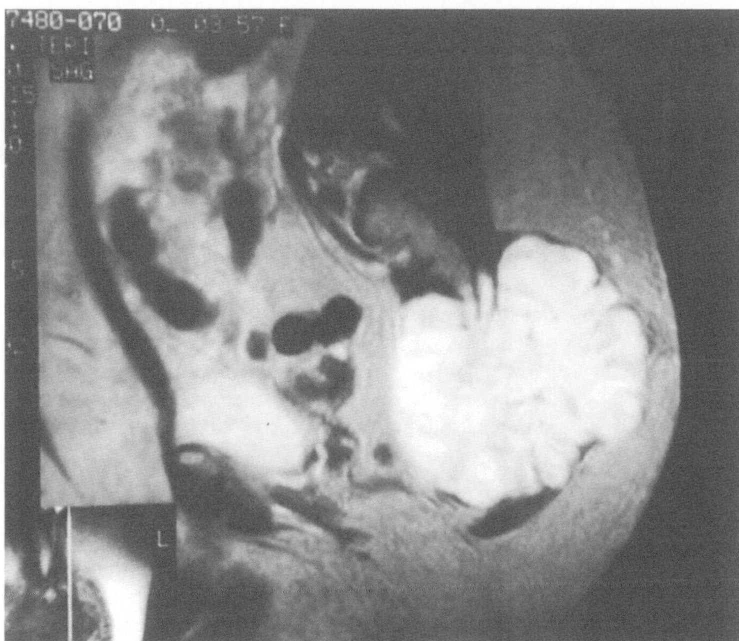

A

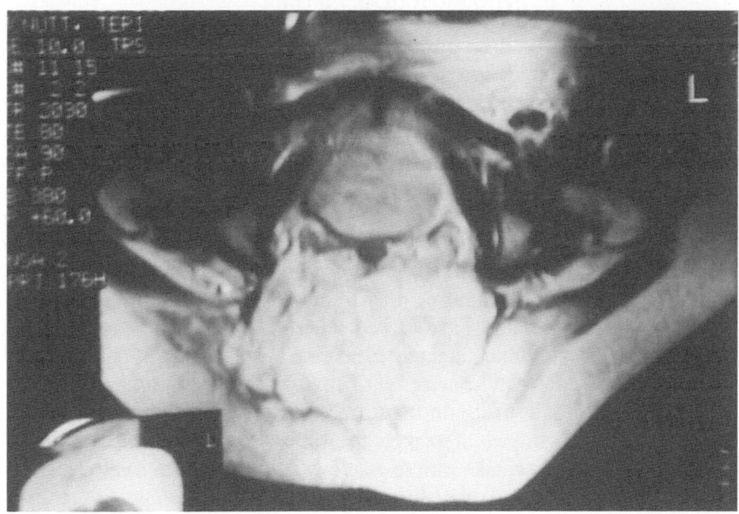

B

Figure 6–52. Sacral chordoma in middle-age woman: T_2 sagittal image (**A**), T_2 transverse image (**B**).

Kaya M et al: Vascular endothelial growth factor expression in untreated osteosarcoma is predictive of pulmonary metastasis and poor prognosis. Clin Cancer Res 2000;6(2):572. [PMID: 10690541]

Khanna C et al: The membrane-cytoskeleton linker ezrin is necessary for osteosarcoma metastasis. Nat Med 2004;10(2):182. [PMID: 14704791]

Kilpatrick SE et al: Clinicopathologic analysis of HER-2/neu immunoexpression among various histologic subtypes and grades of ostesosarcoma. Mod Pathol 2001;14(12):1277. [PMID: 11743051]

Kloen P et al: Expression of transforming growth factor-beta (TGF-beta) isoforms in osteosarcomas: TGF-beta3 is related to disease progression. Cancer 1997;80(12):2230. [PMID: 9404699]

Lewis VO et al: Parosteal osteosarcoma of the posterior aspect of the distal part of the femur. Oncological and functional results following a new resection technique. J Bone Joint Surg Am 2000;82-A(8):1083. [PMID: 10954096]

Maitra A et al: Aberrant expression of tumor suppressor proteins in the Ewing family of tumors. Arch Pathol Lab Med 2001; 125(9):1207. [PMID: 11520274]

Mandahl N et al: Cytogenetic aberrations and their prognostic impact in chondrosarcoma. Genes Chromosomes Cancer 2002; 33(2):188. [PMID: 11793445]

Oberlin O et al: Study of the French Society of Paediatric Oncology (EW88 study). Br J Cancer 2001;85(11):1646. [PMID: 11742482]

Ogose A et al: Elevation of serum alkaline phosphatase in clear cell chondrosarcoma of bone. Anticancer Res 2001;21(1B):649. [PMID: 11299821]

Park YK et al: Overexpression of p53 and absent genetic mutation in clear cell chondrosarcoma. Int J Oncol 2001;19(2):353. [PMID: 11445851]

Pring ME et al: Chondrosarcoma of the pelvis. A review of sixty-four cases. J Bone Joint Surg Am 2001;83-A(11):1630. [PMID: 11701784]

Reddick WE et al: Dynamic MR imaging (DEMRI) of microcirculation in bone sarcoma. J Magn Reson Imaging 1999; 10(3):277. [PMID: 10508287]

Rizzo M et al: Chondrosarcoma of bone: Analysis of 108 cases and evaluation for predictors of outcome. Clin Orthop 2001; (391):224. [PMID: 11603673]

Roland Durr H et al: Multiple myeloma: Surgery of the spine: Retrospective analysis of 27 patients. Spine 2002;27(3):320. [PMID: 11805699]

Scully SP et al: Pathologic fracture in osteosarcoma: Prognostic importance and treatment implications. J Bone Joint Surg Am 2002;84-A(1):49. [PMID: 11792779]

Sluga M et al: The role of surgery and resection margins in the treatment of Ewing's sarcoma. Clin Orthop 2001;(392):394. [PMID: 11716413]

Smith SE et al: Primary musculoskeletal tumors of fibrous origin. Semin Musculoskelet Radiol 2000;4(1):73. [PMID: 11061693]

Tallini G et al: Correlation between clinicopathological features and karyotype in 100 cartilaginous and chordoid tumours. A report from the Chromosomes and Morphology (CHAMP) Collaborative Study Group. J Pathol 2002;196(2):194. [PMID: 11793371]

Tian E et al: The role of the Wnt-signaling antagonist DKK1 in the development of osteolytic lesions in multiple myeloma. N Engl J Med 2003;349(26):2483. [PMID: 14695408]

Weisstein JS et al: Detection of c-fos expression in benign and malignant musculoskeletal lesions. J Orthop Res 2001;19(3): 339. [PMID: 11398843]

Zhou H et al: Her-2/neu staining in osteosarcoma: Association with increased risk of metastasis. Sarcoma 2001;5(S1):9.

BENIGN SOFT-TISSUE TUMORS

Soft tissue can be defined as nonepithelial, extraskeletal mesenchymal exclusive of the reticuloendothelial system and glia. This definition would include fat, fibrous tissue, muscle, and the relating neurovascular structures.

Benign soft-tissue tumors, by definition, represent a differentiated neoplastic process with a limited capacity for autonomous growth. They generally demonstrate a marginal capacity to invade locally with infrequent local recurrence. Because of the extensive numbers of benign soft-tissue tumors, discussion is limited here to the more common entities.

Lipomas

The lipoma is by far the most common soft-tissue tumor and has a large number of variants. Some examples include the superficial subcutaneous lipoma; the intramuscular lipoma; the spindle-cell lipoma; the angiolipoma; the benign lipoblastoma; and the lipomas of tendon sheaths, nerves, synovium, periosteum, and the lumbosacral area.

A. Superficial Subcutaneous Lipoma

The most frequently seen type of lipoma is the superficial subcutaneous type, which can be solitary or multiple. Subcutaneous lipomas occur with equal frequency in men and women and seem to arise spontaneously during the fifth and sixth decade of life. The most common locations are the back, shoulder, and neck.

On palpation this tumor is soft and ballotable. Although it is found more commonly in obese patients, the size of the lipoma does not correlate with the weight of the patient. Lipomas do not reduce in volume with weight loss. They generally grow to a limited size and sarcomatous degeneration does not occur. Surgical treatment is usually cosmetic in nature, and the recurrence rate is less than 5%.

B. Intramuscular Lipoma

The deep intramuscular lipoma is seen in adults between 30 and 60 years of age, affects men more frequently than women, and is commonly found in the large muscles of the extremities. The lesions are slow growing and painless. The intramuscular lipoma has a characteristic radiolucency that contrasts with the surrounding muscle (Figure 6–53). On MRI this tumor demonstrates a uniform high-signal image on the T_1-weighted spin-echo sequence. On gross examination, the tumor can appear quite infiltrative in surrounding muscle and has a faint yellow color on sectioning. Histologic studies show that the intramuscular lipoma, like the subcutaneous lipoma, is composed of benign lipocytes with small pyknotic nuclei that are difficult to see on the surface of the large fat-laden cell. When samples are taken for biopsy purposes, the pathologist must take care to rule out a low-grade, well-differentiated liposarcoma that can coexist with a benign lipoma. On rare occasions, a lipoma can have chondroid or osseous hamartomatous elements that have caused it to be classified as a mesenchymoma in the past. In other cases, evidence of hemorrhage or necrosis can be found in a lipoma and creates low-signal changes on the MRI that are similar to the changes seen in liposarcoma.

A marginal surgical excision is indicated for treatment of intramuscular lipoma. Local recurrence rates of 15–60% are reported.

C. Spindle-Cell Lipoma

The spindle-cell lipoma is seen typically in the posterior neck and shoulder area in men between 45 and 64 years

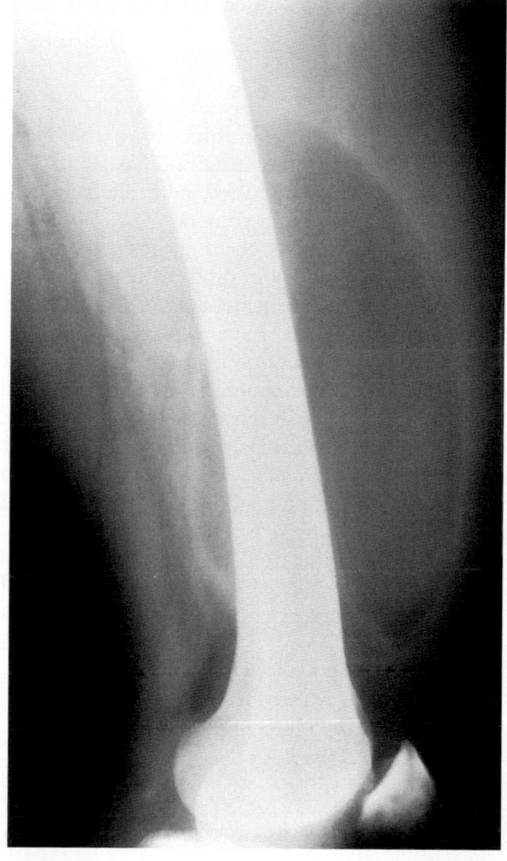

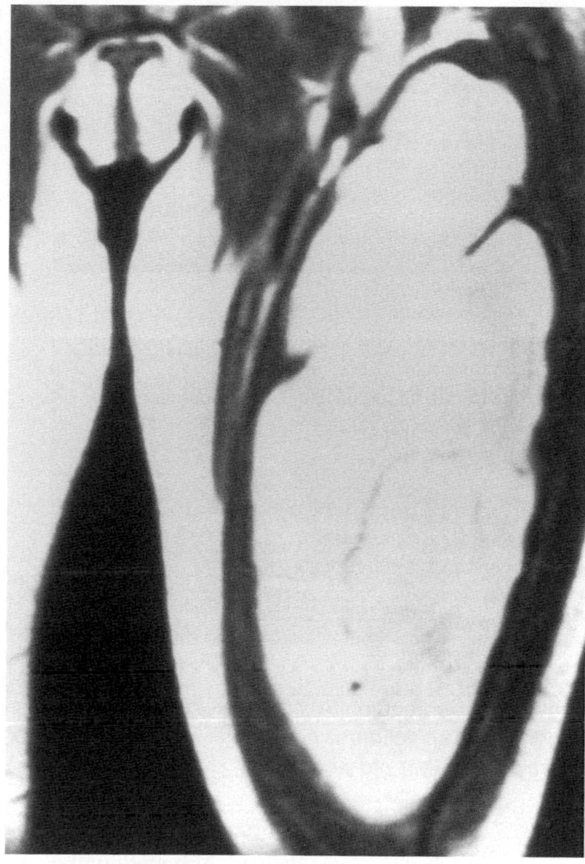

Figure 6–53. Radiograph (**A**) and coronal view T_1-weighted MRI (**B**) of an intramuscular lipoma in the quadriceps muscle of a 72-year-old man.

of age. On gross examination, the spindle-cell lipoma has the appearance of an ordinary lipoma but with areas of gray-white gelatinous foci streaking through it. Microscopic examination of these areas reveals the presence of benign fibroblasts. Thus, with imaging studies, dense areas are scattered throughout the normal radiolucent areas of a lipoma. On MRI, findings generally consist of a low-signal streaking through the typical high-signal pattern of a benign lipoma.

The treatment for this lesion is a simple marginal resection. The chance for local recurrence is minimal.

D. Angiolipoma

The angiolipoma (Figure 6–54) is a subcutaneous lesion seen in young (see Table 6–6) adults, usually on the forearm. Multiple lesions are frequently present and usually painful because of their vascularity. Grossly, the lobular lipoma demonstrates vascular channels.

Treatment of angiolipoma consists of marginal excision.

E. Diffuse Lipomatosis

An extremely rare variant of the lipoma is diffuse lipomatosis, characterized by the presence of multiple superficial and deep lipomas that involve one entire extremity or the trunk and usually have their onset during the first 2 years of life. Histologically, an individual lesion in a patient with diffuse lipomatosis looks no different from a typical solitary lipoma. An involved limb may become massive in size, sometimes making it impossible to remove the fatty tumors surgically. If this is the case, amputation may be indicated.

F. Lumbosacral Lipoma

The lumbosacral lipoma occurs in the lumbosacral area posterior to a spina bifida defect. It is frequently associated with both intradural and extradural lipomas and

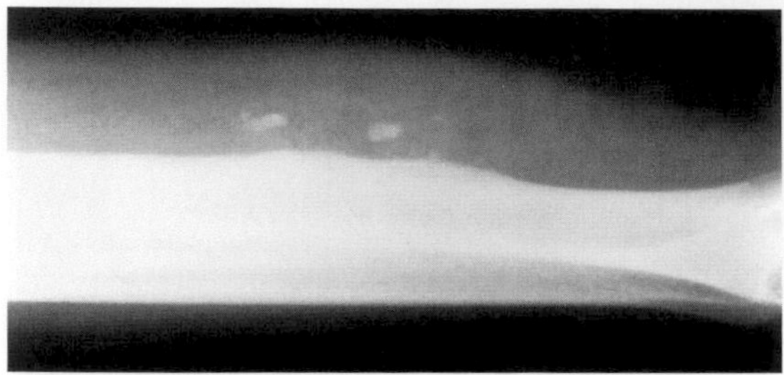

A

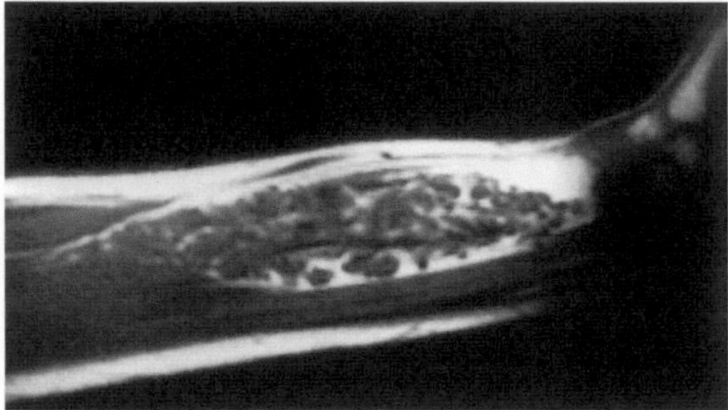

B

Figure 6–54. Radiograph (**A**) and T_1-weighted MRI (**B**) of a soft-tissue angiolipoma in the volar aspect of the forearm of a 27-year-old woman.

thus can result in neurologic deficits. Although lumbosacral lipoma is generally considered a pediatric tumor, it can be seen in adults (Figure 6–55).

Surgical treatment consists of a marginal resection of the entire lipoma, including the portion arising from the vertebral canal and lumbosacral roots.

G. Benign Lipoblastoma and Diffuse Lipoblastomatosis

The benign and diffuse types of lipoma are seen in the extremities of infants. The lesions, solitary or multiple, can be superficial or deep in muscle tissue. They demonstrate cellular immaturity, with lipoblasts similar to the myxoid form of liposarcoma. Even with the cellular aggressiveness of the lesions, the prognosis is excellent following simple surgical resection.

H. Hibernoma

Hibernoma, a rare lipoma usually seen in young (see Table 6–6) adults, commonly occurs in the scapular and interscapular regions, is painless and slow growing, and ranges between 10 and 15 cm in diameter. The hibernoma is composed of finely granular or vacuolated cells characteristic of brown fat and contains a considerable amount of glycogen. The treatment is marginal surgical resection with a low potential for recurrence.

Benign Vascular Tumors

Benign vascular proliferative tumors are the second most common benign tumor after lipomas. Three types of vascular tumors are discussed here: hemangiomas, lymphangiomas, and glomus tumors.

Like lipomas, angiomas occur in a wide variety of clinical conditions seen more often in females than in males. The most common type of angioma is the hemangioma, which can be a superficial cutaneous lesions or a deep and intramuscular one. The lymphatic counterpart of the hemangioma is known as the lymphangioma or hygroma. In most cases, the lesion is solitary or localized. If it is extensive and involves an entire limb, the term *angiomatosis* is used. Because most hemangiomas and lymphangiomas are congenital, the term *hamartomatous* or *arteriovenous malformation* is applied in their classification. Hemangiomas and lymphangiomas arise from developmental dysplasias of the endothelial tube, whereas glomus tumors and heman-

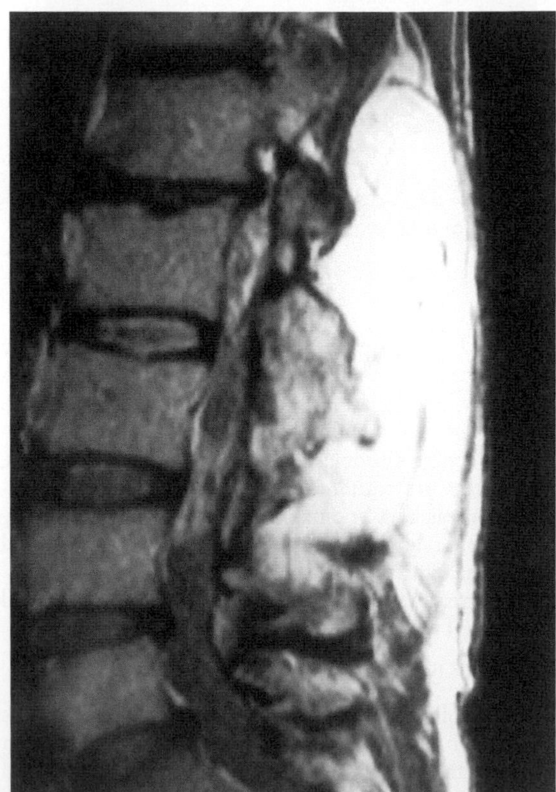

Figure 6–55. T_1-weighted MRI of a lumbosacral lipoma.

giocytomas arise from hemangiopericytes, which are cells that lie outside the endothelial tube. Most vascular anomalies arise sporadically, but some familial, autosomal-dominant inheritance patterns are also described. Genetic analysis of these families identified specific gene mutations supporting the genomic role in the regulation of angiogenesis.

A. Hemangioma

Hemangiomas are the most frequently seen tumors of childhood and account for 7% of all benign tumors.

1. Solitary capillary hemangioma—The most common type of hemangioma is the solitary capillary type, which appears as an elevated red to purple cutaneous lesion on the head or neck. The lesion occurs during the first few weeks after birth, grows rapidly over a period of several months, and regresses over a 7-year period in 75–90% of cases.

Because of the spontaneous regression, no treatment is needed in most cases. In the past, treatment consisted of cryosurgery, sclerotherapy, or irradiation, but frequently this treatment was worse than the disease itself. Today, lasers are used with good preliminary results. This may prove to be the treatment of choice in selected cases.

2. Cavernous hemangioma—The cavernous hemangioma is larger and less common than the capillary hemangioma. The enlarged vascular spaces of the cavernous lesion give it the appearance of a cluster of purple grapes. It lies deep in the extremity, with common involvement of muscles and even the synovial membrane of the joints.

Imaging may be characteristic (Figure 6–56). In some patients with deep intramuscular forms of hemangioma, the skin shows no abnormalities and no phleboliths are apparent on radiograph. With MRI, deep intramuscular hemangiomas can be easily detected by the characteristic mixed-signal serpiginous pattern seen in the T_1-weighted image.

The muscle lesions are usually asymptomatic until intralesional hemorrhage occurs either spontaneously or after a minor injury. The pain symptoms are usually short lived but recur infrequently. In some patients, the pain is more severe and associated with muscle contracture and joint deformity. These patients may require surgical resection of the scarred-down lesion to allow for better joint function and to reduce the pain. In rare cases of multiple hemangiomas involving the entire limb, amputation may be indicated. Vascular embolization of the feeder vessels can be attempted but may lead to a significant compartment syndrome, with severe contractures or with loss of muscle strength and limitation of joint movement.

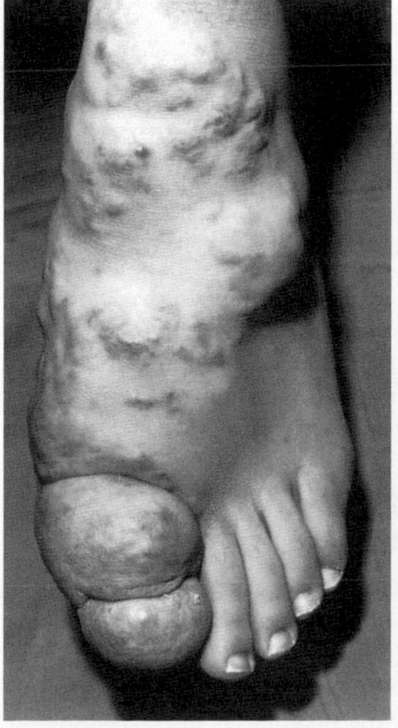
A

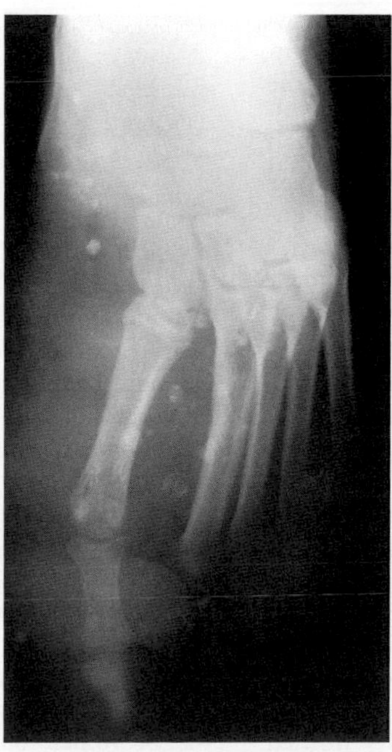
B

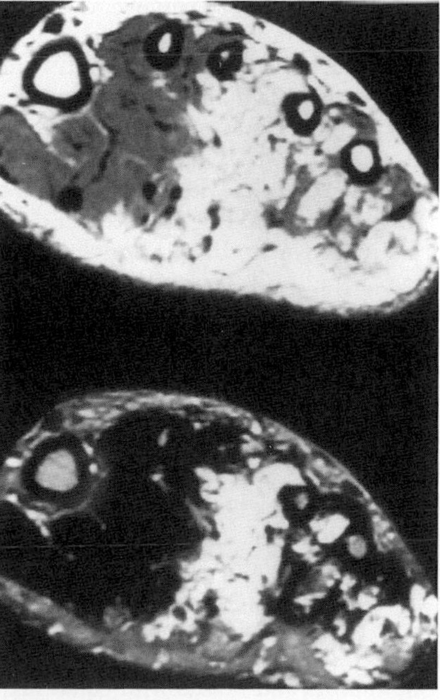
C

Figure 6–56. Clinical appearance (**A**) and radiographic appearance (**B**) of a cavernous hemangioma in the foot of one patient, and T_1-weighted and T_2-weighted MRIs (**C**) of a cavernous hemangioma in the foot of another patient.

3. Arteriovenous hemangioma—The arteriovenous hemangioma is seen in young patients (see Table 6–6) usually in the head, neck, or lower extremity. It is associated with significant arteriovenous shunting in the tumor, which creates increased perfusion. This results in increased local temperature, pain, and continuous thrill or bruit over the mass. In the extremity, it also results in an overgrowth of the limb.

If shunting is excessive, surgical removal of the hemangioma may be necessary to prevent increased pulse pressure from leading to high-output heart failure. Arteriograms are helpful in determining the degree of shunting prior to treatment. Embolization or surgical ligation of feeder vessels is frequently not a successful form of treatment.

4. Epithelioid hemangioma (Kimura disease)—This cutaneous hemangioma is found on the head or neck in women between 20 and 40 years old. It is associated with inflammatory changes and eosinophilia, and it sometime ulcerates. Its name is derived from the epithelial appearance of the endothelia-lined capillary structures.

5. Pyogenic granuloma—The pyogenic granuloma is a polypoid capillary hemangioma that affects the skin or mucosal surfaces of males and females in all age groups. It may be associated with trauma and is found about the mouth, gingivae, or fingers. The lesions have a purple-red color, bleed easily, and ulcerate.

B. Lymphangioma

The lymphangioma is nothing more than an angioma composed of lymphatic endothelial tubes filled with lymphatic fluid, rather than being filled with blood, as the hemangioma is. Lymphangiomas can be localized, which occurs with the cystic hygroma, and they are usually seen about the head, neck, or axilla of young boys and girls (see Table 6–6). As with hemangiomas, the larger lymphomas are cavernous lesions seen in older patients with deeper involvement. In both lymphangioma and hemangioma, because of increased regional perfusion, bony overgrowth can occur (Figure 6–57).

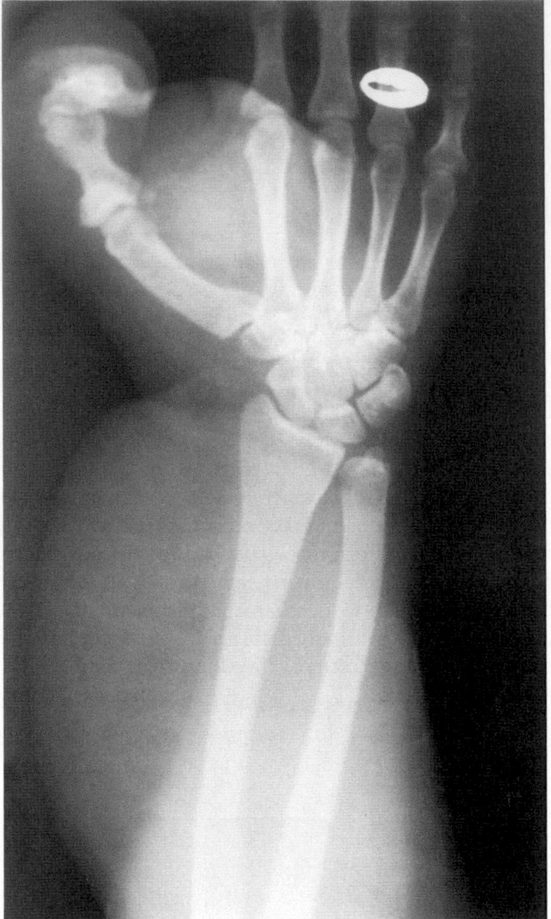

Figure 6–57. Radiograph of a lymphangioma in the forearm and hand of a 23-year-old woman.

C. Glomus Tumor

The glomus tumor arises from the hemangiopericyte, which is a cell seen at the periphery of the capillary vascular network and normally involved with the regulation of blood flow through the capillary system. Microscopic examination of the tumor reveals large vascular spaces surrounded by a homogeneous field of round epithelioid hemangiopericytes, with no evidence of mitotic activity.

The glomus tumor is a pink lesion that measures less than 1 cm in diameter. It represents 1.6% of all soft-tissue tumors and occurs with equal frequency in men and women, usually between 20 and 40 years of age. Although the tumor is found most commonly in the subungual area of a digit, where it is readily visible, it also occurs subcutaneously on the hand, wrist, forearm, or foot, where it may be invisible and thus difficult to diagnose until localized lancinating pain leads to a surgical exploration. After the lesion is surgically removed, the pain subsides, and recurrence is unlikely.

Extraabdominal Desmoid Tumors (Aggressive Fibromatosis)

In comparison with the infantile fibrous lesions mentioned earlier, the desmoid tumor is seen in older children and young adults up through 40 years of age. Whereas abdominal desmoids are seen in the abdominal wall of women following pregnancy, the extraabdominal desmoids usually occur in men and are more common in proximal areas about the shoulder and buttock, followed next by the posterior thigh, popliteal area, arm, and fore-

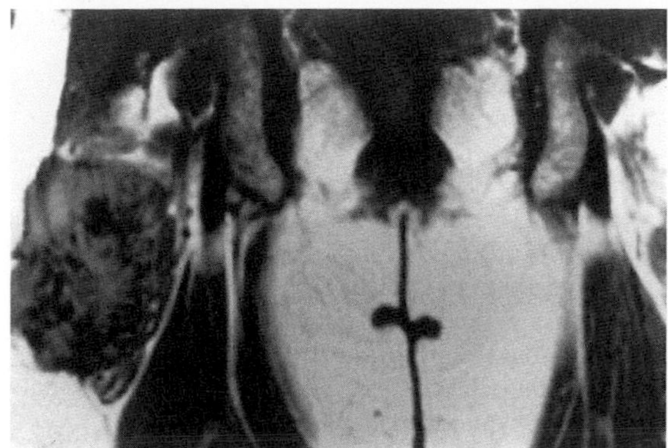

Figure 6–58. T_1-weighted MRI of a desmoid tumor in the gluteal area of a 45-year-old woman.

arm. In most cases, it presents as a solitary tumor. Multicentric involvement is seen at times, however, and can be associated with Gardner syndrome, which is characterized by polyposis of the large bowel and by craniofacial osteomas. In patients with familial adenomatous polyposis (FAP), an inherited disease caused by mutations in the *APC* gene, desmoids are a significant source of morbidity and mortality. The *APC* gene, located on chromosome 5, encodes for a 300-kDa protein, in which a germline mutation is an early event in tumor formation.

Desmoids are deep-seated tumors that arise from muscle fascial planes and infiltrate extensively into adjacent muscle tissue, tendons, joint capsules, and even bone. Compared with malignant fibrosarcomas, desmoids are poorly marginated and thus difficult to resect surgically. Desmoids can engulf surrounding vessels and nerves, whereas fibrosarcomas usually push these structures aside. A desmoid may cause local pain and grow quite rapidly, suggesting a malignant tumor. The desmoid tends to grow more longitudinally along muscle planes to a considerable size, frequently resulting in restricted joint motion about the shoulder, hip, or knee. Because the local aggressiveness of desmoids is so similar to that of malignant fibrosarcomas or malignant fibrous histiocytomas, some experts believe the desmoid may be a low-grade fibrosarcoma that has lost its potential to metastasize; however, molecular analyses may suggest otherwise.

On gross examination, a desmoid tumor is firm and heavily collagenized. Microscopically, it has a low mitotic index, similar to that of a plantar or palmar fibromatosis. Radiographically, a desmoid is noncalcified and appears dense in comparison with normal muscle. It is easily seen in soft window CT scanning. More exact presurgical imaging can be obtained with MRI (Figure 6–58). As with an abdominal desmoid, an extraabdominal desmoid physical injury may play a role in the activation of a preexisting oncogene located in the damaged fibroblast.

Desmoids are usually treated surgically with an aggressive wide resection similar to that used in treating a primary sarcoma. Even following a clean resection of the desmoid, the recurrence rate may approach 50%. For this reason, it is common to administer 50 Gy of radiation to the surgical site starting 2 weeks postoperatively. With radiation therapy, the recurrence rate decreases to 15%. In rare cases an amputation may be necessary after multiple recurrences. A few cases of spontaneous involution of desmoid tumors are reported after 40 years of age.

Based on clinical and experimental evidence, estrogen may play a role in the development of desmoid tumors. Accordingly, agents such as tamoxifen are being used in some centers because of their antiestrogen effects. NSAIDs were also implemented in attempts to treat aggressive cases. In selected patients with progressive disease, low-dose vinblastine and methotrexate chemotherapy may be used.

Benign Tumors of Peripheral Nerves

Benign tumors of peripheral nerve sheaths are common and take their origin from Schwann cells, which normally produces myelin and collagen fiber.

A. Neurilemoma

The neurilemoma (neurinoma or benign schwannoma) is the least common of the benign tumors of peripheral nerve sheaths. It usually affects individuals between 20 and 50 years of age and occurs with equal frequency in men and women. It has a predilection for spinal roots and for superficial nerves on the flexor surfaces of both upper and lower extremities. In most cases, the lesion is solitary, but multiple lesions are occasionally seen in Recklinghausen disease. The neurinoma is slow growing and rarely causes pain or a neurologic deficit.

Unlike the neurofibroma, which has a fusiform appearance, the neurilemoma is round (Figure 6–59). Micro-

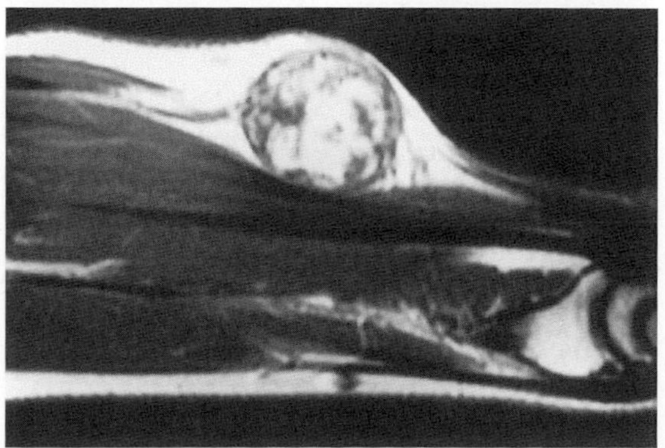

Figure 6–59. T_1-weighted MRI of a neurilemoma of the ulnar nerve in a 69-year-old man.

scopic studies reveal the presence of a characteristic Verocay body, which consists of palisading Schwann cells and is found in the fibrotic Antoni A substance of the tumor. Other areas reveal a more mucinous Antoni B substance. Neurilemomas may occur in an axial fashion involving spinal roots, often presenting as a dumbbell-shaped extradural defect (Figure 6–60). In comparison with the less restricted peripheral lesions, the nerve root lesions are more apt to cause pain associated with neurologic deficiency because of their bony constriction.

In some cases, simple excision of the neurilemoma is clinically indicated, which often can be performed without serious damage to the nerve. If the patient is asymptomatic, observation is appropriate because there is little chance for malignant degeneration.

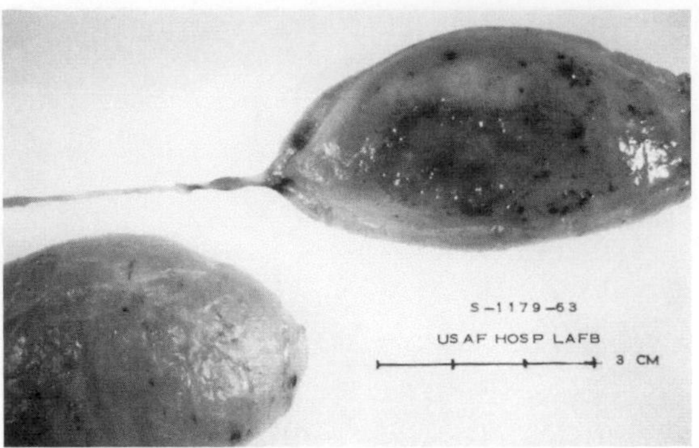

Figure 6–61. Photographic appearance of a solitary neurofibroma.

B. Solitary Neurofibroma

The solitary neurofibroma is a fusiform fibrotic tumor arising centrally from a smaller peripheral nerve (Figure 6–61). The tumor is seen with equal frequency in men and women, usually between 20 and 30 years of age. It is 10 times more common than the multiple form seen in Recklinghausen disease, is usually smaller, and carries less chance of malignant degeneration. Microscopic examination of the solitary neurofibroma shows interlacing bundles of elongated spindle cells with benign-appearing nuclei and occasionally with areas resembling the Antoni A tissue seen in the neurilemoma.

Treatment of the solitary neurofibroma consists of simple excision.

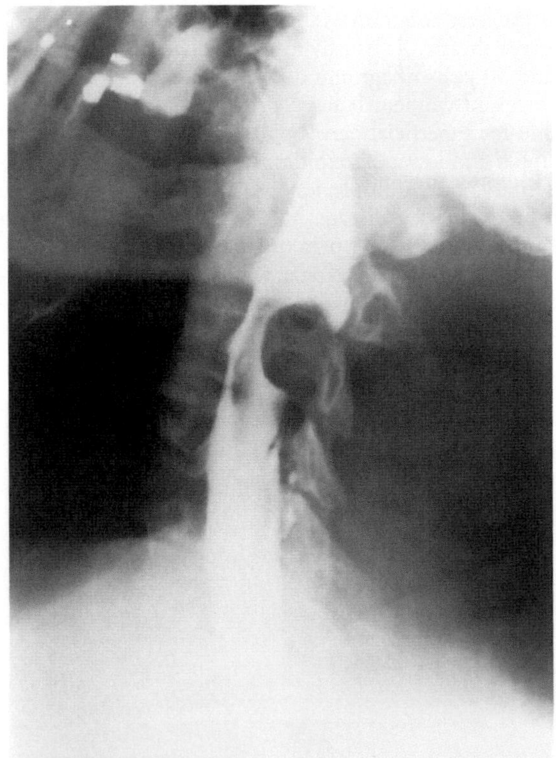

Figure 6–60. Myelogram of a neurilemoma in the cervical spine.

C. Neurofibromatosis (Recklinghausen Disease)

Recklinghausen disease is a familial dysplasia, inherited as an autosomal-dominant trait, with an incidence of approximately 1 in every 3000 live births. The disease usually begins during the first few years of life with the emergence of small café au lait spots. Over time, these lesions grow in number and size. Unlike the lesions seen in fibrous dysplasia, the lesions in Recklinghausen disease do not have rough edges. If a patient has more than six lesions that have smooth edges and are greater than 1.5 cm in diameter, the diagnosis of Recklinghausen disease is certain.

Later in life, the patient develops multiple neurofibromas, each of which appears as a soft cutaneous nodule (Figure 6–62). This pedunculated skin lesion, which is called fibroma molluscum, can be large and pendulous. More pathognomonic of the disease is the plexiform neurofibroma, which appears in larger nerves and can involve an entire extremity (see Figure 6–62). When the overlying skin of an extremity is loose and hyperpigmented, the condition is called elephantiasis neuromatosa, or "elephant man syndrome." (It is now thought that John Merrick, the so-called elephant man, was actually affected by Proteus syndrome.) Among the bony changes seen in Recklinghausen disease are angular scoliosis, spinal meningocele, scalloping of the vertebra, pseudarthrosis of the tibia, and osteolytic lesions in bone.

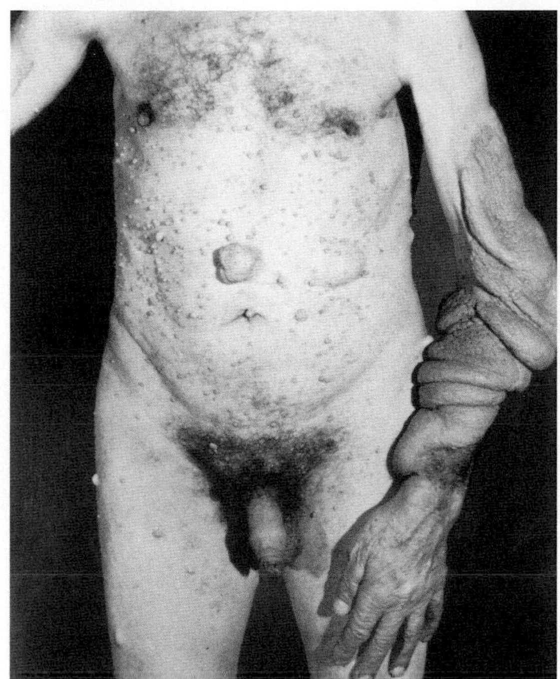

Figure 6–62. Cutaneous manifestations of neurofibromatosis.

A major threat to the patient's life is that a malignant schwannoma will develop from one of the large and deep neurofibromas. This occurs at a later age in 3–5% of patients.

Intramuscular Myxomas

The intramuscular myxoma is a rare tumor seen in patients older than 40 years and affecting the large muscles about the thighs, shoulders, buttocks, and arms. It is a slow-growing well-marginated tumor that has the gelatinous physical quality of a ganglion cyst or myxoid liposarcoma. The intramuscular myxoma causes no pain and can grow to greater than 15 cm in diameter. Although it appears radiolucent on CT scan, MRI demonstrates an intermediate signal on the T_1-weighted image and an extremely high signal on the T_2-weighted image. Multiple myxomas are associated with polyostotic fibrous dysplasia.

The intramuscular myxoma can be resected marginally. After this procedure, the recurrence rate is extremely low.

Azzarelli A et al: Low-dose chemotherapy with methotrexate and vinblastine for patients with advanced aggressive fibromatosis. Cancer 2001;92(5):1259. [PMID: 11571741]

Bertario L et al: Genotype and phenotype factors as determinants of desmoid tumors in patients with familial adenomatous polyposis. Int J Cancer 2001;95(2):102. [PMID: 11241320]

Chun YS et al: Lipoblastoma. J Pediatr Surg 2001;36(6):905. [PMID: 11381423]

Kang HJ et al: Schwannomas of the upper extremity. J Hand Surg [Br] 2000;25(6):604. [PMID: 11106529]

Richards KA et al: The pulsed dye laser for cutaneous vascular and nonvascular lesions. Semin Cutan Med Surg 2000;19(4):276. [PMID: 11149608]

Shields CJ et al: Desmoid tumours. Eur J Surg Oncol 2001; 27(8): 701. [PMID: 11735163]

Sorensen SA et al: Long-term follow-up of von Recklinghausen neurofibromatosis: Survival and malignant neoplasms. N Engl J Med 1986;314:1010. [PMID: 3083258]

Vikkula M et al: Molecular genetics of vascular malformations. Matrix Biol 2001;20(5-6):327. [PMID: 11566267]

MALIGNANT SOFT-TISSUE TUMORS

Sarcomas are capable of invasive, locally destructive growth with a tendency to recur and to metastasize. All sarcomas do not behave the same, however. Some sarcomas, such as dermatofibrosarcoma protuberans, rarely metastasize. Malignant fibrous histiocytoma, in contrast, does so with alacrity.

A. Fibrohistiocytic Tumors

Until recently, MFH was the most common soft-tissue sarcomas seen in adults (Figure 6–63). Strangely, although more frequently encountered than other adult soft-tissue sarcomas, the cell type(s) of origin remain unclear. Current debate is centered on whether MFH is a distinct entity or a diverse group of sarcomas that on histologic evaluation appear similar. The latest World Health Organization classification for sarcomas no longer includes MFH as a distinct entity. The current nomenclature for the majority of MFH is undifferentiated pleomorphic sarcoma.

1. Storiform pleomorphic—Storiform pleomorphic is the most common subtype of MFH. It occurs more frequently in men than in women, primarily affecting individuals between 50 and 70 years of age. Usually it is a deep lesion found in the large muscles about the thigh, hip, and retroperitoneal areas. The tumor may be asymptomatic.

On gross examination, the tumor appears multinodular and may demonstrate several separate satellite lesions in the same muscle belly, especially at the superior and interior poles. It may be necrotic and ranges in color from dirty gray to a reddish tan. Microscopy demonstrates that it is composed of malignant fibroblasts mixed with anaplastic and pleomorphic histiocytes.

The prognosis and treatment vary, depending on the size and location of the tumor. The overall local recurrence potential is 45%, with a 40% incidence of metastasis to the lung and with a 10% incidence of regional lymph node involvement. Tumors smaller than 5 cm in diameter and found in a subcutaneous location in the distal body parts carry a good prognosis, with a 5-year survival rate of 80%, whereas tumors that are 5 cm or more in diameter and located deep in a more proximal

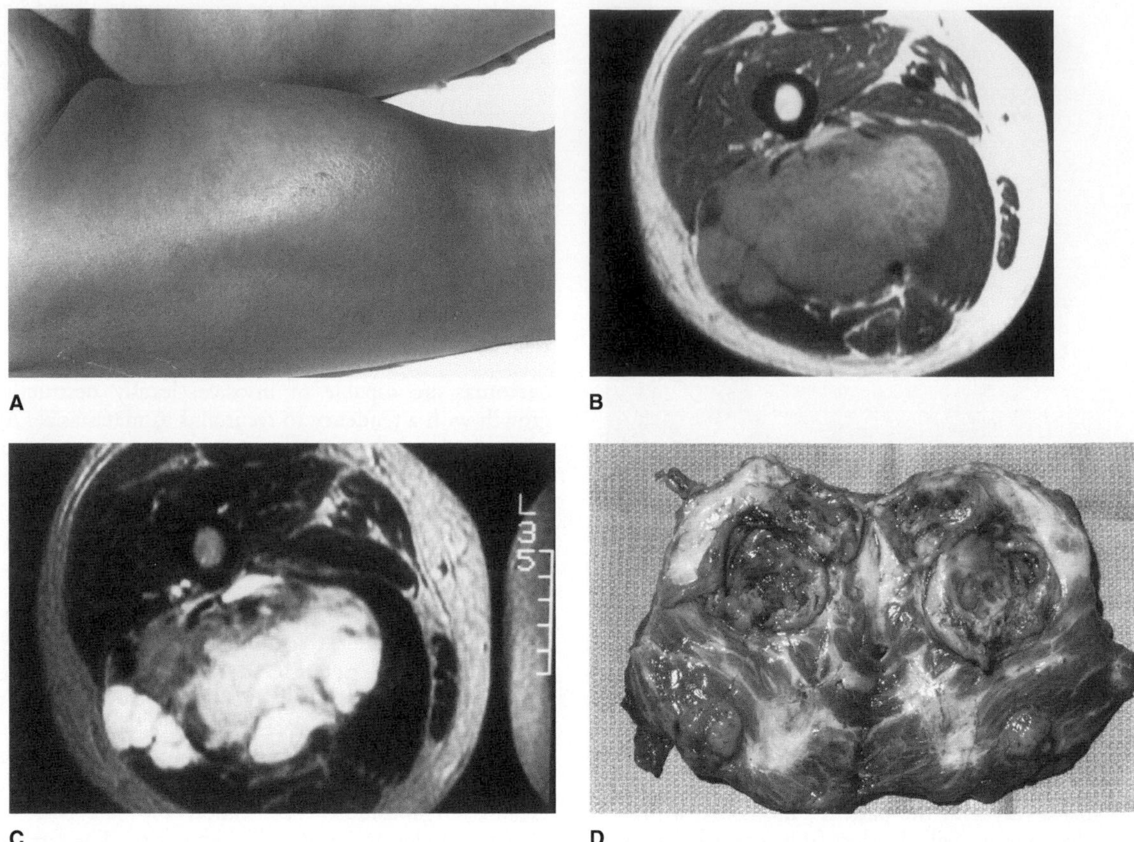

Figure 6–63. Clinical appearance (**A**), T_1-weighted MRI (**B**), T_2-weighted MRI (**C**), and resected surgical specimen (**D**) of a large pleomorphic malignant fibrous histiocytoma in the posterior thigh of a 55-year-old man.

muscle group carry a poor prognosis, with a 5-year survival rate of only 55%.

Although the treatment depends on the clinical situation, it generally consists of an aggressive wide resection after careful preoperative staging, including an MRI of the primary and CT scan of the chest. Amputation is rare, with limb salvage possible in the majority of cases.

The use of adjuvant radiation therapy is important in reducing the local recurrence rate. Most clinicians administer 55 Gy to a wide area, followed by a boost to 65 Gy aimed at the surgical site. An attempt is made to leave a longitudinal strip of tissue out of the field of radiation to reduce the chance of postirradiation edema distal to the treatment site. Some centers advocate preoperative and postoperative radiation with 50 Gy given before resection and approximately 15 Gy postoperatively. Some institutions employ preoperative radiation exclusively. Local recurrence rates are generally between 5% and 25%.

The use of adjuvant chemotherapy is more controversial. Because limited data suggest that chemotherapy results in a significant improvement in survival and because most patients are older individuals who cannot tolerate the high-dose protocols, medical oncologists are divided on whether to advocate the use of chemotherapeutic agents in the treatment of MFH.

2. Myxoid—The myxoid type is the second most common type of MFH and is seen in the same age group of patients and the same locations as the pleomorphic type. On gross examination, myxoid MFH has a multinodular and translucent or gelatinous appearance similar to the appearance of a myxoid liposarcoma or a benign myxoma of muscle. Because of its gelatinous nature, myxoid MFH has a greater chance for local contamination and thus has a higher local recurrence rate than pleomorphic MFH. However, the metastasis rate in cases of myxoid MFH is approximately 25%.

3. Giant cell—The giant cell type of MFH also affects older patients and is seen in large muscle groups, but it is hemorrhagic and carries a 50% chance of pulmonary metastasis.

4. Inflammatory—The inflammatory type of MFH affects the older age groups, is more common in the retroperitoneal areas, and has a 50% metastasis rate.

B. Dermatofibrosarcoma Protuberans

Dermatofibrosarcoma protuberans, a low- to intermediate-grade fibrohistiocytic tumor, is unique because of its nodular cutaneous location. It is seen more commonly in males than females and occurs in young or middle-age (20–40 years) adults. It is typically located about the trunk and proximal extremities. Antecedent trauma is recorded in 10–20% of cases. Dermatofibrosarcoma protuberans begins as a painless subcutaneous nodule or nodules and slowly develops into an elevated multinodular plaque (Figure 6–64). Microscopic examination of the lesion reveals the same storiform or basket-weave pattern of a benign or malignant fibrous histiocytoma but with a very low mitotic index. The pattern tends to infiltrate extensively into surrounding subcutaneous fat and skin, which accounts for the high local recurrence rate, sometimes reported to approach 50%.

Characteristic cytogenetic abnormalities are described with characteristic features such as reciprocal t(17;22)(q22;q13) or, more commonly, supernumerary ring chromosomes containing sequences from chromosomes 17 and 22.

Surgical treatment, consisting of an aggressive resection, is associated with a lower recurrence rate of 20%. Because of the low mitotic index, radiation therapy is not usually indicated, and the chance of pulmonary metastasis is only 1%.

C. Fibrosarcoma

Fifty years ago, fibrosarcoma was considered the most common of the soft-tissue sarcomas, secondary to imprecise pathologic classification of MFH, certain liposarcomas, rhabdomyosarcoma, leiomyosarcomas, and malignant peripheral nerve sheath tumors. Currently, fibrosarcoma is considered one of the least common soft-tissue sarcomas. The diagnosis is reserved for those tumors in which the histology demonstrates a uniform fasciculated growth pattern of spindle cells (malignant fibroblasts). It is clinically similar to MFH, occurs with nearly equal frequency in men and women, is found in patients between 30 and 55 years of age, is sometimes slow growing and painless, and tends to affect deep fascial structures of muscle about the knee and thigh, followed next by the forearm and leg.

On gross examination, fibrosarcoma appears as a firm and lobulated lesion that has a yellowish white to tan color. The lesion may demonstrate a few calcific or osseous deposits on radiographic exam. Microscopy reveals spindle, uniformly shaped fibroblasts that have varying degrees of mitotic activity. Fibrosarcomas contain no malignant histiocytes.

The treatment and prognosis depend on the grade of tumor in a particular patient. Low-grade fibrosarcoma is nearly the same tumor as a benign desmoid tumor and has an extremely low rate of metastasis. However, high-grade fibrosarcoma requires an aggressive wide surgical resection, along with radiation therapy, and has a pulmonary metastasis rate of 50–60%. Lymph node involvement is rare. The use of chemotherapy is considered controversial in patients with fibrosarcoma, as it is in patients with MFH.

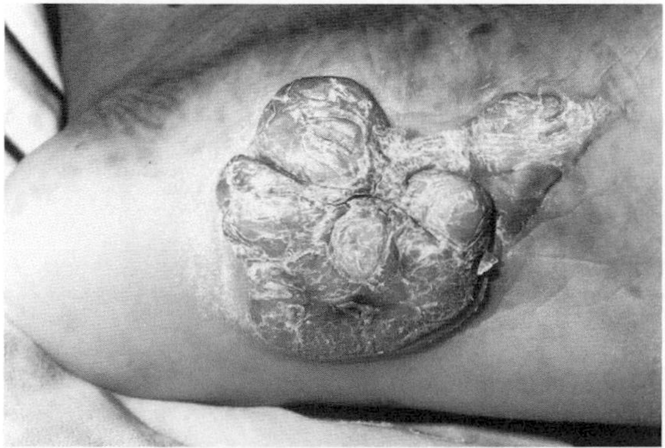

Figure 6–64. Clinical appearance of dermatofibrosarcoma protuberans on the bottom of the heel of a 30-year-old man.

D. Liposarcomas

Liposarcoma is the second most common soft-tissue sarcoma after MFH. Like MFH, liposarcoma is a tumor of older (40–60 years) patients and can be large and deep seated. Four types of liposarcoma are discussed in the following sections. The well-differentiated type and the myxoid type are associated with a low chance for lung metastasis, whereas the round cell and the pleomorphic types tend to behave more aggressively.

1. Well-differentiated liposarcoma—This very low grade tumor affects individuals who are 40–60 years of age and occurs more frequently in men than in women. It grows extremely slowly and reaches a large size without causing pain. The deep-seated tumor is found in the retroperitoneum, buttock, or thigh. In some cases of well-differentiated liposarcoma, findings include inflammation and sclerosis.

On gross examination, this tumor has a fatty lobulated appearance similar to a benign lipoma. Even under the microscope, many large areas of the tumor appear benign. However, with proper sampling, the pathologist will find a few areas of lipoblast activity to suggest the diagnosis of a liposarcoma. MRI findings are sometimes difficult to distinguish from a large deep lipoma (Figure 6–65).

In cases of well-differentiated liposarcoma, a conservative wide resection is performed to avoid local recurrence. Adjuvant radiation therapy is not helpful, and chemo-

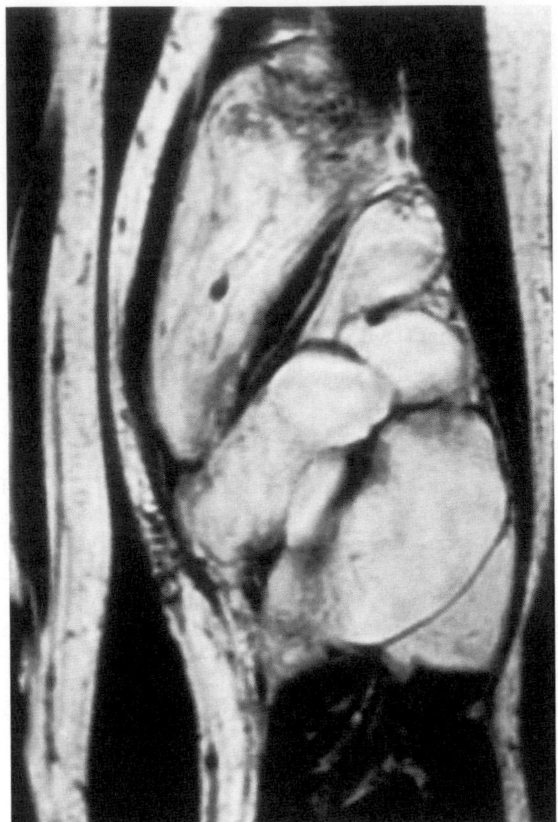

Figure 6–65. T_1-weighted MRI of a well-differentiated liposarcoma in the thigh of a 63-year-old man.

therapy is never used. The chance of metastatic disease is very low, and the prognosis for survival is excellent.

2. Myxoid liposarcoma—Myxoid liposarcoma is the most common fat sarcoma, accounting for 40–50% of all liposarcomas. The myxoid type is low to intermediate grade and seen in older patients (see Table 6–6). The clinical presentation is similar to the well-differentiated liposarcoma.

Gross examination of a myxoid liposarcoma reveals a lobulated pattern with some areas that appear similar to those of a lipoma but with other myxomatous areas. Microscopic examination shows myxoid tissue with areas of signet ring lipoblasts. It is common to find a delicate pattern of capillaries running through the myxoid areas. MRI frequently demonstrates a heterogeneous high- and low-signal pattern typical of myxoid liposarcoma but not present in cases of benign lipoma (Figure 6–66).

Characteristic translocations are also seen in myxoid liposarcoma. The predominant type is t(12;16)(q13;p11); however, t(12;22)(q13;q12) is also described.

Multifocal myxoid liposarcoma is also described. Consideration for additional advanced axial imaging should be entertained with this histologic subtype.

Although myxoid liposarcoma carries a very good prognosis, the tumor should be removed with wide margins, and adjuvant radiation therapy should be given. Chemotherapy is not indicated.

3. Round cell and pleomorphic liposarcoma—These high-grade liposarcomas are seen in the same locations and age group as the well-differentiated and myxoid subtypes. But unlike the latter, the round cell and pleomorphic types are fast-growing tumors that may be painful.

In cases of round cell or pleomorphic liposarcoma, the lesion does not have a fatty appearance on gross examination but instead looks more like an MFH or a fibrosarcoma. Moreover, on MRI, the lesion appears more like an MFH, with a low-signal pattern in the T_1-weighted image and a high-signal pattern in the T_2-weighted image. Microscopically, the round cell type of liposarcoma shows areas of uniformly shaped round cells similar to those found in Ewing sarcoma or lymphoma and also shows areas of myxoid tissue. In the pleomorphic type of liposarcoma, large and bizarre giant cells occur similar to those found in the pleomorphic type of MFH and rhabdomyosarcoma.

In round cell and pleomorphic liposarcoma, there is an early and high rate of pulmonary metastasis. Accordingly, the prognosis for survival is poor. Thus, the treatment should include aggressive resection, adjuvant radiation therapy as necessary, and chemotherapy in selected patients.

E. Rhabdomyosarcomas

Rhabdomyosarcomas account for 20% of all soft-tissue sarcomas. The embryonal and alveolar types of rhabdo-

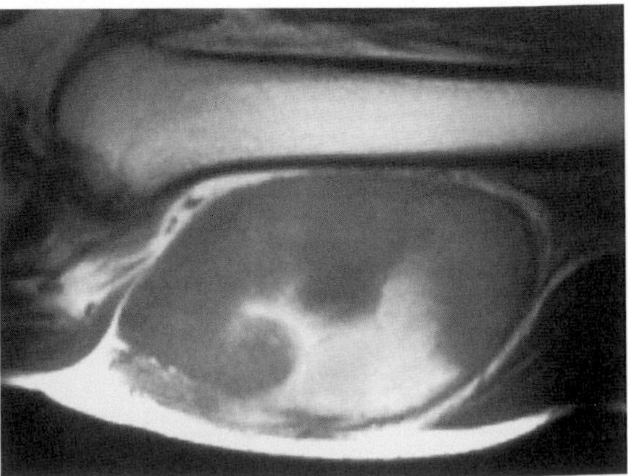

Figure 6–66. Sagittal view T_1-weighted MRI of a myxoid liposarcoma in the thigh of a 32-year-old man.

myosarcoma affect pediatric patients, and the rarer pleomorphic type affects adults.

1. Embryonal rhabdomyosarcoma—The embryonal type is seen in patients from birth to 15 years of age and encountered more frequently in boys than in girls. It is most common in the head and neck area. The so-called botryoid form is seen as a cluster of grapes under mucous membranes in the vagina, bladder, or retroperitoneal area. Histologically, it is a round cell tumor like Ewing sarcoma, but some rhabdomyoblasts with cross striations are present in a few areas.

Embryonal rhabdomyosarcoma is treated with local surgical resection plus preoperative and postoperative chemotherapy consisting of vincristine, dactinomycin, cyclophosphamide, and doxorubicin given in cyclic courses during a 2-year span. If the surgical margins are contaminated, local radiation therapy is used. With this program, the 5-year survival rate is 80%. Prior to the advent of chemotherapy, it was only 10%.

2. Alveolar rhabdomyosarcoma—This type of rhabdomyosarcoma affects individuals between 10 and 25 years of age and is found more commonly in males than in females. Besides affecting the head and neck, it can be seen in the extremities, especially the thigh and calf. Microscopic examination of the lesion reveals a typical alveolar pattern of round cells, with fewer rhabdomyoblasts seen in this type of rhabdomyosarcoma than in the embryonal type. This type of rhabdomyosarcoma is associated with the fusion genes *PAX3-FKHR* and *PAX7-FKHR*. Although not definitive, the presence of the translocation t(2;13)/*PAX3-FKHR* may be an adverse prognostic factor, with molecular screening being implemented in the future. Currently, the treatment is the same as for the embryonal type, but the prognosis is a bit worse.

3. Pleomorphic rhabdomyosarcoma—In the 1940s, pleomorphic rhabdomyosarcoma was a popular histologic diagnosis and MFH was a rare one. Based on today's criteria, most of the old cases classified as pleomorphic rhabdomyosarcoma would now be classified as MFH. Currently, the pleomorphic type of rhabdomyosarcoma is the rarest type.

Pleomorphic rhabdomyosarcoma is a high-grade tumor that affects middle-age and older adults and is seen most commonly in the large muscle groups of the proximal extremities, usually the lower extremities. Microscopic examination of the tumor reveals large atypical giant cells, along with racket- or tadpole-shaped malignant rhabdomyoblasts that stain positive for glycogen, actin, and myosin. The tumor carries a poor prognosis and is associated with a high rate of metastasis to the lung. The treatment for pleomorphic rhabdomyosarcoma is similar to that for MFH and consists of a wide local resection and adjuvant radiation therapy. Chemotherapy is rarely indicated.

F. Leiomyosarcoma

Leiomyosarcoma is a very rare soft-tissue tumor whose cell type of origin is smooth muscle. It is seen in the middle-age (see Table 6–6) adult and is much more common in women than in men. Its usual locations, in order of frequency, are retroperitoneal, intraabdominal, cutaneous, and subcutaneous. In some cases, the lesion has a venous wall origin and is found in the vena cava or large vessels of the leg. On microscopic examination, leiomyosarcoma can demonstrate a palisading, orderly fascicular pattern similar to a malignant schwannoma. A specific immunohistochemical staining for actin may be helpful in the differential diagnosis.

The prognosis and the treatment for leiomyosarcoma are similar to those for fibrosarcoma. However, leiomyosarcomas of venous wall origin have a worse prognosis because they are difficult to resect and have a high rate of pulmonary metastasis.

G. Synovial Sarcomas

Synovial sarcoma (Figure 6–67) is the fourth most common soft-tissue sarcoma. It is seen in young adults between 15 and 35 years of age and affects males slightly more than females. The name of this tumor suggests a synovial cell origin, but only 10% of synovial sarcomas are found in a major joint. Nevertheless, they frequently arise from juxtaarticular structures, especially around the knee, and they can also arise from tendon sheaths, bursal sacs, fascial planes, and deep muscles. Synovial sarcomas can be seen about the shoulder, arm, elbow, and wrist and are the most common soft-tissue sarcoma in the foot.

Synovial sarcomas initially grow slowly and cause pain in approximately half of the affected patients. The tumors may appear after an injury, and because dystrophic calcification or even heterotopic bone formation is seen in half of the cases, the tumors are assumed to be a benign process for 2–4 years before a diagnostic biopsy is performed.

Microscopic examination of the tumor shows a typical biphasic pattern composed of epithelium-like cells that form nests, clefts, or tubular structures surrounded by malignant fibroblastic spindle cells. The epithelium-like cells produce a mucinous material that suggests a synovial cell origin, although this origin is unlikely. A monophasic form of synovial sarcoma is described and reported to consist of a dominant fibroblastic or epithelial cell pattern. If the lesion shows no biphasic component, however, it is difficult to confirm the diagnosis of synovial sarcoma.

Molecular characterization of this tumor reveals a particular translocation, t(X;18), representing the fusion of *SYT* (at 18q11) with either *SSX1* or *SSX2* (both at Xp11). Both *SYT* and *SSX* appear to be transcription regulation factors whose fusion product is seen in the majority of synovial sarcomas.

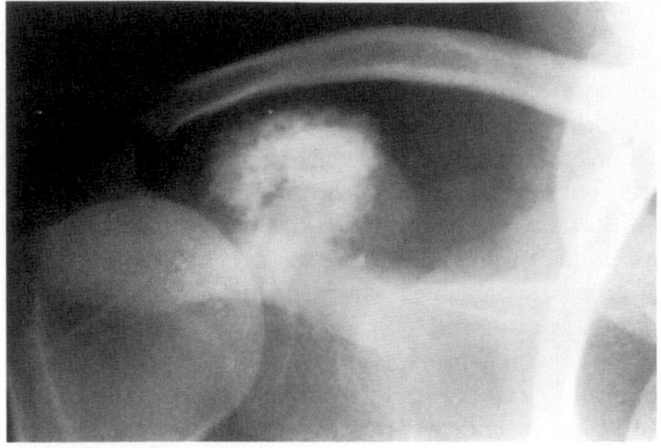

A

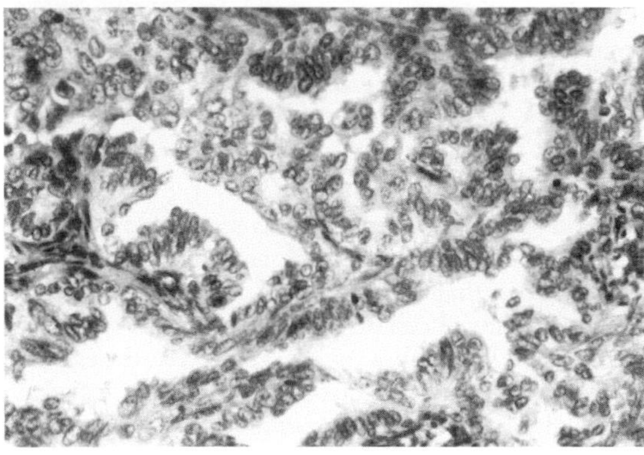

B

Figure 6–67. Radiograph (**A**) and microscopic appearance (**B**) of a synovial sarcoma in the shoulder of a 20-year-old woman.

Despite the slow growth of synovial sarcoma, the 5-year and 10-year survival rates are only 50% and 25%, respectively. In cases in which the tumors are heavily calcified, the 5-year survival rate is 80%. Because of the poor prognosis, the treatment plan should include aggressive wide resection, along with both radiation therapy and chemotherapy. Lymph node involvement is seen in 20% of affected patients and may require a surgical excision followed by local radiation therapy.

H. Malignant Peripheral Nerve Sheath Tumor

A malignant peripheral nerve sheath tumor can arise from a preexisting benign solitary neurofibroma but more frequently arises from the multiple lesions of neurofibromatosis type 1. In both cases, the tumor mass is usually larger than 5 cm in diameter and may arise from a large deep neurogenic structure such as the sciatic nerve (Figure 6–68) or one of the spinal roots. Smaller nerves, even cutaneous branches, however, can give rise to these sarcomas. Malignant degeneration from a solitary neurofibroma usually occurs after 40 years of age with a 5-year survival rate of 75%. In contrast, patients whose schwannoma arose from the lesions of neurofibromatosis type 1 are generally younger and have a 5-year survival rate of 30%. Surgical treatment consists of a wide resection if possible. Adjuvant radiation and chemotherapy are used in selected cases.

I. Malignant Vascular Tumors

1. Kaposi sarcoma—Of the malignant vascular tumors, Kaposi sarcoma is the most common with four specific subtypes: (1) chronic, (2) lymphadenopathic, (3) transplant associated, (4) AIDS related. It is found directly beneath the skin, generally in the lower extremity of adults, is seen more often in men than in women, and is endemic in central Africa. The cutaneous lesions seen frequently in the foot and ankle area are purplish in color and are nodular (Figure 6–69). Microscopic examination of Kaposi sar-

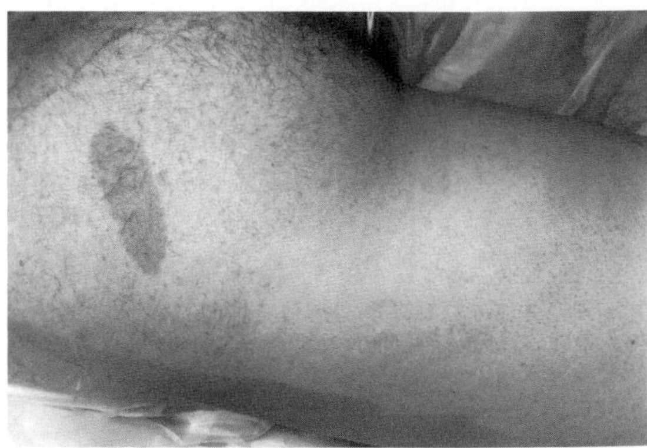

A

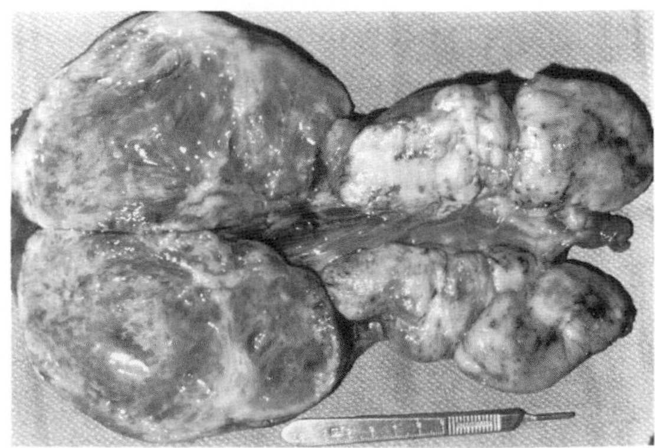

B

Figure 6–68. Clinical appearance of a café au lait defect in the skin overlying a malignant schwannoma in the buttock area of a 42-year-old man (**A**), and gross appearance of the tumor in resected sciatic nerve (**B**).

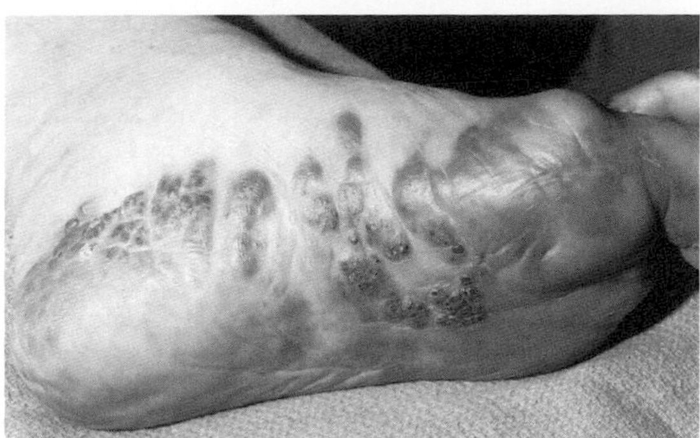

Figure 6–69. Clinical appearance of Kaposi sarcoma of the foot.

coma shows an aggressive vascular pattern with rare mitosis. However, over a period of many years, the tumor progresses into a full-blown angiosarcoma or fibrosarcoma. It is associated with AIDS and other immunosuppressive disorders and is also seen with lymphomas and multiple myeloma. Although the behavior of Kaposi sarcoma is a function of the immunologic status of the patient and other variables, the overall mortality rate is 10–20%.

2. Angiosarcoma—Soft-tissue angiosarcoma is rare, accounting for less than 1% of all sarcomas. Although angiosarcomas are usually cutaneous lesions and tend to affect men more than women, they sometimes take the form of a deep tumor, and they are typically seen in the upper extremities of women who have chronic lymphedema following radical breast surgery and radiation therapy. Histologic examination of angiosarcoma shows anaplastic endothelial cells surrounded by reticulum fiber. Prognosis for the older patient is poor. Smaller lesions in younger (less than 50 years) patients have a distinctively better outcome. The treatment is wide resection, sometimes with radiation therapy.

3. Hemangiopericytoma—This rare perivascular tumor arises from pericytes. Pericytes are highly arborized perivascular cells that line capillaries and venules. The lesion, which affects male and female adults with equal frequency, is usually found deep in muscle bellies and generally located in the thigh or retroperitoneal area of the pelvis. Microscopic examination of the malignant hemangiopericytoma reveals tightly packed cells with round nuclei with moderate amounts of cytoplasm with poorly defined borders. The bifurcating sinusoidal vessels have a typical staghorn appearance. Cytogenetic analysis reveals multiple chromosome translocations including t(12:19) and t(13:22). Treatment consists of a wide surgical resection, followed by local radiation therapy. Some authors recommend preoperative embolization or afferent vessel ligation (or both) intraoperatively.

MISCELLANEOUS SOFT-TISSUE SARCOMAS

The remaining soft-tissue sarcomas are rare and only a brief description of their clinical patterns is summarized.

A. Soft-Tissue Chondrosarcoma

There are three types of soft-tissue chondrosarcomas.

1. Myxoid chondrosarcoma—The myxoid chondrosarcoma is sometimes referred to as a chordoid sarcoma because it looks like a chordoma. It is a slow-growing tumor seen in adults, usually in deep structure of the leg. It has a myxoid appearance, does not calcify, and is low grade. Like the chordoma, the myxoid chondrosarcoma responds only to surgical removal.

2. Mesenchymal chondrosarcoma—This tumor affects individuals between 15 and 40 years of age, is found deep in the lower extremity and neck areas, is fast growing, and carries a poor prognosis because of the high risk of pulmonary metastasis. Calcification may be seen on radiograph, and microscopic examination reveals round cells scattered in a chondroid matrix. Treatment consists of a wide resection in conjunction with chemotherapy and radiation therapy.

3. Synovial chondrosarcoma—The conversion of a synovial chondromatosis to a malignant synovial chondrosarcoma is an extremely rare phenomenon. It can occur with lesions of the hip or knee region in older (more than 60 years) adults.

B. Ewing Sarcoma

Extraskeletal Ewing sarcoma can be found in individuals between 10 and 30 years of age and is usually located in the paravertebral area, thorax, or deep muscle area of the lower extremity. It is a fast-growing tumor with minimal pain symptoms. It carries the same prognosis as its counterpart in bone and is treated with the same combination of surgery, chemotherapy, and radiation therapy.

C. Alveolar Soft Part Sarcoma

This round cell sarcoma affects more females than males, is usually found in patients between 15 and 35 years of age, and arises in the deep muscle tissue of the lower extremity, usually the thigh. Alveolar soft part sarcoma is a slow-growing tumor but carries a poor prognosis because of early pulmonary metastasis. The tumor has increased vascularity and is thought to originate from a neurogenic stem cell. It derives its name from its alveolar pattern, which is seen on microscopic examination and can cause this tumor to be mistaken for an alveolar form of rhabdomyosarcoma. A cytogenetic, unbalanced abnormality, t(x;17)(p11.2;q25), is described. Treatment of alveolar soft part sarcoma consists of a wide surgical resection plus radiation therapy and chemotherapy.

D. Epithelioid Sarcoma

Although this superficial skin lesion is seen most commonly in the palm of the hand, it can also be found on the dorsum of the forearm or on the plantar aspect of the foot. It is a slow-growing tumor that affects patients between 20 and 30 years of age, causes minimal pain symptoms, and is associated with ulceration.

Because epithelioid sarcoma has a whitish color that under the microscope demonstrates cords of epithelium-like cells, it can be mistaken for a synovial sarcoma. Moreover, because of its firm multilobulated presentation, the epithelioid sarcoma may be mistaken for a plantar of palmar fibromatosis (Figure 6–70).

Epithelioid sarcoma spreads as a lumpy nodularity along tendon sheaths or fascial planes and frequently involves local lymph nodes. Local surgical resection is followed by a high local recurrence rate, and a late pulmonary metastasis is common. For this reason, early treatment should consist of an aggressive wide surgical resection.

E. Clear Cell Sarcoma

The clear cell sarcoma is thought to be a deep, noncutaneous variant of the well-known cutaneous melanoma. It is extremely rare, affects women more often than men, and commonly occurs between 20 and 40 years of age. It arises in tendon sheaths and fascial planes, most frequently in the foot and ankle but also in the knee and arm. Clear cell sarcoma starts slowly as a painless lump and has a high potential to spread to local lymph nodes. The lesion in many cases demonstrates evidence of melanin and melanosomes and may be of neural crest origin. The microscopic clear cell appearance can cause this sarcoma to be confused with epithelioid sarcoma and synovial sarcoma.

The prognosis is poor because of a high rate of pulmonary metastasis. This tumor may spread via lymphatics as well. Treatment consists of early aggressive wide resection and may include chemotherapy and local radiation therapy.

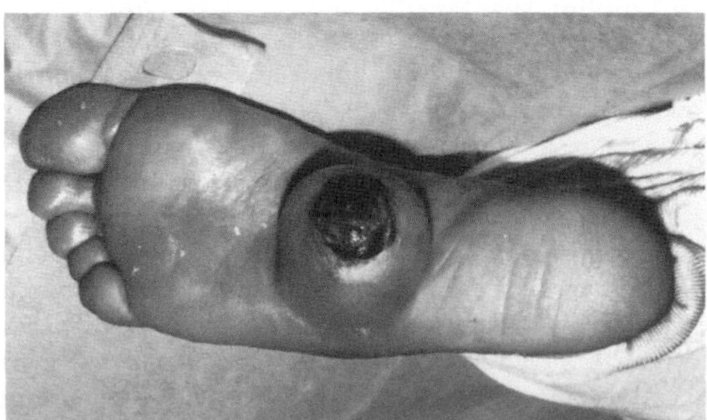

Figure 6–70. Clinical appearance of epithelioid sarcoma on the plantar aspect of the foot of a 36-year-old man.

Ahmad SA et al: Extraosseous osteosarcoma: Response to treatment and long-term outcome. J Clin Oncol 2002;20(2):521. [PMID: 11786582]

Anderson J et al: Detection of the PAX3-FKHR fusion gene in paediatric rhabdomyosarcoma: A reproducible predictor of outcome? Br J Cancer 2001;85(6):831. [PMID: 11556833]

Antonescu CR et al: Monoclonality of multifocal myxoid liposarcoma: Confirmation by analysis of TLS-CHOP or EWS-CHOP rearrangements. Clin Cancer Res 2000;6:2788. [PMID: 10914725]

Bowne WB et al: Dermatofibrosarcoma protuberans: A clinicopathologic analysis of patients treated and followed at a single institution. Cancer 2000;88(12):2711. [PMID: 10870053]

Cormier JN et al: Concurrent ifosfamide-based chemotherapy and irradiation. Analysis of treatment-related toxicity in 43 patients with sarcoma. Cancer 2001;92(6):1550. [PMID: 11745234]

Dei Tos AP: Liposarcoma: New entities and evolving concepts. Ann Diagn Pathol 2000;4(4):252. [PMID: 10982304]

dos Santos NR et al: Molecular mechanisms underlying human synovial sarcoma development. Genes Chromosomes Cancer 2001;30(1):1. [PMID: 11107170]

Gibbs J et al: Malignant fibrous histiocytoma: An institutional review. Cancer Invest 2001;19(1):23. [PMID: 11291552]

Hayes-Jordan AA et al: Nonrhabdomyosarcoma soft tissue sarcomas in children: Is age at diagnosis an important variable? J Pediatr Surg 2000;35(6):948; discussion 953. [PMID: 10873042]

Ladanyi M: Fusions of the SYT and SSX genes in synovial sarcoma. Oncogene 2001;20(40):5755. [PMID: 11607825]

Meis-Kindblom JM et al: Cytogenetic and molecular genetic analyses of liposarcoma and its soft tissue simulators: Recognition of new variants and differential diagnosis. Virchows Arch 2001; 439(2):141. [PMID: 11561754]

Nishio J et al: Supernumerary ring chromosomes in dermatofibrosarcoma protuberans may contain sequences from 8q11.2-qter and 17q21-qter: A combined cytogenetic and comparative genomic hybridization study. Cancer Genet Cytogenet 2001; 129(2):102. [PMID: 11566338]

Orvieto E et al: Myxoid and round cell liposarcoma: A spectrum of myxoid adipocytic neoplasia. Semin Diagn Pathol 2001; 18:267. [PMID 11757867]

Spillane AJ et al: Synovial sarcoma: A clinicopathologic, staging, and prognostic assessment. J Clin Oncol 200015;18(22):3794. [PMID: 11078492]

MANAGEMENT OF CARCINOMA METASTASIZED TO BONE

Incidence & Natural History of Metastases

A. Common Metastatic Carcinomas and Areas of Skeletal Involvement

Metastatic involvement of the musculoskeletal system is one of the most significant clinical issues facing orthopedic oncologists. The number of patients with metastasis to the skeletal system from a carcinoma is 15 times greater than the number of patients with primary bone tumors of all types. Approximately a third of all diagnosed adenocarcinomas include skeletal metastases, resulting in approximately 300,000 cases per year. Furthermore, 70% of patients with advanced terminal carcinoma demonstrate bone metastases at autopsy. The carcinomas that commonly metastasize to bone are prostate, breast, kidney, thyroid, and lung carcinomas. One study showed that nearly 90% of patients with these types of carcinoma had bone metastases. Among the carcinomas that less commonly metastasize to bone are cancers of the skin, oral cavity, esophagus, cervix, stomach, and colon.

The spine is the most frequent area of bone metastasis. Other common skeletal sites include the pelvis, femur, rib, proximal humerus, and skull, in that order. Metastatic lesions are rarely found distal to the elbow or knee. If lesions are found in these areas, the lung is the most common source. Solitary bone lesions comprise only approximately 10% of cases of bone metastasis.

B. Clinical Course of Metastases

The mechanism of metastases is accounted for in a modified "seed/soil" theorem. Less then 1 in 10,000 neoplastic cells that escape into the circulation from the primary site are able to set up a metastatic focus, a complex multistep process by which the cell must first break free. This is a function of *degradative* enzymes such as collagenases, hydrolases, cathepsin D, and proteases. Once the cell invades the vascular channel, it circulates through the body. It is theorized that the cell is protected by a fibrin platelet clot. However, clinical trials with heparin do not show a significant change in metastatic outcome. Local factors such as integrins are instrumental in attracting the circulating metastatic cell to a particular remote tissue site. Once within the new tissue, the metastatic cell releases factors such as tumor angiogenesis factor, inducing neovascularization, which in turn facilitates growth of the metastatic focus.

Patients with advanced metastatic disease frequently experience dysfunction of their hematopoietic and calcium homeostases systems. Patients may develop a normochromic, normocytic anemia with leukocytosis. In response to the anemia, the increased production of immature cells is noted on the peripheral blood smear. This is termed the *leukoerythroblastic reaction.* Hypercalcemia may result in up to 30% of cases with extensive metastases. This is most frequently seen in myeloma, breast cancer, and non–small cell lung cancer.

Blastic metastases are frequently painless and associated with a lower incidence of pathologic fracture because the bone is not as severely weakened (Figures 6–71 and 6–72). Not all tumors that metastasize from the prostate to the bone are blastic. The lytic variants are painful and can cause pathologic fractures.

Most tumors that metastasize from the breast to the bone are blastic, but some demonstrate mixtures of blastic and lytic areas in the same bone. By taking serial radiographs and noting the appearance of bone metastases, it is possible to follow the progress of treatment consisting of systemic therapy with hormones or chemotherapeutic agents plus local radiation therapy. A favorable response may show a gradual conversion from a lytic to a blastic appearance as the pain decreases.

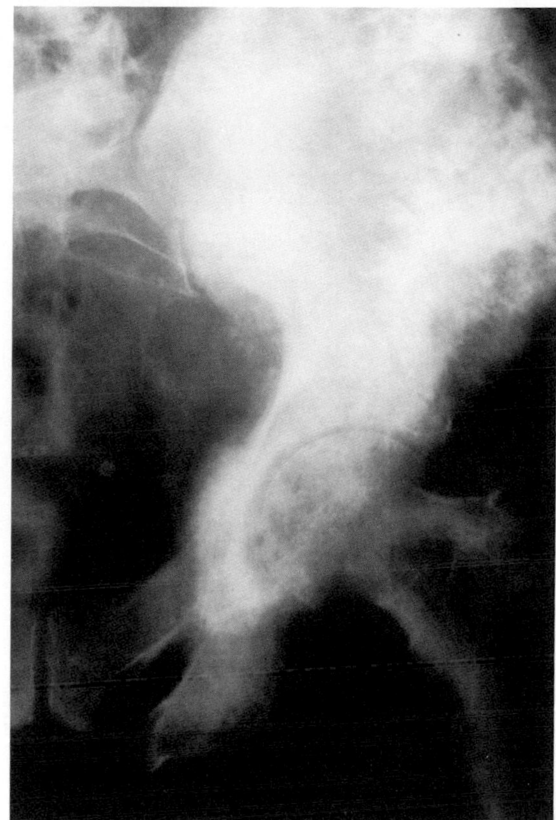

Figure 6–71. Radiograph of a blastic carcinoma that metastasized from the prostate to the pelvis in an 85-year-old man.

Bone destruction in lytic lesions is a response by native osteoclasts to the tumor. Neovascularity is common. Among the tumors that are characteristic for this hemorrhagic response are thyroid carcinomas (Figure 6–73), renal cell (Figure 6–74), and multiple myeloma. Before a surgical intervention, it is beneficial to perform a prophylactic embolization of the area to reduce perioperative bleeding. If a lesion is unexpectedly found to be aneurysmal at the time of surgical exploration, it is best to debulk the friable tumor mass rapidly down to normal bone and then pack the area until it can be stabilized with bone cement.

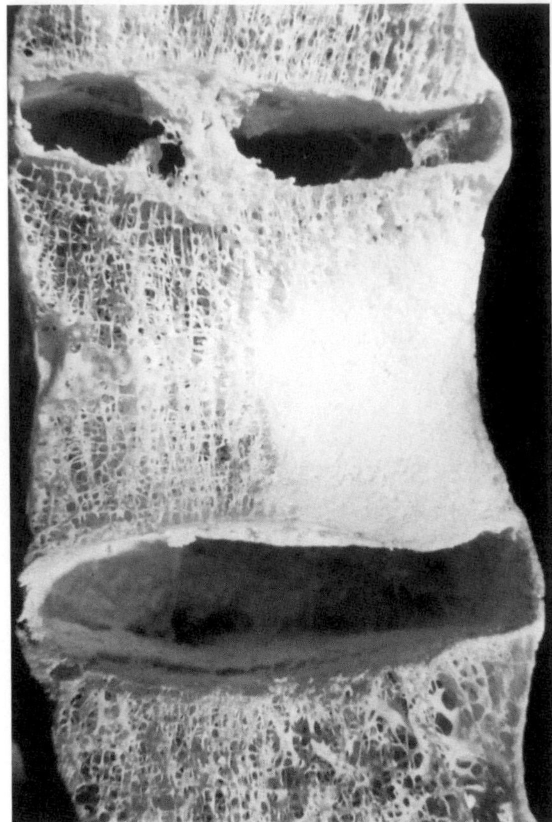

Figure 6–72. Skeletal specimen of a blastic carcinoma that metastasized from the prostate to the lumbar spine.

Diagnosis

A. General Approach

A methodical approach is mandatory in the workup of a patient with presumed metastatic disease to bone to locate the primary tumor. A thorough biopsy and physical examination must be completed prior to laboratory and radiographic analysis. Eight percent of patients may have their primary carcinoma detected on physical exam. Laboratory analysis should include complete blood count, ESR, renal and liver panels, alkaline phosphate, and serum protein electrophoresis.

Radiographic examination should follow with a plain chest radiograph and radiographs of known involved bones. Approximately 45% of primaries are detected in the lung on the chest radiograph. The workup should also include a staging bone scan. If this is negative, myeloma should be suspected. Furthermore, a lesion at a more convenient biopsy site may be found. Bone scan is also more sensitive than plain radiographs in detecting early lesions. CT scans of the chest, abdomen, and pelvis should be performed. Lung CT can detect up to 15% of primaries missed on the plain radiograph.

These studies in conjunction with a well-planned biopsy detect the majority of cases. Routine radiographic screening studies in search of early metastatic disease are not very helpful (Figure 6–75). Lytic changes become evident on routine radiographs only when cortical destruction approaches 30–50% (Figure 6–76).

Treatment & Prognosis

A. Nonsurgical Treatment

Nonsurgical management of metastatic carcinoma to bone includes observation, radiation treatment, and hormonal/cytotoxic chemotherapy. Radiation is reserved for palliative management. Each patient must be carefully evaluated as a candidate for radiation therapy. The histologic type of disease, extent of disease, prognosis, marrow reserve, and overall constitution must be assessed.

After sustaining a pathologic fracture secondary to metastatic carcinoma, the average survival time is 19 months. Each histologic type has varying lengths of survival (prostate, 29 months; breast, 23 months; renal, 12 months; lung, 4 months). Furthermore, each type of carcinoma exhibits varying radiosensitivity. Prostate and lymphoreticular types demonstrate excellent sensitivity. Breast is intermediate, and renal and gastrointestinal are poor. When used, appropriately 90% of patients gain at least minimal relief, with up to two thirds obtaining complete relief. Seventy percent of patients who are ambulatory retain this function after radiation therapy to the lower extremities. Systemic radioisotopes may also be used. Strontium-89 mimics calcium distribution in the body and shows promise in clinical applications.

When a patient has sustained a true pathologic fixation (rather than an impending lesion) surgical stabilization is usually indicated with subsequent radiation therapy. Because of poor bone quality, augmentation of fixation with bone cement may be necessary.

Hormonal therapy has an important role in the management of metastatic breast and prostate cancer. Fortunately, these agents are easy to administer and have few side effects.

For breast cancer, medical hormonal manipulation can be done by use of antiestrogens, progestins, luteinizing hormone-releasing hormone, or adrenal-suppressing agents. Tamoxifen is effective in 30% of all breast cancer cases but increases to 50–75% of cases when the tumor is known to be estrogen receptor, progesterone receptor positive. Surgical ablation (oophorectomy) may also have a role in certain cases.

For prostate cancer, reduction in testosterone levels via bilateral orchiectomy or administration of estrogens or antiandrogens may produce dramatic results in cer-

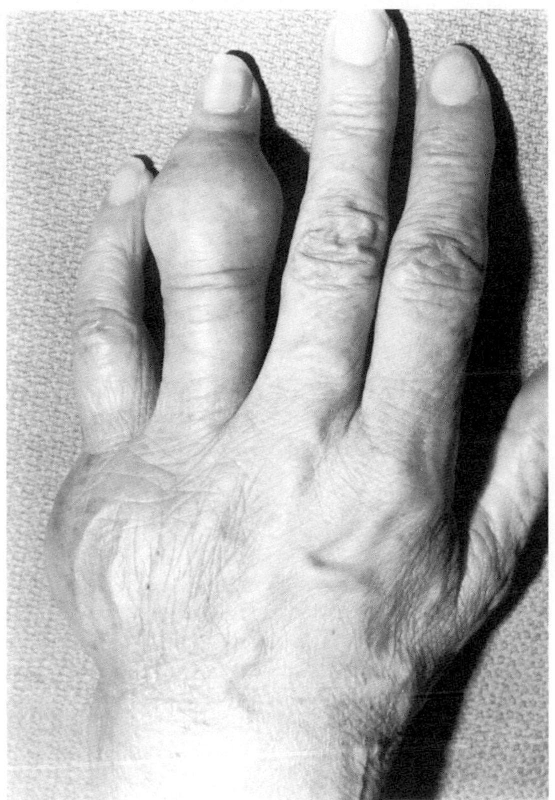

A

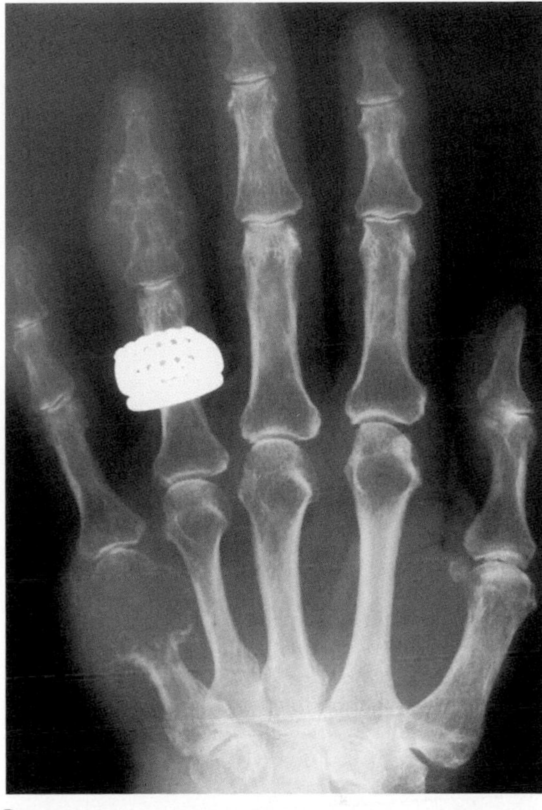

B

Figure 6–73. Clinical appearance (**A**) and radiographic appearance (**B**) of aneurysmal lesions in a case of carcinoma that metastasized from the thyroid to the hand.

tain cases. Estrogens are no longer used as a first agent because of the risk of cardiovascular complication.

Cytotoxic chemotherapy is used in adenocarcinoma treatment quite extensively. In older (more than 60 years) patients with advanced disease, however, the side effects of the drugs may be too severe.

B. Surgical Treatment

The goals for surgical intervention in the patient with metastatic carcinoma to bone are relief of pain; prevention of impending pathologic fixations; stabilization of true fixations; enhancement of mobility, function, and quality of life; and perhaps improvement of survival. It is generally agreed that a patient must have a life expectancy of at least 6 weeks to warrant operative intervention. Special considerations to surgical management include noting that bone quality is attenuated and healing will be delayed if even possible. Cancer patients, irrespective of their age, may have increased difficulty protecting their fixation device/prothesis secondary to systemic debilitation. Accordingly, rigid fixation, with polymethylmethacrylate (PMMA) augmentation as needed, is mandatory.

1. Hip—Seventy-five percent of all surgery for cancer that has metastasized to bone is performed in the hip area (Figure 6–77). Prior to 1970, surgeons attempted to stabilize these fractures with conventional hip nails

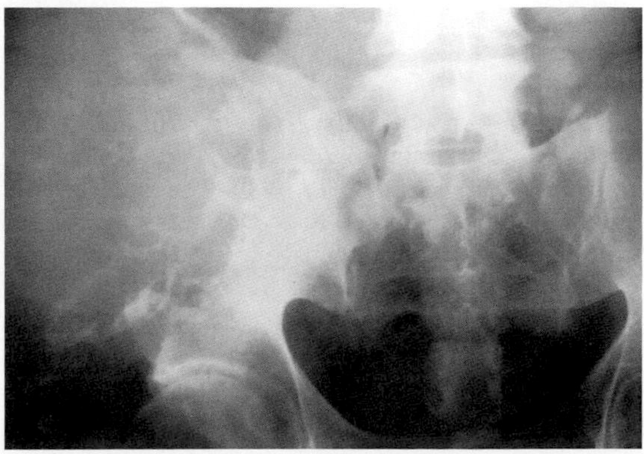

Figure 6–74. Radiograph of a metastatic hypernephroma in the ilium.

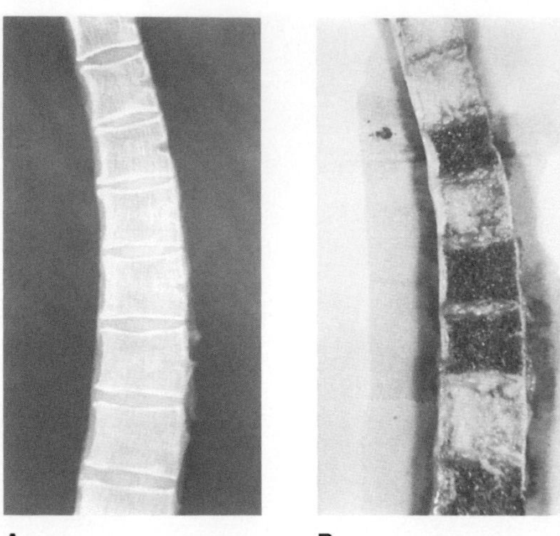

Figure 6–75. Radiograph (**A**) and gross appearance (**B**) of bone in a case of carcinoma that metastasized from the lung to the spine.

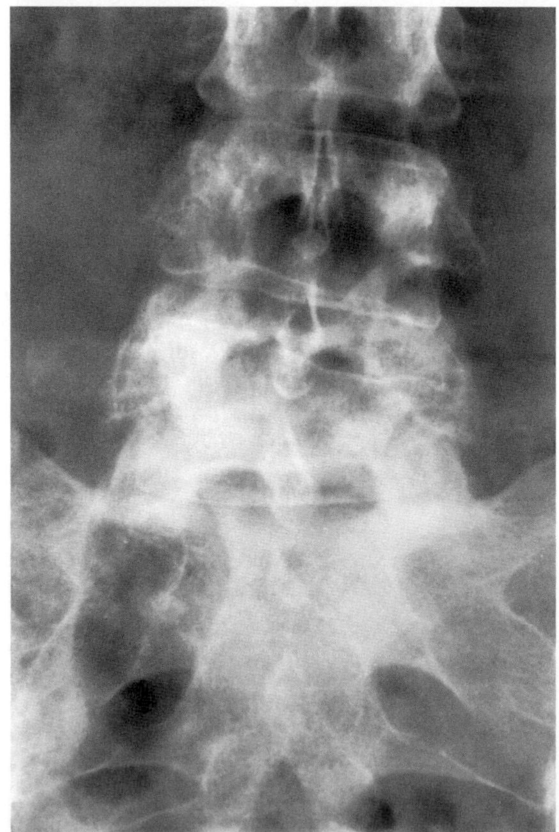

Figure 6–76. Radiograph of the spine of a 45-year-old woman whose cancer had metastasized from the breast.

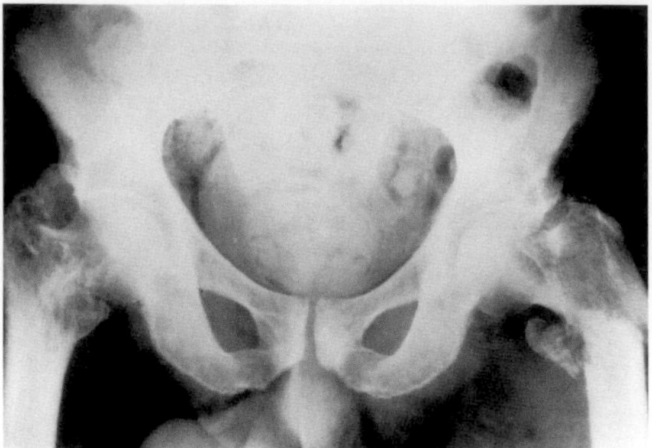

Figure 6–77. Radiograph of the pathologic fractures of both hips in a 55-year-old man with lung carcinoma.

or Austin Moore prostheses, but results were poor because of deficient local bone stock. After 1970, with the advent of bone cement as an adjuvant form of therapy, these same devices could be used, with improved results in most cases, along with local radiation therapy starting 2 weeks after the surgery. This technique allowed for early ambulation with less pain. However, as time passed and survival times increased, more failures were noted after 1–2 years with the hip nail and cement technique. For this reason, most surgeons currently use a cemented bipolar hemiarthroplasty for the femoral neck fractures and a longer stem calcar replacement hemiarthroplasty for the intertrochanteric fractures. Before these procedures are performed, it is wise to evaluate the entire shaft of the femur and the supraacetabular area for other lytic lesions that might require a longer stem femoral component for the shaft or a modified cemented acetabular component with a total hip replacement for acetabular lesions.

In many cases, the diagnosis of metastasis to the proximal femur is made before a fracture occurs. In these cases, it is the responsibility of the orthopedic surgeon to decide whether the patient should receive some form of internal stabilization prior to radiation therapy. A CT scan of the involved area helps make this decision. Criteria for the performance of a prophylactic stabilization procedure include the following: (1) 50% cortical lysis, (2) a femoral lesion greater than 2.5 cm in diameter, (3) an avulsion fracture of the lesser trochanter, and (4) persistent pain in the hip area 4 weeks following the completion of radiation therapy. These criteria are not perfect, however, and large errors arise in estimation of the load-bearing capacity of the bone.

2. Supraacetabular area—In the case of a small supraacetabular lesion with intact cortical bone, a

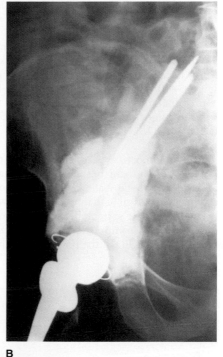

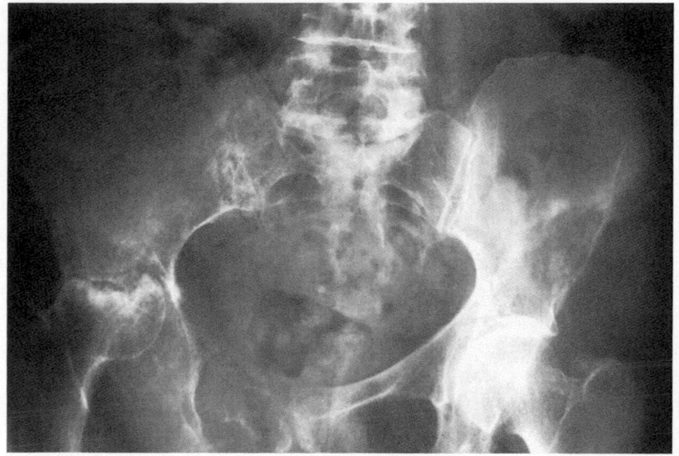

Figure 6–78. Preoperative (A) and postoperative (B) radiographs of the pelvis of a 73-year-old woman whose cancer had metastasized from the breast.

cemented cup with a total hip system is generally most appropriate. Augmentation of the fully cemented reconstruction with threaded Steinmann pins or similar anchoring screws may be necessary in advanced cases (Figure 6–78). The principles of treatment are always the same, irrespective of the extent of disease: aggressive intralesional curettage of the area back to healthy bone, followed by the placement of large (4.76 mm) threaded Steinmann pins into the sacroiliac area. The pins are placed with an initial foundation batch of cement, leaving them exposed for a second batch of cement, on top of which the cup is placed. A routine femoral component is then cemented.

3. Femoral shaft—Diaphyseal lesions that affect the femur but spare the peritrochanteric area are best handled with some form of intramedullary nail (Figure 6–79). Fixation of the entire femur, including the peritrochanteric area, with a reconstruction type nail is preferable in the event the disease progresses within the bone. Current intramedullary fixation devices often do not need cement augmentation. However, in cases of severe bone deficiency, PMMA introduction, either directly into the defect or indirectly at the nail insertion site, is preferable.

4. Humerus—The principle for the management of metastatic disease to the humerus is no different from that for the femur. In the case of diaphyseal lesions,

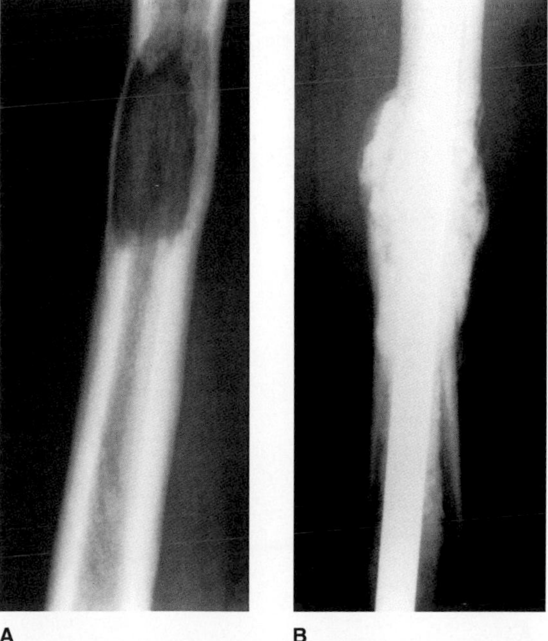

Figure 6–79. Preoperative (A) and postoperative (B) radiographs of the midshaft of the femur of a patient whose treatment involved fixation with a cemented intramedullary nail.

surgeons either use a conventional intramedullary rod or they plate the lesion. PMMA may be used with either technique.

In the case of the proximal humerus involving a large amount of the humeral head and neck, it is frequently necessary to cement a long-stem prosthesis (Figure 6–80). Just as with the proximal femur, in the proximal humerus there is no need to widely resect the tumor, and the rotator cuff is usually left intact.

5. Spine—In most cases of metastasis to the spine, the patient's pain can be managed adequately with local radiation therapy and medication. However, in cases of mechanical collapse associated with bony protrusion into the vertebral canal and cord compromise, surgical decompression and stabilization are frequently indicated. In the past, most of these problems were treated with posterior decompression by laminectomy alone. The results were poor because the spine was further destabilized, which resulted in increased kyphosis and anterior cord compression. With advances in the area of spinal instrumentation, the treatment shifted toward a more aggressive anterior decompression and stabilization if the patient's general condition allows. Even in cases in which the patient's general health does not tolerate the larger anterior approach, a less aggressive alternative might include posterior decompression supplemented by posterior spinal fixation.

The midthoracic spine is the most common area for paraplegia secondary to metastasis because of the narrow vertebral canal at this level of the spine. The ideal surgical approach to the problem in a patient with a reasonable prognosis consists of an anterior thoracotomy and anterior decompression by verte-

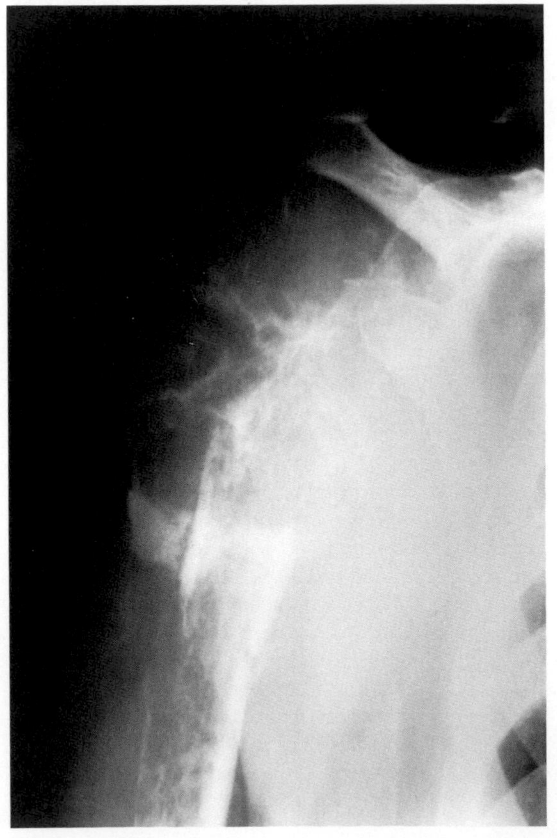

A

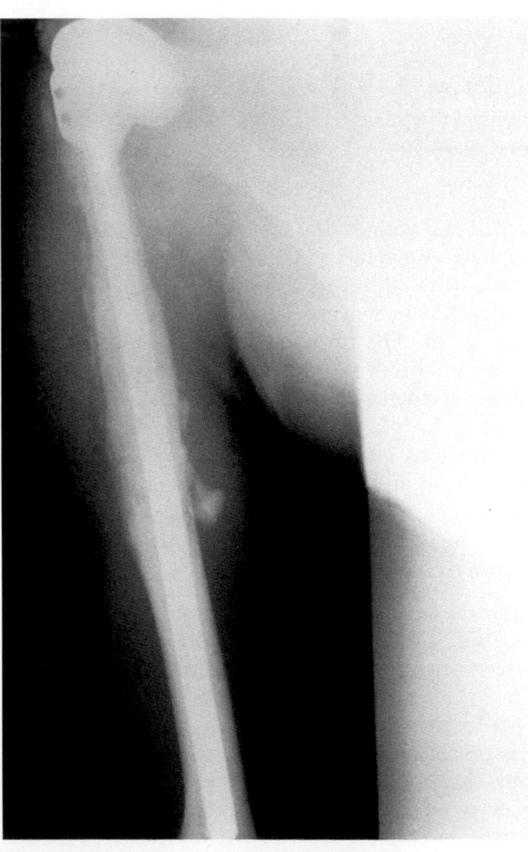

B

Figure 6–80. Preoperative (**A**) and postoperative (**B**) radiographs of the proximal humerus of a patient whose treatment involved the use of a cemented long-stem Neer prosthesis.

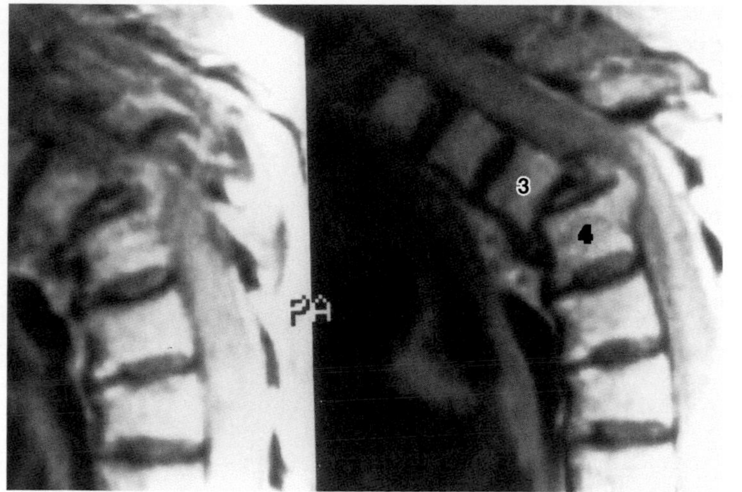

A

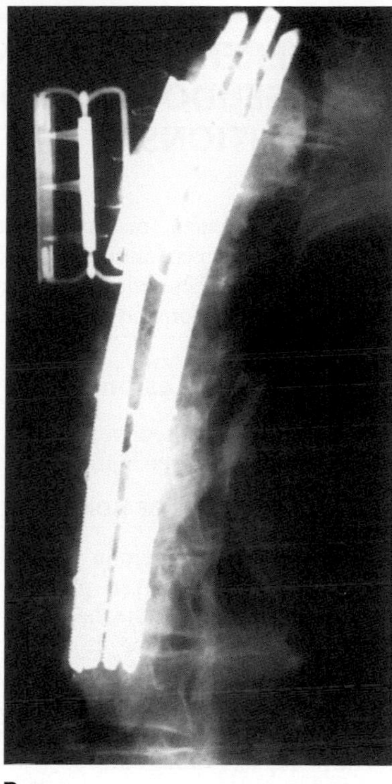

B

Figure 6–81. Preoperative T_1-weighted MRI (**A**) and postoperative radiograph (**B**) of the spine of a patient whose treatment involved use of posterior rods and sublaminal wires for stabilization.

brectomy, followed by anterior stabilization. As an alternative approach in a patient with a worse prognosis and a circumferential cord compression, a posterior decompression stabilization can be considered (Figure 6–81).

The second most common site for cord compression is the thoracolumbar region. The anterior reconstruction is the same in the thoracolumbar area as in the midthoracic area. A posterior stabilization may be advisable, especially in cases in which the prognosis is good.

The cervical spine is the least likely area for surgical treatment, mainly because the vertebral canal is wide at this level and cord compromise is uncommon. If surgery is needed, an ideal reconstruction is an anterior decompression and stabilization.

Radiation therapy is required postoperatively with all of these reconstructions. The use of bone graft is therefore undesirable because of inhibited osteoblastic healing.

Beauchamp CP: Errors and pitfalls in the diagnosis and treatment of metastatic bone disease. Orthop Clin North Am 2000; 31(4):675. [PMID: 11043105]

Hipp JA et al: Predicting pathologic fracture risk in the management of metastatic bone defects. Clin Orthop 1995;312:120. [PMID: 7634597]

Hortobagyi GN et al: Efficacy of pamidronate in reducing skeletal complications in patients with breast cancer and lytic bone metastases. N Engl J Med 1996;24:1785. [PMID: 8965890]

Mirels H: Metastatic disease in long bones. A proposed scoring system for diagnosing impending pathologic fractures. Clin Orthop 1989;(249):256. [PMID: 2684463]

Mundy GR: Mechanisms of bone metastasis. Cancer 1997;80S: 1546. [PMID: 9362421]

Rougraff BT et al: Skeletal metastases of unknown origin: A prospective study of a diagnostic strategy. J Bone Joint Surg AM 1993;75:1276. [PMID: 8408149]

Wedin R: Surgical treatment for pathologic fracture. Acta Orthop Scand Suppl 2001;72(302):2p. [PMID: 11582636]

Wedin R et al: Surgical treatment for skeletal breast cancer metastases: A population-based study of 641 patients. Cancer 2001;92(2):257. [PMID: 11466677]

DIFFERENTIAL DIAGNOSIS OF PSEUDOTUMOROUS CONDITIONS

In addition to benign, malignant, and metastatic neoplasms, a group of pseudotumors masquerade as bone and soft-tissue tumors. These lesions actually appear with greater frequency than either primary bone or soft-tissue tumors.

Stress-Reactive Lesions

The most common pseudotumors are those related to either bone or soft-tissue injury.

A. Stress Fracture of Bone

Stress fractures are common in young (less than 30 years) athletic individuals and can produce radiographic features that might suggest the diagnosis of a bone-forming sarcoma or Ewing sarcoma. It is important to obtain a careful history from patients regarding their physical activity both at work and at play. There will be no history of a single injury if the bone symptoms are caused by repetitive impact loading stress such as occurs with working out for cross-country running. The stress fracture usually occurs several weeks after a sudden increase of physical activity for which the patient is not properly conditioned. This is a common situation in the military, particularly during initial training.

Stress fractures are commonly located in the metaphyseal-diaphyseal areas of long weight-bearing bones. Early radiographs frequently appear normal before periosteal new bone begins to form. The most sensitive early diagnostic tool is a bone scan, which can appear hot or abnormal in the case of stress fractures, neoplasms, and infections. The MRI is sensitive to early fluid shifts in the periosteum overlying a stress fracture, but it is also sensitive to neoplastic and infectious conditions. One of the best methods to help rule out tumors and infection is to simply stop all physical stress to the injured bone for a period of 4 weeks. In patients with stress fracture, the pain should resolve spontaneously during this period, and a follow-up radiograph taken after this period reveals a typical fusiform circumferential periosteal callous formation. In patients with a tumor or infection, the pain persists, and the radiographic signs of permeative osteolysis predominate, in which case a biopsy and culture are indicated.

At times, the clinical picture of a stress fracture is confused by the preexistence of a benign stress raiser, such as a nonossifying fibroma or fibrous cortical defect (Figure 6–82).

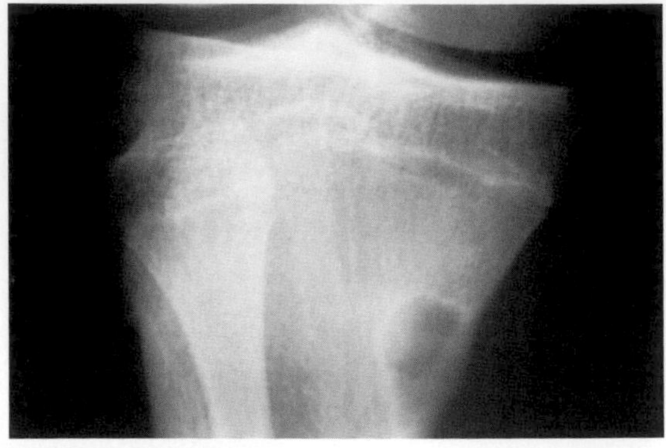

A

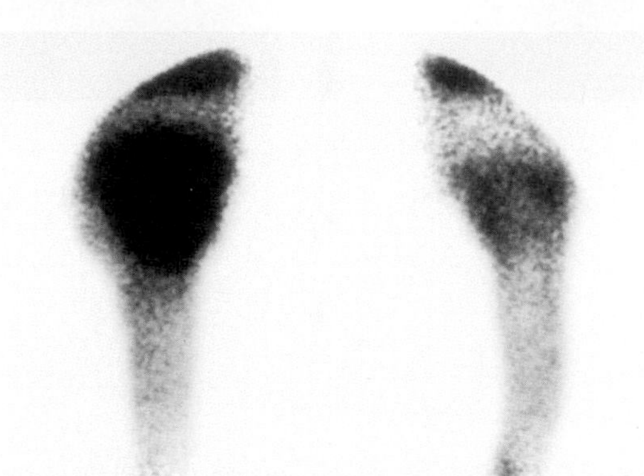

B

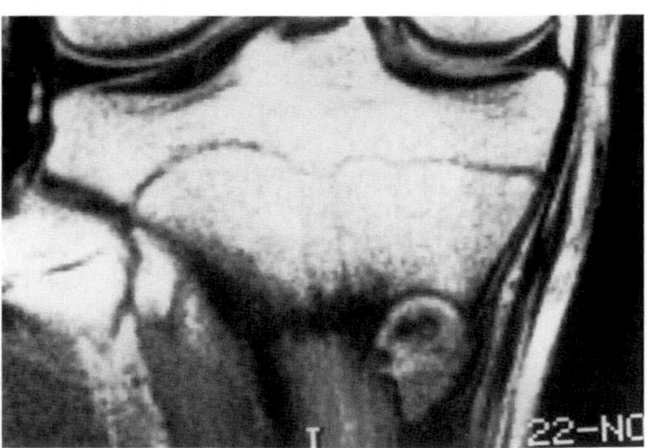

C

Figure 6–82. Radiograph (**A**), isotope bone scan (**B**), and T_1-weighted MRI (**C**) of the proximal tibia in a 16-year-old boy with a stress fracture.

In older patients, especially in postmenopausal women, stress fractures can occur with minimal physical activity. The circumstances under which the fracture occurred might not come out in a routine history. A common location of osteoporotic stress fractures is in the sacrum (Figure 6–83).

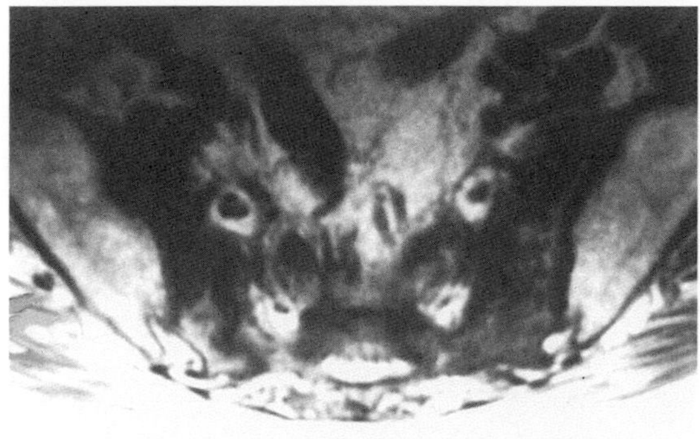

A

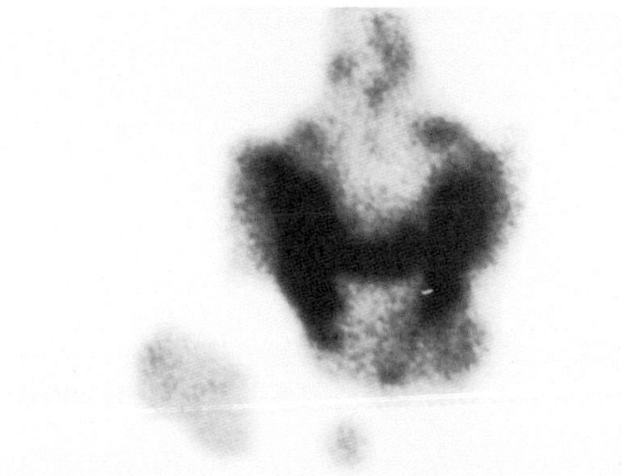

B

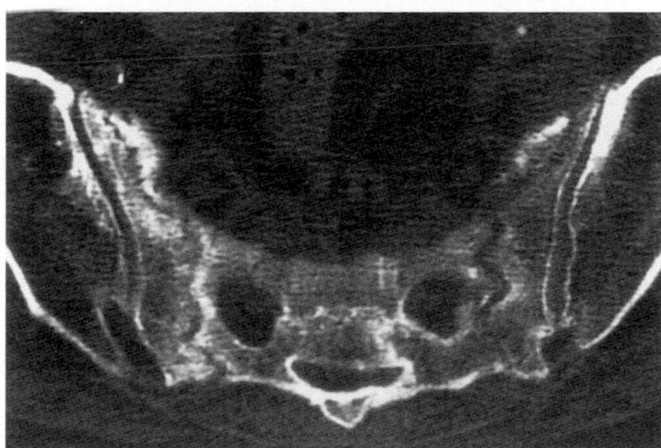

C

Figure 6–83. T_1-weighted MRI (**A**), isotope bone scan (**B**), and CT scan (**C**) of the sacrum in a 71-year-old woman with stress fracture.

B. Myositis Ossificans

Another common stress-reactive pseudotumor seen in the extremity is myositis ossificans, which occurs most frequently in the lower extremity in young men. The quadriceps muscle is commonly involved because of direct blows or tearing injury to this muscle. The pseudotumor mass may not arise for several months after the injury and may not be related to a specific injury. In older (more than 40 years), more sedentary patients, there may be no history of stress injury.

Early radiographs may not reveal soft-tissue calcification. With maturation, ossification occurs in the traumatized muscle fascial planes, which may suggest the diagnosis of a synovial sarcoma or other calcifying sarcoma. If the myositis pseudotumor is attached to the subjacent bone, it can mimic a parosteal osteosarcoma (Figure 6–84).

Infectious Diseases

Bacterial, viral, tuberculous, or fungal infections of the bone or soft tissue can frequently mimic a neoplastic process. This is particularly the case with infections that are not highly virulent, do not create systemic symptoms or a febrile response, and do not cause a large alteration in acute-phase reactant laboratory work. If a tender mass is present on examination and a bone or soft-tissue tumor is suggested by imaging studies, a biopsy may be indicated and should include a tissue culture to make the correct diagnosis. Inflammatory pseudotumors can be seen in any age group but are more common in children and frequently affect the lower extremity.

A. Bacterial Infection

Bacterial infections of bone can take on the appearance of a round cell tumor such as Ewing sarcoma in children or lymphoma in adults (Figure 6–85). In contrast, tuberculous and fungal infections are less inflammatory and thus have more localized, well-marginated lesions that take on the imaging appearance of a benign tumor.

B. Tuberculous or Fungal Infection

A tuberculous or fungal infection of the spine or extremity can present as a pseudotumor in children or young adults, especially in Asian or Mexican patients (Figure 6–86). The incidence of tuberculous and fungal infections, which are low-grade infections that typically have an insidious onset, is also increased in patients with AIDS.

C. Caffey Disease

Caffey disease can mimic a neoplastic process. It is an idiopathic form of periostitis that is seen in infants younger than 6 months and affects the extremities, shoulder girdle, and mandible (Figure 6–87). It may have a viral origin and is currently much rarer than it was 30 years ago. The bony changes are osteoblastic and could suggest the diagnosis of an osteosarcoma, which is rare in infants. Caffey disease is self-

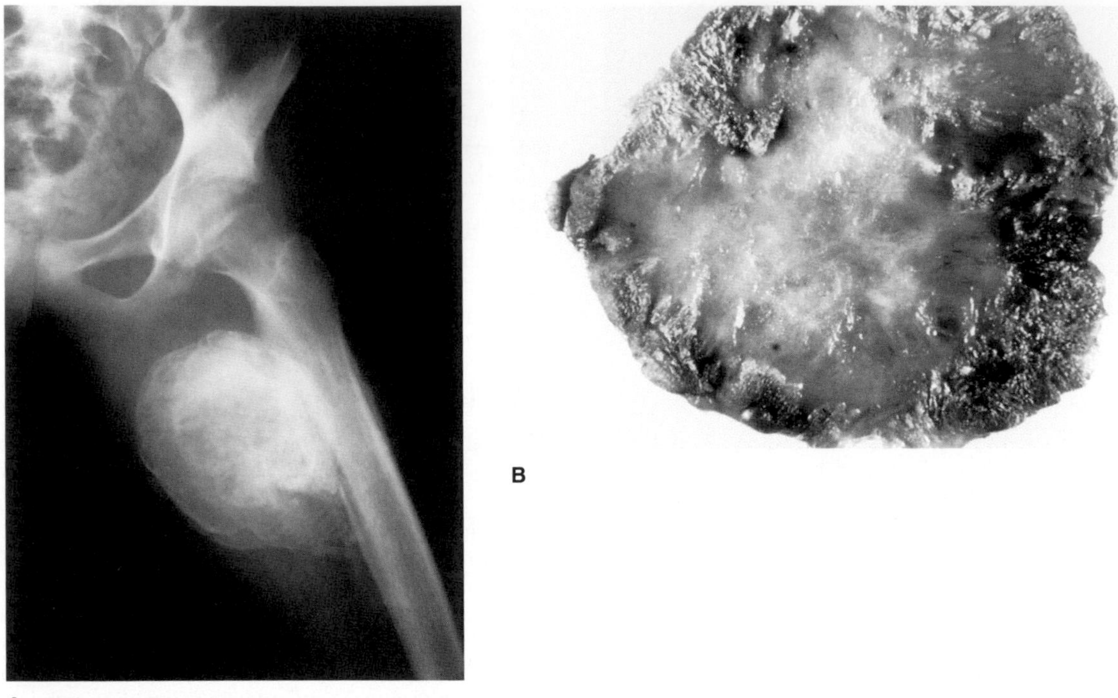

Figure 6–84. Radiograph (**A**) and gross appearance of a resected specimen (**B**) of myositis ossificans in the adductor muscles of a 12-year-old girl.

limiting and usually clears spontaneously without disability.

Metabolic Disorders

A. Brown Tumor of Primary Hyperparathyroidism

Brown tumor is the most common metabolic disorder that mimics a neoplastic process in bone. The lytic giant cell lesions occur symmetrically in metaphyseal-epiphyseal bone as the result of increased parathyroid hormone production by a solitary parathyroid adenoma, by hyperplastic parathyroid glands, or by a solitary parathyroid carcinoma. Brown tumors occur three times more often in females than in males and are usually seen between 15 and 70 years of age. They are most common in the ends of the long bone, followed next in frequency in the pelvis, long bone diaphysis, maxillary bone, cranium, rib, and hand. Brown tumors are rarely seen in the spine. Symptoms of pain are related to the local bone destruction, but widespread pain may result from generalized osteomalacia. The hyperparathyroid condition can lead to weight loss, psychologic disorders, gastrointestinal disorders, renal stones, polyuria, and polydipsia.

The radiographic features of the brown tumor in bone include a round lytic area that may be multicentric and may suggest the diagnosis of metastatic carcinoma, multiple myeloma, or histiocytic lymphoma (Figure 6–88). In the case of a solitary lesion, it may suggest the diagnosis of a nonossifying fibroma, fibrous dysplasia, giant cell tumor, or aneurysmal bone cyst. At the time of biopsy, the brown tumor has the reddish brown appearance of a giant cell tumor. Microscopically, it looks like a giant cell tumor except that the background stromal cells are more fibroblastic and the bone trabeculae demonstrates abnormally thick and poorly mineralized osteoid seams. Because of the marked similarity between the brown tumor and the giant cell tumor, clinicians should routinely order an analysis of serum calcium, phosphorus, and alkaline phosphatase levels in all patients with bone lesions that produce giant cells.

In patients with brown tumors, the treatment consists of removing the source of the excessive parathyroid hormone. After this, the bony defects usually heal spontaneously. Bone grafting is rarely required. Although the secondary hyperparathyroidism seen in renal failure patients does not usually develop into brown tumors, it does produce pseudotumor-

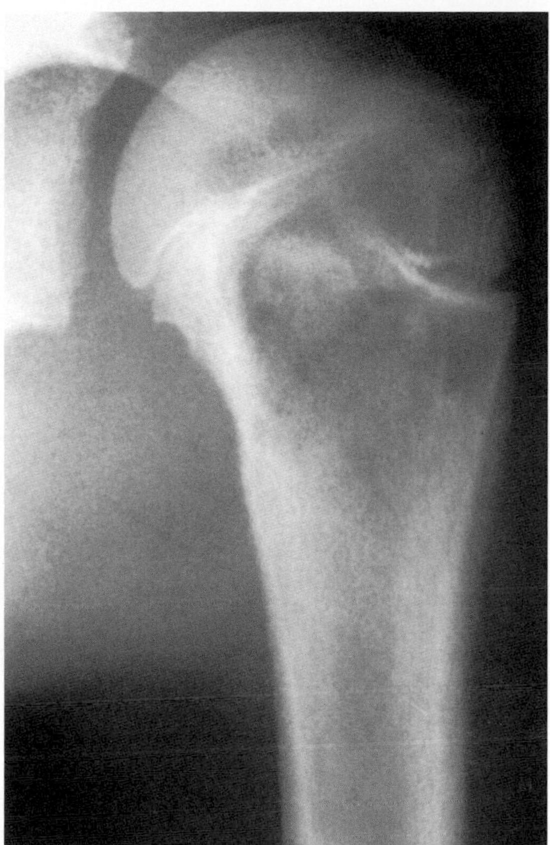

Figure 6–85. Radiograph of acute osteomyelitis caused by *Staphylococcus aureus* in the proximal humerus of a 13-year-old boy.

ous calcification in soft tissue, a condition similar to tumoral calcinosis, which is discussed later in this section.

B. Paget Disease

Paget disease is frequently included in discussions of metabolic bone disorders, although the demonstration of cytoplasmic and nuclear inclusion bodies in osteoclasts of pagetic bone similar to paramyxovirus infections may suggest a viral origin. Most clinicians are familiar with the late changes in Paget disease, which include the bowing of long bones and the finding of dense blastic changes on radiographic examination. However, many are unfamiliar with the early lytic phase of Paget disease when the radiographic findings are more suggestive of metastatic carcinoma, histiocytic lymphoma, primary sarcoma, or even primary hyperparathyroidism (Figure 6–89).

C. Gaucher Disease

Gaucher disease is a rare familial disorder in which accumulation of glucocerebroside causes enlargement of the liver, spleen, and marrow tissues. The marrow infiltration in children and young adults causes a gradual loss of bone that can mimic a neoplastic condition. The most common areas involved include the distal femur, tibia, humerus, vertebral column, skull, and mandible. Isolated focal destructive changed with endosteal scalloping and moth-eaten patterns may suggest the diagnosis of metastatic disease, myelomatosis, primary sarcoma, or fibrous dysplasia (Figure 6–90).

Hemorrhagic Conditions

A. Pseudotumor of Hemophilia

A hematoma in the soft tissue or bone under the periosteum may be difficult to distinguish from a tumor.

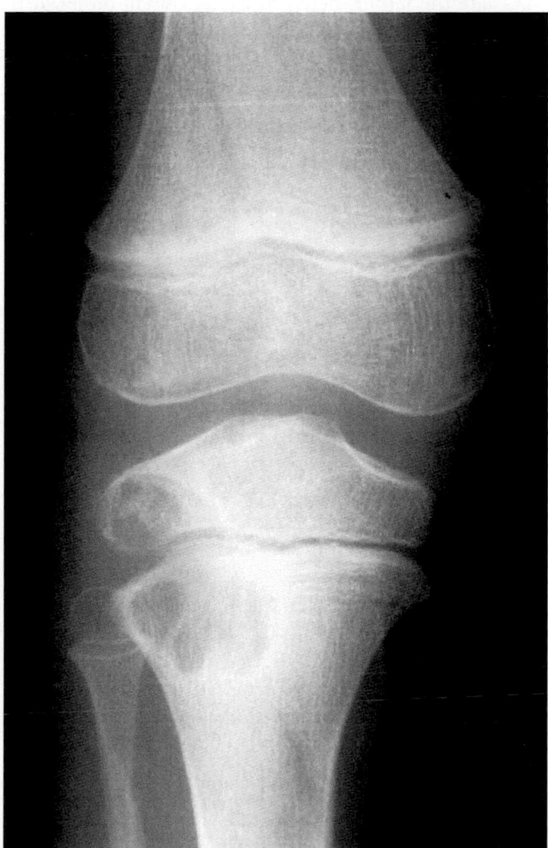

Figure 6–86. Radiograph of tuberculous osteomyelitis in the proximal tibia of a 10-year-old girl.

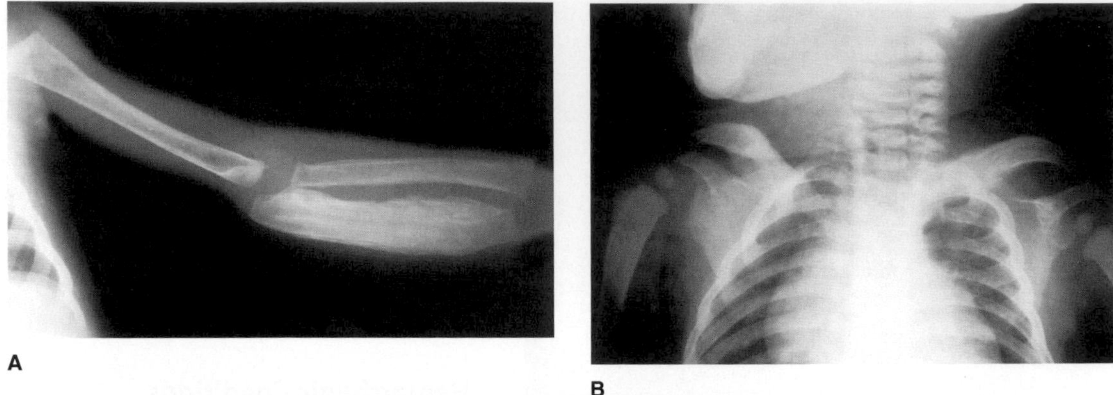

Figure 6–87. Preoperative (**A**) and postoperative (**B**) radiographs of Caffey disease in the upper extremity and shoulder of a 5-month-old infant.

Hematoma formation is frequently precipitated by some form of trauma, and the bones most commonly involved are the femur, pelvis, tibia, and small bones of the hand. It is rare to see multiple lesions. The bony lesions can be central or eccentric. The finding of lytic destruction followed by sclerotic reaction at the periphery may mimic the radiographic picture of an aneurysmal bone cyst or a giant cell tumor. In the hand bones, the osseous pseudotumors take on the appearance of a giant cell reparative granuloma or an osteoblastoma. The subperiosteal lesions

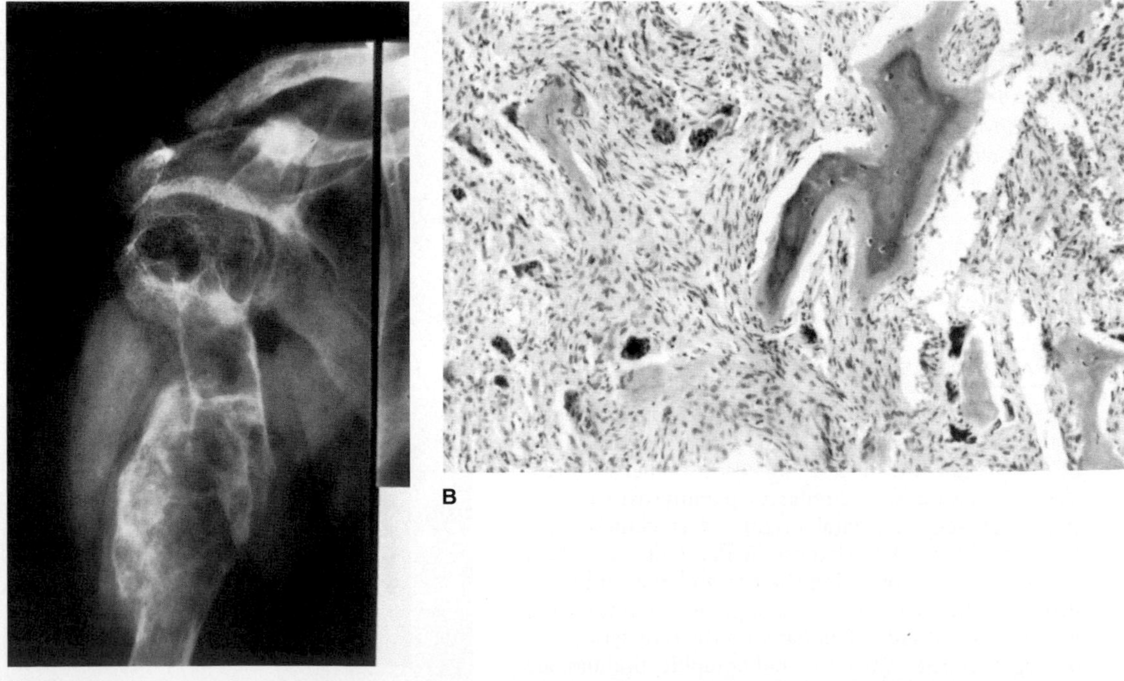

Figure 6–88. Radiograph (**A**) and photomicrograph (**B**) of a brown tumor of hyperparathyroidism in the proximal humerus of a 40-year-old woman.

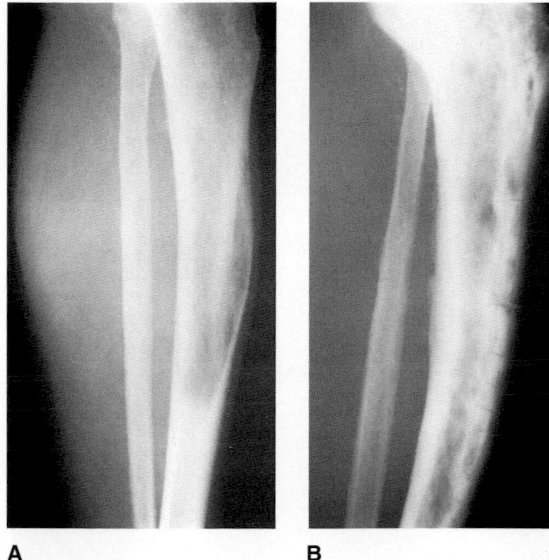

Figure 6–89. Early and late radiographs of Paget disease of the tibia, taken when the male patient was 45 years of age (**A**) and when he was 65 years of age (**B**).

bulge into the surrounding soft tissue and show reactive periosteal new bone formation and subjacent cortical erosion that may mimic Ewing sarcoma or hemorrhagic osteosarcoma (Figure 6–91).

B. Intramuscular Hematoma

Another hemorrhagic disorder that can produce a pseudotumor of soft tissue is the intramuscular hematoma. It is similar to the soft-tissue pseudotumor of hemophilia but without a bleeding abnormality. Intramuscular hematomas are almost always related to blunt trauma, but they occasionally result from a traction injury that may subsequently produce myositis ossificans. There may be no superficial signs of bruising in the overlying skin, and sometimes the hematoma grows in size at a later date, even as long as several years after the initial injury. The radiographic examination is of little help because no calcification or bony abnormality is evident. The MRI is the best imaging study, but unfortunately, the appearance of an intramuscular hematoma on MRI can mimic that of a deep soft-tissue sarcoma such as a malignant fibrous histiocytoma (Figure 6–92).

Ectopic Calcification

Ectopic calcification in soft tissue has many causes, most of which are related to chronic degenerative disorders in collagenous structures such as tendons or ligaments about a joint. However, in cases in which the dystrophic calcification is associated with a soft-tissue mass, the clinician must rule out the diagnosis of a soft-tissue sarcoma such as synovial sarcoma.

A. Tumoral Calcinosis

Tumoral calcinosis, seen about the hip, shoulder, and elbow, is characterized by extensive calcium phosphate deposition in a benign fibrous mass. It is an idiopathic condition that affects patients between 10 and 30 years of age and occurs more frequently in males than in females. Multiple lesions occur, and the lesions cause minimal pain and tenderness.

In cases of tumoral calcinosis, the extensive central fluffy calcification might suggest the diagnosis of a synovial sarcoma, soft-tissue chondrosarcoma, or tuberculosis (Figure 6–93). At biopsy, a chalky white paste exudes from a spongelike fibrous mass. Microscopic findings include extensive amorphous calcium phosphate deposits in a fibrous stroma speckled with macro-

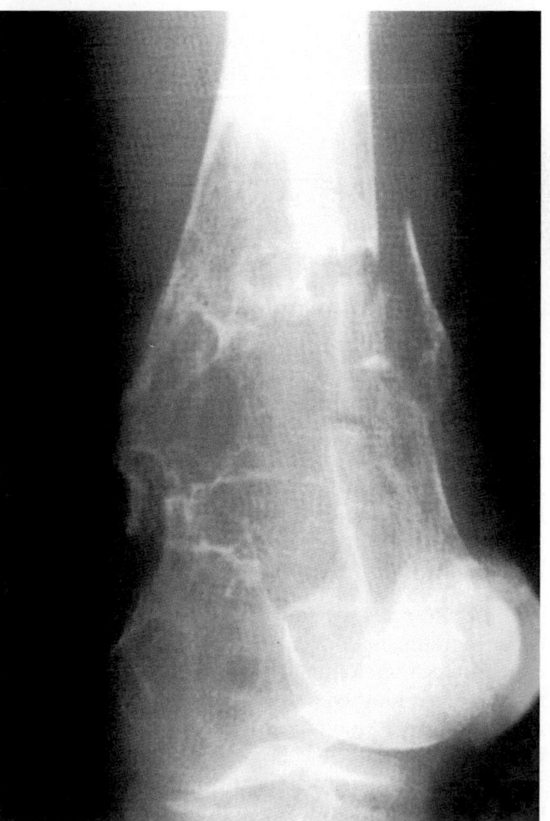

Figure 6–90. Radiograph of a pathologic fracture secondary to Gaucher disease involving the distal femur in a 29-year-old man.

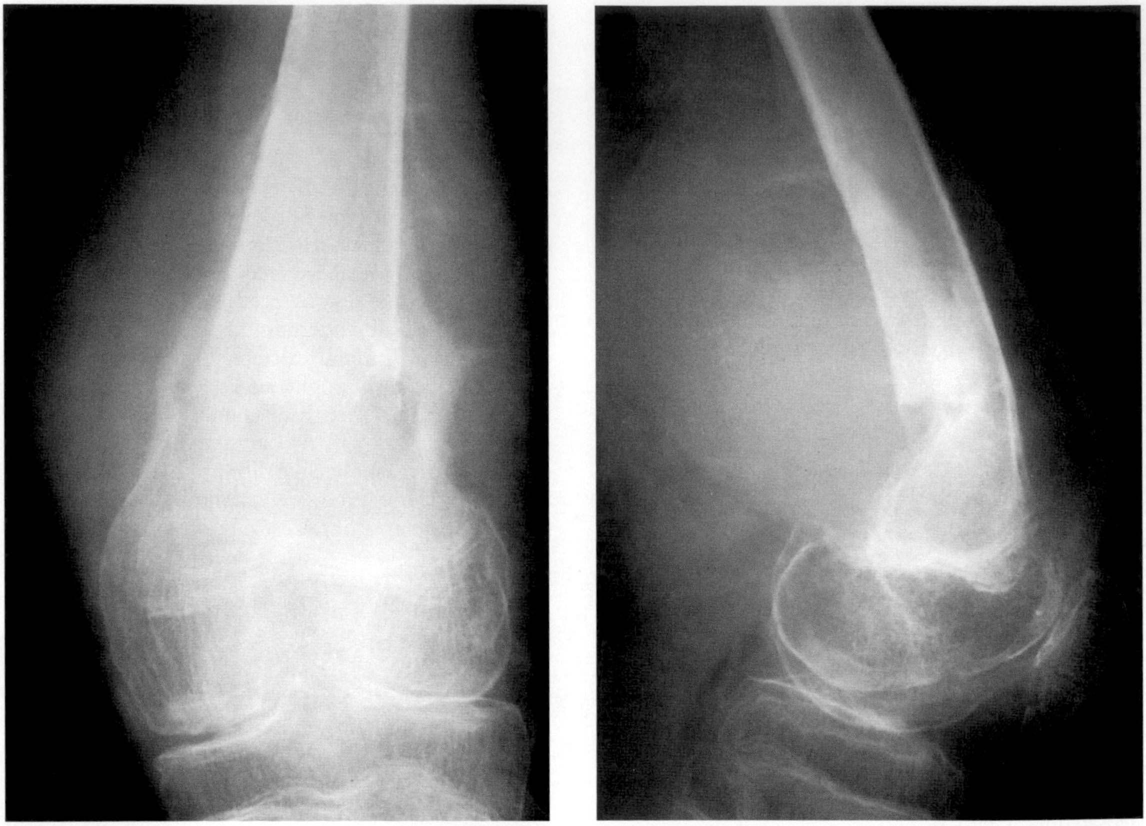

A B

Figure 6–91. Anteroposterior (**A**) and lateral (**B**) radiographs of a pseudotumor of hemophilia in the distal femur of a 14-year-old boy.

phages and inflammatory cells. If the pseudotumor is not completely removed, a recurrence is very likely.

A similar condition is seen in patients with renal osteodystrophy with secondary hyperparathyroidism, and the mechanism for the deposition in this case is a high level of calcium phosphorus production.

B. Compartment Syndrome

The ischemic calcification and even ossification that occur in traumatic compartment syndromes in the lower extremity can often mimic a tumor. The initial injury is usually a crushing type that causes increased compartment pressure from muscle swelling. This pressure eventually leads to ischemic necrosis of the compartment muscle, which several years later becomes calcific or even ossified. Because the muscle appears firm and calcified on radiographic examination, the clinician may not relate the finding to an old injury and may suspect a calcifying sarcoma such as synovial sarcoma. The most common place for this pseudotumor is in one of the

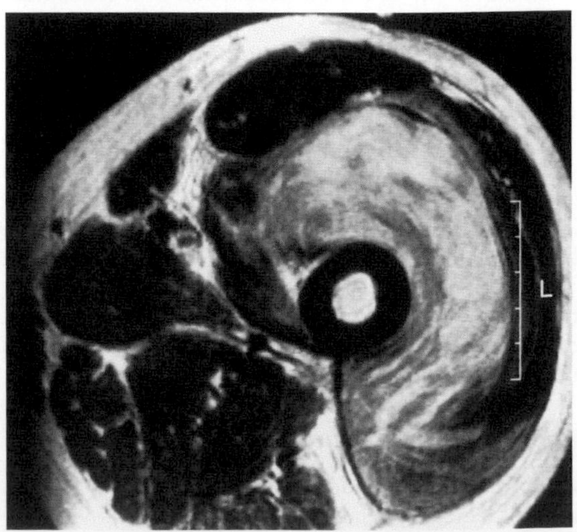

Figure 6–92. Axial view T_2-weighted MRI of a hematoma in the quadriceps muscles of a 46-year-old man.

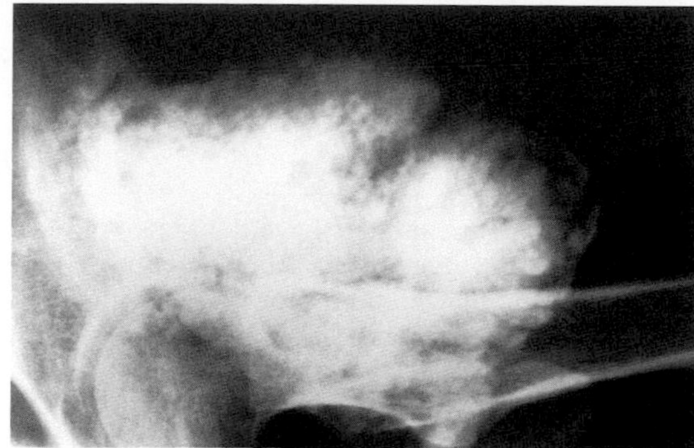

A

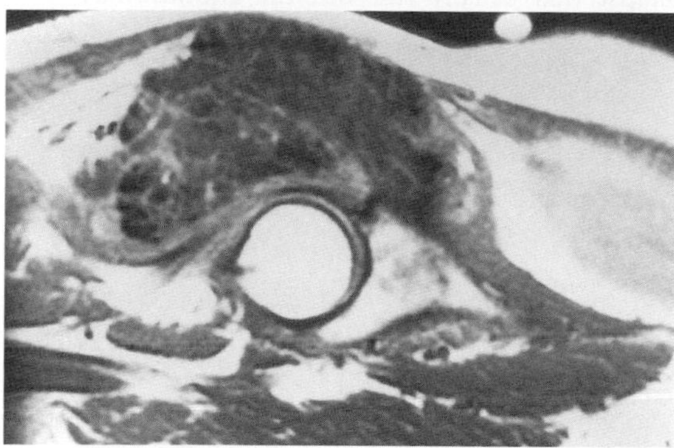

B

Figure 6–93. Radiograph (**A**) and T_1-weighted MRI (**B**) of tumoral calcinosis in the hip of a 54-year-old woman.

muscle compartments of the leg, and it causes stiffness and muscle weakness at the ankle and foot area (Figure 6–94). This process can mimic soft-tissue calcifications secondary to a neoplastic process (Figure 6–95).

Dysplastic Disorders

Many developmental or dysplastic conditions can create bony abnormalities, which, on radiographic examination, can mimic a bone tumor. These are usually focal defects in enchondral bone formation that result from a failure to remodel primary woven bone forming at the metaphyseal end of the physis.

A. Osteoma

Osteoma commonly occurs in the skull or maxilla and is composed of dense unorganized woven bone seen just beneath the cortex. There is no lytic component in or around the dense bone, and no symptoms are associated with the presence of osteomas. Because the lesions are commonly seen in the metaphyseal areas about the knee, the clinician may become concerned about the diagnosis of an early osteosarcoma. However, the lack of periosteal response and minimal uptake on an isotope bone scan help rule out sarcoma (Figure 6–96). In such cases, there should be no concern about future problems from the lesion, and usually no intervention is necessary.

B. Bone Island

The bone island is an even more sharply marginated dysplastic process than the osteoma. It is most commonly located in the pelvis. It can mimic a blastic metastatic lesion in patients with prostate cancer. However, with a bone island, as with an osteoma, the bone scan shows minimal and very focal activity, and the CT scan and MRI show no reaction in the surrounding

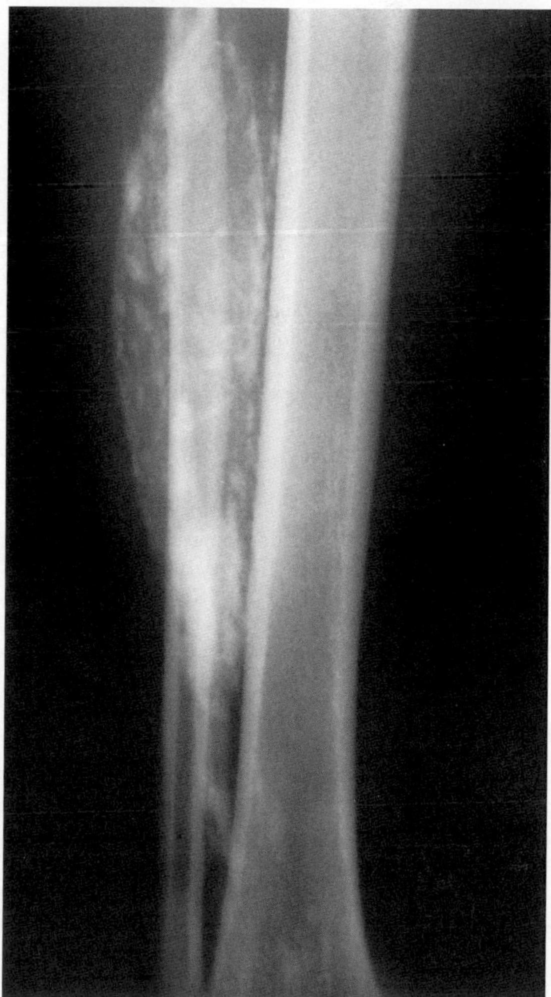

Figure 6–94. Radiograph of an old compartment syndrome in the flexor hallucis longus.

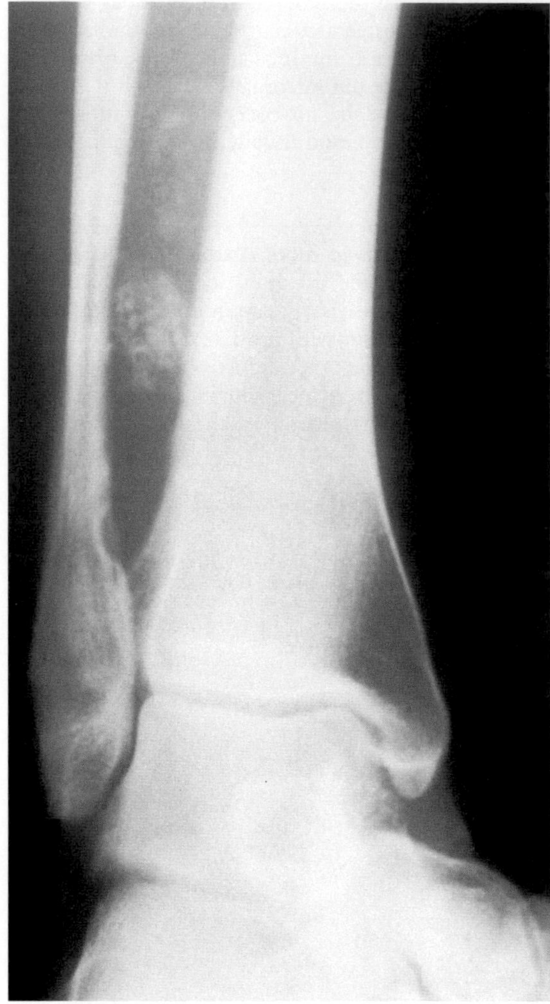

Figure 6–95. Radiograph of calcification in synovial sarcoma of the leg.

marrow. Figure 6–97 shows the findings of a bone island through the pelvis of a 35-year-old man.

Bone Infarcts

The two types of bone infarcts that can mimic bone tumors are the metaphyseal type and the epiphyseal type. They can be idiopathic in origin or secondary to increased alcohol consumption or corticosteroid use.

A. Metaphyseal Bone Infarct

The most common bone infarct is in the metaphyseal region, which is typically seen about the knee, hip, and shoulder in adults. Radiographically, the infarct can mimic a low-grade cartilaginous tumor such as an enchondroma. An infarct presents with a sclerotic honeycombed pattern (Figure 6–98), whereas a cartilaginous lesion presents with central flocculated calcification (Figure 6–99).

B. Epiphyseal Bone Infarct

Although epiphyseal bone infarcts have the same etiology as those in the metaphysis, these are most commonly found in the femoral condyles and the proximal femoral and humeral epiphyses. In these locations, the lytic change seen in the epiphyseal bone can mimic a chondroblastoma. The differential diagnosis can be difficult before the appearance of a crescent sign or other radiographic signs of subchondral collapse that usually rule out the chondroblastoma (Figure 6–100).

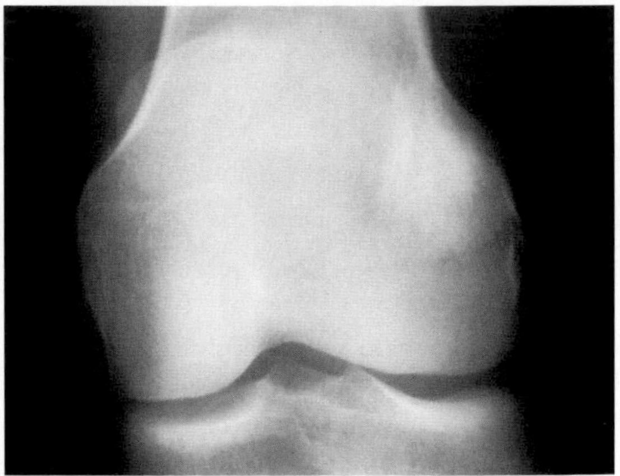

A

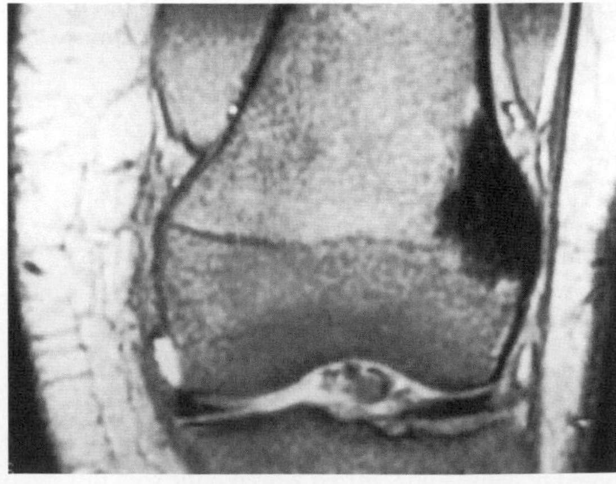

B

Figure 6–96. Radiograph (**A**) and T_2-weighted MRI (**B**) of a dysplastic process in the distal femur of a 64-year-old woman.

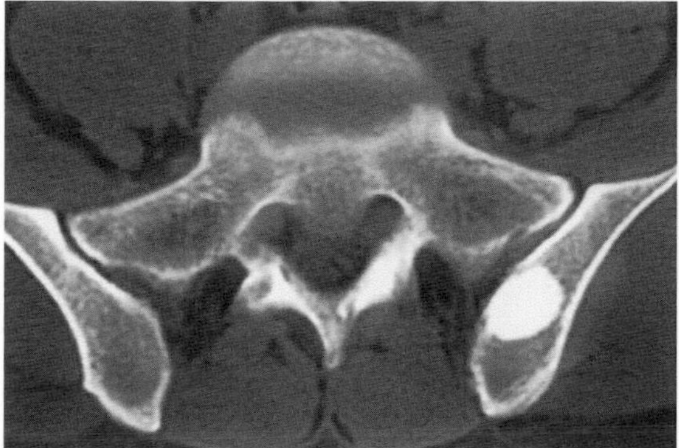

A

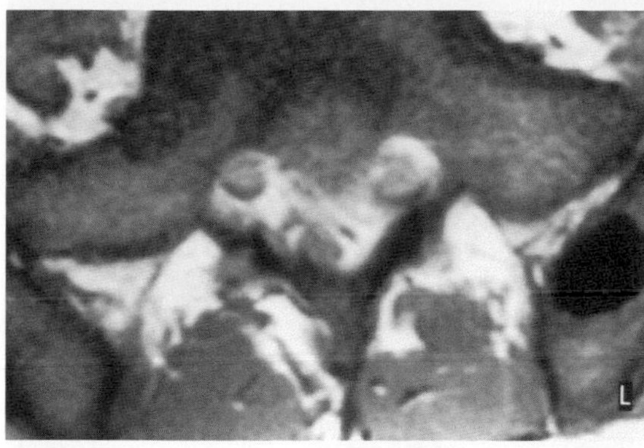

B

Figure 6–97. CT scan (**A**) and T_2-weighted MRI (**B**) of a bone island through the pelvis of a 35-year-old man.

Histiocytic Disorders

A. Langerhans Cell Histiocytosis

Sometimes inappropriately called histiocytosis X, Langerhans cell histiocytosis can present in a variety of ways. Previously considered distinct diseases, including eosinophilic granuloma, Hand-Schüller-Christian disease, and Letterer-Siwe disease, they are now considered part of the same spectrum of histiocytosis presentation. Of these, the localized granulomatous form, which is called eosinophilic granuloma or Langerhans cell granulomatosis, is the one that mimics a tumor radiographically. Eosinophilic granuloma is seen twice as often in boys as in girls and commonly occurs between 5 and 15 years of age. It is usually monostotic but in 10% of cases involves two or three separate areas. It is a histiocytic process of unknown cause but may have a viral origin. It causes local inflammatory pain and may result in low-grade fever associated with an elevated sedimentation rate. Although the most common location of eosinophilic granuloma is the skull, it is also seen in the rib, pelvis, maxilla, vertebral body (vertebra plana), clavicle, and scapula, listed in the order of frequency. Besides affecting flat bones, it can arise in the diaphysis of long bones, followed next by the metaphysis, and it is least common in the epiphysis.

Eosinophilic granuloma can be extremely permeative and destructive, especially in long bones (Figure 6–101) and vertebrae (Figure 6–102), thereby mimicking a more aggressive process, such as Ewing sarcoma, metastatic neuroblastoma, or osteomyelitis. It can also produce a so-called onionskin periostitis of the type seen in Ewing sarcoma. The lesion has a more aggressive pattern in younger children and later becomes more focal and granulomatous. Microscopic findings include large pale-staining histiocytes speckled with small bright-staining eosinophils and an occasional giant cell.

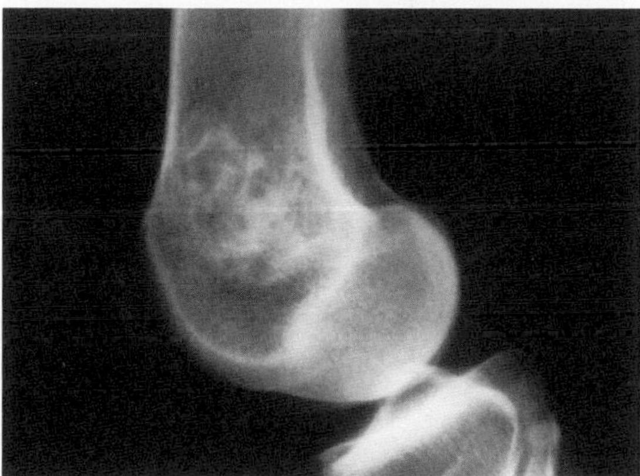

A

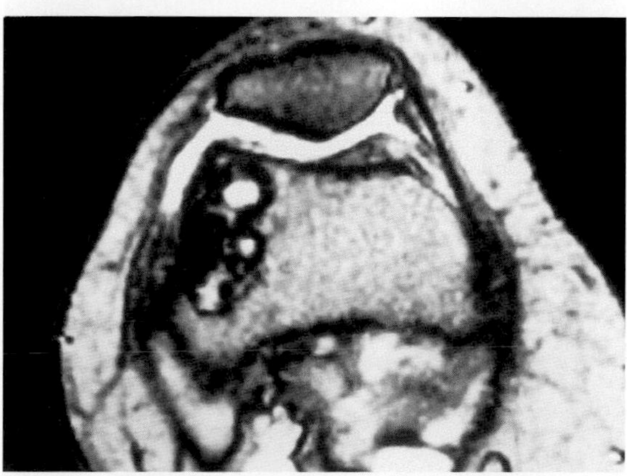

B

Figure 6–98. Radiograph (**A**) and T_1-weighted MRI (**B**) of a metaphyseal infarct in the distal femur of a 52-year-old woman.

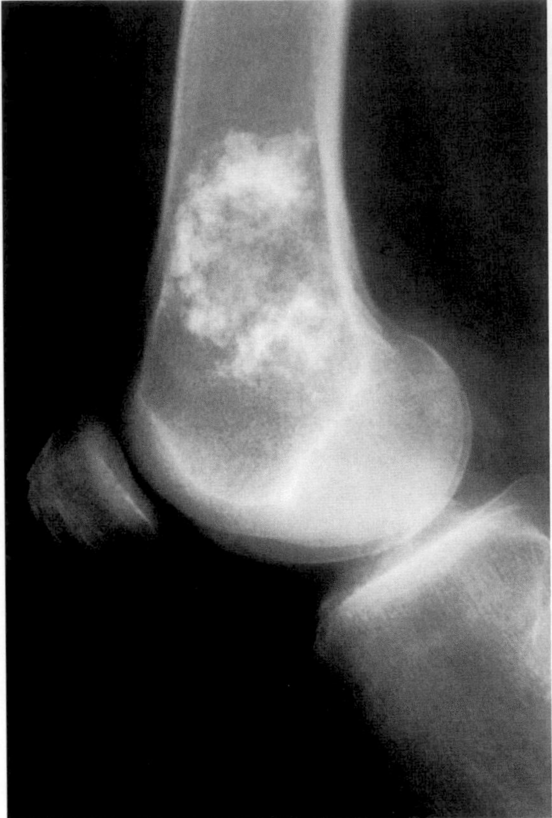

Figure 6–99. Radiograph of a large enchondroma in the distal femur.

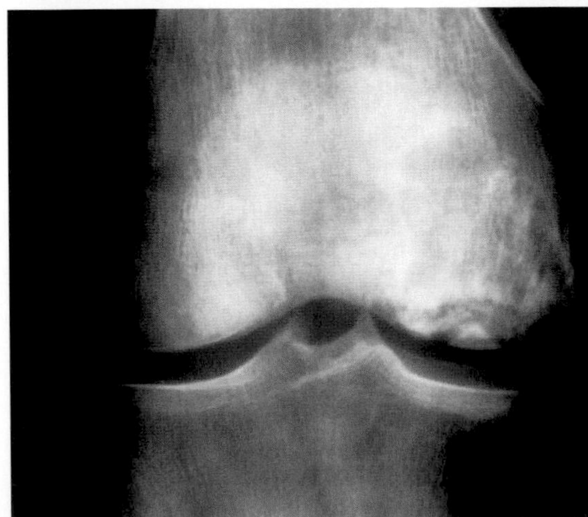

Figure 6–100. Radiograph of an epiphyseal infarct in the femoral condyle of a 45-year-old woman.

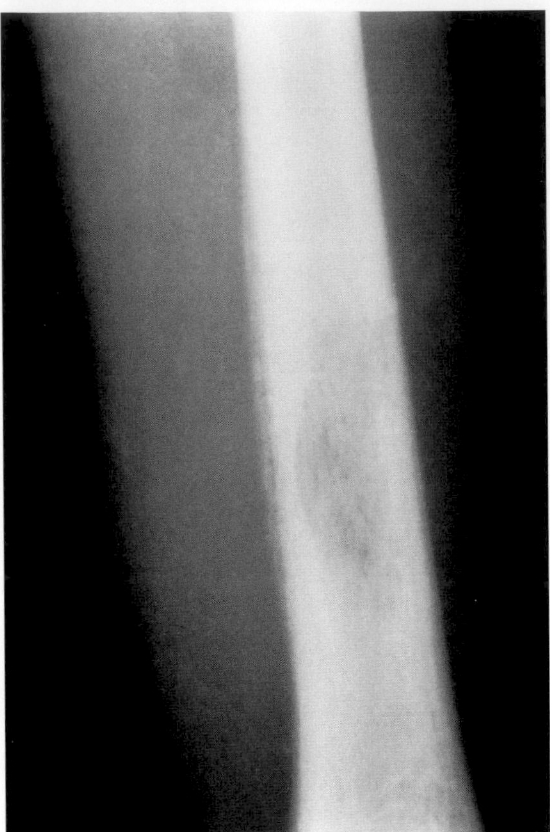

Figure 6–101. Radiograph of an eosinophilic granuloma of the humerus in a 12-year-old boy.

Eosinophilic granulomas tend to involute spontaneously without treatment, and therefore treatment should be conservative. Simple curettement and corticosteroid injections are beneficial. In difficult areas such as the spine or pelvis, low-dose radiation treatment (10 Gy) can be considered. In more disseminated cases that do not respond to simple treatment, low-dose chemotherapy is appropriate.

B. Pigmented Villonodular Synovitis

Although this form of synovitis can mimic a histiocytic tumor, it is thought to be a nonneoplastic condition involving histiocytic proliferation. It occurs in the subsynovial tissue about major joints of the lower extremity in patients between 20 and 40 years of age. The knee joint is the most common site of involvement, followed next by the hip, ankle, and foot. Involvement of the upper extremity is rare.

The histopathology of pigmented villonodular synovitis is similar to that of a giant cell tumor of the tendon

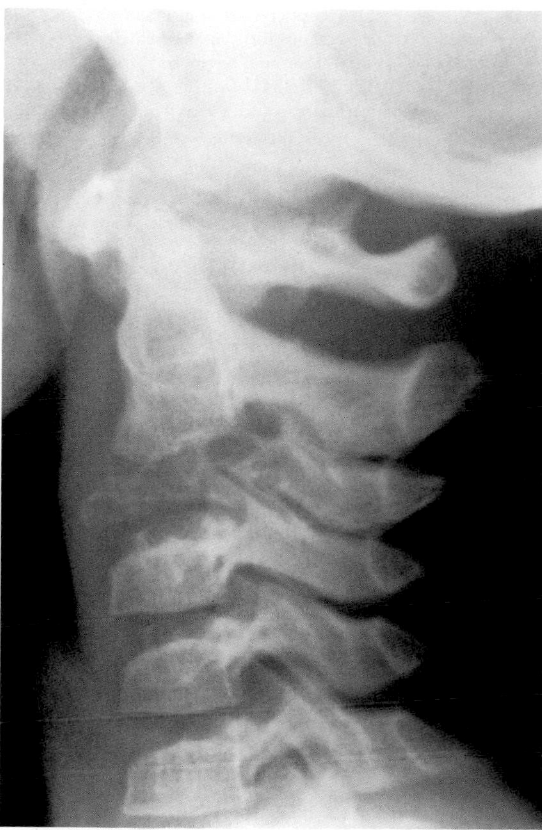

Figure 6–102. Radiograph of an eosinophilic granuloma in the body of the C3 vertebra in a 5-year-old girl.

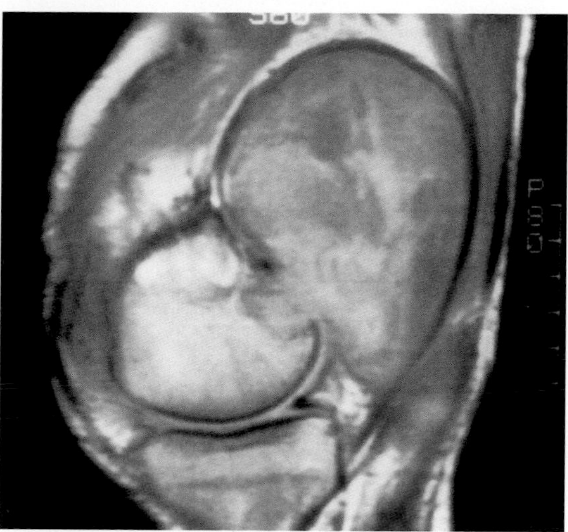

Figure 6–103. T_1-weighted MRI of pigmented villonodular synovitis in the popliteal space of a 50-year-old man.

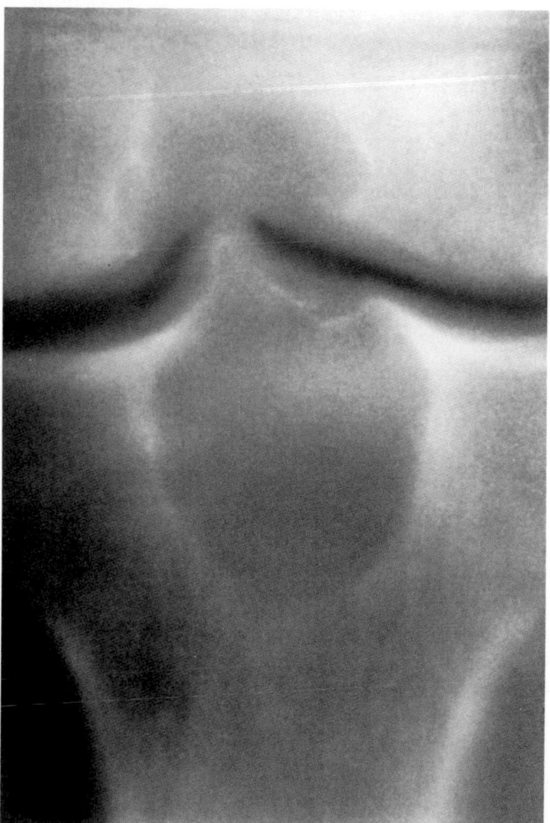

Figure 6–104. Laminagram of pigmented villonodular synovitis in the proximal tibia of a young man.

sheath, which presents with soft-tissue tumors about the ankle and on the fingers of the hand. The usual situation involves spontaneous swelling of one knee secondary to synovial hypertrophy. The swelling can grow gradually to a massive amount and be associated with intermittent hemarthroses. The inflamed synovium can cause juxtaarticular erosion into bone at the point of attachment of the joint capsule, as is seen in any chronic proliferative synovitis, including hemophilia and coccidioidomycosis.

In fewer than 10% of cases, pigmented villonodular synovitis is more localized and presents as a focal soft-tissue mass high in the suprapatellar pouch or in the popliteal space, and no generalized swelling of the knee occurs. In these cases, the mass can mimic a soft-tissue sarcoma such as a synovial sarcoma (Figure 6–103). Cortical erosion with secondary bony changes can also be appreciated frequently (Figure 6–104).

Mankin HJ et al: Gaucher disease. New approaches to an ancient disease. J Bone Joint Surg Am 2001;83-A(5):748. [PMID: 11379747]

Roodman GD: Studies in Paget's disease and their relevance to oncology. Semin Oncol 2001;28(4 Suppl 11):15. [PMID: 11544571]

Shidham V et al: Evaluation of crystals in formalin-fixed, paraffin-embedded tissue sections for the differential diagnosis of pseudogout, gout, and tumoral calcinosis. Mod Pathol 2001; 14(8):806. [PMID: 11504841]

Zelger B: Langerhans cell histiocytosis: A reactive or neoplastic disorder? Med Pediatr Oncol 2001;37(6):543. [PMID: 11745894]

Adult Reconstructive Surgery

7

Robert S. Namba, MD, Harry B. Skinner, MD, PhD, & Ranjan Gupta, MD

Adult reconstructive surgery in orthopedics has rapidly evolved over the past 30 years. Prior to the successful development of so-called low-friction arthroplasty of the hip in the late 1960s, reconstructive options for the hip and the knee were limited. Reconstructive procedures with high success rates are now available for a variety of disorders, from marked degenerative hip disease to rotator cuff tears of the shoulder. Research done in the last 30 years has increased the understanding of major joint function and contributed to the success of reconstructive surgical procedures in almost all cases, and there is now a tremendous demand for these procedures. In 1997, total knee arthroplasty and total hip arthroplasty procedures numbered 338,000 and 289,000, respectively, the result of their great success in returning patients to active lifestyles. Millions of Americans are now benefiting from these procedures for extended periods. Because their cumulative procedure failure rate is approximately 1% per year, 10 years after their operation, patients have approximately a 90% chance of still having a successful, well-functioning joint replacement.

Statistics from American Academy of Orthopedic Surgeons: *Arthroplasty and Total Joint Replacement Procedures in the United States 1990 to 1997.* http://www.aaos.org/wordhtml/press/arthropl.htm

ARTHRITIS & RELATED CONDITIONS

Evaluation of Arthritis

To treat arthritic conditions of the joints appropriately, an understanding of the disease process is essential. This begins with accurate diagnosis and a history of the progression of the disease, so that the future progression can be predicted and appropriate decisions regarding treatment can be made. The physician must evaluate the possibility of traumatic, inflammatory, developmental, idiopathic, and metabolic causes of the arthritis (Table 7–1). Evaluation of the history, physical examination, and laboratory data is helpful in arriving at a diagnosis.

A. History

Clearly the history is important in defining the disease process. The time course, including duration and behavior of symptoms since onset, is a key factor. Gradual rather than acute onset implies a nontraumatic cause. Swelling in the joints is an important sign, as is the distribution of joints if more than one is involved. The degree of interference with activities indicates the seriousness of the disorder.

The presence and extent of pain are valuable pieces of information. Constant pain, night and day, implies infection, cancer, or a functional disorder. Pain only with activity such as walking, standing, or running suggests joint loading. Pain that awakens the patient is considered severe and requires evaluation. Location helps distinguish referred pain from joint pain.

Knowledge of the age distribution of the various arthritic disorders can be very helpful to the student in diagnosing the disease. A hip disorder in the patient under age 40 is unlikely to be OA unless a predisposing condition is present, such as trauma. A more likely diagnosis is osteonecrosis. Similarly, a chronic condition of the knee in the 45-year-old man is likely to be a degenerative meniscus tear, unless the patient had a meniscectomy in his early 20s. This concept can be extended to all age groups for the common disorders of the hip and knee (Figures 7–1 and 7–2). Further, a history of one of these disorders at an earlier age predisposes a patient to earlier osteoarthrosis.

Hip pain is felt typically in the groin or in the lateral aspect of the hip or anterior thigh but seldom in the buttock. Pain arising from the spine may be appreciated in the buttock and less often in the groin and anterior thigh. Acetabular pain or femoral head pain is frequently felt in the groin. Proximal femur pain is usually appreciated in the anteroproximal thigh.

Knee pain is frequently anterior (patellofemoral), medial (medial compartment), or lateral (lateral compartment). It may also be poorly localized by the patient. Pain in the back of the knee may result from a popliteal cyst (Baker cyst) or a torn meniscus. A swol-

Table 7–1. Causes of arthritic conditions.

Traumatic causes	Traumatic arthritis, osteonecrosis (posttraumatic)
Inflammatory causes	Infectious arthritis, gout, pseudogout, rheumatoid arthritis, systemic lupus erythematosus, ankylosing spondylitis, juvenile rheumatoid arthritis, Reiter syndrome
Developmental causes	Developmental dysplasia of the hip, hemophilic arthritis, following slipped capital fermoral epiphysis, following Legg-Calvé-Perthes disease
Idiopathic causes	Osteoarthritis, osteonecrosis
Metabolic causes	Gout, calcium pyrophosphate deposition disease, ochronosis, Gaucher disease

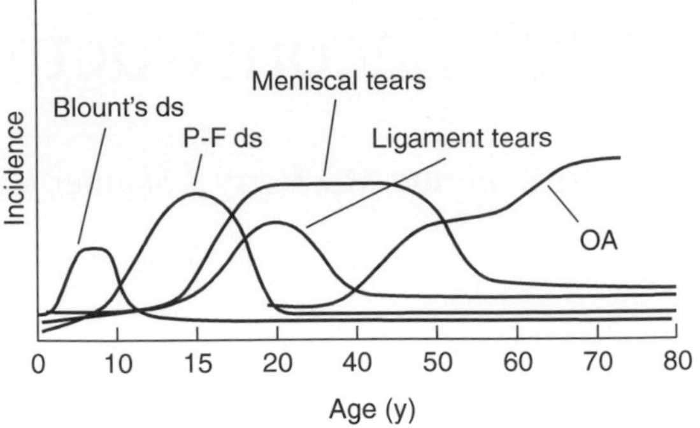

Figure 7–2. The age distribution of knee disorders is given schematically as a function of age. Blount's ds = tibia vara; P-F ds = patellofemoral arthralgia; and OA = osteoarthrosis. Meniscal tears can be either medial or lateral and are traumatic in the younger age group and degenerative in the older age group. Osteoarthrosis shows an earlier onset with the knee than with the hip because there is an incidence of medial gonarthrosis in the 40s and 50s caused by medial meniscectomy in the late teens and early 20s.

len knee may be painful because of pressure. Pain with any motion may indicate a septic joint or possibly a gouty joint. Arthritic pain in the elbow and shoulder is less clearly defined by patients, and in such cases the physical examination is important. Shoulder pain may be caused by cervical, cardiac, or even diaphragmatic disorders.

B. Physical Examination

1. Hip—The physical examination of the hip is important to verify that the reported pain arises from the hip joint and to determine the severity of the pain. It is also useful to document range of motion (ROM), gait, leg-length discrepancy, and muscle weakness. Pain arising from the hip is typically elicited at the extremes of ROM. Active straight leg raising or resisted straight leg raising may produce pain (Figure 7–3). Log rolling (internal and external rotation of the hip in extension) usually elicits hip pain if pain is severe. Frequently, internal rotation of the hip in flexion is limited; this condition is one of the first signs of osteoarthritis (OA) of the hip. Abduction of the hip against gravity loads the hip and may produce hip pain of arthritis, but does not do so if pain in the buttock or thigh is referred from the spine. Increased loading may be achieved by applying resistance to abduction. In the young (under age 40) patient with groin pain, provocative maneuvers can be used to diagnose labral tears. Flexion of the hip with external rotation (ER) and abduction (ABD) is followed by extension, adduction (ADD), and internal rotation (IR). Clicking or catching is observed in patients with anterior labral tears. Posterior tears of the labrum are identified by moving the hip from extension, ABD, and ER to flexion, ADD, and IR.

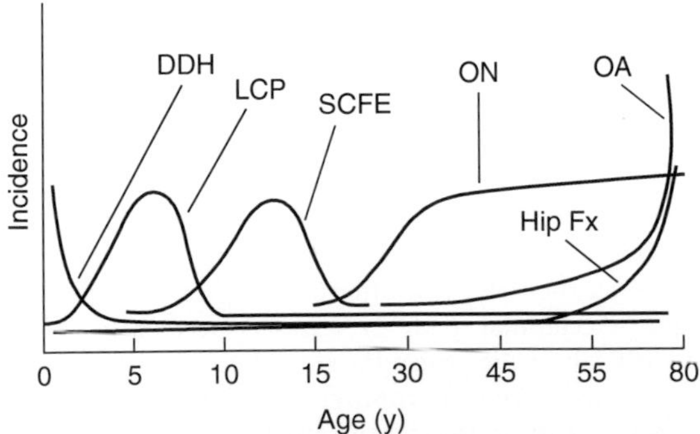

Figure 7–1. The age distribution of hip disorders is given in a schematic representation. DDH = developmental dysplasia of the hip; LCP = Legg-Calvé-Perthes disease; SCFE = slipped capital femoral epiphysis; ON = osteonecrosis; OA = osteoarthrosis; and Hip Fx = hip fracture.

The ROM in flexion, extension (flexion contracture), ABD, ADD, and IR and ER is measured. Decreased IR is an early finding in OA.

2. Knee—The physical examination of the knee localizes the pain to the knee and to the specific involved compartment. ROM of the hip should be evaluated to rule out referred hip pain. Ligamentous stability is discerned in the mediolateral and anteroposterior (AP) planes (see Chapter 4). Instability is not common in osteoarthritis but is often seen in rheumatoid arthritis.

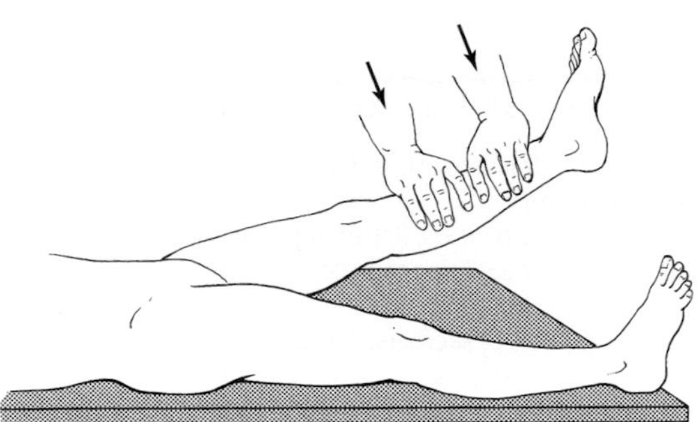

Figure 7–3. Resisted straight leg–raising test. The examiner asks the patient to actively raise the straight leg to approximately 30 degrees. This produces hip pain in severe arthritis. If no pain is produced, the examiner applies pressure to the thigh, which the patient resists. This increased joint loading uncovers mild to moderate hip pain.

Alignment of the knee (varus or valgus) while standing is measured. Varus and valgus alignment increase the odds of progression of OA fourfold and fivefold, respectively, in 18 months. ROM of the knee is measured, and any flexion contracture or extensor lag is noted. Flexion contracture is an inability to come to full extension passively, whereas an extensor lag indicates an inability to extend the knee actively as far as it will extend passively. The contracture is common in advanced OA, whereas the lag is generally a quadriceps muscle or tendon problem. The medial and lateral compartments are loaded during flexion and extension with varus and valgus stress, respectively, to elicit pain arising from arthritis in each compartment. The patellofemoral joint may be assessed for pain and bone-on-bone crepitation by flexion and extension with pressure on the patella. The presence of fluid, synovitis, and erythema is also important.

3. Shoulder—After the cervical spine is ruled out as the source of pain, examination of the shoulder begins with visual inspection for obvious asymmetry of bone and muscle contours. Palpation of muscle tone and of the clavicle, as well as the acromioclavicular and sternoclavicular joints, follows. Tenderness over the anterolateral humeral head is often found with rotator cuff disorders. Tendinitis of the long head of the biceps is easily demonstrated by palpation of the tendon over the anteromedial humeral head. Active ROM is then assessed in flexion and abduction. External rotation is reproducibly measured by keeping the elbow on the waist and rotating the hand away from the body. Internal rotation is best recorded by measuring how high the thumb can be positioned along the spine. Most individuals can position the thumb to the midthoracic area (eg, T6 or T7). When internal rotation is limited, the thumb may only be elevated to L5. If active ROM is at all limited, passive ROM should be assessed. Strength of the upper extremity muscle is then evaluated along with sensation and deep tendon reflexes. Decreased strength in external rotation with the elbow at the side indicates significant rotator cuff weakness. Provocative tests can help evaluate the cause of pain, particularly with instability. The apprehension test is positive, indicating anterior instability, when abduction, extension, and external rotation of the shoulder elicit anxiety or discomfort. Impingement signs are present with rotator cuff disorders and produce pain with passive flexion or internal rotation of the flexed and adducted arm.

4. Elbow—Inspection of the elbow includes measurement of the "carrying angle," the normal 5–7 degree angle of valgus inclination between the humerus and forearm. Scars and obvious deformities are noted, as well as swelling or masses. Bony prominences are palpated, including the mediolateral epicondyles, radial head, and olecranon. Active and passive motion is recorded for both flexion and extension and pronation and supination. Tenderness over the lateral epicondyle exacerbated by resisted wrist dorsiflexion is often seen in lateral epicondylitis (tennis elbow). Tenderness over the medial epicondyle with pain elicited by resisted wrist flexion is seen in medial epicondylitis. Limitation of flexion and extension is seen with arthritis and posttraumatic stiffness.

C. Imaging Studies

Radiologic data, synovial fluid analysis, and blood testing may be beneficial in confirming the diagnosis of arthritis. The most fundamental radiographic data can be provided by a plain radiograph with a minimum of two views. Evaluation of joint pain includes ruling out fracture, joint space narrowing, osteophyte formation, or osteopenia. Views of the hip include a modified AP view of the pelvis (which clips the iliac wings to show the proximal femora) and a lateral view of the affected hip (either "frog," an AP view with the hip externally rotated and abducted, or a true lateral view). Views of the knee should include a 10 degrees down-angled beam posteroanterior radiograph of the bent knee (30–45 degrees of flexion) taken while the patient is standing, a lateral view, and a tangential patellar view (Merchant view, 45 degrees of flexion) (Table 7–2). Views of the shoulder should include AP, axillary, and lateral views of the scapula. Supraspinatus outlet views may be helpful in revealing acromial bone spurs, which produce impingement. The elbow usually can be visualized with AP and lateral radiographs.

D. Laboratory Findings

Basic blood testing should include a complete blood count and sedimentation rate. These are indicated in a suspected septic process or in the evaluation of a painful

Table 7–2. Radiographic findings in arthritis.

Disease State	Findings in Hip or Knee
Osteoarthritis	Joint space narrowing, subchondral sclerosis, osteophytes, subchondral cysts Hip: Superior or medial narrowing Knee: Early narrowing on Rosenberg views; flattening of femoral condyles
Rheumatoid arthritis or sytemic lupus erythematosus	Uniform joint narrowing, erosion near joint capsule
Ankylosing spondylitis	Osteopenia, osteophytes, ankylosis of sacroiliac joints
Gout	Tophi, erosions
Calcium pyrophosphate deposition disease	Calcification of menisci and hyaline cartilage
Osteonecrosis	Crescent sign, spotty calcification
Gaucher disease	Erlenmeyer flask appearance, distal femora
Neuropathic joint	Four *Ds*: destruction, debris, dislocation, densification (sclerosis, hypertrophy)
Hemophilic arthropathy	Epiphyseal widening, sclerosis, cysts, joint space narrowing

joint replacement. A normal white cell count may be helpful in the diagnosis of gout, especially in an inflamed joint other than the first metatarsophalangeal joint.

Synovial fluid analysis is indicated at any time to rule out infection, and it may also be quite helpful in the diagnosis of other arthritides. Table 8–4 shows the significance of yellow and clear synovial fluid. Aspiration of synovial fluid may reveal hemorrhagic fluid. If this is the result of a traumatic tap, it should be so noted and the fluid should be sent for analysis. If the fluid is grossly hemorrhagic, several diagnoses must be entertained, including hemophilia, neuropathic arthropathy, pigmented villonodular synovitis, hemangioma, or trauma. A finding of fat floating on the bloody fluid in the setting of a traumatic injury suggests the presence of an intraarticular fracture.

The combined history, physical examination, and appropriate laboratory studies should narrow the diagnoses to a relative few, if not the definitive one. It is helpful to consider diagnoses in categories, which, despite some overlap, provide a framework for further workup. Many of these arthritic conditions are described in the following pages.

Sharma L et al: The role of knee alignment in disease progression and functional decline in knee osteoarthritis. JAMA 2001; 286:188.

Solomon DH et al: Does this patient have a torn meniscus or ligament of the knee? Value of physical exam of the knee. JAMA 2001;286:1610.

1. Noninflammatory Arthritis

The term **osteoarthritis** is a misnomer, because inflammation is not the primary pathologic process observed in this form of articular joint disruption. More accurately described as degenerative joint disease, the disease represents a final common pathway of injury to articular cartilage. Although the true nature and cause of OA are unclear, radiographic findings and gross and microscopic pathologic features are fairly typical in most cases.

Categorization of primary and secondary forms of OA, although still useful, are blurred. A designation of primary or idiopathic OA was made when no identifiable predisposing conditions could be recognized. OA is considered secondary when an underlying cause such as trauma, previous deformity, or systemic disorder exists. Although many cases of hip OA were considered idiopathic when the end-stage changes were observed, careful analysis indicated predisposing conditions such as slipped capital femoral epiphysis and mild forms of acetabular dysplasia in many cases.

The joints most commonly involved include the hip; knee; distal interphalangeal, proximal interphalangeal, and first carpometacarpal joints of the hand; and cervical, thoracic, and lumbar spine.

Primary Osteoarthritis

A. Epidemiologic Features

OA is a widespread joint disorder in the United States, significantly affecting approximately 40 million people. Though autopsy studies show degenerative changes of weight-bearing joints in 90% of people older than 40 years, clinical symptoms are usually not present. The prevalence and severity of OA increase with age.

When all ages are considered, men and women are equally affected. Younger than 45 years, the disease is more prevalent in men; older than 55 years, women are more commonly afflicted. The pattern of joint involvement commonly includes the joints of the hands and knees in women and the hip joints in men.

The incidence of hip OA is higher in European and American white males than in Chinese, South African blacks, and East Indian persons. Primary hip OA in Japanese persons is rare, but secondary OA is common because of developmental dysplasia of the hip.

Evidence indicates that some distinct forms of OA may be inherited as a dominant trait with a mendelian pattern. These include a primary generalized OA in which Heberden nodes and Bouchard nodes are a prominent feature, and symmetric and uniform loss of articular cartilage of the knee and hip joints is evident. Other types of inherited OA include familial chondrocalcinosis (with deposition of calcium pyrophosphate dihydrate crystals in cartilage), Stickler syndrome (characterized by vitreoretinal degeneration), hydroxyapatite deposition disease, and multiple epiphyseal dysplasias. Certain inherited forms are caused by mutations in the gene for cartilage-specific type II procollagen.

B. Pathologic Features

Early features of OA include focal swelling and softening of the cartilage matrix. Mild loss of metachromatic staining ability represents loss of proteoglycans in the extracellular matrix. Surface irregularities in the form of fibrillation occur. Diffuse hypercellularity of the chondrocytes can be seen. The tidemark, an interface plane between hyaline cartilage and the zone of calcified cartilage, is thin and wavy early in OA.

Later features of OA include progressive loss of proteoglycans manifesting as reduction in safranin-O staining. Fibrillations in the surface deepen into fissures and later into deeper clefts. Chondrocyte cloning is seen and also reduplication of the tidemark, with discontinuous parallel lines indicating progression of calcification of the basal portion of the articular cartilage. Regions of eburnated bone represent complete loss of cartilage.

New bone formation occurs in a subchondral location as well as at margins of the articular cartilage. Areas of rarefaction of bone below eburnation are represented by "cysts" on radiographs and on gross inspection.

C. Laboratory Findings

Specific diagnostic tests for OA are currently not available. Routine blood tests, urinalysis, and even synovial fluid analysis do not provide useful information, except for exclusion of inflammatory or infectious arthritis. Experimental work on identification of markers of cartilage degradation in OA may provide diagnostic tests in the future. These include sensitive and specific assays for synovial fluid cytokines, proteinases and their inhibitors, matrix components and their fragments, serum antibodies to cartilage collagen, and identification of proteoglycan subpopulations.

D. Imaging Studies

Typical radiographic features indicate late pathologic changes in OA. Specifically, narrowing of the joint space, subchondral sclerosis, bony cysts, and marginal osteophytes are seen. End-stage disease is complicated by bony erosions, subluxation, loose bodies, and deformity.

Heberden nodes are commonly seen in primary OA, represented by bony and cartilaginous enlargement of the distal interphalangeal joints of the fingers. Similar enlargements of the proximal interphalangeal joints of the fingers are called **Bouchard nodes.**

Secondary Osteoarthritis

The term **secondary osteoarthritis** is applied when an underlying recognizable local or systemic factor exists. These include conditions leading to joint deformity or destruction of cartilage, followed by signs and symptoms typically seen with primary OA. Examples of preexisting conditions leading to secondary osteoarthritic changes in joints include acute and chronic trauma, Legg-Calvé-Perthes disease, developmental dysplasia of the hip, rheumatoid arthritis, bleeding dyscrasias, achondroplasia, infection, crystal deposition disease, neuropathic disorders, overuse of intraarticular steroids, and multiple epiphyseal dysplasias. Radiographic features of secondary OA reflect the underlying pathologic changes plus the changes resulting from the primary OA.

Bjell A: Cartilage matrix in hereditary pyrophosphate arthropathy. J Rheumatol 1981;8:959.

Hoaglund FT, Steinbach LS: Primary osteoarthritis of the hip: Etiology and epidemiology. J Am Acad Orthop Surg 2001;9(5):320.

Kellgren JH et al: Genetic factors in generalized osteoarthrosis. Ann Rheum Dis 1963;22:237.

Knowlton RG et al: Genetic linkage analysis of hereditary arthro-ophthalmopathy and the type II procollagen gene. Am J Hum Genet 1989;65:681.

Lawrence RC et al: Estimates of the prevalence of arthritis and selected musculoskeletal disorders in the United States. Arthritis Rheum 1999;42(2):396.

Lowman EW: Osteoarthritis. JAMA 1955;157:487.

Marcos JC et al: Idiopathic familial chondrocalcinosis due to apatite crystal deposition. Am J Med 1981;71:557.

Mukhopadhaya B, Barooah B: Osteoarthritis of hip in Indians. Indian J Orthop 1975;1:55.

Palotie A et al: Predisposition to familial osteoarthrosis linked to type II collagen gene. Lancet 1989;1:924.

Reginato AJ: Articular chondrocalcinosis in the Chiloé islanders. Arthritis Rheum 1976;19:396.

Solomon L et al: Rheumatic disorders in the southern African Negro. S Afr Med J 1975;49:1737.

Spranger J: The epiphyseal dysplasias. Clin Orthop 1975;114:46.

Stickler GB et al: Hereditary progressive arthro-ophthalmopathy. Mayo Clin Proc 1965;40:433.

2. Inflammatory Arthritis

Rheumatoid Arthritis

A chronic systemic inflammatory disorder, rheumatoid arthritis (RA) is a crippling disease affecting approximately 1% of the population in the United States. Although similar synovial histopathologic and joint abnormalities are identifiable in all patients, the articular and systemic manifestations, outcomes, and differences in genetic makeup and serologic findings vary widely in individual patients. The cause is unknown, although the disease probably occurs in response to a pathogenic agent in a genetically predisposed host. Possible triggering factors include bacterial, mycoplasmal, or viral infections, as well as endogenous antigens in the form of rheumatoid factor, collagens, and mucopolysaccharides.

Joint involvement is typically symmetric, affecting the wrist, metacarpal, phalangeal, proximal, interphalangeal elbow, shoulder, cervical spine, hip, knee, and ankle joints. The distal interphalangeal joints are typically spared. Extraarticular manifestations include vasculitis, pericarditis, skin nodules, pulmonary fibrosis, pneumonitis, and scleritis. The triad of arthritis, lymphadenopathy, and splenomegaly, known as **Felty syndrome,** is associated with anemia, thrombocytopenia, and neutropenia.

A. Epidemiologic Features

RA occurs two to four times more often in women than men. The disease occurs in all age groups, but increases in incidence with advancing age, with a peak between the fourth and sixth decades.

Evidence for a genetic basis is provided by the association of RA with a certain haplotype of class II gene products of the major histocompatibility complex. Seventy-five percent of patients with RA carry circulating rheumatoid factors, which are autoantibodies against portions of the IgG antibody. In rheumatoid factor–positive patients, there is a high incidence of HLA-DR4, except in black patients. Only a minority of individuals with HLA-DR4 develop RA, however. (See Chapter 13, especially Tables 13–5 and 13–6.)

B. Pathologic Features

Early rheumatoid synovitis consists of a local inflammatory response with accumulation of mononuclear cells. The antigen-presenting cell (macrophage) activates T lymphocytes, resulting in cytokine production, B-cell proliferation, and antibody formation. Chronic inflammation results in formation of a pannus, a thickened synovium filled with activated T and B lymphocytes and plasma cells, as well as fibroblastic and macrophagic types of synovial cells. Joint destruction begins with exposed bone at the margins of articular cartilage denuded of hyaline cartilage. Eventually, the cartilage itself is destroyed by inflammatory byproducts of the pannus. The synovial fluid, in contrast to the mononuclear cell infiltrate seen in the synovial membrane, has neutrophils forming 75–85% of the cells.

Rheumatoid factors are antibodies specific to antigens on the Fc fragment of IgG. The antibodies include IgM, IgG, IgA, and IgE classes, but the IgM rheumatoid factor is typically measured. Rheumatoid factor may be a triggering factor for RA and may contribute to the chronic nature of the disease. Rheumatoid factor is also frequently found in patients with other inflammatory diseases, however, as well as in 1–5% of normal patients.

C. Laboratory Findings

No specific laboratory test exists for RA, but a series of test results help in the diagnosis. A high titer of rheumatoid factor (more than 1:160) is the most significant diagnostic finding. Anemia is moderate, and leukocyte counts are normal or mildly elevated. Acute-phase reactants reflect the degree of inflammation nonspecifically and are often elevated in RA. These include the erythrocyte sedimentation rate (ESR) and levels of C-reactive protein and serum immune complexes. Antinuclear antibodies are often positive in patients with severe RA (up to 37% in one study) but are not specific for the disease.

D. Imaging Studies

Early radiographic changes in RA include swelling of the small peripheral joints and marginal bony erosions. Joint space narrowing occurs later and is uniform, unlike the focal narrowing seen in OA. Regional osteoporosis occurs, unlike the sclerosis seen in OA. Advanced changes include bone resorption, deformity, dislocation, and fragmentation of affected joints. Protrusio acetabuli may be seen in the hips, and ulnar subluxation is common in the metacarpophalangeal joints.

Lipsky PE et al: The role of cytokines in the pathogeneis of rheumatoid arthritis. Springer Semin Immunopathol 1989;11:123. [PMID: 2479111]

Saulsbury FT: Prevalence of IgM, IgA, and IgG rheumatoid factors in juvenile rheumatoid arthritis. Clin Exp Rheumatol 1990;8:513. [PMID: 2261713]

Sutton B et al: The structure and origin of rheumatoid factors. Immunol Today 2001;21:177.

Winchester RG: Genetic aspects of rheumatoid arthritis. Springer Semin Immunopathol 1981;4:89.

Zvaifler NJ: Etiology and pathogenesis of rheumatoid arthritis. In McCarty DJ, ed: *Arthritis and Allied Conditions.* Lea & Febiger, 1989.

Ankylosing Spondylitis

A seronegative (negative rheumatoid factor) inflammatory arthritis, ankylosing spondylitis consists of bilateral sacroiliitis with or without associated spondylitis and uveitis. An insidious disease, the diagnosis is often delayed because of vagueness of the early symptom of low back pain. Diagnostic clinical criteria include low back pain, limited lumbar spine motion, decreased chest expansion, and sacroiliitis.

Joint involvement is primarily axial, including all portions of the spine, sacroiliac joint, and hip joints. Extraskeletal involvement includes dilation of the aorta, anterior uveitis, and restrictive lung disease secondary to restriction of thoracic cage mobility.

A. Epidemiologic Features

The association of HLA-B27 and ankylosing spondylitis is strong, with 90% of patients testing positive for this haplotype; however, only 2% of HLA-B27-positive patients develop ankylosing spondylitis. First-degree family members of a patient who has ankylosing spondylitis and is positive for HLA-B27 have a 20% risk of developing the disease. Clinical and experimental evidence shows that *Klebsiella* infection may be a triggering factor for arthritis in patients positive for HLA-B27.

B. Laboratory Findings

During the active phase of the disease, the ESR is increased. Testing for rheumatoid factor and antinuclear antibodies is negative.

C. Imaging Studies

Early in the course of ankylosing spondylitis, the sacroiliac joints may be widened, reflecting bony erosions of the iliac side of the joint. Later, the inflamed cartilage is replaced by ossification, resulting in ankylosis of the bilateral sacroiliac joints. Vertebrae of the thoracolumbar spine are squared off, with bridging syndesmophytes, forming a so-called bamboo spine. Ankylosis of peripheral joints may be seen. MRI may provide sensitive and specific radiographic evidence of sacroiliitis.

Ebringer RW et al: Sequential studies in ankylosing spondylitis: Association of *Klebsiella pneumoniae* with active disease. Ann Rheum Dis 1978;37:146.

Geczy AF et al: A factor in *Klebsiella* filtrates specifically modifies an HLA-B27 associated cell-surface component. Nature 1980; 283:782.

Luong AA, Salonen DC: Imaging of the seronegative spondyloarthropathies. Curr Rheumatol Rep 2000;2(4):288.

Moll JMH, Wright V: New York clinical criteria for ankylosing spondylitis: A statistical evaluation. Ann Rheum Dis 1973; 32:354.

Van der Linden S et al: The risk of developing ankylosing spondylitis in HLA-B27 positive individuals: A family and population study. Br J Rheum 1983;22(Suppl):18.

Psoriatic Arthritis

A seronegative inflammatory arthritis associated with psoriasis, psoriatic arthritis was long considered a variant of RA. The discovery of rheumatoid factor led to the division of inflammatory arthritides into seropositive and seronegative diseases, separating psoriatic arthritis from RA.

Although psoriatic arthritis is characterized by a relatively benign course in most patients, up to 20% develop severe joint involvement. The distal interphalangeal joints of the fingers are commonly affected, but several patterns of peripheral arthritis exist, including an asymmetric oligoarthritis, a symmetric polyarthritis (similar to RA), arthritis mutilans (a destructive, deforming type of arthritis), and a spondyloarthropathy (similar to ankylosing spondylitis, with sacroiliac joint involvement).

In addition to the dry erythematous papular skin lesions, nail changes are found. These include pitting, grooves, subungual hyperkeratosis, and destruction.

A. Epidemiologic Features

A third of patients with psoriasis have arthritis, with joint symptoms delayed as long as 20 years after onset of skin lesions. Both sexes are affected equally.

B. Laboratory Findings

There are no specific laboratory tests for psoriatic arthritis. Nonspecific inflammatory markers may be elevated, including the ESR. Rheumatoid factor is usually negative but is present in up to 10% of patients.

C. Imaging Studies

Coexistence of erosive changes and bone formation is seen in peripheral joints, with absence of periarticular osteoporosis. Gross destruction of phalangeal joints (so-called pencil-in-cup appearance) and lysis of terminal phalanges are seen. Bilateral sacroiliac joint ankylosis and syndesmophytes of the spine are seen, as in ankylosing spondylitis.

Gladman DD et al: HLA antigens in psoriatic arthritis. J Rheum 1986;13:586.

Hohler T, Marker-Hermann E: Psoriatic arthritis: Clinical aspects, genetics, and the role of T cells. Curr Opin Rheumatol 2001;13(4):273.

Mader R, Gladman D: Psoriatic arthritis: Making the diagnosis and treating early. J Musculoskel Med 1993;10:18.

Juvenile Rheumatoid Arthritis

Juvenile rheumatoid arthritis (JRA) is an inflammatory arthritic syndrome with a variety of symptoms. Early diagnosis is often difficult. Criteria for JRA include distinction of mode of onset as systemic, polyarticular, or pauciarticular. Systemic onset (also known as **Still disease**) occurs in 20% of patients and is characterized by high fever, rash, lymphadenopathy, splenomegaly, carditis, and varying degrees of arthritis. Polyarticular onset occurs in 30–40% of patiemnts and is notable for fewer systemic symptoms, low-grade fever, and synovitis of four or more joints. Pauciarticular onset develops in 40–50% of patients and involves one to four joints; there are no systemic signs, but there is an increased incidence of iridocyclitis. Iridocyclitis is an insidious complication that requires early ophthalmologic slit-lamp evaluation, if JRA is suspected, to prevent blindness.

A. Epidemiologic Features

The two peak ages of onset are between 1 and 3 years and between 8 and 12 years. Females are affected twice as often as males.

B. Laboratory Findings

Leukocytosis up to 30,000/mL is seen with systemic-onset JRA, with mild elevations in polyarticular-onset disease and normal values in pauciarticular-onset disease. White blood cell counts in synovial fluid range from 150 to 50,000/mL. The ESR rate is elevated, as are other acute-phase reactants.

Rheumatoid factor is typically negative in JRA. As many as 50% of patients have positive antinuclear antibodies, a finding correlated with iridocyclitis and pauciarticular-onset disease.

C. Imaging Studies

Soft-tissue swelling and premature closure of physes may be seen early, as well as juxtaarticular osteopenia. Erosive changes are seen late and resemble those of RA.

Falcini F, Cimaz R: Juvenile rheumatoid arthritis. Curr Opin Rheumatol 2000;12(5):415.

Schaller JG: The association of antinuclear antibodies with the chronic iridocyclitis of juvenile rheumatoid arthritis. Arthritis Rheum 1974;17:409.

Systemic Lupus Erythematosus

Systemic lupus erythematosus (SLE) is a chronic inflammatory disease that may affect multiple organ systems. It is an autoimmune disorder in which autoantibodies are formed. The large variety of clinical appearances and laboratory findings may mimic many disorders. The diagnosis is based on the presence of 4 of the following 11 criteria: (1) malar rash; (2) discoid rash; (3) photosensitivity; (4) oral ulcers; (5) arthritis; (6) serositis; (7) renal disorders (proteinuria or casts); (8) neurologic disorders (seizures or psychosis); (9) hematologic disorders (hemolytic anemia, leukopenia, lymphopenia, thrombocytopenia); (10) immunologic disorders (positive lupus erythematosus [LE] cell preparation, anti-DNA antibody, anti-Sm antibody, false-positive serologic test for syphilis); and (11) abnormal titer of antinuclear antibody.

A. Epidemiologic Features

Females are affected eight times as often as males. An increased risk for SLE is noted for Asians and Polynesians over whites in Hawaii. Black females are also associated with an increased risk over white females. Genetic susceptibility is demonstrated with increased frequency (5%) among relatives of patients with the disease. An inherited complement deficiency is inferred from the absence, or near absence, of individual complement components, the most common being C2.

B. Laboratory Findings

Antinuclear antibody determination is the most helpful screening test for SLE. The LE cell preparation was the first immunologic test for SLE, but it is laborious, insensitive, and difficult to interpret. In patients with untreated active disease, 98% have positive antinuclear antibody tests. The higher the titer of antinuclear antibodies, the more likely is the diagnosis of SLE or related rheumatic syndrome. A low value for the antinuclear antibody test is 1:320; values greater than 1:5120 are considered high.

If antinuclear antibody levels are positive, more specific tests may be performed, including testing for anti-DNA antibodies, antibodies to extractable nuclear antigens, and complement levels. High titers of antibodies to double-stranded DNA are highly suggestive for SLE. Low complement levels (C3, C4, and total hemolytic complement levels) are found in the disease but are also seen in related illnesses.

Anemia, leukopenia, and thrombocytopenia are seen, as well as elevations in the ESR. Renal function tests and muscle and liver enzyme tests are often abnormal, reflecting multiple organ system involvement.

C. Imaging Studies

The radiographic features of arthritis in SLE are similar to those of RA. Much of the joint pain may be related to osteonecrosis, particularly of the femoral and humeral heads.

Agnello V: Association of systemic lupus erythematosus and systemic lupus erythematosus-like syndromes with hereditary and acquired complement deficient states. Arthritis Rheum 1978;21:S146.

Block SR et al: Immunologic observations on 9 sets of twins either concordant or discordant for systemic lupus erythematosus. Arthritis Rheum 1976;19:545.

Kaine JL, Kahl LE: Which laboratory tests are useful in diagnosing SLE? J Musculoskel Med 1992;9:15.

Serdula MK, Rhoads GG: Frequency of systemic lupus erythematosus in different ethnic groups in Hawaii. Arthritis Rheum 1979;22:328.

Tan EM et al: Revised criteria for classification of systemic lupus erythematosus: ARA subcommittee. Arthritis Rheum 1982; 25:1271.

Arthritis Associated with Inflammatory Bowel Disease

Peripheral arthritis and spondylitis are associated with ulcerative colitis and Crohn disease. Joint involvement is typically monarticular or oligoarticular and often parallels the activity of the bowel disease. The arthritis, frequently migratory, is self-limiting in most cases, with only 10% of patients having chronic arthritis. The joints most commonly affected are the knees, hips, and ankles, in order of prevalence. Spondylitis associated with inflammatory bowel disease occurs in two forms. One is very similar to ankylosing spondylitis, including the increased incidence of the HLA-B27 haplotype. The other form has no identifiable genetic predisposition.

A. Epidemiologic Features

Up to 25% of patients with inflammatory bowel disease develop arthritis. There is no difference between the sexes in incidence.

B. Laboratory Findings

There is no specific diagnostic test. Synovial fluid analysis reveals an inflammatory process, with leukocyte counts of 4000–50,000/mL.

C. Imaging Studies

Peripheral arthritis is nonerosive, with juxtaarticular osteopenia and joint space narrowing. Spondylitis associated with inflammatory bowel disease resembles ankylosing spondylitis.

Enlow RW et al: The spondylitis of inflammatory bowel disease. Arthritis Rheum 1980;23:1359.

Morris RI et al: HLA-B27, a useful discriminator in the arthropathy of inflammatory bowel disease. N Engl J Med 1974; 290:1117.

Wollheim FA: Enteropathic arthritis: How do the joints talk with the gut? Curr Opin Rheumatol 2001:13(4):305.

Reiter Syndrome

The classic triad of conjunctivitis, urethritis, and peripheral arthritis is known as **Reiter syndrome. Reactive arthritis** is becoming accepted as a more precise term because the initiating condition may be enteritis as well as a sexually transmitted disease. The peripheral arthritis is polyarticular and asymmetric, with knees, ankles, and foot joints most commonly affected.

A. Epidemiologic Features

Nongonococcal urethritis caused by *Chlamydia* accounts for the precipitating event in approximately 20% of cases. Patients who test positive for HLA-B27 are predisposed to developing arthritis after contracting nongonococcal urethritis. A reactive arthritis following enteric infection with *Salmonella, Shigella, Yersinia,* and *Campylobacter* is also noted. For enteric infections with *Shigella,* the risk of developing arthritis in individuals positive for HLA-B27 is close to 20%.

B. Laboratory Findings

There are no specific diagnostic tests for Reiter syndrome. Anemia, leukocytosis, and thrombocytosis occur, and the ESR is often elevated.

C. Imaging Studies

The radiographic features of Reiter syndrome are similar to those of ankylosing spondylitis, with calcifications of ligamentous insertions and ankylosing of joints. The sacroiliitis is unilateral, unlike in ankylosing spondylitis.

Bradshaw CS et al: Etiologies of nongonococcal urethritis, bacteria, viruses, and the association with orogenital exposure. J Infect Dis 2006;193:366. [PMID: 16388480]

Caelin A, Fries JF: An "experimental" epidemic of Reiter's syndrome revisited: Follow-up evidence on genetic and environmental factors. Ann Intern Med 1976;85:563.

Ford DK: Reiter's syndrome: Reactive arthritis. In McCarty DJ, ed: *Arthritis and Allied Conditions.* Lea and Febiger, 1989.

Grayston JT, Wan SP: New knowledge of chlamydiae and the diseases they cause. J Infect Dis 1975;132:87.

3. Metabolic Arthropathy

Gout

Deposition of monosodium urate crystals in the joints produces gout. Although most patients with gout have hyperuricemia, few patients with hyperuricemia develop gout. The causes of hyperuricemia include disorders resulting in overproduction or undersecretion of uric acid or a combination of these two abnormalities. Examples of uric acid overproduction include enzymatic mutations, leukemias, hemoglobinopathies, and excessive purine intake.

The first attack involves sudden onset of painful arthritis, most often in the first metatarsophalangeal joint, but also in the ankle, knee, wrist, finger, and elbow. The intensity of the pain is comparable to that from a septic joint, and differentiation is necessary because the treatment is different. Coexistence of a septic joint is unusual but possible. Rapid resolution with colchicine or indomethacin is seen. Chronic gouty arthritis is notable for tophaceous deposits, joint deformity, constant pain, and swelling. Definitive diagnosis is made upon demonstration of intracellular monosodium urate crystals in synovial cell leukocytes.

A. Epidemiologic Features

Primary gout has hereditary features, with a familial incidence of 6–18%. It is likely that the serum urate concentration is controlled by multiple genes.

B. Laboratory Findings

The key diagnostic test is detection of monosodium urate crystals in white blood cells in synovial fluid. Negative birefringence of the needle-shaped crystals is seen by their yellow coloration on polarized light microscopy.

Hyperuricemia is usually seen, but up to a fourth of gout patients may have normal uric acid levels. Uric acid levels are elevated when they exceed 7 mg/dL. An elevated white blood cell count and sedimentation rate can be seen in acute gout, and thus these tests cannot be used to differentiate between the two processes. Aspirates should be sent for culture to rule out coexisting infection.

C. Imaging Studies

Tophi may be seen when they are calcified. Soft-tissue swelling is seen, as well as erosions. Chronic changes consist of extensive bone loss, joint narrowing, and joint deformity.

Abubaker MY et al: The management of gout. N Engl J Med 1996;334:445.

Agudelo CA, Wise CM: Gout: Diagnosis, pathogenesis, and clinical manifestations. Curr Opin Rheumatol 2001;13(3):234.

Emmerson BT: Coexistence of acute gout and septic arthritis. Arthritis Rheum 2000;43:S189.

Kelley WN et al: Gout and related disorders of purine metabolism. In Kelly WN et al, eds: *Textbook of Rheumatology.* WB Saunders, 1989.

Levinson DJ: Clinical gout and the pathogenesis of hyperuricemia. In McCarty DJ, ed: *Arthritis and Allied Conditions.* Lea & Febiger, 1989.

Calcium Pyrophosphate Crystal Deposition Disease

Calcium pyrophosphate crystal deposition disease, a goutlike syndrome, is also known as pseudogout or chondrocalcinosis. Crystals of calcium pyrophosphate dihydrate are deposited in a joint, most commonly the knee and not the first metatarsophalangeal joint, as in gout. The diagnosis is made by demonstration of the crystals in tissue or synovial fluid and by the presence of characteristic radiographic findings.

Aging and trauma are associated with this disorder, as well as conditions such as hyperparathyroidism, gout, hemochromatosis, hypophosphatasia, and hypothyroidism.

A. Epidemiologic Features

Hereditary forms of calcium pyrophosphate dihydrate deposition disease are reported, with transmission as an autosomal trait. Idiopathic cases were not rigorously examined for genetic factors or association with other diseases.

B. Pathologic Features

Calcification of multiple joint structures occurs, including hyaline cartilage and capsules, with heaviest deposition in fibrocartilaginous structures such as the menisci. The crystals are more difficult to see than urate crystals but have weak positive birefringence.

C. Imaging Studies

Calcification of menisci and hyaline cartilage is seen as punctate or linear radiodensities, which delineate these normally radiolucent structures. Bursas, ligaments, and tendons may have calcifications as well. Bony signs include subchondral cyst formation, signs of carpal instability, sacroiliac joint erosions with vacuum phenomenon, and crowning of the odontoid process.

Kohn NN et al: The significance of calcium phosphate crystals in the synovial fluid of arthritis patients: The "pseudogout syndrome." II. Identification of crystals. Ann Intern Med 1982;56:738.

McCarty DJ et al: The significance of calcium phosphate crystals in the synovial fluid of arthritis patients: The "pseudogout syndrome." I. Clinical aspects. Ann Intern Med 1962;56:711.

Resnick D: Rheumatoid arthritis and pseudorheumatoid arthritis in calcium pyrophosphate dihydrate crystal deposition disease. Radiology 1981;140:615.

Rosenthal AK: Calcium crystal-associated arthritides. Curr Opin Rheumatol 1998;10(3):273.

Ochronosis

A hereditary deficiency in the enzyme homogentisic acid oxidase is present in the disease known as **alkaptonuria.** The presence of unmetabolized homogentisic acid results in a brownish black color of the urine (thus the name of the disease). The term **ochronosis** describes the clinical condition of homogentisic acid deposited in connective tissues, manifested by bluish black pigmentation of the skin, ear, and sclera, and in cartilage.

The diagnosis is made when the triad of dark urine, degenerative arthritis, and abnormal pigmentation is present. Freshly passed urine is normal in color but turns dark when oxidized. Spondylosis is common, with knee, shoulder, and hip joint involvement also seen.

A. Epidemiologic Features

Transmission of alkaptonuria is by a recessive autosomal gene.

B. Imaging Studies

Spondylosis is seen, with calcification of intervertebral disks with few osteophytes. Joint involvement is similar in appearance to that of OA, except for protrusio acetabuli.

Schumacher HR, Holdsworth DE: Ochronotic arthropathy: Clinicopathologic studies. Semin Arthritis Rheum 1977;6:207.

4. Osteochondroses

Osteonecrosis of the Femoral Head

A variety of conditions and diseases are associated with femoral head osteonecrosis, but the pathogenesis is unknown in most cases. Direct injury to the blood supply of the femoral head is implicated in traumatic causes of avascular necrosis such as subcapital femoral neck fracture and dislocation of the hip. The disorder is bilateral in more than 60% of cases and affects other bones in approximately 15% of cases. The leading nontraumatic causes of osteonecrosis of the femoral head include alcoholism, idiopathic causes, and systemic steroid treatment. The mechanism by which steroids cause osteonecrosis may be by adipogenesis because the effects may be reduced, at least in an animal model, by using lovastatin.

Other associated conditions include hemoglobinopathies, Gaucher disease, caisson disease, hyperlipidemia tobacco use, hypercoagulable states, irradiation, and diseases of bone marrow infiltration such as leukemia and lymphoma.

A. Pathologic Features

Regardless of underlying causes, the early lesions in femoral head osteonecrosis include necrosis of marrow and trabecular bone, usually in a wedge-shaped area in the region of the anterolateral superior femoral head. The overlying articular cartilage is largely unaffected because it is normally avascular, obtaining nutrition from the synovial fluid. The deep calcified layer of cartilage, however, does derive nutrition from epiphyseal vessels and also undergoes necrosis. Histologically, necrotic marrow and absence of osteocytes in lacunae are seen.

Leukocytes and mononuclear cells collect around necrotic and fibrovascular tissue and eventually replace necrotic marrow. Osteoclasts resorb dead trabeculae, and osteoblasts then attempt to repair the damaged tissue; during attempted repair, the necrotic trabeculae are susceptible to fatigue fracture. Grossly, a subchondral fracture forms, with deformation of overlying hyaline cartilage. With time, fragmentation of articular cartilage ensues, resulting in degenerative arthritis.

B. Imaging Studies

Ficat created a classification based on the plain radiographic appearance of femoral head osteonecrosis in progressive stages. Stage I represents normal or minimal changes (mild osteopenia or sclerotic regions) in an asymptomatic hip. In stage II, subchondral sclerosis and osteopenia are evident, often in a well-demarcated wedge in the anterolateral femoral head seen best with radiographs taken with the patient in the frog-leg position from the lateral views. Stage III is heralded by collapse of subchondral bone, known as the crescent sign, and is pathognomonic for femoral head osteonecrosis. Femoral head flattening is often seen, but the joint space is preserved. Stage IV consists of advanced degenerative arthritic changes, with loss of joint space and bony changes in the acetabulum.

A newer classification system, devised by Steinberg, is popular and based on extent of head involvement as determined by MRI. This system, called the University of Pennsylvania system, has seven stages from normal (stage 0) to stage VI in which advanced degenerative changes are evident. Stages I to V are divided into three subcategories of mild, moderate, and severe. Stage III of the Steinberg system corresponds to stage III of the Ficat system.

Cui Q et al: The Otto Aufranc Award: Lovastatin prevents steroid-induced adipogenesis and osteonecrosis. Clin Orthop 1997;344:8.

Ficat RP: Idiopathic bone necrosis of the femoral head: Early diagnosis and treatment. J Bone Joint Surg Br 1985;67:3.

Lavernia CJ et al: Osteonecrosis of the femoral head. J Am Acad Orthop Surg 1999;7:250.

Steinberg ME et al: A quantitative system for staging avascular necrosis. J Bone Joint Surg 1995;77B:34.

5. Other Disorders Associated with Arthritis

Hemophilia

Hemophilia A is a heritable bleeding disorder produced by deficiency of factor VIII. Hemophilia B is a disease caused by lack of clotting factor IX. Both hemophilia A (classic hemophilia) and hemophilia B (Christmas disease) are sex-linked recessive disorders, although 30% of patients may have no family history of the disease. Hemophilic arthropathy primarily involves the knee joint, with the elbow and ankle joints affected less frequently.

A. Pathologic Features

Recurrent hemarthrosis produces deposits of hemosiderin and synovitis. In the acute phase, hypertrophy of synovium occurs, causing a higher risk of repeated bleeding. A pannus may form, as in RA, with underlying cartilage destruction. With time, synovial fibrosis occurs, resulting in joint stiffness.

B. Imaging Studies

Soft-tissue swelling, seen early, is associated with hemarthroses. Later stages include widening of epiphyseal regions caused by overgrowth from increased vascularity. Skeletal changes are manifested as subchondral sclerosis and cyst formation early, with later loss of cartilage and secondary osteophyte formation. Squaring of the patella is seen, possibly resulting from overgrowth.

Luck JV, Kasper CK: Surgical management of advanced hemophilic arthropathy. Clin Orthop 1989;242:60.

Gaucher Disease

A rare familial disorder, Gaucher disease is an inborn error of metabolism caused by a deficiency of the lysosomal hydrolase enzyme β-glucocerebrosidase. Accumulation of glucosylceramidase in phagocytic cells of the reticuloendothelial cells occurs, including the liver, spleen, lymph nodes, and bone marrow.

The femur is the most commonly affected bone, but the vertebrae, ribs, sternum, and flat bones of the pelvis may also be affected. The manifestations of skeletal disease are the result of mechanical effects of infiltration of the abnormal cells, leading to erosion of cortices and interference with the normal vascular supply. Expansion of bone and areas of osteolysis predispose affected bones to pathologic fracture, and vascular interruption leads to avascular necrosis of the femoral hip.

A. Epidemiologic Features

Inherited in an autosomal recessive manner, Gaucher disease is the most common inherited disorder of lipid metabolism. The disease is especially common in the Ashkenazi Jewish community.

B. Pathologic Features

Histologic examination of involved reticuloendothelial tissues demonstrates foam cells, which are large lipid-laden macrophages.

C. Imaging Studies

Early stages of skeletal involvement in Gaucher disease include diffuse osteoporosis and medullary expansion. The distal femur may expand to form a characteristic Erlenmeyer flask deformity. Localized erosions and sclerotic areas are seen. Osteonecrosis may be seen in the femoral head, humeral head, and distal femur. Secondary degenerative changes follow collapse of necrotic articular bone.

Amstutz HC, Carey EJ: Skeletal manifestations and treatment of Gaucher's disease. J Bone Joint Surg Am 1966;48:670.

Goldblatt J et al: The orthopaedic aspects of Gaucher's disease. Clin Orthop 1978;137:208.

Hip Labral Tears

The hip has a cartilaginous extension of the bony acetabulum called the labrum that deepens the acetabulum and stabilizes the hip. Labral tears were newly rediscovered as a source of pain and a cause of osteoarthrosis, partially because of the relative ease of evaluating their presence and subsequently treating them. Arthroscopy can be used to remove the torn labrum, similar to torn menisci.

A. Pathologic Features

The normal labrum is triangular in shape and variable in size from 1 to 10 mm in length. The pathologic labrum is classified into types A and B, depending on whether the labrum is traumatic (triangular: A) or degenerative (thick and rounded: B) and three stages: (1) intrasubstance degeneration, (2) partial tear, and (3) complete tear.

B. Imaging Studies

MRI arthrography is the test of choice for suspected labral tears. Contrast is seen going into the tear, which is frequently in the weight-bearing area of the acetabulum. CT arthrography and MRI are not as sensitive.

Plotz GM et al: Magnetic resonance arthrography of the acetabular labrum. J Bone Joint Surg Br 2000;82:426.

MEDICAL MANAGEMENT

Nonsteroidal Antiinflammatory Drugs

The use of nonsteroidal antiinflammatory drugs (NSAIDs) in the management of OA is widespread but controversial. Because only minimal inflammatory changes are present in joints with OA, the use of acetaminophen is advocated as a first-line drug. In a short-term study of patients treated for OA, acetaminophen (4000 mg/d) was found to be as effective as ibuprofen (2400 mg/d).

The therapeutic effect of NSAIDs can be dramatic in the osteoarthritic patient, even with severe disease. The main problems with routine NSAID therapy are the gastrointestinal (GI) and renal complications and the inhibition of normal platelet function. Thus, alternative therapies should be carefully considered, and therapy should be closely monitored. Current NSAIDs work by altering prostaglandin synthesis through nonspecific inhibition of both cyclooxygenase isoforms 1 (COX-1) and 2 (COX-2). COX-1 inhibition can have deleterious effects on hemostasis and the GI tract.

Patients treated with NSAIDs have a three times greater relative risk of developing GI complications than nonusers. In one study, NSAIDs were associated with acute hospital admissions of 30% of elderly patients. Patients at high risk for developing ulcers with use of NSAIDs are those with any of the following characteristics: age older than 65 years, history of prior ulcer disease, use of multiple dose or high-dose NSAIDs, or use of concomitant corticosteroids. The antiprostaglandin effects of NSAIDs can reduce renal blood flow, leading to acute and chronic renal insufficiency. Patients at risk for acute renal insufficiency because of NSAIDs are elderly patients, those with atherosclerotic cardiovascular disease, and those with preexisting renal impairment. The platelet effects of these drugs are variable, depending on the NSAID half-life, on whether the NSAID inhibits thromboxane A, and on whether that inhibition is reversible. Aspirin, for example, is permanent for the life of the platelet. Many patients report increased bruising as a result of taking these drugs.

Table 7–3 compares the toxicities of currently available NSAIDs. Because the effects are not caused solely by the inhibitory effects on prostaglandin synthesis, the various chemical origins of these drugs may lead to slightly different clinical effects in different patients.

The chemical families of these drugs are noted in Table 7–4 with their half-lives and their dosing frequency. Dosing frequency is important because patient compliance with use of these drugs goes up with less frequent dosing, such as daily or twice daily.

Much anticipated is the development of COX-2-selective NSAIDs, which are now available. Most of the side effects attributable to NSAIDs are caused by inhibition of COX-1, an isoform that is normally present ("constitutive") in renal and GI tissues. COX-2-selective NSAIDs inhibit the isoenzyme that develops ("inducible") as a response to inflammation. By selectively inhibiting COX-2, the efficacy of NSAIDs is retained with much less side effects.

Although COX-2-selective NSAIDs are purportedly safe, they are not without side effects. Celecoxib did not exhibit statistically significant decreased rates of complicated upper GI events in a randomized controlled trial. Rofecoxib was shown to decrease complicated upper GI events significantly compared with conventional NSAIDs, but the rate of myocardial infarction was increased, possibly related to loss of the antiplatelet effect normally present in NSAIDs.

The choice of an appropriate NSAID should be based on the following factors: clotting problems, compliance of the patient, GI symptom history, renal function, drug cost, and the effect on the patient with previously used NSAIDs. Patients taking warfarin would probably be better treated with a drug having no platelet effect that is COX-2-specific. Patients with a poor response to one type of NSAID may benefit from a trial with one from another chemical family. A patient with a history of poor drug compliance with other medications would benefit from daily dosing, whereas a patient

Table 7–3. Toxicity profiles of currently available NSAIDs.

Generic Name	Proprietary Name	Gastrointestinal Toxicity	Renal Toxicity	Platelet Effects (d)[a]	Other Toxicity[b]
Diclofenac	Voltaren	Moderate	Moderate	1	Hepatitis
Etodolac	Lodine	Low[c]	Moderate	NA	—
Indomethacin	Indocin	High	Moderate	1	Headache
Nabumetone	Relafen	Low[c]	Moderate	NA	Hepatitis
Sulindac	Clinoril	Moderate	Low	1	Dermatitis
Tolmetin	Tolectin	Moderate	Moderate	2	—
Meclofenamate	Meclomen	Moderate	Moderate	1	Diarrhea
Piroxicam	Feldene	Moderate	Moderate	14	—
Fenoprofen	Nalfon	Moderate	Moderate	1	—
Flurbiprofen	Ansaid	Moderate	Moderate	1	—
Ibuprofen	Motrin	Moderate	Moderate	1	—
Ketoprofen	Orudis	Moderate	Moderate	2	—
Naproxen	Naprosyn	Moderate	Moderate	4	—
Oxaprozin	Daypro	Moderate	Moderate	NA	—
Ketorolacq	Toradol	High	Moderate	1	—
Salicylsalicylic acid[d]	Disalcid	None	None	None	—
Sodium salicylate[d]	—	None	None	None	—
Aspirin	—	High	Moderate	10	Tinnitus
Diflunisal[e]	Dolobid	Low	Low	None	—
Celecoxib	Celebrex	Low	Low	None	Sulfa allergies

[a]Average time to normal platelet function after discontinuation of drug.
[b]Other NSAIDs may have similar toxicity, but the effects are more prevalent with these agents.
[c]Simultaneous efficacy comparisons in inflammatory disease not available.
[d]No prostaglandin inhibition.
[e]Weak prostaglandin inhibitor.
NA = data not available.

Table 7–4. Dosage data of currently available NSAIDs.

Generic Name	Proprietary Name	Largest Unit Dose (mg)	Half-Life (h)	Dosing Frequency[a]	Family
Diclofenac	Voltaren	75	2	bid	Acetic acid
Etodolac	Lodine	300	6	qid	Acetic acid
Indomethacin	Indocin	50	4	tid	Acetic acid
Nabumetone	Relafen	500	20–30	2 qd	Acetic acid
Sulindac	Clinoril	200	8–14	bid	Acetic acid
Tolmetin	Tolectin	400	1–2	tid	Acetic acid
Meclofenamate	Meclomen	100	2	tid	Fenamates
Piroxicam	Feldene	20	30–86	qd	Oxicams
Fenoprofen	Nalfon	600	2–3	qid	Proprionates
Flurbiprofen	Ansaid	100	6	tid	Proprionates
Ibuprofen	Motrin	800	2	qid	Proprionates
Ketoprofen	Orudis	75	3	tid	Proprionates
Naproxen	Naprosyn	500	14	bid	Proprionates
Oxaprozin	Daypro	600	40–50	2 qd	Proprionates
Ketorolac	Toradol	10	5	qid	Pyrrolo-pyrrole
Salicylsalicylic acid	Disalcid	750	1	qid	Salicylates
Sodium salicylate	—	650	0.5	q4h	Salicylates
Aspirin	—	325	0.25	2q4h	Salicylates
Diffunisal	Dolobid	500	10	bid	Salicylates
Celecoxib	Celebrex	200	11	bid	Sulfonamide

[a]Dosage required for treatment of inflammation.
bid = twice a day; qd = each day; q4h = every 4 hours; qid = four times a day; tid = three times a day.

already taking another drug three times daily would probably find three-times-daily dosing more convenient. Obviously, a patient with renal disease should be treated with a drug having not only low renal toxicity, but also probably a short half-life to minimize the accumulation of the drug in the body because of lack of renal excretion. The COX-2-selective NSAIDs will not eliminate the need for the other drugs. The vast majority of patients tolerate the side effects of the older drugs, and the risk-benefit ratio for these drugs is quite favorable, especially for short courses of treatment.

The advent of the COX-2-specific NSAIDs adds to their safety as analgesics for acute pain because the COX-2 inhibitors block the pain, fever, and inflammatory response while not affecting clotting. Thus, their use in the perioperative setting is significantly increased.

Surgical intervention is generally indicated for patients who have failed conservative therapy with NSAIDs. For patients who are not surgical candidates, a long-term regimen of narcotic medication may be considered.

Batchlor EE, Paulus HE: Principles of drug therapy. In Moskowitz RW et al, eds: *Osteoarthritis: Diagnosis and Medical Surgical Management.* WB Saunders, 1993.

Berger RG: Nonsteroidal anti-inflammatory drugs: Making the right choice. J Am Acad Orthop Surg 1994;2:255.

Bombardier C et al: Comparison of upper gastrointestinal toxicity of rofecoxib and naproxen in patients with rheumatoid arthritis. VIGOR Study Group. N Engl J Med 2000;343(21):1520.

Bradley JD et al: Comparison of an anti-inflammatory dose of ibuprofen, an analgesic dose of ibuprofen, and acetaminophen in the treatment of patients with osteoarthritis of the knee. N Engl J Med 1991;325:87.

Gabriel SE et al: Risk for serious gastrointestinal complications related to use of nonsteroidal anti-inflammatory drugs. Ann Intern Med 1991;115:787.

Hochberg MC et al: Guidelines for the medical management of osteoarthritis: I. Osteoarthritis of the hip. Arthritis Rheum 1995;38:1535.

Hochberg MC et al: Guidelines for the medical management of osteoarthritis: II. Osteoarthritis of the knee. Arthritis Rheum 1995;38:1541.

Hosie J et al: Meloxicam in osteoarthritis: A 6-month, double-blind comparison with diclofenac sodium. Br J Rheumatol 1996;35(Suppl 1):39.

Silverstein FE et al: Gastrointestinal toxicity with celecoxib vs nonsteroidal anti-inflammatory drugs for osteoarthritis and rheumatoid arthritis: The CLASS study: A randomized controlled trial. Celecoxib long term arthritis safety study. JAMA 2000;284(10):1247.

Simon LS et al: Preliminary study of the safety and efficacy of SC-58635, a novel cyclooxygenase 2 inhibitor: Efficacy and safety in two placebo-controlled trials in OA and rheumatoid arthritis, and studies of gastrointestinal and platelet effects. Arthritis Rheum 1998;41:1591.

Disease-Modifying Agents in Rheumatoid Arthritis

Three new disease-modifying antirheumatic drugs (DMARDs) are now available for the medical treatment of rheumatoid arthritis. Although the experience of these new agents is limited, the mechanisms of their actions may guide orthopedic surgeons with respect to their potential effect on the surgical procedures. Etanercept is an artificially bioengineered molecule that binds to the receptor of TNF (tumor necrosis factor), preventing activation of the inflammatory cascade. Infliximab is a chimeric antibody that also targets TNF. Both of these drugs probably have little effect on healing and most likely can be continued up to any surgical procedure. Leflunomide inhibits an enzyme, decreasing levels of pyrimidine nucleotides, inhibiting clonal expansion of T cells in RA. This DMARD should probably be discontinued 1 week prior to surgery, similar to methotrexate.

Kremer JM: Rational use of new and existing disease-modifying agents in rheumatoid arthritis. Ann Intern Med 2001;134:695.

OTHER THERAPIES

Nutritional Supplements

The nutritional supplements glucosamine sulfate and chondroitin sulfate are popular as nonprescription products for arthritis therapy. This popularity arises from the concept that these products may serve as substrate for the reparative processes in cartilage. Glucosamine sulfate is found as an intermediate product in mucopolysaccharide synthesis, and an elevated urinary excretion is seen in patients with OA and RA. Oral administration of glucosamine sulfate was compared with analgesic doses of ibuprofen in a 4-week trial in patients with OA of the knee. Ibuprofen was found to provide pain relief more quickly, but the response rates were similar at 4 weeks.

Chondroitin sulfate is another glycosaminoglycan present in articular cartilage; its oral administration in one study resulted in no change in serum levels. In another study, patients with OA of the hip and knee used fewer NSAIDs when given chondroitin sulfate compared with a placebo control group. Although glucosamine sulfate and chondroitin sulfate are unproven therapies at this time, their use may provide safe and effective symptomatic relief in some patients with OA. Newer reports indicate improved symptoms of OA with oral glucosamine and chondroitin sulfate, but the mechanisms of action are unknown.

Brief AA et al: Use of glucosamine and chondroitin sulfate in the management of osteoarthritis. J Am Acad Orthop Surg 2001;9:71.

Houpt JB et al: Effect of glucosamine hydrochloride (GHCl) in the treatment of pain of osteoarthritis of the knee. J Rheumatol 1998;25(Suppl 52):8.

Hughes RA, Carr AJ: A randomized double-blind placebo-controlled trail of glucosamine to control pain in osteoarthritis of the knee. Arthritis Rheum 2000;43(Suppl 9):S384.

Leffter CT et al: Glucosamine, chondroitin, and manganese ascorbate for degenerative joint disease of the knee or low back: A randomized, double-blind, placebo-controlled pilot study. Mil Med 1999;164(2):85.

Mazieres B et al: Chondroitin sulfate in the treatment of gonarthrosis and coxarthrosis. Five-month results of a multicenter double-blind controlled prospective study using placebo. Rev Rhum Mal Osteoartic 1992;59:466.

McAlindon TE et al: Glucosamine and chondroitin for treatment of osteoarthritis: A systemic quality assessment and meta-analysis. JAMA 2000;283:1469.

Muller-Fabender H et al: Glucosamine sulfate compared to ibuprofen in osteoarthritis of the knee. Osteoarthritis Cartilage 1994;2:61.

Reginster JY et al: Long term effects of glucosamine sulphate on osteoarthritis progression: A randomized, placebo-controlled clinical trial. Lancet 2001;357:251.

Rindone JP et al: Randomized, controlled trial of glucosamine for treating osteoarthritis of the knee. West J Med 2000; 172(2):91.

Injections

One of the mainstays of the treatment of osteoarthrosis and RA is the cortisone injection, which can be used for joints, bursae, and trigger points. Generally, shoulders, elbows, wrists, finger joints, knees, ankles, and joints of the foot can be given in the office without radiographic control. Hips and some joints of the foot and hand are best done with radiographic control to ensure location of the injection. The injections can be therapeutic with steroids or diagnostic with local anesthetic. For example, differentiation between the amount of a patient's pain coming from the back and the proportion coming from the hip can be ascertained with a lidocaine injection into the hip. This reliably informs the patient as to the realistic expectations of pain relief after a hip replacement. Similarly, an ankle injection predicts pain relief after ankle fusion. Intraarticular administration of hyaluronic acid is now available for treatment of OA of the knee with products of different molecular weight. The treatment protocols for these drugs call for weekly injections for 3–5 weeks to obtain a therapeutic effect.

Hyaluronic acid is a long-chain polysaccharide responsible for the viscoelastic properties of synovial joint fluid. In pathologic states, such as OA and RA, both the concentration and molecular size of hyaluronic acid is diminished. In animal experimental models, evidence indicates that hyaluronic injections may retard progression of OA. Serial injections of hyaluronic acid in patients with osteoarthritic knees are reported to reduce pain for up to 10 months, but the mechanism of action is unknown.

Because of the short half-life of hyaluronic acid, it is unlikely that the injections significantly boost lubrication of arthritic joints. Rather than being a disease-modifying therapy, the injectable hyaluronic acid products should be considered long-acting pain-relieving drugs.

Adams ME et al: The role of viscosupplementation with hylan G-F 20 (Synvisc) in the treatment of osteoarthritis of the knee: A Canadian multicenter trial comparing hylan G-F 20 alone, hylan G-F 20 with nonsteroidal anti-inflammatory drugs (NSAIDs) and NSAIDs alone. Osteoarthritis Cartilage 1995;3(4):213.

Altman RD, Moskowitz R: Intraarticular sodium hyaluronate (Hyalgan) in the treatment of patients with osteoarthritis of the knee: A randomized clinical trial. Hyalgan Study Group. J Rheumatol 1998;25(11):2203.

Marshall KW et al: Amelioration of disease severity by intraarticular hylan therapy in bilateral canine osteoarthritis. J Orthop Res 2000;18(3):416.

Watterson JR, Esdaile JM: Viscosupplementation: Therapeutic mechanisms and clinical potential in osteoarthritis of the knee. J Am Acad Orthop Surg 2000;8:277.

Orthotic Treatment

The use of orthotics can ameliorate the symptoms of osteoarthrosis in the knee, the ankle, and possibly the elbow, but other joints are not really amenable to this treatment. The medial compartment of the knee is more commonly affected than the lateral, leading to, or resulting from varus deformity. Thus, this disorder lends itself to orthotic treatment to remove the deformity. Heel wedges and valgus braces can be helpful in relieving the pain and improving the ambulatory function of patients with medial gonarthrosis. Similarly, orthotics to control varus and valgus forces at the ankle can be very helpful for ankle arthrosis.

Draper ERC et al: Improvement of function after valgus bracing of the knee. J Bone Joint Surg Br 2000;82:1001.

Pollo FE: Bracing and heel wedging for unicompartmental osteoarthritis of the knee. Am J Knee Surg 1998;11:47.

SURGICAL MANAGEMENT

PROCEDURES FOR JOINT PRESERVATION

A joint can potentially deteriorate for the following reasons: (1) trauma, which may distort the joint so abnormal loads are applied; (2) hemophilia, which forces the joint to dispose of blood on multiple occasions, causing synovitis; (3) rheumatoid arthritis, which causes a proliferation of the synovium, which may destroy the hyaline joint cartilage; and (4) osteonecrosis, which may result in fatigue fractures and collapse of the joint, with subsequent incongruity or (5) rotator cuff tear, leading possibly to cuff arthropathy. Certain procedures can slow progression of the deterioration and prolong the useful service of the joint. These include synovectomy, core decompression, osteotomy, and rotator cuff repair.

Rotator Cuff Repair

Chronic rotator cuff tears of the shoulder can lead to a degenerative condition called **cuff arthropathy.** The rotator cuff functions to counter the upward shear force on the articular cartilage exerted by the unopposed deltoid musculature. By repairing a torn rotator cuff, kinematic balance can be restored, preventing degeneration of the glenohumeral joint. Rotator cuff tears are repaired by mobilizing the rotator cuff and debriding the degenerated margins. These freshened edges are then sutured into bone at their insertion to restore function of the rotator cuff muscles. Removal of acromial spurs and excision of the coracoacromial ligament are also performed at the time of repair.

Synovectomy

Synovectomy is a treatment that may prolong the life of the hyaline joint surface through removal of proliferative synovitis, which damages cartilage. Synovectomy is indicated for chronic but not acute synovitis. Chronic synovitis is a clinical entity characterized by proliferation of the synovium and may be monarticular, as in pigmented villonodular synovitis, or polyarticular, as in RA or hemophilia. The term **synovitis** is relatively nonspecific, and the disorder is usually the result of a reaction to joint irritation.

A. Indications and Contraindications

The most common indication for synovectomy is RA, but the procedure may be beneficial in many other conditions, such as synovial osteochondromatosis, pigmented villonodular synovitis, and hemophilia, and occasionally following chronic or acute infection.

More specific indications for synovectomy include the following conditions:

1. synovitis with disease limited to the synovial membrane with little or no involvement of the other structures of the joint;
2. recurrent hemarthroses in conditions such as pigmented villonodular synovitis or hemophilia;
3. imminent destruction of the joint by lysosomal enzymes derived from white blood cells that may be liberated from infection; and
4. failure of an adequate trial of conservative management.

Contraindications include reduced ROM, significant degenerative arthrosis of the involved joint or other joint, or cartilage involvement.

B. Technique

Synovectomy is most commonly performed on the knee and also often on the elbow, ankle, and wrist. Three main techniques are available: open synovectomy, synovectomy with use of the arthroscope, and radiation synovectomy.

1. Open synovectomy—Open synovectomy is becoming less common because of pain that causes difficulty in obtaining full motion following surgery. Continuous passive motion may be beneficial in these cases. Open synovectomy may be necessary in cases of pigmented villonodular synovitis or synovial osteochondromatosis, although these diseases may also be treated by arthroscopy, which permits noninvasive complete removal of the synovium in many cases.

2. Synovectomy with use of arthroscope—Synovectomy with use of the arthroscope may be tedious, especially in large joints such as the knee, because complete treatment requires removal of the entire synovium in many cases.

A study of pigmented villonodular synovitis of the knee treated by total and partial arthroscopic synovectomy demonstrated that total synovectomy resulted in a low recurrence rate, whereas partial synovectomy resulted in symptomatic and functional improvement but a fairly high recurrence rate. Arthroscopic synovectomy was recommended only for localized lesions.

3. Radiation synovectomy—Radiation synovectomy is a technique that is becoming much more popular. It is used in knee joints affected by RA. An injection of dysprosium-165-ferric hydroxide macroaggregates is given and leads to improvement in a significant percentage of patients. Proliferation of synovium decreases following this procedure, and there is less pain, blood loss, and expense than with more invasive procedures.

A similar technique is used in the knee joint in hemophiliacs. Phosphorus-32 chromic phosphate colloid is used and can be given on an outpatient basis. This is a safer technique for health care personnel, who have less contact with the blood of the hemophiliac patients, many of whom have become HIV positive through contaminated blood factor replacement.

Cartilage Transplant Techniques

Defects of hyaline cartilage were long considered permanent injuries, and the irrevocable sequelae were gradual deterioration of the architecture of the tissue. The treatment of cartilaginous diseases and injuries was limited by the slow and poorly understood metabolism of articular chondrocytes. Current development of cartilage repair procedures pertain only to focal defects of full-thickness cartilage loss. Such injuries occur typically in young (less than 40 years) patients during athletic activities or in patients with osteochondritis dissecans.

Because cartilaginous tissues are avascular, prior surgical treatment consisted of chondroplasty, where underlying subchondral bone was either drilled, burred, or microfractured to produce bleeding and an inflammatory response. Although multiple growth factors may be released with bleeding, the ensuing repair tissue is essentially fibrous scar tissue with inferior load-bearing capabilities compared with hyaline articular cartilage. As a result, the repair tissue eventually degrades, leaving the defect little better than if left alone.

Much enthusiasm followed the procedure described by Brittberg and colleagues, in which viable articular chondrocytes are harvested from a patient with a focal cartilaginous defect and cultured in a laboratory. The population of chondrocytes is expanded and placed back in the patient at the site of the cartilage injury. The cells are held in place with a flap of periosteum sutured to surrounding healthy cartilage. Although encouraging early clinical results were reported with this method, similar results are shown using only the flap of periosteum. Further, the procedure using cells failed to demonstrate reconstitution of normal hyaline cartilage in a canine model experiment.

Another method of dealing with focal defects of cartilage includes transplantation of small plugs of mature cartilage and bone. Small cylinders of cartilage and bone are removed from non–weight-bearing portions of cartilage and transplanted into focal femoral defects. Although encouraging short-term results are reported, whether the reconstructed cartilage endures remains to be seen.

In contrast, OA is a more prevalent affliction of cartilage, affecting more than 40 million patients in the United States. The early pathologic observations of OA indicate structural degradation of the superficial layers of the cartilage architecture. Meaningful spontaneous repair of injuries limited to cartilage are not observed clinically, but a variety of experimental evidence suggests a latent ability to effect some degree of healing after injury and possibly in OA. These suppositions include observation of increased DNA synthesis and proteoglycan synthesis in chondrocytes during intermediate stages of OA. The procedures just described for cartilage repair do not apply for osteoarthritic involvement of any significant portions of a joint.

Brittberg M et al: Treatment of deep cartilage defects in the knee with autologous chondrocyte implantation. N Engl J Med 1994;331:889.

Hangody L et al: Mosaicplasty for the treatment of articular defects of the knee and ankle. Clin Orthop 2001;391(Suppl):S328.

Rodrigo JJ et al: Improvement of full-thickness chondral defect healing in the human knee after debridement and microfracture using continuous passive motion. Am J Knee Surg 1994;7:109.

Core Decompression with or without Structural Bone Grafting

A. Indications and Contraindications

Core decompression with or without bone grafting is a surgical treatment primarily used for the femoral head because the hip is the joint most commonly affected by osteonecrosis. The knee and the shoulder may also be affected. Osteonecrosis results from loss of blood supply to the bone and is associated with a variety of conditions. Under repetitive stress, microfractures occur, are not repaired, and eventually lead to collapse of the necrotic bone and disruption of the joint surface.

The treatment of osteonecrosis is controversial because the outcome is frequently unsatisfactory. Spontaneous repair of the osteonecrotic lesion may occur but is an exception to the usual natural history of osteonecrosis. Core decompression, core decompression with electrical stimulation and bone grafting, and core decompression with structural bone grafting are considered acceptable forms of treatment for this disorder. Another treatment involves use of a free vascularized fibula transplant after core decompression.

B. Technique

The goal of core decompression is to alleviate hypertension in the bone caused by obstructed venous egress from the affected area. The theory is that drilling a hole in an involved bony area diminishes pressure and permits the ingrowth of new blood vessels, which allow repair of the avascular bone and prevent joint destruction. Corticocancellous bone grafting is considered an alternative to simple core decompression because some evidence indicates this would place the femoral head at less risk of collapse in the postoperative period before new bone formation can occur. Core decompression or structural bone grafting is indicated in early osteonecrosis prior to collapse of the femoral head (Ficat stage I or II).

Core decompression is usually performed on the hip but may also be done on the knee or the shoulder. A lateral approach is used for the hip, and a pin is placed into the osteonecrotic area under fluoroscopic control. A reamer or core device is then passed over the pin to achieve decompression, and a sample of bone may be obtained for pathologic analysis. If structural bone grafting is to be performed, the graft may be placed over the pin (allograft or autograft fibula). Again, placement is performed under direct radiograph control.

The results of core decompression are mixed, possible as a result of poor technique, lack of standardization of staging, and factors causing the osteonecrosis. The major complication of the procedure in the hip is torsional failure resulting from the stress concentration site in the lateral aspect of the cortex. Reports of structural bone grafting by some investigators are highly favorable, with a high percentage of asymptomatic hips showing no evidence of progression of necrosis or collapse. One series reported a relatively high rate of postoperative or intraoperative fracture (4 of 31 cases).

Osteotomy

Osteotomy should be considered part of the armamentarium of the orthopedic surgeon in the treatment of biomechanical disorders of the knee and the hip. Osteotomy of the hip for OA is less frequently performed than osteotomy of the knee. Abnormal distribution of load may be alleviated by osteotomy. Femoral head coverage may be improved with osteotomy of the pelvis, orientation of the femoral head may be improved with osteotomy of the proximal femur, and realignment of the load on the medial and lateral condyles of the tibia may be improved with osteotomy of the femur and the tibia. The most common procedure is high tibial osteotomy, sometimes referred to as **Coventry osteotomy,** which corrects varus deformity of the knee by removal of a wedge of bone from the lateral side of the tibia. Other osteotomies are performed for residual deformity for fracture. These are tailored to the particular problem presented by the patient. Either intraarticular (ie, condylar osteotomy of the medial compartment [Figure 7–4]) or extraarticular osteotomies can be done to correct deformity.

A. High Tibial Osteotomy

Alleviation of abnormal stress through high tibial osteotomy prevents osteoarthrosis or, alternatively, reduces pain caused by unicompartmental gonarthrosis. The procedure is indicated in relatively young (less than 55 years) patients who have unicompartmental degeneration with relative sparing of the patellofemoral joint. The knee should have a good ROM, preferably with no flexion contracture. The knee must be stable, with no demonstrated medial or lateral subluxation. The ideal patients are younger than 65 years, not obese, and wish to continue an active lifestyle, including activities such as skiing or tennis. These activities are contraindicated in total joint replacement or unicompartmental replacement. Evaluation of the uninvolved compartment (either medial or lateral) may be accomplished by arthroscopy or with a technetium bone scan. A cold scan of the uninvolved compartment indicates relative normalcy. The normal anatomic axis of 5–7 degrees (angle between the shaft of the femur and the shaft of the tibia) on the standing AP film must usually be overcorrected to 10 degrees. High tibial osteotomy is usually indicated for patients with medial gonarthrosis, although it can be performed in patients with a valgus angulation of less than 12 degrees. If the angle is outside of this range, the patient may be a candidate for distal femoral supracondylar osteotomy. A high tibial osteotomy that results in a joint line that is not parallel to the ground indicates that the osteotomy should probably be performed through the distal femur.

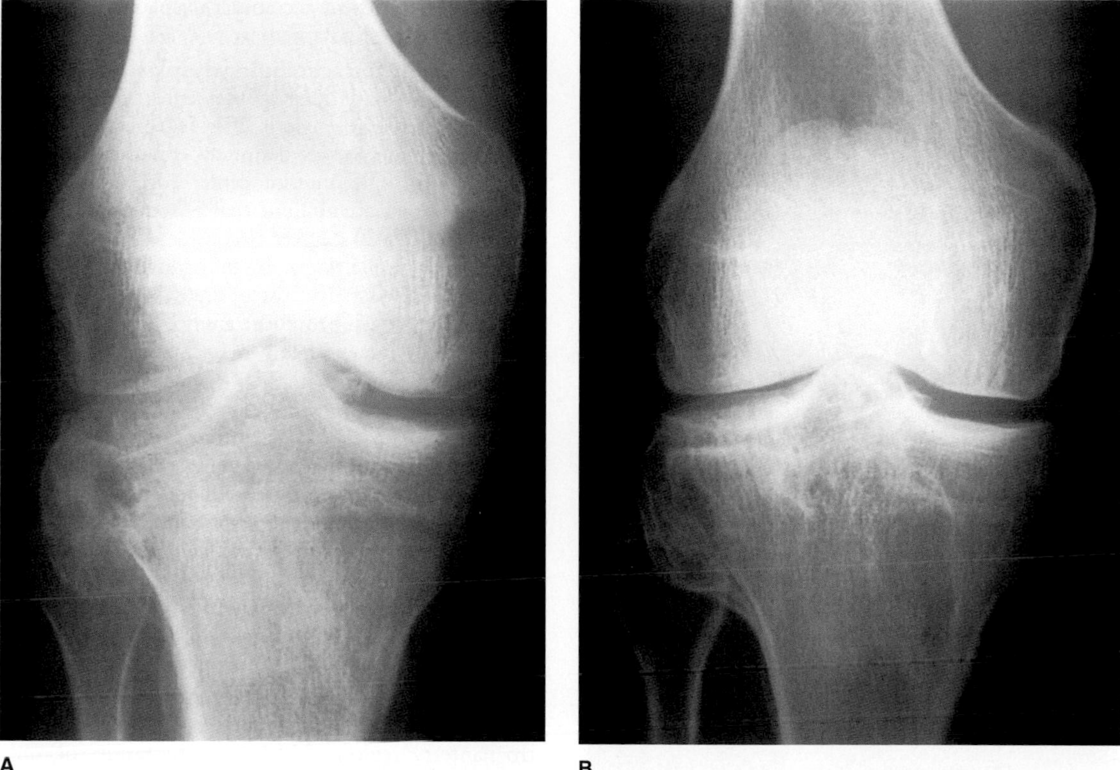

Figure 7–4. An intraarticular osteotomy can be of benefit in tibial plateau fractures. **A:** Preoperative radiograph of an intracondylar fracture of the tibial plateau. **B:** Postoperative view after osteotomy of the medial tibial condyle.

Proximal tibial osteotomy is performed through a lateral hockey-stick incision or a straight lateral incision. Exposure of the lateral, anterior, and posterior aspects of the tibia is made, and a closing wedge osteotomy is performed. The proximal portion of this osteotomy is made parallel to the joint surface under image intensifier control (Figure 7–5). With the help of guide pins, the appropriate distal cut is made, as determined from preoperative standing radiographs, to provide the necessary correction, which in the average case is approximately 1 mm per degree of correction as measured on the lateral cortex. This technique should only be used to double-check previous calculations, however. Resection of the fibular head or the proximal tibiofibular joint allows correction of the valgus angle. Fixation can reliably be obtained with staples, and other commercial fixation devices are available. Care must be taken to avoid damage to the peroneal nerve. Other problems that may be encountered include fracture of the proximal fragment or avascular necrosis of this fragment, which may occur if care is not exercised in performing the procedure.

The results of high tibial osteotomy are not as predictable as unicompartmental knee replacement or total knee replacement. Although pain is relieved in a high percentage of patients, this relief deteriorates over time. Clinical reports indicate that approximately 65–85% of patients have a good result after 5 years. Results of series vary because of the differences in patient population, surgical technique, and preexisting pathologic factors. The procedure should be considered in a patient who wants to maintain a more active lifestyle and would be willing to accept the possibility of some pain or loss of pain relief over time.

Lateral gonarthrosis from genu valgum is a relatively frequent result of lateral tibial plateau fractures, although RA, rickets, and renal osteodystrophy may also produce this disorder. There has been limited success in using varus tibial osteotomy in treating genu valgum because the procedure frequently produces a joint line that is not parallel to the ground, resulting in medial subluxation of the femur. Several reports of distal femoral osteotomy for genu valgum demonstrated this is a viable alternative for treating painful lateral gonarthrosis.

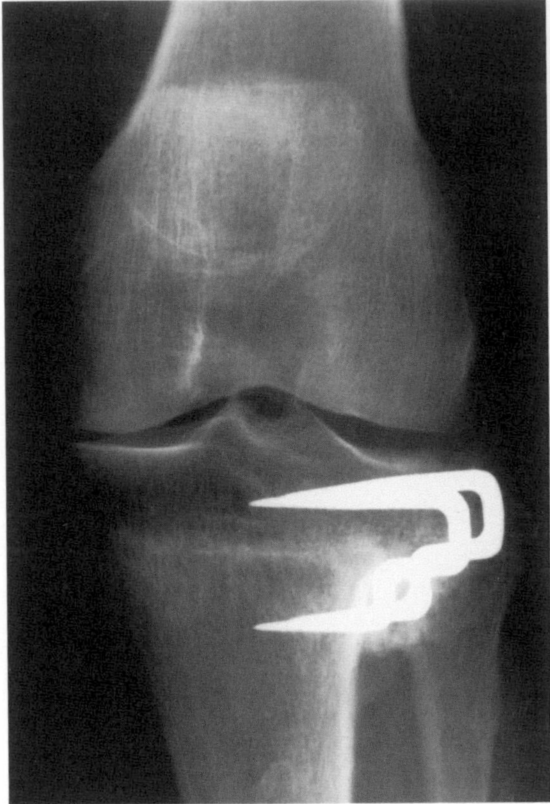

Figure 7–5. High tibial osteotomy, showing staples holding the osteotomy in place.

B. Osteotomy of the Hip

Certain unusual conditions of the hip can be treated with osteotomy to prevent or retard coxarthrosis. These include osteochondritis dissecans and other traumatic conditions that produce localized damage to the surface of the hip. Various biomechanical theories are proposed regarding the benefit of osteotomy of the pelvis and hip in decreasing the load on the hip. Although the theoretical arguments may be correct, in practical terms the two reasons for performing this procedure are (1) a normal viable cartilage surface is moved to the weight-bearing area where previously there was degenerated, thinned articular cartilage; and (2) the biomechanical loads on the joints that cause pain are reduced. These can be reduced either through alteration of moment arms for muscles or, alternatively, by releasing or weakening the muscles. Significantly lengthening or shortening a muscle reduces the force it can apply across a joint. In hip disorders, disease on one side of the hip joint cannot be addressed by an operation on the other side. For example, although it is tempting to use femoral osteotomy to treat acetabular dysplasia, only temporary relief may be obtained.

1. Treatment for acetabular dysplasia—Acetabular dysplasia may be defined by the center edge angle. The normal center edge angle is 25–45 degrees; an angle of less than 20 degrees is definitely considered dysplastic (Figure 7–6). The anterior center edge angle can also demonstrate an acetabulum that is too open anteriorly; an angle of 17–20 degrees is considered the lower limit on the false profile view. In individuals with a mature skeleton, limited pelvic osteotomies such as the Salter innominate or shelf procedure are not appropriate. These measurements are probably best considered in a three-dimensional view with CT.

To improve coverage and hip biomechanics significantly, an acetabular-reorienting procedure that also permits medialization is ideal. The Wagner spherical osteotomy permits complete redirection of the acetabulum but does not permit medialization and is technically demanding. A triple osteotomy is useful in positioning the acetabulum but causes severe pelvic instability. The periacetabular osteotomy described by Ganz permits acetabular redirection and medialization but preserves the posterior column, minimizing instability.

2. Treatment of femoral disorders—Osteotomy of the femur can safely and reliably be performed in the intertrochanteric region, with the expectation of union. Osteotomy of the femoral neck is likely to compromise the blood supply to the femoral head. Intertrochanteric

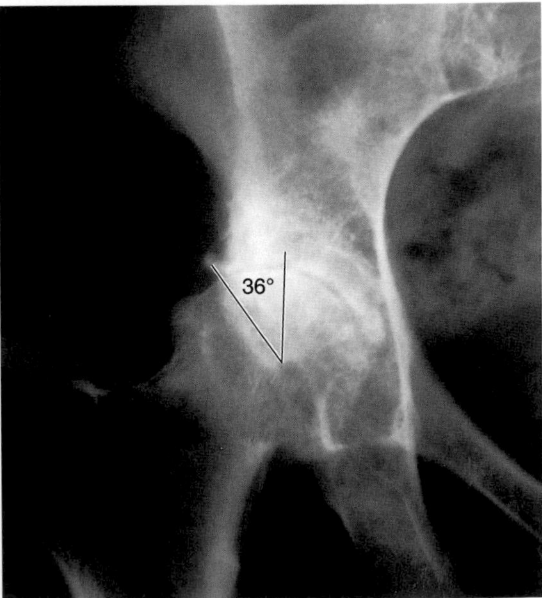

Figure 7–6. Anteroposterior pelvis film demonstrating the center edge angle.

osteotomies of the femur of various types are described. The goal of osteotomy is removal of degenerated articular cartilage from the weight-bearing dome and replacement of it with more viable cartilage. This procedure may involve any of the three degrees of freedom: varus and valgus angle, internal and external rotation, and flexion and extension. It is necessary when planning these procedures to be sure the osteotomy will provide an adequate ROM for the patient. These osteotomies have usefulness in very specific cases for osteoarthrosis, but their usefulness for osteonecrosis is extremely limited in the United States.

Bonfiglio M, Voke EM: Aseptic necrosis of the femoral head and nonunion of the femoral neck: Effect of treatment by drilling and bone-grafting (Phemister technique). J Bone Joint Surg Am 1968;50:48.

Buckley PD et al: Structural bone-grafting for early atraumatic avascular necrosis of the femoral head. J Bone Joint Surg Am 1991;73:1357.

Coventry MB: Osteotomy about the knee for degenerative and rheumatoid arthritis: Indications, operative technique, and results. J Bone Joint Surg Am 1973;55:23.

Crockarell JR et al: The anterior center-edge angle: A cadaver study. J Bone Joint Surg Br 2000:82.532.

Edgerton BC et al: Distal femoral varus osteotomy for painful genu valgum: A five-to-11-year follow-up study. Clin Orthop 1993; 288:263.

Fairbank AC et al: Long-term results of core decompression for ischaemic necrosis of the femoral head. J Bone Joint Surg Br 1995;77:42.

Haddad FS et al: CT evaluation of periacetabular osteotomies. J Bone Joint Surg Br 2000:82;526.

Mont MA et al: Core decompression versus nonoperative management for osteonecrosis of the hip. Clin Orthop 1996;324:169.

Morita S et al: Long-term results of valgus-extension femoral osteotomy for advanced osteoarthritis of the hip. J Bone Joint Surg Br 2000:82:824.

Ogilvie-Harris DJ et al: Pigmented villonodular synovitis of the knee: The results of total arthroscopic synovectomy, partial arthroscopic synovectomy, and arthroscopic local excision. J Bone Joint Surg Am 1992;74:119.

Ohashi H et al: Factors influencing the outcome of Chiari pelvic osteotomy: A long-term follow-up. J Bone Joint Surg Br 2000: 82;517.

Shoji H, Insall J: High tibial osteotomy for osteoarthritis of the knee with valgus deformity. J Bone Joint Surg Am 1973;55:963.

Sledge CB et al: Synovectomy of the rheumatoid knee using intra-articular injection of Dysprosium-165-ferric hydroxide macroaggregates. J Bone Joint Surg Am 1987;69:970.

Urbaniak JR, Harvey EJ: Revascularization of the femoral head in osteonecrosis. J Am Acad Orthop Surg 1998;6(1):44.

JOINT SALVAGE PROCEDURES

1. Arthrodesis

Arthrodesis is the creation of a bony union across a joint. The creation of a fibrous union across a joint with no motion is ankylosis. With bony union across a joint, motion of one bone on another is eliminated, relieving pain caused by arthritis. Although ankylosis may prevent observable motion, micromotion may be associated with significant pain. Ankylosis or arthrodesis may occur spontaneously, as in infection or ankylosing spondylitis, or may be surgically produced. The functional results of spontaneous arthrodesis are not ideal because the patient typically holds the joint in the position that causes minimum pain, which frequently is an inappropriate angle for function. Although surgical arthrodesis can be created in almost any joint, including the spine, the most common joints fused are the ankle, knee, shoulder, and hip. The technique used in any of the joints follows the same general pattern. The articular surfaces are denuded of remaining hyaline cartilage and then placed together in the optimal position of function after shaping to achieve maximum contact between the two opposing surfaces. Bone grafting is frequently used, and some form of fixation, either internal (plates, rods, or screws) or external (external fixators or a cast), is used to immobilize the arthrodesis site in the optimal position (Table 7–5). After adequate healing, the rehabilitation process is begun. Multiple techniques of arthrodesis are described for each joint.

Ankle Arthrodesis

The orthopedic community generally considers arthrodesis of the tibiotalar joint to be a good operation for treatment of tibiotalar arthrosis. A well-done ankle arthrodesis results in freedom from pain and nearly normal walking ability. Perhaps the main reason that the ankle arthrodesis is regarded so highly, however, is that other options, such as total ankle replacement, are less viable.

The indications for ankle arthrodesis are as follows:

1. degenerative arthrosis;
2. rheumatoid arthritis;
3. posttraumatic arthritis;
4. avascular necrosis of the talus;
5. neurologic disease resulting in an unstable ankle; and
6. neuropathic ankle joint.

The relative contraindications include degenerative joint disease in the subtalar and midtarsal joints.

The ankle arthrodesis can be performed through an anterior, lateral, or medial approach, and even posterior approaches are described. Arthroscopic techniques are now employed. The most common techniques are probably external fixation or internal screw fixation to achieve compression. Preparation of the ankle for arthrodesis is performed as mentioned earlier. Positioning of the ankle is important, with the talus in a neutral position or at an angle of 5 degrees of dorsiflexion. The midtarsal joints have a greater ROM in plantar flexion than in dorsiflex-

Table 7–5. Optimal position of joints after arthrodesis.

Joint	Angle	Length	Other Consideration
Ankle	0° dorsiflexion 0–5° valgus of hindfoot 5–10° external rotation	Slight shortening	Talus displaced posteriorly.
Knee	15° flexion 5–8° flexion	Slight shortening	—
Shoulder	20–30° flexion 20–40° abduction (lateral border of scapula) 25–40° internal rotation	—	Patient's hand should be able to touch the head and face.
Hip	25° flexion 0–5° abduction (measured between the shaft and a line through the ischia) 0–5° external rotation	Slight shortening	Do *not* destroy abductor mechanism.

ion, resulting in a more flexible foot. The talus is also displaced slightly posteriorly to make it easier for the patient to roll the foot over at the completion of the stance phase. A varus position is to be avoided because this restricts mobility at the midtarsal joints.

Kitaoka HB, Patzer GL: Arthrodesis for the treatment of arthrosis of the ankle and osteonecrosis of the talus. J Bone Joint Surg 1998;80:370.

Scranton PE: An overview of ankle arthrodesis. Clin Orthop 1991;268:96.

Knee Arthrodesis

Knee arthrodesis is seldom done for primary problems and generally done as the last resort for other problems. Indications for the procedure include infection, such as tuberculosis, neuropathic joint secondary to syphilis or diabetes, and loss of quadriceps function. The latter is a relative indication for arthrodesis because joint mobility can be maintained without quadriceps function, and joint stability can be obtained through the use of orthosis, which locks the joint in the fully extended position but can be unlocked for sitting. Although knee arthrodesis is usually successful and provides pain-free weight bearing, it is associated with other problems, especially in tall people. Sitting in airplanes, movie theaters, and even automobiles may be difficult. The most common indication for knee arthrodesis at the present time is failed total knee arthroplasty, usually because of infection. In a patient who wishes to maintain an active lifestyle, such as hunting on rough ground or performing manual labor, a knee arthrodesis is a viable alternative. The relative contraindications include bilateral disease or a problem such as an above-knee amputation of the other leg. In such a case, it would be extremely difficult for a person to arise from a chair with an arthrodesis on the contralateral side.

The technique of arthrodesis varies with the problem being treated. After infection, particularly when it is associated with total knee replacement, bone loss is often moderate to severe. Cancellous bone from the distal femur and proximal tibia may be nearly nonexistent, and external fixation may be necessary to obtain adequate immobilization for arthrodesis. For less severe cases, intramedullary rod fixation may be indicated, particularly if the infection is under control. Similarly, use of double plates at 90 degrees is a viable method of immobilization. Frequently, iliac crest bone grafting is necessary to stimulate healing. Although bone loss often makes it necessary to shorten the extremity, some shortening (2–3 cm) is desirable to prevent a circumduction gait after fusion. The knee should be positioned at 10–15 degrees of flexion and at the normal valgus alignment of 5–8 degrees, if possible.

Donley BG et al: Arthrodesis of the knee with an intramedullary nail. J Bone Joint Surg Am 1991;73:907.

Nichols SJ et al: Arthrodesis with dual plates after failed total knee arthroplasty. J Bone Joint Surg Am 1991;73:1020.

Papilion JD et al: Arthroscopic assisted arthrodesis of the knee. Arthroscopy 1991;7:237.

Elbow Arthrodesis

Elbow arthrodesis is an uncommon procedure. Loss of elbow motion may be particularly disabling. Thus, the indications for arthrodesis are few, and few are performed because fusion causes severe functional limitations. To perform activities of daily living, a flexion arc of 100 degrees from 30 degrees of extension to 130 degrees of flexion is required. A range of 100 degrees for pronation and supination is also required. Painful arthrosis in a patient who is willing to accept the tradeoff between stability and loss of motion is the indication for arthrodesis. Infectious processes, such as tuberculosis or fungus, are also indications for arthrodesis.

Several techniques are described, but the relative rarity of the operation prevents recommendation of one particular method. One report recommends screw fixation. Resection of the radial head may be necessary to allow for pronation and supination. The position of fusion is 90 degrees.

Irvine GB, Gregg PJ: A method of elbow arthrodesis: Brief report. J Bone Joint Surg Br 1989;71:145.

Morrey BF et al: A biomechanical study of normal elbow motion. J Bone Joint Surg Am 1981;62:872.

Shoulder Arthrodesis

Paralysis of the deltoid muscle and sepsis after an arthroplasty are possible indications for shoulder arthrodesis. Obtaining fusion may be a relatively difficult process because of the very long lever arm on the shoulder joint. This is accentuated by the position of fusion, which places the arm in abduction. Before the advent of comprehensive internal fixation devices, intraarticular and extraarticular arthrodeses were performed to provide a reasonable probability of obtaining fusion.

The AO technique (Arbeitsgemeinschaft für Osteosynthesefragen technique) is the most promising because it provides rigid internal fixation and the potential for immobilization without postoperative external immobilization. The patient is placed in the lateral decubitus position. The incision is made over the spine of the scapula, over the acromion, and down the lateral aspect of the humerus. The surface of the glenohumeral joint and the undersurface of the acromion are cleaned of residual cartilage and cortical bone to provide as much contact as possible with the arm in the appropriate position (see Table 7–5). A broad bone plate or pelvic reconstruction plate is then used to fix the humerus to the scapula. The bone plate is fixed to the spine of the scapula and the shaft of the humerus and bent into the appropriate position. Additional fixation may be obtained by placing another plate posteriorly. Bone grafting may be necessary for defects. Rigid fixation must be obtained. After surgery, a soft dressing is used until pain is controlled. A shoulder spica cast is preferred for immobilization by some surgeons. Exercises are begun to gently obtain scapular motion if no cast is used.

A modification of the AO technique that uses an external fixator to neutralize forces on interfragmentary screws has good results. Functional results are varied and depend on the position of fusion. Overhead work or work with the arm abducted is not possible. Excessive internal and external rotation must be avoided.

Johnson CA et al: External fixation shoulder arthrodesis. Clin Orthop 1986;211:219.

Muller ME et al: *Manual of Internal Fixation.* Berlin: Springer-Verlag, 1970.

Richards RR et al: Shoulder arthrodesis using a pelvic-reconstruction plate. J Bone Joint Surg Am 1988;70;416.

Riggins RS: Shoulder fusion without external fixation: A preliminary report. J Bone Joint Surg Am 1976;58:1007.

Hip Arthrodesis

Arthrodesis of the hip, as of other joints, produces a relatively pain-free stable joint that allows the patient to perform heavy labor. The disadvantage of hip arthrodesis in a young person who performs heavy labor is that over a period of time, degenerative disk disease of the lumbar spine and degenerative arthrosis of the ipsilateral knee frequently occur, even with optimal position of the arthrodesis. In fact, an indication for converting a hip fusion to a total hip arthroplasty is incapacitating back or knee pain.

The most obvious indication for arthrodesis of the hip is tuberculosis. Chronic osteomyelitis is a relative indication. Contraindications to arthrodesis include limited motion of the ipsilateral knee or degenerative arthrosis of the ipsilateral knee, as well as significant degenerative lumbar spine disease and arthrosis of the contralateral hip. Perhaps the biggest problem in performing a hip arthrodesis in a patient with adequate indications is obtaining agreement from the patient. Because joint replacement offers mobility, early rehabilitation, and a less extensive operation, patients are reluctant to consider the potential problems of hip arthrodesis. This is particularly true when total hip arthroplasty is performed in professional athletes, permitting some of them to continue in sports. Because of these factors, hip arthrodesis is now a relatively uncommon operation.

Multiple techniques are described for performing hip arthrodesis. Truly rigid fixation is difficult to achieve, and cast immobilization after surgery is usually needed. During the fusion procedure, care should be taken to preserve the abductors, so future reconstructive procedures may be performed if desired. The crucial aspect of the operation is fusing the hip in the appropriate position. The optimal position is slight flexion (25 degrees) from the normal position of the pelvis and spine, slight external rotation (5 degrees), and neutral abduction and adduction. Previously, the hip was placed in abduction, producing a very abnormal gait with additional stress on the lumbar spine. A position of neutral to slight abduction minimizes this problem because the body's center of gravity when the patient is in a one-legged stance is moved closer to the foot. Too much flexion makes both walking and lying in bed difficult, and too little flexion makes sitting difficult. Too much external rotation forces the knee joint to move in a plane oblique from that defined by the collateral and cruciate ligaments.

Blasier RB, Holmes JR: Intraoperative positioning for arthrodesis of the hip with the double bean bag technique. J Bone Joint Surg Am 1990;72:766.

Callaghan JJ et al: Hip arthrodesis: A long-term follow-up. J Bone Joint Surg Am 1984;67:1328.

2. Resection Arthroplasty

Resection arthroplasty, or excisional arthroplasty, is a procedure that is applied primarily to the hip, the elbow, and, more recently, the knee. Resection arthroplasty, or a modification called **fascial arthroplasty,** was a procedure used in the elbow for many years. Resection arthroplasty of the hip is also called **Girdlestone pseudoarthrosis** and dates back to 1923. Resection arthroplasty of the knee is a relatively new procedure that is used when infection compromises total knee replacement. Similarly, Girdlestone pseudoarthrosis is performed with increasing frequency as an intervening, sometimes permanent treatment for infection following total hip arthroplasty.

Hip Arthroplasty

Resection arthroplasty of the hip produces a relatively pain-free joint with reasonably good motion. It is indicated as a primary procedure when ankylosis causes the hip to be placed in an unsuitable position; such patients would otherwise be at high risk for dislocation or infection with a total hip arthroplasty. Spinal cord injury, head injury, and, perhaps, severe Parkinson disease would be diagnoses that might warrant primary resection arthroplasty. Disadvantages of the procedure result from lack of mechanical continuity between the femur and the pelvis; this causes an abnormal gait and the need for support with a cane or other device, and shortening occurs with each step. Patients who previously had infection following total hip replacement usually have the most stable hip joints because dense scar tissue has formed. The procedure can be very helpful in reambulating wheelchair-bound patients in whom peroneal care is very difficult.

For infection compromising total hip replacement, resection arthroplasty is accomplished by removing all of the cement, the prosthesis, any necrotic bone, and the soft tissue. In primary resection arthroplasty, the procedure is more of a reconstructive procedure in which the femoral head and neck are removed flush with the intertrochanteric line and the capsule is reconstructed to help provide some stability of the hip. Traction with a pin in the tibia is frequently used for variable periods to maintain leg length.

Knee Arthroplasty

Resection arthroplasty of the knee has a much less satisfactory functional result. After removal of an infected knee prosthesis, there is usually significant bone loss and the knee is quite unstable. Bracing improves the condition only modestly, and the patient still requires crutches or a walker to ambulate.

Elbow Arthroplasty

Resection arthroplasty or fascial arthroplasty of the elbow is one means of managing ankylosis after trauma or infection. Resection arthroplasty may be performed for failure of total elbow arthroplasty resulting from sepsis. Resection arthroplasty in the patient with RA should be discouraged because one of the problems associated with the procedure is instability. The rheumatoid patient frequently depends on the upper extremity to ambulate with walking aids. Interpositional arthroplasty, using fascia or split-thickness skin grafts, was thought to reduce resorption of bone, but the additional benefit of the interpositional tissue is doubtful. Although resection arthroplasty frequently relieves pain, instability is a major problem, and bracing is required in most cases. With the availability of elbow arthroplasty, this procedure is rarely performed.

Milgram JW, Rana NA: Resection arthroplasty for septic arthritis of the hip in ambulatory and nonambulatory adult patients. Clin Orthop 1991;272:181.

Thornhill TS et al: Alternatives to arthrodesis for failed total knee arthroplasty. Clin Orthop 1982;170:131.

JOINT REPLACEMENT PROCEDURES

1. Hemiarthroplasty

Hemiarthroplasty is the replacement of only one side of a diarthrodial joint. The procedure is indicated for displaced fractures of the femoral neck or four-part fractures of the humeral head, but there are other indications in adult reconstructive surgery. In both the shoulder and the hip, osteonecrosis may result in collapse of the humeral or femoral articulating surface, with sparing of the glenoid or acetabulum. In the hip, nonunion of the femoral neck after open reduction and internal fixation may also be an indication for endoprosthetic replacement. In either joint, pathologic fracture or tumor may be an indication. Contraindications include active infection, RA, and possibly the patient's age. Endoprosthetic replacement in a young individual is certain to result, with time, in destruction of the articular surface of the acetabulum. This may, however, take many years, and the patient may have a serviceable joint in the intervening period.

The choice of prosthesis depends on factors such as life expectancy, cost, and physiologic demand. For the shoulder, a cemented prosthesis should probably be modular to permit conversion to total shoulder replacement at a later date without removal of the stem, should that become necessary. Similar concerns for the hip apply. The femoral head can be replaced with a unipolar or bipolar prosthesis. The bipolar prosthesis allows motion to occur between the acetabulum and the prosthesis, as well as between the prosthesis and the articulating surface of the metal femoral head. This articulation is metal or ceramic on plastic and certain to produce debris from wear that may be detrimental to the durability of the hip prosthesis. Selection of a monopolar prosthesis, however, must not compromise conversion of the hemiarthroplasty to a total hip arthroplasty, should this become necessary.

The operative technique is quite similar to that of total joint replacement for each joint. The main difference in the hip is that the capsule is usually repaired after hemiarthroplasty. A posterolateral approach is most commonly used in the hip, although an anterolateral approach may be preferred in a patient with associated mental problems that may limit postoperative cooperation. If the posterolateral approach is used in such patients, a knee immobilizer may be necessary to prevent hip flexion that might lead to dislocation.

2. Total Joint Arthroplasty

Joint replacement surgery became a viable treatment for arthritic afflictions of joints when the low-friction hip arthroplasty was developed by Sir John Charnley in the 1960s. This procedure consisted of the articulation of a metal femoral head on an ultrahigh-molecular-weight polyethylene (UHMWPE) acetabular component, with both components fixed in place with acrylic cement (polymethylmethacrylate [PMMA]). The long-term results are quite satisfactory, and the concept is now applied to other joints with variable success. The knee replacement, shoulder replacement, and elbow replacement have evolved to the point that satisfactory results are routine when the indications for surgery are appropriate. Other arthroplasties, such as the ankle, wrist, and first metatarsophalangeal joint, are less successful. In fairness, the application of technology to these joints is not at the level applied to other joints. Success of all arthroplasties depends on the skill of the surgeon, the surgeon's understanding of the basic biomechanics underlying the joint function, the design of the prosthesis, and the technical equipment used to insert the prosthesis.

The design of the prosthesis is an evolutionary process that depends on laboratory and clinical experience. Hip replacement surgery, performed often, is highly successful. Less frequently performed arthroplasties, such as elbow replacement, are associated with less clinical and laboratory experience.

Total Hip Arthroplasty

The original Charnley total hip arthroplasty was a stainless steel femoral prosthesis with a small collar, a rectangular cross section, and a 22-mm femoral head. The acetabular component was a UHMWPE cup (Figure 7–7). Both components were cemented into place with acrylic bone cement. Since then, an entire industry has evolved to produce new designs for hip components, including different head sizes (22, 25, 25.4, 28, 32, and 35 mm); different femoral component lengths (ranging from 110 mm to 160 mm for standard prostheses); different cross sections (square, round, oval, I-beam); a porous coating for bone ingrowth attachment; and metal backing for the acetabulum (cemented or porous coated). The two generic designs that evolved from experience with bone attachment technique are the porous ingrowth and cement fixation prostheses.

A. Indications

The indications for hip arthroplasty are incapacitating arthritis of the hip combined with appropriate physical and roentgenographic findings. The historical data that justify consideration of hip replacement surgery include pain requiring medication stronger than aspirin, inability to walk more than a few blocks without stopping, pain following activity, pain that wakes the patient at night, difficulty with shoes and socks or foot care such as cutting nails, and difficulty in climbing stairs. It is good practice to use a clinical rating score to evaluate these historical data (Table 7–6).

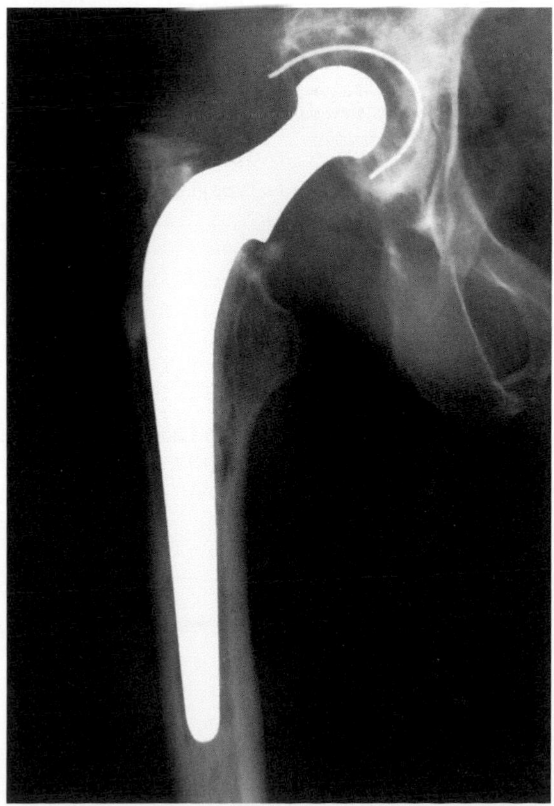

Figure 7–7. Radiograph of a Charnley arthroplasty.

Table 7–6. Harris hip evaluation (modified).

I. Pain (44 possible)
- A. None or ignores it 44
- B. Slight, occasional, no compromise in activities 40
- C. Mild pain, no effect on average activities, rarely moderate pain; with unusual activity may take aspirin 30
- D. Moderate pain, tolerable, but makes concessions to pain; some limitation of ordinary activity or work; may require occasional pain medicine stronger than aspirin 20
- E. Marked pain, serious limitation of activities 10
- F. Totally disabled, crippled, pain in bed, bedridden 0

II. Function (47 possible)
- A. Gait (33 possible)
  - 1. Limp
    - a. None 11
    - b. Slight 8
    - c. Moderate 5
    - d. Severe 0
  - 2. Support
    - a. None 11
    - b. Cane for long walks 7
    - c. Cane most of the time 5
    - d. One crutch 3
    - e. Two canes 2
    - f. Two crutches 0
    - g. Not able to walk (specify reason) 0
  - 3. Distance walked
    - a. Unlimited 11
    - b. Six blocks 8
    - c. Two or three blocks 5
    - d. Indoors only 2
    - e. Bed and chair 0
- B. Activities (14 possible)
  - 1. Stairs
    - a. Normally without using a railing 4
    - b. Normally using a railing 2
    - c. In any manner 1
    - d. Unable to do stairs 0
  - 2. Shoes and socks
    - a. With ease 4
    - b. With difficulty 2
    - c. Unable 0
  - 3. Sitting
    - a. Comfortably in ordinary chair 1 hour 5
    - b. On a high chair for one-half hour 3
    - c. Unable to sit comfortably in any chair 0
    - 4. Enter public transportation 1

C. Range of Motion	R	L
Flexion	_____	_____
Flexion contracture	_____	_____
Abduction	_____	_____
Adduction	_____	_____
External rotation	_____	_____
Internal rotation	_____	_____
D. Location of pain		
Groin	_____	_____
Thigh	_____	_____
Buttock	_____	_____

Physical examination typically demonstrates a limited ROM, pain at extremes of motion, a positive Trendelenburg test, a limp, and groin or anterior thigh pain with active straight leg raising.

Radiographs demonstrate loss of joint space and other findings consistent with the cause of the disorder. Noteworthy features requiring special considerations for surgery are dysplasia of the acetabulum, protrusio acetabuli, and proximal femoral deformity or the presence of metal implants from previous operations.

After consideration of the lifestyle requirements of the patient, the surgeon may suggest this procedure as a means of alleviating pain, which is the main indication for hip replacement surgery. Other reconstructive procedures should be considered, including arthrodesis, osteotomy, and hemiarthroplasty. When selecting a procedure, one should consider the patient's goals in terms of work and leisure activity. A young person who performs heavy labor and has unilateral traumatic arthritis may be best served by arthrodesis. A 50-year-old bank executive who does not ski, play tennis, or ride horses but does swim and bicycle will probably have best results with hip arthroplasty.

A choice must be made between cemented and uncemented arthroplasty, with the uncemented acetabular component nearly universally indicated. Its advantages include a consistently pain-free result, long-lasting fixation, and modularity to permit latitude in selecting head size and acetabular polyethylene component offset designs. Its disadvantages include the need for metal backing of the polyethylene liner, which may increase wear, and the possibility of dissociation of the plastic component from the metal. A cemented acetabular component manufactured from UHMWPE is usually reserved for an individual with a life expectancy of 10 years or less. The indications for an uncemented femoral component vary with the surgeon but usually depend on the age of the patient, with younger patients most likely to benefit from the porous-coated prosthesis.

B. Surgical Technique

Certain aspects of hip replacement surgery apply to all arthroplasty techniques, including cement technique and bone surface preparation.

1. Posterolateral approach—The most common approach for total hip arthroplasty is the posterolateral approach. After administration of anesthesia and placement of a thromboembolic stocking and intermittent compression stocking on the unaffected limb, the patient is rolled into the lateral decubitus position, with the affected side superior. Draping should leave the entire leg free and extending above the iliac crest. Kidney rests are used to support the pelvis at the pubis and the sacrum, and bony prominences should be protected. The incision is outlined on the skin before the skin is completely covered with an adhesive drape. By flexing the hip to 45 degrees, the incision can be made in line with the femur from approximately 10 cm proximal to the tip of the trochanter to 10 cm distal to the tip of the trochanter.

Alternatively, with the hip in the extended position, the incision is made from 10 cm distal to the tip of the trochanter extending proximally along the line of the trochanter and then curving posteriorly at approximately a 45-degree angle for another 10 cm. The incision is deepened to show the fascia lata and the gluteus maximus. An incision is made in the fascia lata directly lateral and extended proximally into the gluteus maximus, which is split in line with its fibers. A Charnley retractor is placed, and fat overlying the external rotators is removed. After putting the femur into internal rotation, the external rotators (piriformis, gemelli, obturator internus, and quadratus femoris) are tagged with sutures for reattachment and removed from their attachments at the trochanter. The gluteus minimus is separated from the capsule and preserved and protected, and a capsulectomy is performed. Alternatively, portions of the posterior capsule can be reflected for later reattachment. If the patient is not paralyzed with nondepolarizing muscle relaxant agents, excision of the capsule with electrocautery signals whether the sciatic nerve is particularly closely applied to the posterior of the acetabulum. The sciatic nerve must be identified and protected throughout the procedure if there is electrical transmission. Internal rotation of the flexed hip dislocates the hip, and the femoral head is delivered into the operative field. Using an appropriate template, the femoral head is resected with an oscillating saw. The femur is then externally rotated, and Taylor retractors are placed anteriorly and posteriorly to permit visualization of the acetabulum. The acetabulum is medialized if appropriate when medial osteophytes are present. Anterior osteophytes, if present, are removed under direct visualization. Reaming of the acetabulum is performed until a good bed of bleeding subchondral bone is obtained; progressive reamers are usually used. At this point, techniques diverge based on whether a cemented or an uncemented cup is used.

If a cemented cup is used, multiple holes with a diameter of $^{1}/_{4}$–$^{3}/_{8}$ inch are drilled in the acetabulum to provide firm cement interdigitation. One of the commercially available techniques that prevents bottoming out of the acetabular cup should be used, so the medial cement mantle will be adequate. The position of the cup is determined with trials, using the native acetabulum for guidance and radiograph if there is any concern about positioning. The cup is cemented into place after the acetabular bone is prepared with pulsatile lavage, epinephrine-soaked sponges, and pressurization of the cement.

If an uncemented cup is used, reaming progresses to a diameter 1–2 mm smaller than the actual size of the cup to be implanted. The cup is impacted into place, ensuring appropriate positioning. Fixation is achieved with screws or pegs, as specified by the manufacturer. A trial plastic component is inserted, and attention is returned to the femur.

The hip is internally rotated, flexed to approximately 80 degrees, and adducted, so the cut femoral neck is presented to the surgeon. Homan retractors may be used to help elevate the amputated femoral neck into the wound. A box chisel is then used to remove the femoral neck laterally. The canal is broached with a curet to provide an indication of the direction of the intramedullary canal. The femoral canal is then broached with increasing sizes of broaches, until all weak cancellous bone is removed. The prosthesis size is determined, and a cement restrictor is placed 2 cm distal to the final position of the stem tip. The canal is prepared for cementing with pulsatile lavage, medullary canal brushing, and sponges soaked with hydrogen peroxide or epinephrine. The cement is prepared and centrifuged or vacuum mixed and inserted into the femoral canal with a cement gun. The cement is pressurized, and the prosthesis is inserted into appropriate anteversion (approximately 10 degrees) and held in position until the cement cures. When the appropriate broach, as indicated by preoperative templating, is reached, a trial femoral prosthesis is inserted, the neck length is checked, and the prosthesis is reduced into position. Range of motion is tested at 90 degrees of flexion and should be stable to 40–45 degrees of internal rotation. External rotation to 40 degrees in the fully extended position must be obtained without impingement on the femoral neck posteriorly. Proper myofascial tension is assessed by telescoping the hip at 45 degrees (approximately 3 or 4 mm). Proper leg length is usually achieved when the rectus femoris tightness (flexion of the knee with the hip extended) is similar to prior to surgery. A further check on leg lengths can be made by comparing the center of the femoral head preoperatively with the proximal tip of the trochanter to trochanter-prosthesis center distance with the prosthesis in place. Measuring devices are designed to measure leg lengths, but up to a centimeter of discrepancy can still occur. An extended lip on the UHMWPE component may provide additional stability but may form a fulcrum on which the head may be levered out. The prosthesis trial is removed, and the permanent polyethylene component is put into place in the acetabular metallic shell. The femoral canal is then prepared for cementing.

After the cement hardens, a trial femoral head is used to put the hip through a second ROM. The optimal neck length is selected, and the appropriate prosthetic component is impacted into place. When combining modular components held together with a Morse-type taper, the manufacturers' components should not be mixed. It is mandatory that the surfaces be clean and dry. The bore in the femoral head is placed on the trunnion and twisted and impacted into place with several sharp blows. The acetabulum is cleaned of debris, the femoral head is reduced, and the wound is closed. The external rotators are reattached with sutures placed through bone while the hip is in external rotation and abduction. The fascia is closed with interrupted sutures.

The design and insertion technique of the uncemented femoral components are quite variable and therefore are not described here.

Abbreviated mini incisions for the posterolateral approach to the hip are described. These generally use a small portion of the routine incision but are carefully placed to optimize visualization of the hip.

2. Lateral approach—The lateral approach to the hip is performed with a trochanteric osteotomy after the fascia of the tensor fascia lata and gluteus maximus are entered. The patient may be in the supine position with a bump under the hip or in the lateral position. Prior to osteotomy, the trochanter is mobilized, and the trochanteric osteotomy is performed with an osteotome or a Gigli saw. The gluteus minimus is peeled off the capsule as the trochanter is mobilized proximally. After capsulectomy, the femoral head is dislocated anteriorly. The procedure is essentially identical from this point on until the trochanter is reattached. Various modifications of trochanteric osteotomy techniques are described. The abductor mechanism is extremely important in preserving the stability of the hip as well as the gait. Thus, extreme care must be taken to reattach the trochanter when the procedure is completed, so reliable union is achieved. Even in the best of hands, approximately 1 in 20 trochanters fails to unite, although the number of people who have disability or pain from a fibrous union is much lower. If wires are used to reattach the trochanter, they should be biocompatible with the prosthetic component, and a minimum of three should be used to achieve adequate fixation.

3. Anterolateral approach (Watson-Jones approach)—The interval between the gluteus medius muscle and the tensor fascia lata is utilized proximally to gain access to the femoral neck and hip joint. The patient is in the supine position, with a bump under the buttock. The skin incision follows the shaft of the femur distally and curves slightly anteriorly proximally. The fascia is incised in line with the skin incision and proximally splits the interval between the tensor fascia lata and the gluteus medius. The tensor fascia lata is then retracted anteriorly, and the gluteus medius is retracted superiorly and laterally. Because the fibers of the gluteus medius and minimus tend to run anteriorly, particularly in the osteoarthritic hip with destruction and shortening, these fibers must be released to provide access to the hip joint. The hip is externally rotated. The anterior capsule is incised, and the hip joint can then be dislocated. Osteotomy of the femoral neck proceeds at the appropriate level. Capsulotomy is performed, retractors are placed to provide acetabular exposure, and hip replacement is performed. The femur during this procedure is externally rotated. Care must be taken in exposing the acetabulum to prevent damage to the femoral nerve and femoral muscles.

4. Other approaches—Other approaches are used for hip replacement, some of which are successful according to the skill of the individual surgeon. Some approaches, including the direct lateral approach, may be fraught with problems such as abductor weakness after surgery, and the result may be disappointing to the patient as well as the surgeon.

C. Implants

The two basic types of total hip replacement are cemented and uncemented. The bearing surfaces for both are the same, either cobalt chromium alloy or ceramic (alumina or zirconia), articulating with a UHMWPE bearing surface. The femoral stem replacement may be cobalt chromium or titanium alloy, either of which is also used for the metal backing of the acetabulum. Cobalt chromium alloy is associated with much less stress on the bone–cement interface because of its higher modulus; this prolongs fixation. The femoral component should be designed to provide intrinsic torsional stability without having sharp edges that would create stress concentration sites in the bone cement. A matte surface should be created to allow some mechanical interlocking with the cement, although currently this is controversial, and some surgeons recommend a polished surface. Adequate offset is necessary to restore the mechanical advantage of the abductors.

The choice of material for the femoral head is a trade-off between cost and theoretical advantages. The harder, wettable surface of ceramic heads theoretically results in less production of debris from wear and longer service of the hip replacement without loosening, but the cost is two to three times that of an equivalent-sized cobalt chromium (Co/Cr) head. Thus, in most individuals undergoing total hip arthroplasty, a Co/Cr head is probably optimal. In younger patients, the increased cost of a ceramic head may be warranted. Femoral heads are available now in 22-, 26-, 28-, and 32-mm sizes. One clinical investigation of total hip replacements showed that 26- and 28-mm heads are associated with the least amount of linear and volumetric wear. A head of 22 mm may be necessary for patients with smaller acetabular sockets to provide adequate thickness of the polyethylene bearing surface. A minimum of 6 mm, preferably 8 mm or more, is suggested to lower the contact stress on the polyethylene and thereby reduce wear.

New bearing surfaces for the articulation of the hip joint are becoming popular. The possibilities include ceramic on ceramic, Co/Cr on Co/Cr, and ceramic or Co/Cr on radiation cross-linked polyethylene. The impetus for this change is the possibility of lower wear debris. These articulation couples require long-term follow-up to determine if they will live up to their promise.

No evidence justifies use of a metal backing on the cemented acetabular component. Other design considerations to avoid are deep grooves that might evolve into cracks in the PMMA. The surface must be rough enough to allow the cup to bond to the cement through mechanical interlock.

Uncemented acetabular components have a spherical outer surface with at least one hole to permit the surgeon to determine if the prosthesis is fully impacted into place. The shell should have a minimum of 3 mm of metal to reduce the risk of fatigue failure. Cobalt chromium alloy or titanium alloy appears to be equally efficacious. The inner surface should lock the polyethylene in some fashion to reliably limit rotation and dissociation. The inner surface should be the mate of the polyethylene outer surface to reduce the chance of cold flow of the plastic as well as wear from relative motion. Recommended materials are listed in Table 7–7.

Table 7–7. Preferred materials for total hip replacement.

Component	Material	Alternative Material
Uncemented femoral component	Titanium alloy	Cobalt chromium alloy
Cemented femoral component	Cobalt chromium alloy (forged)	Cast cobalt chromium alloy, titanium alloy
Femoral head	Cobalt chromium alloy	Zirconia, alumina
Cemented acetabulum bearing surface	Ultrahigh-molecular-weight polyethylene component (no metal backing)	—
Uncemented acetabulum bearing surface	Ultrahigh-molecular-weight polyethylene component	—
Acetabulum ingrowth surface	Titanium alloy, cobalt chromium alloy	—

Design considerations for the uncemented femoral component are unclear at present. Use of porous coating, hydroxyapatite, or tricalcium phosphate coating is driven by manufacturing concerns and prosthesis strength requirements rather than an understanding of the biologic principles of hip replacement. Two design factors are important: (1) If a prosthesis is excessively stiff in relation to the bone to which it is attached, proximal osteopenia may result from "stress shielding" or "stress bypassing" of the bone; and (2) stiffer prostheses also seem to be associated with more pain in the thigh. Therefore, strategies to reduce stiffness seem appropriate. Both of these factors are addressed by using titanium alloy as opposed to cobalt chromium alloy, but other factors may surface to affect this choice. Creating slots or grooves to reduce the torsional and bending stiffness also seems to be effective in reducing stiffness and resulting thigh pain.

D. Complications

Any major surgery is associated with a certain incidence of complications, which is certainly true for total hip arthroplasty. The surgeon must recognize these complications in a timely manner and treat them appropriately. The most common complications include deep venous thrombosis (DVT), fracture or perforation of the femoral shaft, infection, instability (dislocation), heterotopic bone formation, and nerve palsies.

1. Deep venous thrombosis—Although some morbidity results from DVT, the real risk is pulmonary embolism, which is occasionally fatal. The incidence of DVT is high, but the incidence of fatal pulmonary emboli fortunately is low, in the range of 0.3%. The high incidence of DVT during hip replacement surgery is related to femoral vein damage from manipulation or retraction, intraoperative or postoperative venous stasis caused by immobility and limb swelling, and a hypercoagulable state directly resulting from the surgical trauma to the patient. Certain factors are recognized as predisposing the patient to higher risk for DVT, including a prior history of pulmonary embolus, estrogen treatment, preexisting cancer, older (more than 60 years) age of the patient, and length of the operative procedure, one factor that is under the surgeon's control.

Pharmacologic and mechanical measures are used to reduce the risk of DVT. Some surgeons prefer surveillance through clinical or laboratory tests such as duplex scanning, venograms, and fibrinogen scans, followed by anticoagulation therapy in patients with clot formation. The National Institutes of Health Consensus Conference concluded that mechanical measures such as intermittent pneumatic compression provide adequate prophylaxis for patients who are mobilized quickly, whereas anticoagulation therapy is recommended for those expected to undergo prolonged bed rest. Pharmacologic prophylaxis includes sodium warfarin, subcutaneous heparin, and aspirin. The efficacy of subcutaneous minidose heparin and aspirin is controversial. The first low-molecular-weight heparin (enoxaparin) is administered subcutaneously and was approved by the Food and Drug Administration (FDA) for prophylaxis in total hip arthroplasty patients. This drug offers the benefit of twice-daily administration without the need for coagulation monitoring. Its indications were extended to total knee replacement prophylaxis. Other similar low-molecular-weight heparin products are now available and may permit single daily dosing. These include such products as dalteparin sodium and tinzaparin sodium. These drugs offer higher factor Xa inhibition in relation to factor IIa inhibition than unfractionated heparin, which prevents clotting without affecting the activated partial thromboplastin time (PTT). Other chemotherapeutic agents include fondaparinux, a pentasaccharide that is a factor Xa inhibitor, also given by injection once daily. On the horizon are oral thrombin (IIa) inhibitors that may be more convenient for outpatient use.

Because DVT can lead to a catastrophic outcome, preventative measures are indicated starting in the presurgical area. The patient should wear an antiembolic stocking on the unaffected extremity, and both extremities can be treated with intermittent pneumatic compression during the operative procedure. Following surgery, a low-molecular-weight heparin (enoxaparin or dalteparin) is the treatment of choice. Patients who develop pulmonary embolus should receive routine treatment with heparin followed by warfarin.

2. Nerve palsies—Three degrees of nerve injury are recognized. In order of increasing severity, these are neurapraxia, in which conduction is disrupted; axonotmesis, in which the neuron is affected but not the myelin sheath; and neurotmesis, in which the nerve is completely disrupted, as in laceration. In total hip arthroplasty, the most common injuries are neurapraxia and axonotmesis. Neurotmesis is unlikely to occur, except when severe scar tissue predisposes the nerve to laceration. Early nerve recovery (days to weeks) indicates neurapraxia; while longer recovery (months) indicates axonotmesis.

Nerve palsies after total hip arthroplasty are relatively infrequent, but the incidence increases as the complexity of the surgical procedure increases. The sciatic nerve is most commonly involved, with the peroneal division of the sciatic nerve at the greatest risk (80% of cases). The femoral nerve is involved less frequently. An early study indicated an overall prevalence of 1.7%, with total hip arthroplasty for congenital hip dysplasia having a rate of 5.2% and for osteoarthrosis 1%, but a subsequent review suggested that the overall rate of palsy was reduced to approximately 1%. Revision surgery was associated with a rate of 3.2%. The type of injury most likely to produce nerve palsy is stretching or compression, although other mechanisms, such as ischemia, intraneural hemorrhage, dislocation of the femoral component, and cement extrusion, are also suggested as causes.

Nerve injury may be prevented by identifying high-risk cases, protecting the sciatic nerve from compression, and evaluating the sciatic nerve for possible stretching before the wound is closed. Stretching the sciatic nerve by as little as 2 cm increases the risk of palsy significantly. Palpation of the sciatic nerve for tautness with the hip and knee extended and with the hip flexed and knee extended (straight leg–raising test) indicates whether there is danger of stretching the sciatic nerve. Shortening the femoral neck is one means of addressing this problem. If any doubt exists about whether stretching occurred, the patient should be placed in the hospital bed following operation with the hip extended and the knee flexed to relieve tension of the nerve, until the patient is awake and function of the nerve can be monitored.

Management of nerve palsy is generally conservative, with observation when the nerve is known to be in continuity and not stretched. Electromyograms and nerve conduction studies may be helpful but may not show changes until 3 weeks after injury. Recovery of some motor function in the hospital heralds a good prognosis, and if complete return is to occur, it does so by 21 months, according to one study.

3. Vascular complications—Significant vascular complications are reported to occur in approximately 0.25% of total hip replacements. These may be caused by placement of retractors and acetabular screws and by damage to atherosclerotic vessels. Early recognition is important in these injuries.

4. Fracture or perforation—The typical fracture associated with total hip arthroplasty involves the femoral shaft, but other fractures do occur. Fatigue fractures of structures such as the pubic ramus may occur following increased activity after hip replacement relieves pain. The intraoperative problem of fracture or perforation of the femur is relatively uncommon in primary arthroplasty. Perforation may occur in disorders such as sickle cell anemia and osteopetrosis or following previous internal fixation. These conditions may have resulted in sclerotic bone, which may direct the broach astray. Perforations are relatively easily managed by extending the prosthesis past the area of perforation. This distance is generally considered to be two femoral diameters for a perforation with a cemented arthroplasty, but longer distances may be necessary with uncemented arthroplasties, depending on the size of the perforation. An alternative is to use a structural allograft held in place with cerclage wires. In either case, cancellous bone grafting is prudent to facilitate healing.

After total hip arthroplasty, the stress state of the bone is definitely changed, and there is a stress concentration area at the tip of the prosthesis. Fractures in the periprosthetic area are relatively common. These fractures are classified as type A, involving the greater or lesser trochanter; type B1, B2, B3, around or just below the stem, with the stem well fixed (B1), stem loose (B2), or poor bone stock in the proximal femur (B3); or type C, well below the stem. Type A fractures are treated nonoperatively unless the cause is osteolysis, which may predispose the femur to more serious injury. Type B and C fractures are generally treated surgically. Revision is usually the treatment of choice if the prosthesis demonstrates loosening on plain radiographs. Bone grafting is generally necessary with bone deficiencies, and bicortical onlay grafting techniques may be necessary with poor bone stock. Open reduction and internal fixation may be indicated if the prosthesis is tight (types B1 and C), but generous bone grafting and careful observation are necessary to ensure healing. Fracture fixation devices applied in the vicinity of the femoral component may be tenuous, and these devices must not compromise the integrity of the cement mantle or prosthesis.

5. Dislocation following total hip arthroplasty—The incidence of dislocation following total hip arthroplasty varies somewhat from series to series, but ranges from 1% to 8% and averages 2–2.5%. Several factors are associated with higher rates of dislocation, including female sex of the patient and nonunion of the trochanteric osteotomy, revision surgery, and use of the posterior approach. Dislocation after revision surgery in one series was 10% after the first revision and 26.7% after two or more revisions. An ununited trochanter after revision was associated with a 25% rate of dislocation.

Factors important in preventing dislocation are proper placement of components, adjustment of myofascial tension, component design, and patient compliance. Variables found to have no effect on the dislocation rate include the ROM of the hip and the femoral head size. A 32-mm head has a theoretic advantage over a 22-mm head because a neck of the same diameter would impinge earlier with a 22-mm head. At the time of surgery, the myofascial tension is tested by traction on the femur. Displacement of 1 cm or more suggests an increased probability of dislocation after surgery.

The risk of dislocation after total hip arthroplasty diminishes as time passes without dislocation. A first dislocation often occurs within 6 weeks following surgery and is frequently a result of patient noncompliance with postsurgical guidelines. For a first dislocation, closed reduction is used, and careful assessment of the cause of dislocation should be made. If component position appears to be adequate, bracing for 3 months is recommended, along with careful explanation of hip dislocation precautions to the patient. Alternatively, removal of the acetabular component with replacement by a bipolar into the reamed acetabulum may be the best salvage procedure. Recurrent dislocation should be examined carefully for cause, with radiographs taken to evaluate the abduction and anteversion of the cup as well as the anteversion of the femoral head (Figure 7–8). Examination under fluoroscopy may reveal impingements, and push-and-pull films may reveal inadequate myofascial tension.

After careful evaluation of the cause(s) of dislocation, surgical correction may be undertaken. Possible solutions include reorienting the offset lip of the acetabulum, changing the anteversion or abduction of the acetabulum, changing the anteversion of the femoral component, or advancing the trochanter to tighten the muscle envelope. Failure of these methods may require the use of a constrained acetabulum to prevent dislocation. This treatment should be considered a last resort because the reduced ROM resulting from the design of these cups can predispose the patient to dislocation as a result of levering out of the cup from neck impingement. Long-term bracing is a possible solution for recurrent dislocation in a patient with limited goals for activity. Recurrent dislocation causes significant anxiety, which encourages patients to seek surgical correction. The recurrence rate in such patients is as high as 20% after surgical correction.

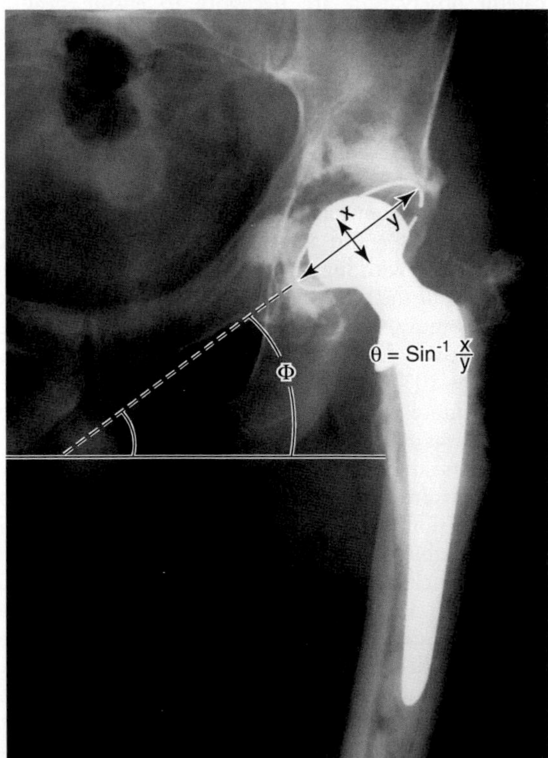

Figure 7–8. Approximate determination of the abduction-adduction angle and angle of anteversion of the cup. Exact measurement requires careful control of the direction of the x-ray beam.

6. Leg-length discrepancy—During hip replacement surgery, an attempt is made to maintain the preoperative length of the affected leg, so it is as long as the unaffected leg. This goal, however, is sometimes incompatible with (and therefore subservient to) myofascial tension in the ligamentously lax individual or may be a potential cause of damage to nerve or vascular structures. Hence, most surgeons advise their patients that the leg may be longer or shorter than normal after operation.

7. Trochanteric nonunion—The rate of trochanteric nonunion after a primary total hip arthroplasty is approximately 5%. The percentage of patients who develop symptoms from this complication is smaller. Usually, migration of less than 1 cm is not associated with functional symptoms or pain.

The rate of nonunion after revision surgery is much higher, as much as 40%, particularly if there has been nonunion following the primary procedure. Diminished function, as evidenced by weakness in abduction and a limp that cannot be compensated for with a cane, is an indication for an attempt at reattachment of the trochanter. The surfaces should be freshened and rigidly fixed together; bone grafting may be necessary. Subperiosteal release of the iliac wing muscles may be necessary to allow the trochanter to be reattached to the femur.

Pain after trochanteric nonunion may be the result of a painful pseudoarthrosis or, alternatively, to fixation wires that may form a painful bursa.

8. Heterotopic ossification—The incidence of significant heterotopic ossification after total hip arthroplasty is 5% or 10%, although it is present to a lesser degree in perhaps 80% of patients. Definite risk factors include previous heterotopic ossification, ankylosing spondylitis, diffuse idiopathic skeletal hyperostosis or spinal ostosis (Forestier disease), unlimited hip motion preoperatively, head injury, and male sex of the patient. Other possible risk factors include trochanteric osteotomy, interoperative fracture, bone grafting, or localized muscle damage or hematoma.

Heterotopic bone is classified by either the Brooker or the Mayo classification (Table 7–8). Patients identified as being at risk for heterotopic ossification should undergo prophylactic treatment, careful surgical treat-

Table 7–8. Heterotopic bone classification systems.

Stage	Mayo Classification	Brooker Classification
I	5 mm or less	Islands of bone
II	< 50% bridging laterally	Bone spurs 1 cm or greater gap
III	> 50% bridging laterally	Bone spurs less than 1 cm
IV	Apparent ankylosis	Apparent ankylosis

Reprinted, with permission, from Brooker AF et al: Ectopic ossification following total hip replacement. J Bone Joint Surg Am 1973; 55:1629; and Morrey BF, Adams RA, Cabanela ME: Comparison of heterotopic bone after anterolateral, transtrochanteric, and posterior approaches for total hip arthroplasty. Clin Orthop 1984;188:160.

ment, wound drainage, and irrigation of the wound prior to closing. In patients at risk, low-dose radiation, 6–8 cGy in the first 3 days after surgery, prevents grade 3 or 4 heterotopic ossification. Indomethacin is effective, although it may be poorly tolerated by some patients. Early studies indicate that the bone inhibition is a COX-1 function, suggesting that COX-2 inhibitors may not prevent heterotopic bone. Diphosphonates are not effective in prevention of heterotopic ossification and should not be used. Indomethacin may not be optimal for prophylaxis in uncemented total hip arthroplasty because ingrowth may be retarded. Irradiation may cause problems if ingrowth components are not appropriately shielded.

If heterotopic ossification causes symptoms (pain, decreased ROM), surgical excision may be considered after the ossification is fully mature. Irradiation and NSAIDs are recommended postoperatively to prevent recurrence.

9. Infection—Prevention of infection after total hip arthroplasty is important because of the grave consequences. Frequently, the only way to treat an infected total hip arthroplasty is to remove the components and control the infection with antibiotics. Reinsertion of the components is then required 1.5–6 months later.

An innovation in the treatment of infected total hips and knees is the prosthetic antibiotic-loaded acrylic cement (PROSTALAC) technique. The prostheses are removed, sterilized, and reinserted as press-fit components with a layer of antibiotic-impregnated bone cement covering all surfaces except the bearing surface. This procedure is performed at the initial meticulous debridement, to provide a spacer for subsequent, definitive joint replacement.

Prevention is much more desirable than subsequent treatment of infection. Total joint arthroplasty implants are such large foreign bodies that all reasonable prophylactic measures should be employed. Laminar flow and ultraviolet lights are used in operating rooms to reduce the number of viable particles per volume of air in the room. Because bacteria are shed from people, keeping the number of people in an operating room to a minimum and reducing the exposed skin area may be beneficial. Antimicrobial therapy may be the single most important prophylaxis against infection. Good surgical technique and minimal operating times also contribute to lowering of infection rates. Infections occurring 6 weeks to 3 months after surgery probably originate from intraoperative contamination. Careful surveillance in this period for signs of infection, including pain, elevated white blood cell count, fever, and wound drainage, allows for early identification of deep wound infection, and early debridement is then indicated to eradicate the infection. Similarly, large hematomas should be debrided because they may cause chronic drainage and constitute a culture media for infectious agents. One report indicates that prophylactic antibiotics given in the period before and immediately after significant dental procedures may be beneficial in preventing hematogenous infection of total joints, despite recent recommendations that routine prophylaxis 2 years after joint arthroplasty is not necessary.

Amoxicillin, 3 g taken 1 hour before and 1.5 g taken 6 hours after a dental procedure, is recommended to reduce the risk of hematogenous infection. For penicillin-allergic patients, erythromycin, 1 g before and 500 mg after the procedure, is recommended.

Barrack RL, Harris WH: The value of aspiration of the hip joint before revision total hip arthroplasty. J Bone Joint Surg Am 1993;75:66.

Callaghan JJ et al: Charnley total hip arthroplasty with cement: Minimum twenty-five year follow-up. J Bone Joint Surg Am 2000;82:487.

Coventry MB: Late dislocations in patients with Charnley total hip arthroplasty. J Bone Joint Surg Am 1985;67:832.

Daly P, Morrey BF: Operative correction of an unstable total hip arthroplasty. J Bone Joint Surg Am 1992;74:1334.

DeHart MM and Riley LH: Nerve injuries in total hip arthroplasty. J Am Acad Orthop Surg 1999;7:101.

Dorr LD et al: Total hip arthroplasty with use of the Metasul metal-on-metal articulation: Four to seven year results. J Bone Joint Surg Am 2000;82:789.

Harris WH: Traumatic arthritis of the hip after dislocation and acetabular fractures: Treatment by mold arthroplasty. J Bone Joint Surg Am 1969;51:737.

Harris WH, Barrack RL: Contemporary algorithms for evaluation of the painful total hip replacement. Orthop Rev 1993;22:531.

Huddleston HD: An accurate method for measuring leg length and hip offset in hip arthroplasty. Orthopedics 1997;20:331.

Khan MAA et al: Dislocation following total hip arthroplasty. J Bone Joint Surg Br 1981;63:214.

Lester DK, Helm M: Mini-incision posterior approach for hip arthroplasty. Orthop Traumatol 2001;4:245.

Lewinnek GE et al: Dislocations after total hip replacement arthroplasties. J Bone Joint Surg Am 1970;60:217.

Markolf KL et al: Mechanical stability of the greater trochanter following osteotomy and reattachment by wiring. Clin Orthop 1979;141:111.

McDonald DJ, Fitzgerald RH Jr: Two-stage reconstruction of a total hip arthroplasty because of infection. J Bone Joint Surg Am 1989;71:828.

Mont MA et al: Total hip replacement without cement for noninflammatory osteoarthrosis in patients who are less than forty-five years old. J Bone Joint Surg Am 1993;75:740.

Ritter MA: A treatment plan for the dislocated total hip arthroplasty: Treatment with an above-knee hip spica cast. Clin Orthop 1980;153:153.

Schmalzried TP et al: Update on nerve palsy associated with total hip replacement. Clin Orthop 1997;344:188.

Waldman BJ et al: Total knee arthroplasty infections associated with dental procedures. Clin Orthop 1997;343:164.

Revision Total Hip Arthroplasty

The clinical success of revision total hip arthroplasty (THA) procedures historically was greatly inferior to the results of primary hip arthroplasty procedures. Loosening rates from 13% to 44% of cemented femoral revision procedures were reported at follow-ups of less than 5 years.

Improved techniques of cementing femoral stems led to improved results with cemented femoral revision. Pressurization of cement delivered, in a doughy stage, with a cement gun; pulsatile lavage; and an intramedullary plug permitted reproducible creation of adequate cement mantles. Only 14% of revised cemented femoral components were loose radiographically in one series after an average of 6 years. Other series indicate a revision rate of approximately 10% at 10 years, which is much improved from earlier series but inferior to those obtained with primary cemented stems.

Estok DMD II, Harris WH: Long-term results of cemented femoral revision surgery using second-generation techniques: An average 11.7 years follow-up evaluation. Clin Orthop 1994;299:190.

Katz RP et al: Cemented revision total hip arthroplasty using contemporary techniques: A minimum ten-year follow-up study. J Arthroplasty 1994;9:103.

Kavanagh BF et al: Revision total hip arthroplasty. J Bone Joint Surg 1985;67:517.

Pellicci PM et al: Revision total hip arthroplasty. Clin Orthop 1982;170:34.

Rubash HE, Harris WH: Revision of nonseptic, loose, cemented femoral components using modern cementing techniques. J Arthroplasty 1988;3:241.

Cementless reconstructions of failed femoral components were developed in response to the early high rates of failure with cemented revision procedures. However, early cementless revision series were generally unsuccessful, with failure rates of 4–10% at follow-ups less than 4 years. The use of proximally porous coated stems with inadequate stabilization, in the setting of deficient femoral bone stock, led to unreliable bone ingrowth fixation. Encouraging reports were obtained with modular proximally coated stems, such as the S-ROM (Johnson and Johnson, Raynham, MA) prosthesis, and extensively porous coated stems, such as the AML and Solution (Depuy, Warsaw, IN). Re-revision rates from 1.5% to 6% were achieved with use of these types of cementless femoral component at follow-ups from 5 to 8.4 years.

Gustilo RB, Pasternak HS: Revision total hip arthroplasty with titanium ingrowth prosthesis and bone grafting for failed cemented femoral component loosening. Clin Orthop 1988;235:111.

Harris WH et al: Results of cementless revisions of total hip arthroplasties using the Harris-Galante prosthesis. Clin Orthop 1988;235:120.

Hedley AK et al: Revision of failed total hip arthroplasties with uncemented porous-coated anatomic components. Clin Orthop 1988;235:75.

Lawrence JM et al: Revision total hip arthroplasty: Long term results with cement. Orthop Clin North Am 1993;24:635.

McCarthy JC et al: Revision of the deficient femur with a modular femoral component. Orthop Trans 1993;17:966.

Paprosky WG et al: Cementless femoral revision in the presence of severe proximal bone loss using diaphyseal fixation. Orthop Trans 1993;17:965.

In the situation where inadequate femoral bone stock exists, the use of allograft bone is advocated. For extended loss of proximal femoral bone stock, cementing a smooth tapered femoral stem in a bed of impacted particulate allogenic bone produces promising short-term clinical results. When deficiency of proximal bone stock is severe, use of structural femoral allografts may be required, and short-term reports suggest good clinical results.

Gie GA et al: Impacted cancellous allografts and cement for revision total hip replacement. J Bone Joint Surg 1993;75:14.

Gross AE et al: Proximal femoral allografts for reconstruction of bone stock in revision arthroplasty of the hip. Clin Orthop 1995;319:151.

Similar to early experience with cemented revisions of the femoral component, acetabular revision with cement was generally unsuccessful. Because of the difficulty of interdigitating cement into a sclerotic and often deficient acetabular bone stock, failure rates of loosening were reported from 53% to 93% at follow-ups from only 2–4.5 years.

Kavanagh BF et al: Charnley total hip arthroplasty with cement: Fifteen-year results. J Bone Joint Surg 1985;71:1496.

Snorrason F, Karrholm J: Early loosening of revision hip arthroplasty: A roentgen stereophotogrammetric analysis. J Arthroplasty 1990;5:217.

The introduction of cementless porous-coated acetabular implants for revision of failed cemented cups greatly facilitated early clinical results. Large hemispherical cementless acetabular implants can accommodate most bone defects encountered after removal of failed cemented cups. Where an adequate press-fit cannot be obtained, adjuvant fixation of the implant with screws or spikes can provide adequate stability to permit bone ingrowth fixation. Re-revision rates are reported from 0% to 1.6% with follow-up of 2–4 years.

Engh CA et al: Results of cementless revision for failed cemented total hip arthroplasty. Clin Orthop 1988;235:91.

Harris WH et al: Results of cementless revision of total hip arthroplasties using the Harris-Galante prosthesis. Clin Orthop 1988;235:120.

Hedley AK et al: Revision of failed total hip arthroplasties with uncemented porous-coated anatomic components. Clin Orthop 1988;235:75.

Padgett DE et al: Revision of the acetabular component without cement after total hip arthroplasty: Three- to six-year follow-up. J Bone Joint Surg 1993;75A:663.

Where inadequate bone stock of the acetabulum precludes reconstructions with conventional hemispherical implants, structural allografts fixed to the pelvis with screws can provide acceptable middle-term results. Other alternatives include the use of eccentric shaped cementless implants and cemented reconstructions with particulate allografting and antiprotrusio cages.

Berry DJ, Muller M: Revision arthroplasty using an antiprotrusio cage for massive acetabular bone deficiency. J Bone Joint Surg 1992;74:711.

Garbuz D et al: Revision of the acetabular component of a total hip arthroplasty with a massive structural allograft. J Bone Joint Surg 1996;78:693.

Peters CL, Curtain M, Samuelson KM: Acetabular revision with the Burch-Schnieder antiprotrusio cage and cancellous allograft bone. J Arthroplasty 1995;10:307.

Sutherland CJ: Early experience with eccentric acetabular components in revision total hip arthroplasty. Am J Orthop 1996;25:284.

Total Knee Arthroplasty

A. Indications

As with other joints, the primary indication for total knee arthroplasty is pain. Absolute contraindications to total knee arthroplasty include active sepsis, absence of an extensor mechanism, and neuropathic joint. Relative contraindications include a patient's young (less than 40 years) age, heavy demand for activity, or a patient's unreliability.

When both hips and knees are involved with painful arthritis, the joint causing the most discomfort should be replaced first. If hips and knees are equally painful, hip arthroplasty should precede knee arthroplasty. Rehabilitation following total hip arthroplasty is easier and less affected by a painful knee than vice versa. Additionally, motion of the hip joint greatly facilitates surgery for the knee.

B. Implants

Early designs of total knee arthroplasty were developed in Europe and may be categorized as constrained or resurfacing. Constrained devices consisted of fixed hinges, and resurfacing devices relied on ligaments for stability. Constrained devices predictably loosened, although they were used primarily in severe bone or ligamentous deficiency states. Early resurfacing implants were flat, roller pin–shaped implants or unicondylar devices that replaced only the medial or lateral compartment. Early knee replacements did not resurface the patellofemoral joints.

Contemporary total knee replacements represent a convergence of two major designs developed in the United States during the early 1970s: the total condylar and the duopatellar prostheses. The total condylar prosthesis had a femoral component made of Co/Cr and an all-polyethylene tibial component with a central peg. Excision of the posterior cruciate ligament was required because the entire surface of the tibial plateau was resurfaced. The patellar component was a dome-shaped polyethylene implant. All components were fixed with acrylic cement.

The Duocondylar knee replacement was the forerunner of the duopatellar prosthesis and did not resurface the patellofemoral joint. Extension of the anterior flange of the Co/Cr femoral component provided an articulation surface for an all-polyethylene dome-shaped patellar component. The tibial component was originally designed with separate medial and lateral runners, allowing preservation of the central insertion of the posterior cruciate ligament. Later, the two components were joined together, but a cutout was made posteriorly to permit retention of the posterior cruciate ligament.

Retention of the posterior cruciate ligament permitted increased flexion over that with the total condylar design because the normal femoral rollback during knee flexion was retained. Shifting of the center of rotation posteriorly during knee flexion greatly improves the lever arm of the quadriceps mechanism. The ability to climb stairs was superior when the cruciate ligament was retained. Central to the design of a cruciate ligament–retaining prosthesis is avoidance of excessive constraint by the tibial surface to permit rollback.

To overcome limitations in flexion and stair-climbing function, the total condylar prosthesis was modified with a cam mechanism (posterior-stabilized condylar prosthesis). The central cam design permits substitution of the function of the posterior cruciate ligament, providing a mechanical recreation of femoral rollback.

The differences in ROM and stair-climbing function achieved with cruciate-retaining and posterior-stabilized knee replacements are now considered negligible. Arguments in favor of the posterior-stabilized implant include technical ease in reconstructing severely deformed knees and less shear force at the articular bearing because sliding is reduced. The arguments in favor of cruciate-retaining designs are reduction of bone–cement interface forces because of less constraint, improved stability in flexion, less removal of bone from the intercondylar region, and absence of patellofemoral impingement syndrome (formed by scar tissue in the intercondylar recess of the posterior stabilized femoral component).

Problems with high-contact, stress-inducing fatigue wear of the polyethylene surfaces stimulated a new design concept in knee replacement. This design uses a polyethylene component that can move in relation to the tibial base plate. Thus, the surface of polyethylene in contact with the femoral component can be made to be more conforming because it can change positions during flexion and extension of the knee. Two types have evolved: the rotating platform, which only allows rotation of the polyethylene around an axis approximating the axis of the tibia, and variations on the "meniscal bearing" knee. In this design, the individual medial and lateral poly components can rotate (tibial axis) and translate (AP direction), or the entire poly plateau can rotate and translate in the AP direction. The latter concept seems to better address the biomechanical aspects of the knee, but results are early or limited on all designs.

C. Surgical Technique

Total knee replacement surgery is greatly facilitated by use of a thigh tourniquet. Following exsanguination of the lower limb with an elastic wrap, the tourniquet is inflated to 250–300 mm Hg. An anterior midline skin incision is made, followed most commonly by a deep medial parapatellar approach. The lateral flap containing the patella is everted to allow exposure of the tibiofemoral joint. Remnants of menisci and anterior cruciate ligament are excised, with careful release of contracted soft-tissue structures as needed.

Instrumentation systems guide the surgeon to create bone cuts with a saw that match the prosthetic fixation surface and reproduce anatomic alignment of the knee joint. Typically, in the coronal plane, the tibial plateau is cut horizontally to be at a right angle with the shaft of the tibia. The distal femur is usually cut at 5–7 degrees of valgus from the shaft of the femur. Such bone cuts provide a neutral mechanical alignment in the coronal plane so a line can be drawn from the center of the femoral head, through the middle of the knee joint, and through the center of the ankle joint. In the sagittal plane, the femoral cut is at right angles to the femoral shaft, but the tibial cut is made with 3–5 degrees of posterior slope. Slight external rotation of the femoral component allows symmetric tension of collateral ligaments during knee flexion and facilitates tracking of the patellar component.

Retention or sacrifice of the posterior cruciate ligament depends on the design of the implant used. When the cruciate ligament is sacrificed, bone from the intercondylar notch is removed to accommodate the box that houses the cam mechanism.

When the patellar surface is replaced, a saw is used to create a flat surface with symmetric bone thickness. Inadequate resection predisposes to subluxation because excessive extensor mechanism length is used, and the lateral ligamentous structures are relatively tightened. Many patellar components are 10 mm thick; thus, adequate resection must be almost 10 mm, within the limits of the anatomy of the patella. At least 10 mm and preferably 15 mm of patella (AP thickness) should remain. Patellar tracking is assessed by using trial components and ranging the knee from full extension to full flexion. In knees with valgus deformity, it is common to have lateral subluxation of the patella. In such cases, a careful lateral retinacular release that preserves the superior lateral geniculate vessels is performed. Positioning the patellar implant slightly medially on the patellar bone surface also improves tracking.

After appropriate trials are used to confirm accurate sizes of the components as well as ligamentous stability, cementing is performed. Careful cleansing of the bone surfaces with pulsatile lavage facilitates interdigitation of doughy-stage methylmethacrylate cement. The prosthetic components must be seated in the correct orientation, and excess acrylic cement must be removed. Before closure of the knee, it is prudent to lavage fragments of bone and cement and release the tourniquet to obtain hemostasis. At surgery, little bleeding is seen in the flexed knee. Thus, many surgeons close the wound and maintain the knee in flexion for periods up to 24 hours to decrease blood loss.

D. Clinical Results

Long-term results of contemporary cemented total knee arthroplasty designs are excellent. Survivorship of the total condylar prosthesis is calculated to be 90–95% at 15 years. Excellent functional results of posterior stabilized total knee replacements are also reported, with a 12-year survival rate of 94% for functional prostheses. Similarly, excellent function and only a 1% rate of loosening of the tibial or femoral component was reported with a cruciate ligament–retaining knee replacement when followed up at 10–14 years.

E. Complications

Complications are infrequent with total knee arthroplasty but include many of the same problems encountered with total hip arthroplasty. Additional problems arise from wound healing, fracture, extensor mechanism problems, and stiffness of the knee.

1. Deep vein thrombosis—DVT is common following knee arthroplasty, occurring in more than 50% of patients in one study. Further, 10–15% of patients develop DVT in the contralateral leg after unilateral knee arthroplasty. The use of the tourniquet during surgery does not have a clear detrimental effect on thrombus formation. The incidence of pulmonary embolism is lower than that reported in hip arthroplasty. This may be caused by the greater propensity to form calf thrombi after total knee arthroplasty; these thrombi may be less likely to cause emboli than thigh thrombi. Antithrombotic prophylactic measures include use of pulsatile compression stockings and administration of warfarin or low-molecular-weight heparin.

2. Wound problems—Wound problems can arise from incision-related issues and from patient-related risk factors. The skin incision should optimally be midline and longitudinal, and the skin should have minimal undermining. Preexisting skin incisions should be used when possible. Because wound healing is crucial to the success of the procedure, preoperative plastic surgery consultation may be beneficial if multiple scars, burns, or previous irradiation to the skin are present. Patient-related risk factors include chronic corticosteroid use, obesity, malnutrition, tobacco use, diabetes, and hypovolemia.

Treatment of wound problems depends on the type of problem. Drainage of serous material that does not clear in 5–7 days is an indication for open debridement. Hematoma formation (without drainage) is treated nonoperatively unless there are signs of impending skin necrosis or compromise of ROM. Small areas of superficial necrosis at the wound edge are treated with routine local wound care. Full-thickness soft-tissue necrosis places the joint space at high risk of infection and must be treated aggressively. Debridement with flap closure is frequently required. The medial gastrocnemius flap is useful because the tissue necrosis is frequently medial.

Prevention of wound problems through careful planning, gentle handling of soft tissues, and patient education to minimize risk factors is preferable to subsequent treatment of the problems.

3. Nerve palsy—Nerve palsies are a rare complication of total knee arthroplasty. The peroneal nerve is believed to be at increased risk for injury from surgery performed on valgus knees with flexion contractures or other significant deformity, ischemia from stretching small vessels in the surrounding soft tissue, and compression resulting from a tight dressing or splint. The risk is reported to be approximately 0.6%.

4. Femoral fracture—Notching of the anterior femoral cortex may predispose to distal femoral fracture. A technical error, notching can be prevented by careful femoral sizing before use of the anterior distal femur cutting block and by avoidance of posterior displacement or extension of the cutting block. Use of an intramedullary stem extension is advised if notching occurs. Fracture of the medial or lateral condyle may occur, particularly in patients with poor bone stock, such as those with RA or osteoporosis or in patients with cruciate-sacrificing femoral components. Large intercondylar boxes in these prostheses can cause weakening of the distal femur. Prevention is the rule, facilitated by vigilance during exposure of a stiff knee. Useful techniques to avoid avulsion include a V turndown quadricepsplasty, quadriceps "snip," tibial tubercle osteotomy, and placement of a Steinmann pin in the tubercle to prevent excessive traction on the patellar tendon. Treatment of the disruption is similar to the treatment in a normal knee. The patellar tendon is attached to bone, and the repair is protected with a wire around the patella and the tibial tubercle, holding the patella at the correct length from the tibial tubercle.

Patellar complications include maltracking, loosening of the patellar component, fractures, and impingement. The patellofemoral forces are among the highest anywhere in the body, and avoidance of intraoperative technical errors may minimize patellar complications. Patellar tracking should be assessed intraoperatively during flexion and extension of the prosthetic knee. Lateral patellar subluxation or dislocation may be caused by internal rotation of the femoral or tibial component, as well as a tight lateral patellar retinaculum. Careful release of the lateral patellar retinaculum may correct maltracking. Subluxation can predispose to patellar component loosening, as can abnormal stress caused by uneven patellar bone resection. Excessive bone resection and avascularity, caused by damage to the superior lateral geniculate artery during lateral release, can predispose to fractures. When using a posterior stabilized prosthesis, maintaining the inferior pole of the patella within 10–30 mm of the joint line may prevent impingement syndrome, which is characterized by pain or clicking when peripatellar synovial scar tissue impinges against the intercondylar box of the femoral component during flexion and extension.

In some studies, patellar complications are the cause for as many as half of the knee revisions performed. For this reason, some surgeons do not resurface the patella when the appearance is relatively normal. Because most patellofemoral replacement problems are attributed to technical errors, inferior prosthetic design, and excessive loads, replacement will probably become more prevalent as these problems are resolved.

5. Extensor mechanism complications—Many extensor mechanism problems can be prevented by careful surgical technique because many of these arise from technical problems, such as quadriceps (or patellar) tendon rupture, patellofemoral instability, and patella fracture.

Intraoperative rupture of the patellar or quadriceps tendon at the time of arthroplasty can be repaired, but a repair complicates the postoperative ROM regimen, at least to some extent. The incidence ranges from 0.2% to 2.5%.

6. Knee stiffness—Knee stiffness is a common problem in the early postoperative period. Methods to reduce stiffness include physical therapy (active or active-assisted ROM) and continuous passive motion (CPM). The CPM machine moves the knee through a preset passive ROM This modality is generally accepted and even liked by patients but does not affect the final ROM or reduce hospital stay. An acceptable ROM is 90–95 degrees of flexion with less than 10 degrees of flexion contracture, but the activities of daily living, such as getting out of a chair or climbing stairs, should be painless. Postoperative stiffness should generally subside by 6–8 weeks after surgery, and improvement in ROM should occur for 1 year with most gain in the first 3 months. The preoperative ROM is an important indicator of the ROM to be expected postoperatively.

Prevention of significant flexion contracture at the time of surgery and in the early postoperative period is important because improvement with manipulation is unrewarding. Manipulation with or without steroid injection can be beneficial in the first 3 months. Arthroscopic debridement may be necessary after intraarticular fibrosis occurs. Decreases in ROM after initial gains should alert the surgeon to possible infection, reflex sympathetic dystrophy, or mechanical problems, such as loose components or interposed soft tissue.

Ayers DC et al: Common complications of total knee arthroplasty. J Bone Joint Surg Am 1997;79:278.

Barrack RL, Wolfe MW: Patellar resurfacing in total knee arthroplasty. J Am Acad Orthop Surg 2000;8:75.

Callaghan JJ et al: Cemented rotating-platform total knee replacement: A nine to twelve year follow-up study. J Bone Joint Surg Am 2000;82:705.

Callaghan JJ et al: Mobile-bearing knee replacement: Concepts and results. J Bone Joint Surg 2000;82:1020.

Figgi HF et al: The influence of tibial-patellofemoral location on function of the knee in patients with the posterior stabilized condylar knee prosthesis. J Bone Joint Surg Am 1986;68: 1035.

Hahn SB et al: A modified Thompson quadricepsplasty for stiff knee. J Bone Joint Surg Br 2000;82:992.

Rinonapoli E et al: Long-term results and survivorship analysis of 89 total condylar knee prostheses. J Arthroplasty 1992;7: 241.

Scuderi GR et al: Survivorship of cemented knee replacements. J Bone Joint Surg Br 1989;71:798.

Ververeli PA et al: Continuous passive motion after total knee arthroplasty: Analysis of cost and benefits. Clin Orthop 1995; 321:208.

Total Shoulder Arthroplasty

A. Indications

The primary indication for shoulder arthroplasty is severe pain that was treated unsuccessfully with nonsurgical management. The underlying causes for the loss of articular cartilage and the incongruent osseous surfaces of the glenohumeral joint are usually OA, RA, posttraumatic arthritis, and dislocation arthropathy. The functional status of the soft tissues is vitally important because they provide a significant component of the joint stabilizing force through the concavity-compression mechanism. Techniques for replacement of the glenoid remains controversial based on the glenoid wear pattern. Newer reports suggest that asymmetric loading with excessive or repetitive overhead activities may eventually lead to posterior glenoid erosion. Most surgeons currently still recommend that glenoid replacement may be performed if and only if the rotator cuff is intact or reparable at the time of surgery. Although still controversial, a shoulder hemiarthroplasty is performed for patients with rotator cuff arthropathy and osteonecrosis. In this subset of patients, a surface replacement arthroplasty is an option to preserve bone stock. For patients with rotator cuff arthropathy or severe glenohumeral arthritis with an irreparable rotator cuff, a "reverse" or "inverted" shoulder prosthesis was reintroduced to improve function. With this design, the socket is placed in the humerus and the ball is placed in the glenoid with hopes of resisting glenohumeral subluxation. There is currently not enough follow-up data available to determine the efficacy of these devices. If RA has caused profound bony erosion of the glenoid medially to the level of the coracoid process, hemiarthroplasty may be the only viable option because the glenoid may not be able to support a prosthetic component. Contraindications to shoulder arthroplasty include active sepsis, neuropathic arthropathy, and the absence of a functional deltoid.

B. Surgical Technique

A deltopectoral surgical approach is performed, with careful retraction of the conjoined tendon medially to avoid injury to the musculocutaneous nerve. Although some suggest releasing the subscapularis tendon 1 cm lateral to its humeral insertion because it may facilitate later repair, most currently recommend detaching the subscapularis directly off the humeral insertion. Attachment of the subscapularis to the edge of the humeral osteotomy lengthens the muscle-tendon unit so a coronal Z-plasty is not required to improve external rotation of the glenohumeral joint. Palpation of the axillary nerve medially along the inferior border of the subscapularis is recommended to avoid injury to this vital nerve. A capsulotomy is then performed from the humeral attachment, and the humeral head is delivered out of the wound, with extension and external rotation of the arm. The humeral head is carefully resected to protect the rotator cuff insertion, and the humeral component is placed in 30–35 degrees of retroversion. Preparation of the humeral intramedullary canal is followed by insertion of a trial stemmed humeral component. After the appropriate thickness of the humeral head and stem is determined, the trial humeral head component is removed, and the stem is left in place to tamponade the intramedullary bleeding and to provide strength to the humerus during glenoid preparation. Posterior displacement of the proximal humerus is performed using a humeral head retractor, such as a Fukuda retractor, for exposure of the glenoid vault. Minimal bone is removed from the glenoid bone with a motorized burr to preserve cortical bone for support of the glenoid component. Long-term follow-up studies show that both bone grafting of deficient glenoid bone and building up defects with cement are not routinely recommended. With posterior glenoid wear, bone is removed form the glenoid anteriorly to match the posterior aspect of the glenoid. A keel or drill holes for peg insertion are made for cemented applications. To date, the FDA has not approved any noncemented glenoid components. There are glenoid components with trabecular metal for bony ingrowth that are currently in clinical trials. The humeral component is then implanted with or without cement, depending on surgeon preference and quality of bone stock. The closure must include a robust repair of the subscapularis tendon so that physical therapy may be initiated in the immediate postoperative period.

C. Implants

Early total shoulder arthroplasties were designed with constrained articulations between the humeral and glenoid components. Predictably, glenoid loosening and implant failures were commonplace, leading to development of unconstrained designs. Currently, nonconstrained resurfacing devices are primarily used with stemmed metal humeral components. Options include modular head and neck assemblies as well as a porous coating for cementless implantation. Although most commonly used glenoid components are made of high-density polyethylene, some designs of metal backing with porous coating and screw fixation for cementless applications are being explored.

D. Clinical Results

Shoulder arthroplasty has made significant progress, similar to the advances in hip and knee arthroplasty. The current so-called third-generation prosthetic designs incorporate variable offset and inclination, anatomic humeral heads, precision instruments, and variable glenoid curvature in their designs. Pain relief is reliably achieved with shoulder arthroplasty in more than 90–95% of patients. Pain relief obtained from hemiarthroplasties is equivalent to total shoulder replacement in selected patients younger than 50 years. As would be expected, shoulder arthroplasty performed in a high-volume hospital or high-volume surgeons are more likely to have a better outcome than their counterparts who perform the surgery infrequently.

Functional results are variable, however, depending largely on the underlying cause. A ROM three quarters to four fifths of normal can be expected in patients treated for OA or osteonecrosis. For RA, one half to two thirds of normal motion is usually obtained. For patients with cuff tear arthropathy, the ROM achieved may be only one third to one half of normal. Furthermore, the results for either hemiarthroplasty or total shoulder arthroplasty for patients younger than 50 years show higher failure rates. As such, alternative solutions in these younger patients may be explored.

The major complication associated with total shoulder arthroplasty involves loosening of the glenoid component; instability and late rotator cuff tears are next in frequency. Less common complications are humeral component loosening, sepsis, nerve injury, and humeral fractures. The incidence of shoulder arthroplasty infection is less than 0.5% and usually attributed to the abundant blood supply and surrounding musculature of the joint.

Radiolucent lines were observed around the glenoid component in 30–90% of cases in most published series, but the rate of definite and probable radiographic loosening is between 0% and 11%. Despite this, the revision rate for glenoid loosening is approximately 6% at 12 years. A higher failure rate caused by glenoid component loosening is associated with deficiency of the rotator cuff. Superior migration of the humeral articulation leads to eccentric loading and a rocking-horse effect on the glenoid component and loosening. Most surgeons currently perform hemiarthroplasty for rotator cuff tear arthropathy. In certain cases of cuff tear arthropathy or of significant medial glenoid erosion, a large-diameter humeral head or bipolar hemiarthroplasty may be used to lateralize the joint center, thereby facilitating the mechanical advantage of the deltoid. Alternatively, the so-called reverse or inverted shoulder prosthesis is being offered at certain centers for rotator cuff arthropathy, but it should be entertained in only select patients.

Baumgarten KM et al: Glenoid resurfacing in shoulder arthroplasty: Indications and contraindications. Instr Course Lect 2004;53:3.

Gupta R, Lee TQ: Positional-dependent changes in glenohumeral joint contact pressure and force: Possible biomechanical etiology of posterior glenoid wear. J Shoulder Elbow Surg 2005;14:S105.

Harman M et al: Initial glenoid component fixation in "reverse" total shoulder arthroplasty: A biomechanical evaluation. J Shoulder Elbow Surg 2004;14:S162.

Jain N et al: The relationship between surgeon and hospital volume and outcomes for shoulder arthroplasty. J Bone Joint Surg Am 2004; 86-A:496.

Levy O et al: Copeland surface replacement arthroplasty of the shoulder in rheumatoid arthritis. J Bone Joint Surg Am 2004;86-A:512.

Lyman S et al: The association between hospital volume and total shoulder arthroplasty outcomes. Clin Orthop 2005;432:132.

Sperling J et al: Minimum fifteen-year follow-up of Neer hemiarthroplasty and total shoulder arthroplasty in patients aged fifty years or younger. J Shoulder Elbow Surg 2004;13:604.

Total Elbow Arthroplasty

A. Indications

Although total elbow arthroplasty (TEA) may be an appropriate method of restoring joint function and stability, its primary goal is pain relief. With increased surgical experience, improvement of prosthetic designs, and evolving biomechanical knowledge, the indications for TEA have broadened to include the following, in order of frequency:

1. rheumatoid arthritis (RA);
2. posttraumatic arthritis;
3. juvenile rheumatoid arthritis (JRA);
4. distal humeral nonunions and severe comminuted distal humeral fractures, especially in the elderly; and
5. primary OA.

The severity of the disease and the choice of prosthesis in all of these situations are critical to the final outcome. TEA achieves its best results in individuals who do not tax the functional design of the prosthesis and who do not expect to use their upper limb beyond the level of basic daily functional activities such as combing hair, eating, and drinking. Active sepsis is an absolute contraindication to total elbow arthroplasty. Relative contraindications for TEA include previously open wound associated with trauma around the elbow, a previous infection of the elbow associated with prior TEA, arthrodesis, paralysis of the biceps or triceps, severe joint capsule contracture, and poor patient compliance. Lifting limitations after TEA remain 2.25 kg for repetitive lifting and 4.5 kg for single-episode lifting. Because most devices have higher failure rates approximately 10 years after implantation, alternative therapeutic interventions such as interpositional arthroplasty should be considered for younger (less than 60 years) patients. Thus, patient selection, compliance, and age become critical factors in determining the successful long-term outcome of prosthetic elbows.

B. Surgical Technique

Attention to the soft tissue, including the triceps insertion, collateral ligaments, and the ulnar nerve, is of vital importance when performing a TEA. Although the direct posterior approach is routinely recommended, especially early in the surgeon's learning curve, failures in TEA are attributed to this approach. After the flap of triceps muscle is turned down, the tissue may be devascularized and lead to overlying skin necrosis and weakness of the triceps muscle. If this approach is used, careful reattachment of the triceps insertion to the ulna is mandatory.

Because maintenance of the collateral ligaments is of vital importance when a nonconstrained device is used, the Kocher posterolateral approach allows preservation of the ulnar collateral ligament. This ligament provides the major restraint against valgus forces in the flexed elbow, and so it must be preserved when a nonconstrained device is used. The surgical plane is between the anconeus and extensor carpi ulnaris muscles distally and proximally between the triceps and brachioradialis muscles.

The Bryan posteromedial approach is routinely used for implantation of semiconstrained devices. The surgical plane is between the medial triceps and forearm flexors proximally and between the flexor carpi ulnaris and flexor carpi radialis distally. This approach allows direct visualization of the ulnar nerve and facilitates transposition of the nerve. Great care should be taken when encountering Sharpey fibers during elevation of the triceps from its olecranon insertion to prevent discontinuity with the forearm fascia. Release of the medial collateral ligament is required to proceed with implantation.

C. Implants

Early TEA designs included constrained devices, which predictably failed because of early aseptic loosening. In response to these failures, devices with less constraint and those permitting more normal elbow kinematics were developed. The two currently available types of elbow implants include resurfacing nonconstrained devices and semiconstrained devices. The most popular semiconstrained devices are the Coonrad Morrey, Pritchard-Walker, and GSB III (Geschwend-Scheier-Bahler III) prostheses. These implants have a linked hinge that provides stability but less constraint than early designs. The sloppy fit of these hinges permits varus, valgus, and rotatory forces to the implant and fixation to be dissipated. The inherent stability of these designs permits application in cases of soft-tissue and bony insufficiency, but theoretically there is increased risk of loosening. Excision of the radial head is also recommended during implantation of semiconstrained total elbow arthroplasties. Nonconstrained devices are widely used outside the United States, and the most popular devices are the Souter-Strathclyde, Roper-Tuke, and the Kudo implants. These nonconstrained implants permit restoration of the center of rotation of the ulnotrochlear joint with a metal-on-polyethylene articulation. The humeral and ulnar components are not linked, minimizing stresses to the fixation of these components. Because these implants lack intrinsic stability, they should not be used in cases of ligamentous instability or deficiency of supporting bone.

D. Clinical Results

Ten-year follow-up studies for TEA are currently only available for two semiconstrained linked devices—the Coonrad-Morrey and the GSB III designs—as well as for three nonconstrained devices: the Kudo, the Souter-Strathclyde, and the Roper-Tuke designs. Most of the experience using resurfacing devices in the United States was with the capitellocondylar design. Although no consistent 10-year studies exist for the capitellocondylar device, supporters of these implants report functional outcome of TEAs with nonconstrained devices comparable to those with semiconstrained device. Nevertheless, most of the reported past experiences suggest that high complication rates, particularly joint subluxations and dislocations, are associated with the use of these devices. The currently available 10-year long-term studies, as well as previous intermediate follow-up results, seem to suggest that the better semiconstrained designs may be associated with smaller numbers of revisions and aseptic loosening and greater success in maintaining pain relief and joint stability compared with the best nonconstrained devices.

Although previous radial head resection and synovectomy does not increase the rate of revision surgery for the subsequent elbow arthroplasty, this prior procedure did increase the complication rate when the elbow arthroplasty was performed. Newer data support the use of interpositional arthroplasty for younger patients because a semiconstrained arthroplasty remains a viable option at a later date. Although not as effective for pain relief, debridement arthroplasty and ulnohumeral arthroplasty are also options in active, younger high-demand patients who are not ready to accept the limitations of an elbow prosthesis.

Common complications encountered following TEA include aseptic loosening and joint instability, ulnar neuropathy, and infections. Ulnar neuropathies do not tend to require additional procedures, usually manifesting as paraesthesias and rarely showing signs of motor weakness. Many cases resolve or ameliorate over time. Many patients with RA already have preoperative evidence of ulnar neuropathy and the TEA did not contribute significantly to postoperative ulnar nerve dysfunction. Aseptic loosening of the cement–stem interface, polyethylene bushing wear (in semiconstrained devices), metallosis, and infections are major reasons for reoperation. For these patients that require revision procedures for aseptic loosening, the use of a longer stem prosthesis may be required. Alternatively, impaction grafting into the distal humerus or proximal ulna may be an option. These remain extremely challenging procedures with significant morbidity and often require multiple subsequent procedures. Infections are the most serious complications among these indications and have the potential to develop further into devastating local and systemic complications.

Blaine TA et al: Total elbow arthroplasty after interposition arthroplasty for elbow arthritis. J Bone Joint Surg Am 2005;87-A:286.

Chafik D, Lee TQ, Gupta R: Total elbow arthroplasty: Current indications, factors affecting outcomes, and follow-up results. Am J Orthop 2004;33:496.

Kelly EW et al: Five- to thirteen-year follow-up of the GSB III total elbow arthroplasty. J Shoulder Elbow Surg 2004;13:434.

Loebenberg MI et al: Impaction grafting in revision total elbow arthroplasty. J Bone Joint Surg Am 2005;87-A:99.

Malone AA et al: Successful outcome of the Souter-Strathclyde elbow arthroplasty. J Shoulder Elbow Surg 2004;13:548.

Sarris I et al: Ulnohumeral arthroplasty: Results in primary degenerative arthritis of the elbow. Clin Orthop 2004;420:190.

Wada T et al: Debridement arthroplasty for primary osteoarthritis of the elbow. J Bone Joint Surg Am 2005;87-A:95.

Whaley A et al: Total elbow arthroplasty after previous resection of the radial head and synovectomy. J Bone Joint Surg Br 2005;87:47.

Total Ankle Arthroplasty

The total ankle arthroplasty was under development for many years as a result of the success with total joint replacement of the knee and the hip. Initial designs met with modest short-term success and caused almost an abandonment of the procedure because of the comparison to ankle arthrodesis. The longevity of present total ankle joint replacements is somewhat erratic for a variety of reasons. The articular surface that must be replaced is unlike any other joint, and thus, experience cannot be carried directly from the knee or the hip to the ankle. Joint loads and requirements are less well characterized, and surgical technique is less well developed and, therefore, less reliable. For these reasons, total ankle replacement remains a developmental procedure indicated for patients with low activity demand and the need for ankle motion.

Encouraging early reports with newer designs of total ankle arthroplasty have emerged and are being closely observed. Results with the Scandinavian total ankle replacement (STAR) prosthesis in short-term follow-up are promising. Total ankle replacement is desirable because of the drawbacks of ankle arthrodesis, which include a significant pseudoarthrosis rate of 10–20%, despite extended cast immobilization to achieve arthrodesis. Furthermore, extended arthrodesis results in osteopenia and diminished motion in the subtalar and midtarsal joints. The additional stress on these joints from the ankle arthrodesis predisposes them to degenerative changes over the long term, as is seen fre-

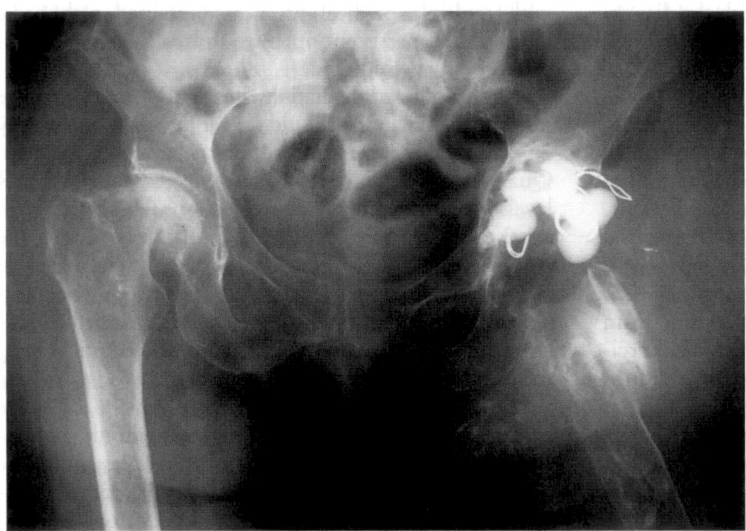

Figure 8–2. Anteroposterior pelvic radiograph depicting the Girdlestone arthroplasty and retained antibiotic beads in the left hip area and a painless malunion of a subcapital fracture of the right hip.

therapy. PICC lines can be inserted by qualified nursing personnel in an outpatient setting, and the placement of the line can be confirmed by a chest radiograph. Specialized personnel in the radiology department can also place PICC lines using ultrasound to identify suitable veins and fluoroscopy to ensure appropriate catheter placement with the tip of the catheter in the superior vena cava. A subclavian central line such as a Hickman catheter is used as a backup if peripheral access cannot be established. These catheters are generally placed in an operating room setting with the patient heavily sedated or under general anesthesia.

Most home health agencies are expert in managing PICC lines and administering antibiotics to patients in a home setting. Portable computerized IV pumps with replaceable drug cartridges are often used to automate the delivery of antibiotics throughout a 24-hour period.

3. Methicillin-resistant *Staphylococcus aureus/epidermidis*—Methicillin-resistant *Staphylococcus aureus* (MRSA) is the most common resistant bacteria encountered in orthopedic practice. *S. epidermidis* is rapidly becoming a concern as isolates start to demonstrate methicillin resistance. This is particularly important because one study showed the methicillin-resistant *Staphylococcus epidermidis* (MRSE) rate on routine screening for total joint replacement was 55% of samples that grew *S. epidermidis.* A 6-week course of vancomycin (1 g IV every 12 hours) is the current standard treatment for MRSA. However, this drug has relatively poor bone penetration, and it requires close monitoring because, rarely, it can be the cause of nephrotoxicity and ototoxicity. Establishing therapeutic drug levels by adjusting the dose and interval of treatment should be performed based on drug peak and trough levels. Generally, if the peak level is too high, the dose has to be lowered; and if the trough is too high, the interval between doses has to be lengthened. Dosing has to be adjusted in patients with renal insufficiency based on creatinine clearance, and one daily dose or one dose every other day is not uncommon in this setting. Toxicity is more likely to occur if the trough level remains above the acceptable range. Many infectious disease experts treat MRSA with a two-drug regimen, often adding rifampin to vancomycin. There are reports of vancomycin-resistant MRSA. Newer antibiotics such as linezolid (Zyvox) are now being introduced for MRSA and can be administered orally.

B. Surgery

1. Septic arthritis—Complete surgical evacuation of a purulent effusion offers the best protection against cartilage destruction in patients with acute infectious pyarthrosis. The greatest risk of cartilage damage comes from proteolytic enzymes produced by the recruited polymorphonuclear leukocytes rather than from direct action of the bacteria. Although serial needle aspirations may accomplish this goal in the acute setting, surgical drainage, irrigation, and drain tube placement are more efficient and better tolerated by the patient. Whenever technically possible arthroscopy is preferred, especially when dealing with septic arthritis of the knee joint. Limited open arthrotomy may also be used because the synovium need not be extensively debrided in acute infections.

In chronic septic arthritis, a pannus of hypertrophic synovium forms that must be surgically debrided to ensure successful treatment. Debridement debulks the bacterial load and decreases the production of inflammatory agents that destroy cartilage.

2. Osteomyelitis—Successful treatment of bone and soft-tissue infections requires the surgical removal of all nonviable tissue and foreign debris. Necrotic tissue shelters bacteria from access by white blood cells and from therapeutic concentrations of antibiotics. In acute open fractures, all devitalized soft tissue and all free bony fragments that are completely denuded of periosteum must be removed from the wound. Although buckshot and isolated bullets do not need to be removed from gunshot victims, thorough exploration of the bullet wounds is necessary to remove any embedded bullet wadding and clothing fragments. In chronic osteomyelitis, the sequestrum must be completely removed, although the involucrum should be left in place. Involucrum is viable reactive tissue that has a generous vascular supply and contributes to the mechanical stability of the bone.

Skin, subcutaneous fat, and muscle should be sharply debrided until they bleed freely. The appearance of viable cancellous bone is easily discerned by the presence of bleeding trabecular surfaces. It is more difficult to tell the viability of cortical bone because of its normally sparse vascularity. Biologic dyes such as fluorescein and isosulfan blue and flow Doppler examination are used intraoperatively to estimate the vascularity of cortical bone. However, visual inspection for punctate bleeding remains the simplest and most popular method of determining the viability of cortical bone. The so-called paprika sign should be apparent after water-cooled high-speed burring of all exposed cortical surfaces to ensure that all dead bone tissue was removed (Figure 8–3).

Infections occasionally are so severe or are located in such unforgiving anatomic locations that amputation is the best method of curing the infection surgically. For example, a 60-year-old man with insulin-dependent diabetes and extensive peripheral vascular disease developed a rapidly worsening heel infection that exposed his calcaneus (Figure 8–4). During physical examination, a cotton swab could easily probe exposed cancellous bone of the calcaneus and subtalar joint. A subtotal calcanectomy with free flap coverage after peripheral arterial bypass would have been necessary for any chance of infection control and limb salvage. The patient elected to proceed with a recommended below-knee amputation.

3. Implantable antibiotics—An excellent method to supplement the IV administration of systemic antibiotics is to implant local antibiotics into the wound using polymethylmethacrylate bone cement as a carrier. Antibiotic "spacers" and "beads" have the added advantage of provisionally filling dead spaces so that bacteria-rich fluids do not accumulate and thwart the host's defenses. Intraoperatively, methacrylate powder is thoroughly mixed with powdered antibiotics and then made into a dough by adding the liquid methacrylate monomer. The antibiotic dough can be fashioned into a string of beads using gauge-5 wire or number 5 nonabsorbable suture (Figure 8–5). Antibiotic-laden cement spacers can be molded into a disk shape like a hockey puck for the knee joint after removal of a total knee prosthesis. Also cement spacers can be molded into the shape of a femoral head and secured to the femur using a rush rod placed in the femur. Alternatively, hip and knee joint prostheses made of antibiotic bone cement are now commercially available. Palacos cement has superior

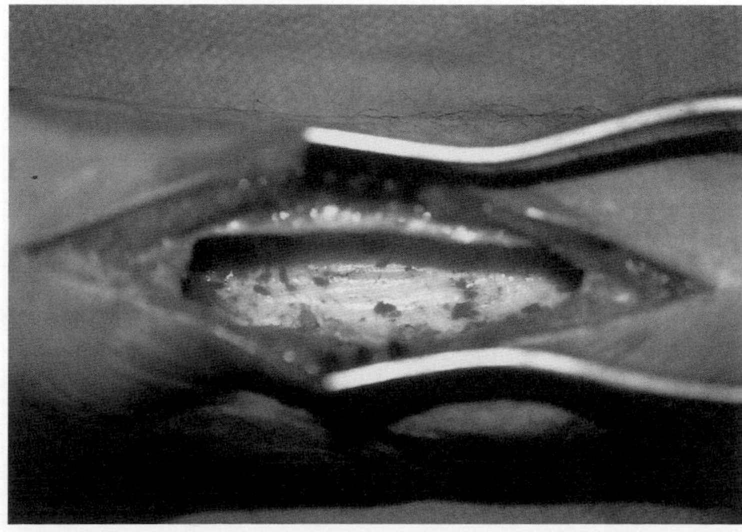

Figure 8–3. Intraoperative photograph of the so-called paprika sign, representing punctate bleeding from the endosteal surface of a tibia that has just undergone aggressive debridement with a high-speed burr.

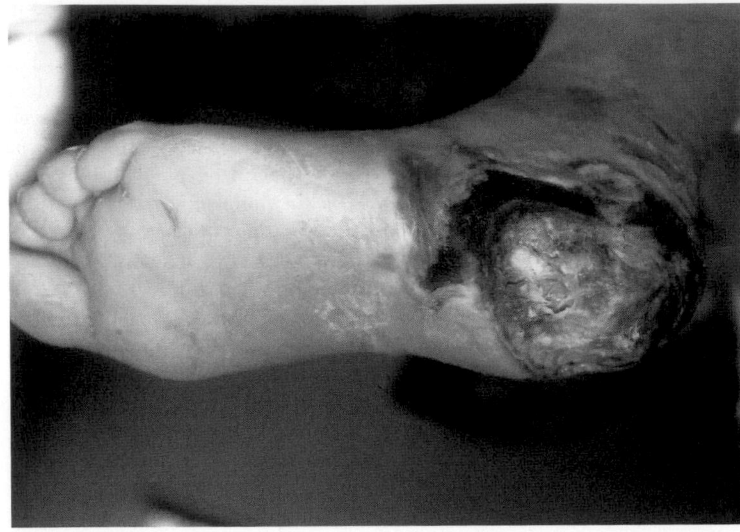

Figure 8–4. Calcaneus ulcer with exposed bone and blackened eschar.

antibiotic elution characteristics when compared with other bone cements. Vancomycin and tobramycin are commonly used in combination to treat presumed staphylococcal infections. A standard recipe in a patient without renal insufficiency is to mix one full bag of Palacos with 2 g of vancomycin and 3.6 g of tobramycin. Scoring the surface of a spacer and using numerous small beads rather than a few large beads increases the overall surface area of the antibiotic cement implant, enhances the elution of the antibiotics, and results in higher local concentrations of antibiotics. Initially the local serum concentrations may be as much as 100 times the minimal inhibitory concentration for *Staphylococcus.* After 3 weeks the antibiotic concentrations drop below the minimal inhibitory concentration. Although spacers and beads are left in place indefinitely, it is a good practice to remove them after the infection is treated to ensure that the cement does not act as a foreign body and precipitate a new infection.

4. Soft-tissue and bone reconstruction—Assuming musculoskeletal infections were treated comprehensively with antibiotics and debridement, bone reconstruction can proceed in a standard fashion. Total joints can be reimplanted, and structural bone defects can be filled with bone graft. Intercalary long bone defects can

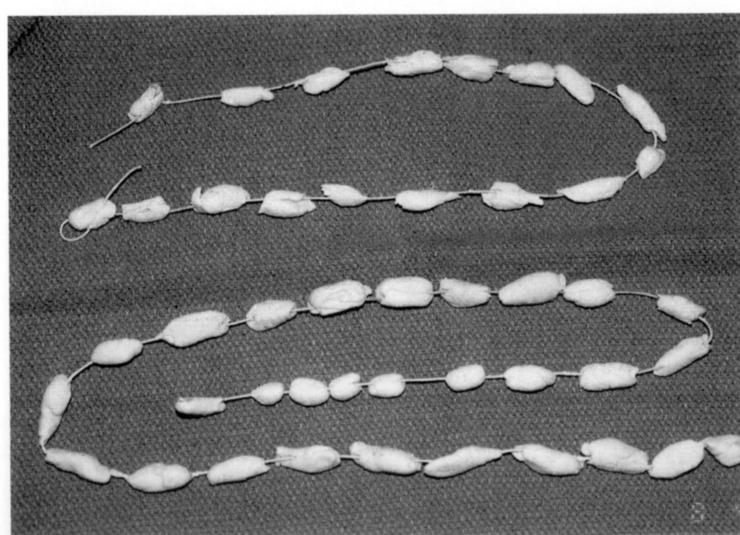

Figure 8–5. Two strings of antibiotic beads were molded onto a number 5 braided nonabsorbable suture with the knotted ends incorporated into the outermost beads.

be spanned with bone transport techniques, vascularized structural bone autotransplants supported by external fixators, or even structural allografts secured with intramedullary rods.

Expeditious soft-tissue coverage is the first reconstructive priority in the contemporary management of acute open fractures. Rotation, pedicled, or free flaps are used to accomplish wound closure. Early flap reconstruction also ensures a good vascular supply to the injured area that promotes bone healing and resistance to local infection. If definitive bone fixation must be delayed until after complete debridement and soft-tissue coverage is accomplished, provisional stabilization of the bone can be achieved with orthotics, skeletal traction, or external fixation.

An acute infection occasionally develops after orthopedic fixation of a fracture. Assuming good soft-tissue coverage of the fracture area, the patient is treated with antibiotics, and the implanted hardware is left in place until the fracture heals. Once biologic union of the fracture is achieved, surgical debridement of the wound and removal of the fixation hardware can be performed without having to be concerned about a mechanically unstable bone. Alternatively, debridement of dead bone and removal of hardware with the placement of an external fixator can provide stabilization until the infection is under control. Bone graft for small defects or bone transport for segmental defects can successfully achieve union.

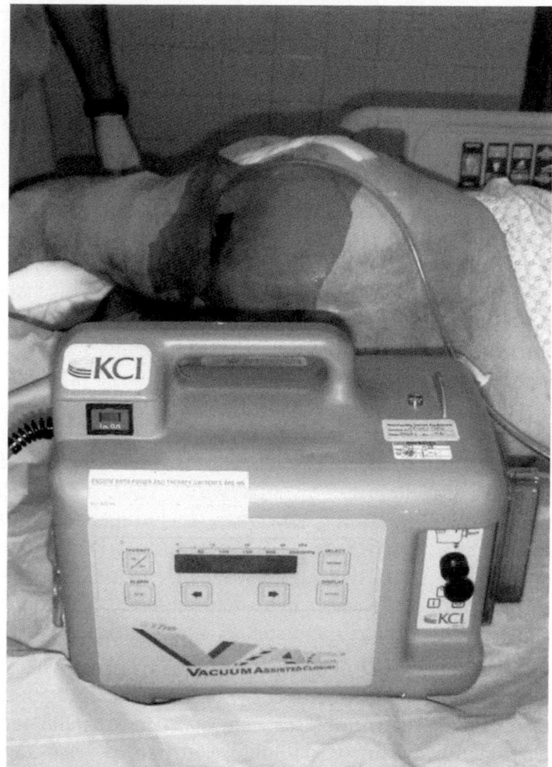

Figure 8–6. Portable wound suction pump (also known as a wound vacuum-assisted closure device, or VAC). Note the tubing that runs from the pump to a black sponge placed in a patient's ischial decubitus.

C. Adjunctive Therapies

1. Local wound care—Newer alginate dressing materials are more absorbant and may be left in place for 24 hours. Saline wet-to-dry dressings can be used for initial mechanical debridement of wounds that contain necrotic material and must be changed every 6 hours. Antiseptic solutions such as hydrogen peroxide, povidone-iodine, isopropyl alcohol, and sodium hypochlorite (Dakin solution, 5% NaClO) are now used only for the first few days until the bacterial load is reduced and necrotic tissue is debrided. Extended use of these caustic agents inhibits fibrogenesis. Instead, petroleum gel or topical antibiotic cream are placed on the wounds to keep the tissues from desiccating and to promote fibroblast growth.

Treatment of open wounds is now transformed using a new method that employs a sealed sponge dressing to which a negative pressure is applied using a portable pump (Figure 8–6). An open-cell sponge is cut to fit the shape of the wound and secured by an airtight plastic dressing (see Figure 8–12D and E). The sponge is connected to a vacuum pump by way of a plastic tube. When the pump is activated, a partial vacuum is generated within the wound. The porous sponge partially collapses, causing contraction of the walls of the wound. All drainage fluids are sucked out through the sponge and tubing and collected in a container located in the pump unit. The wound is kept quite clean, and the dressing is changed every 2–3 days. The units are portable and can be serviced by visiting nurses in an outpatient setting.

2. Hyperbaric oxygen—Hyperbaric oxygen (HBO) therapy is used to treat a variety of orthopedic disorders. Specialized diving chambers developed for medical purposes expose patients to 100% oxygen at 2 or more atmospheres of pressure. During an HBO treatment, superphysiologic concentrations of oxygen from the lungs are dissolved into the serum. These high serum oxygen levels stimulate neoangiogenesis, sustain hypoxic tissues, support the activity of phagocytic white blood cells, and inhibit infections caused by anaerobic bacteria. It does not cause oxygen to be absorbed from the skin or wound surface, and it does not revitalize tissue that is already necrotic. Therefore, an adequate vascular inflow to the wound is necessary for HBO to work. When appropriately indicated, HBO can be a useful adjunct to good medical and surgical wound management.

Acute problems that can be helped by HBO include severe crush injury, compromised muscle flaps, and necrotizing fasciitis. Each of these conditions is characterized by soft tissues that have become acutely hypoxic and are at risk for infection. So-called acute HBO protocols usually require higher pressures (2.4–3 atm) and more frequent sessions (two to three times a day) for several days. To be effective, an acute HBO treatment protocol must be started as soon as possible after the injury because a 48-hour delay in initiating HBO can render it ineffective.

Chronic wounds that can be helped by HBO are primarily related to chronic ischemic ulcers that are not caused by peripheral vascular disease, venous stasis disease, or pressure necrosis. Diabetic foot ulcers in particular may benefit from HBO protocols with a reduction in risk for major amputation. The older literature includes uncontrolled studies that expound the use of treating chronic osteomyelitis with HBO. However, newer reconstruction techniques, including free flaps for soft-tissue coverage and bone transport for bone defect restoration, have empowered the surgeon to perform more comprehensive debridement and more aggressive wound closure. Better surgical management results in better cure rates for chronic osteomyelitis.

3. Nutritional support—Patients with severe infections and large wounds have increased nutritional and caloric needs. Nutritional depletion can be measured using the following tests: albumin, prealbumin, total protein, total lymphocyte count, and anergy panel (see Table 8–2). Dietary supplementation to restore normal healing in a compromised host may be accomplished using enteral tube feedings or parenteral infusions.

Antony SJ, Diaz-Vasquez E, Stratton C: Clinical experience with linezolid in the treatment of resistant gram-positive infections. J Natl Med Assoc 2001;93:386. [PMID: 11688919]

Centers for Disease Control and Prevention: Vancomycin-resistant *Staphylococcus aureus*—Pennsylvania, 2002. JAMA 2002;288: 2116.

Connolly LP et al: Acute hematogenous osteomyelitis of children: Assessment of skeletal scintigraphy-based diagnosis in the era of MRI. J Nucl Med 2002;43:1310. [PMID: 12368368]

Gristina AG et al: The glycocalyx, biofilm, microbes, and resistant infection. Semin Arthroplasty 1994;5:160. [PMID: 10155159]

Hanssen AD, Spangehl MJ: Practical applications of antibiotic-loaded bone cement for treatment of infected total joint replacements. Clin Orthop 2004;427:79. [PMID: 15552141]

Herscovici D Jr et al: Vacuum-assisted wound closure (VAC therapy) for the management of patients with high-energy soft tissue injuries. J Orthop Trauma 2003;17:683. [PMID: 14600567]

Hiramatsu K: Vancomycin-resistant *Staphylococcus aureus*: A new model of antibiotic resistance. Lancet Infect Dis 2001;1:147. [PMID: 11871491]

Jenson JE et al: Nutrition in orthopaedic surgery. J Bone Joint Surg Am 1982;64:1263. [PMID: 7142234]

Jones S et al: Cephalosporins for prophylaxis in operative repair of femoral fractures. Levels in serum, muscle, and hematoma. J Bone Joint Surg Am 1985;67:921. [PMID: 4019541]

Kartsonis N et al: Efficacy of caspofungin in the treatment of esophageal candidiasis resistant to fluconazole. J Acquir Immune Defic Syndr 2002;31:183. [PMID: 12394797]

Ledermann HP et al: Pedal abscesses in patients suspected of having pedal osteomyelitis: Analysis with MR imaging. Radiology 2002;224:649. [PMID: 12202694]

Mazza A: Ceftriaxone as short-term antibiotic prophylaxis in orthopedic surgery: A cost-benefit analysis involving 808 patients. J Chemother 2000;12(Suppl 3):29. [PMID: 11432680]

Mohanty SS, Kay PR: Infection in total joint replacements: Why do we screen MRSA when MRSE is the problem? J Bone Joint Surg Br 2004;86:266. [PMID: 15046444]

Neut D et al: Biomaterial-associated infection of gentamicin-loaded PMMA beads in orthopaedic revision surgery. J Antimicrob Chemother 2001;47:885. [PMID: 11389124]

Perea S, Patterson TF: Antifungal resistance in pathogenic fungi. Clin Infect Dis 2002;35:1073. [PMID: 12384841]

Petty W et al: The influence of skeletal implants on the incidence of infection: Experiments in a canine model. J Bone Joint Surg Am 1985;67:1236. [PMID: 3802846]

Roeckl-Wiedmann I, Bennett M, Kranke P: Systematic review of hyperbaric oxygen in the management of chronic wounds. Br J Surg 2005;92:24. [PMID: 15635604]

Schmidt AH, Swiontkowski MF: Pathophysiology of infections after internal fixation of fractures. J Am Acad Orthop Surg 2000;8:285. [PMID: 11029556]

Segreti J: Efficacy of current agents used in the treatment of Gram-positive infections and the consequences of resistance. Clin Microbiol Infect 2005;11(Suppl 3):29. [PMID: 15811022]

Shirtliff ME, Mader JT: Acute septic arthritis. Clin Microbiol Rev 2002;15:527. [PMID: 12364368]

Stewart PS, Costerton JW: Antibiotic resistance of bacteria in biofilms. Lancet 2001;358:135. [PMID: 11463434]

Stott NS: Review article: Paediatric bone and joint infection. J Ortho Surg (Hong Kong) 2001;9:83. [PMID: 12468850]

Stratton RJ et al: Malnutrition in hospital outpatients and inpatients: Prevalence, concurrent validity and ease of use of the "malnutrition universal screening tool" ("MUST") for adults. Br J Nutr 2004;92:799. [PMID: 15533269]

Stumpe KD et al: FDG positron emission tomography for differentiation of degenerative and infectious endplate abnormalities in the lumbar spine detected on MR imaging. AJR Am J Roentgenol 2002;179:1151. [PMID: 12388490]

Tarkowski A et al: Current status of pathogenetic mechanisms in staphylococcal arthritis. FEMS Microbiol Lett 2002;217:125. [PMID 12480095]

Tomas MB et al: The diabetic foot. Br J Radiol 2000;73:443. [PMID: 10844873]

Turpin S, Lambert R: Role of scintigraphy in musculoskeletal and spinal infections. Radiol Clin North Am 2001;39:169. [PMID: 11316353]

van de Belt H: Infection of orthopedic implants and the use of antibiotic-loaded bone cements. A review. Acta Orthop Scand 2001;72:557. [PMID: 11817870]

Vandecasteele SJ et al: New insights in the pathogenesis of foreign body infections with coagulase negative staphylococci. Acta Clin Belg 2000;55:148. [PMID: 10981322]

Webb LX: New techniques in wound management: Vacuum-assisted wound closure. J Am Acad Orthop Surg 2002;10:303. [PMID: 12374481]

Zhuang H et al: Exclusion of chronic osteomyelitis with F-18 fluorodeoxyglucose positron emission tomographic imaging. Clin Nucl Med 2000;25:281. [PMID: 10750968]

Zhuang H et al: Persistent non-specific FDG uptake on PET imaging following hip arthroplasty. Eur J Nucl Med Mol Imaging 2002;29:1328. [PMID: 12271415]

OSTEOMYELITIS

Classification Systems

Several classification systems are used to describe osteomyelitis. The traditional system divides bone infections according to the duration of symptoms: acute, subacute, and chronic (Table 8–5). Acute osteomyelitis is identified within 7–14 days of onset. Acute infections are most frequently associated with hematogenous seeding of bones in children. However, adults may also develop acute hematogenous infections, especially around implanted metal prostheses and fixation hardware. The duration of subacute osteomyelitis is between several weeks and several months. Chronic osteomyelitis is a bone infection that is present for at least several months. It is associated with an epicenter of bone necrosis called a sequestrum that is generally encased in vascular reactive bone called an involucrum.

Another system, developed by Waldvogel, categorizes bone infections based on etiology and chronicity: hematogenous, contiguous spread (with or without concomitant vascular disease), and chronic (see Table 8–5). Hematogenous and contiguous spreading infections may be acute, although the latter is associated with trauma or preexisting localized soft-tissue infections such as diabetic foot ulcers. Compromise in soft-tissue vascular supply may inhibit the immunological response to an infection. Therefore, Waldvogel created this subcategory to acknowledge the increased difficulty in treating infections in hosts with compromised vascularity.

Cierny and Mader developed a staging system for osteomyelitis that is classified by the anatomic extent of the infection and by the physiologic status of the host rather than by chronicity or etiology (see Table 8–5 and Box 8–1). The four stages are characterized by the pattern of bony involvement of the infection in order of increasing complexity: stage 1—medullary only, stage 2—superficial cortex only, stage 3—localized medullary and cortical, and stage 4—diffuse medullary and cortical (see Box 8–1). The latter two categories are best distinguished by the presence or absence of mechanical compromise of the involved bone. Localized infections have not created an unstable bone. However, diffuse infections have sufficiently weakened the bone that surgical stabilization of the bone is necessary.

Table 8–5. Classification systems for osteomyelitis.

Traditional system	
Type	**Time of onset**
Acute	≤ 2 weeks
Subacute	Weeks to months
Chronic	≥ 3 months
Waldvogel system	
Hematogenous	
Arising from contiguous infection	
No vascular disease	
Vascular disease present	
Chronic	
Cierny-Mader system	
Anatomic extent of infection	
1. Medullary only (acute hematogenous)	
2. Superficial cortex (contiguous spread or soft tissue trauma)	
3. Localized (cortical and medullary, mechanically stable)	
4. Diffuse (cortical and medullary, mechanically unstable)	
5. Subtype by host's physiologic status	
A	Healthy
Bs	Compromised because of systemic factors
B1	Compromised because of local factors
B1s	Compromised because of both local and systemic factors
C	Treatment worse than the disease

Host factors that mitigate healing are subcategorized into three groups: A—healthy host, B—compromised host, and C—"incurable" host (the treatments necessary to cure the disease are worse than living with the symptoms of the disease itself). A good example is an ambulatory diabetic smoker with peripheral vascular disease who has a stage 3 infection in a mechanically stable femur. Appropriate local wound care and suppressive antibiotic therapy may indeed be preferable to extensive surgical debridement that would risk destabilizing the bone, worsening a nonhealing soft-tissue wound, and increasing the risk of an above-knee amputation.

Systemic factors that compromise the host include diabetes mellitus, immunosuppression (eg, corticosteroid or cyclosporin usage), immune disease (eg, AIDS), malnutrition (often associated with alcohol or IV drug abuse), renal or hepatic failure, chronic hypoxia, and extremes of age. Local factors include peripheral vascular disease, venous stasis disease, chronic lymphedema, extensive soft-tissue scarring, radiation fibrosis, arteritis, diabetic dysvascularity of small vessels, neuropathy, and tobacco use.

BOX 8-1. THE CIERNEY AND MADER STAGING SYSTEM.

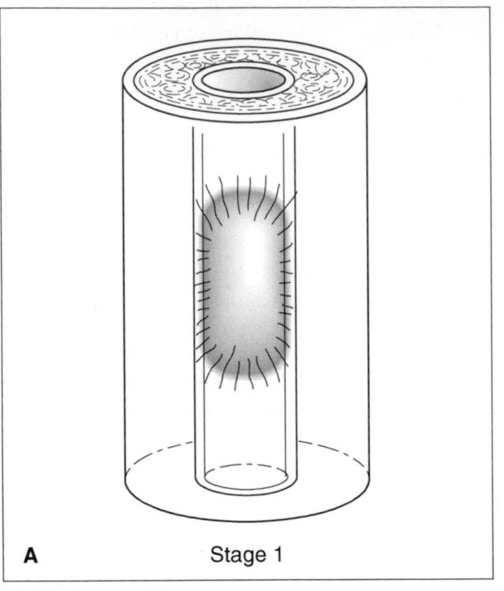
A Stage 1

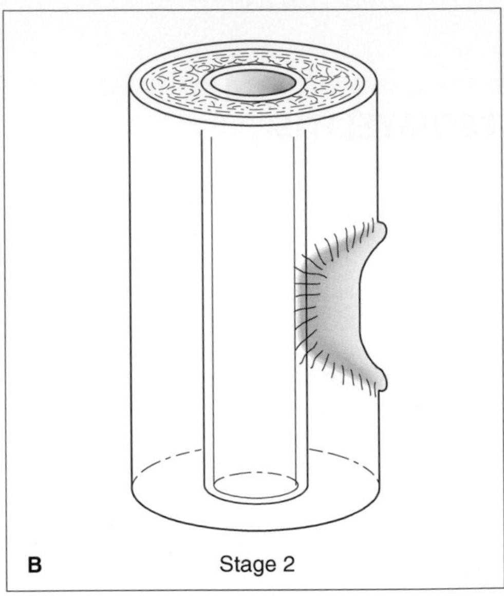
B Stage 2

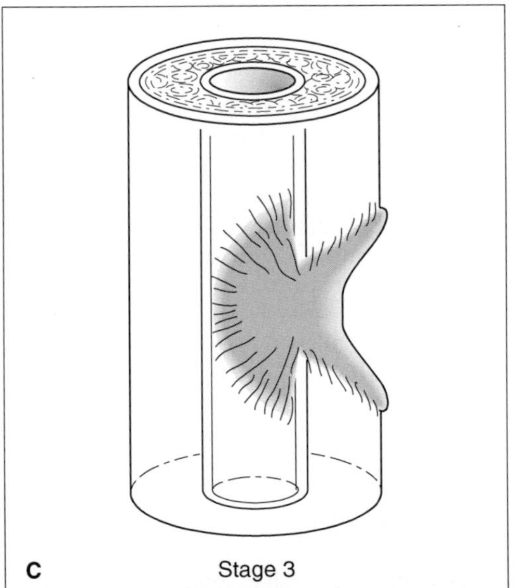
C Stage 3

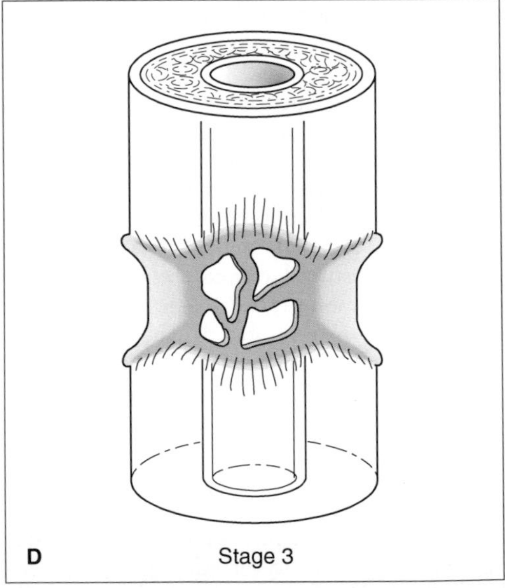
D Stage 3

The Cierny and Mader staging system for osteomyelitis is classified by the anatomic extent of the infection and by the physiologic status of the host rather than by chronicity or etiology. The four stages are characterized by the pattern of bony involvement of the infection in order of increasing complexity: stage 1—medullary only, stage 2—superficial cortex only, stage 3—localized medullary and cortical, and stage 4—diffuse medullary and cortical.

Belzunegui J et al: Musculoskeletal infections in intravenous drug addicts: Report of 34 cases with analysis of the microbiological aspects and pathogenic mechanisms. Clin Exp Rheumatol 2000;18:383. [PMID: 10895378]

Casado E et al: Musculoskeletal manifestations in patients positive for human immunodeficiency virus: Correlation with CD4 count. J Rheumatol 2001;28:802. [PMID: 11327254]

Gilad J et al: Polymicrobial polyarticular septic arthritis: A rare clinical entity. Scand J Infect Dis 2001;33:381.

Lazzarini L, Mader JT, and Calhoun JH: Osteomyelitis of long bones. J Bone Joint Surg Am 2004;86:2305. [PMID: 15466746]

ACUTE OSTEOMYELITIS

1. Acute Hematogenous Osteomyelitis

Acute hematogenous osteomyelitis (AHO) is most frequently encountered in the metaphysis of long bones in children. Clinically, patients have the signs and symptoms of an acute inflammation. Pain is usually localized, although it may radiate to adjacent regions of the body. For example, if a child complains of knee pain, the hip joint must be thoroughly evaluated for the possibility of septic arthritis. If a bone in the leg is infected, the child may limp or stop walking altogether. Children may also demonstrate guarding of an infected arm, refusing to use it and holding it to their side. Exam usually reveals local tenderness and occasionally limited motion of an adjacent joint, but swelling and redness are less frequent. Systemic signs of fever and chills may be present, and infants may be irritable or lethargic and uninterested in eating.

Serology characteristically shows dramatic elevations in the CRP and the ESR. The WBC is usually elevated, and a left shift may be apparent. Peripheral blood cultures grow the offending organism in up to half of acutely infected children.

Plain radiographs taken early in the course of disease are usually negative. After a week or two, radiographs may reveal a radiolucent lesion and periosteal elevation. Reactive sclerosis is absent because it is encountered only in chronic bone infections. Technetium bone scan shows increased activity on soft tissue and delayed bone images. CT may show a radiolucent area in cancellous bone and signs of periosteal elevation. MRI shows early inflammation of bone marrow with inflammation of the periosteum and adjacent soft tissues as the infection progresses. In later stages abscess formation may be seen as a signal void on gadolinium contrast images.

The clinical and radiologic appearance of AHO may be similar to inflammatory neoplasms such as acute lymphocytic leukemia, Ewing sarcoma, and Langerhans cell histiocytosis (also known as eosinophilic granuloma). Therefore, a biopsy may be required to distinguish an infection from a tumor.

Standard evaluation of a patient with suspected AHO includes a needle or open biopsy to obtain tissue for culture *and* histology and subsequent initiation of empirical antibiotics. If an abscess is identified, thorough irrigation and local debridement through a small cortical window should be performed. Once the culture results and sensitivities are obtained, the final antibiotic regimen may be selected. Six weeks of antibiotic therapy are usually indicated. In pediatric patients with sensitive staphylococcal infections, 2 weeks of parenteral antibiotics may be followed by 4 weeks of oral antibiotic therapy. Close clinical follow-up is necessary to ensure that the patient's inflammatory symptoms are resolving. Serial ESR and CRP should return to normal within the treatment period.

If the patient does not improve, temporary discontinuation of antibiotics may be necessary prior to performing a surgical exploration to culture the infected site. Often antibiotics, even those to which the bacteria are resistant, may suppress the bacteria enough that they will not grow in culture. Although a 2-week waiting period off antibiotics, which is customary for cases of chronic osteomyelitis, may not be tolerated by patients with acute osteomyelitis, even waiting for several days may increase the culture yield. This further highlights the potential problems of beginning an empirical regimen using inappropriate antibiotics and then having difficulty obtaining productive cultures. Either a delay in treatment occurs or the patient has to be placed on several antibiotics to cover all possible organisms.

In patients with stable prosthetic joints who acquire an acute hematogenous infection because of a sensitive organism, thorough soft-tissue debridement, exchange of the polyethylene liner or temporary substitution of the polyethylene with a molded antibiotic spacer, and 6 weeks of IV antibiotic therapy confer a salvage rate approaching 50%.

Clinical Example

A 13-year-old girl complained of acute knee pain beginning 7 days earlier when arising from sleep. Her pain worsened to the point where she had to stay at home from school because she could not walk. On exam her thigh was tender, and her hip and knee motion severely restricted because of pain, but there was no knee effusion. Her temperature was 38.2°C (100.9°F). The serum white blood cell count was 17,000 with a left shift, and the ESR was four times normal. Plain films of the femur were normal. An MRI of the thigh showed significant inflammation of the marrow and adjacent soft tissues on T_2-weighted images (Figure 8–7A). Intraoperatively the midfemur was exposed, a hole was drilled in the femur, and a collection of pus was aspirated from the marrow cavity (Figure 8–7B). Irrigation was performed through the drill hole and the wound closed over a drain. *Staphylococcus aureus* was cultured, and the patient was successfully treated with 6 weeks of IV antibiotics.

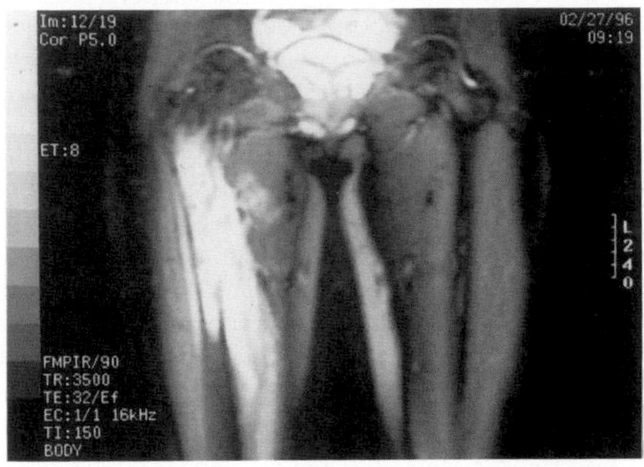

A

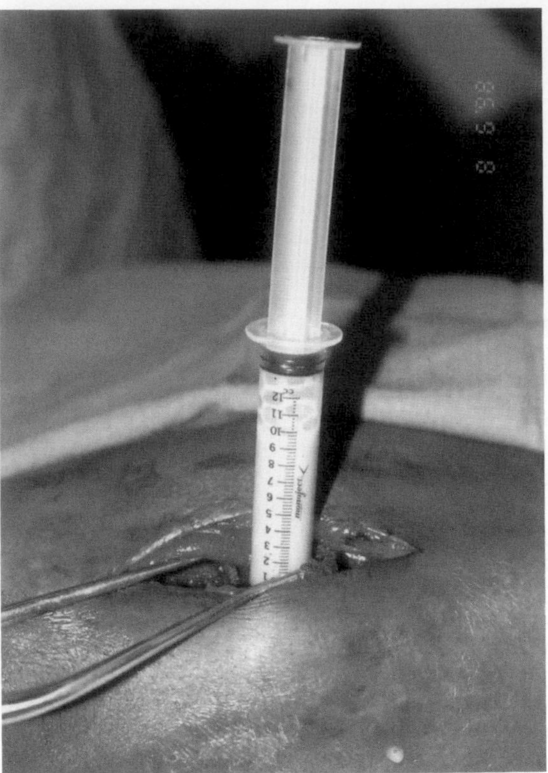

B

Figure 8–7. **A:** T_2-weighted MRI of the thigh, showing marrow edema in the femur and surrounding musculature. **B:** Aspiration of the medullary cavity of the femur produces 10 mL of pus in the syringe.

2. Acute Osteomyelitis Caused by Puncture Wound

Acute osteomyelitis must be considered in the evaluation of a patient who has suffered a deep puncture wound. The feet and hands are the most frequent sites of these injuries. The soft tissue wound may appear insignificant. It may be difficult to detect a foreign body made of wood or plastic on plain radiography, and wound exploration for a foreign body in a clinic setting is frequently unrewarding. Refer to Chapter 9 (Foot & Ankle Surgery) and Chapter 10 (Hand Surgery) for further information.

Clinical Example

An 11-year-old boy punctured his foot when he stepped on a sharp object. Initial radiographs of the foot showed no evidence of a foreign body (Figure 8–8A). In retrospect, a small puncture wound can be visualized in the middistal diaphysis. He was initially treated with a limited irrigation and debridement in the emergency department and discharged on oral antistaphylococcal antibiotics. Two weeks later. the arch of his foot became swollen and drainage emanated from the puncture wound (Figure 8–8B). He was admitted to the hospital and placed empirically on triple IV antibiotics. Superficial swabs of the wound grew *Pseudomonas.*

A technetium bone scan identified a significant uptake of radiotracer in the distal aspect of the first metatarsal compared with the opposite normal foot (Figure 8–8C). New radiographs of the foot depicted a circular region of osteolysis with a slight elevation of the adjacent periosteum (Figure 8–8D). The patient underwent a thorough irrigation and debridement in the operating room. No foreign body was identified. Deep cultures of the wound revealed *Mycobacterium fortuitum,* a rapidly growing mycobacteria other than tuberculosis (MOTT). He clinically improved within several days of beginning oral clarithromycin and continued this treatment for 9 months.

This case illustrates the need to obtain accurate wound cultures in order to choose appropriate antibiotic therapy. Superficial cultures often reveal skin con-

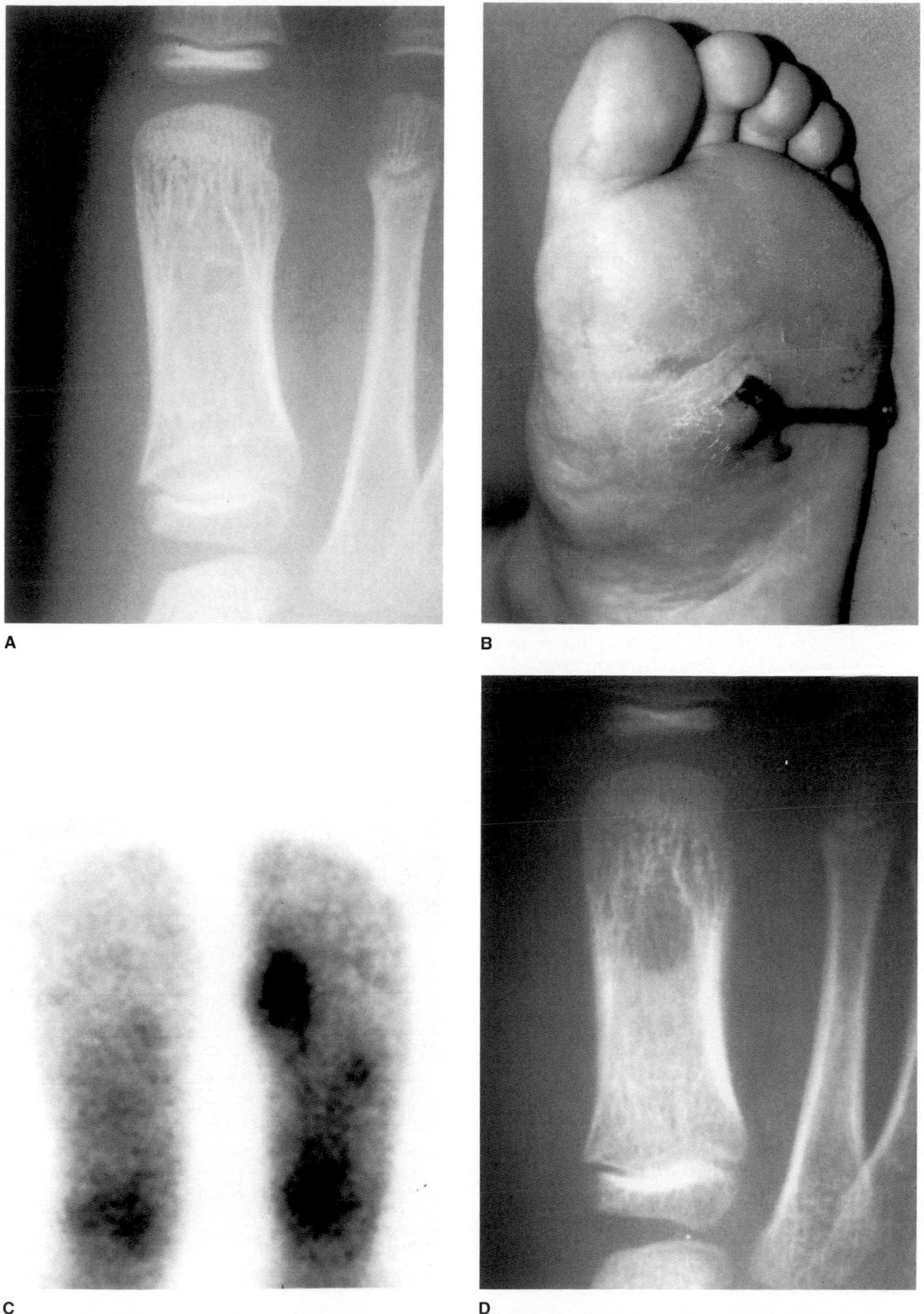

Figure 8–8. **A:** Initial plain radiograph of the first metatarsal. **B:** Preoperative view of the puncture wound. **C:** Bone phase of a technetium bone scan of the feet. **D:** Follow-up radiograph of the first metatarsal taken 2 weeks after Figure 8–8A.

taminants that are not representative of the organisms actually causing the infection. When infections do not respond to routine empirical antibiotic therapy, it is always important to consider surgical exploration to obtain deep cultures of the wound for mycobacterium and fungal organisms as well as for aerobic and anaerobic organisms.

Agrawal A et al: Cryptococcal arthritis in an immunocompetent host. J S C Med Assoc 2000;96:297. [PMID: 10933007]

Babhulkar SS, Pande SK: Unusual manifestations of osteoarticular tuberculosis. Clin Orthop 2002;398:114. [PMID: 11964639]

Blumberg HM, Leonard MK Jr, Jasmer RM: Update on the treatment of tuberculosis and latent tuberculosis infection. JAMA 2005;293:2776. [PMID: 15941808]

Caspofungin: New preparation. A last resort for invasive aspergillosis. Prescrire Int 2002;11:142. [PMID: 12378745]

Centers for Disease Control and Prevention: Trends in Tuberculosis—United States, 2004. MMWR Morb Mortal Wkly Rep 2005;54:149. [PMID: 15772584]

Dhillon MS et al: Tuberculosis of the sternoclavicular joints. Acta Orthop Scand 2001;72:514. [PMID: 11728080]

Hansen BL, Andersen K: Fungal arthritis. A review. Scan J Rheumatol 1995;24:248. [PMID: 7481591]

Nolan CM, Goldberg SV: Treatment of isoniazid-resistant tuberculosis with isoniazid, rifampin, ethambutol and pyrazinamide for 6 months. Int J Tuberc Lung Dis 2002;6:952. [PMID: 12475140]

Silber JS et al: Insidious destruction of the hip by *Mycobacterium tuberculosis* and why early diagnosis is critical. J Arthroplasty 2000;15:392. [PMID: 10794239]

SUBACUTE OSTEOMYELITIS

Subacute infections are often associated with pediatric patients. These infections are usually caused by organisms of low virulence and associated with muted symptoms. Ultimately, the infection appears to reach a stalemate with the host's defenses and does not progress. Subacute osteomyelitis shares some of the radiographic characteristics of both acute and chronic infections. Like acute osteomyelitis, regions of osteolysis and periosteal elevation may be present. Like chronic osteomyelitis, a circumferential zone of reactive sclerotic bone may be visualized. When subacute osteomyelitis affects the diaphysis of a long bone, it may be particularly difficult to distinguish from Langerhans cell histiocytosis (also known as eosinophilic granuloma) or Ewing sarcoma.

Clinical Example

A 14-year-old boy presented with a 2-month history of left ankle pain and swelling that occurred when he jumped off a farm trailer. His symptoms persisted, although some improvement was reported. He denied any fever, chills, or night sweats and could walk without assistance. On exam he was still tender and focally erythematous over the anterior region of the ankle. His WBC was normal and the ESR was only slightly elevated.

Anteroposterior (AP) and lateral radiographs of the tibia show mixed areas of radiodensity and radiolucency in the metaphysis and a slightly raised periosteum (Figures 8–9A and B). Axial T_2-weighted MRI shows marrow edema and periosteal elevation—identified as the outer dark ring just superficial to the cortex. A halo of inflammation surrounds the raised periosteum (Figure 8–9C). Coronal T_2-weighted MRI shows the periosteal elevation along the metadiaphysis and the marrow edema extending as far proximally as the midtibia (Figure 8–9D). During open surgical biopsy, purulent material was encountered within the metaphysis but not along the periosteal surface or in the ankle joint. Thorough irrigation and debridement of the area was performed with primary closure of the incision over a drain. The patient was subsequently cured of his subacute nonresistant *S. aureus* infection with 6 weeks of IV nafcillin.

Lazzarini L, Lipsky BA, Mader JT: Antibiotic treatment of osteomyelitis: What have we learned from 30 years of clinical trials? Int J Infect Dis 2005;9:127. [PMID: 15840453]

Mader JT et al: Antibiotic therapy for musculoskeletal infections. Instr Course Lect 2002;51:539. [PMID: 12064145]

Vinod MB et al: Duration of antibiotics in children with osteomyelitis and septic arthritis. J Paediatr Child Health 2002;38: 363. [PMID: 12173997]

CHRONIC OSTEOMYELITIS

Chronic osteomyelitis is the result of untreated acute or subacute osteomyelitis. It can occur hematogenously, iatrogenically, or as a result of penetrating trauma. Chronic infections are often associated with orthopaedic metal implants used to replace joints, fuse spine segments, or fix fractures. Direct intraoperative inoculation or subsequent hematogenous seeding of metal or dead bone surfaces may provide a haven for the bacteria, protecting them from white blood cells and effective concentrations of antibiotics. Therefore, removal of the metal and dead bone are necessary in addition to appropriate antibiotics to eradicate chronic osteomyelitis.

Surgical debridement of necrotic bone for infection control is akin to curettage of a benign bone tumor. A study validating the Cierny-Mader classification system substaging A and B was reported. Debridements were wide marginal or intralesional.

Clinical Example

A 62-year-old man sustained a closed femur fracture when he fell from a ladder 40 years ago. His fracture was fixed with an intramedullary rod that was subsequently removed after the fracture healed. Unfortunately, the patient's leg became infected postoperatively

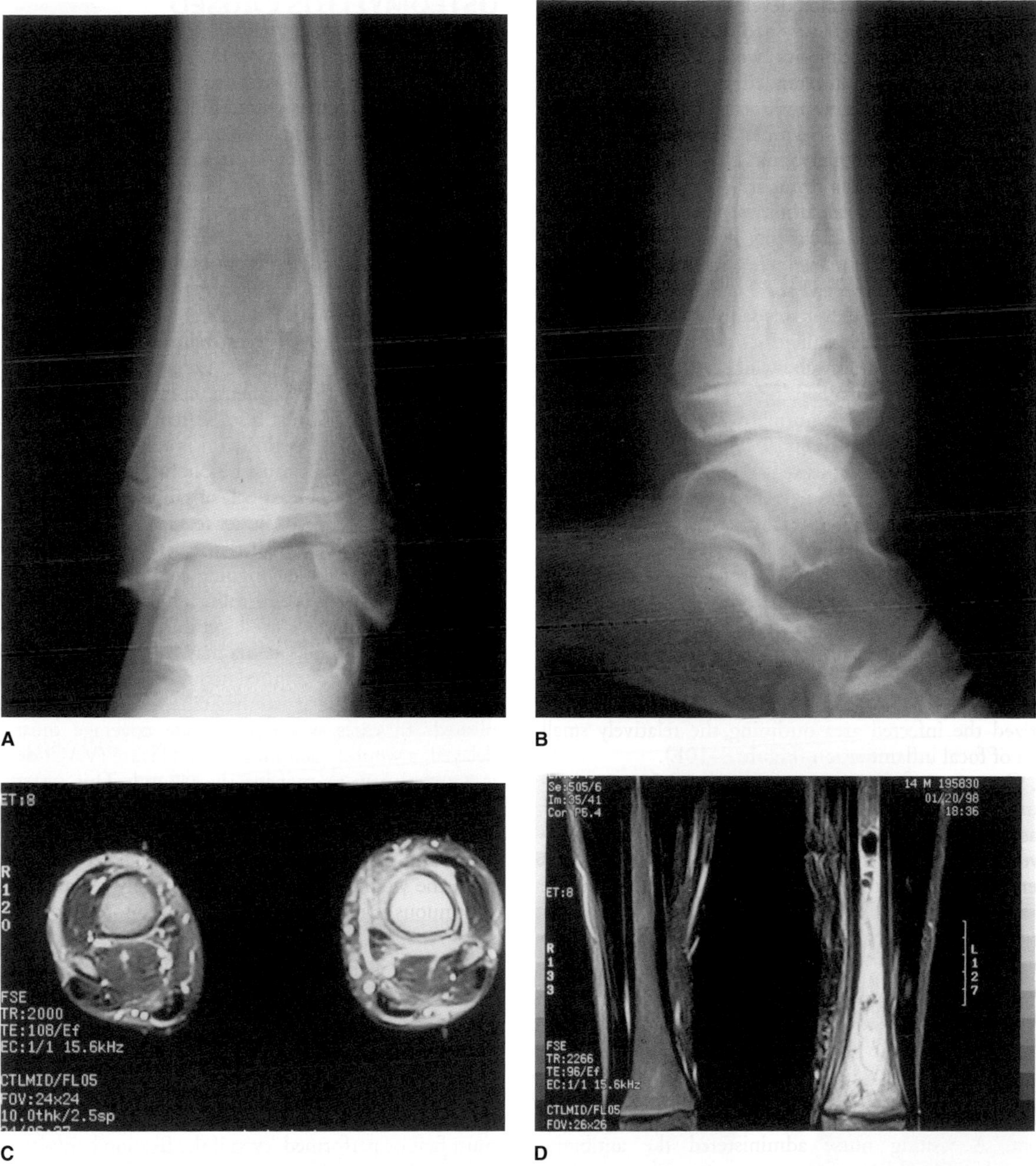

Figure 8–9. **A:** Anteroposterior radiograph of the distal tibia. **B:** Lateral radiograph of the distal tibia. Notice focal region of osteopenia immediately above the growth plate. **C:** Axial T_2-weighted MRI of both tibias in the region of the distal metaphysis shows marrow edema and periosteal elevation and inflammation on the affected left side. **D:** Coronal T_2-weighted MRI of both tibias shows extensive marrow edema and periosteal inflammation ascending to the midtibia on the affected side.

tinely complain of severe pain with passive motion of the affected joint. Rest pain, guarding, swelling, erythema, and heat become more pronounced as the infection progresses. Fever and chills are not sensitive indicators of septic arthritis.

The most common joint affected by hematogenous septic arthritis is the knee. The hip, ankle, wrist, shoulder, and elbow follow in frequency of involvement. The differential diagnosis includes Charcot joint, gout, pseudogout, RA, and other inflammatory arthropathies. The diagnosis is tentatively made on joint fluid analysis (see Table 8–4).

Although infections often spread from joints to affect adjacent metaphyseal bone, tumors seldom do except at the sacroiliac joint. Surgical decompression and irrigation of all large joints is preferred to serial needle aspirations. In the acute setting, arthroscopy is ideal for culturing synovial tissue, thoroughly irrigating the joint space, and for placement of an indwelling drainage tube.

Clinical Example

A 53-year-old woman with RA and a painful left hip presented with a 3-week history of rapidly worsening groin pain, slight fever, and lethargy. Degenerative narrowing of the hip joint is seen on a prior AP radiograph (Figure 8–13A). Although the patient's WBC was normal, the hematocrit was only 18! Her groin was extremely tender, and any motion of the hip joint elicited excruciating pain. The patient was admitted to the hospital directly from the clinic. A bone scan showed intense activity in the region of the hip (Figure 8–13B). A CT of the pelvis outlines a loculated soft-tissue mass anterior to the femoral head displacing the femoral artery and vein medially (Figure 8–13C). Using CT guidance, the region was aspirated, and a pigtail catheter was inserted to drain the abscess cavity. MRI with T_1 fat-saturated sequences and gadolinium contrast further characterized the infection, revealing significant inflammation in the femoral head and an effusion of the hip joint (Figure 8–13D). A plain radiograph at that time showed a dramatic collapse of the femoral head (Figure 8–13E). A Girdlestone arthroplasty was performed, and the remainder of the femoral head was submitted for histologic analysis (Figure 8–13F). An antibiotic spacer was orthotopically placed to stabilize the femur, and the wound was closed over drains (Figure 8–13G). A 6-week course of IV antibiotics was given. Afterward, the hip was surgically reexamined, and no evidence of persistent infection was seen grossly or by frozen section analysis. At that time a total hip prosthesis was successfully implanted.

CHRONIC SEPTIC ARTHRITIS

Unlike acute septic arthritis, which is intensely painful, chronic septic arthritis presents with indolent joint symptoms that are often muted by oral or intraarticular injections of antiinflammatory medications and may be attributed to coexistent chronic joint arthritis. Immunocompromised patients are susceptible to less virulent and slower growing organisms such as atypical mycobacteria and fungus. These organisms may solicit a subdued chronic inflammatory response that generates less pain and joint effusion, resulting in a delay in diagnosis.

Clinical Example

A 52-year-old man with AIDS on retroviral therapy presented with a 4-month history of arthritic pain and effusion in his knee and a 1-week history of an enlarging painful mass on the medial aspect of his knee (Figure 8–14A). One year earlier he was diagnosed with a large popliteal abscess in the same leg caused by *S. epidermidis* that was successfully treated with surgical drainage and 6 weeks of IV antibiotics. Exam revealed focal swelling, warmth, erythema, and restricted motion because of pain. During arthrotomy, the medial swelling was found to communicate directly with the knee joint. Intraoperative findings included a large quantity of pus, extensive erosion of cartilage, and chronic proliferative synovial tissue (Figure 8–14B). After irrigation and debridement, the wound was primarily closed over drainage catheters. Cultures grew *Candida albicans,* and the patient was treated with fluconazole (Diflucan).

Even though this patient's symptoms appeared acute, he actually had chronic septic arthritis that likely began 4 months previously when he began having arthritic pain. Because he was immunocompromised, his inflammatory symptoms were muted, causing a delay in clinical presentation. Unusual pathogens are a hallmark of immunocompromised patients. Therefore, it is essential to acquire mycobacterial and fungal cultures in addition to aerobic and anaerobic bacterial cultures. Unless the cause of immunosuppression is known, a comprehensive diagnostic survey must be undertaken to identify the underlying causes, including cancer, severe malnutrition, immune disorders, and chronic viral infection.

Aubry A et al: Sixty cases of *Mycobacterium marinum* infection: Clinical features, treatment, and antibiotic susceptibility of the causative isolates. Arch Intern Med 2002;162:1746. [PMID: 12153378]

Biviji AA et al: Musculoskeletal manifestations of human immunodeficiency virus infection. J Am Acad Orthop Surg 2002;10: 312. [PMID: 12374482]

Le Dantec C et al: Occurrence of mycobacteria in water treatment lines and in water distribution systems. Appl Environ Microbiol 2002;68:5318. [PMID: 12406720]

Laine M, Luukkainen R, Toivanen A: Sindbis viruses and other alpha viruses as a cause of human arthritic disease. J Intern Med 2004;256:457. [PMID: 15554947]

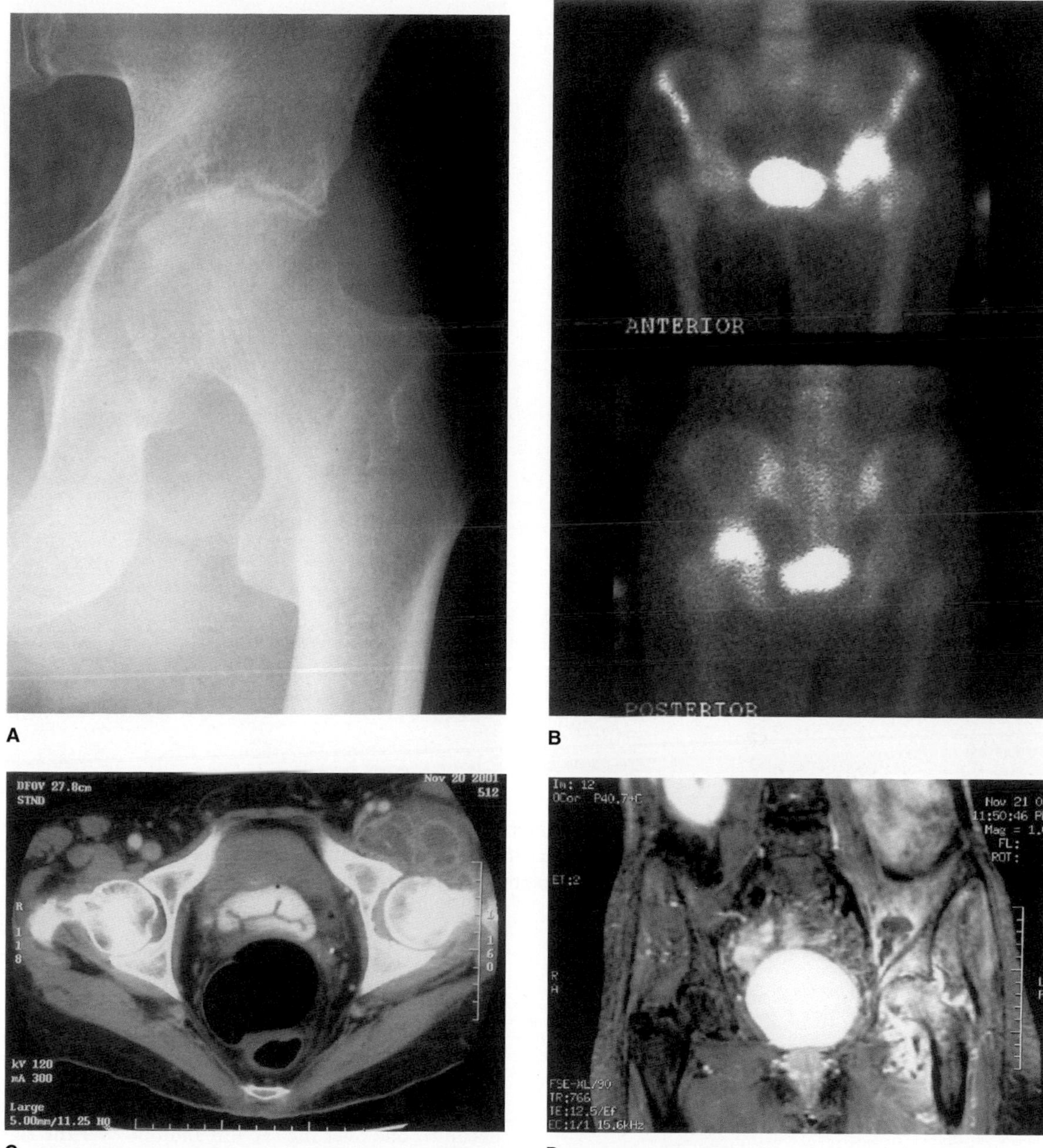

Figure 8–13. **A:** Initial anteroposterior radiograph of hip joint with narrowed cartilage caused by rheumatoid arthritis. **B:** Technetium bone scan shows intense activity in region of left hip. **C:** CT scan shows loculated soft-tissue mass anterior to the femoral head displacing the femoral artery and vein medially. **D:** T_1-weighted fat-saturated MRI with gadolinium contrast shows intense inflammation around hip joint and in acetabulum and femoral head. A retroperitoneal abscess is depicted in the enlarged iliopsoas muscle by a dark central area of signal void surrounded by a halo of bright inflammation. *Continued.*

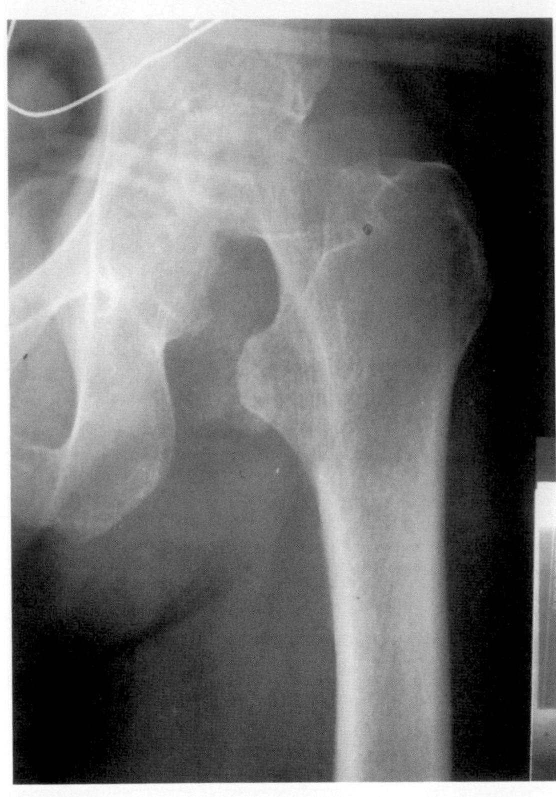

E

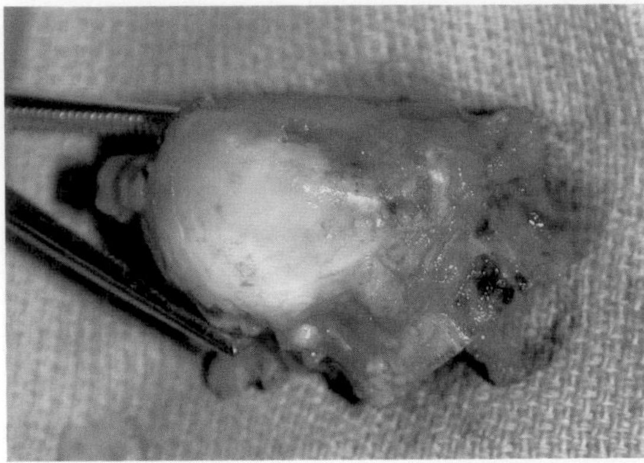

F

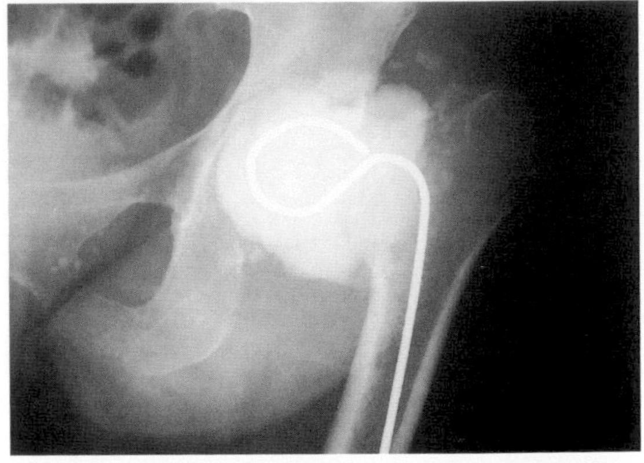

G

Figure 8–13. (Continued) **E:** Preoperative plain radiograph showing extensive collapse of the weight bearing portion of the femoral head. **F:** Surgical specimen showing flattened femoral head (upper portion). Note the cut surface of the neck (lower right). **G:** Radiograph of an antibiotic spacer molded around a rush rod that was implanted in the femoral canal.

Mylonas AD et al: Natural history of Ross River virus-induced epidemic polyarthritis. Med J Aust 2002;177:356. [PMID: 12358577]

Stahl HD et al: Detection of multiple viral DNA species in synovial tissue and fluid of patients with early arthritis. Ann Rheum Dis 2000;59:342. [PMID: 10784515]

SEPTIC ARTHRITIS CAUSED BY ADJACENT INFECTION

Contiguous spread of infection to a joint most commonly occurs in pediatric patients with AHO or in adults with chronic wounds such as ischial decubiti and diabetic foot ulcers. Chronic soft-tissue and bone infections may extend into joints in adults as well. Of particular concern is occurrence in patients who are immunocompromised or insensate.

Clinical Example

A 28-year-old man with paraplegia and a long-standing history of sacral and ischial decubiti presented with a 2-week history of fevers, anemia, and increased spasticity of the lower extremities. Two large fist-sized decubiti, one over the sacrum and one over the right ischium, were observed (Figure 8–15A). The underlying bone was easily palpated at the base of both of these ulcers. Further examination with a probing finger revealed a deep sinus that tracked to the posterior aspect of the femoral head. Plain films revealed a chronically dislocated hip with cephalad migration of the femur and concomitant destruction of the ilium (Figure 8–15B). Axial CT scan showed air within and surrounding the dislocated femoral head (Figure 8–15C). MRI with inversion recovery sequenc-

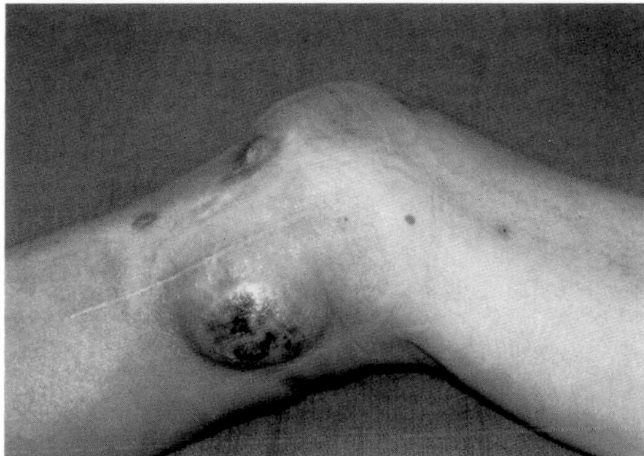

A

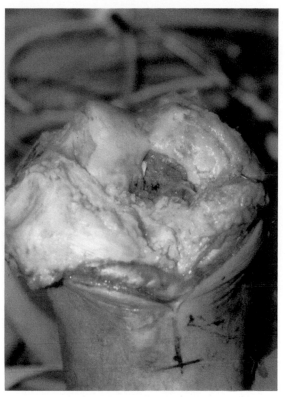

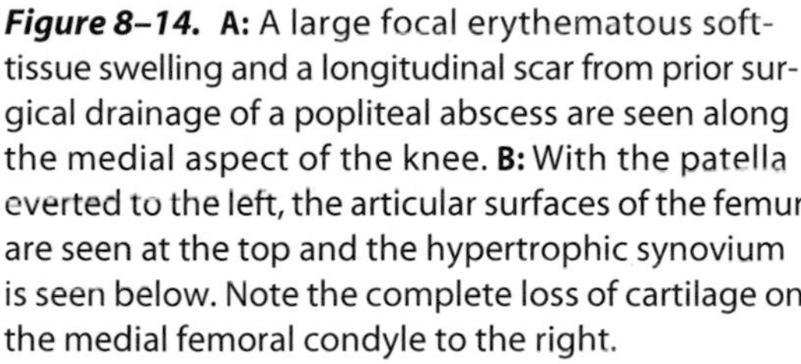

B

Figure 8–14. **A:** A large focal erythematous soft-tissue swelling and a longitudinal scar from prior surgical drainage of a popliteal abscess are seen along the medial aspect of the knee. **B:** With the patella everted to the left, the articular surfaces of the femur are seen at the top and the hypertrophic synovium is seen below. Note the complete loss of cartilage on the medial femoral condyle to the right.

ing depicted extensive inflammation of the femur, the ilium, and the surrounding gluteal musculature (Figure 8–15D). An extensive surgical debridement of the acetabulum and removal of the proximal femur was performed through the lateral ulcer. A wound VAC was placed on both ulcers, and culture-specific antibiotics were administered. The patient refused a hip disarticulation with an anterior thigh flap that would close both ischial and sacral decubiti, and he was subsequently treated with chronic oral antibiotic suppression and daily wound packing.

Goergens ED et al: Acute osteomyelitis and septic arthritis in children. J Pediatr Child Health 2005;41:59. [PMID: 15670227]

Li SF et al: Laboratory tests in adults with monoarticular arthritis: Can they rule out a septic joint? Acad Emerg Med 2004; 11:276. [PMID: 15001408]

Salter RB, Bell RS, Keeley FW: The protective effect of continuous passive motion on living articular cartilage in acute septic arthritis. Clin Orthop 1981;159:223. [PMID: 7285461]

Shirtliff ME, Mader JT: Acute septic arthritis. Clin Microbiol Rev 2002;15:527. [PMID: 12364368]

Swan A, Amer H, Dieppe P: The value of synovial fluid analysis in the diagnosis of joint disease: A literature survey. Ann Rheum Dis 2002;61:493. [PMID: 12006320]

Yu KH et al: Concomitant septic and gouty arthritis—An analysis of 30 cases. Rheumatology (Oxford) 2003;42:1062. [PMID: 12730521]

SOFT-TISSUE INFECTIONS

CELLULITIS

Skin infections are common, and it is important to distinguish cellulitis from noninfectious rashes and from deeper infections that have a component of cellulitis, such as osteomyelitis, septic arthritis, myositis, and necrotizing fasciitis. Stasis dermatitis may visually mimic cellulitis. Patients often present with a rash over areas of increased peripheral edema.

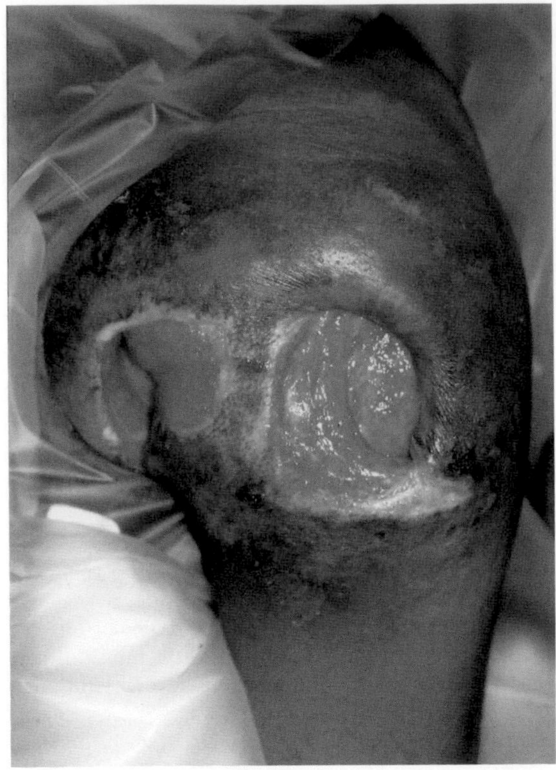

A

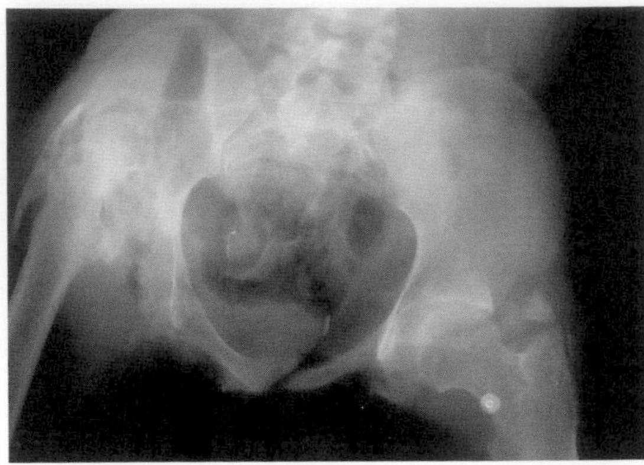

B

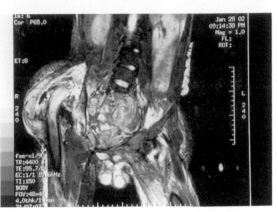

D

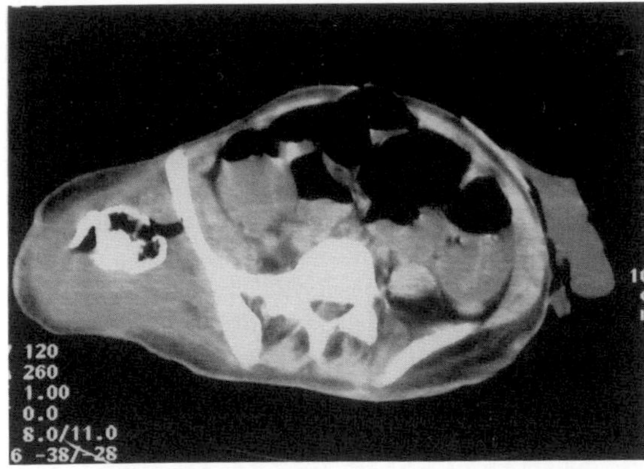

C

Figure 8–15. **A:** Large sacral and right ischial ulcer. **B:** Anteroposterior radiograph of the pelvis. **C:** CT scan of pelvis. **D:** MRI with inversion recovery sequence of the pelvis.

Unlike patients with cellulitis, these patients do not have a fever or elevated WBC.

Clinical Example

A 43-year-old man fell 3 weeks ago, injuring his leg. He presented with progressively worsening pain and swelling in his thigh. On examination, cellulitis of the anterior and lateral thigh was manifested by erythema, diffuse and tense swelling with shiny skin, and dramatic pain with knee flexion and tenderness with light palpation (Figure 8–16A). No swelling or erythema of the calf or foot was noted, and distal pulses and sensation were intact. Plain radiographs of the femur were

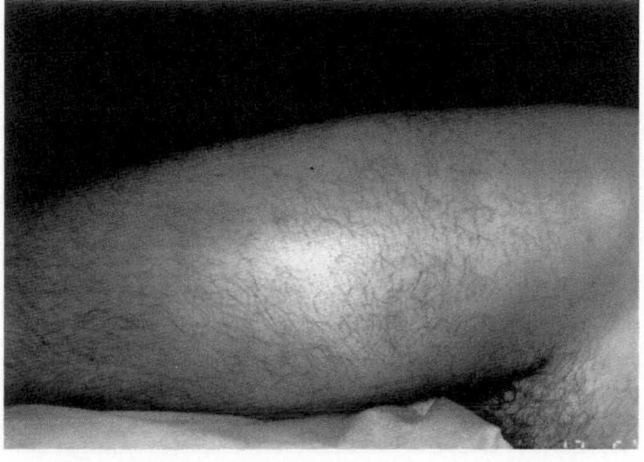

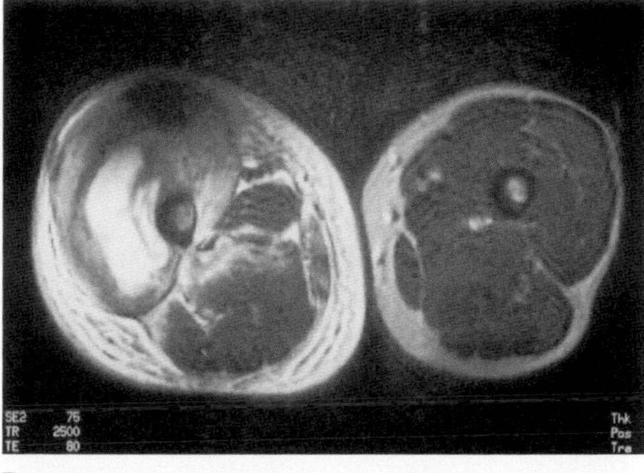

Figure 8–16. **A:** Cellulitis and diffuse thigh swelling. **B:** Axial T_2-weighted MRI of the thigh.

normal. Doppler ultrasound ruled out a deep venous thrombosis but identified diffuse swelling of the muscle compartment. A T_2-weighted MRI depicted characteristic expansion of the subcutaneous tissues with feathery streaks of increased water content circumferentially. It also revealed an underlying fluid collection within the vastus lateralis and intermedius (Figure 8–16B). Surgical inspection of this fluid revealed pus from an underlying myositis. An intramuscular hematoma from nonpenetrating trauma to the thigh had become hematogenously seeded with *S. aureus.* The infection caused an expanding abscess with myositis and superficial cellulitis. Culture acquisition, serial irrigation and debridement with open packing, and antibiotic therapy were started. Delayed primary closure and 6 weeks of culture-sensitive IV antibiotics cured the patient's infection. It should be noted in this case that the cellulitis was manifested after the leg began to swell, indicating clinically that the cellulitis was a secondary finding. In this circumstance a search for an underlying cause was necessary to understand the source of infection.

PYOMYOSITIS

Pyomyositis is usually caused by hematogenous spread of bacteria rather than direct inoculation via penetrating trauma. Usually there is very limited muscle necrosis, and a very vascular fibrous reactive capsule contains the abscess. Open exploration with copious irrigation, limited debridement, and primary wound closure over a surgical drain is the surgical treatment of choice. Evaluation for contiguous spread to bone or joint must be performed. Aspiration for culture and insertion of a pigtail catheter for drainage can be done with ultrasound or CT guidance.

Clinical Example

A 6-year-old boy presented with a 2-week history of a posterior thigh mass. Focal tenderness and swelling were present, but no erythema was noted (Figure 8–17A). Further inspection revealed numerous insect bites around his ankle and leg that had become open pustules because of vigorous scratching. A T_1-weighted fat-saturated MRI with gadolinium clearly characterized a fluid collection represented by a black signal void (Figure 8–17B). A halo of increased signal uptake along the rim of the fluid collection represents intense localized inflammation. The patient underwent surgical exploration, and pus was easily expressed from the thigh. The wound was debrided, irrigated, and a surgical drainage tube was placed. The wound was primarily closed. Staining revealed gram-positive cocci in clusters, and cultures grew a sensitive *S. aureus.* IV antibiotics were initiated, and the patient's symptoms rapidly improved. A week later he was discharged to home with 5 weeks of oral antibiotics that cured his infection.

BURSITIS

A bursa occasionally becomes infected by hematogenous spread or because of open trauma to the overlying skin. The patient complains of pain and stiffness and possibly a fever. A tender, inflamed bursal region is seen clinically with significant erythema and swelling. Because these findings may also occur in acute exacerbations of rheumatism and flare-ups of gout, the patient must be carefully questioned regarding a possible history of these diagnoses. For example, aspiration of a soft, inflamed olecranon tophus may yield fluid that is strikingly similar to pus. Gram stain and polarized microscopy are necessary to identify negatively birefringent crystals.

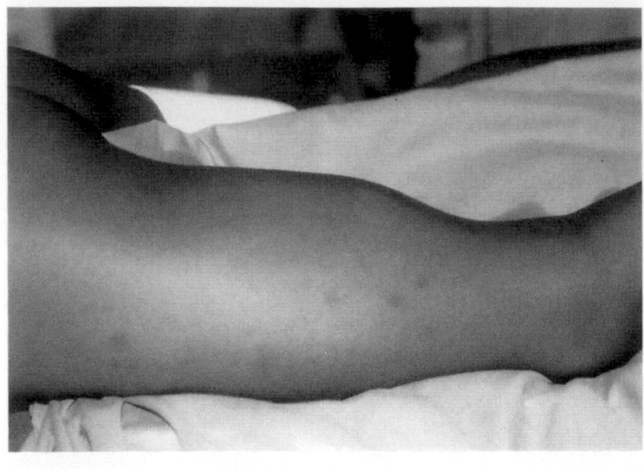

A

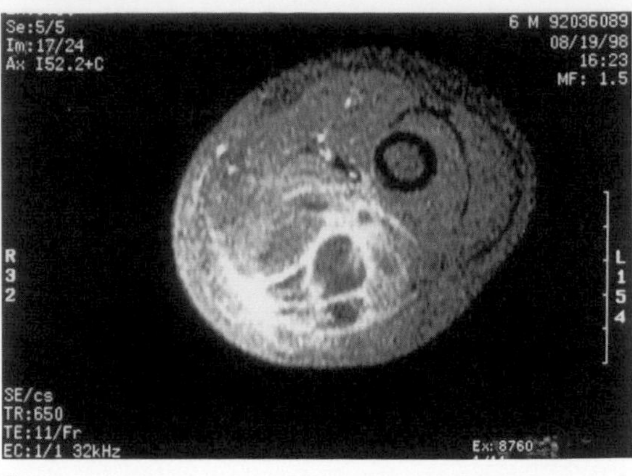

B

Figure 8–17. **A:** Prone patient with focal swelling of the posterior region of the midthigh. Note the insect bites scarring the skin. **B:** T_1-weighted MRI with gadolinium contrast showing dark signal void in center of abscess.

If infectious bursitis is identified within the first several days, an oral course of antibiotics may successfully treat the infection. If skin erythema spreads and the bursa fills with fluid, the patient must be admitted to the hospital to aspirate and culture the bursal fluid and to begin empirical IV antibiotics. If the infection does not begin to resolve clinically within 48 hours, surgical bursectomy and primary closure of the wound over a drain should be performed.

Clinical Example

An 18-year-old woman skinned her knee on the gym floor during a game of basketball 1 week prior to presentation. She was noted on exam to have a dramatically painful, swollen, and erythematous prepatellar region with only slight loss of knee motion. A small central eschar, indicative of a floor burn, was observed (Figures 8–18A and B). Gram stain of the aspirate from the prepatellar bursa revealed gram-positive cocci in clusters. Despite 2 days of IV antistaphylococcal antibiotic therapy, the inflammation worsened. A complete bursectomy was performed (Figure 8–18C). A layer of normal appearing fatty tissue was left to cover the surface of the patella (Figure 8–18D), and the wound was closed over a surgical drain. The inflammation quickly improved within 3 days, and the patient was sent home with 3 weeks of culture-specific antibiotics.

NECROTIZING FASCIITIS

Necrotizing fasciitis is a rare but extremely aggressive, life-threatening soft-tissue infection of the subcutaneous and fascial tissues often encountered in diabetic patients. The muscle tissues are generally spared. Clinical examination of the skin reveals streaking erythema and sometimes small blisters, arising in the region of an incidental puncture wound. Local induration is always found, and occasionally subcutaneous crepitation caused by gas in the soft tissues is encountered. Air in the soft tissues can usually be seen on plain radiographs in gas-producing clostridial infections (see Figure 8–1). Serial exams are necessary to track the leading edge of the infection, which rapidly progresses in the direction of venous drainage. Emergent surgical debridement of devitalized tissues (sometimes necessitating amputation) along with antibiotics and intensive care treatment for hypotension are required to prevent death.

Clinical Example

A 38-year-old woman with a history of insulin-dependent diabetes mellitus sustained a penetrating trauma to the dorsum of her wrist while using scissors. Two days later she presented to the emergency room with a very painful arm and an infected stab wound that was draining serous fluid, an erythematous rash that extended from the wound to her elbow, and an increase of her forearm circumference of 6 cm compared with the other arm. She had a temperature of 38.6°C (101.5°F), a serum WBC of 22,000 with a left shift, and normal plain radiographs of the forearm.

The patient was admitted to the hospital and started empirically on a ticarcillin with clavulanate potassium (Timentin) and gentamicin. After 24 hours, however, the arm pain progressively worsened, and the rash advanced above the elbow (Figure 8–19A). MRI showed significant soft-tissue edema in the subcutaneous tissues but not in the muscle compartments (Fig-

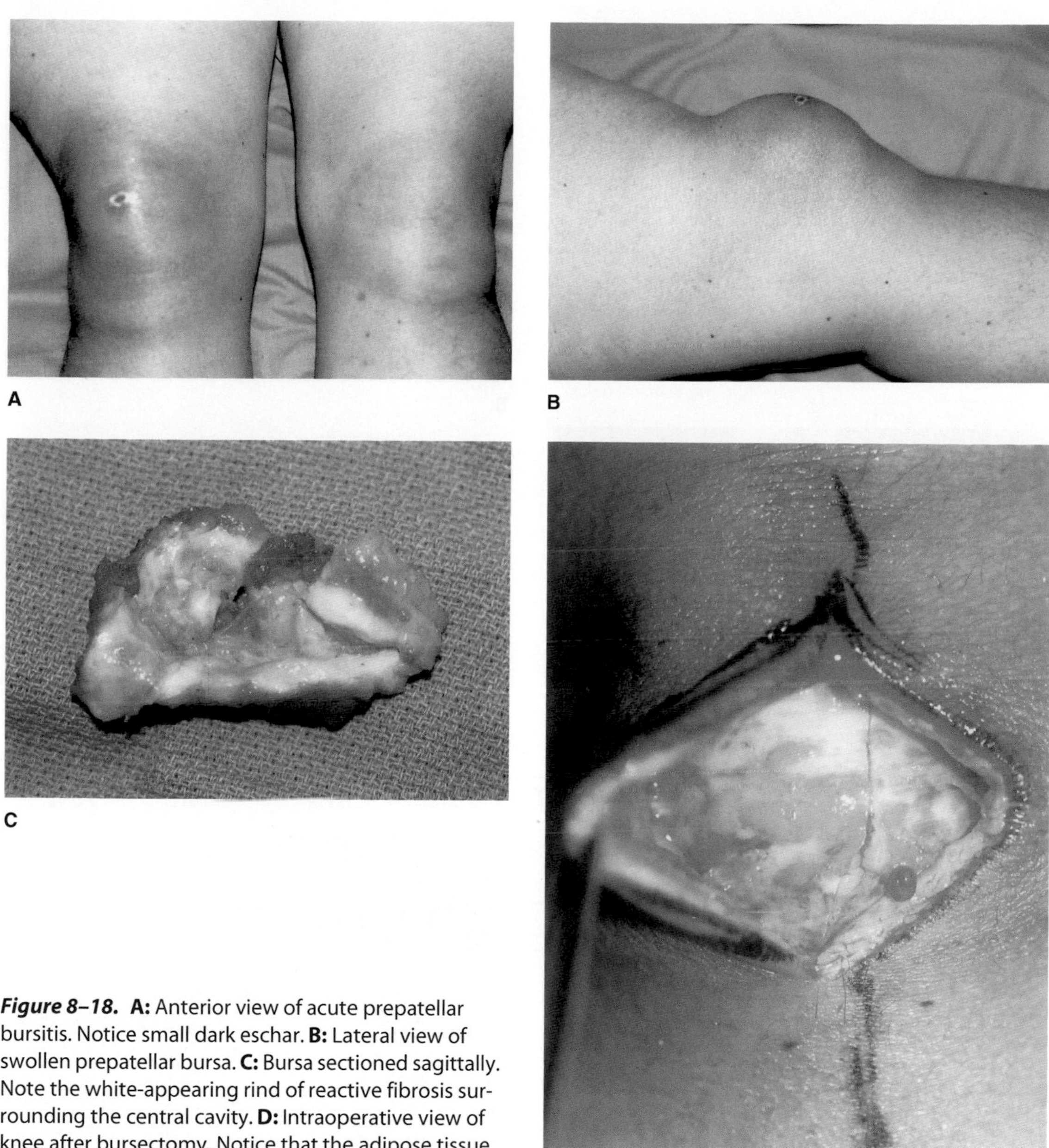

Figure 8–18. **A:** Anterior view of acute prepatellar bursitis. Notice small dark eschar. **B:** Lateral view of swollen prepatellar bursa. **C:** Bursa sectioned sagittally. Note the white-appearing rind of reactive fibrosis surrounding the central cavity. **D:** Intraoperative view of knee after bursectomy. Notice that the adipose tissue covering periosteum of patella was retained.

ures 8–19B and C). Concerned about an uncontrolled necrotizing fasciitis, surgical exploration was emergently performed. Although most of the skin and all of the muscle tissues were viable, necrosis of the subcutaneous tissues and fascia was extensive (Figures 8–19D and E). All necrotic tissue was sharply excised. The necrotic tissue could easily be distinguished because it was friable to palpation. Normal-appearing tissue was firmer, and a finger could not easily dissect the plane between the subcutaneous tissue and the fascia. The wound was copiously irrigated with a pulsatile lavage device and packed open with moist gauze dressings secured with sterile rubber bands and staples in a shoelace fashion (Figure 8–19F). Gram-positive cocci in chains were identified intraoperatively, and the antibiotics were switched to oxacillin and clindamycin.

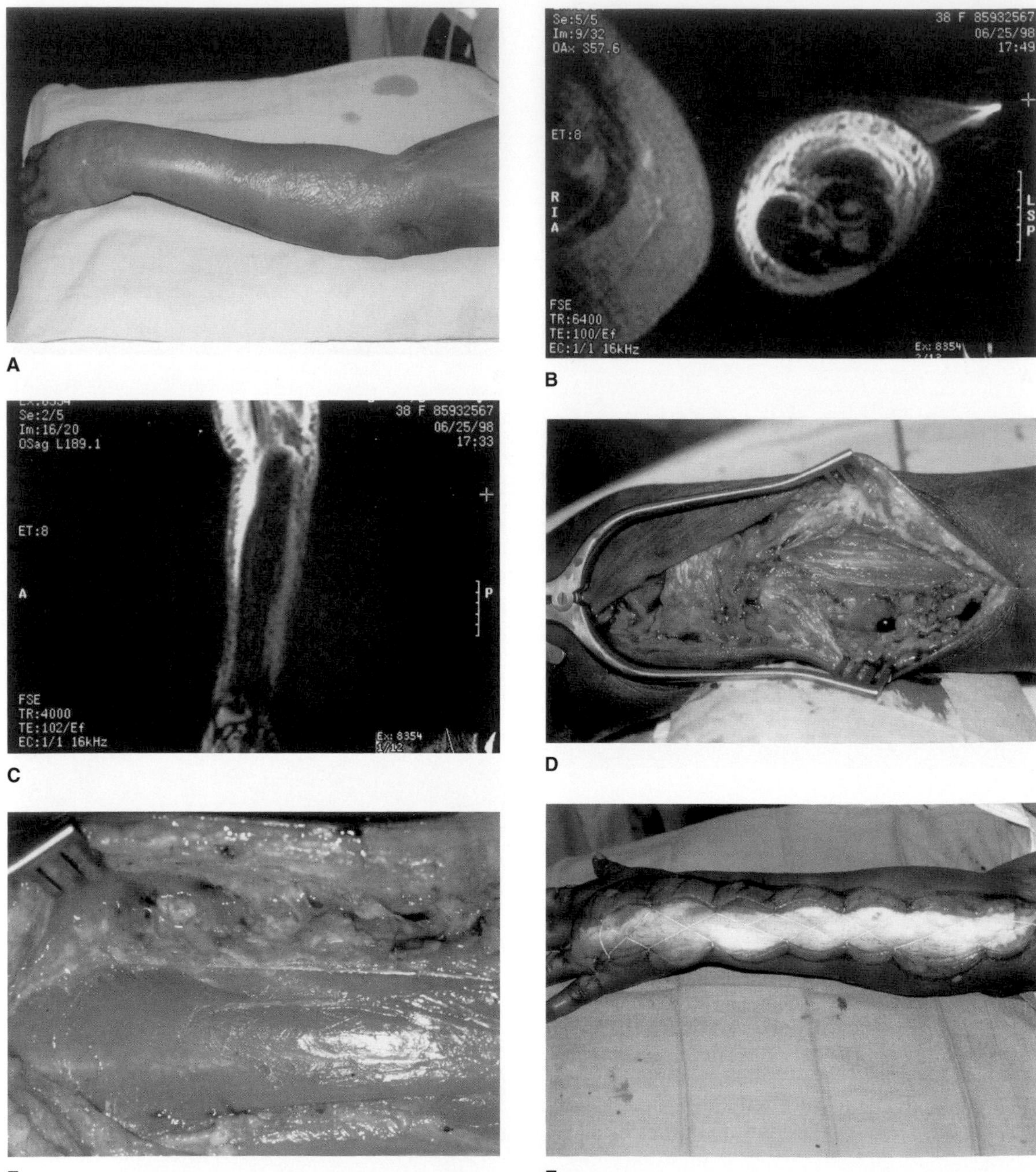

Figure 8–19. **A:** A small draining puncture wound is noted at the middorsum of the hand, and an extensive erythematous rash covers the forearm. **B:** Axial MRI inversion recovery sequence showing circumferential subcutaneous inflammation. **C:** Sagittal MRI inversion recovery sequence showing subcutaneous inflammation but absence of inflammation in muscle tissue. **D:** Dorsal forearm incision revealing extensive subcutaneous necrosis. **E:** Necrosis in subcutaneous tissues but not in muscle tissue. **F:** Open packing of wound with saline-dampened gauze sponges secured with staples and sterile rubber bands in a shoelace fashion. *Continued.*

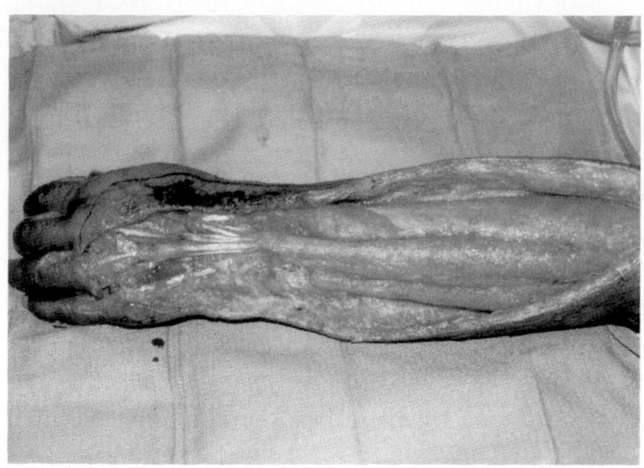

G

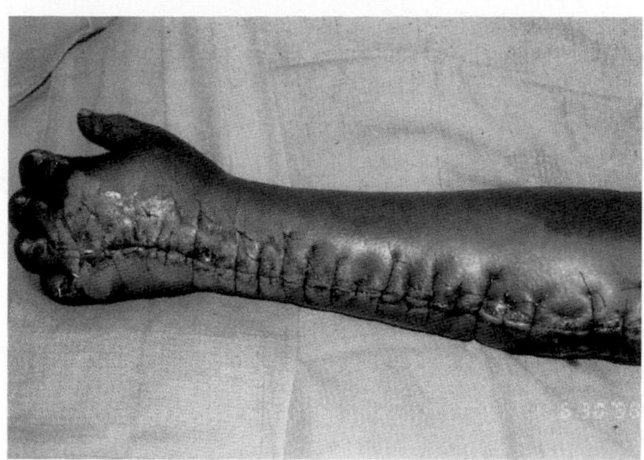

H

Figure 8–19. (Continued) **G:** Appearance of viable wound after 1 week of serial debridements, antibiotics, and hyperbaric oxygen treatments. **H:** Delayed primary closure with interrupted retention sutures.

Hyperbaric oxygen treatments using an acute protocol of 2.4 atm for 90 minutes three times daily was begun, and daily surgical debridements were performed for 3 days (Figure 8–19G). Some skin died and was debrided. The patient's infection cleared, and the wound was left to heal by delayed primary closure with use of split-thickness skin grafts where necessary (Figure 8–19H).

Tiu A et al: Necrotizing fasciitis: Analysis of 48 cases in South Auckland, New Zealand. ANZ J Surg 2005;75:32. [PMID: 15740513]

Foot & Ankle Surgery

9

Jeffrey A. Mann, MD, Loretta B. Chou, MD, & Steven D. K. Ross, MD

BIOMECHANIC PRINCIPLES OF THE FOOT & ANKLE

The following is a limited discussion of the biomechanic principles governing the foot and ankle during the gait cycle. The physician must have a clear understanding of these principles to evaluate problems affecting the foot and ankle accurately. Once normal biomechanic function is understood, anatomic and functional abnormalities are more easily detected.

Gait

Gait is the orderly progression of the body through space while expending as little energy as possible. As the body moves through a gait cycle, forces are generated actively, by action of the body's muscles, and passively, by the effects of gravity on the body. To accommodate these forces, the foot is flexible at the time of heel strike, when it must absorb the impact of the body against the ground, and rigid at the time of toe-off, when it must assist in moving the body forward. The magnitude of the forces on the foot increases significantly as the speed of gait increases. For example, when an individual is walking, the initial force with which the foot meets the ground is approximately 80% of body weight, whereas when an individual is jogging, it is approximately 160%. The peak force against the foot during walking is approximately 110% of body weight, whereas for jogging it is approximately 240%. This marked increase probably contributes to some of the injuries seen in runners.

The Walking Cycle

The walking cycle is discussed more extensively in Chapter 1, but pertinent aspects relating to the foot are discussed here (Figure 9–1).

Observation of the patient while walking may give the clinician insight into the cause of a gait anomaly (Figure 9–2). For example, equinus deformity resulting from spasticity or contracture may cause the toe to make initial contact with the ground rather than the heel. At 7% of the gait cycle, the foot is usually flat on the ground, but spasticity or tightness of the Achilles tendon causes this to be delayed. At 12% of the cycle, the opposite foot toes off and the swing phase begins. Heel rise of the standing foot begins at 34% of the cycle as the swinging leg passes the standing limb. Heel rise may be premature in spasticity or prolonged in weakness of the gastrocsoleus muscle. Heel strike of the opposite foot occurs at 50% of the cycle, ending the period of single-limb support; this may occur sooner if there is weakness of the contralateral calf muscle. Toe-off of the opposite foot occurs at 62% of the cycle, at the beginning of the swing phase. These markers of the gait cycle should be kept in mind when observing gait, so pathologic conditions may be identified.

Motions of the Foot & Ankle

The names for various motions about the foot and ankle may be confusing and used incorrectly. The motions that occur at the ankle joint are dorsiflexion and plantar flexion. The motions of the heel medially and laterally, which occur at the subtalar joint, are inversion (varus) and eversion (valgus), respectively. The motion occurring at the transverse tarsal joint (talonavicular and calcaneocuboid) is adduction, which is movement toward the midline, and abduction, which is movement away from the midline.

Supination and *pronation* are terms for two different combinations of movements, but unfortunately these terms are sometimes used in the literature interchangeably. *Pronation* refers to dorsiflexion of the ankle joint, eversion of the subtalar joint, and abduction of the transverse tarsal joint. *Supination* is the opposite; namely, plantar flexion of the ankle joint, inversion of the subtalar joint, and adduction of the transverse tarsal joint.

The nomenclature may also be confusing when such terms as *forefoot varus* and *forefoot valgus* are used (Figure 9–3). Forefoot varus or valgus is an anatomic deformity that is observed when the hindfoot is placed in neutral position. Neutral position is achieved when the calcaneus is aligned with the long axis of the tibia and the head of the talus is covered with the navicular bone. Forefoot varus deformity is present when the lateral aspect of the forefoot is in greater plantar flexion than the medial aspect. With a flexible deformity, the foot lies flat on the floor during stance, but with a fixed deformity, excessive weight is borne on the lateral side of the foot. As a result,

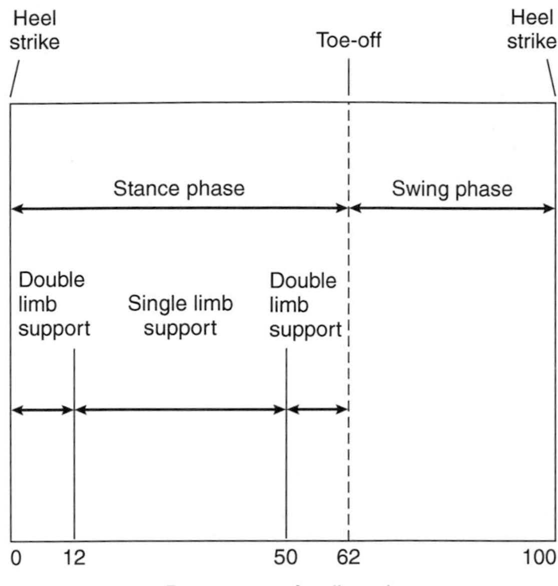

Figure 9–1. Phases of the walking cycle. Stance phase constitutes approximately 62% and swing phase 38% of the cycle. (Reproduced, with permission, from Mann RA, Coughlin MJ: *The Video Textbook of Foot and Ankle Surgery.* Medical Video Productions, 1991.)

as the weight passes onto the forefoot region, the calcaneus goes into valgus position, and this may result in lateral impingement of the calcaneus against the fibula if severe. In forefoot valgus deformity, the medial side of the foot has greater plantar flexion than the lateral side and results in excessive weight bearing by the first metatarsal head. To accommodate for this deformity, the calcaneus assumes a varus position, which may result in a feeling of instability at the ankle joint.

Mechanisms of the Foot during Weight Bearing

As mentioned previously, the normal foot is flexible at the time of heel strike to absorb the impact of striking the ground. As a result, the subtalar joint literally collapses into a position of valgus, causing internal rotation of the tibia and resulting distally in unlocking of the transverse tarsal (talonavicular and calcaneocuboid) joint. Thus, the forefoot is more flexible. The only muscle group that is functioning about the foot and ankle during heel strike is the anterior compartment muscle group, which helps control the initial rapid plantar flexion following heel strike by an eccentric or lengthening contraction. The flexibility of the foot is greatest at approximately 7% of the cycle, and a series of changes is then initiated. With the foot fixed to the ground, the body passes over the foot, which lifts the heel up and forces the metatarsophalangeal joints into extension. As this occurs, the foot is converted into a rigid lever that supports the body at the time of toe-off. The mechanisms that bring about conversion of the foot from a flexible to a rigid structure are (1) the tightening of the plantar aponeurosis, the windlass mechanism, (2) the progressive external rotation of the lower extremity, which begins at the pelvis and is passed distally across the ankle joint into the subtalar joint, and (3) the stabilization of the transverse tarsal joint, which results from the progressive inversion of the subtalar joint.

Joints About the Foot & Ankle

A. Ankle Joint

The ankle joint consists of the articulation of the talus with the tibia and fibula, with a range of motion (ROM) of 15 degrees of dorsiflexion and 55 degrees of plantar flexion. There is also a small amount of motion in the transverse plane, approximately 15 degrees. The anterior compartment muscles of the leg, the tibialis anterior and the toe extensors, control the amount of plantar flexion of the ankle joint at the time of heel ground contact to 10% stance. In addition, these muscles provide dorsiflexion of the ankle joint during swing phase. If this muscle group does not function, a footslap is observed at the time of heel strike, and a dropfoot occurs during swing phase. The greatest force across the ankle joint during walking is calculated to be approximately 4.5 times body weight; this force is present at 40% of the walking cycle.

B. Subtalar Joint

The subtalar joint is the articulation between the talus and the calcaneus. The primary joint surface is the

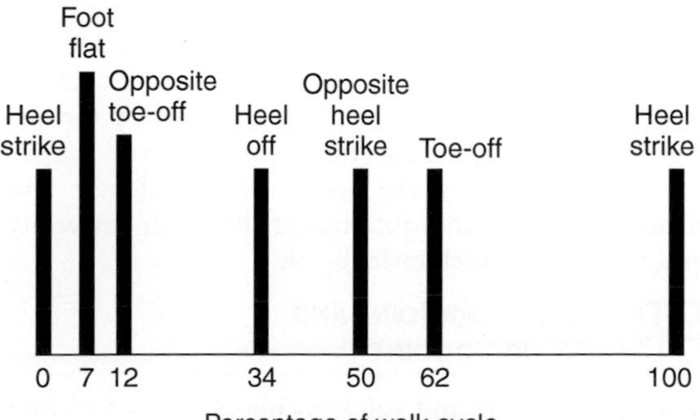

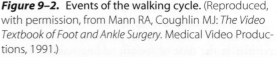

Figure 9–2. Events of the walking cycle. (Reproduced, with permission, from Mann RA, Coughlin MJ: *The Video Textbook of Foot and Ankle Surgery.* Medical Video Productions, 1991.)

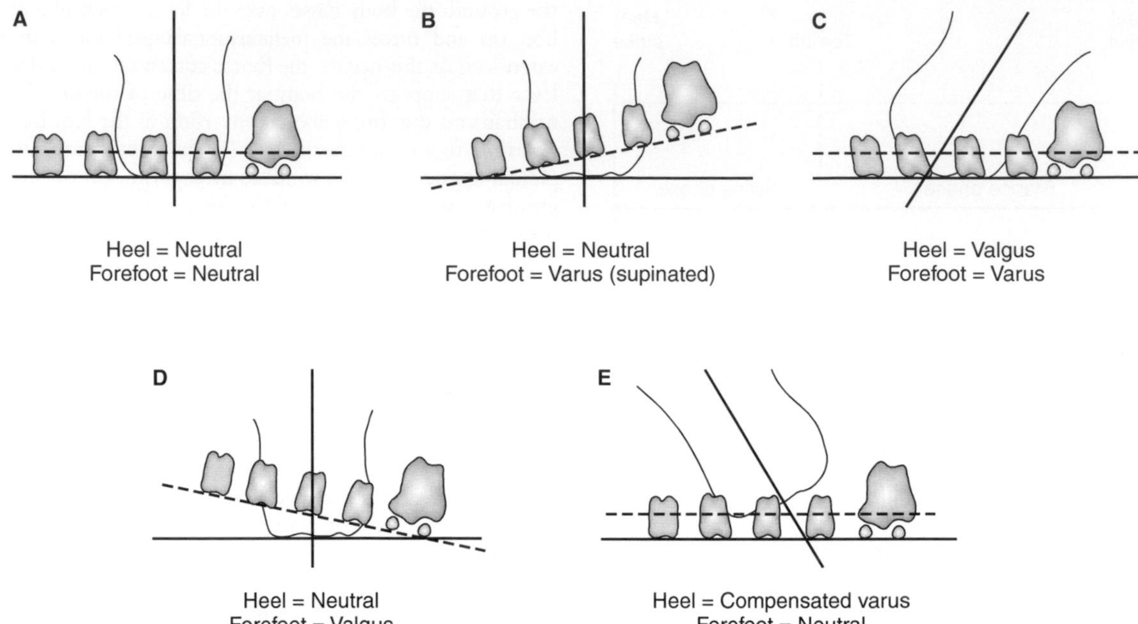

Figure 9–3. Biomechanics of foot posture. **A:** Normal alignment: forefoot perpendicular to heel. **B:** Forefoot varus (uncompensated): lateral aspect of forefoot plantar flexed in relation to medial aspect. **C:** Forefoot varus (compensated): With the forefoot flat on the floor, the heel assumes a valgus position. **D:** Forefoot valgus (uncompensated): medial aspect of forefoot plantar flexed in relation to lateral aspect. **E:** Forefoot valgus (compensated): With the forefoot flat on the floor, the heel assumes a varus position. (Reproduced, with permission, from Mann RA, Coughlin MJ: *The Video Textbook of Foot and Ankle Surgery*. Medical Video Productions, 1991.)

posterior facet, with much smaller middle and anterior facets. The motion of this joint is inversion of approximately 30 degrees and eversion of approximately 10 degrees. The tibialis posterior causes inversion and the peroneus brevis eversion at the subtalar joint. At the time of initial ground contact, eversion is a passive mechanism and occurs because of the shape of the articulations and their ligamentous support. Inversion occurs both actively and passively at the time of toe-off. Active control is achieved by the gastrocsoleus and posterior tibial muscles, and passive inversion occurs by the action of the plantar aponeurosis, the external rotation of the lower extremity, and the oblique metatarsal break.

C. Talonavicular Joint and Calcaneocuboid Joint

The talonavicular and calcaneocuboid joints functionally act as a unit known as the *transverse tarsal joint.* Motion at the transverse tarsal joint is approximately 10 degrees of abduction and approximately 15 degrees of adduction. The head of the talus is firmly seated into the navicular at the time of toe-off, adding stability to the foot. The stability of the transverse tarsal joint is controlled by the position of the subtalar joint. When the subtalar joint is in an inverted position, the axes of these two joints are nonparallel, giving rise to increased stability of the hindfoot. When the calcaneus is in an everted position at the time of heel strike, these joints are parallel to one another, thereby giving rise to increased flexibility of these joints (Figure 9–4). The clinical implication is that when carrying out a subtalar arthrodesis, placement of the subtalar joint into a varus position locks the transverse tarsal joint, causing increased stiffness of the forefoot and, frequently, discomfort. When the hindfoot is everted into a position of 5–7 degrees of valgus, the flexibility of the transverse tarsal joint is maintained. This allows the forefoot to be more supple and makes ambulation easier.

D. Metatarsophalangeal Joints

The motion at the metatarsophalangeal joints is between 50 and 70 degrees of dorsiflexion (extension) and 15 and 25 degrees of plantar flexion (flexion). The role of the metatarsophalangeal joints during gait is discussed in the section on deformities of the first toe.

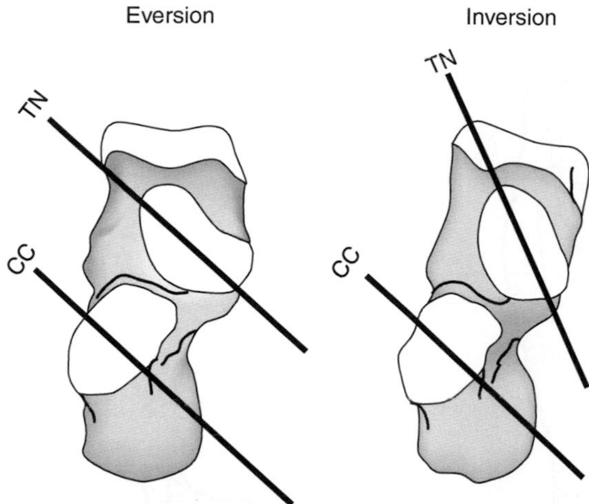

Figure 9–4. The function of the transverse tarsal joint as described by Elftman demonstrates that when the calcaneus is in eversion, the resultant axes of the talonavicular and calcaneocuboid joints are parallel or congruent. When the subtalar joint is in an inverted position, the axes are incongruent, giving increased stability to the midfoot. (Reproduced, with permission, from Mann RA, Coughlin MJ: *The Video Textbook of Foot and Ankle Surgery.* Medical Video Productions, 1991.)

E. The Plantar Aponeurosis

Although the plantar aponeurosis is not an articulation per se, it probably plays the predominant role in the overall stability of the foot. The plantar aponeurosis arises from the tubercle of the calcaneus and passes distally to insert into the base of each proximal phalanx (Figure 9–5). As the metatarsophalangeal joints pass into dorsiflexion in the last half of the stance phase, the rigidity of the plantar aponeurosis forces the metatarsal heads into a plantarward direction, which raises the longitudinal arch. This is known as a windlass mechanism. It also increases the effect that a tensile force in the tendo Achilles has on the tensile force in the plantar fascia. The now-rigid foot provides support to the body for the push-off phase of gait. Secondarily, this mechanism also helps bring about inversion of the subtalar joint.

F. Gait Abnormalities

The following is a brief description of the more common gait abnormalities.

1. Dropfoot gait—Patients with dropfoot gait lack ankle dorsiflexion, resulting in plantar flexion at the ankle joint. When walking, these patients adopt a steppage-type gait. This gait pattern is manifested by increased flexion of the hip and knee to enable the swinging leg to clear the ground. If this compensatory mechanism does not occur, the patient may catch the toes on the ground and fall.

2. Equinus gait—In an equinus gait pattern, the ankle joint is fixed in plantar flexion throughout the entire gait cycle. This situation may result from a stroke or head injury, trauma to the lower extremity, or a congenital deformity, and it often is associated with tightness of the posterior capsule. This gait pattern is characterized by forefoot floor contact (no heel contact). The anterior loading of the foot results in a back knee thrust, which may, over a long period of time, result in a hyperextension deformity of the knee. A weak quadriceps muscle may accentuate this problem.

3. Cavus deformity—A cavus deformity is an excessive elevation of the longitudinal arch. A moderate decrease in the ROM of the foot usually accompanies this deformity. In addition, the hindfoot is often in a varus posture and the forefoot in valgus posture. This is most frequently observed in Charcot-Marie-Tooth disease but may also be seen in poliomyelitis and occasionally as a late result of calf compartment syndrome. The deformity significantly diminishes the overall surface available for weight bearing in these patients. Clawing of the toes may further reduce contact with the ground. Thus, the gait pattern in these patients is altered, with increased pressure on the heel at initial ground contact, followed by increased pressure along the lateral side of the foot and underneath the first metatarsal head as the gait cycle progresses.

4. Pes planus deformity—Usually, the patient with a pes planus deformity demonstrates just the opposite of cavus deformity; the foot is too flexible. At the time of initial ground contact, there is excessive valgus of the hindfoot and in severe cases breaking down of the longitudinal arch with an associated abduction of the forefoot. This results in an increased weight-bearing surface and often easy fatigability because of the lack of adequate support of the longitudinal arch.

Carlson RE, Fleming LL, Hutton WC: The biomechanical relationship between the tendoachilles, plantar fascia and metatarsophalangeal joint dorsiflexion angle. Foot Ankle Int 2000;21:18–25. [PMID: 10710257]

Hunt AE, Smith RM, Torode M: Extrinsic muscle activity, foot motion and ankle joint moments during the stance phase of walking. Foot Ankle Int 2001;22:31–41. [PMID: 11206820]

Mann RA: Biomechanics of the foot and ankle. In Mann RA, Coughlin MJ, eds: *Surgery of the Foot and Ankle.* Mosby-Year Book, 1993.

Nester CJ, Findlow AF, Bowder P et al: Transverse plane motion at the ankle joint. Foot Ankle Int 2003;24:164. [PMID: 12627625]

Saunders JB, Inman VT, Eberhart HD: The major determinants in normal and pathologic gait. J Bone Joint Surg Am 1953;3 5:543. [PMID: 13069544]

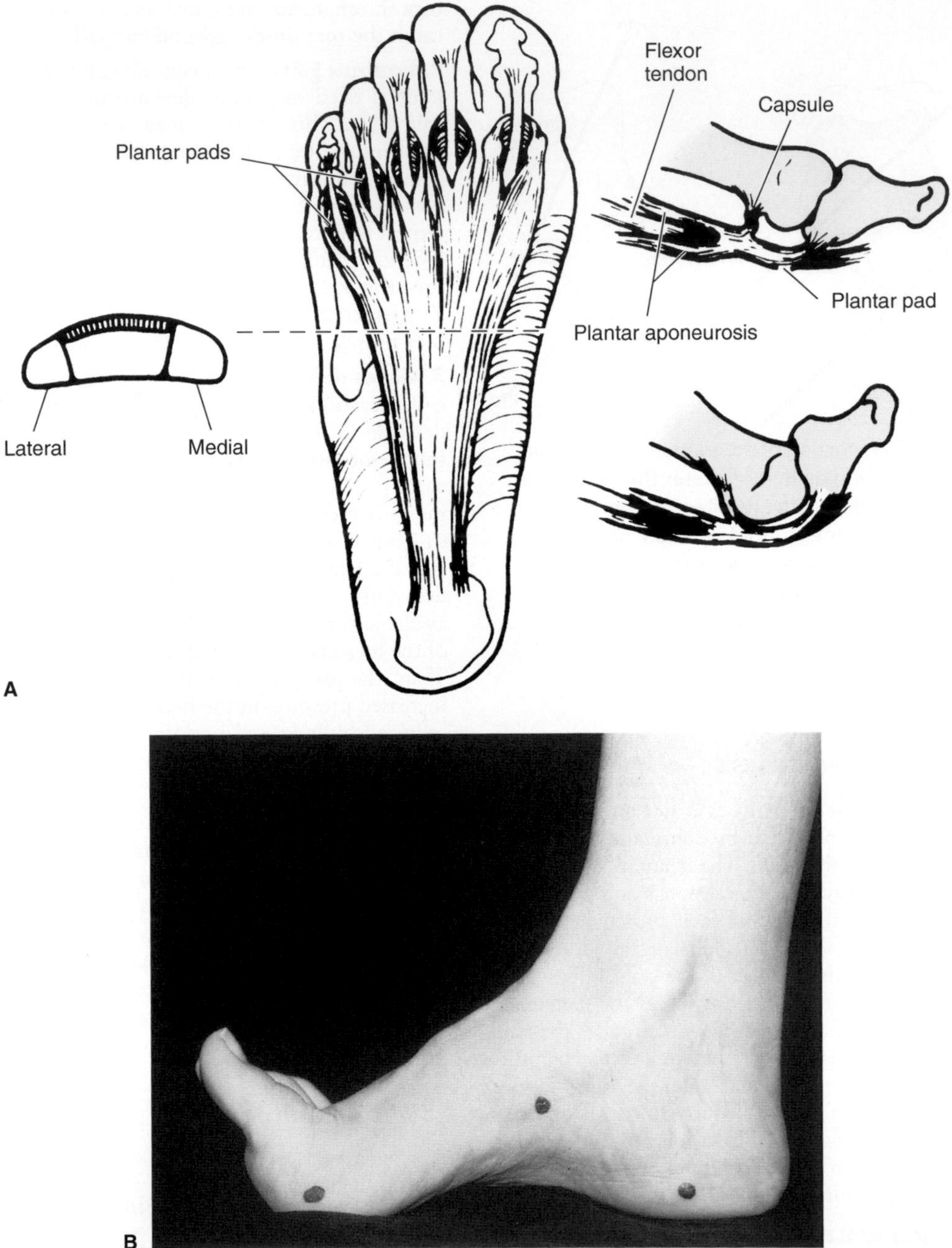

Figure 9–5. Windlass mechanism. **A:** The plantar aponeurosis, which arises from the tubercle of the calcaneus, divides and inserts into the base of each of the proximal phalanges. **B:** Dorsiflexion of the metatarsophalangeal joints wraps the plantar aponeurosis around the metatarsal head, depressing the metatarsal heads and elevating the longitudinal arch. (Reproduced, with permission, from Mann RA, Coughlin MJ: *The Video Textbook of Foot and Ankle Surgery*. Medical Video Productions, 1991.)

DEFORMITIES OF THE FIRST TOE

Biomechanic Principles

The first metatarsophalangeal joint functions mainly as a weight-bearing structure and stabilizer of the medial aspect of the longitudinal arch. The static stability of the first metatarsophalangeal joint is provided by the collateral ligaments and the strong plantar plate, which consists of the plantar aponeurosis and the joint capsule. Added dynamic stability is provided by the abductor hallucis and adductor hallucis muscles, which insert along the medial and lateral sides of the metatarsal head, respectively. No muscle inserts into the metatarsal head per se, and therefore it is suspended in a sling of muscles and tendons. This allows the metatarsal head to be pushed in a medial or lateral direction, depending on the deviation of the proximal phalanx.

As previously discussed, the plantar aponeurosis forces the metatarsal heads into plantar flexion during the last third of the stance phase of the walking cycle. As a result, pressure that is present under the metatarsal heads is transferred to the toes, especially the hallux (see Figure 9–5). If this windlass mechanism for the hallux is lost as occurs in a bunion deformity, pressure is no longer transferred to the toes but remains beneath the metatarsal heads. Metatarsalgia results from this transfer of load, especially beneath the lesser metatarsal heads. The second metatarsal frequently bears the load because the weight-bearing ability of the first metatarsal is disrupted.

Any type of surgical procedure that disrupts this mechanism may result in the development of transfer lesions as well. This problem can be seen after the Keller arthroplasty, in which the base of the proximal phalanx is removed, or after prosthetic replacement of the first metatarsal joint. Metatarsal osteotomy with excessive shortening (more than 5–7 mm) or dorsiflexion of the first metatarsal may also cause this problem.

Normal Anatomy

The first metatarsophalangeal joint consists of the articulating surfaces of the metatarsal head and the base of the proximal phalanx. On the plantar aspect of the foot beneath the metatarsal head are the two sesamoid bones, which are embedded in the dual tendons of the flexor hallucis brevis and lie on either side of the crista. Medially and laterally, the collateral ligaments stabilize the metatarsophalangeal joint, and toward the plantar surface, they blend with the adductor and abductor hallucis tendons along the lateral and medial sides of the joint. Further toward the plantar surface, the sesamoids are stabilized by the firm attachment of the encapsulating plantar aponeurosis, which inserts into the base of the proximal phalanx. Plantar to the sesamoids passes the flexor hallucis longus tendon. Dorsally, the extensor hallucis longus tendon is stabilized by a medial and lateral hood mechanism similar to that present in the hand, and the extensor digitorum brevis muscle inserts into the proximal phalanx along the lateral aspect of the joint. Normal motion of the metatarsophalangeal joint consists of dorsiflexion and plantar flexion.

Hallux Valgus

The most common deformity of the metatarsophalangeal joint is hallux valgus or the so-called bunion deformity, which results from the lateral deviation of the proximal phalanx and the resultant medially directed pressure exerted against the metatarsal head. The medial eminence becomes prominent as the proximal phalanx drifts into a valgus position. Attenuation of the medial joint capsule and contracture of the lateral joint capsule occur. As the metatarsal head is pushed medially, the sesamoids, which are firmly anchored by the adductor hallucis tendon and transverse metatarsal ligament, slowly erode the crista. Eventually the sesamoids subluxate from underneath the first metatarsal, with the fibular sesamoid lying in the first web space. The extensor hallucis longus and flexor hallucis longus, which insert into the base of the distal phalanx, also deviate in a lateralward direction and contribute to the progressive hallux valgus deformity. As the deformity becomes more severe, both the extrinsic and intrinsic muscles lie lateral to the longitudinal axis of the first metatarsophalangeal joint, thereby further enhancing the deformity. As the deformity progresses, pronation of the great toe occurs. Attenuation of the weakest portion of the capsule (the dorsomedial aspect) allows the abductor hallucis tendon to slide beneath the metatarsal head and rotate the proximal phalanx into a position of pronation. More rapid progression of the deformity may occur in a small percentage of patients whose first metatarsocuneiform joint demonstrates a significant degree of instability.

Etiology of Hallux Valgus Deformity

Hallux valgus deformity occurs in women approximately 10 times more frequently than in men. The incidence is also significantly higher in persons who wear shoes than in those who do not. The conclusion can therefore be made that a major contributing cause of hallux valgus deformity is wearing tight pointed-toed shoes that women often wear. Other factors that may contribute to hallux valgus are congenital deformity or predisposition, severe flatfoot deformity, chronic tightness of the Achilles tendon, spasticity, hypermobility of the first metatarsocuneiform joint, and systemic disease such as rheumatoid arthritis (RA).

Clinical Findings

A. History

The clinical evaluation of hallux valgus deformity begins with a careful history to obtain the chief complaint, which may be primarily medial eminence pain, plantar first metatarsal or lesser metatarsal head pain, impingement upon the second toe, resultant deformities of the lesser toes, or the inability to wear certain shoes. The examiner should ask about factors that seem to aggravate the discomfort, the patient's occupation and level of athletic endeavors, and what type of shoe is most commonly worn.

B. Physical Examination

The physical examination starts with the patient in a standing position to observe the degree of deformity of the great toe and lesser toes. The overall posture of the foot is noted. The patient's gait is observed, looking for evidence of abnormal ground contact or early heel rise, which would indicate possible tightness of the Achilles tendon. In the seated position, the ROM of the ankle, subtalar, transverse tarsal, and metatarsophalangeal joints is noted. The neurovascular status of the foot is carefully assessed, noting venous stasis changes. Doppler studies are obtained if there is any question regarding the circulatory status of the foot. The plantar aspect of the foot is examined for abnormal callus formation, particularly beneath the metatarsal head and along the medial aspect of the great toe.

The motion of the first metatarsophalangeal joint is carefully observed in its deformed position and after the toe is carefully brought back toward normal alignment. Restriction of motion gives the clinician insight into the degree of surgical correction that can be obtained at the joint without impairing motion of the joint. The first metatarsocuneiform joint is examined for hypermobility by moving it in a dorsomedial and plantolateral direction.

C. Imaging Studies

The radiographic evaluation consists of weight-bearing anteroposterior, lateral, and oblique radiographs. From these radiographs, the following measurements are made:

1. The hallux valgus angle is the angle created by the intersection of the lines that longitudinally bisect the proximal phalanx and first metatarsal. A normal angle is less than 15 degrees (Figure 9–6A).
2. The intermetatarsal angle is defined as the angle created by the intersection of the lines bisecting the first and second metatarsal shafts. This angle should be less than 9 degrees.
3. The distal metatarsal articular angle measures the relationship of the distal articulating surface of the first metatarsal to the long axis of the metatarsal. Normally there is less than 10 degrees of lateral deviation (Figure 9–6B).
4. A determination is made as to whether or not the first metatarsophalangeal joint is congruent or incongruent. A congruent joint is one in which no lateral subluxation of the proximal phalanx occurs on the metatarsal head; an incongruent joint is one in which lateral subluxation of the proximal phalanx on the metatarsal head does occur (Figure 9–7).
5. The shape of the metatarsocuneiform joint is observed, looking for evidence of excessive medial deviation of this articulation. This observation alerts the examiner to the fact that hypermobility may be present.
6. The presence of arthrosis of the metatarsophalangeal joint is evaluated, as characterized by narrowing or osteophyte formation about the joint.
7 The size of the medial eminence is measured by a line drawn down the medial aspect of the first metatarsal shaft.
8. The presence of a hallux valgus interphalangeus is characterized by lateral deviation of the proximal or distal phalanx, or both, in relation to a line drawn across the base of the proximal phalanx. Normal is considered up to approximately 10 degrees of lateral deviation.

Treatment

A. Nonoperative Treatment

The patient should be encouraged to wear shoes of adequate size and shape. This simple form of management may relieve most symptoms.

A variety of pads are available to address symptoms that occur because of the bunion deformity. Pads may be placed in the first web space or over the median eminence to help take pressure off a painful median eminence. Pads are also available that can be placed underneath the metatarsal heads to take pressure off painful calluses or sesamoids.

If after adequate conservative management the patient continues to have discomfort, surgical intervention may be considered. Surgery is not performed for cosmetic reasons or to allow patients to wear fashionable shoes, but rather to correct a symptomatic structural deformity.

Juvenile hallux valgus deformity presents a significant problem in management, but as a general rule, conservative management should be continued until

A

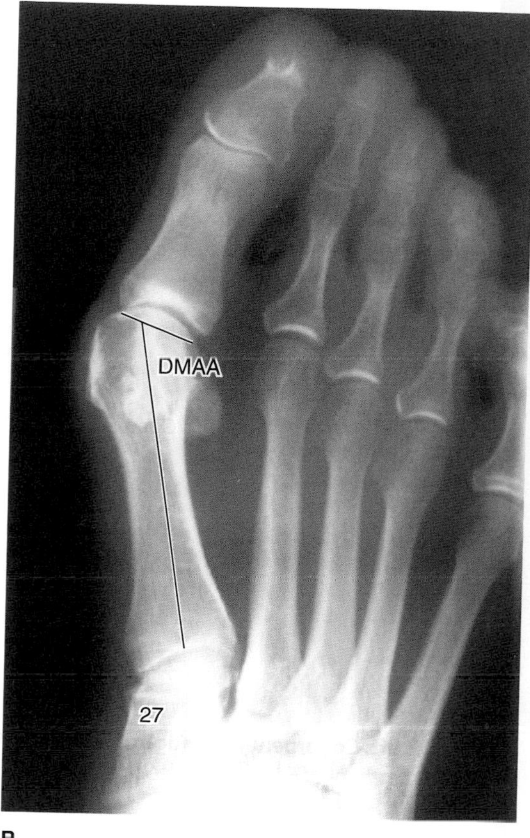

B

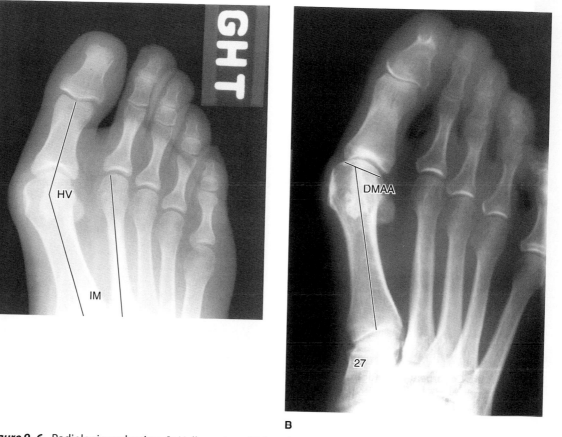

Figure 9–6. Radiologic evaluation. **A:** Hallux valgus (HV) and intermetatarsal (IM) angles. **B:** Distal metatarsal articular angle (DMAA = 27). (Reproduced, with permission, from Mann RA, Coughlin MJ: *The Video Textbook of Foot and Ankle Surgery*. Medical Video Productions, 1991.)

growth is completed, after which surgery may be considered. Extra care must be taken into consideration in the juvenile population where cosmetic appearance may play a greater role in the patient's or parents' desire for surgery.

Hallux valgus surgery is generally contraindicated in high-performance athletes or dancers until they are no longer able to perform at the level necessary to continue in their vocation or avocation. Premature surgery in these individuals may diminish their special abilities.

B. Surgical Treatment

1. Algorithm for surgical treatment—If surgery is being considered, the patient's chief complaint, the physical findings, and the radiographic measurements must be correlated to enable the surgeon to select the best procedure. No single procedure succeeds for all hallux valgus deformities, and careful preoperative planning is essential.

The following factors need to be considered in the decision-making process:

1. patient's chief complaint;
2. physical findings;
3. degree of hallux valgus and intermetatarsal angle;
4. distal metatarsal articular angle;
5. congruency or incongruency of the metatarsophalangeal joint;
6. presence of arthrosis of the joint;
7. degree of pronation of the hallux;
8. age of the patient;
9. circulatory status; and
10. patient expectations for outcome of operation.

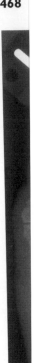

made over the dorsal aspect of the distal interphalangeal joint. Along with the ellipse of skin, the extensor tendon is excised, the collateral ligaments released, and the distal portion of the middle phalanx removed. The distal phalanx is reduced and held in place either with a 0.045-in. K-wire for 4 weeks or with Telfa bolsters (Figure 9–14).

Good results may be expected following this procedure. The most common complication occurs because a contracture of the flexor digitorum longus tendon was not appreciated prior to surgery or because insufficient bone was removed from the middle phalanx to decompress the deformity adequately.

2. Hammer Toe Deformity

A hammer toe deformity is a plantar flexion deformity of the proximal interphalangeal joint, which may either be fixed or flexible. It is frequently associated with varying degrees of hyperextension of the metatarsophalangeal joint. A flexion deformity of the distal interphalangeal joint usually accompanies a hammer toe, but an extension deformity is occasionally observed.

Clinical Findings

A. Symptoms and Signs

Clinical evaluation is similar to that of a mallet toe deformity, with care taken to distinguish between a fixed or flexible deformity. Also, the metatarsophalangeal joints of each toe are evaluated for hyperextension deformities. Callus formation or even an ulcer may be present over the extensor surface of the proximal interphalangeal joint. Metatarsophalangeal joint correction may be necessary to alleviate the hammer toe. Similarly, a significant hallux valgus deformity that is impinging on the second toe may require treatment to make room for correction of the hammer toe.

B. Imaging Studies

Radiographs help in the evaluation of proximal interphalangeal flexion deformity, hyperextension deformity at the metatarsophalangeal joint, and hallux valgus deformity. It is critical that all joints be assessed when hammer toe correction is being considered.

Treatment

A. Conservative Management

The conservative management of hammer toe deformities is foremost that of proper shoe wear, as previously emphasized. In addition, toe sleeves are available that pad the painful callus.

Conservative management becomes more difficult if a significant fixed deformity is present, particularly if it is associated with extension of the metatarsophalangeal joint or a significant hallux valgus deformity.

B. Surgical Treatment

Surgical decision making regarding the hammer toe hinges on whether (1) the deformity is fixed or flexible, (2) any deformity of the metatarsophalangeal joint needs to be corrected concomitantly, and (3) a space must be created for the toe by correcting the hallux valgus deformity.

1. Flexible hammer toe deformity—A flexible hammer toe deformity is corrected with the Girdlestone flexor tendon transfer. In this procedure, the long flexor tendon is harvested from the plantar aspect of the foot, brought up on either side of the extensor hood mechanism, and sutured into the extensor hood with the toe held in approximately 5 degrees of plantar flexion and the ankle in plantar flexion (Figure 9–15). This causes the long flexor tendon to act as an extensor of the interphalangeal joints and a flexor of the metatarsophalangeal joint, thereby correcting the deformity. A soft

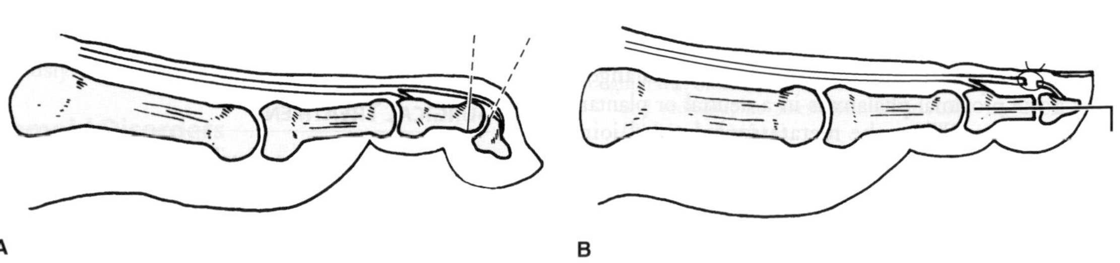

Figure 9–14. Mallet toe repair. **A:** Resection of condyles of the middle phalanx. **B:** Intramedullary K-wire fixation. (Reproduced, with permission, from Mann RA, Coughlin MJ: *The Video Textbook of Foot and Ankle Surgery*. Medical Video Productions, 1991.)

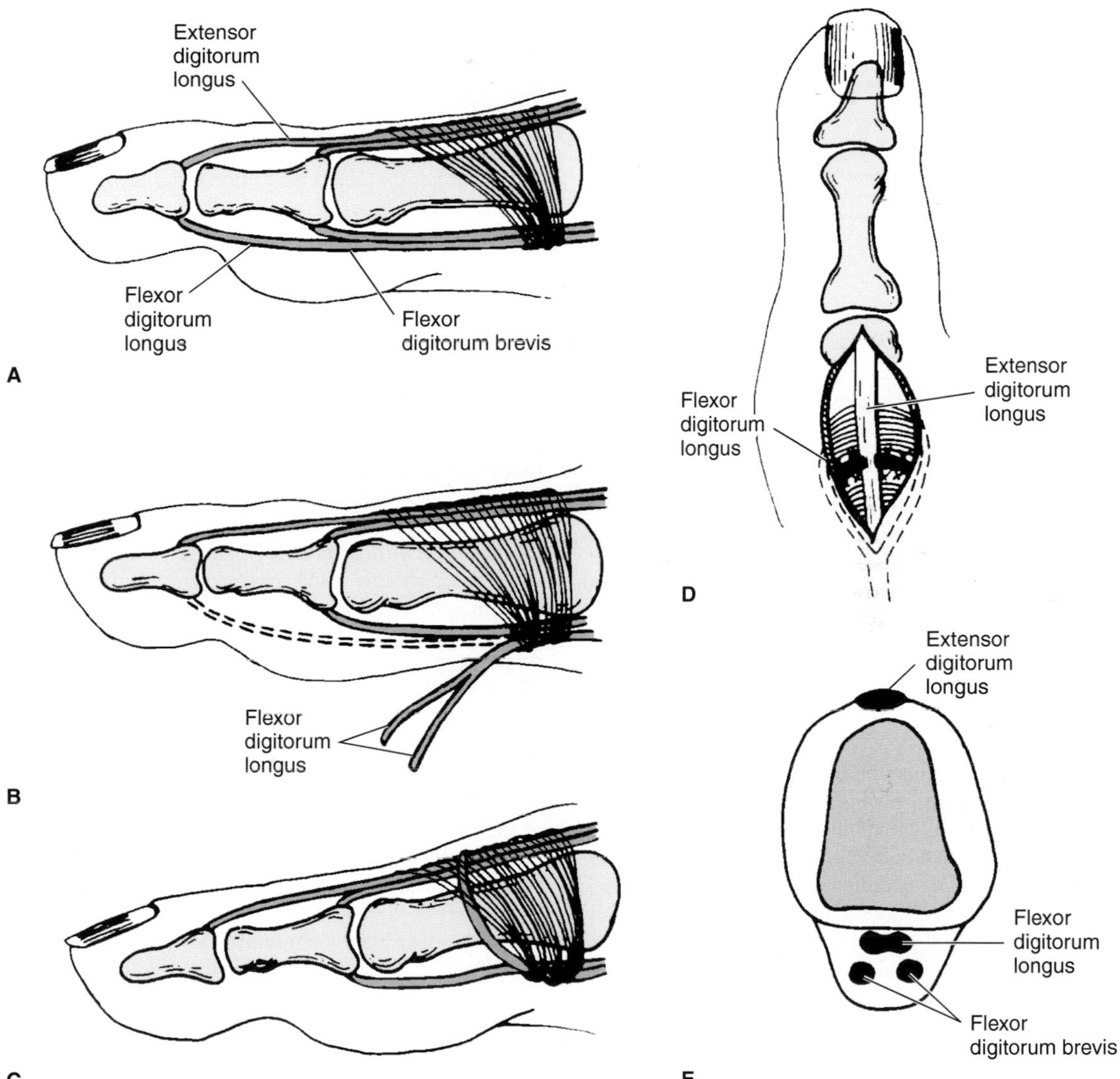

Figure 9–15. Flexor tendon transfer for flexible hammer toe deformity. **A:** Lateral view of lesser toe. **B:** The long flexor is detached from its insertion and delivered through the proximal plantar wound. It is split longitudinally along the median raphe. **C:** Each limb is transferred dorsally on either side of the proximal phalanx and secured on the dorsal aspect. **D:** Dorsal view after tendon transfer. **E:** Cross section showing flexor digitorum longus tendon in sheath. (Reproduced, with permission, from Mann RA, Coughlin MJ: *The Video Textbook of Foot and Ankle Surgery.* Medical Video Productions, 1991.)

dressing is applied and a postoperative shoe is worn for 4 weeks, after which ambulation is allowed.

2. Fixed hammer toe deformity—The DuVries proximal phalangeal condylectomy is used for the fixed deformity. This procedure, which is identical to that described for treatment of the mallet toe deformity, involves the proximal interphalangeal joint instead of the distal interphalangeal joint (Figure 9–16). Clinical results show a majority of patients were satisfied and a low risk of recurrence of deformity.

3. Complications—The main complication observed with either procedure is inadequate correction of the deformity, usually because of failure to appreciate a contracture of the flexor digitorum longus tendon at the time of surgery.

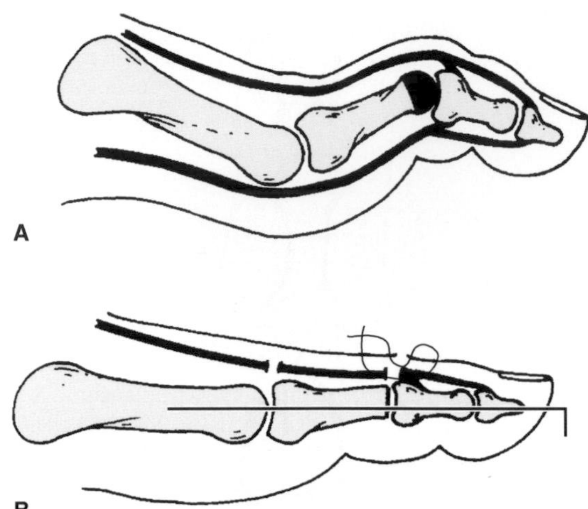

Figure 9–16. Fixed hammer toe repair. **A:** Resection of the head of the proximal phalanx. **B:** Intramedullary K-wire fixation. (Reproduced, with permission, from Mann RA, Coughlin MJ: *The Video Textbook of Foot and Ankle Surgery*. Medical Video Productions, 1991.)

3. Clawtoe Deformity

Clawtoe deformity involves both the metatarsophalangeal and interphalangeal joints and may be flexible or fixed. Clawtoe deformity can be disabling, particularly in the patient with a neuromuscular disorder. This deformity is characterized by marked dorsiflexion of the metatarsophalangeal joint, which results in pain secondary to chafing over the interphalangeal joints against the shoe and pain beneath the metatarsal heads because the metatarsal heads are forced into plantar flexion. In contrast to hammer toe or mallet toe deformities, which usually involve a single toe, clawtoe deformity usually involves all of the lesser toes. An associated deformity of the great toe may occur as well.

Clinical Findings

A. Symptoms and Signs

The clinical evaluation is similar to that described for the previous lesser toe deformities. The metatarsal heads are palpated because the fat pad may be displaced distally and the skin beneath the metatarsal heads may be atrophic. Callosities may be present on the extensor surface of the proximal interphalangeal joints and on the plantar aspect of the metatarsophalangeal joints.

B. Imaging Studies

Radiographs demonstrate the deformity, which is present at the metatarsophalangeal and interphalangeal joints. The posture of the entire foot needs to be evaluated, looking for the presence of a cavus-type foot deformity, characterized by increased dorsiflexion pitch of the calcaneus and increased plantar flexion of the first metatarsal.

Treatment

A. Conservative Management

An extra-depth shoe reduces the pressure on the lesser toes, and arch supports placed under the metatarsal head area may relieve the pain. Flexible mild deformities can be treated with shoe inserts placed immediately proximal to the metatarsophalangeal joints. These can have the effect of balancing the extensors and flexors of the toes.

B. Surgical Treatment

The type of operative intervention depends upon the nature of the deformity. Flexible deformities can be treated with the Girdlestone flexor tendon transfer. In addition, however, the extensor tendons usually must be lengthened to permit correction of the metatarsophalangeal joints to neutral plantar flexion.

A concomitant fixed contracture of the proximal interphalangeal joint requires a DuVries proximal phalangeal condylectomy as well as the Girdlestone tendon transfer procedure. Furthermore, release of the dorsal capsule, collateral ligaments, and extensor tendon is performed at the metatarsophalangeal joint. Postoperative management for the patient with clawtoe deformity is the same as discussed earlier for hammer toe deformity.

Following this surgical procedure no active motion of the toes occurs. The toes are usually well aligned in a plantigrade position. The marked deformity of the proximal interphalangeal joints is relieved so they no longer strike the top of the shoe. The main problems that can occur after surgery are (1) failure to correct a fixed hammer toe deformity adequately by use of the tendon transfer and (2) failure to release the fixed deformity adequately at the metatarsophalangeal joint, resulting in recurrence of the deformity.

4. Hard Corn & Soft Corn (Clavus Durum & Clavus Mollum)

A corn is a keratotic lesion that forms over a bony prominence on the lesser toes because of excessive pressure on the skin. A hard corn occurs most commonly over the dorsal and lateral aspect of the fifth toe, usually over the lateral condyle of the proximal phalanx. A soft corn represents a keratotic lesion in a web space and is so named because maceration results from moisture between the toes. The soft corn may occur anywhere along the toe where a bony excrescence is present and frequently occurs in the fourth web space between the base of the proximal phalanx of the fourth toe and the medial condyle of the head of the proximal phalanx of the fifth toe. At times, an ulceration may occur because of the extent of the maceration.

Treatment

A. Conservative Management

The main objective of conservative management is reducing pressure on the bony prominences. Footwear with a large toe box can relieve this pressure. Debridement or shaving of the lesion reduces pain. The procedure can frequently be carried out by younger patients without assistance but becomes increasingly difficult in older individuals because of decreasing flexibility and poor eyesight. Skin compromise, especially in the diabetic patient, must be avoided. At times, soft pads or lamb's wool can be placed around the toe to minimize pressure on the involved area, but the patient must wear a shoe with an adequate toe box to accommodate such modalities.

B. Surgical Treatment

1. Surgical treatment of the hard corn—The hard corn, over the fifth toe, is managed surgically by removing the distal portion of the proximal phalanx and occasionally the dorsolateral aspect of the proximal portion of the middle phalanx. The longitudinal incision is made over the dorsal aspect so the scar will not chafe against the shoe. The extensor tendon is split, the collateral ligaments cut, and the condyle exposed. With a bone cutter, the distal portion of the proximal phalanx is generously removed and the edges smoothed with a rongeur. Following closure, a compression dressing is applied for several days. The toe is taped to the adjacent fourth toe for 8 weeks. Long-term results show a high level of patient satisfaction and a low recurrence rate. Removal of excessive bone is the major complication, which causes the small toe to become too floppy, creating a nuisance for the patient.

2. Surgical treatment for the soft corn—Soft corns are treated surgically by making an incision over the lesion and using a small rongeur to remove the underlying bony excrescence. This is a simple procedure and almost invariably results in satisfactory resolution of the problem.

3. Syndactyly—Because the soft corn is caused by pressure on the skin, removal of the skin between the toes can resolve the problem. Syndactyly is a procedure by which the skin is removed between the fourth and fifth toes and the two toes are sutured together to eliminate the problem of a soft corn in the web space. Although the soft corn can usually be managed with a condylectomy, as described earlier, occasionally a great deal of maceration or ulceration precludes treating it only with a condylectomy. In these cases, syndactyly is indicated. Occasionally, a floppy fifth toe from previous surgery can be stabilized by syndactyly.

5. Subluxation & Dislocation of the Metatarsophalangeal Joint

Dorsal subluxation or dislocation of the metatarsophalangeal joint occurs because of weakening of the supporting plantar capsule and collateral ligament structures, which maintain the stability of the metatarsophalangeal joint. Secondary changes such as hammer toe may occur in the toe itself. Pain usually occurs either beneath the metatarsophalangeal joint or over the dorsal aspect of the toe as it strikes the top of the shoe.

Etiologic Findings

The most common cause of a subluxed or dislocated joint is probably a progressive hallux valgus deformity pressing against the second toe. Over time, subluxation and eventual dislocation of the second metatarsophalangeal joint can occur.

A nonspecific synovitis, isolated to the metatarsophalangeal joint and usually involving the second metatarsophalangeal joint, is the next most common cause. The clinical picture is one of generalized swelling about the metatarsophalangeal joint that subsides over a period of 3–6 months, followed by progressive subluxation and eventual dislocation of the joint. Occasionally, subluxation or dislocation of the metatarsophalangeal joint may result from trauma.

Arthritic conditions such as rheumatoid or psoriatic arthritis can cause subluxation or dislocation at multiple joints. Advanced neuromuscular disorders may cause severe subluxation of the metatarsophalangeal joint, but dislocation is unusual.

A variant of this condition results from attenuation of collateral ligaments on one side of the metatarsophalangeal joint. The cause may be idiopathic but occasionally may follow a steroid injection into the area. The metatarsophalangeal joint, instead of subluxing in a dorsalward direction, deviates medially or occasionally laterally, crossing over the adjacent toe. This again is most common in the second metatarsophalangeal joint. When the toe deviates in a medialward direction and crosses over the great toe, the patient may have difficulty wearing shoes.

Clinical Findings

A. Symptoms and Signs

Patients complain of pain on the dorsal and plantar aspects of the affected joint. They may note swelling as well and complain of an associated hammer toe or lateral deviation of the toe if present. The degree of deformity is evaluated with the patient in a standing and sitting position. The affected metatarsophalangeal joint is palpated for active synovitis, flexibility of the joint, and degree of subluxation.

The dorsal-plantar stability of the joint is evaluated by holding the proximal phalanx between the examiner's fingers and moving it dorsally and plantarward, similar to a Lachman test of the knee. If a significant hallux valgus deformity is associated with crossover of the second toe on the first toe, the hallux valgus requires evaluation.

B. IMAGING STUDIES

The radiographs of the foot reveal the extent of the subluxation or dislocation. The severity of the hallux valgus is evaluated, and changes about the articular surface of the joint are observed. In RA, multiple joint involvement is noted.

Treatment

A. CONSERVATIVE MANAGEMENT

Conservative management consists of using a shoe with a wide enough toe box to accommodate the deformity and prescribing a well-molded, soft orthotic device to relieve pressure on the metatarsal head. Unfortunately, this may raise the forefoot, causing impingement on the toe box area of the shoe and some discomfort. A series of cortisone injections into the affected joint may be performed. No more than three injections are given, and at least 1 month is allowed between injections. If the patient cannot be accommodated adequately with these modalities, surgical intervention may be indicated. A significant hallux valgus deformity indicates the need for correction to make a space for second toe correction. Failure to treat both problems results in recurrence.

B. SURGICAL TREATMENT

The subluxed metatarsophalangeal joint with a flexible hammer toe is treated by releasing the dorsal contracture of the extensor tendons and joint capsule, followed by a Girdlestone flexor tendon transfer, as previously described. This technique usually brings the toe into better alignment, although the patient loses some selective voluntary control of the toe, which is usually not of any significance. If a fixed hammer toe is present, a proximal phalanx condylectomy is added to the procedure.

The more severe complete dorsal dislocation of the metatarsophalangeal joint is a difficult surgical problem. In the past it was treated by an aggressive release of the dorsal joint capsule and collateral ligaments and a synovectomy of the metatarsophalangeal joint. The distal third of the metatarsal head is removed to decompress the joint. Accompanying hammer toe procedures are performed to correct the invariably present fixed hammer toe.

A longitudinal K-wire stabilizes the correction for 2 weeks. After pin removal, motion is started at the metatarsophalangeal joint. This procedure results in significant joint stiffness and possible resubluxation of the joint.

An osteotomy of the metatarsal neck is now used to treat dislocated or advanced subluxation of the metatarsophalangeal joint. An oblique osteotomy is performed, starting at the metatarsal neck and aimed proximally at a shallow angle to the metatarsal shaft, creating a long osteotomy site. Once the osteotomy is complete, the metatarsal head is allowed to slide proximally to the appropriate level that will allow the joint to assume a reduced position. The amount of shortening is usually between 4.0 mm and 6.0 mm. The osteotomy is fixed with a single 2.5-mm or smaller diameter cortical screw. Accompanying hammer toe procedures are then performed if necessary. Good short-term results are noted with this procedure without the complication of joint stiffness as occurs with the previously described procedures. Common complications include plantar penetrating hardware and floating-toe deformity (extension contracture of the metatarsophalangeal joint causing the toe not to touch the ground).

Repair of the medially or laterally dislocated metatarsophalangeal joint can be a technically difficult problem. Satisfactory correction can be achieved with one of two techniques. A soft-tissue release of the joint capsule can be performed on the side to which the toe deviates, allowing realignment of the toe. Alternatively, a closing-wedge osteotomy at the base of the proximal phalanx can also achieve good realignment of the toe. Severe deformities can be corrected with an oblique metatarsal neck osteotomy, previously described for treatment of dorsally subluxated metatarsophalangeal joints. The technique is identical, although some soft-tissue balancing may need to be added to the procedure.

Coughlin MJ: Lesser toe abnormalities. Instr Course Lect 2003; 52:421. [PMID: 12690869]

Coughlin MJ, Kennedy MP: Operative repair of fourth and fifth toe corns. Foot Ankle Int 2003;24:147. [PMID: 12627623]

Dhukaram V, Hossain S, Sampath J et al: Correction of hammer toe with an extended release of the metatarsophalangeal joint. J Bone Joint Surg Br 2003;84:986. [PMID: 12358391]

Migues A, Slullitel G, Bilbao F et al: Floating-toe deformity as a complication of the Weil osteotomy. Foot Ankle Int 2004; 25:609. [PMID: 15563380]

Trnka HJ, Gebhard C, Muhlbauer M et al: The Weil osteotomy for treatment of dislocated lesser metatarsophalangeal joints: Good outcome in 21 patients with 42 osteotomies. Acta Orthop Scand 2002;73:190. [PMID: 12079018]

REGIONAL ANESTHESIA FOR FOOT & ANKLE DISORDERS

Regional anesthesia is becoming more commonly used because many foot and ankle procedures are performed in the outpatient setting. Most procedures below the ankle can be performed without general anesthesia, eliminating the hazards of central nervous system depression. Pain develops gradually as the anesthesia wears off, and the analgesic requirements of the patient are thereby reduced significantly. Efficacy, safety, and high patient satisfaction are demonstrated.

Digital Block

A. INDICATIONS

Digital block is suitable for procedures used in the toes, such as treatment of nail disorders, correction of hammer toe or mallet toe, tendon releases, and some metatarsophalangeal joint procedures.

B. Technique

Short- and longer-term anesthesia is provided by digital block using a 1:1 mixture of 1% lidocaine hydrochloride and 0.25% bupivacaine. A short 25-gauge needle is used to inject approximately 1.5 mL on either side of the toe within the subcutaneous layer between the skin and deeper fascia. The needle is then passed toward the plantar aspect of the toe to anesthetize the digital nerves. Both sides of the toe should be anesthetized. Anesthesia should be administered before the operative site is prepared to allow approximately 15 minutes necessary for the block to take effect before starting a procedure.

Ankle Block

A. Indications

Ankle block anesthesia is commonly used for operations on the forefoot and midfoot, such as bunion procedures, neuroma excision, metatarsal osteotomies, and tarsometatarsal fusions. If more than one lesser toe procedure is being performed, an ankle block is preferred to multiple digital blocks. Ankle block anesthesia is not recommended for hindfoot or ankle procedures, such as hindfoot fusions or ankle arthroscopy.

B. Technique

The successful ankle block must anesthetize the posterior tibial nerve, superficial branch of the deep peroneal nerve, sural nerve, saphenous nerve, and superficial peroneal nerve. The posterior tibial nerve requires a larger 3-cm, 22- or 25-gauge needle and approximately 7–10 mL of a 1:1 mixture of 1% lidocaine hydrochloride and 0.25% bupivacaine. The landmark for the posterior tibial nerve behind the malleolus is approximately two finger breadths proximal to the tip of the malleolus and along the medial border of the Achilles tendon (Figure 9–17). The needle is inserted perpendicular to the shaft of the tibia until the posterior cortex of the tibia is palpated with the tip of the needle. The needle is then withdrawn approximately 2 mm. Approximately 5 mL of anesthetic agent is injected into this area after aspiration is done to confirm that the needle is not in a vessel.

To anesthetize the deep peroneal nerve, the site of the injection is located by palpating the extensor hallucis and extensor digitorum longus tendons at the level of the navicular. The deep peroneal nerve lies just lateral to the dorsalis pedis artery. The 25-gauge needle is inserted and advanced to bone and then withdrawn 1–2 mm, aspiration is attempted, and approximately 5 mL of anesthetic is injected.

The saphenous nerve is identified one to two finger breadths proximal to the tip of the medial malleolus and just posterior to the saphenous vein. A 25-gauge needle is inserted and 5 mL of anesthetic injected.

The sural nerve is blocked approximately 1–1.5 cm distal to the tip of the lateral malleolus and can often be palpated in the subcutaneous fat. A 25-gauge needle is inserted and approximately 5 mL of anesthetic injected.

The superficial peroneal nerve branches are blocked starting two finger breadths proximal and anterior to the tip of the lateral malleolus, and the injection is carried out below the subcutaneous veins but above the long extensor tendons in a ring-type block. Approximately 5 mL of anesthetic agent is used. The anesthesia for ankle block takes effect within 15–20 minutes.

Popliteal Block

A. Indications

The popliteal block is used for major foot or ankle procedures. These include ankle arthrodesis, hindfoot arthrodesis, calcaneal osteotomy, tarsometatarsal arthrodesis, posterior tibial tendon reconstruction, and surgical treatment of calcaneal or ankle fractures. The popliteal block can be placed by the anesthesiologist or surgeon, and it can be used with general anesthesia, sedation, or as the sole anesthetic technique.

B. Technique

The patient is placed in the lateral decubitus position with a pillow between the knees. The landmarks of the popliteal fossa are identified, using the horizontal popliteal skin crease that divides the fossa into superior and inferior quadrants (Figure 9–18). Approximately 7–8 cm superior to the popliteal skin crease and 1 cm lateral to the midline is where the common peroneal branch separates from the tibial branch of the sciatic nerve. A nerve stimulator is set at 3 mA to assist in locating the nerve. When a twitch is found, the stimulator is decreased until there is loss of twitch at 0.8 to 1.0 mA (Figure 9–19). Following aspiration, 30 mL of 0.5% bupivacaine with 1:200,000 epinephrine are slowly injected. The saphenous nerve can be infiltrated with 3–5 mL of 0.5% bupivacaine proximal to the ankle.

Delgado-Martinez AD, Marchal-Escalona JM: Supramalleolar ankle block anesthesia and ankle tourniquet for foot surgery. Foot Ankle Int 2001;22:836. [PMID: 11642537]

Jarrett GJ, Rongstad KM, Snyder M: Popliteal nerve block by surgeon in the lateral decubitus position. Foot Ankle Int 2004;25:37. [PMID: 14768963]

Provenzano DA, Viscusi ER, Adams SB Jr et al: Safety and efficacy of the popliteal fossa nerve block when utilized for foot and ankle surgery. Foot Ankle Int 2002;23:394. [PMID: 12043982]

METATARSALGIA

Metatarsalgia is a general term for pain arising from the metatarsal head region. The center of pressure during nor-

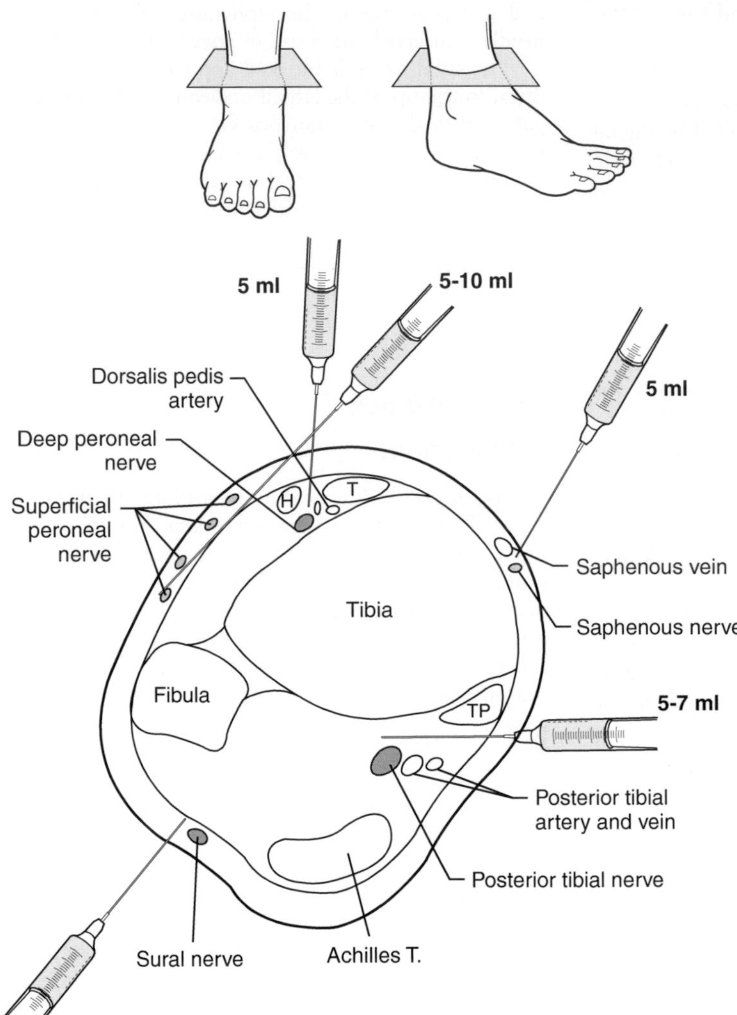

Figure 9–17. Anesthetic technique for ankle block. H: extensor hallucis longus tendon; T: tibialis anterior tendon; TP: tibialis posterior tendon. (Reproduced, with permission, from Delgado-Martinez AD, Marchal-Escalona JM: Supramalleolar ankle block anesthesia and ankle tourniquet for foot surgery. Foot Ankle Int 2001.)

mal gait is initially applied to the heel and progresses along the plantar aspect of the foot. For more than 50% of the stance time, the pressure is concentrated beneath the metatarsal head area. This extended period of pressure can cause bothersome pain. A precise diagnosis is necessary in metatarsalgia to direct treatment toward the specific cause.

Etiologic Findings

Metatarsalgia encompasses a broad spectrum of conditions with various causes arising out of the anatomic structures in the area. It may be associated with abnormalities of the metatarsal head subluxation or dislocation of the metatarsophalangeal joints, systemic diseases, dermatologic lesions, soft-tissue disorders, or iatrogenic causes. Table 9–1 lists the various causes of metatarsalgia and the differential diagnoses that should be considered in evaluating these patients.

Clinical Findings

A. Symptoms and Signs

The clinical evaluation begins with a careful history directed toward delineating the precise location of the pain. The physical examination of the foot and lower extremity begins with the patient standing. Any deformities of the toes are noted, such as clawing of the toes, a long second ray, or swelling around any of the joints. The patient should be evaluated for a postural problem of the foot, such as a flat foot or cavus foot. The plantar aspect of the foot is carefully evaluated for evidence of callus formation. The metatarsal heads are palpated individually to assess for generalized plantar fat pad atrophy, a prominent fibular condyle, synovitis, or possibly a transfer lesion beneath a metatarsal head resulting from previous forefoot surgery.

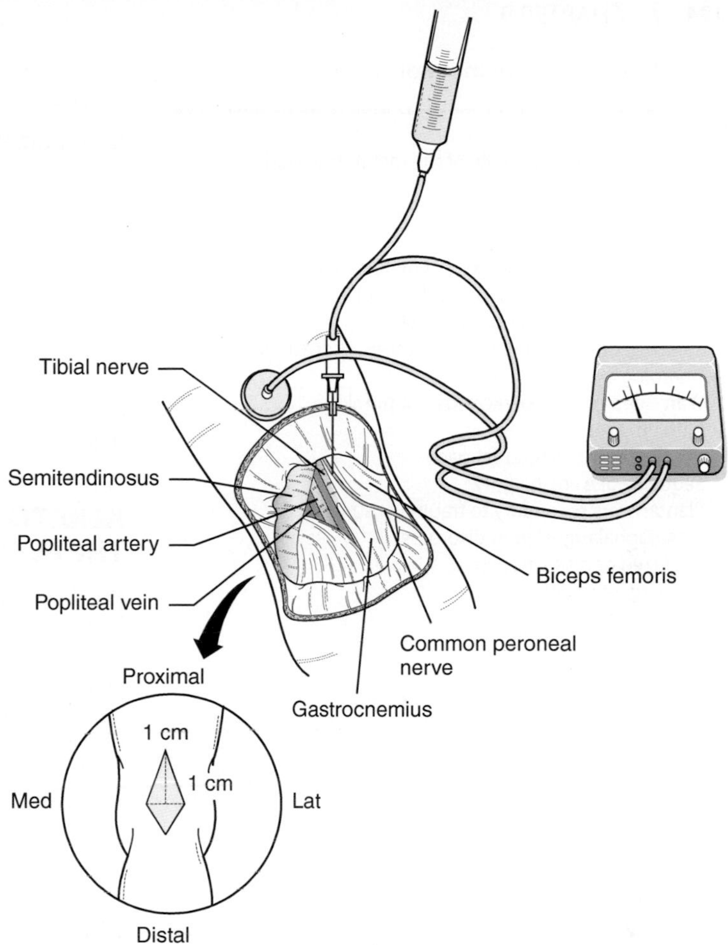

Figure 9–18. **Anesthetic technique. The popliteal block is performed with the needle tip inserted 7–8 cm above the popliteal crease and 1 cm lateral to the midline.** (Reproduced, with permission, from Rongstad KM, Mann RA, Prieskorn D et al: Popliteal sciatic nerve block for postoperative analgesia. Foot Ankle Int 1996.)

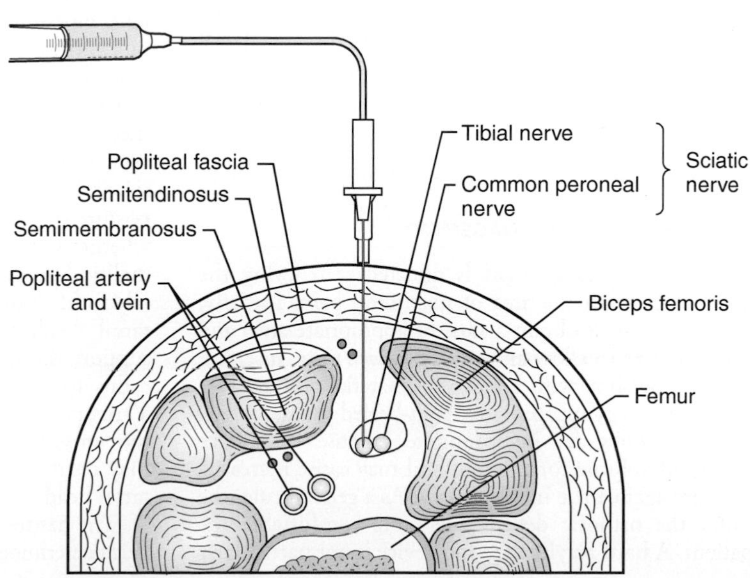

Figure 9–19. **Anesthetic technique for the popliteal block. The needle tip is positioned to localize the sciatic nerve, and aspiration ensures no vascular penetration.** (Reproduced, with permission, from Rongstad KM, Mann RA, Prieskorn D et al: Popliteal sciatic nerve block for postoperative analgesia. Foot Ankle Int 1996.)

Table 9–1. Causes of metatarsalgia.

Bone causes
Prominent fibular condyle of the metatarsal head
Long metatarsal
Morton foot
Hypermobile first ray
Posttraumatic malalignment of metatarsals
Abnormal foot posture such as forefoot varus or valgus, cavus foot, or equinus deformity
Systemic disease, rheumatoid arthritis, psoriatic arthritis
Dermatologic lesions
Wart, seed corn, hyperkeratosis of the skin
Soft tissue disorders
Atrophy of the plantar fat pad
Sequelae of a crush injury
Plantar scars secondary to trauma or surgery
Metatarsophalangeal joint disorders
Subluxed or dislocated joint
Freiberg infraction
Nonspecific synovitis
Iatrogenic causes
Residuals of metatarsal surgery
Transfer lesion due to previous surgery
Hallux valgus surgery (eg, shortening or dorsiflexion of the metatarsal)

B. Imaging Studies

The radiographic evaluation includes weight-bearing anteroposterior, lateral, and oblique views of the foot. Occasionally, the so-called skyline view of the metatarsal heads (obtained with the metatarsophalangeal joints in dorsiflexion) is helpful to evaluate their overall alignment, particularly in cases resulting from previous surgery, by demonstrating the height of the metatarsal heads. MRI can be useful in the diagnosis of metatarsalgia, such as distinguishing among a neuroma, cyst, bursa, or synovitis.

Treatment

A. Conservative Management

Conservative management is directed at relieving the pressure beneath the area of maximum pain. Initially, the patient must obtain a shoe of appropriate style and adequate size to allow an orthotic device to be inserted. A lace-type shoe with a soft sole material and an adequate toe box is appropriate. High-heeled shoes, loafers, or tight shoes are inappropriate because they have decreased volume for the foot and may cause increased pressure against the involved area. As a general rule, the softer the orthotic device, the more comfortable the patient. A hard acrylic orthotic device is not particularly comfortable for the patient and should usually be avoided.

B. Surgical Treatment

The surgical management of metatarsalgia depends on the cause and is discussed in different sections of this chapter. In general, pain from a bony prominence can be relieved by a partial ostectomy or osteotomy, dermatologic lesions such as warts can often be burned off with liquid nitrogen or excised, or pain caused by a subluxated metatarsophalangeal joint can be corrected with tendon transfer. The outcome depends on the severity of the problem and the type of surgical intervention required to correct it.

KERATOTIC DISORDERS OF THE PLANTAR SKIN

Friction and pressure over bony prominences, particularly on the plantar skin, can often result in callus formation. Modest callus formation is normal, but more extensive callus formation, particularly on the plantar aspect of the foot, may become symptomatic and occasionally quite disabling.

Etiologic Findings

Many of the intractable plantar keratoses arise from the bony abnormalities presented in Table 9–1.

Clinical Findings

A. Symptoms and Signs

A careful history of the problem is extremely important, especially if the patient has had multiple surgical procedures. The patient's activities, type of shoes that exacerbate or relieve the pain, how often the lesion needs to be trimmed, and the type of orthotic devices used are all important. The physical examination, however, is the most important single factor in the diagnosis of intractable plantar keratoses. First, the overall posture of the foot needs to be evaluated to determine whether the condition is the result of a postural abnormality. Specifically, a rigid plantar-flexed first metatarsal could cause a diffuse callus beneath the first metatarsal head, or a hypermobile first ray that fails to support the medial forefoot may result in generalized callus formation beneath the lesser metatarsal heads. Varus posture of the forefoot (the lateral aspect of the foot in greater plantar flexion than the medial aspect) may result in callus formation beneath the fifth metatarsal head.

The nature of the callus itself is important because it helps determine the cause of the problem. A well-localized lesion beneath the metatarsal head is often caused by a prominent fibular condyle on the second or third metatarsal. A diffuse callus is usually associated with a long metatarsal. The callus may have arisen after trauma or surgery in which an adjacent metatarsal was dorsiflexed, thereby increasing the weight-bearing load of the metatarsal. A callus on the bottom of the foot must be differentiated from a plantar wart, which can occasionally mimic a plantar callosity. Shaving the lesion reveals bleeding from end arteries in a plantar wart, whereas a keratotic lesion consists only of hyperkeratotic tissue.

B. Imaging Studies

Routine weight-bearing radiographs of the foot are performed and correlated with the clinical findings in evaluation of these patients.

Treatment

A. Conservative Management

A wide, soft lace-up shoe is recommended, often with the addition of a soft metatarsal support. The orthotic device usually consists of a soft pad (Figure 9–20). It is

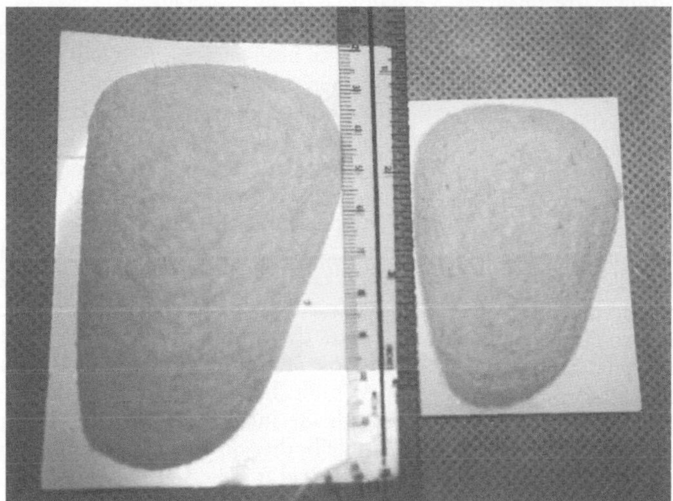

A

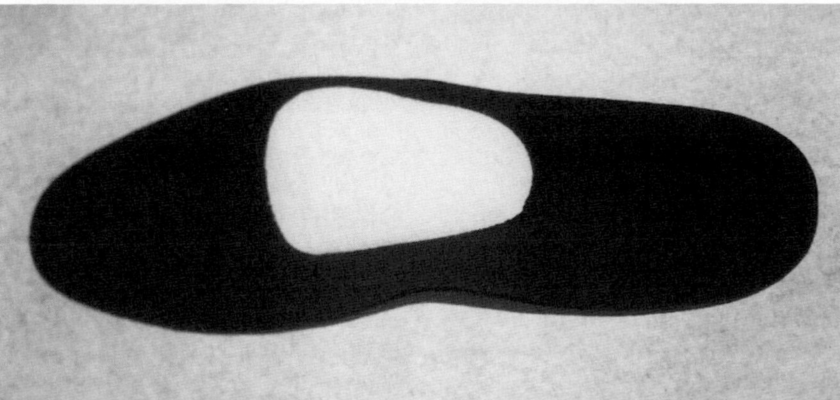

B

Figure 9–20. **A:** A metatarsal pad may help redistribute weight bearing and relieve symptoms. **B:** A soft insole may be added to help absorb pressure and allow transfer of the metatarsal pad from one shoe to another. (Reproduced, with permission, from Mann RA, Coughlin MJ: *The Video Textbook of Foot and Ankle Surgery*. Medical Video Productions, 1991.)

usually not necessary for an orthotic device to be fabricated early in the treatment of metatarsalgia because the less expensive, commercially available pads are sufficient in most cases.

B. Surgical Treatment

The surgical management of metatarsalgia depends on the cause of the condition. The following causes of intractable plantar keratoses may respond to surgical intervention.

Localized intractable plantar keratosis beneath a metatarsal head is usually caused by a prominent fibular condyle. It occurs most frequently underneath the second metatarsal but may also be found underneath the third and fourth metatarsals. Surgical treatment is accomplished through a dorsal hockey stick incision over the metatarsophalangeal joint. The toe is plantar flexed to allow removal of 30% of the plantar condyle of the metatarsal head, thereby removing the sharp bony prominence (Figure 9–21). This procedure results in predictable pain relief of the affected toe, although 5–10% of patients develop a transfer lesion beneath the adjacent metatarsal head.

A diffuse callus beneath the second metatarsal that is the result of a dorsiflexed or hypermobile first metatarsal can be treated with dorsiflexion osteotomy done at the base of the second metatarsal. If the lesion is the result of an excessively long metatarsal, it may be shortened to the level of a line drawn between the adjacent metatarsal heads, thereby reestablishing a smooth metatarsal pattern. If the callus is a result of a dislocated metatarsophalangeal joint, the joint must be surgically reduced, using one of the techniques previously described, to alleviate the chronic downward pressure against the metatarsal head. All of these surgical procedures to eliminate a callus are fairly successful, although the possibility of a transfer lesion developing is approximately 5–10%.

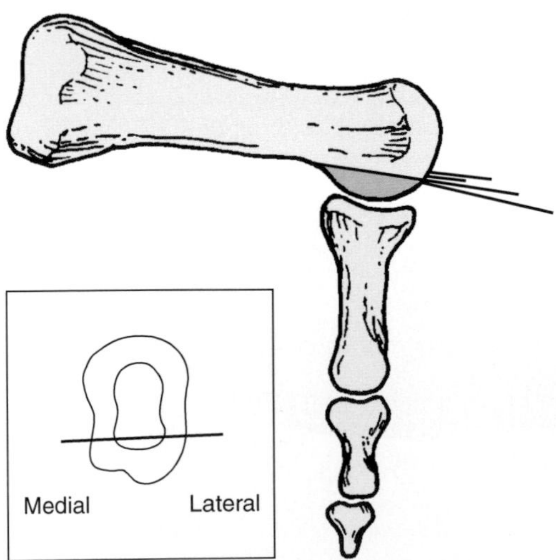

Figure 9–21. A plantar condylectomy is performed with resection of one fourth to one third of the plantar surface of the metatarsal head. (Reproduced, with permission, from Mann RA, Coughlin MJ: *The Video Textbook of Foot and Ankle Surgery*. Medical Video Productions, 1991.)

Occasionally, a well-localized callus is present beneath the tibial sesamoid, which can be treated surgically by shaving the plantar third of the sesamoid. This alleviates the callus in almost all cases, with the only significant complication being caused by inadvertent disruption of the plantar medial cutaneous nerve during the surgical approach to the sesamoid.

Bunionettes are caused by prominence of the fifth metatarsal head and may lead to metatarsalgia. A diffuse callus beneath the fifth metatarsal head can be treated with a midshaft metatarsal osteotomy to bring it out of its plantar-flexed position, which usually alleviates the condition. It is unusual for a transfer lesion to occur beneath the fourth metatarsal head.

At times, the fifth metatarsal head is too prominent on the lateral aspect of the foot rather than the plantar aspect. In these cases, a chevron osteotomy of the fifth metatarsal head, displacing it in a medialward direction, alleviates the condition (Figure 9–22), sometimes with slight loss of motion of the metatarsophalangeal joint.

A subhallux sesamoid can cause a small callus beneath the interphalangeal joint of the great toe and be quite bothersome to the patient. Surgical excision of the sesamoid is indicated, with good results and little or no disability.

Mann RA, DuVries HL: Intractable plantar keratosis. Orthop Clin North Am 1973;4:67.

Mann RA, Mann JA: Keratotic disorders of the plantar skin. AAOS Instr Course Lect 2004;53:287. [PMID: 15116622]

Yu JS, Tanner JR: Considerations in metatarsalgia and midfoot pain: An MR imaging perspective. Semin Musculoskelet Radiol 2002;6:91. [PMID: 12077699]

DIABETIC FOOT

Approximately 22 million people in the United States are diabetic, and foot problems are the most common cause for hospitalization, accounting for 20% of all inpatient days in this population. More than half of all nontraumatic amputations are performed on diabetics. One report showed a 68% incidence of foot disorders in a large diabetic clinic, and the cost of care of these problems approaches $100 million per year. Treatment of the diabetic, who presents with foot problems, can be complex and require a team approach, involving the primary care physician, vascular surgeon, orthopedic surgeon, infectious disease specialist, orthotist, diabetic

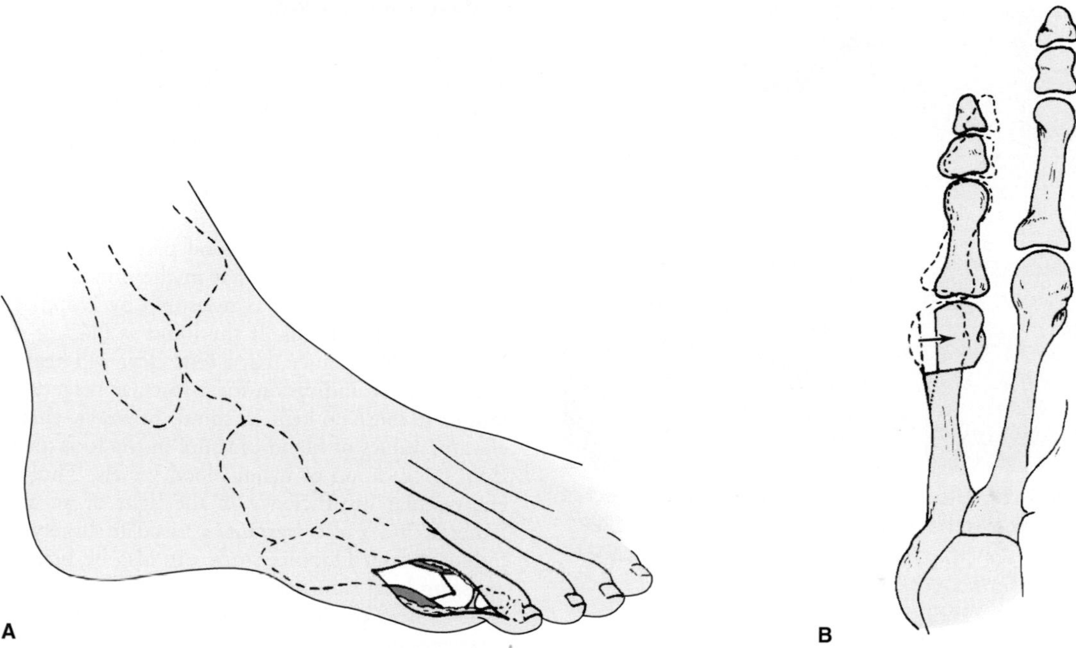

Figure 9–22. **A:** Lateral view of chevron fifth metatarsal osteotomy. **B:** Diagram following completion of this procedure. (Reproduced, with permission, from Mann RA, Coughlin MJ: *The Video Textbook of Foot and Ankle Surgery.* Medical Video Productions, 1991.)

nurse specialist, and, whenever possible, the patient's family members.

Pathophysiologic Findings

Diabetes is a metabolic disorder that involves all the organ systems. Those of primary interest to the orthopedist are integumentary with the risk of ulceration, neurological with the loss of protective sensation, vascular with diminished perfusion, and immunologic with limited ability to fight infection. The most frequent problem faced by the diabetic is breakdown of the skin of the foot (Figure 9–23). The cause of foot ulcers is multifactorial but stems from diminished sensation resulting from neuropathic disease. Unappreciated local stresses are placed on the skin externally by poorly fitting shoes and internally by skeletal deformity. Autonomic neuropathy causes dry skin and cracks in the dermis, which may become portals of entry for infection. Reactive hyperemia, which normally helps clear infections, is blunted by autonomic neuropathy. Motor neuropathy affects the intrinsic muscles of the foot and may lead to clawtoe deformities with metatarsal heads and proximal interphalangeal joints becoming prominent and predisposed to ulcerations. (Figure 9–24). Hyperglycemia can impair wound healing strength as well as damage vascular endothelium, which is a precursor to atherosclerosis and leads to diminished extremity blood flow and limited healing potential. Elevated blood glucose levels over a long period also leads to glycation of the body's proteins and is commonly measured by the hemoglobin A1c. Glucose covalently binds to lycine in proteins in a reversible process. It is believed that the addition of glucose molecules changes the flexibility of tissues, especially fibrous tissue, making tissues such as skin less able to handle shear stresses. The neuropathy in diabetics is caused by the loss of myelinated and unmyelinated nerve fibers. Other factors that affect healing in diabetics include nutritional deficiencies, diminished microcirculation, and lowered resistance to infection.

History

When a diabetic patient presents to an orthopedist, the four areas of impact are ulcers and their prevention, amputations, Charcot arthropathy, and toenail abnormalities. With an infected foot ulceration, it is essential to obtain a history that will help delineate why the ulcer occurred and how to optimize the patient's healing potential. A past history of foot surgery is sought, previous or current antibiotic usage is detailed, and any recent trauma to the foot is noted. A history is taken about the severity of the patient's diabetes, including

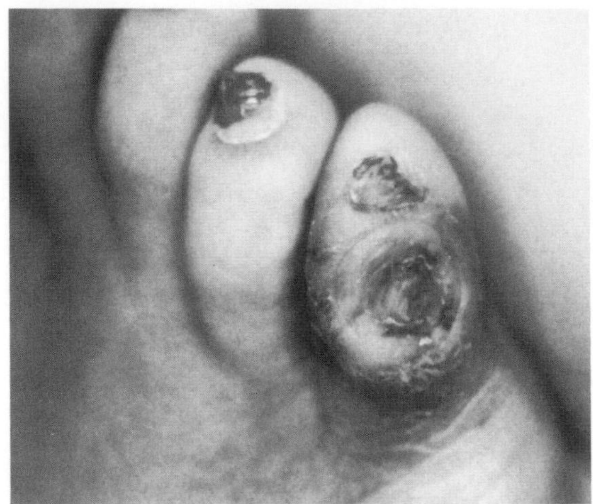

Figure 9–23. Ulceration over the dorsolateral aspect of the fifth toe as the result of pressure from a shoe. (Reproduced, with permission, from Mann RA, Coughlin MJ: *The Video Textbook of Foot and Ankle Surgery*. Medical Video Productions, 1991.)

how long ago the diabetes was diagnosed, whether the patient is taking insulin, the recent level of control, what other organ systems are involved, and the degree of neuropathy present in the patient's feet.

Clinical Findings

A. General Examination

Examination of the diabetic patient should begin with inspection of the shoe for internal and external wear patterns. The leg and foot are inspected for overall appearance of the skin, hair growth, perfusion, pulses, and color.

B. Foot Examination

Any bony prominences are recognized as areas of potential skin breakdown. The most common prominences are located at the apex of deformities. Neurologic examination should test for the presence of protective sensation, as defined by the patient's ability to feel the 10-g Semmes-Weinstein monofilament as well as motor function. Ulcers should be carefully documented and evaluated for evidence of infection in the adjacent soft tissues. Wounds should be measured for length, width, and depth as well as documenting their location. Open wounds should be probed with a sterile cotton swab or other appropriate instrument to evaluate the extent of involvement of deeper structures, such as tendons, joints, and bone. A positive probe-to-bone test usually indicates the presence of osteomyelitis.

C. Vascular Findings

Vascular evaluation is essential to ensure that the patient has adequate perfusion to allow healing. The patients with palpable pedal pulses and normal capillary filling have adequate blood supply and usually do not require further vascular evaluation. For those patients with less perfusion, one method of assessing the overall potential for healing of foot lesions is the ischemic index, obtained by dividing the blood pressure measurement in the brachial artery by that in the dorsalis pedis and posterior tibial arteries, as measured by Doppler ultrasound with a calf cuff. If the index is 0.45 or greater, there is a 90% chance that a foot ulcer will heal. Lower indexes are an indication for a vascular surgery consultation. It must be kept in mind, however, that falsely elevated values of blood pressure in the foot may result from calcification of major blood vessels. Thus, apparent vascular insufficiency in the light of an adequate ischemic index also warrants a vascular surgery consultation. A laser Doppler study can also be beneficial in assessing local skin perfusion. This information can be used to help predict the patient's response to surgical intervention.

D. Imaging Studies

Radiographic studies should include weight-bearing radiographs of both feet and ankles as indicated. Plain radiographs can help identify bony prominences that predispose the patient to ulcer formation, and osteomyelitis or changes consistent with a neuropathic foot may be identified. Early Charcot (neuropathic) joint changes may be difficult to differentiate from osteomyelitis. The

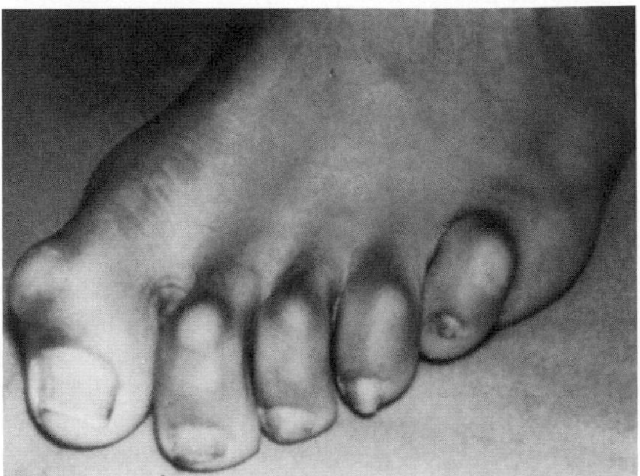

Figure 9–24. Clawtoe deformity involves hammer toe deformity associated with dorsiflexion of metatarsophalangeal joint. (Reproduced, with permission, from Mann RA, Coughlin MJ: *Surgery of the Foot and Ankle*, 6th ed. Mosby-Year Book, 1993.)

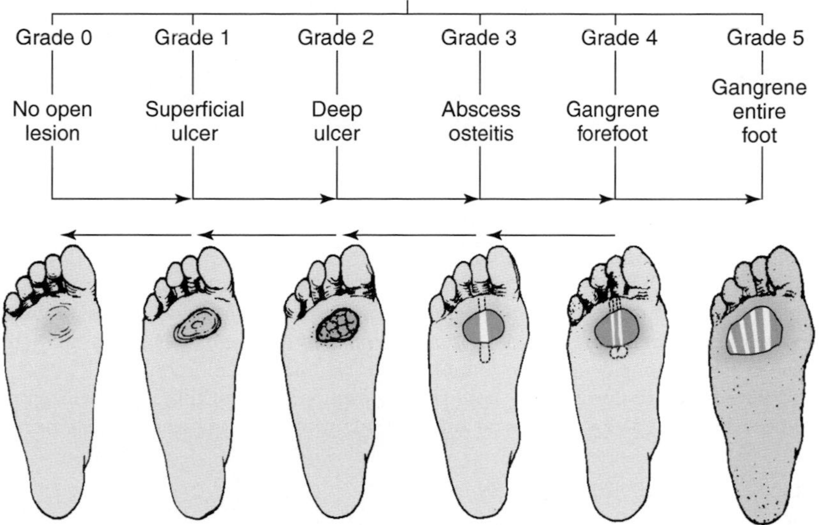

Figure 9–25. The original Rancho Los Amigos classification by Wagner and Meggitt presented the first widely referenced classification of diabetic foot lesions. Two concepts included in this classification are now in need of revision, in light of further experience. The first is the concept that all lesions of the diabetic foot from grade 1 ulcers to grade 5 gangrene occur along a natural continuum. Although this may often be true for the grade 1 ulcer, which progresses to the grade 3 lesion of osteomyelitis, this is not the case with grades 4 and 5. Grades 4 and 5 are vascular lesions or descriptions of the vascular status of the foot and not necessarily related to the progression of the lesser grades. The ischemic lesions of grades 4 and 5 may exist separately from the lesser grades or coincide with any of them, including a forefoot that is otherwise grade 1 (ie, a superficial lesion). Vascular pathologic changes can and should be graded also, but there is not necessarily a relationship between the depth of ulcerative lesions (ie, grades 0, 1, 2, and 3) and the dysvascularity of the foot (ie, grades 4 and 5). Moreover, the grade 5 foot is truly no longer a foot problem but belongs in the domain of salvage of the proximal portion of the leg. The second concept that needs to be refined is that there are not necessarily pathways backward and forward from each grade of lesion (eg, grade 4 feet [partial gangrene] cannot be reversed to grade 3). (Reproduced, with permission, from Brodsky JW: The diabetic foot. In Mann RA, Coughlin MJ, eds: *Surgery of the Foot and Ankle,* 6th ed. Mosby-Year Book, 1993.)

four D's of neuropathic joints are helpful in delineating more advanced cases: debris, destruction, dislocation, and densification.

The presence of bony infection may be delineated on serial radiographs as progressive osteolysis, realizing that changes on plain films are late findings and suggesting the infection was present for weeks. A technetium bone scan is sensitive in detecting early osteomyelitis but quite nonspecific. MRI can demonstrate bone and soft-tissue changes, such as edema or the extent of an abscess cavity, and can be helpful in distinguishing Charcot changes from osteomyelitis.

Classification & Treatment of Diabetic Foot Ulcers

The Rancho Los Amigos Hospital classification of diabetic foot ulcers (Figure 9–25) is based on the depth of tissue affected and extent of the foot involved. Treatment choice depends on the grade of ulcer (Figure 9–26). Table 9–2 shows treatment based on classification of foot ulcers.

As a general rule in treating infections of the foot, a balance must be struck between salvage of tissue and foot function. A healed amputation at a more proximal level is

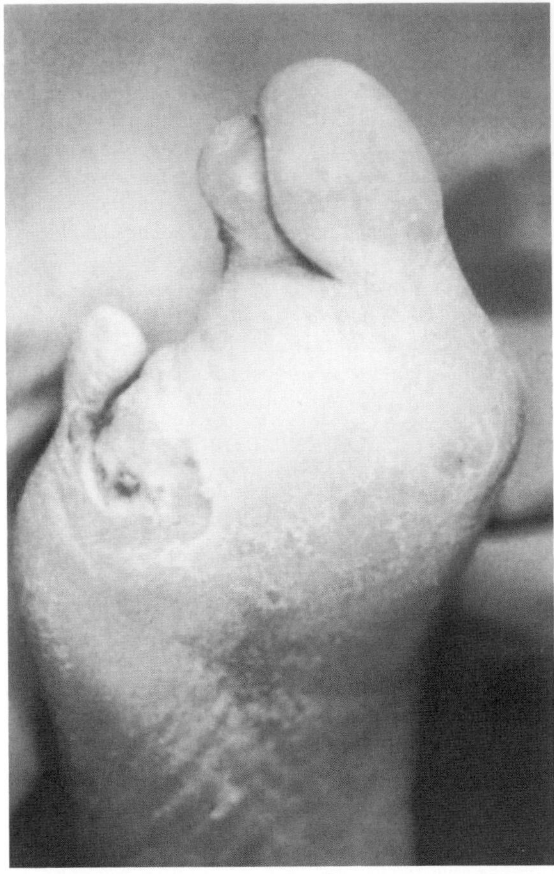

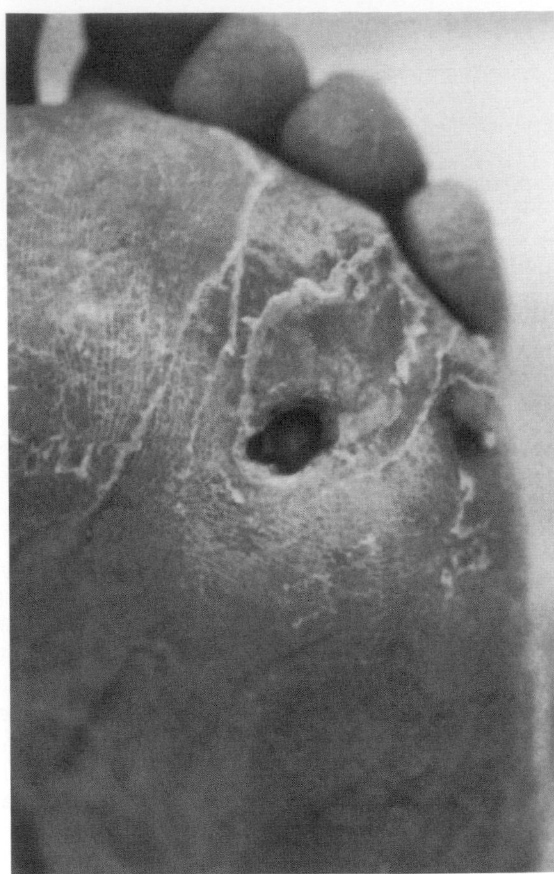

A B

Figure 9–26. Comparison of grade 1 (**A**) and grade 2 (**B**) ulcers (new depth and ischemia classification). Note the exposed deep tissues of the grade 2 ulcer. (Reproduced, with permission, from Brodsky JW: The diabetic foot. In Mann RA, Coughlin MJ, eds: *Surgery of the Foot and Ankle,* 6th ed. Mosby-Year Book, 1993.)

Table 9–2. Classification and treatment of diabetic foot ulcers.

Grade	Classification	Treatment
0	Foot is "at risk" for developing ulcer. Skin remains intact, but underlying bone deformity places foot at risk for skin breakdown.	Proper footwear plus other preventive measures such as patient education and surgical correction as described in text.
1	Lesion affects skin only	Outpatient dressing changes or total contact cast. Antibiotics usually not necessary.
2	Deep lesions that involve underlying tendons, bones, or ligaments (Figure 9–25).	Surgical debridement and hospitalization for aggressive wound care and intravenous antibiotics. Goal is conversion to grade 1 ulcer.
3	Abscess or osteomyelitis present as complication of ulcer.	Emergency surgery for drainage of acute infection. Wound often left open, with dressing changes performed until definitive closure or amputation is done at a later date.
4	Gangrene is present in the toes or forefoot.	Appropriate amputation.
5	Entire foot is gangrenous.	Appropriate amputation.

more advantageous to the patient than leaving a marginally viable area of the foot that requires constant wound care.

Large wounds heal slowly with the risk of secondary infection, and if possible, they should not be left to heal by secondary intention. Split-thickness skin grafts, especially on the sole of the foot or over an amputation site, are prone to breakdown.

A. Surgical Treatment for Relieving Bony Prominences

As previously stated, a major goal of treatment in the ulcerated or at-risk foot is to relieve bony prominences that cause pressure on the skin. Treatment consists of measures to relieve the pressure. Many appropriate measures are available to relieve pressure on the skin from the outside. Examples include extradepth shoes for clawtoes and accommodative foot orthoses with metatarsal pads to relieve pressure under a prominent metatarsal head. If these measures fail or are inappropriate, the pressure should be relieved from the inside by correcting the bony deformity. These prominences are located at several common sites.

The hallux may have a prominence beneath the metatarsal head, on the plantar-medial aspect of the interphalangeal joint, or over the median eminence secondary to a bunion deformity (Figure 9–27). A prominence caused by the medial sesamoid can be relieved by complete or partial removal of the sesamoid. If this does not relieve the prominence adequately, a dorsiflexion osteotomy or resection of the metatarsal head can be performed. Ulcers found over the plantarmedial aspect of the interphalangeal joint can often be relieved by simple excision of the prominent medial condyles or by resection of the

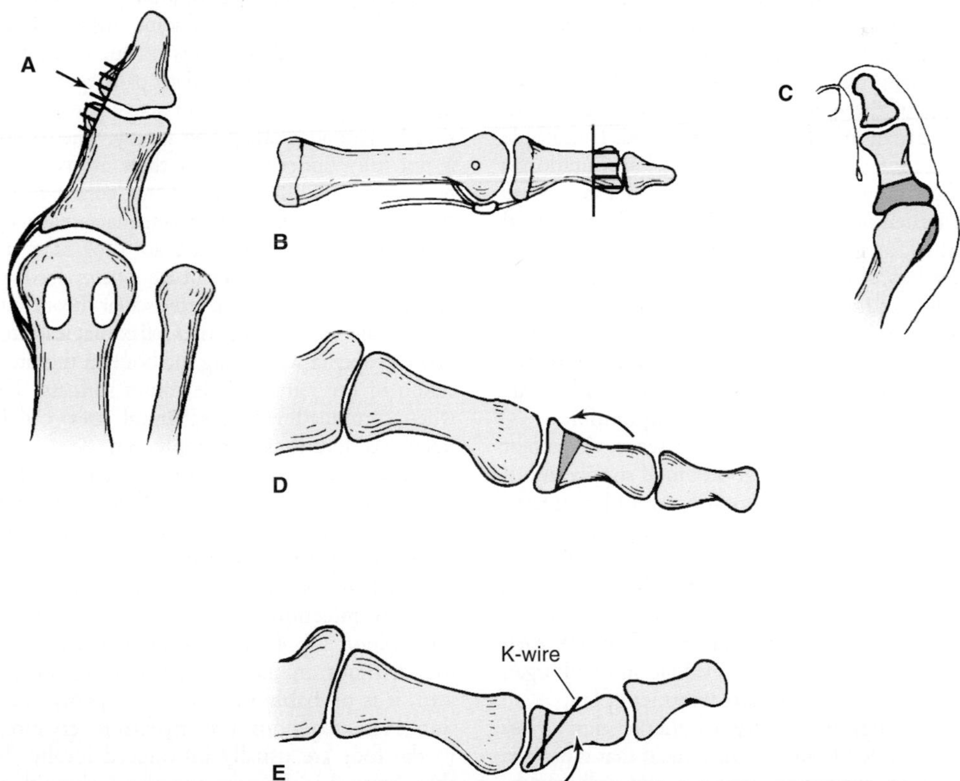

Figure 9–27. Four procedures for recalcitrant ulceration over the condyles of the interphalangeal joint of the hallux. **A:** Reduction of the condyles of the joint. **B:** Resection of the interphalangeal joint. **C:** Modified Keller procedure (resection of the base of the proximal phalanx). **D:** Dorsiflexion osteotomy of the base of the proximal phalanx. **E:** K-wire fixation of dorsiflexion osteotomy. (Reproduced, with permission, from Brodsky JW: The diabetic foot. In Mann RA, Coughlin MJ, eds: *Surgery of the Foot and Ankle,* 6th ed. Mosby-Year Book, 1993.)

entire joint. A prominence over the median eminence can be addressed with a routine bunion procedure.

The diabetic patient is subject to clawtoe deformities resulting from motor neuropathy, causing prominences under the metatarsal heads and over the dorsum of the proximal interphalangeal joints. Depending on the severity, treatment varies from reduction of the metatarsophalangeal joints and proximal interphalangeal arthroplasties to resection of the metatarsal heads and interphalangeal fusions.

A collapsed longitudinal arch from Charcot changes causes the classic rocker-bottom foot with prominences along the plantar and medial aspects of the midfoot. This can be addressed with a simple exostectomy for a mild deformity, or an appropriate osteotomy and arthrodesis for a more complex deformity.

B. Treatment of Osteomyelitis

Osteomyelitis is a common complication present in a grade 3 diabetic foot ulcer. The infection is seldom eradicated without surgical debridement of the bone. Frequently, more radical treatment than simple exostectomy is required. For example, infection of a proximal phalanx is usually treated by resection of the phalanx. Osteomyelitis of the metatarsal may require ray amputation if more than just the head is involved. If multiple metatarsals are infected, a transmetatarsal amputation is often the best treatment with the reminder to always consider lengthening the tendo Achilles to decrease load on the residual forefoot.

Osteomyelitis of the midfoot is a complication of a collapsed Charcot foot. The treatment options for such an infection include wide local debridement with exostectomy or a more proximal amputation. Similarly, osteomyelitis of the calcaneus can be treated with a partial calcanectomy or a more proximal amputation.

Treatment of ulcers should make sense. A patient with a superficial wound with good blood supply, minimal infection, and protective sensation would be treated with topical wound care, a shoe to accommodate the dressing, and limited activity to control swelling. A patient with an infected deep wound with osteomyelitis and nonreconstructable dysvascularity would probably be best served with early amputation. Of course, each patient is unique and deserves an evaluation of all organ systems to develop an appropriate treatment plan.

Wound dressings should try to mimic skin. They should try to provide a healing environment that is bacteria free, warm, moist, strain free, nontoxic, and well oxygenated. There is nothing that will provide all of these. Dressings should be chosen based on the needs of the wound, possibly needing infection control and debridement in the initial phases but later only requiring protection and absorption of wound drainage. The gold standard for treating plantar ulcers is a total contact or healing cast. This protective cast provides wound protection, edema control, and a moist environment, and it decreases plantar loading to the ulcer. When the wound is draining, the cast does require frequent changing or the odor can be intolerable.

Biological wound healing products that provide wound healing factors can be helpful in the patient with marginal healing potential. Larger wounds, especially those with considerable drainage, can benefit from vacuum-assisted closure where a constant negative suction pressure is applied to a sealed wound, thereby decreasing its size and pulling away wound drainage.

A small number of patients who are marginal wound healers benefit from hyperbaric oxygen treatment. When placed at 2 atm of pure oxygen, the serum becomes supersaturated and benefits some patients who receive serial treatments.

C. Charcot Foot

A Charcot joint is also referred to as a neuropathic, neurotrophic, or neuroarthropathic joint. Diabetes is by far the leading cause of Charcot joints. A Charcot foot is characterized by destruction of joint surfaces, fractures often accompanied by dislocations of one or more joints in a patient with an inappropriate pain response (Figure 9–28).The requirements are an active patient who has neuropathy and adequate blood supply. The pathophysiology is not fully understood, but there are two theories. The neurotraumatic theory claims that cumulative mechanical strains in a patient with inadequate sensory protection leads to stress fractures that are progressive because the patient does not have adequate sensory feedback to limit his or her activity. The neurovascular theory suggests there is a neurally initiated vascular reflex that leads to juxtaarticular osteopenia weakening the bone in this area while glycation of the joint capsule causes stiffness. These factors when combined with mechanical stress can lead to the fracture dislocations commonly seen.

Eichenholtz defined three stages in Charcot arthropathy. Stage 1 is the acute inflammatory phase where there is swelling, redness, and increased warmth. Radiographs likely show fractures and dislocations and the involved area is unstable. The concern in this stage is to rule out infection. If the patient is neuropathic with good blood supply and has an acute, red, hot, swollen foot without an ulcer or a history of an ulcer in that area, it is probably Charcot arthropathy and not infection. Hematogenous osteomyelitis is very rare; infections in the foot are usually introduced locally through the skin. Stage 2 is the subacute phase where there are signs of healing, less swelling, warmth, and radiographic signs of new bone formation. Stage 3 is the chronic phase with consolidation and resolution of inflammation. Typical locations include the midfoot with the creation of the rocker-bottom foot deformity as the arch collapses, the hindfoot, and the ankle with the risk of collapse into varus or valgus that can lead to ulcerization.

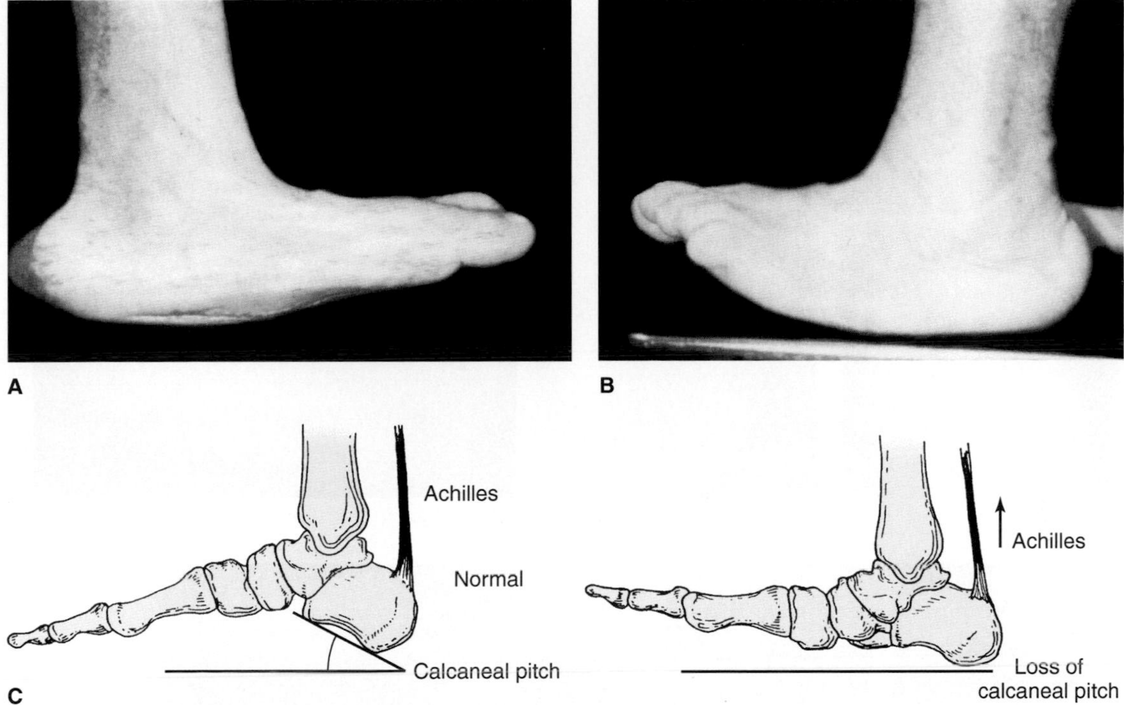

Figure 9–28. **A, B:** The classic rocker-bottom Charcot foot, with collapse and then reversal of the longitudinal arch. **C:** Loss of the normal calcaneal pitch, or angle relative to the floor, in patients with Charcot collapse of the arch. This leads to a mechanical disadvantage for the Achilles tendon. (Reproduced, with permission, from Brodsky JW: The diabetic foot. In Mann RA, Coughlin MJ, eds: *Surgery of the Foot and Ankle,* 6th ed. Mosby-Year Book, 1993.)

1. Principles of treatment—There are several important principles to follow in the treatment of Charcot joints. The primary goal is to limit joint destruction and preserve a stable plantigrade foot that protects the soft tissues and prevents ulceration.

2. Treatment of acute phase—For a patient who presents in the acute phase of Charcot joint, the initial treatment should be immobilization and elevation of the foot. This can best be achieved with a non–weight-bearing total contact cast for those patients who can be placed in a plantigrade position. The skin must be checked at weekly intervals initially to look for breakdown. Surgery is rarely attempted on the acute Charcot foot, unless necessitated by the inability to obtain a stable plantigrade position. Even in those patients who require acute stabilization to obtain a plantigrade foot, it is best to allow the swelling and inflammation to diminish by offloading and immobilization prior to surgical intervention. Once the acute phase subsides and the fractures heal, immobilization can be accomplished by means of an ankle-foot orthosis (AFO) or other appropriate removable support. Custom-made shoes can then be fitted to accommodate for the bony prominences.

3. Treatment of subacute phase—In this phase the foot has stabilized, and there is no ongoing bony destruction. Operations address the bony prominences that were created by Charcot destruction and collapse. Simple removal of a prominence is often all that is required, and, sometimes, fusion of one or several joints is necessary. One of the most common foot deformities is a collapsed arch and rocker-bottom deformity from subluxation of multiple joints in the midfoot. An exostectomy of the prominent bones on the plantar aspect of the midfoot usually is sufficient. Alternatively, an osteotomy and arthrodesis of the midfoot can be performed to realign the foot and reconstitute the arch in cases where a simple exostectomy is inadequate (Figure 9–29). This procedure has a high complication rate and an extended time to achieve union. In the case of Charcot involvement of the ankle joint, the goal is a stable and plantigrade foot, which often requires arthrodesis. Retrograde intramedullary nailing is successful in achieving union but also has significant complication rates.

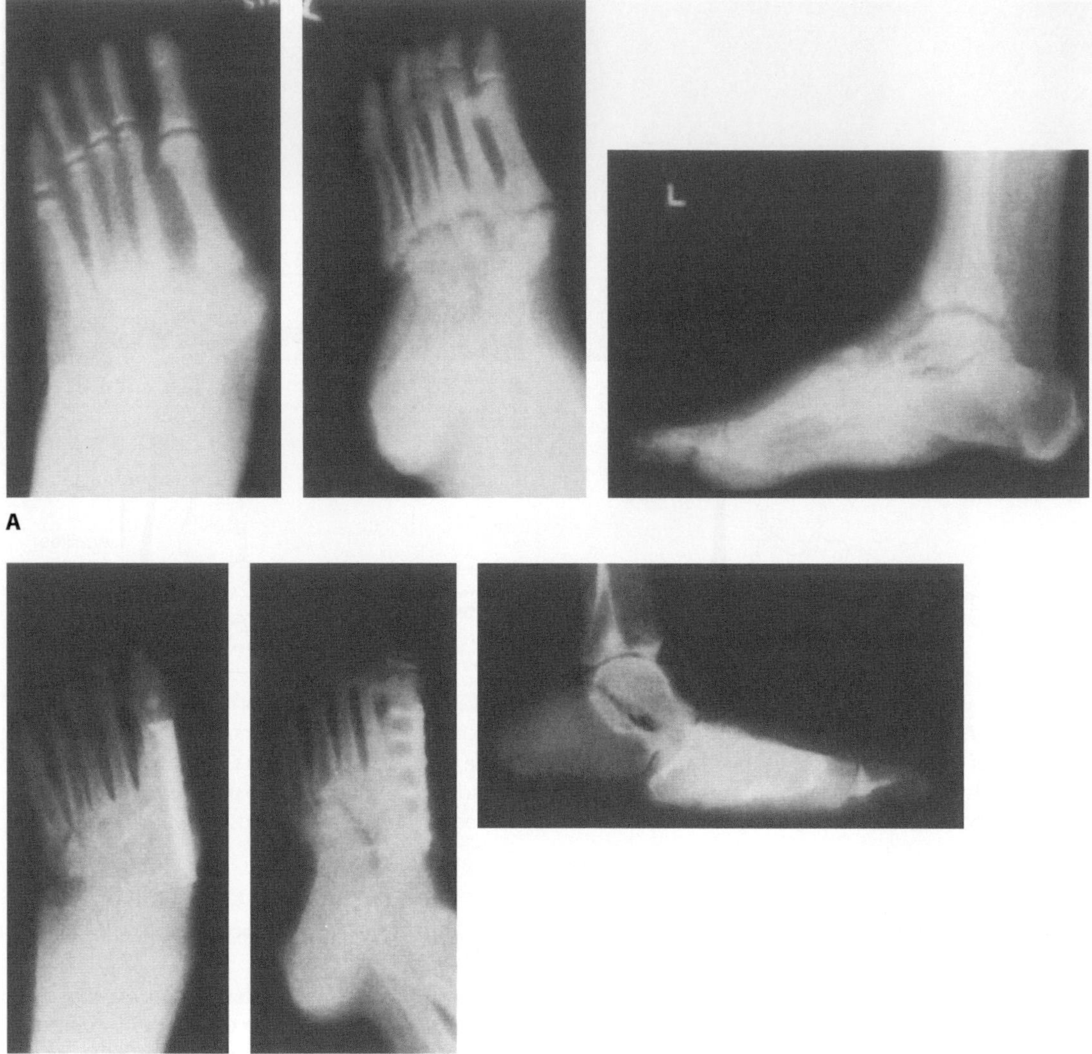

Figure 9–29. **A:** Patient with advanced midfoot Charcot deformity and soft-tissue breakdown over an extruded medial cuneiform. **B:** Limited arthrodesis with internal fixation and iliac grafting to relieve pressure on soft tissue and reestablish weight bearing of the first ray. (Reproduced, with permission, from Brodsky JW: The diabetic foot. In Mann RA, Coughlin MJ, eds: *Surgery of the Foot and Ankle,* 6th ed. Mosby-Year Book, 1993.)

Andros G: Diagnostic and therapeutic arterial interventions in the ulcerated diabetic foot. Diabetes Metab Res Rev 2004;20 (Suppl 1):S29. [PMID: 15150810]

Brem H, Sheehan P, Boulton AJ: Protocol for the treatment of diabetic foot ulcers. Am J Surg 2004;187(5)(Suppl 1):S1. [PMID: 15147985]

Eldor R et al: New and experimental approaches to treatment of diabetic foot ulcers: A comprehensive review of emerging treatment strategies. Diabet Med 2004:21:1161. [PMID: 15498081]

Gil H, Morrison WB: MR imaging of diabetic foot infection. Semin Musculoskelet Radiol 2004;8(3):189. [PMID: 15478022]

Lipsky B: Medical treatment of diabetic foot infections. Clin Infect Dis 2004;39:S104. [PMID: 15306988]

Perry JE et al: The use of running shoes to reduce plantar pressures in patients who have diabetes. J Bone Joint Surg 1995;778: 1819. [PMID: 8550649]

Pinzur M: Surgical versus accommodative treatment for Charcot arthropathy of the midfoot. Foot Ankle Int 2004;25(8):545. [PMID: 15363375]

Pinzur MS, Kelikian A: Charcot ankle fusion with a retrograde locked intramedullary nail. Foot Ankle Int 1997;18:699. [PMID: 9391814]

Wagner FW Jr: A classification and treatment program for diabetic, neuropathic, and dysvascular foot problems. Instr Course Lect 1979;28:143.

DISORDERS OF THE TOENAILS

Toenail problems in younger (less than 20 years) patients usually involve trauma, such as stubbing the toe or, more frequently, improper nail care, which can contribute to ingrown toenails. This is usually the result of tearing off a toenail, which leaves the nail too short and predisposes it to become ingrown.

Toenail problems in the older age group are more varied, including an incurvating nail, a thickened hypertrophied nail associated with a chronic fungal infection, an ingrown nail resulting from improper nail cutting, and on rare occasions a subungual exostosis.

Etiologic Findings

The anatomy of the toenail is demonstrated in Figure 9–30. The nail unit consists of four components: the proximal nail fold, the nail matrix, the nail bed, and the hyponychium. The area in which most of the problems occur is the lateral or medial nail groove, where an ingrown nail occurs at the level of the nail bed or hyponychium.

Clinical Findings

A. Symptoms and Signs

The history of most nail problems is not complex and usually quickly defines the nature of the problem.

1. Infection of the toenails—Infection of the toenails usually begins slowly, with erythema and swelling along the margin of the nail, followed by increasing pain and drainage, and finally the development of granulation tissue, usually in response to the foreign body reaction of the nail itself.

2. Mycotic nail—In the case of the mycotic (fungal) nail, there is usually a long, slow history of development of deformation of the nail, often with medial or lateral deviation of the nail, marked hypertrophy, and increased pain when wearing shoes. At times, an incurvated nail condition develops in which one or both edges of the nail slowly curve inward, resulting in pinching of the nail plate. This may cause a localized infection, or just the sheer pressure of the nail against the skin may be the cause of the pain. Medical therapy is based on direct microscopy (KOH [potassium hydroxide]) and culture studies.

3. Subungual exostosis—The patient who develops subungual exostosis usually notes pain evolving beneath the toenail over a long period. Erosion of the nail from below occurs because of the pressure of the exostosis against the nail itself. The patient often does not seek help until there is actual breakdown of the tissue, giving rise to a rather ugly-appearing lesion that seems much more ominous than the condition itself.

B. Imaging Studies

Radiographs are necessary when evaluating a toenail problem for subungual exostosis, which is clearly seen with a lateral view. In patients with long-standing infected ingrown toenails, a radiograph can be important to rule out underlying osteomyelitis.

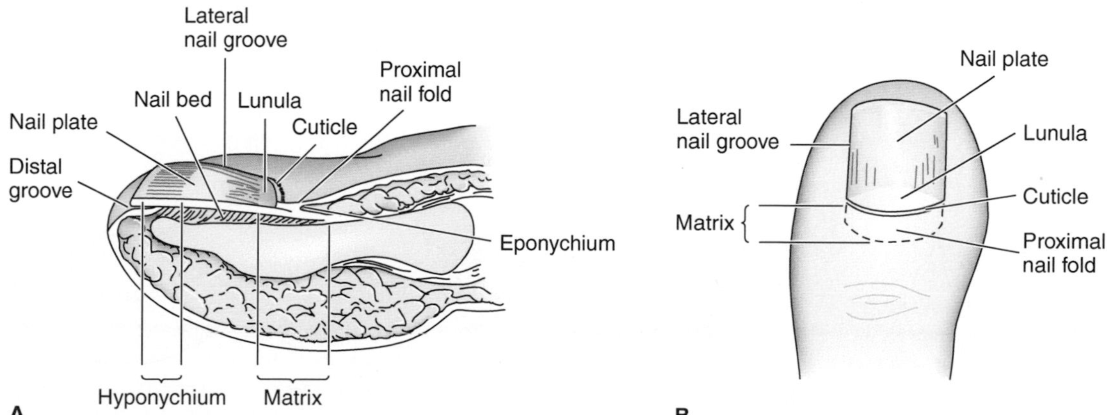

Figure 9–30. **A:** Cross section of the toe demonstrates the components of the toenail and supporting structures. **B:** The proximal nail is covered by the proximal nail fold and cuticle. The lunula is the main germinal area. (Reproduced, with permission, from Mann RA, Coughlin MJ: *The Video Textbook of Foot and Ankle Surgery*. Medical Video Productions, 1991.)

Treatment

A. Conservative Management

1. Chronic ingrown toenail—For the chronic ingrown toenail, the margin of the nail is removed to relieve the pressure of the nail against the skin. This procedure, along with local care and occasionally systemic antibiotics, usually permits the condition to resolve. It is important, however, to explain to the patient the necessity of permitting the nail to grow out over the ungual labia, to depress it and prevent the ingrown nail from recurring.

2. Chronic onychophosis of the nail—Chronic onychophosis of the nail must be kept debrided. If an ingrown nail occurs, the margins must be trimmed to relieve the pressure against the skin.

3. Subungual exostosis—Subungual exostosis that is symptomatic is treated by excision.

B. Surgical Treatment

1. Ingrown toenail—The surgical management of the recurrent ingrown toenail consists of the Winograd procedure, in which the medial or lateral margin of the offending nail plate is removed along with the underlying nail matrix. The nail matrix is removed as thoroughly as possible to prevent the possible growth of a nail horn, which occurs in approximately 5% of cases. The nail matrix can be removed by sharp dissection or ablated with a laser or treated with phenol to kill the nail matrix.

2. Chronic infection—If chronic infections has caused severe distortion of the nail, the nail and the nail bed can be removed in their entirety. This usually results in a horny base where the nail existed, often a satisfactory outcome. The terminal Syme amputation can be carried out to eliminate the nail and matrix completely (Figure 9–31). Although results are usually satisfactory, some patients do not like the appearance of the toe or absence of the toenail because of its somewhat bulbous appearance. The terminal Syme procedure can be carried out under digital block in most patients. An elliptical incision is made over the distal end of the toe, removing the nail and its matrix in their entirety. The distal portion of the distal phalanx is removed and the edges smoothed, thus shortening the toe. The tip of the toe is defatted and loosely sutured. In this manner, the nail is completely removed and soft tissue covers the area of the former nail bed. The only significant complication associated with this procedure is the regrowth of some nail matrix beneath the healed flap, which results in an inclusion cyst that must be drained and the residual nail matrix excised.

3. Subungual exostosis—Surgical management of subungual exostosis requires lifting the nail, identification of the exostosis, and complete removal of the exostosis and its stalk. The dissection must be carefully carried out and the entire exostosis removed to prevent recurrence. The nail bed is repaired to cover the defect.

Baran R, Dawber RPR: *Diseases of the Nails and Their Management.* Blackwell Scientific Publications, 1984.

Coughlin MJ: Toenail abnormalities. In Mann RA, Coughlin MJ, eds: *Surgery of the Foot and Ankle.* Mosby-Year Book, 1993.

Mann RA, Coughlin MJ: Toenail abnormalities. In Mann RA, Coughlin MJ, eds: *The Video Textbook of Foot and Ankle Surgery.* Video Medical Productions, 1990.

Mayeaux EJ: Nail disorders. Prim Care 2000;27:333. [PMID: 10815047]

Rounding C, Hulm S: Surgical treatments for ingrowing toenails. Cochrane Database Syst Rev 2000;(2):CD001541. [PMID: 10796808]

Summerbell RC, Cooper E, Bunn U et al: Onychomycosis: A critical study of techniques and criteria for confirming the etiologic significance of nondermatophytes. Med Mycol 2005;43:39. [PMID: 15712607]

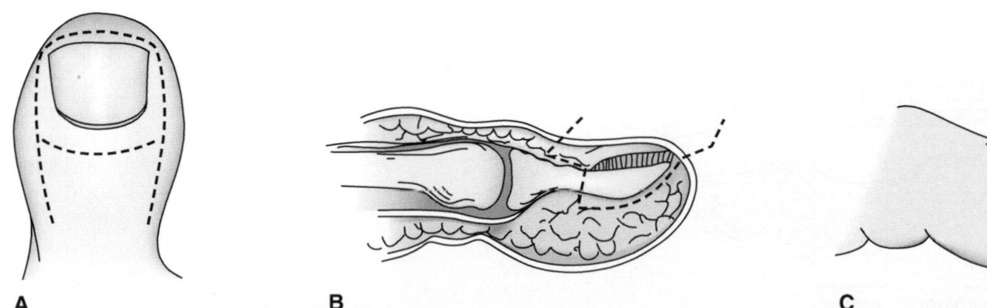

Figure 9–31. Syme amputation of toenail. **A:** Elliptical or rectangular incision is centered over the nail bed and matrix. **B:** The distal half of the distal phalanx is resected. **C:** Excess skin is resected, and skin edges are approximated. (Reproduced, with permission, from Mann RA, Coughlin MJ: *The Video Textbook of Foot and Ankle Surgery.* Medical Video Productions, 1991.)

NEUROLOGIC DISORDERS OF THE FOOT

1. Interdigital Neuroma (Morton Neuroma)

An interdigital neuroma is a painful affliction involving the plantar aspect of the forefoot. It usually involves the third interspace and is characterized by a well-localized area of pain on the plantar aspect of the foot that radiates into the web space. The symptoms are usually aggravated by ambulation and relieved by rest. As a rule, wearing a tight-fitting shoe aggravates the pain, and walking barefoot often relieves it.

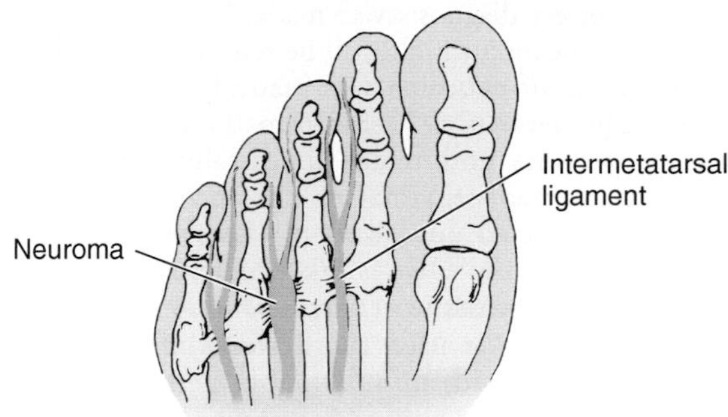

Figure 9–32. An interdigital neuroma impingement occurs beneath the intermetatarsal ligament. (Reproduced, with permission, from Mann RA, Coughlin MJ: *The Video Textbook of Foot and Ankle Surgery.* Medical Video Productions, 1991.)

Etiologic Findings

The precise cause of interdigital neuroma is not determined. It occurs in women approximately 10 times more frequently than men, and, as a result, high-fashion shoe wear is implicated. Several studies demonstrate that the changes in the nerve appear to occur just distal to the transverse metatarsal ligament. This finding has given rise to the hypothesis that the neuroma results from the constant traction of the nerve against the ligament as the toes are brought into a dorsiflexed position, a theory that explains the higher incidence in women wearing high-heeled shoes. Although this condition is called **interdigital neuroma,** it is not a true neuroma. The pathologic changes involve actual degeneration of the nerve fibers associated with deposition of amorphous eosinophilic material that is felt to be consistent with an entrapment neuropathy (Figure 9–32).

Clinical Findings

A. Symptoms and Signs

Patients with an interspace neuroma usually present with a complaint of localized pain in the metatarsal head region that is increased by walking and relieved by rest and by removing the shoe. Palpation of the involved interspace produces sharp pain that often radiates into the toes. There can be a palpable mass, and squeezing the forefoot, thereby narrowing the intermetatarsal space while compressing the mass, often reproduces the patient's symptoms. If this maneuver produces a snapping sensation, it is referred to as a Mulder click. The third interspace is more frequently involved than the second, and it is extremely rare to have involvement of the first or fourth web space. Pain over the metatarsophalangeal joint itself is caused by disease involving the metatarsophalangeal joint, and pain in the interspace must be distinguished from pain associated with pathology in the metatarsophalangeal joint. The differential diagnosis of metatarsalgia includes avascular necrosis (Freiberg disease), synovitis caused by mechanical instability, synovial cysts, or even referred pain from tarsal tunnel compression or lumbar disk disease.

B. Imaging Studies

Radiographs are not helpful in the diagnosis of an interdigital neuroma but may reveal pathology at the metatarsophalangeal joint as the cause of the patient's symptoms. There are several reports regarding the use of ultrasound to evaluate the presence of nerve enlargement, but this is very user dependent. MRI can be used effectively but is rarely necessary.

Treatment

A. Conservative Management

Conservative management begins with wearing a wider soft-soled shoe to accommodate the foot without mediolateral compression and lowering the heel. A soft metatarsal support is placed in the shoe proximal to the area of the neuroma, thereby spreading the metatarsal heads and lifting them. Approximately a third of patients respond to this treatment. Steroid injection into the web space can be helpful in resolving the symptoms but is not without the hazard of local fat atrophy, which can lead to diminished padding under the metatarsal heads or local skin thinning and discoloration.

B. Surgical Treatment

Surgical excision of the nerve is indicated if conservative treatment fails. A dorsal incision is made in the midline of the involved web space and carried down to the transverse metatarsal ligament, which is cut. The nerve is noted to lie just beneath the transverse metatarsal ligament. A quite thickened nerve is reassuring evidence that the correct diagnosis was made; however, a nerve of normal thickness should still be removed if the clinical diagnosis of neuroma was made from other evidence. The nerve is delivered into the interspace by plantar pressure and freed up distally and proximally, transected proximal to the metatarsal head, and then dissected out distally, where it is cut just past its bifurcation. Care is taken not to disrupt the surrounding fatty tissue or intrinsic muscles. A compression dressing is used for 3 weeks after routine wound closure, and ambulation is permitted in a postoperative shoe. Decreased sensation in the toes on either side of the web space is expected postoperatively. Approximately 80% of patients are totally satisfied with the results of the procedure; 20% obtain little or no relief. The precise cause of this failure rate is a bit of an enigma. Obviously in some patients, the diagnosis was made incorrectly, and the metatarsophalangeal joint was actually involved.

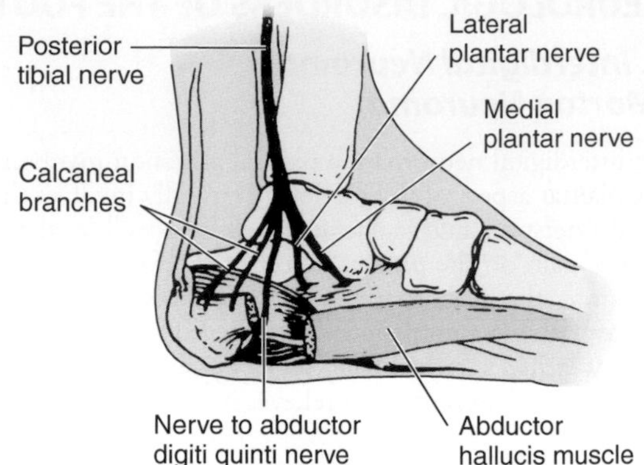

Figure 9–33. Posterior tibial nerve and major branches. (Reproduced, with permission, from Mann RA, Coughlin MJ: *The Video Textbook of Foot and Ankle Surgery.* Medical Video Productions, 1991.)

C. Recurrent Neuroma

A recurrent neuroma is indeed a true surgical bulb neuroma that resulted following the transection of the common digital nerve on the plantar aspect of the foot. True neuritic symptoms occur in some cases in which transection was not proximal enough or the nerve became adherent and trapped beneath the metatarsal head. Careful percussion of the plantar aspect to elicit the Tinel sign can frequently localize the cut end of the nerve (bulb neuroma). If the severed nerve can be clinically well localized, reexploration for the neuroma is carried out either through a dorsal or plantar approach. The neuroma is identified and transected to a more proximal level or implanted into muscle, and symptoms are relieved in 60–70% of patients.

2. Tarsal Tunnel Syndrome

Tarsal tunnel syndrome is a compressive or traction neuropathy of the posterior tibial nerve as it passes behind the medial malleolus. The tarsal tunnel is formed by the fibroosseous tunnel resulting from the flexor retinaculum as it wraps around the posterior aspect of the medial malleolus (Figure 9–33). Tarsal tunnel syndrome causes poorly localized dysesthesias on the plantar aspect of the foot. The symptom complex is often aggravated by activity and relieved by rest. Some patients complain mainly of nocturnal dysesthesias.

Etiologic Findings

Tarsal tunnel syndrome may arise from a space-occupying lesion within the tarsal tunnel (eg, a ganglion, synovial cyst, or lipoma) or distally against one of the two terminal branches: the medial or lateral plantar nerve. It occasionally follows severe trauma to the lower extremity, probably because of edema or scarring. Other causes are severe venous varicosities, tenosynovitis, or a tumor within the nerve. Traction neuropathy can occur in those patients who have an excessively valgus hindfoot position, especially those that are unstable. As the patient walks, the posterior tibial nerve is subjected to stretching as it courses around the convex side of the deformity. In more than half of the cases, however, the precise cause cannot be determined.

Clinical Findings

A. Symptoms and Signs

The diagnosis is entertained after obtaining a history of paresthesias or burning in the posterior tibial nerve distribution. Careful evaluation of the patient in the standing and sitting positions is necessary to check posture and increased fullness, thickening, or swelling in the involved tarsal tunnel area. Careful percussion may elicit a Tinel sign over the posterior tibial nerve in the tarsal tunnel or distally along the divisions of the posterior tibial nerve (the medial calcaneal nerve and medial and lateral plantar nerves). Muscle weakness is usually not observed, but loss of sensation and two-point discrimination may be occasionally detected.

Electrodiagnostic studies should be carried out to help confirm the diagnosis of tarsal tunnel syndrome. Nerve conduction velocities along the medial plantar nerve to the abductor hallucis muscle (latency less than 6.2 ms) and of the lateral plantar nerve to the abductor digiti quinti (latency usually less than 7 ms) should be within 1 ms of each other, otherwise indicating nerve compression in the tarsal tunnel. Motor-evoked potentials that demonstrate a decreased amplitude and increased duration are also indicative of tarsal tunnel syndrome. The most accurate study for tarsal tunnel syndrome appears to be sensory nerve conduction velocity, although this is also the least reproducible study.

The definitive diagnosis of tarsal tunnel syndrome should be based on (1) the clinical history of ill-defined burning, tingling pain in the plantar aspect of the foot, (2) positive physical findings of Tinel sign along the course of the nerve, and (3) electrodiagnostic studies. If all three factors are not positive, the diagnosis of tarsal tunnel syndrome should be suspect. MRI may be quite useful in demonstrating the presence of a space-occupying lesion.

Treatment

A. Conservative Management

The tarsal tunnel syndrome should be managed with NSAIDs and an occasional steroid injection into the tarsal tunnel area. Aspiration and injection of a cyst or ganglion may be attempted but is rarely successful. Immobilization in a polypropylene AFO may also be useful, especially in the patient with unstable valgus.

B. Surgical Treatment

Surgical intervention can be considered if conservative management fails. Approximately 75% of patients operated on for tarsal tunnel syndrome are satisfied with the result. The other 25% may continue to have varying degrees of discomfort. The surgical release uses an incision behind the medial malleolus that is carried distally to about the level of the talonavicular joint. The investing retinaculum is exposed and released. The posterior tibial nerve is identified proximal to the tarsal tunnel area and carefully traced distally behind the medial malleolus. The division into its three terminal branches is identified. Because the medial calcaneal branch passes from the posterior aspect of the lateral plantar nerve, the dissection should be carried out along its dorsal aspect. There may be one or more medial calcaneal branches. The medial plantar nerve should be traced distally until it passes through the fibroosseous tunnel in the abductor hallucis muscle. The lateral plantar nerve should be traced behind the abductor hallucis muscle until it passes toward the lateral aspect of the foot. A preoperative Tinel sign distal to the tarsal tunnel area requires that the area be carefully explored to determine whether there is a ganglion or cyst within the tendon sheath as a cause of the tarsal tunnel syndrome.

Postoperatively, a compression dressing is applied and weight bearing is prohibited for 3 weeks, before progressive ambulation is permitted.

The results following tarsal tunnel release depend on the pathology found at the time of surgery. Removal of a space-occupying lesion usually relieves all of the symptoms. Involvement of a single nerve branch, such as the medial or lateral plantar nerve, also portends good results after surgery. If more diffuse pain is felt throughout the foot before surgery and no definite constriction on the nerve is found at exploration, only one half to two thirds of patients can be expected to experience pain relief. Patients with traction neuropathy caused by the unstable valgus foot are treated by correction of the instability, usually with arthrodesis, and not with soft tissue tarsal tunnel release.

3. Traumatic Neuromas About the Foot

A traumatic neuroma about the foot presents a difficult problem in management because footwear can cause constant irritation of the neuroma. The most frequent cause of traumatic neuroma in the foot is previous surgery. Despite caution in making incisions about the foot, many lesser and occasionally major nerve trunks can be injured. The dorsal aspect of the foot is most frequently involved (Figure 9–34).

Clinical Findings

The clinical evaluation begins with a careful history of the problem and an evaluation of the area involved to determine the precise location of the neuroma, which is essential for proper treatment. Rarely is any type of electrodiagnostic study indicated, and radiographs are not usually necessary.

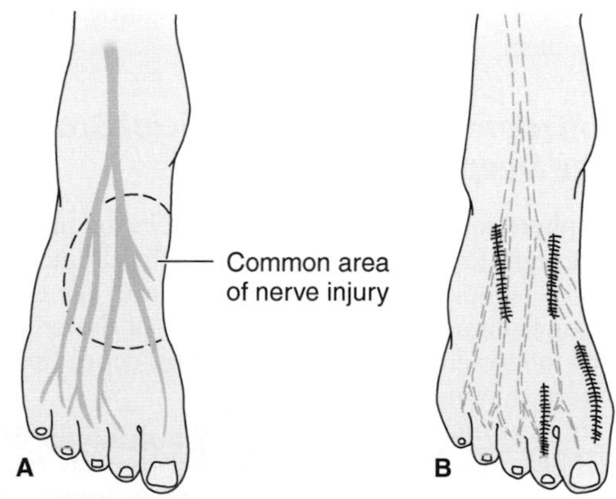

Figure 9–34. **A:** Common area of traumatic nerve entrapment. **B:** Frequent incisions that may lead to entrapment of dorsal sensory nerves. (Reproduced, with permission, from Mann RA, Coughlin MJ: *The Video Textbook of Foot and Ankle Surgery.* Medical Video Productions, 1991.)

Treatment

A. Conservative Management

Attempts to relieve pressure on the neuroma with a large shoe or a carefully designed pad may be of benefit. A cortisone injection into the area occasionally may help, particularly when a small nerve is involved. Surgical intervention is indicated if conservative measures fail.

B. Surgical Treatment

Careful planning must be undertaken prior to the excision of a traumatic neuroma. The exact location of the neuroma and the area of sensitivity proximal to it must be determined. The incision must be made as precisely as possible to identify the neuroma and trace the nerve proximally into an area that would not be affected by pressure from shoes and boots. The neuroma is excised, leaving enough nerve to bring the cut end into an area of minimal pressure. The cut end is buried into an excavation in bone, if possible, or beneath a muscle such as the extensor digitorum brevis muscle. When carrying out a resection of the sural nerve, it is important, particularly in an individual who wears heavy work boots, that the end of the nerve is brought proximally enough so the top of the boot will not press on the nerve, resulting in continued symptoms.

The results following resection of a traumatic neuroma are quite variable. Initial relief from removing the traumatic neuroma is routine, but unless the nerve is buried where it will not be exposed to pressure, the symptoms may recur in time. It is therefore preferable to bury the end of the nerve into bone, if possible. Resection of most neuromas accentuate a sensory deficit, which is usually not a significant clinical problem.

4. Entrapment of the Superficial Branch of the Deep Peroneal Nerve

Osteophyte formation at the talonavicular or metatarsocuneiform joint may entrap the superficial branch of the deep peroneal nerve as it passes beneath the extensor retinaculum. Patient complaints are of dysesthesias on the foot or difficulty in wearing shoes, depending on the location of the entrapment.

The superficial branch of the deep peroneal nerve passes onto the dorsum of the foot between the extensor hallucis longus and extensor digitorum longus tendons. It continues beneath the extensor retinaculum, coursing along the dorsal surface of the talus and navicular and more distally across the metatarsocuneiform joints. Osteophyte formation at any point along the course of the nerve may cause sufficient pressure against the nerve to cause an entrapment problem.

Clinical Findings

A. Symptoms and Signs

The clinical evaluation begins with a careful history regarding the patient's complaint of dysesthesias over the dorsum of the foot. The physical examination demonstrates tingling along the course of the superficial branch of the deep peroneal nerve, which radiates into the first web space. Often the precise location of the nerve entrapment can be identified by careful palpation and by rolling the nerve across the involved bony prominence.

B. Imaging Studies

Radiographs usually reveal the offending osteophytes, often along the area of the talonavicular or metatarsocuneiform joints. Placing a radiographic marker at the area of maximum tenderness can help identify the offending bony prominence.

Treatment

A. Conservative Management

Conservative management consists of attempting to keep the pressure off the involved area, either by padding the tongue of the shoe or by trying to create a pad that will not put pressure directly on the nerve. If these measures fail, decompression of the nerve usually brings about satisfactory resolution of the condition.

B. Surgical Treatment

Depending on the area of entrapment (talonavicular or metatarsocuneiform), a slightly curved incision is made and carried down through the retinaculum to expose the nerve. Great caution must be taken during the approach so the nerve is not inadvertently damaged. The nerve is carefully lifted off of its bed, exposing the osteophytes, which are removed with a rongeur. The bone surfaces are coated with bone wax prior to laying the nerve back on its bed. After wound closure in layers, the foot is immobilized for approximately 3 weeks in a postoperative shoe.

The results following release of the superficial portion of the deep peroneal nerve are usually satisfactory. Because the nerve itself usually is not damaged by the entrapment, a favorable outcome is expected.

Bailie DS, Kelikian AS: Tarsal tunnel syndrome: Diagnosis, surgical technique, and functional outcome. Foot Ankle Int 1998; 2:65. [PMID: 9498577]

Beskin JL: Nerve entrapment syndromes of the foot and ankle. J Am Acad Orthop Surg 1997;5:261. [PMID: 10795062]

Coughlin M et al: Concurrent interdigital neuroma and MTP joint instability: Long-term results of treatment. Foot Ankle Int 2002;23:1018. [PMID: 12449407]

Okafor B, Shergill G, Angel J: Treatment of Morton's neuroma by neurolysis. Foot Ankle Int 1997;5:284. [PMID: 9167928]

Stamatis ED, Myerson MS: Treatment of recurrence of symptoms after excision of an interdigital neuroma. J Bone Joint Surg Br 2004;86:48. [PMID: 14765865]

RHEUMATOID FOOT

The foot is involved in 90% of patients with long-standing RA, and the involvement is almost always bilateral. The forefoot is most commonly involved, and these joints are often the first joints to be affected, but deterioration of the subtalar joint is noted in approximately 35% of patients and of the ankle joint in approximately 30%.

Etiologic Findings

The changes in the forefoot are caused by chronic synovitis, which destroys the supporting structures about the metatarsophalangeal joints. The joint capsules are distended and the ligaments destroyed. When these structures no longer function to provide stability for the joint, progressive dorsal subluxation and eventual dislocation of the metatarsophalangeal joints occur. As the metatarsophalangeal joints progress from subluxation to dislocation, the plantar fat pad is drawn distally, and the base of the proximal phalanx eventually comes to rest on the metatarsal head. Thus, the metatarsals are forced into a position of plantar flexion, which results in significant callus formation beneath the metatarsal heads. The changes at the metatarsophalangeal joints result in imbalance of the intrinsic muscles, and severe hammer toe and clawtoe deformities usually result.

Significant midfoot and hindfoot pathology is also found in patients with RA. A severely flattened longitudinal arch can result from long-standing subtalar joint involvement with subluxation. Pain with less severe deformity is present in isolated talonavicular involvement of the midfoot.

Clinical Findings

A. Symptoms and Signs

The clinical evaluation of the rheumatoid patient begins with a careful history of the disease and the medications the patient is taking and an attempt to ascertain whether the disease process is currently in an active or a quiescent stage. It is important to obtain some indication of the patient's wound-healing capacity in the foot or elsewhere in the body.

The vascular status of the foot and quality of the skin is noted. The feet are assessed with the patient standing, which often demonstrates marked deformities of multiple joints or localized involvement of only one or two joints. The patient is then seated and a careful evaluation of all the joints about the foot and ankle is carried out to determine precisely the degree to which they are affected. Careful palpation of the metatarsophalangeal joints often demonstrates the degree of the synovial activity as well as the degree of stability of the joints. The plantar aspect of the foot is inspected for the callus formation and past or present ulcerations. Flattening of the longitudinal arch and any hindfoot valgus are evaluated with a careful assessment of joint stability to determine the risk of deformity progression.

B. Imaging Studies

Radiographs help assess the number of joints involved and the degree of involvement. Bilateral involvement is frequently asymmetric. Standing radiographs are beneficial in assessing the effect of joint stability on the severity of deformity.

Treatment

A. Conservative Management

Conservative management includes medical management, carried out by the patient's rheumatologist. The patient with sufficient deformity should wear an extra-depth shoe with a soft accommodative liner to reduce pressure on the metatarsal heads and the toes, which may be severely contracted dorsally. Frequently, the patient is quite comfortable in this shoe and does not require further treatment. With significant hindfoot involvement, an AFO may be required to help relieve pain by providing adequate stabilization.

B. Surgical Treatment

The main goal of surgical management of the forefoot is to create a stable foot that will alleviate the pain beneath the metatarsal head region (Figure 9–35). Arthrodesis of the first metatarsophalangeal joint is the procedure most commonly used, with the joint placed in approximately 15 degrees of dorsiflexion in relation to the floor and approximately 15 degrees of valgus position. The lesser metatarsophalangeal joints are corrected by release of the soft-tissue contracture and resection arthroplasty. The metatarsal heads are excised to decompress the metatarsophalangeal joints, and the fat pad is brought back down onto the plantar aspect of the foot by realigning and securing the plantar plates of the joints under the residual metatarsals. The hammer toes can be corrected by closed osteoclasis, which often results in satisfactory realignment. Open hammer toe procedures are also very effective in correcting residual deformities. The toes and metatarsophalangeal joint area are stabilized with longitudinal K-wires postoperatively for approximately 4 weeks.

The results of this rheumatoid forefoot repair are most gratifying in that approximately 90% of patients are satisfied with the results. There are few complica-

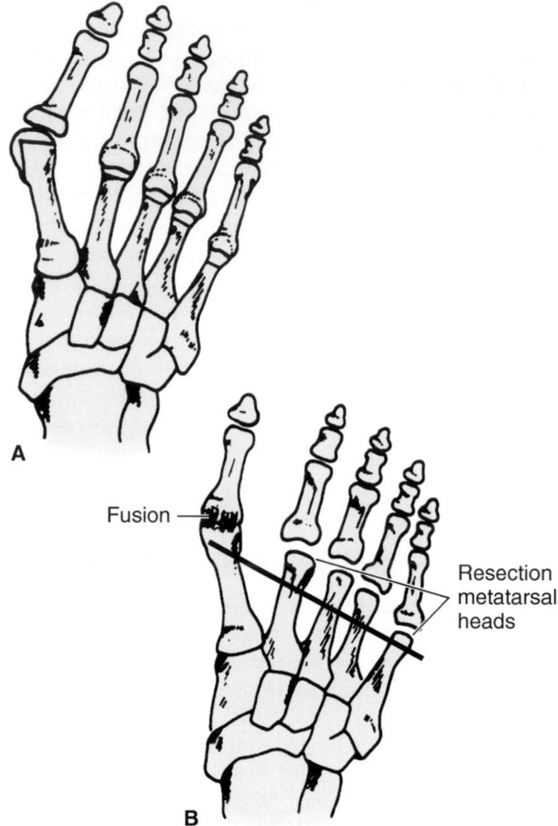

Figure 9–35. **A:** Resection of metatarsal heads. **B:** Symmetric resection of metatarsal heads minimizes recurrence of intractable plantar keratoses. (Reproduced, with permission, from Mann RA, Coughlin MJ: *The Video Textbook of Foot and Ankle Surgery.* Medical Video Productions, 1991.)

tions, although the blood supply to the toes is always of concern because the procedure is extensive. Occasionally, wound healing is delayed, particularly if the patient is taking high dosages of corticosteroids or the antimetabolite drugs.

Hindfoot and ankle disease is usually managed medically unless there is instability and progressive deformity. Orthotic support or bracing can be beneficial, but if the deformity is increasing and the patient's thin skin cannot tolerate further pressure, surgical stabilization with arthrodesis is necessary. If only a single joint is involved with the rheumatoid process, a less extensive procedure is carried out. For isolated talonavicular RA with no significant deformity of the arch, an isolated talonavicular fusion is adequate. If significant deformity is present because of subtalar joint subluxation, a triple arthrodesis is required. Ankle joint involvement is treated with ankle joint fusion or total ankle arthroplasty. The details of the surgical procedures are described elsewhere in this chapter.

Cracchiolo A III: Surgery for rheumatoid disease. Part I. Foot abnormalities in rheumatoid arthritis. Instr Course Lect 1984;33:386. [PMID: 6400419]

James D et al: Orthopaedic intervention in early rheumatoid arthritis. Occurrence and predictive factors in an inception cohort of 1064 patients followed for 5 years. Rheumatology 2004;43:369. [PMID: 14722346]

Kavlak Y et al: Outcome of orthoses intervention in the rheumatoid foot. Foot Ankle Int 2003;24(6):494. [PMID: 12854671]

Mann RA, Schakel ME: Surgical correction of rheumatoid forefoot deformities. Foot Ankle Int 1995;16:1. [PMID: 7697146]

McGarvey SR, Johnson KA: Keller arthroplasty in combination with resection arthroplasty of the lesser metatarsophalangeal joints in rheumatoid arthritis. Foot Ankle 1988;9:75. [PMID: 3224902]

Ostendorf B et al: Diagnostic value of magnetic resonance imaging of the forefeet in early rheumatoid arthritis when findings on imaging of the metacarpophalangeal joints of the hands remain normal. Arthritis Rheum 2004;50(7):2094. [PMID: 15248206]

HEEL PAIN

Heel pain can be caused by several distinct entities. When evaluating the patient for heel pain, the clinician must attempt to define as precisely as possible the location and hence the cause of the pain.

Table 9–3 presents the causes of heel pain, which are quite variable and need to be carefully defined, so the proper treatment can be chosen.

Table 9–3. Causes of heel pain.

Causes of plantar heel pain
Plantar fascitis
Atrophy of heel pad
Posttraumatic (eg, calcaneal fracture)
Enlarged calcaneal spur
Neurologic conditions such as tarsal tunnel syndrome or entrapment of nerve to abductor digiti quinti
Degenerative disk disease with radiation toward heel
Systemic disease (eg, Reiter syndrome, psoriatic arthritis)
Acute tear of plantar fascia
Calcaneal apophysitis
Causes of posterior heel pain
Retrocalcaneal bursitis
Achilles tendinitis
Haglund deformity
Degeneration of Achilles tendon insertion

Clinical Findings

A. Symptoms and Signs

The clinical evaluation begins with a careful history of the onset and location of the pain. The patient's activities and types of footwear that aggravate and relieve the pain are discussed. Specific inquiry regarding radiation of pain proximally in the lower extremity may suggest lumbar disk disease as the cause. Patients active in sports should be questioned regarding significant changes in their level of activity because heel pain often is the result of increased stress on the foot. The cause of the patient's heel pain can usually be determined by palpating the area of maximum tenderness.

Plantar fasciitis, the most common cause of plantar heel pain, usually has an area of maximum tenderness along the plantar medial aspect of the heel, which corresponds to the origin of the plantar fascia at the medial calcaneal tuberosity. In most cases the pain is most severe with the first steps upon arising. The pain is usually aggravated by dorsiflexion of the toes, the so-called windlass stretch, because this applies more tension on the damaged plantar fascia.

Achilles tendonitis/tendinosis typically occurs at one of two discrete sites: at the calcaneal insertion or centered 3–4 cm proximal to the insertion. Insertional Achilles tendinitis/tendinosis is characterized by pain and swelling that is increased by activity. There is usually tenderness in the posterior midline with local increased warmth. Noninsertional Achilles tendinitis/tendinosis is usually associated with a thickened tendon and often quite severe pain to palpation of the thickened area in the midportion of the tendon. Both of these are more degenerative than true inflammatory processes and more properly referred to as tendinosis.

Heel pain can also be caused by inflammation of the retrocalcaneal bursa, which sits between the tendo Achilles and the posterior calcaneus and is often associated with the Haglund heel deformity.

Tarsal tunnel syndrome with involvement of the medial calcaneal branches should be investigated by careful percussion of the posterior tibial nerve. Evidence of degenerative disk disease requires careful testing of motor function and sensation more proximally in the calf.

B. Imaging Studies

Radiographs may demonstrate calcaneal spur formation or calcification at either the insertion of the Achilles tendon or the origin of the plantar fascia. Alternatively, the posterosuperior aspect of the calcaneus may be too prominent and protrude into the Achilles tendon, a condition known as Haglund disease or Haglund deformity, with the symptoms coming from the inflamed retrocalcaneal bursa. A bone scan sometimes reveals increased activity diffusely about the calcaneus, as may be seen in systemic diseases such as Reiter syndrome or a discrete area of uptake as in a stress fracture. MRI scan may help delineate the degree of the Achilles tendon degeneration present in cases of Achilles tendinosis and can help identify rupture of the tendon if this is in question.

Treatment

A. Conservative Management

The conservative management of heel pain depends on the specific cause. Because many causes are related to abnormal stress on the foot, the basic principles involve reducing the stress on the involved area. Activity modification, footwear with a softer, more resilient heel, and use of a soft orthotic device under the longitudinal arch to relieve some of the pressure on the region of pain can be helpful. NSAIDs are often useful as is physical therapy to teach stretching exercises of the Achilles tendon and plantar fascia. Plantar fasciitis is treated initially with stretching exercises, soft cushioned heel shoes, NSAIDS if they are tolerated, and avoidance of strong toe-off activities such as running and jumping. The use of a night splint to help keep the Achilles tendon and plantar fascia stretched often relieves the acute pain patients experience when they first get up in the morning. Patients refractory to treatment may benefit from a steroid injection into the plantar fascia origin, although there is a risk of plantar fascia rupture. Cast immobilization also benefits these refractory patients.

In general, the treatment of heel pain is often prolonged, requiring a great deal of patience on the part of the physician and patient. It is important to explain to the patient the nature of the problem and the fact that it is often a chronic condition requiring many months to resolve.

Achilles tendinosis is treated with stretching exercises, activity modification, NSAIDS, and a heel lift. If these modalities are inadequate, bracing or casting provides more strain relief to the damaged tissue.

B. Surgical Treatment

Patients with plantar fasciitis, in whom symptoms cannot be controlled after 9–12 months of conservative management, may become candidates for surgery. The options include orthotripsy or surgical release of the medial half of the plantar fascial origin. With surgical release, the success rate is approximately 75%. Caution must be exercised with the approach to the medial side of the heel to avoid damage to the medial calcaneal branch of the posterior tibial nerve. Disruption of this nerve causes an area of heel numbness and possibly a troublesome neuroma along the medial side of the heel. An endoscopic approach for plantar fascia release is described in patients who do not have a plantar heel spur that requires removal. Orthotripsy, although less invasive, still has conflicting literature about its effectiveness.

Surgical treatment of Achilles tendinosis is offered if 6–9 months of conservative measures do not help eliminate symptoms. Insertional Achilles tendinosis is treated with debridement of degenerative tendon and excision of bone spurs with repair of the Achilles insertion. If a Haglund deformity is present, it is also resected. Noninsertional Achilles tendinosis is treated with debridement of the degenerative tendon. In either case, if the majority of the tendon is nonviable, it must be repaired, often requiring a graft such as the flexor hallucis longus tendon.

Baxter DE, Pfeffer GB: Treatment of chronic heel pain by surgical release of the first branch of the lateral plantar nerve. Clin Orthop 1992;279:229. [PMID: 1600660]

Boyle RA, Slater GL: Endoscopic plantar fascia release: A case series. Foot Ankle Int 2003;24:176. [PMID: 12627628]

Erdimir A Piazza SJ: Changes in foot loading following plantar fasciotomy: A computer modeling study. J Biomech Eng 2004;126:237. [PMID: 15179854]

Jerosch J et al: Indication, surgical technique and results of endoscopic fascial release in plantar fasciitis (E FRPF). Knee Surg Sports Traumatol Arthrosc 2004;12:471. [PMID: 15088083]

Ogden J et al: Plantar fasciopathy and orthotripsy: The effect of prior cortisone injection. Foot Ankle Int 2005;26:231. [PMID: 15666426]

Williams SK, Brage M: Heel pain-plantar fasciitis and Achilles enthesopathy. Clin Sports Med 2004;23:123. [PMID: 15062587]

Zhu F et al: Chronic plantar fasciitis: Acute changes in the heel after extracorporeal high-energy shock wave therapy—Observations at MR imaging. Radiology 2005;234:206. [PMID: 15564391]

ARTHRODESIS ABOUT THE FOOT & ANKLE

General Considerations

A. Goals of Arthrodesis

Arthrodesis is surgical fixation of a joint to obtain fusion of the joint surfaces. Arthrodesis about the foot and ankle can be effective in achieving the following goals:

1. elimination of joint pain;
2. correction of deformity;
3. stabilization of the foot or ankle when adequate muscle function or ligamentous support is lacking, as in residual poliomyelitis or the acquired flat foot caused by peritalar instability; and
4. restoration of function by salvaging a situation in which no reasonable reconstructive procedure is available, as in fusion of the first metatarsophalangeal joint after failed hallux valgus repair.

B. Principles of Arthrodesis

An arthrodesis about the foot and ankle requires adherence to these general principles:

1. To be effective, the arthrodesis must produce a plantigrade foot.
2. Broad, cancellous bony surfaces must be placed into apposition.
3. The arthrodesis site should be stabilized with rigid internal fixation, preferably with interfragmentary compression.
4. When correcting malalignment of the foot, it is imperative that the hindfoot be placed into 5–7 degrees of valgus and the forefoot in neutral position with regard to abduction, adduction, pronation, and supination.
5. The surgical approaches should be carried out in such a way as to minimize the risk of damage to the nerves.

C. Effects of Arthrodesis on Joint Motion

Following ankle arthrodesis, residual dorsiflexion and plantar flexion movement occurs within the subtalar and transverse tarsal joints, and additional, compensatory motion may develop over time. Arthritic changes in these joints may become symptomatic following ankle arthrodesis, and in time, extension of the fusion may be required.

The subtalar joint and transverse tarsal joints must be viewed as a joint complex similar to the universal joint of a car. Movement in these joints is interrelated. After subtalar arthrodesis, inversion and eversion is lost, but transverse tarsal joint motion is minimally affected. Arthrodesis of the talonavicular joint, however, eliminates most of the subtalar joint motion because rotation must occur around the head of the talus for subtalar motion to occur.

A triple arthrodesis eliminates the subtalar and transverse tarsal joint motion, causing increased stress on the ankle joint and the midtarsal joints distal to the fusion site. A small percentage of patients develop degenerative changes in the ankle joint following triple arthrodesis. It is imperative, therefore, to evaluate the ankle joint carefully prior to carrying out a triple arthrodesis.

Arthrodesis of the tarsometatarsal joints does not significantly affect motion of the foot and ankle, but a certain degree of stiffness is noted through the midtarsal area following this fusion. Fusion of the first metatarsophalangeal joint places added stress on the interphalangeal joint of the great toe, particularly with poor alignment. Although up to 40% of patients may develop degenerative changes in this joint, they are rarely of clinical significance.

D. Disadvantages of Arthrodesis

Although arthrodesis is an effective reconstructive tool, the resulting loss of motion places increased stress on the surrounding joints, making them more prone to developing arthritis or worsening preexisting degenerative changes. Thus, correction of a problem without arthrodesis is preferable whenever possible, such as with an osteotomy, tendon transfer, or both.

Ankle Fusion

A. Indications

The main indications for ankle arthrodesis are the following:

1. arthrosis of the ankle joint usually secondary to a previous ankle fracture, although primary arthrosis does occur;
2. arthritis secondary to rheumatoid disease; and
3. instability with malalignment of the ankle joint as the result of an epiphyseal injury or previous fracture.

B. Technique

The surgical approach preferred by the authors is a transfibular approach (Figure 9–36). The incision begins along the fibula, approximately 10 cm proximal to the tip of the fibula, and is carried distally along the shaft of the fibula and then curves toward the base of the fourth metatarsal. In this way, the incision avoids the sural nerve posteriorly and the superficial peroneal nerve dorsally. The flaps created are full thickness, to lessen the possibility of wound-healing problems. The dissection is carried across the anterior aspect of the ankle joint, to the medial malleolus and along the lateral aspect of the neck of the talus. Posteriorly, the fibula and the posterior aspect of the ankle joint are exposed; distally, the subtalar joint and sinus tarsi area are exposed. The fibula is removed approximately 2 cm proximal to the joint, after which the residual cartilage and subchondral bone are removed from the distal tibia (Figure 9–37). This cut should be made as perpendicular as possible to the long axis of the tibia and should extend to the medial malleolus but not through it. The foot is placed into a plantigrade position and a cut made in the dome of the talus parallel to the cut in the tibia, thereby creating two flat surfaces and correcting any malalignment. At this point, the ankle should be aligned in neutral position, insofar as dorsiflexion and plantar flexion are concerned, and at approximately 5 degrees of valgus. The degree of rotation should be equal to that of the opposite extremity, which is usually 5–10 degrees of external rotation. If the two joint surfaces do not easily oppose each other, it is because the medial malleolus is too long, and the malleolus should be exposed through a dorsomedial incision and the distal centimeter removed.

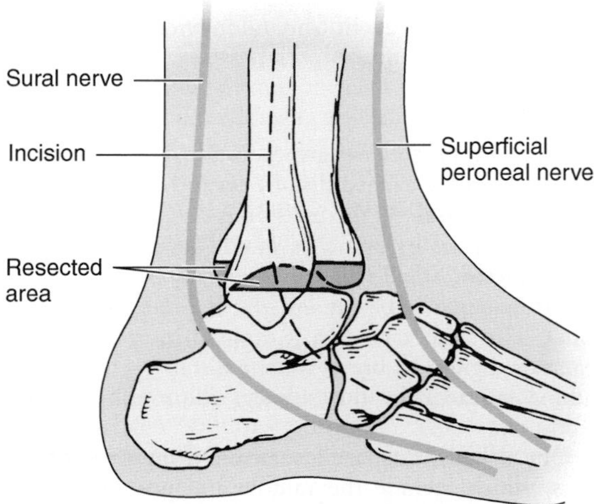

Figure 9–36. **Technique for ankle arthrodesis. Skin incision is placed between superficial peroneal nerve and sural nerve.** (Reproduced, with permission, from Mann RA, Coughlin MJ: *The Video Textbook of Foot and Ankle Surgery.* Medical Video Productions, 1991.)

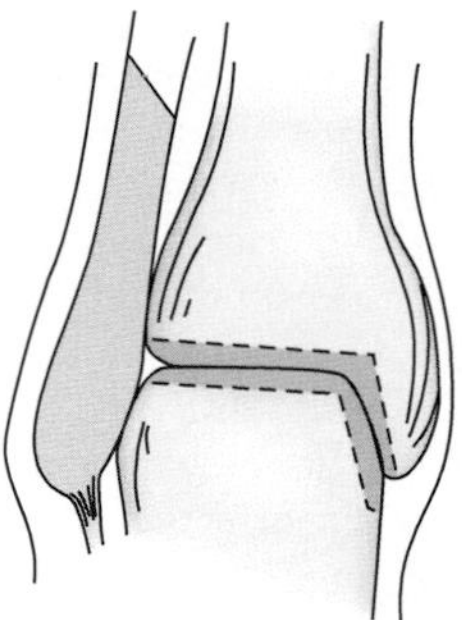

Figure 9–37. **The fibula is excised approximately 2–2.5 cm proximal to the ankle joint, and the distal portion of the tibia is cut, producing a flat cut perpendicular to the long axis of the tibia.** (Reproduced, with permission, from Mann RA, Coughlin MJ: *The Video Textbook of Foot and Ankle Surgery.* Medical Video Productions, 1991.)

The two flat surfaces should now be in total apposition, with little or no pressure being exerted. Temporary fixation is obtained by inserting two 0.062 K-wires. Interfragmentary compression is gained with at least two 6.5-mm cancellous screws. These screws should be placed to gain adequate interfragmentary compression (Figure 9–38). Following insertion of the screws, there should be rigid fixation of the arthrodesis site. Because

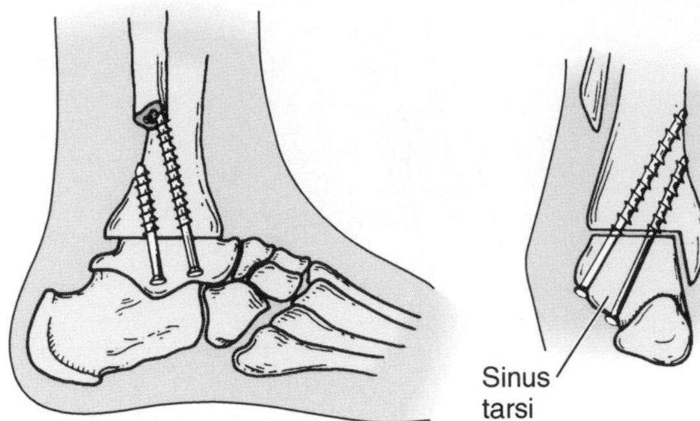

Figure 9–38. **Diagram demonstrating placement of the 6.5-mm screws across the arthrodesis site.** (Reproduced, with permission, from Mann RA, Coughlin MJ: *The Video Textbook of Foot and Ankle Surgery.* Medical Video Productions, 1991.)

the joint surfaces are fully opposed, there is no room for bone grafting. In the immediate postoperative period, a firm compression dressing incorporating plaster splints is applied. After swelling is decreased, a short leg cast is applied and weight bearing is not allowed for 6 weeks. Weight bearing is then allowed with the short leg cast in place for another 6 weeks. Arthrodesis generally occurs following 12 weeks of immobilization.

C. Complications

Nonunion of the ankle joint, although uncommon, does occur. Using the surgical technique described earlier, a fusion rate of 90% can be anticipated. If nonunion occurs, bone grafting and further internal fixation may be required.

Malalignment of the ankle joint with the foot in too much internal rotation is poorly tolerated and often requires revision surgery. Excessive plantar flexion causes a back knee thrust and eventually some knee discomfort; excessive dorsiflexion causes increased stress on the heel (which can usually be treated with adequate padding); varus deformity may cause subtalar joint instability; excessive valgus causes stress on the medial aspect of the knee joint. It is extremely important not to place any pin or screw across the subtalar joint for fear of damaging the posterior facet, which may lead to arthrosis.

D. Special Considerations

Avascular necrosis of the talus requires excision and tibiocalcaneal fusion or a fusion that bypasses the necrotic bone. Bone grafting may also be necessary when attempting to carry out a fusion after a severely comminuted pilon fracture because there are often defects that affect stability because of the previous crushing of cancellous bone.

Total Ankle Arthroplasty

Total ankle arthroplasty is an alternative to ankle arthrodesis for painful arthrosis of the ankle joint. Advantages include maintenance of some ankle joint motion with a more normal gait and thus less stress on adjacent joints. Unfortunately, the procedure is technically difficult with a steep learning curve, there is a higher complication rate than arthrodesis, and the long-term survival rate is unknown. The intermediate-term survival rate of the Agility total ankle reported by Saltzman suggests the outcome is durable in selected patients. Several other prostheses, including the STAR and the HINTEGRA, used primarily in Europe, have reported promising early results. The long-term results are necessary before widespread use is advocated.

Subtalar Arthrodesis

A. Indications

The main indications for subtalar arthrodesis are the following:

1. arthrosis of the subtalar joint, usually following a calcaneal fracture, but occasionally for primary arthrosis of the joint;
2. varus or valgus deformity secondary to RA;
3. varus deformity secondary to residual clubfoot or possibly following compartment syndrome;
4. unstable subtalar joint secondary to poliomyelitis, a neuromuscular disorder, or tendon dysfunction, such as posterior tibial tendon dysfunction; and
5. symptomatic talocalcaneal coalition without secondary changes in the talonavicular or calcaneocuboid joints.

B. Technique

The incision for subtalar arthrodesis begins at the tip of the fibula and is carried distally toward the base of the fourth metatarsal. As the incision is deepened, the sural nerve or one of its branches should be carefully noted and retracted. Small twigs of nerve may be present that unfortunately may be cut and give rise to a painful neuroma. The sinus tarsi area is exposed by reflecting the extensor digitorum brevis muscle distally. The use of a lamina spreader in the subtalar joint enhances the exposure.

The articular cartilage is removed from the joint surfaces, which include the middle and posterior facets. The bony joint surfaces are then deeply feathered or scaled using a small osteotome. These cuts through the subchondral bone greatly enhance the possibility of fusion. The area around the floor of the sinus tarsi and anterior process region can be carefully shaved to obtain local bone graft for the fusion.

The alignment of the subtalar joint is critical. It must be aligned into approximately 5–7 degrees of valgus position, producing a supple transverse tarsal joint. If it is placed in varus position, the foot is stiff and the patient must walk on the side of the foot.

Rigid fixation of the subtalar joint is achieved by using a 7-mm cannulated interfragmentary screw starting at the posterior tip of the calcaneus and passing into the body or neck of the talus. The guide pin is first placed up into the posterior facet, the subtalar joint is then manipulated into proper alignment, and the guide pin is passed into the talus. The alignment of the screw is verified on radiograph, and the screw is inserted.

Following adequate internal fixation, the local bone graft is packed into the sinus tarsi area. Additional bone may be obtained from the area of the medial malleolus, the proximal tibia, or occasionally the iliac crest, although the latter site significantly adds to the morbidity of the procedure.

Postoperatively, a firm compression dressing incorporating plaster splints is applied. A short leg cast is applied, and weight bearing is not allowed for 6 weeks. The cast is changed, and weight bearing is allowed for another 6 weeks. Twelve weeks of immobilization generally achieves an arthrodesis.

C. Complications

Nonunion of the subtalar joint is uncommon, although it can occur. Careful surgical technique and heavy scaling of the joint surfaces can help prevent this complication. If nonunion occurs, bone grafting and added fixation are required to attempt to achieve a solid union.

Misalignment of the subtalar joint may also be a complication. An excessive valgus deformity following subtalar fusion may result in impingement laterally against the fibula or peroneal tendons. It also causes excessive stress along the medial aspect of the midfoot and occasionally the knee joint. A varus deformity of the subtalar joint imparts rigidity to the transverse tarsal joint, resulting in stiffness of the forefoot. This also increases pressure along the lateral aspect of the foot, particularly in the area of the base of the fifth metatarsal.

D. Special Considerations

The patient with RA or posttraumatic complications may have lateral subluxation of the calcaneus in relation to the talus, which usually requires CT scanning for identification. The calcaneus must be displaced medially during surgery to align it with the lateral aspect of the talus and place it under the tibia in a proper weight-bearing position. If the calcaneus is fused with significant lateral deviation, the abnormal alignment places added stress on the ankle and midfoot region.

Special attention to the peroneal tendons is necessary when a subtalar arthrodesis is done to correct an old calcaneal fracture. Protrusion of the lateral wall of the body of the calcaneus from the healed fracture results in impingement on the peroneal tendons beneath the fibula. This protrusion must be carefully excised when the subtalar fusion is carried out, so the lateral aspect of the talus and calcaneus are in line. Further, the peroneal tendon sheath should be dissected subperiosteally off the calcaneus to provide tendon sheath and protect the peroneal tendons from the raw, bony surface of the calcaneus.

Occasionally a bone block distraction arthrodesis of the subtalar joint is performed in cases of severe deformity after a calcaneus fracture. If the talus assumes a horizontal position because of flattening of Böhler's angle, it can cause limited ankle joint dorsiflexion. Placing a tricortical block of iliac crest into the posterior facet of the subtalar joint helps improve the overall alignment of the hind foot and regain ankle joint dorsiflexion.

Talonavicular Arthrodesis

A. Indications

Talonavicular arthrodesis is indicated in the following conditions:

1. posttraumatic injury, RA, or primary arthrosis;
2. unstable talonavicular joint secondary to rupture of the posterior tibial tendon and the peritalar ligaments and RA; and
3. double or triple arthrodesis of the hindfoot.

B. Technique

The talonavicular joint is approached through a medial or dorsomedial incision that starts in the region of the naviculocuneiform joint and extends to the neck of the talus. The soft tissues are stripped from around the joint and the articular cartilage removed with a curet or curved osteotome. Distraction of the joint by placing a towel clip into the navicular often facilitates exposure and debridement of the joint. Correct alignment of the talonavicular joint is extremely critical because this fusion essentially eliminates motion in the subtalar joint. The fusion position of the subtalar joint is 3–5 degrees of valgus with the forefoot in a plantigrade position (Figure 9–39). After the foot is properly aligned to correspond to the opposite foot, fixation of the joint is carried out. Proper alignment of this joint is particularly critical when treating the laterally subluxed talonavicular joint in the patient with a ruptured posterior tibial tendon. The internal fixation is carried out by using interfragmentary compression with a single large screw (6.5 mm), two smaller screws (4.0 mm), or multiple staples.

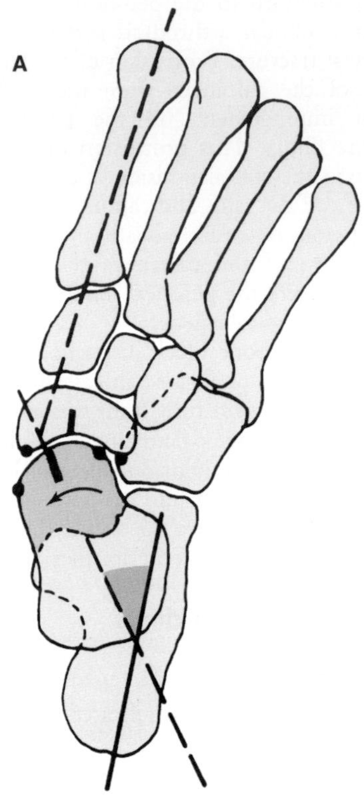

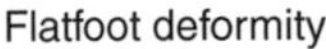

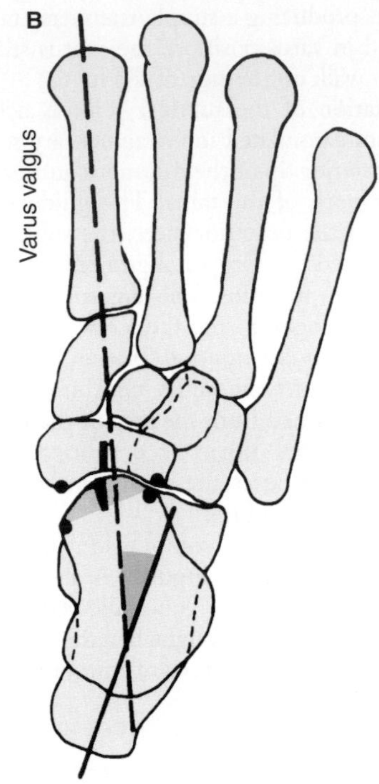

Figure 9–39. Talonavicular fusion. **A:** Changes that occur in the talonavicular joint with a flatfoot deformity. Note that the head of the talus deviates medially as the forefoot deviates laterally into abduction. **B:** The forefoot was brought into adduction so the navicular is once again centered over the head of the talus. (Reproduced, with permission, from Mann RA, Coughlin MJ: *The Video Textbook of Foot and Ankle Surgery*. Medical Video Productions, 1991.)

Postoperatively the patient is immobilized in a non–weight-bearing cast for 6 weeks followed by a weight-bearing cast for an additional 6 weeks.

The talonavicular joint has a relatively high incidence of nonunion, which is probably the result of the difficulty in exposing the joint. If the joint is also approached medially to gain additional exposure, the surfaces can be well scaled, and the fusion rate should approach 90%.

C. Complications

Complications of nonunion and misalignment are similar to those discussed for subtalar joint fusion.

D. Special Considerations

An isolated talonavicular joint fusion usually produces a satisfactory result, particularly in relatively sedentary patients older than 50 years. In younger, more active individuals with no other affliction (eg, RA), consideration should be given to including the calcaneocuboid joint at the same time to obtain a more stable transverse tarsal joint and enhance the fusion of the talonavicular joint through added stability.

Double Arthrodesis (Calcaneocuboid & Talonavicular Joints)

A. Indications

Double arthrodesis today is a procedure that provides the same degree of stability to the foot as a triple arthrodesis (Figure 9–40). By locking the transverse tarsal joint (calcaneocuboid and talonavicular), further subtalar motion is prevented because these three joints function together. This procedure is also indicated in the younger, active patient in whom an isolated talonavicular fusion is contemplated because it gives added stability to the foot.

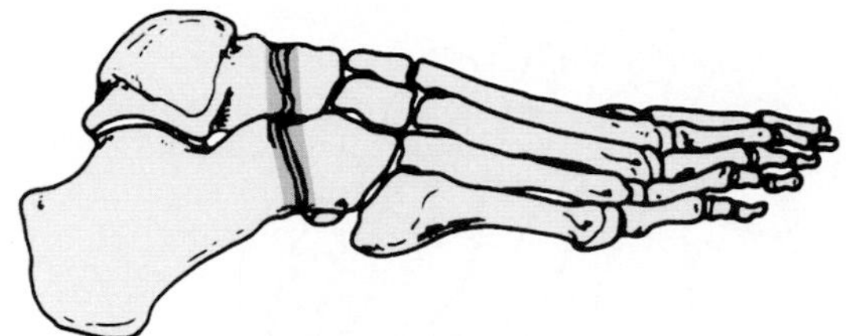

Figure 9–40. **Double arthrodesis consisting of a talonavicular and calcaneocuboid fusion.** (Reproduced, with permission, from Mann RA, Coughlin MJ: *The Video Textbook of Foot and Ankle Surgery.* Medical Video Productions, 1991.)

Indications for double arthrodesis are as follows:

1. arthrosis of the talonavicular and calcaneocuboid joints (eg, following trauma);
2. unstable talonavicular and calcaneocuboid joint following rupture of the posterior tibial tendon or neuromuscular disease when a flexible subtalar joint is present; and
3. arthrosis of the talonavicular joint or calcaneocuboid joint in an active individual, usually younger than 50 years of age, to give the midfoot a greater degree of stability.

B. Technique

The talonavicular joint is approached through a medial or dorsomedial incision, as previously described, and the calcaneocuboid joint is approached through the same incision along the lateral side of the foot as described for subtalar fusion. Once these joints are exposed, the joint surfaces are denuded of articular cartilage and the subchondral bone heavily feathered.

The alignment when carrying out a double arthrodesis is extremely critical because once this fusion is achieved, the subtalar joint or the transverse tarsal joint no longer move. Therefore, the foot must be placed into a plantigrade position prior to the fixation of the arthrodesis site. The desired position is 5 degrees of valgus of the calcaneus, neutral abduction and adduction of the transverse tarsal joint, and correction of any forefoot varus that is present. This alignment creates a plantigrade foot. The fixation of the talonavicular joint is done first with the insertion of a screw (6.5 mm) or screws (4 mm) or possibly the use of multiple staples. The calcaneocuboid joint is then fixed the same way. Postoperative care is the same as for other foot fusions.

C. Complications

Complications of nonunion and malalignment are similar to those discussed for subtalar joint fusion.

Triple Arthrodesis

The triple arthrodesis is a fusion of the talonavicular, calcaneocuboid, and subtalar joints (Figure 9–41). In the past, it was the procedure of choice for all hindfoot problems, before isolated fusions became more accepted. Now, this procedure is still commonly used when limited fusions are inadequate.

A. Indications

Indications for triple arthrodesis are as follows:

1. arthrosis secondary to trauma involving the subtalar, talonavicular, or calcaneocuboid joints;
2. arthrosis or instability of the talonavicular or calcaneocuboid joints in association with a fixed deformity of the subtalar joint;
3. instability of the foot secondary to posterior tibial tendon dysfunction with a fixed subtalar joint that cannot be realigned by a double arthrodesis;
4. unstable hindfoot secondary to poliomyelitis, nerve injury, or RA;
5. symptomatic, unresectable calcaneonavicular bar; and
6. malalignment of the hindfoot secondary to trauma such as a crush injury or compartment syndrome.

B. Technique

The triple arthrodesis is carried out as previously described for subtalar fusion and talonavicular fusion. The foot is fixed after manipulation back into a plantigrade position (3–5 degrees of valgus of the subtalar joint), neutral position as far as abduction and adduction of the transverse tarsal joint, and correction of forefoot varus. Postoperative care is the same as for subtalar fusion.

C. Complications

The main complication is failure of fusion of one of the joints, which is uncommon, because the successful

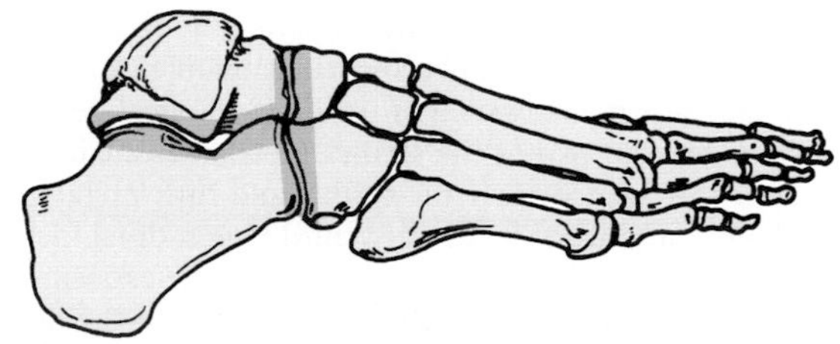

Figure 9–41. **Diagram of a triple arthrodesis.** (Reproduced, with permission, from Mann RA, Coughlin MJ: *The Video Textbook of Foot and Ankle Surgery.* Medical Video Productions, 1991.)

fusion rate exceeds 90%. The talonavicular joint is most likely to have nonunion. Malalignment of the foot or forefoot may require revision and technically is a difficult procedure. The sural nerve may become entrapped or disrupted through the lateral approach.

Tarsometatarsal Arthrodesis

Arthrodesis in the tarsometatarsal area may involve a single tarsometatarsal joint, usually the first joint, or multiple joints. The fusion mass not infrequently extends proximally to include the intertarsal bones and sometimes even the naviculocuneiform joints. A careful determination of the involved joints is important when considering a tarsometatarsal fusion for a patient with posttraumatic disorders. At times, in addition to the plain radiograph, a CT scan and bone scan may be necessary to help define the involved area precisely.

A. Indications

The indications for a tarsometatarsal fusion are as follows:

1. hypermobility of the first metatarsocuneiform joint associated with a hallux valgus deformity in a small percentage of patients with a bunion deformity;
2. arthrosis involving one or more of the tarsometatarsal joints either resulting from trauma or as a primary disease process; and
3. arthrosis associated with a deformity resulting from an old Lisfranc fracture-dislocation.

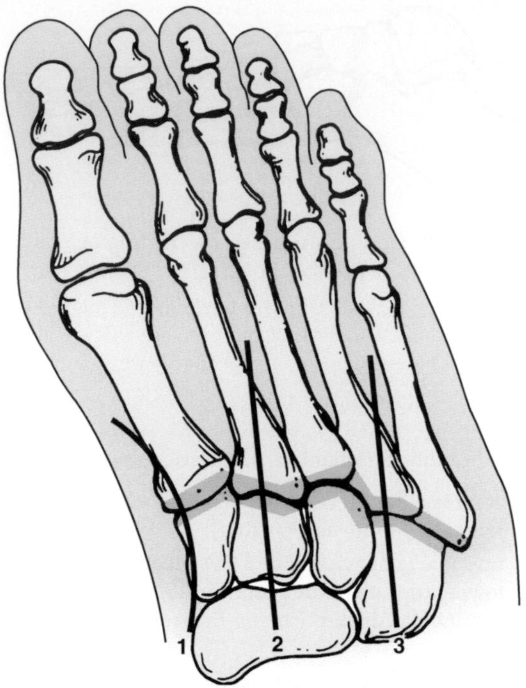

Figure 9–42. Longitudinal incisions used for a tarsometatarsal arthrodesis. (Reproduced, with permission, from Mann RA, Coughlin MJ: *The Video Textbook of Foot and Ankle Surgery*. Medical Video Productions, 1991.)

B. Technique

The surgical approach to the first metatarsocuneiform joint is through a dorsomedial longitudinal incision to expose the joint. If multiple joints are involved, the second incision is centered over the second metatarsal, through which the lateral side of the first and all of the second and third metatarsocuneiform joints can be adequately viewed (Figure 9–42). The incision must be sufficiently long to permit adequate exposure of the joints and must be extended proximally if the naviculocuneiform joints are going to be fused as well. Cautious dissection is necessary because there are numerous superficial nerves as well as the neurovascular bundle (dorsalis pedis and superficial branch of the deep peroneal nerve) passing over the area of the second metatarsocuneiform joint in this approach. If the fourth and fifth metatarsocuboid joints are to be fused, a third longitudinal incision is made over this area to enable adequate exposure. The articular cartilage is carefully removed from the tarsometatarsal and intertarsal joints, depending on the extent of the fusion mass. The bones are heavily feathered to create a good environment for healing. If a deformity is present (usually an abduction deformity of the foot or possibly dorsiflexion), it should be corrected. The first metatarsocuneiform joint is aligned and fixed using 4-mm cancellous screws or a dorsomedial plate. Interfragmentary longitudinal compression of the other joints is obtained to prevent possible nonunion. The screw pattern found to be most useful for the first metatarsocuneiform joint is one brought from the dorsal aspect of the cuneiform directed distally, and a second screw from the dorsal aspect of the metatarsal base directed proximally, crossing the metatarsocuneiform joint. Care must be taken to also correct any dorsiflexion or abduction deformity that is present.

Postoperatively, the joint is placed in a short leg, non–weight-bearing cast for 6 weeks, and then in a weight-bearing cast for another 6 weeks.

C. Complications

The possibility of nonunion exists, but with interfragmentary compression the risk is minimized. If nonunion occurs, bone grafting may be required as well as improved internal fixation. When multiple tarsometatarsal joints are fused, a moderate amount of swelling and tension is placed against the incisions. It is critical postoperatively to use a compression dressing to minimize the risk of swelling and prevent possible wound sloughing. If sloughing occurs, it must be treated appropriately, and, occasionally, skin grafting is required.

A tarsometatarsal fusion involving multiple joints may cause a plantar callus because one of the metatarsals was placed in a position of too much plantar flexion. Osteotomy at the base of the metatarsal may be necessary to realign the metatarsal.

Staples should be avoided as a means of internal fixation of the tarsometatarsal joints because they have a tendency to cause dorsiflexion of the metatarsals, which could result in transfer pressure problems under the uninvolved metatarsal heads.

First Metatarsophalangeal Joint Arthrodesis

See the discussion of hallux valgus at the beginning of the chapter.

Interphalangeal Joint Arthrodesis (Hallux Arthrodesis)

A. Indications

Interphalangeal joint arthrodesis is usually indicated for the following problems:

1. arthrosis, usually secondary to trauma or occasionally following a first metatarsophalangeal joint arthrodesis; and
2. stabilization of the interphalangeal joint when carrying out a transfer of the extensor hallucis longus into the neck of the first metatarsal (first toe Jones procedure).

B. Technique

The interphalangeal joint is approached through a dorsal transverse incision centered over the joint. An ellipse of skin is usually removed, exposing the ends of the involved joints. Using a small power saw, the end of the distal portion of the proximal phalanx and the proximal portion of the distal phalanx are removed, placing the distal phalanx into approximately 5–7 degrees of plantar flexion and 3–4 degrees of valgus position. Internal fixation is achieved by using a longitudinal screw (4 mm) or crossed K-wires, or both. A postoperative shoe is used, with weight bearing allowed but avoiding the toe-off phase of gait until fusion occurs, usually in 8 weeks.

C. Complications

Nonunion of interphalangeal joint fusion is uncommon. If it does occur, it often is asymptomatic and does not require treatment. If it is symptomatic, usually the fusion needs to be revised because the area is too small for adequate bone grafting.

Buchner M, Sabo D: Ankle fusion attributable to posttraumatic arthrosis: A long-term followup of 48 patients. Clin Orthop 2003;406:155. [PMID: 12579015]

Buck P et al: The optimum position of arthrodesis of the ankle. J Bone Joint Surg Am 1987;69:1052. [PMID: 3654697]

Clain MR, Baxter DE: Simultaneous calcanealcuboid and talonavicular fusion: Long term follow up study. J Bone Joint Surg Am 1994;76:133. [PMID: 8300657]

Harper MC: Talonavicular arthrodesis for the acquired flat foot in the adult. Clin Orthop 1999;365:65. [PMID: 10627687]

Hintermann B et al: The HINTEGRA ankle: rationale and short-term results of 122 consecutive ankles. Clin Orthop 2004; 424:57. [PMID: 15241144]

Knecht S et al: The Agility Total Ankle Arthroplasty J Bone Joint Surg AM 2004;86:1161. [PMID: 15173288]

Kofoed H: Scandinavian Total Ankle Replacement (STAR). Clin Orthop 2004;424:73. [PMID: 15241146]

Kofoed H, Sorensen TS: Ankle arthroplasty for rheumatoid arthritis and osteoarthritis. J Bone Joint Surg Br 1998;80;328.

Komenda GA et al: Results of arthrodesis of the tarsometatarsal joints after traumatic injury. J Bone Joint Surg 1996; 78:1665. [PMID: 8934480]

Mann RA, Beaman DN, Horton GA: Isolated subtalar arthrodesis. Foot Ankle Int 1998;19:511. [PMID: 9728697]

Rosenfeld FF, Budgen SA, Saxby TS: Triple arthrodesis: Is bone grafting necessary? The results of 100 consecutive cases. J Bone Joint Surg Br 2005;87:175. [PMID: 15736738]

Robinson JF, Murphy GA: Arthrodesis as salvage for calcaneal malunions. Foot Ankle Clin 2002;7:107. [PMID: 12380384]

Winson IG, Robinson DE, Allen PE: Arthroscopic ankle arthrodesis. J Bone Joint Surg Br 2005;87:343. [PMID: 15773643]

CONGENITAL FLATFOOT

Congenital flatfoot is the term used to describe a flatfoot present since birth. The condition may not be apparent during the early years of life but is usually identified toward the end of the first or during the second decade. The typical asymptomatic flexible flatfoot is probably a normal variant of the longitudinal arch. This deformity must be differentiated from the symptomatic flexible or more rigid flatfoot, which usually becomes symptomatic in the early teen years and is often caused by a tarsal coalition. These individuals have a fairly flexible foot until adolescence, when the foot often becomes somewhat more rigid and symptomatic.

The patient with a tarsal coalition frequently presents with a peroneal spastic flatfoot, usually around the age of 10–12 years. The theory is that the foot is locked in a valgus position by the peroneal muscle spasm that is trying to immobilize the painful peritalar joints. A tarsal coalition is the union of two or more tarsal bones, usually occurring between the calcaneus and the navicular or between the talus and the calcaneus. This process is a congenital failure of segmentation between the bones of the hindfoot. Coalitions are usually not symptomatic until adolescence, with symptoms brought on by increasing stiffness of the hindfoot as the cartilaginous coalition begins to ossify. Flatfoot associated with an accessory navicular bone usually becomes symptomatic in the early to mid teenage years and may be unilateral or bilateral. Residual congenital deformity from conditions such as clubfoot or congenital vertical talus are present from birth and discussed in Chapter 11, Pediatric Orthopedic Surgery.

The patient with generalized dysplasia, such as Marfan syndrome or Ehlers-Danlos syndrome, may present with flatfoot. A generalized ligamentous laxity is present from the time of birth, and the diagnosis is usually already known.

Clinical Findings

A. Symptoms and Signs

The clinical evaluation begins with the patient in a standing position. In all cases of congenital flatfoot, the longitudinal arch flattens when the patient is standing. In the case of tarsal coalition with peroneal spastic flatfoot, the calcaneus is in a severe fixed valgus position. A tarsal coalition or an accessory navicular may be unilateral, as well as the residuals of a congenital deformity such as clubfoot or congenital vertical talus. The symptomatic and asymptomatic flexible flatfoot and the generalized dysplasias are present bilaterally.

The physical examination of these patients is extremely important. The asymptomatic flexible flatfoot usually demonstrates a satisfactory ROM and no contracture of the Achilles tendon. The symptomatic flexible flatfoot, however, almost invariably demonstrates an equinus contracture. To test adequately for tightness of the Achilles tendon, the head of the talus is covered with the navicular, after which the foot is brought up into dorsiflexion with the knee extended. If the foot is brought into dorsiflexion, permitting lateral subluxation of the talonavicular joint, the examiner often is fooled into thinking that dorsiflexion is adequate when indeed it is not.

The patient with tarsal coalition usually demonstrates restricted hindfoot motion secondary to peroneal spasm and to the cartilaginous or bony bar. The peroneal tendons can actually be felt to be bow strung behind the fibula, not permitting any passive or active inversion of the subtalar joint to occur. On occasion, clonus can be elicited. As a rule, stressing of these joints causes the patient increased discomfort. In flatfoot associated with an accessory navicular, pain is present over the prominence. Frequently, stressing of the posterior tibial tendon aggravates the condition. The patient with residual congenital deformity often demonstrates a certain degree of stiffness of the foot and, not infrequently, varying degrees of deformity of the remainder of the foot. The patient with generalized dysplasia demonstrates marked hypermobility of all the joints, with no contractures whatsoever.

B. Imaging Studies

The radiographic evaluation is useful in differentiating the various types of flatfoot. In almost all cases, the lateral view shows a lack of normal dorsiflexion pitch of the calcaneus, which is approximately 20 degrees or more. In symptomatic flexible flatfoot, the calcaneus may even be in a mild degree of equinus position. On the lateral radiograph, a line drawn through the long axis of the talus and first metatarsal demonstrates an angle of more than 30 degrees in severe flatfoot, 15–30 degrees in moderate flatfoot, and 0–15 degrees in mild flatfoot (Figure 9–43).

The calcaneonavicular coalition is best observed on an oblique radiograph and identified as a bridge from

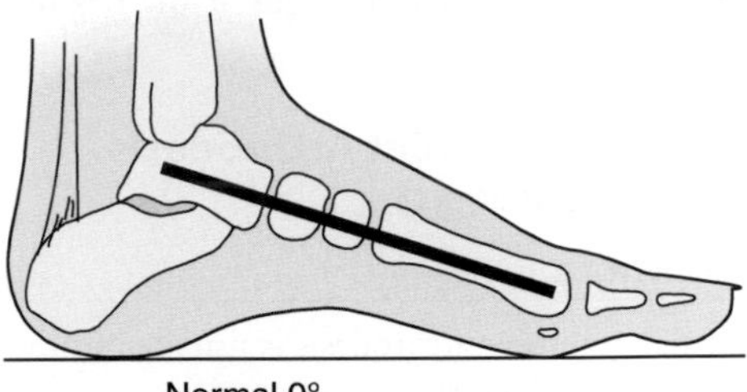

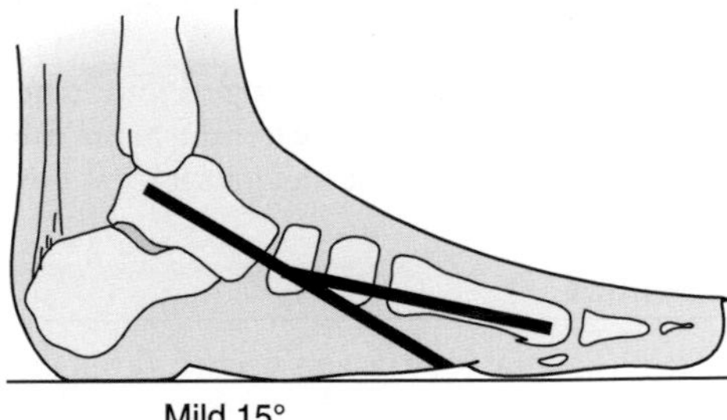

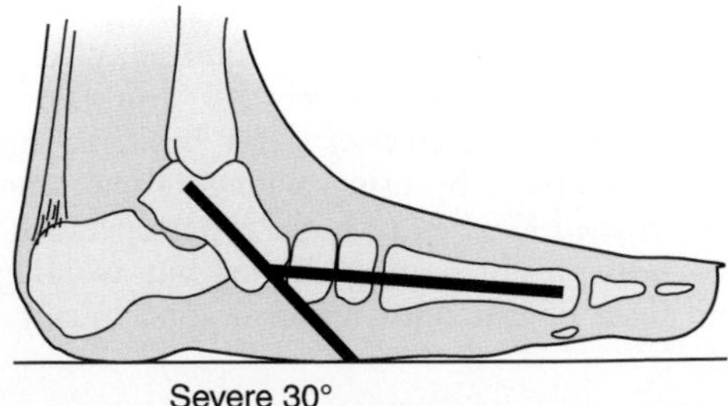

Figure 9–43. **Measurement of flatfoot deformity by using the lateral talometatarsal angle: 0 degrees, normal; 1–15 degrees, mild; 16–30 degrees, moderate; greater than 30 degrees, severe.** (Reproduced, with permission, from Bordelon RL: Correction of hyper mobile flatfoot in children by molded insert. Foot Ankle 1980;1:143.)

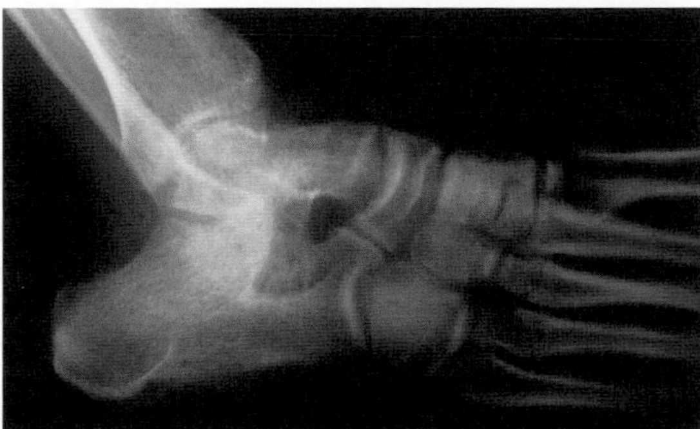

Figure 9–44. **Oblique view of the foot at 45-degree angle demonstrating calcaneonavicular coalition.** (Reproduced, with permission, from Mann RA, Coughlin MJ: *Surgery of the Foot and Ankle,* 6th ed. St. Louis: Mosby-Year Book, 1993.)

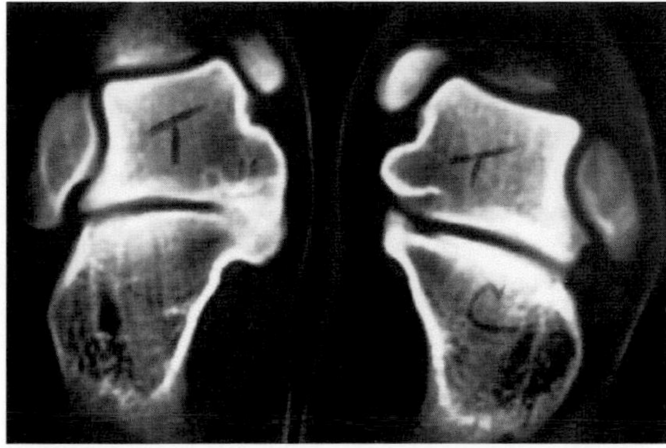

Figure 9–45. **CT scan demonstrating osseous coalition on one side (left) and fibrous coalition on the other (right).** (Reproduced, with permission, from Mann RA, Coughlin MJ, eds: *Surgery of the Foot and Ankle,* 6th ed. Mosby-Year Book, 1993.)

the anterior process of the calcaneus to the inferior lateral aspect of the navicular (Figure 9–44). The subtalar or talocalcaneal bar is best demonstrated on a CT scan taken in the coronal plane (Figure 9–45). Flatfoot associated with an accessory navicular demonstrates the accessory bone along the medial side of the navicular, but occasionally a medial oblique view is necessary to outline the size of the fragment (Figure 9–46). In a patient with a residual congenital deformity, such as a clubfoot or congenital vertical talus, the changes about the foot are often sufficient to make the diagnosis fairly obvious. The patient with generalized dysplasia often demonstrates complete collapse of the longitudinal arch.

Treatment

A. Conservative Management

Conservative management is undertaken for congenital flatfoot deformities. A longitudinal arch support may benefit the patient but is usually not necessary for the

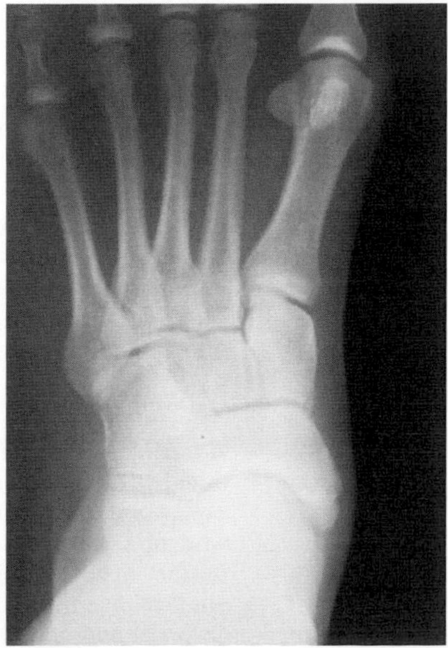

A

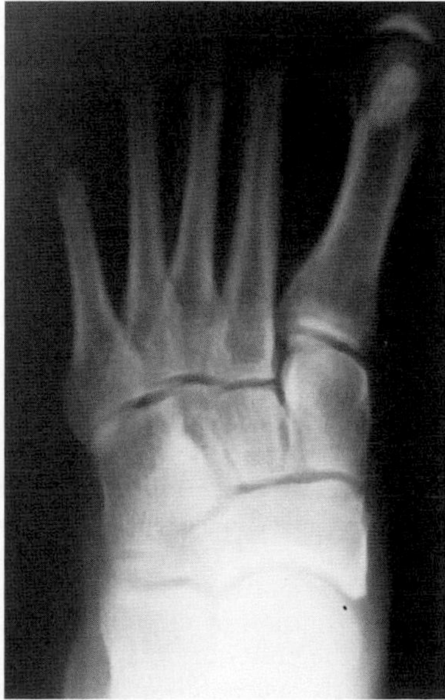

B

Figure 9–46. **Large accessory navicular. A: Preoperatively, a cartilaginous plate is loose and painful. B: One year postoperatively.** (Reproduced, with permission, from Mann RA, Coughlin MJ, eds: *Surgery of the Foot and Ankle,* 6th ed. St. Louis: Mosby-Year Book, 1993.)

asymptomatic flexible flatfoot. For symptomatic flexible flatfoot, a semirigid longitudinal arch support and Achilles stretching exercises may be of some benefit.

The tarsal coalition can be treated conservatively with a short leg walking cast, followed by a polypropylene AFO or a University of California Biomechanics Laboratory (UCBL) insert. If adequate pain relief is achieved, further treatment is not necessary. Flatfoot with an accessory navicular may respond to modification of the shoe to relieve some of the pressure from the involved area. Occasionally, the use of a longitudinal arch support relieves the pressure.

Residual flatfoot resulting from congenital problems can be treated with an AFO or UCBL insert if symptomatic. The patient with generalized dysplasia usually does not require any treatment at all.

B. Surgical Management

Surgical procedures are never appropriate for asymptomatic flatfoot. Symptomatic flexible or semiflexible flatfoot occasionally is treated surgically, particularly if equinus contracture is observed after 5 or 6 years of age. A significant equinus contracture may benefit from lengthening of the Achilles tendon. A lateral column lengthening procedure, such as an Evans calcaneal osteotomy, is indicated in cases of symptomatic flexible flatfoot that fail conservative management. This procedure helps correct heel valgus and forefoot abduction and should be done as late into growth as possible to avoid disturbing open growth centers. A triple arthrodesis should only rarely be carried out because it leaves a young patient with a very stiff foot.

A tarsal coalition that does not respond to conservative management may require resection. The surgical approach to the calcaneonavicular bar is identical to that of the subtalar joint. The bar is carefully outlined and then resected in its entirety. Talocalcaneal coalitions are resectable throughout the adolescent years, if less than 20% of the posterior facet of the subtalar joint is involved or if the coalition is confined only to the middle facet. More extensive involvement of the subtalar joint in an adolescent or any bar in an adult patient is an indication for subtalar arthrodesis. The approach is through a medial incision centered over the middle facet, and caution is taken to carefully reflect the tendons and posterior tibial nerve. The extent of the coalition is identified, and it is resected to expose the area of normal-appearing articular cartilage. Bone wax is applied to the edges or a free fat graft is inserted to prevent reformation of the bar. Flatfoot associated with an accessory navicular may require excision of the accessory navicular and plication of the posterior tibial tendon (Kidner procedure). This fairly successful operation is usually carried out during the late adolescent years.

Residual congenital deformity or generalized dysplasias usually do not require surgical management. In severe cases, a triple arthrodesis is indicated after the foot has matured.

Coleman S: *Complex Foot Deformities in Children.* Lea and Febiger, 1983.

Frischhut B et al: Foot deformities in adolescents and young adults with spina bifida. J Pediatr Orthop B 2000;9:161. [PMID: 10904902]

Giannini S et al: Operative treatment of flatfoot with talocalcaneal coalition. Clin Orthop 2003;411:178. [PMID: 12782874]

Gonzalez P, Kumar SJ: Calcaneonavicular coalition treated by resection and interposition of the extensor digitorum brevis muscle. J Bone Joint Surg 1990;72:71. [PMID: 2104855]

Varner KE, Michelson JD: Tarsal coalition in adults. Foot Ankle Int 2000;21:669. [PMID: 10966365]

ACQUIRED FLATFOOT DEFORMITY

Acquired flatfoot deformity is a condition affecting a foot that at one time had a normal functioning longitudinal arch. Over time, the arch progressively flattens, often causing the foot to become symptomatic. This deformity is different from congenital flatfoot deformity, present since birth. Acquired flatfoot deformity in the adult may be caused by the following conditions:

1. posterior tibial tendon dysfunction;
2. arthrosis of the tarsometatarsal joints, which may be primary or secondary to a previous Lisfranc fracture or dislocation;
3. Charcot changes in the midfoot resulting from a peripheral neuropathy; or
4. talonavicular collapse resulting from trauma or RA.

Acquired flatfoot deformities are complex deformities that affect different areas of the midfoot and hindfoot. The deformities may include dorsal subluxation of the talonavicular joint and tarsometatarsal joints, abduction of the forefoot, valgus deformity of the hindfoot, or all three. The extent of the deformity varies widely and is usually progressive. Depending on the etiology, acquired flatfoot deformity may affect a patient bilaterally.

Clinical Findings

A. Symptoms and Signs

A careful history is important to help distinguish among differing causes of acquired flatfoot deformity. Usually, no specific traumatic event is recalled by the patient who presents with dysfunction of the posterior tibial tendon. In approximately half of patients with tarsometatarsal joint arthrosis, a Lisfranc fracture-dislocation has occurred, whereas the other half has primary arthrosis. The patient with Charcot foot usually gives a relevant history of the cause of the peripheral neuropathy, such as diabetes. The patient with collapse of the talonavicular joint gives a history of prior trauma to the talus or navicular or has RA, which causes disruption of the spring ligament complex.

The physical examination begins by observing the foot with the patient standing, observing for unilateral or bilateral flattening of the longitudinal arch. Varying degrees of abduction of the forefoot and hindfoot valgus should also be evaluated.

The patient with posterior tibial tendon dysfunction demonstrates little or no active inversion strength. Usually, the posterior tibial tendon is thick and swollen and there is increased warmth and pain to palpation over the tendon sheath. When the patient is asked to stand on tiptoe, the involved calcaneus remains in valgus position rather than inverting, as normally occurs. When the patient is viewed from the posterior aspect, more toes are visible laterally on the involved foot than the uninvolved foot, commonly known as the "too many toes sign."

Arthrosis of the tarsometatarsal joints creates a deformity of abduction of the forefoot with varying degrees of dorsiflexion, giving rise to a rather prominent medial cuneiform. Not infrequently, palpable osteophytes are present on the dorsal and plantar aspect of the tarsometatarsal joints.

A Charcot foot presents with varying degrees of swelling and deformity. In the early stages, the foot demonstrates generalized swelling and increased warmth, with loss of sensation in a stocking-glove distribution. Deformity may vary from a mild flat foot to a severe rocker-bottom deformity. It is important to palpate for bony prominences on the medial and plantar aspects of the foot that make it at risk for ulcerations.

In the patient with RA, most of the changes occur within the talonavicular joint. In this case, the head of the talus is often palpable on the plantar medial aspect of the foot. When the subtalar joint is more involved, a fixed hindfoot valgus deformity is usually present as well.

The posttraumatic deformity may vary, depending on precisely which joints are involved. If trauma led to a collapse of the navicular, the longitudinal arch is flattened with little forefoot abduction, and the head of the talus is often palpable on the plantar medial aspect of the foot. There is usually little or no motion in the hindfoot and midfoot joints.

B. Imaging Studies

Radiographs usually differentiate the cause of the problem. In the patient with posterior tibial tendon dysfunction, there is sagging of the talonavicular joint and abduction of the navicular on the head of the talus. The patient with tarsometatarsal joint arthrosis demonstrates typical degenerative changes at the affected joints, along with varying degrees of lateral and dorsal subluxation of the joints. Patients with Charcot foot demonstrate characteristic changes seen in a neuropathic joint, including dramatic bone destruction and joint dislocations (Figure 9–47). The patient with RA demonstrates the typical destructive changes observed with this disease process, with joint space narrowing but little osteophyte formation.

Treatment

A. Conservative Management

Conservative management is aimed at providing support to the longitudinal arch and ankle with a polypropylene AFO. The orthosis must be shaped to accommodate any prominences that might be present. Unfortunately, these prominences present the potential for skin breakdown, particularly in the neuropathic foot. A rocker-bottom-type shoe with an adequate toe box is sometimes indicated to give the patient a smoother gait pattern.

B. Surgical Treatment

The surgical management of these various conditions is specific for each problem. Posterior tibial tendon dysfunction with a satisfactory ROM of the joints of the hindfoot and midfoot can be treated with reconstruction of the posterior tibial tendon, using a flexor digitorum longus tendon transfer. A calcaneal osteotomy is performed as well, if a significant valgus deformity of the heel is present. Alternatively, a lateral column lengthening, consisting of a calcaneal-cuboid distraction arthrodesis, can be used to correct a flexible flat foot with significant abduction of the forefoot. When a fixed deformity is present in the hindfoot or forefoot, a triple arthrodesis is indicated.

The patient with Charcot foot is treated in a short leg cast until the acute process subsides, after which a polypropylene AFO is used. Occasionally, a bony prom-

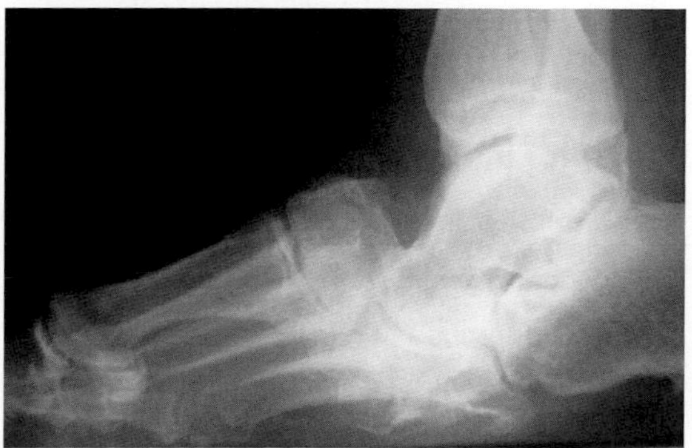

Figure 9–47. Charcot midfoot changes resulting in joint dislocations and a rocker-bottom deformity of the foot.

inence that continues to cause skin breakdown may be excised to permit the patient to use an AFO. In extreme rocker-bottom deformities, midfoot correction with an osteotomy may be required. The rheumatoid patient usually requires stabilization of the involved area with an isolated talonavicular fusion if little deformity is present, or a triple arthrodesis if there is a hindfoot or midfoot deformity.

The posttraumatic foot with involvement of the talonavicular joint requires a triple arthrodesis. The fusion may need to be extended distally to include the naviculocuneiform joints if arthrosis is present at these joints.

The patient with arthrosis of the tarsometatarsal joints responds well to surgical management by realigning the foot and carrying out arthrodesis of the involved joints.

Castro MD: Arthrodesis of the navicular. Foot Ankle Clin 2004;9(1):73. [PMID: 15062215]

Guyton GP et al: Flexor digitorum longus transfer and medial displacement calcaneal osteotomy for posterior tibial tendon dysfunction: A middle-term clinical follow-up. Foot Ankle Int 2001;22:627. [PMID: 11527022]

Mann RA, Thompson FM: Rupture of the posterior tibial tendon causing flatfoot: Surgical treatment. J Bone Joint Surg Am 1985;67:556. [PMID: 3980501]

Thomas RL et al: Preliminary results comparing two methods of lateral column lengthening. Foot Ankle Int 2001;22:107. [PMID: 11249219]

Trepman E et al. Current topics review: Charcot neuroarthropathy of the foot and ankle. Foot Ankle Int 2005;26(1):46. [PMID: 15680119]

Trnka HJ: Dysfunction of the tendon of tibialis posterior. J Bone Joint Surg Br 2004;86(7):939. [PMID: 15446514]

CAVUS FOOT

Cavus foot deformity is characterized by an abnormal elevation of the longitudinal arch, with resulting decrease in the plantar weight-bearing area and stress concentrated on the metatarsal heads. The condition may be aggravated by clawing of the toes, further reducing the forefoot weight-bearing area. Generalized stiffness of the joints is common, causing the patient to avoid prolonged use of the foot.

Etiologic Findings

The various causes of cavus foot deformity include the following:

1. anterior horn cell disease, such as poliomyelitis, diastematomyelia, and spinal cord tumor;
2. nerve disorders, such as Charcot-Marie-Tooth disease and spinal dysraphism;
3. muscular diseases, such as muscular dystrophy;
4. long tract and central diseases, such as Friedreich ataxia and cerebral palsy;
5. idiopathic conditions, such as residual clubfoot, arthrogryposis, and cavus foot of undetermined cause; and
6. posttraumatic disorders following injuries, such as compartment syndrome or crush injury.

Anatomy

Cavus foot deformity is extremely variable in its presentation, from mild to extremely severe degree of cavus. The types of deformities can be classified based on the localizing of the area of deformity:

1. Posterior cavus deformity—This deformity mainly involves the calcaneus, which has a dorsiflexion pitch angle of greater than 40 degrees measured on a weight-bearing lateral radiograph. Normally, the dorsiflexion pitch to the calcaneus is approximately 20 degrees. Some degree of varus deformity of the heel is usually present as well.

2. Anterior cavus deformity—In anterior cavus deformity, there is a forefoot equinus deformity with the hindfoot in a neutral position. The anterior cavus may be localized, mainly involving the first and second metatarsal, or it may be more global, with the entire forefoot in a position of plantar flexion. Some degree of adduction of the forefoot is usually present.

3. Combined cavus deformity—In a combined cavus deformity, which is the most severe, there are both anterior and posterior components.

Clinical Findings

A. Symptoms and Signs

A careful history regarding the onset of the condition and progression is important. A detailed family history should also be obtained because idiopathic cavus deformity does tend to run in families. Progression of deformity should be ascertained, particularly in the adolescent, because it may indicate a spinal cord abnormality or neoplasm. Activity level and ambulation should also be carefully evaluated as markers of progression of neural or muscular disease.

The degree of deformity of the foot must be examined with the patient in a standing position. This also reveals any evidence of atrophy of the calf muscles, as seen in Charcot-Marie-Tooth disease, clubfoot, or arthrogryposis. The active and passive ROM of the joints of the foot and ankle should be carefully measured. The muscle strength of each muscle must be carefully evaluated, especially if considering a tendon transfer. The degree of deformity and flexibility of the rearfoot, forefoot, metatarsophalangeal joints, and lesser toes must be ascertained. The presence of a tight plantar fascia should also be noted. The lateral ankle ligaments must be evaluated for integrity because they often become stretched out with long-standing varus heel deformity.

B. Imaging Studies

Weight-bearing radiographs of the foot and ankle are obtained to help classify the type of cavus deformity and formulate a treatment plan. Any degree of arthrosis or varus tilting of the talus in the ankle mortise is also evaluated.

Treatment

A. Conservative Management

Conservative care is tailored to the severity of the cavus deformity. Mild deformities may only require a softer-soled shoe. Significant clawing of the lesser toes may require an extra-depth shoe. A custom-made Plastazote liner with a built-in arch support helps decrease the stress on the metatarsal heads. A significant motor deficit may require an AFO to stabilize the ankle. Most cases of cavus foot can be managed with conservative modalities.

B. Surgical Treatment

Surgical treatment for the cavus foot is aimed at correcting the site of the deformity. The most frequent pattern consists of plantar flexion of the first metatarsal, contracture of the plantar fascia, and varus deformity of the calcaneus. These problems respond to release of the plantar fascia, dorsiflexion osteotomy of the first and perhaps second metatarsal, and lateral closing-wedge osteotomy (Dwyer procedure) of the calcaneus to correct the varus deformity. Fusion of the joints is avoided to maintain as much flexibility of the foot as possible (Figure 9–48).

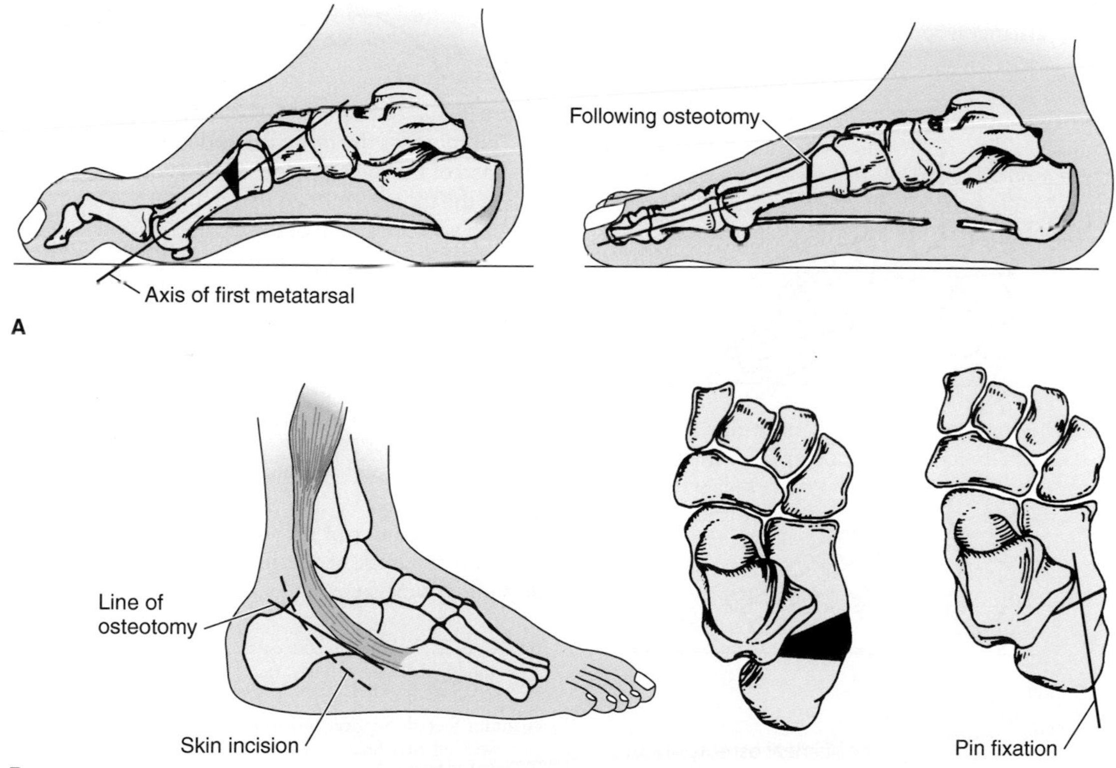

Figure 9–48. Technique for correction of cavus foot. **A:** For first metatarsal osteotomy, a dorsally based wedge of bone was removed approximately 1 cm distal to the metatarsocuneiform joint. The plantar fascia was released. Dorsiflexion of the osteotomy site helps correct the cavus deformity by flattening the arch. **B:** Heel varus is corrected by a closing-wedge calcaneus osteotomy. (Reproduced, with permission, from Mann RA, Coughlin MJ: *The Video Textbook of Foot and Ankle Surgery*. Medical Video Productions, 1991.)

A more severe deformity involving dorsiflexion of the calcaneus can be treated with sliding osteotomy of the calcaneus (Samilson procedure), correcting any varus deformity with a lateral closing-wedge osteotomy and releasing the plantar fascia (Figure 9–49). Forefoot deformity is treated with osteotomy of the first and sometimes second metatarsal. In some patients, transfer of the peroneus longus tendon into the brevis and lengthening of the posterior tibial tendon provides dynamic muscle balance for the foot.

Severe deformities not amenable to procedures that retain joint motion require triple arthrodesis. A Siffert beak-type triple arthrodesis corrects the deformity because the navicular is mortised under the head of the talus to help reduce the elevation of the longitudinal arch (Figure 9–50). A first metatarsal osteotomy may need to be added to the procedure as well.

The lesser toes may have either fixed or flexible clawtoe deformities. Flexible deformity often responds to release of the extensor tendons and a Girdlestone flexor tendon transfer. If a fixed deformity is present, a DuVries phalangeal condylectomy corrects the hammer toe, followed by extensor tendon release and the Girdlestone procedure.

Hyperextension of the first metatarsophalangeal joint is corrected by interphalangeal arthrodesis of the hallux and transfer of the extensor hallucis longus tendon into the neck of the first metatarsal (Jones procedure) (Figure 9–51).

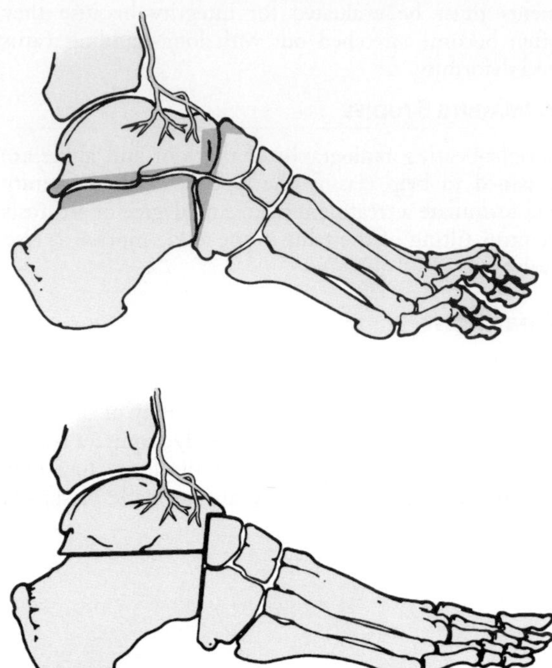

Figure 9–50. **A diagram of a beak-type triple arthrodesis. This mortises the navicular underneath a portion of the head of the talus to allow rotation of the distal portion of the foot, permitting flattening of the longitudinal arch and correction of the cavus deformity.** (Reproduced, with permission, from Mann RA, Coughlin MJ: *The Video Textbook of Foot and Ankle Surgery*. Medical Video Productions, 1991.)

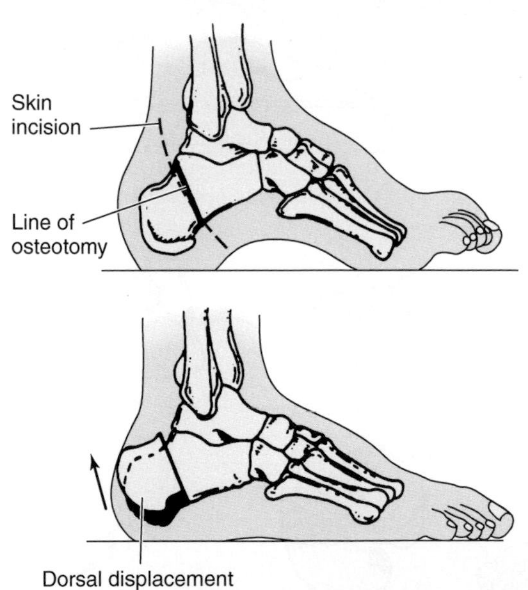

Figure 9–49. **Techniques of calcaneal osteotomy. In the treatment of pes cavus, the osteotomy permits the calcaneus to be moved into a more dorsal position and, if necessary, to be closed laterally to correct heel varus.** (Reproduced, with permission, from Mann RA, Coughlin MJ: *The Video Textbook of Foot and Ankle Surgery*. Medical Video Productions, 1991.)

Breusch SJ et al. Function after correction of a clawed great toe by a modified Robert Jones transfer. J Bone Joint Surg (Br) 2000:82-B:250. [PMID: 10755436]

Giannini S et al. Surgical treatment of adult idiopathic cavus foot with plantar fasciotomy, naviculocuneiform arthrodesis, and cuboid osteotomy. A review of thirty-nine cases. J Bone Joint Surg Am. 2002;84-A Suppl 2:62. [PMID: 12479341]

Siffert RS del Torto U "Beak" triple arthrodesis for severe cavus deformity. Clin Orthop Relat Res 1983;181:64. [PMID: 6641068]

Sammarco GJ, Taylor R Cavovarus foot Treated with combined calcaneus and metatarsal osteotomies. Foot Ankle Int 2001; 22:19. [PMID: 11206819]

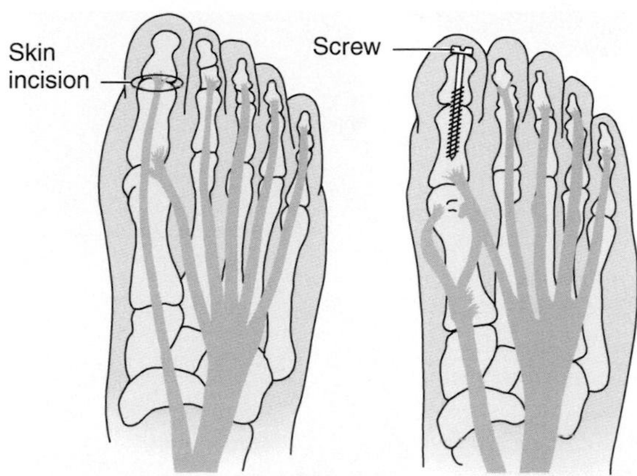

Figure 9–51. Diagram of the first toe Jones procedure. This procedure moves the pull of the extensor hallucis longus tendon from the great toe into the neck of the metatarsal. An interphalangeal arthrodesis of the hallux is carried out. (Reproduced, with permission, from Mann RA, Coughlin MJ, eds: *Surgery of the Foot and Ankle*. Mosby-Year Book, 1993.)

ORTHOTIC DEVICES FOR THE FOOT & ANKLE

Orthotic devices are used to redistribute stresses on the foot as it makes contact with the ground and to accommodate for abnormal function of defective muscles or ligaments. This is achieved by controlling the posture of the foot and padding certain areas to relieve pressure and provide increased comfort for the foot. Orthoses are also used to limit motion in arthritic joints, making them less painful. The orthotic device may be attached to the sole of the shoe, may be inserted inside the shoe as an insole, may cup the foot (UCBL insert), or may extend across the ankle to hold the entire foot and ankle in place (AFO).

Orthotic Shoe Sole Devices

A variety of heel and sole corrections are available to accommodate foot postural abnormalities. A medial or lateral heel or sole wedge (or a combination of both) can help control excessive pronation or supination from weak tendons, ligamentous instability, or fixed deformities. A wide heel is used to increase the stability of the subtalar joint. A rocker sole helps stabilize the forefoot in the case of a fracture or arthritis and also aids a patient with an ankle fusion to allow a more normal gait pattern.

Orthotic Insole Devices

Insole orthotic devices can be used for flexible deformities to alter the posture of the foot and for fixed deformities to redistribute stress. The simplest device is a soft liner for a shoe or boot made out of a high-density foam material. Other simple orthoses include a soft felt pad to relieve pressure on the metatarsal heads or a combination of materials to produce a more rigid support to help control a forefoot deformity such as forefoot varus or valgus deformity. Orthotic devices take up space in the shoe, and the patient may need a larger or deeper shoe.

University of California Biomechanics Laboratory Insert

The principle of the UCBL insert is to correct a foot deformity such as flatfoot by stabilizing the calcaneus in neutral position and molding the orthosis to block abduction of the forefoot. Posting along the medial aspect may compensate for forefoot varus. In theory, this orthotic device is excellent for controlling the rearfoot and forefoot, but two caveats apply to the use of this device. The first is that the foot must be flexible because correction of a rigid deformity is impossible. The second is that a bony prominence can chafe against the polypropylene material, resulting in pain or skin breakdown over the prominence.

Ankle-Foot Orthosis

An AFO is a molded polypropylene device that passes along the posterior aspect of the calf and then onto the plantar aspect of the foot to the metatarsal heads. Alterations are made in a variety of ways to accommodate the patient's problem (Figure 9–52). Ankle problems such as arthrosis or dorsiflexion weakness require adequate rigidity to eliminate ankle joint motion. An orthosis for a subtalar joint problem should have enough flexibility to provide ankle joint motion but must be rigid enough to immobilize the subtalar joint. When the problem involves the transverse tarsal joint, the AFO can be fabricated to permit some ankle joint motion but maintain immobilization of the transverse tarsal joint area, usually by blocking abduction of the forefoot. When managing tarsometatarsal arthritis, the footpiece is carried to the tips of the toes. Again, a significant fixed bony deformity results in pressure points, making fitting of the device difficult. If the patient has loss of sensation, careful construction and padding are essential to minimize the risk of ulcers forming over a bony prominence. In cases of marked instability or discomfort, an anterior shell can be added to the AFO, and the brace is extended proximally to create a patellar tendon bearing surface.

Double Upright Orthosis

The double upright orthosis with a hinged ankle may be used when individuals require stability but are engaged in physically demanding activities. The double upright orthosis is somewhat more cumbersome than the AFO

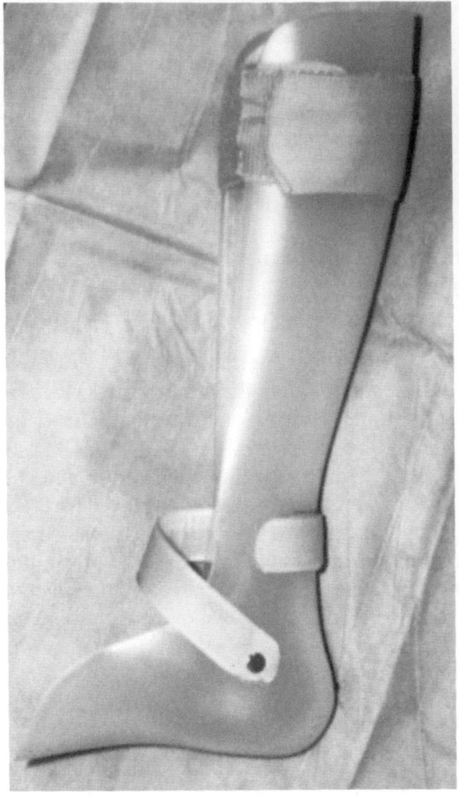

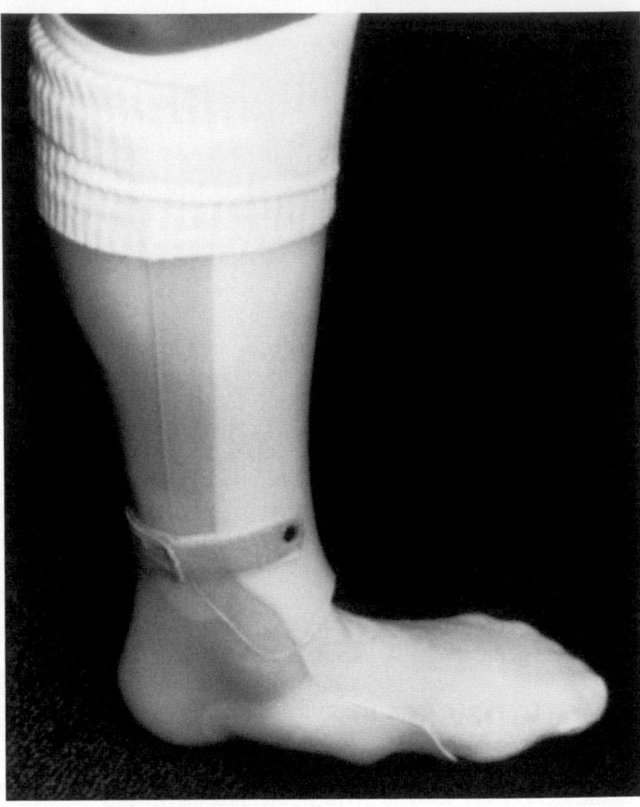

A B

Figure 9–52. Types of ankle-foot orthoses (AFOs). **A:** A standard AFO with a trim-line cut to maximum stability of the ankle joint. If the trim line is cut more posteriorly, there would be some give at the ankle joint. **B:** An anterior shell was added to the AFO to increase the stability of the foot and ankle within the brace. (Reproduced, with permission, from Mann RA, Coughlin MJ, eds: *Surgery of the Foot and Ankle*, 6th. ed. Mosby-Year Book, 1993.)

but provides rigid immobilization. The hinge mechanism of the ankle joint may be changed, depending on the nature of the patient's problem. The ankle joint can be free, which allows dorsiflexion and plantar flexion to occur, or it can be fixed to prevent plantar flexion past 90 degrees. This brace can be modified with a spring load to provide dorsiflexion for the patient with dropfoot resulting from paralysis but should not be used for the patient with spasticity because it may accentuate the spasticity.

Prescriptions for Orthotic Devices

The following are typical prescriptions for orthotic devices.

A. Metatarsalgia or Atrophy of Plantar Fat Pad

1. Treatment—A full-length well-molded orthosis for metatarsal arch support is used to relieve pressure under the metatarsal heads. Soft insole material should be used.

2. Explanation—In the treatment of metatarsalgia or atrophy of the plantar fat pad, a full-length orthosis is needed that is molded to the plantar aspect of the foot and built up just proximal to the metatarsal heads to relieve pressure on them. The material should be soft to provide extra cushioning for the foot.

B. Ruptured Posterior Tibial Tendon with Moderately Severe Flexible Flatfoot Deformity

1. Treatment—AFO with trim-line cut to permit 30% ankle joint motion is molded to reestablish the longitudinal arch and built up on the lateral aspect of the footpiece to block abduction of the forefoot.

2. Explanation—With a moderately advanced flexible flatfoot deformity, an in-shoe orthotic device alone does not provide sufficient support; the AFO is needed to provide adequate stability. Some ankle joint motion is included, which makes ambulation more comfortable for the patient. The longitudinal arch is molded to support the foot in a plantigrade position, and the lateral aspect of the AFO is built up to prevent the forefoot from moving into an abducted position. By blocking abduction, the amount of pressure needed beneath the longitudinal arch to prevent it from collapsing is decreased.

C. Posterior Tibial Tendon Insufficiency with Mild Flatfoot Deformity and 5 Degrees of Forefoot Varus Deformity

1. Treatment—Use a well-molded longitudinal arch support, with a 5-degree varus post and a 3-degree medial heel lift.

2. Explanation—Insufficiency of the posterior tibial tendon that has not produced a significant foot deformity can be treated with a well-molded longitudinal arch support. The 5-degree varus forefoot post compensates for the fixed forefoot varus, and the 3-degree heel lift likewise helps tilt the hindfoot from valgus deformity closer to neutral position.

D. Dropfoot Secondary to Peroneal Nerve Injury

1. Treatment—An AFO with a full footpiece is molded to the longitudinal arch.

2. Explanation—A dropfoot secondary to a peroneal nerve injury responds well to an AFO with a full footpiece. The footpiece supports the toes so they do not drop and makes it easier for the patient to put on shoes.

E. Diabetic Neuropathy with Clawfoot Deformity

1. Treatment—An extra-depth shoe with a molded Plastazote liner is backed with a Pelite material.

2. Explanation—The patient with clawfoot deformity requires a shoe that has extra height in the toe box. The extra-depth shoe provides enough room for the toes, so they do not chafe against the top of the shoe. The molded Plastazote liner is an excellent means of providing full contact to the plantar aspect of the foot. Plastazote has a tendency to bottom out, as it were, and by backing the material with a Pelite liner or some comparable material, the life expectancy of the Plastazote is extended significantly.

Bordelon RL: Orthotics, shoes, and braces. Orthop Clin North Am 1989;20:751. [PMID: 2797761]

Major RE et al: A new structural concept in moulded fixed ankle foot orthoses and comparison of the bending stiffness of four constructions. Prosthet Orthot Int 2004;28:44. [PMID: 15171577]

Pfeffer G et al: Comparison of custom and prefabricated orthoses in the initial treatment of proximal plantar fasciitis. Foot Ankle Int 1999;20:214. [PMID: 10229276]

Pinzur M: Surgical versus accommodative treatment for Charcot arthropathy of the midfoot. Foot Ankle Int 2004;25:545. [PMID: 15363375]

Raikin SM et al: Biomechanical evaluation of the ability of casts and braces to immobilize the ankle and hindfoot. Foot Ankle Int 2001;22:214. [PMID: 11310863]

LIGAMENTOUS INJURIES ABOUT THE ANKLE JOINT

Ankle ligament injuries represent the most common musculoskeletal injury; therefore, accurate assessment and treatment of these injuries are important. The lateral collateral ligament complex is most commonly injured, but damage to other important structures around the ankle joint should not be overlooked, as discussed in this section.

Functional Anatomy

The lateral collateral ligament structure of the ankle consists of three distinct ligamentous bands: the anterior and posterior talofibular ligaments (ATFL and PTFL) and the calcaneal fibular ligament (CFL).

When the ankle joint is in plantar flexion, the ATFL is positioned in line with the fibula and therefore placed under stress with an inversion injury and will be damaged. Conversely, when the ankle joint is in dorsiflexion, the CFL is positioned in line with the long axis of the fibula and is therefore subject to injury. If the applied stress is severe, both the ATFL and the CFL may be torn, no matter the position of the ankle joint. The syndesmosis ligament complex tethers the tibia and fibula together and is injured by an external rotational force to the foot. The deltoid ligament is the sole medial stabilizer of the ankle joint. An isolated deltoid ligament injury can occur with an eversion or external rotation force on the foot. The deltoid ligament can also sustain injury in conjunction with a syndesmosis ligament injury, with lateral ankle sprains, or with a concomitant fibula fracture (known as a Maisonneuve fracture).

Clinical Findings

A. Classification

Lateral collateral ankle ligament injuries are divided into three degrees of severity. A grade I sprain is confined to the ATFL and demonstrates no instability. A grade II sprain involves injury to both the ATFL and CFL, with mild laxity of one or both ligaments. A grade III sprain involves injury and significant laxity of both the ATFL and CFL.

B. Symptoms and Signs

A past history of injuries of the ankle and problems with chronic ankle ligament instability should be ascertained. A careful physical examination is important to evaluate the degree of involvement of each ligament and to rule out injury to any adjacent bony or soft-tissue structures. The ATFL, PTFL, CFL, and syndesmosis ligaments are palpated for tenderness. To rule out fractures, pain should be elicited in the area of the distal fibula, the anterior process of the calcaneus, the lateral process of the talus, and at the base of the fifth metatarsal. Other areas where an injury must be ruled out include the subtalar joint and the peroneal tendon sheath.

A patient with significant medial joint pain with or without lateral ligament pain should be evaluated for an injury to the deltoid ligament complex, the posterior tibial tendon, and the medial talar dome. Assessment of ankle ligament stability requires clinical and radiographic stress examinations. To perform an anterior drawer maneuver, which tests stability of the ATFL, the ankle is placed in 30 degrees of equinus, and the ankle is pulled in an anterior and slightly internally rotated direction (Figure 9–53). A feeling of subluxation is present if a significant ligament injury has occurred. A talar tilt maneuver is performed by placing an inversion stress on the heel. With the foot in plantar flexion, this tests the stability of the ATFL. With the foot in neutral or dorsiflexion, a talar tilt maneuver tests the stability of the CFL. If clinical instability is suggested by either maneuver, radiographic confirmation can be performed, with comparison to the unaffected ankle.

Deltoid ligament insufficiency may cause a feeling of instability and giving way, affecting the medial aspect of the ankle joint. Stress examination is performed by pulling the foot laterally and into valgus while stabilizing the distal tibia.

Injury to the syndesmosis ligament complex is suspected if the region between the distal anterior tibia and fibula is tender to palpation. If extensive swelling is present more than 2 cm proximal to the ankle joint, syndesmosis rupture is a strong possibility. Pain elicited by squeezing the tibia and fibula together in the midcalf is diagnostic of a syndesmosis ligament tear. A syndesmosis ligament injury is also suspected if external rotation of the foot is painful or if lateral translation of the talus in the ankle mortice occurs with direct lateral force on the foot.

C. Imaging Studies

Standard anteroposterior, lateral, and oblique radiographs of the ankle should be obtained to rule out a fracture of the fibula, talus, or calcaneus. If ligament laxity is suggested on clinical examination, stress radiographs should be obtained. An anteroposterior view is taken while a talar tilt maneuver is performed, and a lateral view is taken while an anterior drawer maneuver is performed. More than 10 degrees of tilt and more than 5–7 mm of anterior drawer are considered abnormal.

If a syndesmosis ligament injury is suspected, careful attention must be paid to the joint spaces to rule out

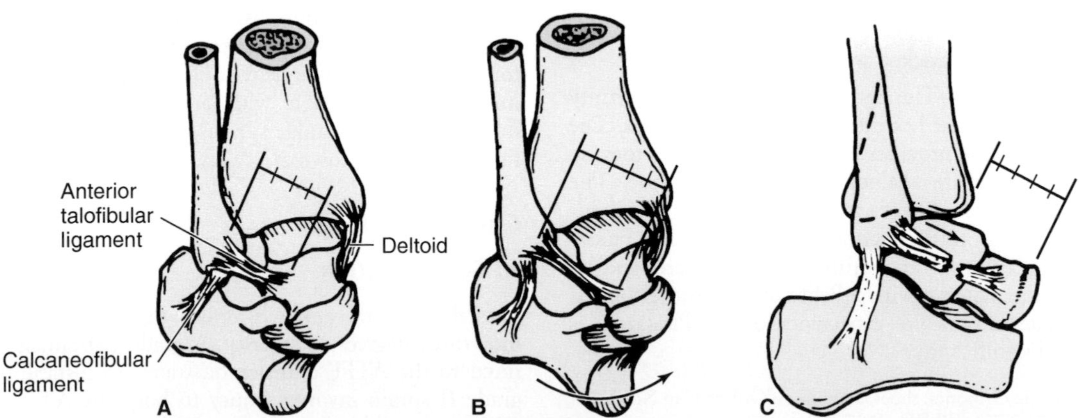

Figure 9–53. Mechanics of carrying out a stress test of the lateral ankle ligaments. **A:** Normal anatomic alignment, which demonstrates the checkrein effect of the anterior talofibular ligament on the talus. **B:** The stress test for the calcaneofibular ligament is carried out by firmly inverting the calcaneus. **C:** The anterior talofibular ligament is tested by placing the ankle joint in neutral position and applying an anterior pull with slight medial rotation. (Reproduced, with permission, from Mann RA, Coughlin MJ, eds: *Surgery of the Foot and Ankle*, 6th. ed. Mosby-Year Book, 1993.)

widening of the ankle mortise. If instability is suspected, a stress radiograph is performed by externally rotating the foot with the tibia held still.

MRI or CT scan may be helpful in some instances if there is a high index of suspicion for an accompanying injury. Osteochondral injuries to the talus should be ruled out with an MRI scan. If a talus or calcaneus fracture is suspected, either MRI or CT scan may be of benefit.

Treatment

A. Conservative Management

Acute grade I ligament tears are treated with a lateral stabilizing ankle brace, ice, and avoidance of painful activities. Immediate full weight-bearing is allowed, as are non–weight-bearing physical activities, such as bicycling and swimming. The brace can be discontinued in 1 month.

Grade II ligament tears are treated with protected weight bearing and a lateral stabilizing ankle brace. The patient can begin non–weight-bearing exercise (stationary bicycle) after 7 days, along with peroneal strengthening exercises. Weight-bearing exercise (jogging) may resume after 2–4 weeks.

In a grade III ligament tear, the ankle is immobilized with a removable walking cast for 3–4 weeks. This is followed by a period of physical therapy consisting of range-of-motion (ROM) exercises, peroneal strengthening, and proprioception training using a biomechanical ankle platform system (BAPS) board.

Treatment of isolated deltoid ligament sprains depends on the severity of the injury and is similar to lateral ligament injuries. Mild injuries can be treated with immediate mobilization and rapid return to activity, whereas more severe injuries should be casted for 3–4 weeks.

Syndesmosis ligament tears, if mild, can be treated with weight bearing in a cast or brace and close follow-up to assess for widening of the ankle joint mortise. If the interosseous membrane is damaged, as evidenced by massive swelling of the leg proximal to the ankle joint, treatment depends on the radiographic appearance of the ankle. If the mortise has not widened, the patient is kept on a non–weight-bearing regime in a cast for 6 weeks, with close radiographic follow-up. If initial or follow radiographs show a widened mortise, the patient requires surgical repair of the syndesmosis ligaments with temporary screw placement until the ligaments heal.

B. Surgical Treatment

The surgical treatment of an acute ligamentous injury is indicated only for the occasional elite athlete. Most ligamentous injuries, even grade III sprains, heal sufficiently with no significant disability if properly treated, as just described. However, even less severe ankle sprains may cause chronic pain or functional instability if left untreated.

The indication for a lateral ligament reconstruction is functional ligament instability. A patient with ligament instability complains of recurrent sprains that occur with sports activities or even with activities of daily living, despite 4–6 months of physical therapy and use of a lateral stabilizing brace. A patient with functional ligament instability also complains of difficulty walking on uneven ground. This history must be found in conjunction with physical examination findings of ligament instability.

Although many lateral ankle reconstruction procedures are described for chronic lateral ankle ligament instability, a Broström repair is generally the procedure of choice. The Broström procedure is a soft-tissue ligamentous repair in which the ATFL and CFL are plicated and reattached to their anatomic positions (Figure 9–54). The repair is reinforced by bringing up a portion of the inferior extensor retinaculum. The Broström procedure is highly effective and has lower morbidity than other procedures that harvest the peroneus brevis tendon. In patients who have severe and long-standing laxity or have failed a Broström repair, revision surgery with an allograft or autograft tendon is indicated.

Chronic lateral ankle pain following an ankle sprain may be caused by a previously undiagnosed condition rather than chronic ankle instability. The differential diagnosis for chronic ankle pain is similar to that following an acute injury and also includes subtalar joint instability, subtalar joint chondral damage or synovitis, and dislocating or torn peroneal tendons. Impingement of scar tissue in the lateral gutter between the talus and fibula may also cause chronic lateral ankle pain. In addition to a careful physical examination, an MRI or CT scan may be helpful for distinguishing among these possible causes of pain.

Surgical treatment may help relieve symptoms of chronic lateral ankle pain, once an accurate diagnosis is made. Chondral or osteochondral fractures involving the ankle or subtalar joints can be treated with arthroscopic or open debridement or pinning. Subtalar joint instability is addressed with a Broström procedure. A fracture of the anterior or lateral process of the talus is either removed if it is small or fixed if it is a large fragment. Tears or dislocations of the peroneal tendons are repaired or stabilized. Scar tissue in the lateral gutter can be treated with arthroscopic debridement.

Chronic instability of the deltoid ligament or syndesmosis ligament is uncommon but can occur after an untreated injury. Diagnosis of either condition is made with stress radiographs. Treatment usually requires a free tendon graft to reconstruct the damaged ligament, with the addition of internal fixation for chronic syndesmosis tears.

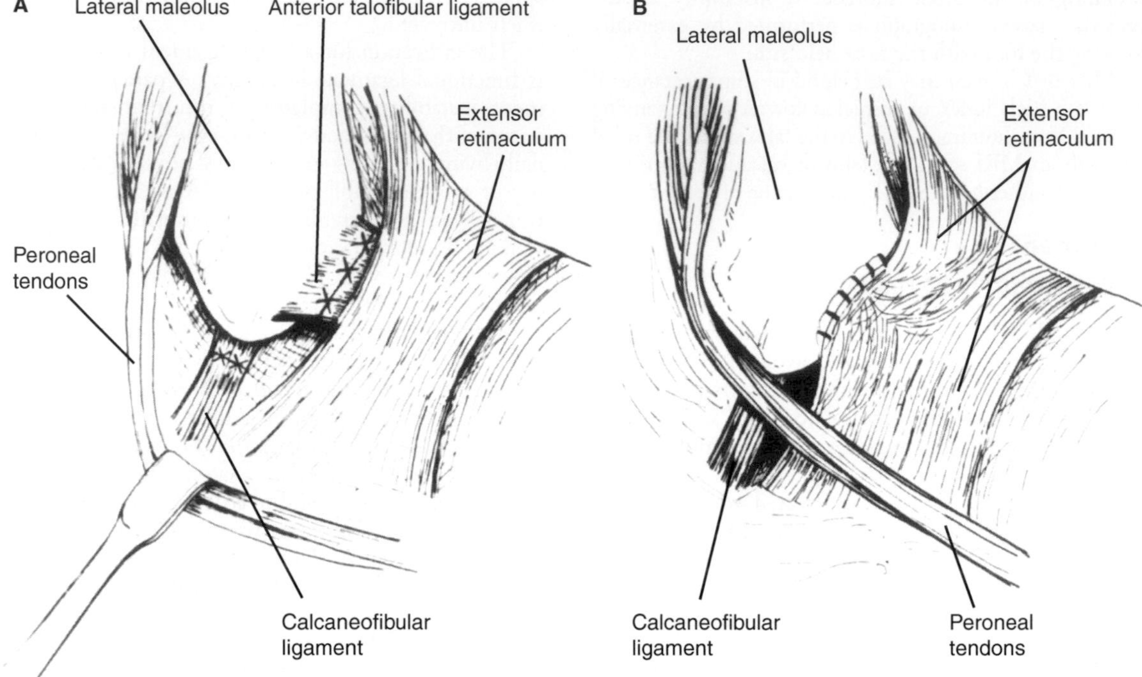

Figure 9–54. Modified Broström anatomic reconstruction. **A:** Imbrication of anterior talofibular and calcaneofibular ligaments. **B:** Imbrication of inferior extensor retinaculum to reinforce the repair. (Reproduced, with permission, from Coughlin MJ, Mann RA, eds: *Surgery of the Foot and Ankle,* 7th ed. Mosby, 1999. Modified from Renstrom PA, Trevino S, eds: *Operative Techniques in Sports Medicine,* Vol. 2. WB Saunders, 1994.)

Coughlin MJ et al: Comprehensive reconstruction of the lateral ankle for chronic instability using a free gracilis graft. Foot Ankle Int 2004;25:231. [PMID: 15132931]

DiGiovanni BF et al: Acute ankle injury and chronic lateral instability in the athlete. Clin Sports Med 2004;23:1. [PMID: 15062581]

Hintermann B et al: Medial ankle instability: An exploratory, prospective study of fifty-two cases. Am J Sports Med 2004; 32:183.

Hoiness P, Stromsoe K: Tricortical versus quadricortical syndesmosis fixation in ankle fractures: A prospective, randomized study comparing two methods of syndesmosis fixation. J Orthop Trauma 2004;18:331. [PMID: 15213497]

Krips R et al: Long-term outcome of anatomical reconstruction versus tenodesis for the treatment of chronic anterolateral instability of the ankle joint: A multicenter study. Foot Ankle Int 2001;22:415. [PMID: 11428761]

Messer TM et al: Outcome of the modified Broström procedure for chronic lateral ankle instability using suture anchors. Foot Ankle Int 2000;21:996. [PMID: 11139039]

Pijnenburg ACM et al: Treatment of ruptures of the lateral ankle ligaments: A meta-analysis. J Bone Joint Surg Am 2000; 82:761. [PMID: 10859095]

ARTHROSCOPIC EXAMINATION OF THE FOOT & ANKLE

Arthroscopy is an important tool for use in diagnosis and treatment of foot and ankle disorders. With developments in instrumentation, more ankle joint conditions can be treated arthroscopically. Arthroscopy of the subtalar joint is also now an accepted method for diagnosing and treating some subtalar joint abnormalities.

Advantages of Ankle Arthroscopy over Ankle Arthrotomy

Arthroscopy of the ankle joint offers distinct advantages over open exploration of the ankle. The entire joint can be visualized using the arthroscope, including the lateral and medial gutters and the posterior aspect of the joint. Dynamic studies can be performed to stress ligaments or identify areas of soft-tissue or bony impingement. Furthermore, the low morbidity of arthroscopy allows rapid rehabilitation.

Table 9–4. Proven indications for ankle arthroscopy.

Loose body removal
Irrigation and debridement for infection
Shaving of small osteophytes
Debridement of localized general synovitis
Debridement of osteochondral fractures
Debridement of osteochondritis dissecans lesions
Debridement of soft-tissue impingement

Indications

Table 9–4 lists the indications for ankle joint arthroscopy. In addition, arthroscopic examination can be used as a diagnostic tool in some instances when the precise cause of ankle pain remains in question.

A. Therapeutic Indications

1. Loose bodies—Intraarticular loose bodies are generally easy to identify and remove arthroscopically. These bony or cartilaginous fragments may occur as a result of a single incident or repetitive trauma, or they may represent a fragment of an osteochondritis dissecans lesion. They cause pain or locking symptoms of the ankle and are diagnosed on plain radiographs, CT, or MRI scan.

2. Ankle joint infection—Arthroscopic irrigation, drainage, and synovectomy is an excellent method of treating ankle joint infections.

3. Synovitis—Synovitis may be present as a result of inflammatory arthritis (RA) or neoplastic diseases (pigmented villonodular synovitis), following trauma, or for unknown reasons (idiopathic). Whether the synovitis is localized or diffuse, arthroscopic debridement of inflamed synovium often relieves symptoms. Synovectomy is more easily and thoroughly performed arthroscopically.

4. Osteophyte formation—Repetitive trauma or early osteoarthritis can lead to osteophyte formation on the anterior lip of the tibia and the neck of the talus. These lesions can cause pain and limited ankle joint dorsiflexion and can be removed arthroscopically with a high-speed burr.

5. Other lesions within the joint—Chondral or osteochondral lesions, whether caused by trauma or osteochondritis dissecans, can be treated arthroscopically. This may involve debridement of loose cartilage flaps, drilling of subchondral bone, or pinning of large osteochondral fragments.

Patients who present with ankle pain over the anterolateral joint line and a history of a severe ankle sprain or recurrent sprains may have impingement of scar tissue in the lateral gutter between the talus and fibula. This entity responds well to arthroscopic debridement of scar tissue from the lateral gutter.

6. Ankle arthrodesis—Techniques for arthroscopically assisted ankle arthrodesis are well detailed, and several published studies discuss this method. The technique causes less morbidity and allows a shorter time to fusion than open methods of ankle fusion. But this is a technically demanding procedure and cannot be used to correct any joint deformity.

7. Ankle arthritis—Arthroscopic debridement of the arthritic ankle joint is not beneficial for generalized arthritis but may help for localized degenerative changes accompanied by early osteophyte formation.

8. Ankle fractures—Arthroscopically assisted fixation of ankle fractures is described and potentially allows for more accurate realignment of the joint surfaces and identification of chondral lesions that might otherwise be missed. However, the use of arthroscopy in the treatment of most routine ankle fractures is probably not indicated.

B. Diagnostic Indications

Ankle arthroscopy can be a valuable diagnostic tool when the cause of symptoms remains unclear (Table 9–5). Chronic ankle pain or swelling that remains refractory to conservative measures and was not diagnosed by conventional imaging studies may warrant arthroscopic exploration to help make a diagnosis. Chondral damage or inflamed synovium are examples of symptomatic lesions that may not be demonstrated on imaging studies, including MRI. Patients with episodes of locking, stiffness, or instability for which a cause cannot be found may be aided by diagnostic ankle arthroscopy. Loose bodies, cartilage flaps, or arthrofibrosis may be contributing to such symptoms, all of which can be treated arthroscopically (see Table 9–5).

Table 9–5. Refractory conditions diagnosed by arthroscopy.

Chondromalacia
Synovitis
Locking of the joint
Chronic stiffness
Instability
Loose bodies
Cartilage flaps
Arthrofibrosis

Technique of Ankle Arthroscopy

The patient is placed supine on the operating table with the foot positioned to allow access from all directions. This can be achieved with the foot placed off the edge of the bed or with the thigh held flexed in a well-padded thigh holder (Figure 9–55). General or spinal anesthesia is necessary for full relaxation of the extremity.

The use of distraction greatly enhances arthroscopic procedures, providing better views of the structures of the joint and allowing tools to be introduced into the joint. Noninvasive distractors with padded straps over the foot and heel are most commonly used (see Figure 9–55) Invasive distractors require placement of pins or screws through the tibia proximally and the calcaneus or talus distally. Stronger distraction forces can be obtained in this manner, but the morbidity is higher when using an invasive distractor.

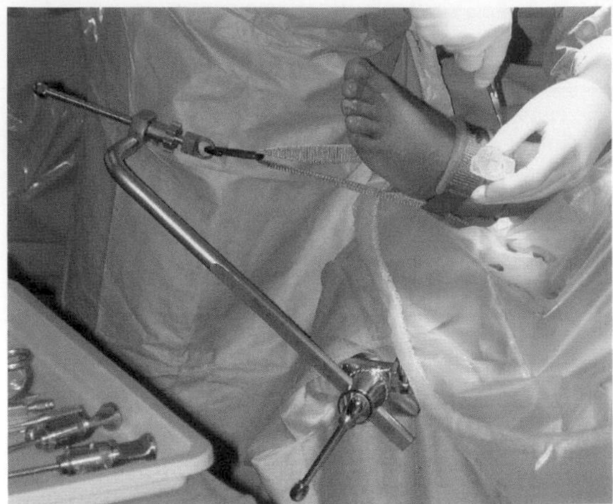

Figure 9–55. Soft strap type of distractor used during ankle arthroscopy.

Most ankle arthroscopies are performed using two anterior portals: anterolateral and anteromedial (Figure 9–56). A posterolateral portal may be helpful for use as outflow or to access the posterior aspect of the joint. Thorough knowledge of the anatomy of the tendons, nerves, and vessels is essential to prevent damage to any of these structures with portal placement. The anterolateral portal is placed just lateral to the tendon of the peroneus tertius muscle, taking care to avoid branches of the superficial peroneal nerve. The anteromedial portal is placed just medial to the anterior tibial tendon, taking care to avoid the saphenous nerve and vein. The posterolateral portal is placed just lateral to the Achilles tendon, to avoid damage to the sural nerve.

Initially, the entire joint is explored systematically, to ensure that abnormalities are not overlooked. The cartilaginous surfaces of the talus and tibia are thoroughly examined for osteochondral defects, unstable cartilage flaps, and areas of softening. The medial and lateral gutters are explored, paying special attention to tibiotalar

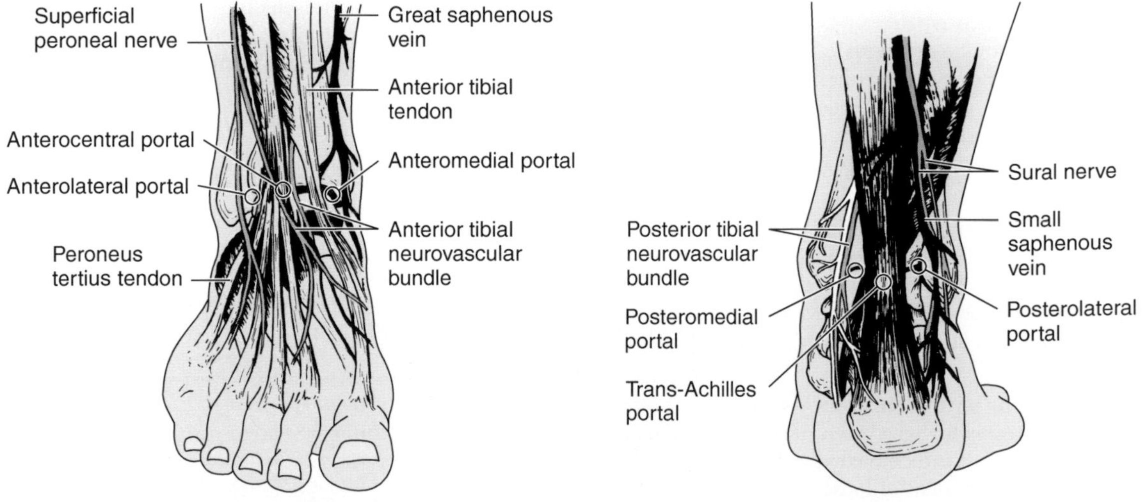

Figure 9–56. **A:** The anterior portals used for ankle arthroscopy are illustrated. The anterocentral portal is not used. **B:** The posterolateral portal is the only posterior portal utilized for ankle arthroscopy. (Reproduced, with permission, from Ferkel RD: Arthroscopy of the ankle and foot. In Mann RA, Coughlin MJ, eds: *Surgery of the Foot and Ankle,* 6th ed. Mosby-Year Book, 1993.)

and talofibular articulations. The synovium is inspected for inflammation. Ligamentous structures are identified, specifically the deltoid and talofibular ligaments, which are observed closely for signs of laxity while varus and valgus forces are applied. Loose bodies are carefully searched for, especially in the anterior and posterior recesses of the joint. The presence of osteophytes on the distal tibia and talar neck is also evaluated.

After a thorough diagnostic examination, surgical procedures are performed. These include synovial biopsy or synovial resection, removal of loose bodies, debridement of abnormal cartilaginous surfaces with subchondral drilling, and removal of bone spurs.

Postoperatively, a compression dressing is applied with a posterior splint for 5 to 7 days to allow the portals to heal. Weight bearing is then progressed as tolerated, and activities are advanced to normal.

Complications

Although several complications are reported, the most common is nerve damage in the form of hypesthesias or neuroma formation associated with portal placement. Postoperative joint infection, draining sinuses, arterial or tendon damage, and infections at the sites of distraction pins are all described but are very uncommon complications of ankle arthroscopy.

Subtalar Joint Arthroscopy

The subtalar joint is technically challenging for arthroscopy, given its complex shape and the difficulty distracting the joint. Subtalar joint arthroscopy is indicated for several conditions involving the subtalar joint. Talocalcaneal interosseous ligament tears, chondral lesions, synovitis, and focal degenerative changes may respond to arthroscopic debridement of the subtalar joint.

For subtalar joint arthroscopy, the patient can either be placed supine with a bump under the ipsilateral hip or in the lateral decubitus position. Two portals are used over the anterolateral subtalar joint, approximately 1.5 cm apart. The anterior and lateral portions of the posterior facet and the interosseous ligament can be visualized from these portals. A third portal is placed posterolaterally, for outflow and for visualization of the posterior aspect of the joint. The references here provide additional details about the technique of subtalar joint arthroscopy.

Frey C et al: Arthroscopic evaluation of the subtalar joint: Does sinus tarsi syndrome exist? Foot Ankle Int 1999;20:185. [PMID: 10195298]

Henderson I, La Valette D: Ankle impingement: Combined anterior and posterior impingement syndrome of the ankle. Foot Ankle Int 2004;25:632. [PMID: 15563385]

Kim SH, Ha KI: Arthroscopic treatment for impingement of the anterolateral soft tissues of the ankle. J Bone Joint Surg Br 2000;82-B;1019. [PMID: 11041593]

Okuda R et al: Arthroscopic findings in chronic lateral ankle instability: Do focal chondral lesions influence the results of ligament reconstruction? Am J Sports Med 2005;33:35. [PMID: 15610997]

Philbin TM et al: Arthroscopy for athletic foot and ankle injuries. Clin Sports Med 2004;23:35. [PMID: 15062583]

Schimmer RC et al: The role of ankle arthroscopy in the treatment strategies of osteochondritis dissecans lesions of the talus. Foot Ankle Int 2001;22:895. [PMID: 11722142]

Stroud CC: Arthroscopic arthrodesis of the ankle, subtalar, and first metatarsophalangeal joint. Foot Ankle Clin 2002;7:135. [PMID: 12380386]

Thordarson DB et al: The role of ankle arthroscopy on the surgical management of ankle fractures. Foot Ankle Int 2001;22:123. [PMID: 11249221]

TENDON INJURIES

Tendon injuries about the foot and ankle are common causes of disability because large forces are acting on these tendons in a repetitive fashion during walking, running, and athletic activities. The tendons cross the ankle joint at an acute angle, which further predisposes them to injury. Injury to tendons may be caused by acute trauma, such as in Achilles tendon ruptures, or may be caused by chronic strain, such as posterior tibial tendon dysfunction.

ACHILLES TENDON INJURIES

Achilles tendon abnormalities are extremely common, especially among active men and women between 30 and 50 years of age. The primary disorders are Achilles tendinitis, either insertional or noninsertional, and Achilles tendon ruptures. Achilles tendinitis was previously discussed in the section on heel pain.

1. Achilles Tendon Rupture

Pathogenesis

The mechanism of injury is usually mechanical overload from an eccentric contraction of the gastrocsoleus muscle complex. This occurs as a sudden, forceful dorsiflexion of the foot as the gastrocsoleus is contracted. The tear usually occurs 3–6 cm proximal to the insertion of the Achilles tendon, at the site of its poorest blood supply (Figure 9–57). At times, a history of intermittent pain in the tendon is elicited, suggestive of a prior tendinitis. The typical patient is between 30 and 50 years of age and a recreational athlete. These factors suggest that insufficient conditioning of the musculotendon unit plays a role in many injuries. The most common sports activities leading to Achilles tendon ruptures are basketball, racket sports, soccer, and softball.

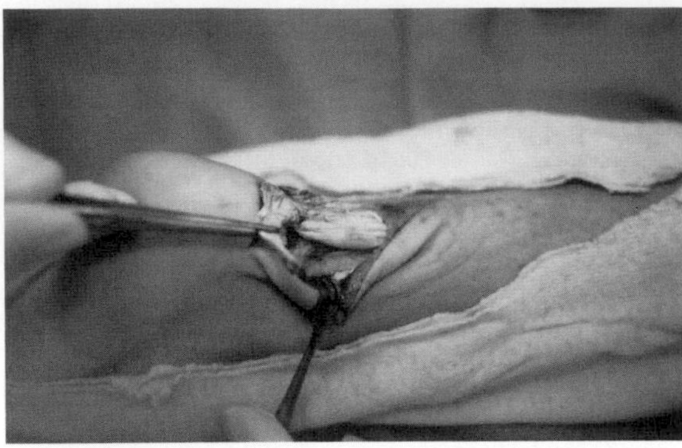

A

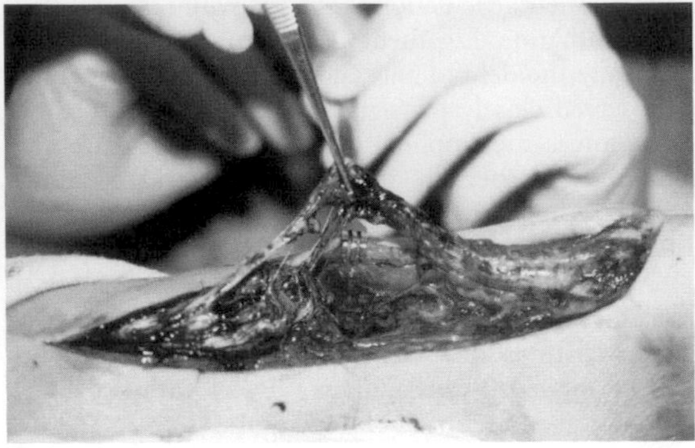

B

Figure 9–57. Examples of acute Achilles tendon ruptures. **A:** Complete rupture with minimal fraying of the tendon. **B:** Achilles tendon rupture with marked fraying of the tendon. (Reproduced, with permission, from Plattner P, Mann RA: Disorders of tendons. In Mann RA, Coughlin MJ, eds: *Surgery of the Foot and Ankle,* 6th ed. Mosby-Year Book, 1993.)

Clinical Findings

A. Symptoms and Signs

The patient describes sudden pain in the calf after attempting a pushing-off movement, often accompanied by an audible pop. Immediate weakness is noted in the affected leg. On physical examination, a palpable defect is often present in the tendon. Ankle plantar flexion is markedly weak compared with the unaffected side. A positive Thompson test, diagnostic of complete Achilles tendon rupture, is performed with the patient prone and the affected knee bent 90 degrees. Squeezing the calf causes plantar flexion of the foot if the Achilles tendon is intact or partially torn but not if there is complete rupture of the tendon.

B. Imaging Studies

Plain radiographs are not helpful in diagnosing Achilles tendon tear, unless there is an avulsion off the calcaneus with a fragment of bone, an uncommon condition. MRI is extremely sensitive in diagnosing this disorder and in determining if some tendon remains in continuity (Figure 9–58). However, MRI is rarely needed because physical exam is usually diagnostic of Achilles tendon rupture.

Treatment

Methods for treating Achilles tendon rupture include primary repair, using open or percutaneous techniques, or cast immobilization. Surgical repair is recommended for active individuals, in the case of a rerupture, or if the injury is older than 2 weeks.

Cast treatment for Achilles tendon ruptures is recommended for more sedentary individuals, patients who are at increased risk of developing wound problems, or high-risk surgical patients. The primary risk of cast immobilization is a higher chance of rerupture. For the vast majority of patients, either treatment method results in a good outcome.

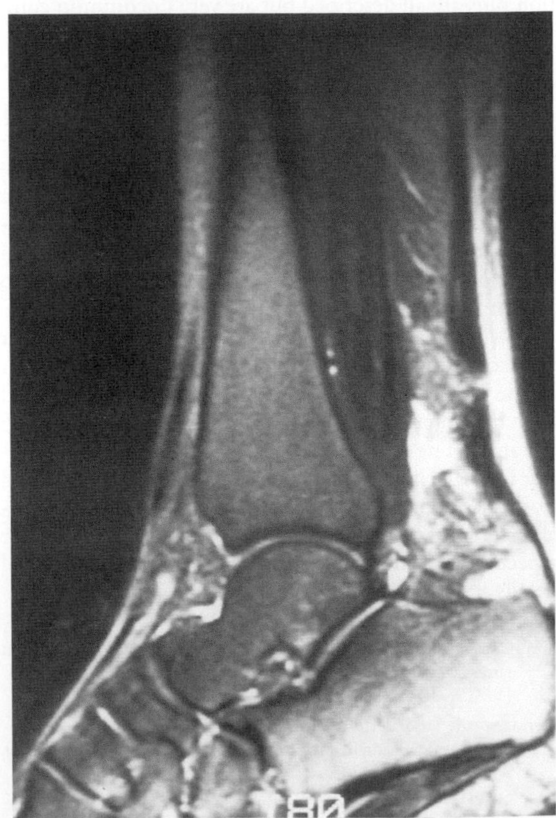

Figure 9–58. MRI of Achilles tendon rupture.

A. Nonsurgical Treatment

Once an acute rupture is diagnosed, the patient should be placed in a gravity equinus cast. A below-knee cast is adequate in a reliable patient. If there is a question of whether the tendon edges are properly apposed in the cast, an MRI scan be done, although this is not routine. After 4 weeks, the cast is changed, with correction of approximately half of the previous equinus. Over the next 4 weeks, the patient is brought down to neutral with serial casts. Once at neutral, the patient is given a removable walking cast for 4 weeks. Supervised strengthening activities then begin.

B. Surgical Treatment

The surgical approach is on the medial side of the Achilles tendon sheath. The frayed edges of the tendon are debrided. The foot is positioned in equinus position equal to the resting equinus of the opposite ankle. Two heavy nonabsorbable sutures are woven through 3–4 cm of each tendon edge using a Bunnell or Kessler stitch (Figure 9–59). The repair can be reinforced with lighter, absorbable sutures at the site of the tear. If the plantaris tendon is intact, it can be harvested and used to reinforce the repair.

Postoperatively, a hard cast is used for 3 weeks, followed by a removable cast with adjustable ankle motion. Over the next 2–3 weeks, the joint should be gradually brought out of equinus. Weight bearing is then allowed, and ROM exercises are begun. The cast is discontinued at 6–8 weeks, and supervised strengthening exercises are performed.

The primary risk of surgical repair is wound healing problems, which occur in approximately 5% of patients. A percutaneous method of Achilles tendon repair is listed in the references.

C. Treatment of Chronic Ruptures or Reruptures

Chronic Achilles tendon ruptures, more than 6 weeks old, or reruptures of previously treated injuries can be challenging reconstruction problems because of retraction and degeneration of the tendon ends. A number of different procedures are described to address this problem, including a variety of synthetic and interpositional grafts (Figure 9–60).

Small defects can be bridged by turning down a strip of gastrocnemius fascia, which is sutured into the distal tendon stump. Larger defects can be treated by using a V-Y lengthening of the gastrocnemius aponeurosis. If the deficit is too large for V-Y lengthening, transfer of the flexor hallucis longus tendon can be performed. The tendon of the flexor hallucis longus is transected distally in the foot, and the distal segment is tenodesed to the flexor digitorum longus to maintain flexion of the great toe. The proximal tendon is secured to the calcaneus through a drill hole or by using an absorbable anchor or screw. A central slip of the Achilles tendon is advanced to bridge the gap, and then the repair is reinforced by securing it to the flexor hallucis (Figure 9–61).

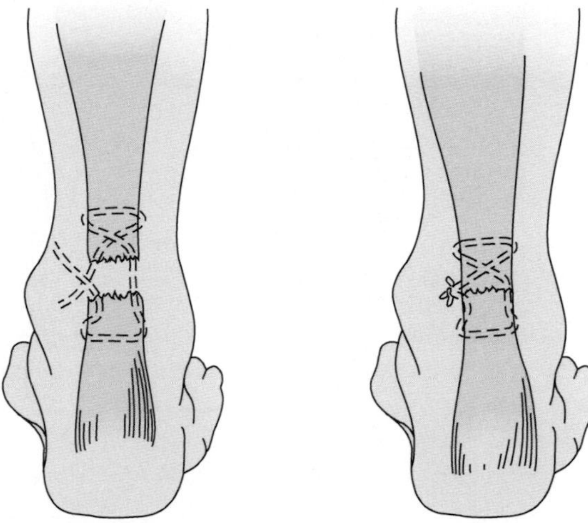

Figure 9–59. Suture techniques used to reapproximate the ruptured Achilles tendon. (Reproduced, with permission, from Mann RA, Coughlin MJ, eds: *Surgery of the Foot and Ankle,* 6th ed. Mosby-Year Book, 1993.)

The postoperative course for these procedures includes 6 weeks of non–weight bearing and a total of 3 months protection in a cast.

POSTERIOR TIBIAL TENDON INJURIES

This topic is covered in the section on acquired flatfoot deformities.

PERONEAL TENDON INJURIES

Peroneal tendon injuries fall into the categories of peroneal tendonitis, peroneal tendon tears, and peroneal tendon subluxation or dislocation.

1. Peroneal Tendonitis

Pathogenesis

Inflammation of the peroneal tendons may be caused by acute trauma, inflammatory arthropathy conditions, or repetitive motion. Traumatic events that may induce tendonitis include a direct blow to the posterolateral ankle, a fracture of the calcaneus or fibula, or a severe inversion sprain of the ankle. Most tendonitis is caused by repetitive motion injury from recurrent rubbing of the peroneal tendons on the distal end of the fibula. Often there is an abnormal bony contour of the distal

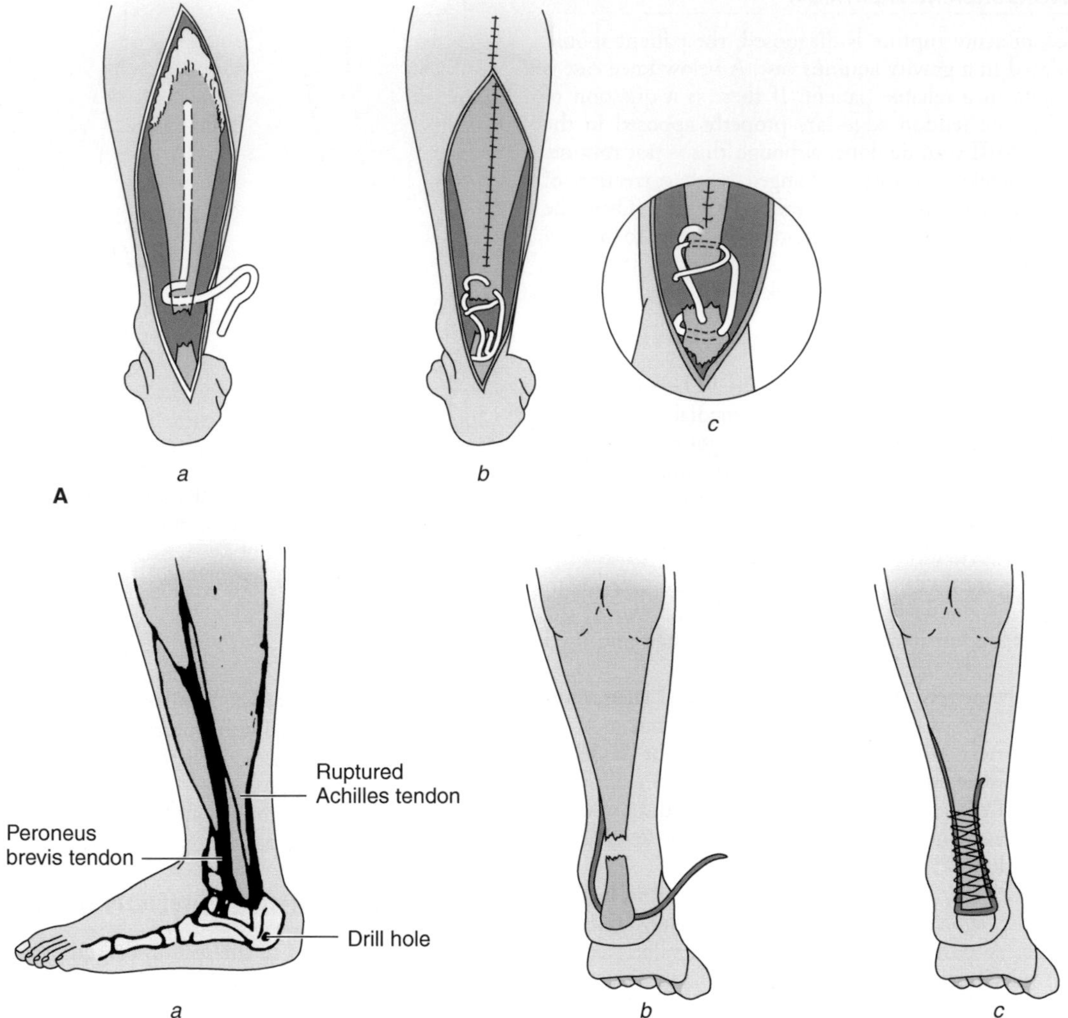

Figure 9–60. Various methods of reconstruction for untreated Achilles tendon ruptures. **A:** Repair using fascial strip from proximal gastrocsoleus complex. *a:* Distally based fascial strip is passed transversely through proximal tendon fragment. *b:* The strip is woven across the gap. *c:* Enlarged diagram of *b*. **B:** Repair using peroneus brevis tendon. The peroneus brevis is isolated and detached from its insertion into the fifth metatarsal. *a:* A transverse drill hole is placed in the calcaneus. *b:* The peroneus brevis is transferred through the drill hole. *c:* The tendon is sutured to itself and to the Achilles tendon proximally and distally. (A: Reproduced, with permission, from Bosworth DM: Repair of defects in the tendo achillis. J Bone Joint Surg Am 1956;38:111. **B:** Reproduced, with permission, from Plattner P, Mann RA: Disorders of tendons. In Mann RA, Coughlin MJ, eds: *Surgery of the Foot and Ankle*, 6th ed. Mosby-Year Book, 1993.)

fibula or the peroneal tubercle. Tendonitis of the peroneus longus may be associated with abnormality of the os peroneum, a small sesamoid bone located in the tendon where it curves around the lateral border of the cuboid.

Clinical Findings

A. Symptoms and Signs

The patient complains of pain over the lateral aspect of the ankle, made worse with activity, and improved with

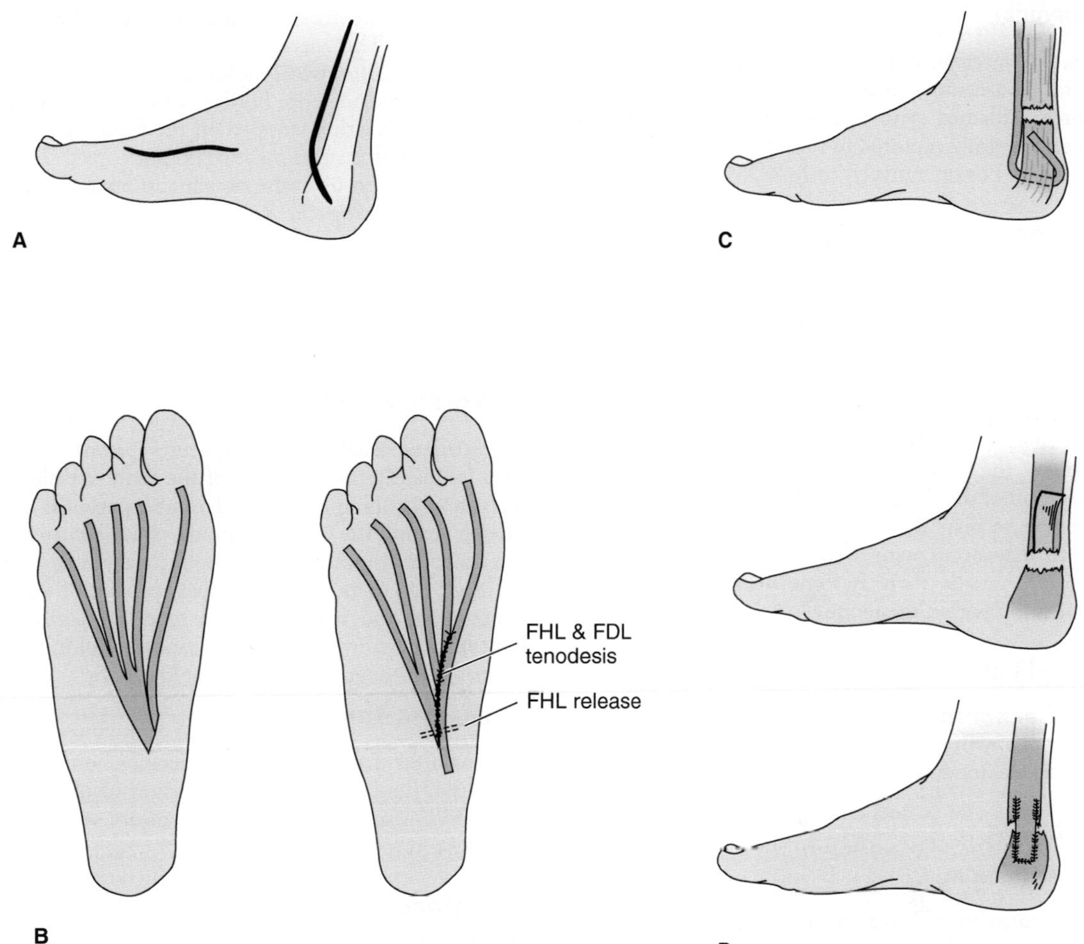

Figure 9–61. Delayed repair of ruptured Achilles tendon using flexor digitorum longus (FDL) transfer. **A:** Operative technique demonstrating incisions. **B:** Tenodesis of the FDL stump to the flexor hallucis longus (FHL). **C:** Flexor digitorum longus pulled through drill hole in calcaneus. **D:** Augmentation of spanned gap by turndown of fascial strip from gastrocsoleus complex. (Reproduced, with permission, from Plattner P, Mann RA: Disorders of tendons. In Mann RA, Coughlin, MF, eds: *Surgery of the Foot and Ankle,* 6th ed. Mosby-Year Book, 1993.)

rest and NSAIDs. The onset may be insidious, or it may be associated with an acute injury. Physical examination usually demonstrates pain located along the course of the peroneal tendons. Pain and weakness is noted with resisted eversion of the foot.

B. Imaging Studies

An MRI scan may help distinguish between tendonitis and a tendon tear, although small tears may not be identified on an MRI.

Treatment

A. Nonsurgical

If symptoms are mild, the recommended treatment includes NSAIDs, activity modification, and an ankle brace. Four to 6 weeks of cast immobilization is used for more advanced symptoms or for patients who do not respond to initial treatment. Occasionally, a diagnostic injection with bupivacaine is given into the tendon sheath.

B. Surgical

Operative intervention is recommended for patients who fail conservative treatment. The tendon sheath is explored, inflamed synovium is removed, and the tendons are carefully explored to look for tears or degenerative lesions. Postoperatively, early ROM is encouraged.

2. Peroneal Tendon Tears

Pathogenesis

The majority of peroneal tendon tears are attritional in nature, caused by mechanical irritation within the fibular groove. The peroneus longus tendon, which lies posterior, places pressure on the brevis tendon. Also, a sharp lateral edge of the fibula may predispose to a longitudinal split of the tendons. Laxity of the tendon sheath and subluxation of the tendons out of the fibular groove may contribute to tears as well. Acute tears of the peroneal tendons may occur with a sudden, severe stress to the ankle, but usually there is some degree of preexisting degeneration within the tendon.

Clinical Findings

Clinical presentation is similar to that of peroneal tendonitis, but with a more acute onset of pain and swelling along the tendon sheath.

Treatment

A. Nonsurgical

Initial treatment is similar to that of peroneal tendonitis, but it is less likely to result in resolution of symptoms if a tear is present.

B. Surgical

Surgical repair of a peroneal tendon tear is indicated when nonoperative treatment fails to relieve symptoms. At surgery, both tendons are carefully examined, the fibula is explored for sharp edges, and the tendon sheath is evaluated for laxity. Small areas of the tendon that demonstrate significant degeneration are removed. The remainder of the tendon is repaired with nylon or polypropylene suture. Postoperatively, the ankle is immobilized for 4 weeks; then weight bearing and gentle ROM is allowed.

3. Peroneal Tendon Subluxation and Dislocation

Pathogenesis

Peroneal tendon dislocation is caused by a sudden forceful dorsiflexion motion of the ankle combined with a simultaneous strong contraction of the peroneal musculature. This mechanism injures the superior peroneal retinaculum, which holds the peroneal tendons in place along the posterior border of the distal fibula. The retinaculum is either stripped off the fibular periosteum or avulsed with a small piece of fibular cortex. This permits the creation of a false pouch and laxity of the retinaculum, allowing the peroneal tendons to dislocate anteriorly. If this condition goes unrecognized, either the tendons remain dislocated, or they relocate with the propensity for recurrent subluxation or dislocation.

Clinical Findings

A. Symptoms and Signs

The patient usually recalls an acute episode of trauma and frequently the sensation of the tendon dislocating. Pain and swelling is localized to the peroneal tendon sheath around the tip of the fibula. With recurrent subluxation or dislocation, the tendons are felt to pop out of place. On examination, resisted eversion of the ankle elicits pain and may cause the tendons to subluxate. Unfortunately, many acute peroneal tendon dislocations go unrecognized as lateral ankle sprains.

B. Imaging Studies

Radiographs may show a small piece of bone lateral to the distal fibula, indicative of avulsion of the retinaculum. MRI scan usually details the injury well if careful attention is paid to this area.

Treatment

A. Nonsurgical

Treatment of acute peroneal tendon dislocations consists of casting in plantarflexion and inversion for 4 weeks, followed by a walking cast for an additional 2 weeks. Cast treatment has at least a 50% failure rate. Once a tendon is chronically dislocated or recurrently subluxates, only surgical treatment will keep it in position.

B. Surgical

Surgical repair is recommended for an athletic individual following an acute dislocation of the peroneal tendons. It is also recommended for patients with recurrent dislocation if their physical activities are significantly restricted. The procedure consists of repairing the superior peroneal retinaculum to the fibula, either through drill holes or with suture anchors. In the case of attenuated retinaculum caused by chronic dislocations, the repair can be reinforced with a strip of Achilles or by rerouting the calcaneofibular ligament over the tendons. At the time of surgical repair, the tendons are inspected for tears and the contour of the posterior fibular groove is evaluated. If a shallow groove is noted, a bony procedure to deepen the groove is necessary to prevent recurrent dislocations. Postoperatively, the patient is immobilized in a cast for 6 weeks.

ANTERIOR TIBIAL TENDON RUPTURE

Pathogenesis

Rupture of the anterior tibial tendon occurs infrequently, and most often in patients older than 60. The mechanism is either chronic rubbing against the inferior edge of the extensor retinaculum or rubbing against an exostosis at the first metatarsocuneiform joint. The rupture usually occurs at the distal 2–3 cm of tendon. Nondegenerative traumatic ruptures of the anterior tibial tendon are rare.

Clinical Findings

A. Symptoms and Signs

Patients with a degenerative rupture present with complaints of pain and swelling over the anterior ankle. They sense the foot slapping down, or they may be catching their toes on the ground when they walk. Patients frequently present after the symptoms have been bothersome for several months. Physical exam is notable for weakness of ankle dorsiflexion, often with a palpable mass over the anterior ankle joint.

B. Imaging Studies

If the diagnosis is in doubt, MRI scan can accurately determine if the tendon is ruptured.

Treatment

A. Nonsurgical

In the case of a less active patient, nonsurgical treatment appears to give equal functional results to surgical repair. Cast immobilization is followed by long-term use of an AFO.

B. Surgical

Acute tendon rupture in an active individual should be surgically repaired. Chronic ruptures that are symptomatic usually require reconstruction using an extensor tendon graft or tendon transfer because the distal stump is usually too degenerated to perform a primary repair.

Brandes CB, Smith RW: Characterization of patients with primary peroneus longus tendinopathy: A review of twenty-two cases. Foot Ankle Int 2000;21:462. [PMID: 10884103]

Haji A et al: Percutaneous versus open tendo Achilles repair. Foot Ankle Int 2004;25:215. [PMID: 15132928]

Jaakkola JI et al: Early ankle motion after triple bundle technique repair vs casting for acute Achilles tendon rupture. Foot Ankle Int 2001;22:979. [PMID: 11783925]

Tan V et al: Superior peroneal retinaculoplasty: A surgical technique for peroneal subluxation. Clin Orthop 2003;410:320. [PMID: 12771847]

van der Linden-van der Zwaag HM et al: Results of surgical versus non-surgical treatment of Achilles tendon rupture. Int Orthop 2004;28:370. [PMID: 15241626]

Wong MW, Ng VW: Modified flexor hallucis longus transfer for Achilles insertional rupture in elderly patients. Clin Orthop 2005;431:201. [PMID: 15685076]

OSTEOCHONDRAL LESIONS OF THE TALUS

Osteochondral lesions of the talus (OLTs) are defects of cartilage and subchondral bone in the talar dome. More sophisticated imaging techniques allow for precise diagnosis of OLTs, and advanced arthroscopic and open methods are available to treat this difficult problem.

Pathogenesis

OLTs, also known as osteochondritis dissecans lesions, are generally located in one of two areas on the talar dome: either posteromedial or anterolateral. The more common posteromedial lesions are usually deeper lesions involving subchondral bone. Their origin is thought to involve ischemia, often with an episode of trauma exacerbating the underlying condition. Anterolateral lesions are a result of a single traumatic episode or repetitive trauma from lateral ankle sprains. These lesions tend to be purely cartilaginous.

Clinical Findings

A. Symptoms and Signs

Patients usually present with several months of ankle pain following a routine ankle sprain. Sometimes they recount a history of recurrent sprains to the ankle. The pain is usually located over the anterior aspect of the ankle on the side of the lesion, but it may be diffuse. Occasionally, there is a sensation of locking in the ankle when a loose flap of cartilage is present. A high index of suspicion is necessary because OLTs can be misdiagnosed as a chronic ankle sprain, as discussed in the section on ligamentous injuries about the ankle joint.

B. Imaging Studies

Radiographs are often normal in OLTs. MRI scan is the imaging procedure of choice for determining the size, location, and extent of bony or cartilaginous involvement (Figure 9–62).

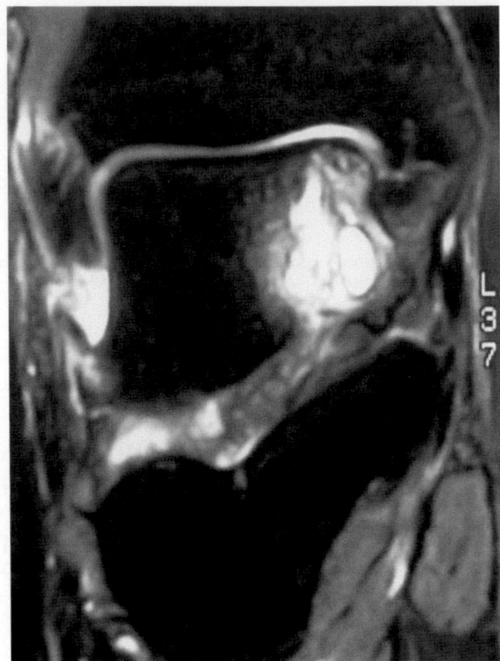

Figure 9–62. MRI scan of extensive osteochondral lesion of the talus.

Treatment

A. Nonsurgical

A 6-week trial of cast immobilization is warranted if the MRI scan shows no evidence of a displaced bone or cartilage fragment.

B. Surgical

The surgical treatment method depends on the type of lesion. Acutely displaced lesions can be reduced and pinned with an absorbable pin by either open or arthroscopic methods. Purely cartilaginous lesions are curetted to a stable rim and drilled to stimulate vascular ingrowth and fibrocartilage formation. OLTs with significant bony involvement require bone grafting in addition to drilling and curettage. A medial malleolar osteotomy is required to access a posteromedial lesion. If a bony lesion has intact overlying cartilage, drilling and bone grafting can be performed under radiographic guidance through the talus, thereby sparing the overlying cartilage. Postoperatively, patients are kept non–weight bearing for 4 weeks, but early ROM is encouraged.

New techniques were developed for larger lesions or ones that fail curettage and drilling. Osteochondral autograft or allograft plugs can be used to replace bone and cartilage defects. Autograft plugs are generally harvested from the ipsilateral knee. Intermediate-term follow-up data shows good results in most patients following this technique. Autologous chondrocyte implantation is also used to a limited extent for OLTs.

Barnes CJ, Ferkel RD: Arthroscopic debridement and drilling of osteochondral lesions of the talus. Foot Ankle Clin 2003; 8:243. [PMID: 12911239]

Hangody L: The mosaicplasty technique for osteochondral lesions of the talus. Foot Ankle Clin 2003;8:259. [PMID: 12911240]

Hunt SA Sherman O: Arthroscopic treatment of osteochondral lesions of the talus with correlation of outcome scoring systems. Arthroscopy 2003;19:360. [PMID: 12671618]

Petersen L et al: Autologous chondrocyte transplantation of the ankle. Foot Ankle Clin 2003;8:291. [PMID: 12911242]

Robinson DE et al: Arthroscopic treatment of osteochondral lesions of the talus. J Bone Joint Surg Br 2003;85:989. [PMID: 14516033]

Takao M et al: Arthroscopic drilling with debridement of remaining cartilage for osteochondral lesions of the talar dome in unstable ankles. Am J Sports Med 2004;32:332. [PMID: 14977656]

Hand Surgery

10

Michael S. Bednar, MD, & Terry R. Light, MD

Function of the Hand

The hand is a vital part of the human body, allowing humans to directly interact with their environment. The functional capabilities of the hand are many because the hand is ultimately an end organ of the human mind. The hand's enormous capacity for adaptability allowed primitive humans to make stone tools and modern humans to pilot complex aircraft.

The human hand is capable of prehension, which involves approaching an object, grasping it, modulating and maintaining grasp, and ultimately releasing the object. When a power grasp is used, the object is pushed by the flexed fingers against the palm while the thumb metacarpal and proximal phalanx stabilize the object. When an object is held with a precision pinch pattern, the object is secured between the pulp of the thumb distal phalanx and the index finger or index and middle fingers.

The hand can touch objects or other human beings while sensing temperature, vibration, and texture. This quality of tactile gnosis is sophisticated enough to allow blind individuals to read the pattern of small elevations that distinguish one Braille letter from another. The hand is also an instrument of communication, whether by making a gesture, playing a musical instrument, drawing, writing, or typing.

General Considerations in Treatment of Hand Disorders

Treatment of hand disorders requires an understanding of normal anatomy and its common variations. Treatment usually attempts to restore the normal anatomy, but when that is not possible, the goal should be restoration of maximal function. The appearance of the hand is vital because the hand is usually uncovered and exposed to the scrutiny of others. Imperfections are often a source of embarrassment. Effective treatment requires a mature balancing of the need for optimal function and normal appearance of the hand. Complex reconstruction that restores prehension but results in a hideous appearance of the hand are ineffective if the patient is so reluctant to expose the hand that he or she avoids using it. Conversely, a functionless stiff finger leading to awkward motion of an otherwise supple hand may cause the patient more embarrassment than amputation.

DIAGNOSIS OF DISORDERS OF THE HAND

History

When a patient seeks evaluation of a hand disorder, the physician should ask many general questions as well as questions specific to hand function and injury. The chief complaint as perceived by the patient should be summarized in one or two sentences. The patient's hand dominance, age, gender, and occupation should be noted, as well as any hobbies that require hand dexterity or strength. The approximate date of onset of symptoms should be recorded. If injury is the cause of discomfort, the exact date and mechanism of injury should be noted and whether the injury occurred at the workplace. The patient should be questioned about prior treatment and his or her perception of its effectiveness.

Complaints should then be further detailed, such as the nature of pain (sharp, aching, dull, or burning), whether night symptoms are present, and whether the pain is worse upon awakening in the morning or after a full day of work. The patient should be asked whether symptoms include numbness or tingling. Specific motor difficulties, such as difficulty in writing or unscrewing jar tops, should be noted. If the patient complains principally of unilateral symptoms, the examiner should ask whether similar symptoms are occurring on the opposite side. Finally, because the hand is an exposed area of the body, the impact of altered appearance should be discussed.

The medical history should include any prior hand injuries and any systemic diseases such as rheumatoid arthritis (RA) or other inflammatory arthropathies, diabetes, other endocrine disorders, renal disease, or vascular disease. Women of childbearing age should be questioned about recent pregnancies. A careful history suggests the correct diagnosis in approximately 90% of patients with hand problems.

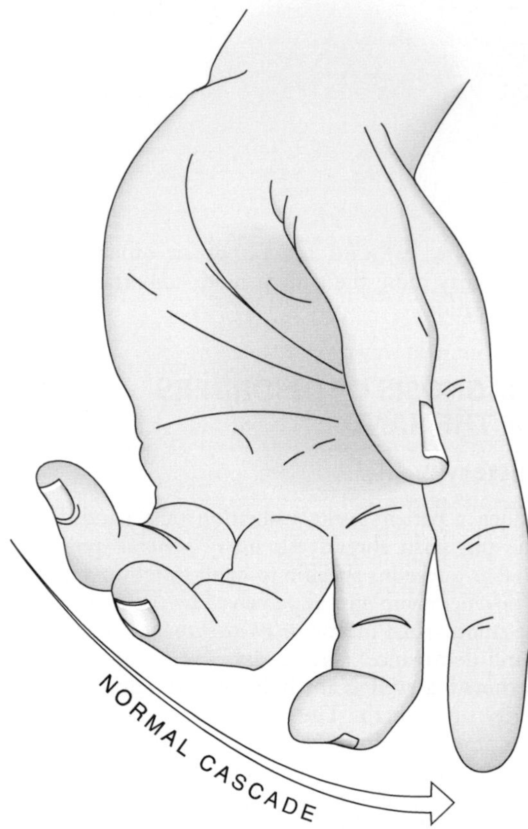

Figure 10–1. Normal cascade of digital flexion posture. When the wrist is in slight extension and the fingers are at rest, there is progressively less flexion from the little finger to the index finger. (Reproduced, with permission, from Carter PR: *Common Hand Injuries and Infections.* WB Saunders, 1983.)

Examination of the Hand

A. General Examination

Examination of the hand should begin with observation. Vascular condition can be assessed by noting the color of the fingers. Some hint of nerve function can be obtained by observing pseudomotor function as revealed by sweatiness or dryness of the finger pulps. The extent and timing of injury is suggested by the degree of swelling and ecchymosis. The posture of the digits and the wrist may signal tendon or bone disruption. Normally, a cascade of increased digital flexion is noted when ulnar digits are observed next to radial digits (Figure 10–1).

A diagram of the hand is often helpful in documenting the abnormality. Laceration sites, previous scars, amputated fingers, and subjective areas of decreased sensation can be noted on the diagram.

Next, the hand, wrist, and forearm are gently palpated. The temperature and moisture of the fingers should be noted. When the skin is blanched in the paronychial region, circulation should return within 3 seconds. Areas of tenderness on palpation are carefully noted.

B. Range of Motion

The passive and active range of motion (ROM) of the shoulder, elbow, forearm, wrist, and hand are evaluated. The normal ROM of the wrist and fingers is indicated in Table 10–1. In documenting ROM, active extension should be to the left and active flexion to the right. When the range of passive extension and flexion is different from that of active motion, the passive ROM values are noted in parentheses next to the corresponding active ROM values. The ROM of a stiff proximal interphalangeal joint could thus be recorded as 20/70 (15/80), indicating an arc of active motion from 20 to 70 degrees and a passive arc of motion from 15 to 80 degrees.

C. Muscle Function

The integrity of individual muscles should be documented. The flexor digitorum profundus to each finger is tested by stabilizing the middle phalanx and asking the patient to flex the distal interphalangeal joint (Figure 10–2). The flexor digitorum superficialis of each finger is tested by keeping all fingers except the one to be tested in full extension. The patient is then asked to flex the finger being evaluated at the proximal interphalangeal joint (Figure 10–3). The function of the flexor

Table 10–1. Normal range of motion in joints of arm and hand.

Joint	Motion
Elbow:	Extension and flexion 0°/135°
Forearm:	Supination and pronation 90°/90°
Wrist:	Flexion and extension 80°/70°
	Radial deviation and ulnar deviation 20°/30°
Finger	
MP:	Extension and flexion 0°/90°
PIP:	Extension and flexion 0°/110°
DIP:	Extension and flexion 0°/65°
Thumb	
CMC:	Extension and flexion 50°/50°
	Abduction and adduction 70°/0°
MP:	Extension and flexion—variable, up to 0°/90°
IP:	Extension and flexion—variable, up to 0°/90°

MP = metacarpal phalangeal; PIP = proximal interphalangeal; DIP = distal interphalangeal; CMC = carpometacarpal; IP = interphalangeal.

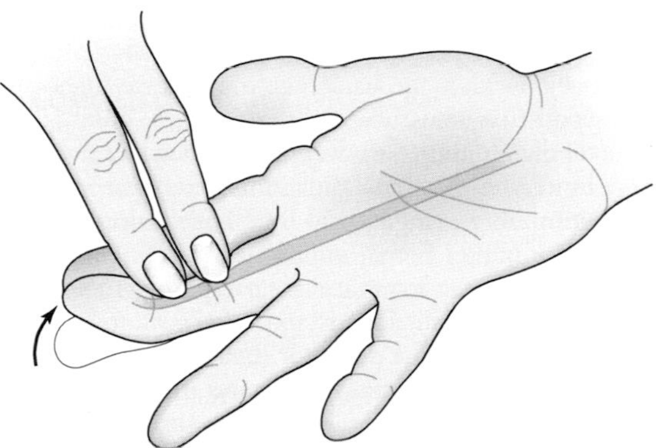

Figure 10–2. Testing of flexor digitorum profundus integrity. If the distal interphalangeal joint can be actively flexed while the proximal interphalangeal joint is stabilized, the profundus tendon is not severed. (Reproduced, with permission, from American Society for Surgery of the Hand: *The Hand: Examination and Diagnosis,* 2nd ed. Churchill Livingstone, 1983.)

pollicis longus is tested by asking the patient to flex the interphalangeal joint of the thumb.

The function of the extrinsic extensors is tested by asking the patient to extend the metacarpophalangeal joints of the fingers. If the examiner simply asks the patient to open the hand, the proximal and distal interphalangeal joints may be extended by contraction of the interosseous muscles, which may mislead the examiner to conclude that digital extension is normal. Interosseous muscle function is screened by asking the patient to abduct the fingers. The examiner assesses the strength of muscle force while palpating the contraction of the hypothenar and the first dorsal interosseous muscles.

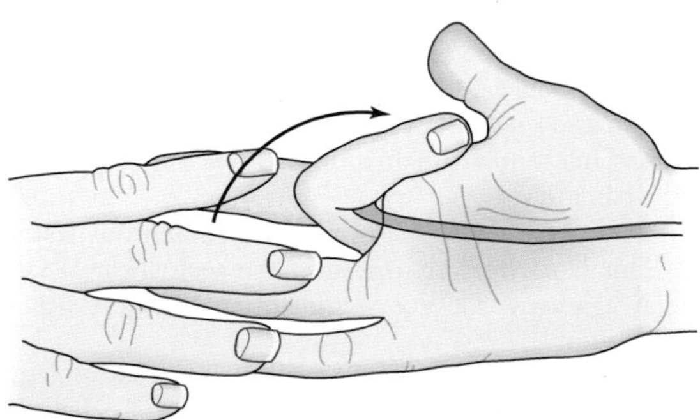

Figure 10–3. Testing of flexor digitorum superficialis integrity. If the proximal interphalangeal joint can be actively flexed while the adjacent fingers are held completely extended, the sublimis tendon is not severed. (Reproduced, with permission, from American Society for Surgery of the Hand: *The Hand: Examination and Diagnosis,* 2nd ed. Churchill Livingstone, 1983.)

D. Sensory Function

Examination of sensory function requires evaluation of the integrity of the median, ulnar, and radial nerves as well as the component proper digital nerves to each side of each finger. Each of the major nerves has an autogenous sensory zone, an area of the hand supplied predominantly by that nerve (Figure 10–4). The autogenous zone of the median nerve is the pulp of the index finger, whereas the ulnar nerve provides sensory fibers from the pulp of the little finger. The skin on the dorsum of the first web space is innervated by the superficial branch of the radial nerve.

1. Two-point discrimination—The integrity of each digital nerve may be evaluated using either a blunt-tipped caliper or an unfolded paper clip to test two-point discrimination. The two points of the testing instrument are held apart at a measured distance. The examiner alternates between touching the skin with one or two

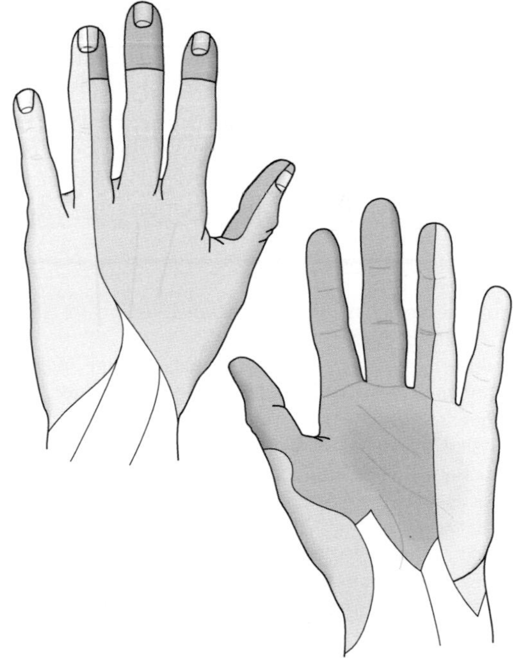

Figure 10–4. Sensory distribution in the hand. Light shading = ulnar nerve; medium shading = radial nerve; darkest shading = median nerve. (Reproduced, with permission, from Way LW, ed: *Current Surgical Diagnosis & Treatment,* 10th ed. Appleton & Lange, 1994.)

points. The points may be either touched (static two-point discrimination) or longitudinally moved (moving two-point discrimination) against the skin on either the radial or ulnar side of the finger. The points should be pressed against the finger until the skin just begins to blanch. The two-point discrimination value is the smallest distance between the two points that the patient can correctly detect in two out of three trials. Because of the increased sensory cues provided by movement, moving two-point discrimination has a value less than or equal to static two-point discrimination. Static two-point discrimination is normal if the distance is less than 7 mm, impaired if 7–14, and absent if 15 mm or greater.

E. Motor Function

Examination of motor function may be organized by considering groups of muscles within specific nerve domains (Table 10–2). Proximally, the median nerve innervates the pronator teres, flexor carpi radialis, palmaris longus, and flexor digitorum superficialis muscles. The anterior interosseous nerve branch of the median nerve innervates the flexor digitorum profundus of the index and middle fingers, flexor pollicis longus, and pronator quadratus muscles. The motor branch of the median to the thenar musculature innervates the opponens pollicis, abductor pollicis brevis, and superficial portion of the flexor pollicis brevis. The index- and long-finger lumbricals are innervated by median motor fibers running with the sensory nerve branches of the median nerve to the index and middle fingers.

Table 10–2. Innervation of the hand and forearm.

Median nerve
- Proximal median nerve: pronator teres, flexor carpi radialis, flexor digitorum superficialis
- Anterior interosseous nerve: flexor pollicis longus, index and middle flexor digitorum profundus, pronator quadratus
- Distal median nerve: index and middle lumbrical, opponens pollicis, abductor pollicis brevis, flexor pollicis brevis

Ulnar nerve
- Proximal ulnar nerve: flexor carpi ulnaris, ring and small flexor digitorum profundus
- Distal ulnar nerve: flexor digiti minimi, abductor digiti minimi, opponens digiti minimi, volar and dorsal interossei, flexor pollicis brevis, adductor pollicis, ring and small lumbricals

Radial nerve: brachioradialis, extensor carpi radialis longus, supinator, anconeus

Posterior interosseous nerve: extensor carpi radialis brevis, extensor digitorum communis, extensor indicis proprius, extensor digiti minimi, extensor carpi ulnaris, abductor pollicis longus, extensor pollicis longus, extensor pollicis brevis

The ulnar nerve innervates the flexor carpi ulnaris and flexor digitorum profundus of the ring and little fingers proximally. Within the hand, the ulnar nerve innervates the hypothenar musculature, flexor digiti quinti, and abductor digiti quinti. The deep motor branch of the ulnar nerve innervates the dorsal and palmar interosseous muscles, lumbricals to the ring and little fingers, deep portion of the flexor pollicis brevis, and adductor pollicis muscles.

The radial nerve innervates the triceps, brachioradialis, extensor carpi radialis longus and brevis, supinator, and anconeus muscles. The posterior interosseous division of the radial nerve then distally innervates the extensor digitorum communis, extensor indicis proprius, extensor digiti minimi, extensor carpi ulnaris, abductor pollicis longus, and extensor pollicis longus and brevis.

Muscle strength should be graded according to the British muscle grading system based on a scale of 0 to 5, with 5/5 being normal strength, 4/5 less than normal strength but with ability to resist a fair amount of resistance, 3/5 resistance against gravity, 2/5 resistance with gravity eliminated, and 1/5 only a trace or flicker of contraction without significant motion.

Diagnostic Studies

A number of studies may be helpful in establishing the proper diagnosis in a patient with hand or wrist pain. The choice of technique should be based on a careful history and physical examination.

A. Imaging Studies

In most instances, radiographic evaluation includes anteroposterior and lateral films. The importance of obtaining a true lateral radiograph of the finger and wrist cannot be overemphasized because many disorders, particularly interphalangeal joint subluxation and carpal instability, are not evident on oblique views. Oblique views may be useful in defining phalangeal fracture patterns. Tangential views are useful in assessing a carpometacarpal boss. The carpal tunnel view may allow visualization of a fracture of the hook of the hamate.

Stress views allow assessment of ligamentous stability. This is particularly useful in the evaluation of collateral ligament stability of the thumb metacarpophalangeal joint.

Ligamentous stability of the wrist may also be evaluated by radial and ulnar deviation views and by clenched-fist grip views. Grip views and ulnar deviation views may demonstrate a gap between the scaphoid and the lunate that is not apparent on simple anteroposterior and lateral studies.

B. Electrodiagnostic Studies

Electrodiagnostic studies include both nerve conduction studies and electromyography. Nerve conduction studies measure both motor (proximal to distal) and sensory (distal to proximal) conduction. Electromyography allows evaluation of muscle function.

C. Computed Tomography Scan

A CT scan allows excellent visualization of the distal radioulnar joint. The relationship of the distal ulna to the sigmoid notch should be viewed in pronation, neutral, and supination. CT scanning may be helpful in evaluating displacement as well as healing of scaphoid fractures.

D. Magnetic Resonance Imaging

MRI provides direct visualization of soft-tissue structures. The integrity of the transverse carpal ligament may be evaluated, which is particularly helpful in patients with persistent symptoms following carpal tunnel release. Evaluation of tumors and avascular necrosis is also facilitated by MRI. MRI scans also allow visualization of many triangular fibrocartilage complex and intercarpal ligament tears.

E. Bone Scan

The technetium-99 MDP bone scan is a useful physiologic test in the evaluation of unexplained hand or wrist pain. This test can rule out bone involvement and can be used to localize inflammatory processes for further study with CT or MRI scans (Figure 10–5).

F. Wrist Arthroscopy

Arthroscopic examination of the wrist allows for direct visualization of articular surfaces, wrist ligaments, and the triangular fibrocartilage complex. The effect of stress maneuvers on intercarpal kinematics may be directly observed. Wrist arthroscopy is particularly helpful in the debridement or repair of the triangular fibrocartilage complex tears. Partial tears of either the scapholunate or lunotriquetral ligaments may be debrided. Intraarticular fracture of the distal radius may be anatomically aligned and pinned under direct observation.

Bernstein MA, Nagle DJ, Martinez A et al: A comparison of combined arthroscopic triangular fibrocartilage complex debridement and arthroscopic wafer distal ulna resection versus arthroscopic triangular fibrocartilage complex debridement and ulnar shortening osteotomy for ulnocarpal abutment syndrome. Arthroscopy 2004;20:392. [PMID: 15067279]

Cerezal L, del Pinal F, Abascal F et al: Imaging findings in ulnar-sided wrist impaction syndromes. Radiographics. 2002;22:105. [PMID: 11796902]

Kocharian A, Adkins MC, Amrami KK et al: Wrist: improved MR imaging with optimized transmit-receive coil design. Radiology 2002;223:870. [PMID: 12034961]

Morley J, Bidwell J, Bransby-Zachary M: A comparison of the findings of wrist arthroscopy and magnetic resonance imaging in the investigation of wrist pain. J Hand Surg 2001; 26B:544. [PMID: 11884109]

Potter HG, Weiland AJ: Magnetic resonance imaging of triangular fibrocartilage complex lesions. J Hand Surg [Am] 2002;27(2): 363. [PMID: 11901408]

Slutsky DJ: Wrist arthroscopy through a volar radial portal. Arthroscopy 2002;18:624. [PMID: 12098124]

SPECIAL TREATMENT PROCEDURES FOR HAND DISORDERS

1. Replantation

Replantation is the reattachment of a body part that was totally severed from the body, without any residual soft-

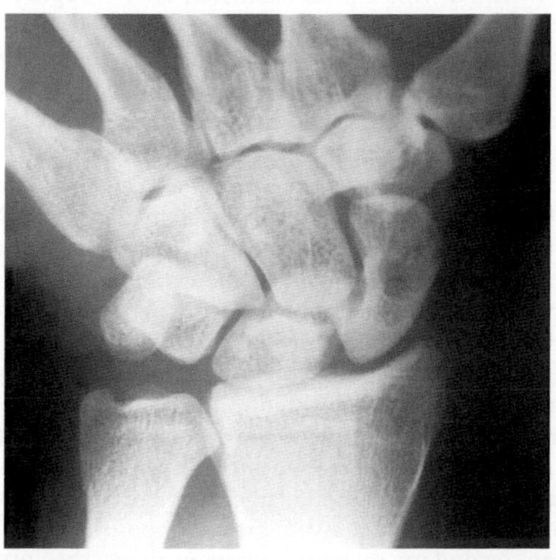

A

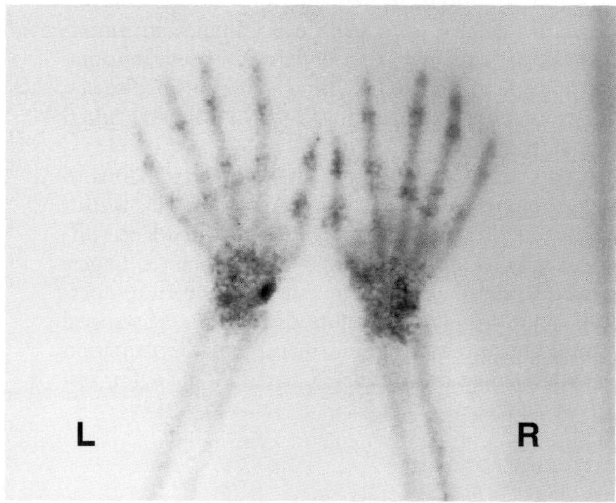

B

Figure 10–5. Radiograph (**A**) and bone scan (**B**) demonstrating increased activity in the region of the scaphoid in a woman with a symptomatic cyst.

tissue continuity. Revascularization is the reconstruction of damaged blood vessels to prevent an attached but ischemic body part from becoming necrotic.

Initial Care of Patient

Effective treatment of the patient and the ischemic or detached body part requires appropriate initial care and prompt referral to a surgeon at a center capable of mobilizing resources for early surgical care. The initial treating physician should place the amputated part in a sponge soaked with either normal saline or Ringer's lactate solution. The wrapped part should then be placed into a plastic bag, which is sealed and immersed in an ice-water solution. Under no circumstances should the amputated part be placed directly into ice water or exposed to dry ice.

A tourniquet is usually not required to control bleeding. A compressive dressing should be applied to the amputation stump. No attempt should be made to ligate bleeding vessels because it might compromise subsequent neurovascular repair. If the amputated part is not cooled, ischemia is poorly tolerated and successful revascularization is unlikely after 6 hours. Cooled parts may be replanted up to 12 hours after injury.

Indications & Contraindications

Replantation is indicated for severed thumbs or multiple digits, transmetacarpal hand amputations, wrist- or distal forearm-level amputations, and amputations of almost any body part in a child. In more proximal levels of amputation, only sharp or moderately avulsed parts can be considered for replantation. The more proximal the amputation, the greater the amount of ischemic muscle mass and the more urgent the need for revascularization.

Contraindications to replantation include severely crushed or mangled parts; multilevel amputation; amputations in patients with arteriosclerotic vessels; amputations in patients with other serious injuries or diseases; and amputations with prolonged warm ischemic times, particularly at proximal levels.

In adults, replantation of a single finger proximal to the insertion of the flexor digitorum superficialis is usually contraindicated because of the likelihood of stiffness. Limited tendon function in these replanted fingers is caused by simultaneous zone 2 flexor digitorum superficialis and profundus tendon disruption, phalangeal fracture, and extensor tendon disruption. Replantation at this level may be considered in children or for aesthetic reasons.

Surgical Procedure

The preferred method of anesthesia is axillary block because this technique provides a sympathetic block resulting in vasodilation. The surgical sequence of replantation begins with a wide surgical exposure that allows identification and isolation of arteries, veins, and nerves. The soft tissue is then meticulously debrided. The bone is shortened and securely internally fixed with sufficient stability to allow institution of early postoperative motion.

The extensor tendons are repaired first and then the flexor tendons. Anastomosis of one or preferably two arteries is then performed, followed by repair of the nerves and anastomosis of the veins. Two veins should be repaired for each artery repaired. Skin should be closed loosely, with care taken to approximate soft tissue over repaired vessels and nerves.

In replantations proximal to the distal forearm, fasciotomies of all muscle compartments should be performed at the time of replantation. The patient should be returned to the operating room in 48–72 hours, so the wound may be reevaluated and any additional necrotic tissue debrided.

Postoperative Care

Postoperatively, the hand is protected in an elevated, loose, bulky dressing. Anticoagulation should be given in the perioperative period to diminish the likelihood of anastomosis thrombosis. Low-molecular-weight dextran for 5–7 days and aspirin are among the recommended regimens. Some patients, particularly children, may require sedation to decrease early postoperative arterial spasm. Vasospastic agents such as nicotine, caffeine, theophylline, and theobromine should be restricted for the first few weeks after replantation or revascularization. The patient should be placed on a broad-spectrum antibiotic for 5–7 days. Clinical monitoring of the replanted or revascularized part may be supplemented with a pulse oximeter, laser Doppler, or temperature probe.

In those replanted or revascularized parts that show impending failure by change in color, capillary refill, or tissue turgor, the dressing should be loosened. Hand position should be changed to relieve pressure on the part. Patients may be given a heparin bolus of 3000–5000 U. The patient must be kept well hydrated and the room warm. If no improvement is seen after 4–6 hours, the patient may be returned to the operating room for exploration of the anastomoses. Vascular revision is most successful when carried out within 48 hours of injury.

Technical problems involving vascular anastomoses are most often caused by thrombosis, an ill-placed suture occluding the lumen, poor proximal flow secondary to spasm, or undetected intimal vessel damage. If vascular damage is found, a larger segment of the vessel should be resected and a vein graft interposed. If failure appears secondary to poor venous outflow, the intermittent application of leeches (*Hirudo* species) for 1–5 days may provide transient venous drainage while adequate venous drainage is reestablished.

Prognosis

Approximately 85% of replanted parts remain viable. Sensory recovery with two-point discrimination of 10 mm or less occurs in approximately 50% of adults. Patients with viable replanted or revascularized parts often complain of cold intolerance during the first 2 or 3 years after replantation. ROM in replanted digits largely depends on the level of injury and averages approximately half of the normal side.

In most children, normal sensation is regained after digital replantation, and the epiphyseal plates remains open and achieves approximately 80% of normal longitudinal growth. Although the functional results are more promising in children, the viability rate is lower in children because of the greater technical demands of the small vessel anastomoses and the greater sympathetic tone.

Because nerves transected in the proximal arm must regenerate over the considerable length of the limb, only limited motor return is seen in the forearm and hand in proximal limb replantations in adults. One potential benefit of a proximal upper limb replantation may be converting a traumatic above-elbow amputation to an assistive limb with elbow control. Replantation may provide dramatic restoration of hand function when the level of initial amputation is either in the distal forearm or at the wrist level (Figure 10–6).

2. Amputation

The purpose of amputation is to preserve maximal function consistent with bone loss and to achieve an aesthetically acceptable appearance. Priority should be given to preserving functional length, minimizing scar and joint contractures, and preventing the development of symptomatic neuromas.

Phalangeal Amputation

Digital amputation may be carried out through a phalanx or an interphalangeal joint. If the amputation is through the proximal or distal interphalangeal joint, the distal articular surface is reshaped to remove the palmar condylar prominences. If the normal insertion of a tendon was amputated, the tendon should be pulled distally, severed proximally, and allowed to retract. The flexor and extensor tendons should never be sewn over the amputation bone end to provide soft-tissue coverage. Nerves should be identified, gently drawn distally, and transected proximally to prevent the development of a neuroma adherent to the skin scar. If possible, the thick well-padded skin of the palmar surface of the finger should be used to cover the amputation stump. A nontender, shortened, well-padded digit is preferable to a poorly covered, slightly longer, tender digit.

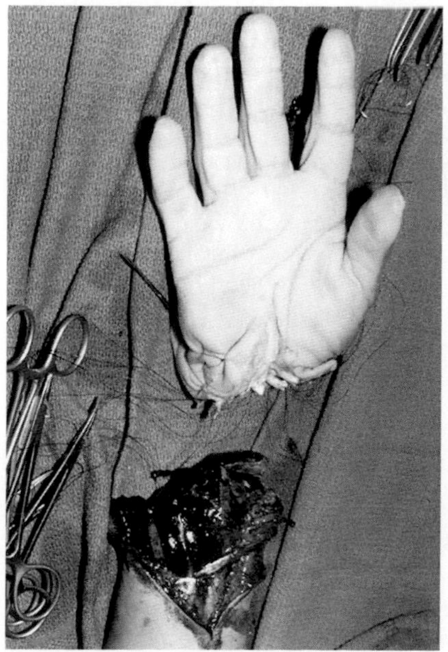

A

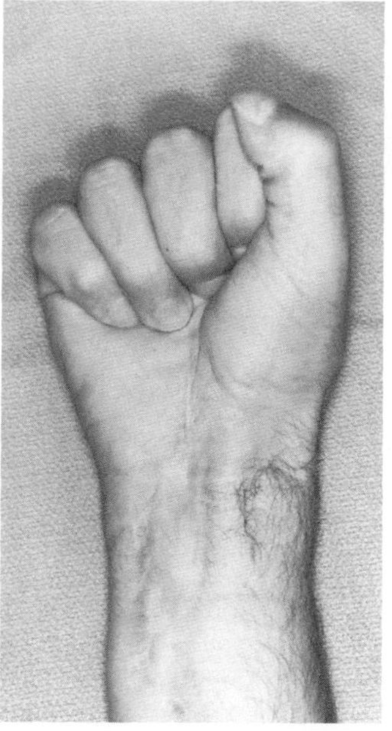

B

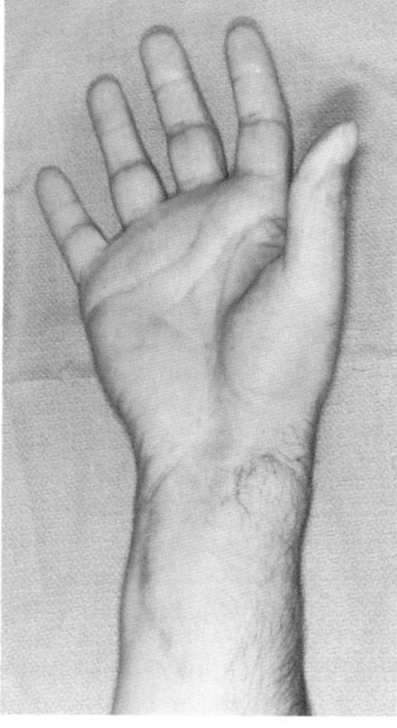

C

Figure 10–6. Replantation of hand. Intraoperative view (**A**). Following operation, flexion (**B**) and extension (**C**) are restored.

Ray Resection

Amputations through the proximal portion of the proximal phalanx or at the metacarpophalangeal joint of the index or little finger may leave an unsightly bony prominence on the border of the palm, and amputations at a similar level in the middle or ring finger may create an awkward interdigital gap that allows small objects to fall through the palm. Ray resection of a digit's phalanges and metacarpal may be employed to close traumatic wounds, remove dysfunctional or dysesthetic digits, or treat malignant tumors. The aesthetic and functional advantages of ray resection must be balanced against the loss of palmar breadth and, hence, diminution of grip strength.

Index-ray resection creates a normal-appearing web between the middle finger and the thumb. Similarly, resection of the little-finger metacarpal leaves a smooth ulnar contour. Little-finger ray resection is contraindicated in patients who prefer maximal grip strength over cosmesis. Resection of the middle- or ring-finger ray should be accompanied by either soft-tissue coaptation or metacarpal transposition. Resection of the middle ray through the proximal metacarpal metaphysis allows transposition of the corresponding distal portion of the index ray to the middle-ray position (Figure 10–7). Ring-finger ray resection may be closed by either osteotomizing the little-finger metacarpal and moving it to the ring-finger base or by pulling the little finger radialward across the hamate by tight repair of the deep transverse intermetacarpal ligament between the middle and little fingers.

Adani R, Marcoccio I, Castagnetti C et al: Long-term results of replantation for complete ring avulsion amputations. Ann Plast Surg 2003;51:564. [PMID: 14646649]

Melikyan EY, Beg MS, Woodbridge S et al: The functional results of ray amputation. J Hand Surg 2003;8:47. [PMID: 12923934]

Nuzumlali E, Orhun E, Ozturk K et al: Results of ray resection and amputation for ring avulsion injuries at the proximal interphalangeal joint. J Hand Surg 2003B;28:578. [PMID: 14599832]

Wilhelmi BJ, Lee WP, Pagensteert GI et al: Replantation in the mutilated hand. Hand Clin 2003;19:89. [PMID: 12683449]

Yu JC, Shieh SJ, Lee JW et al: Secondary procedures following digital replantation and revascularisation. J Plast Surg 2003B; 56:125. [PMID: 12791355]

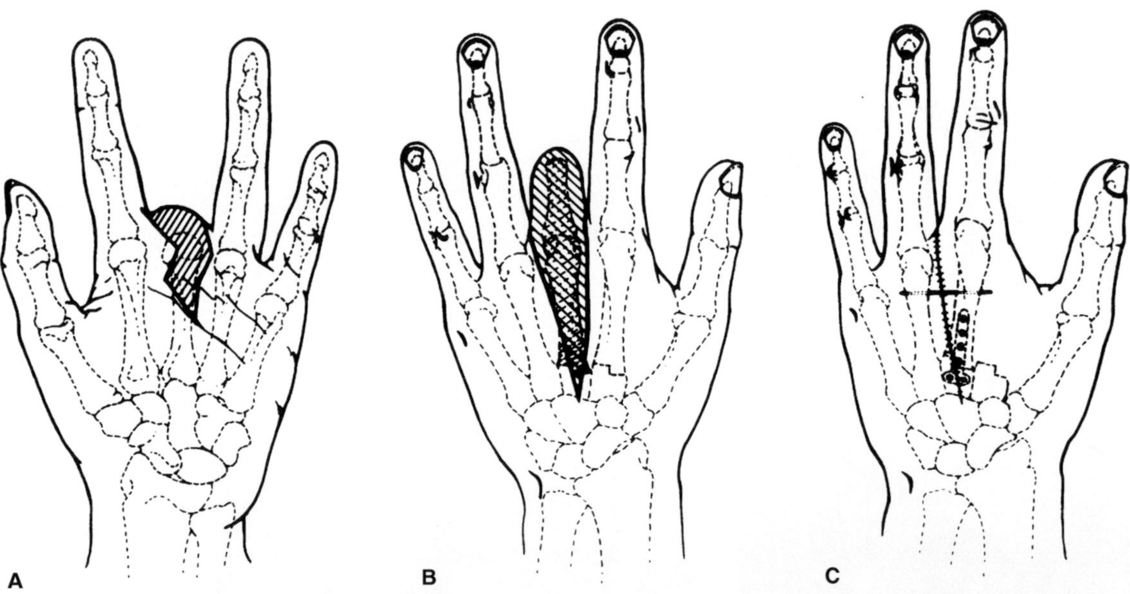

Figure 10–7. Middle-ray resection and index-ray transposition. **A:** Converging chevron incisions reduce palmar skin and soft-tissue redundancy. **B:** Corresponding step-cut osteotomies are fashioned in both the index and middle metacarpal proximal metaphyses. **C:** The transposed index finger is fixed to the middle finger with a plate and further stabilized with K-wire into the ring-finger metacarpal. (Reproduced, with permission, from Chapman MW, ed: *Operative Orthopaedics*, Vol. 2, 3/e, 2001.)

DISORDERS OF THE MUSCULATURE OF THE HAND

Anatomy

Control of digital posture requires a complex balance of extrinsic and intrinsic muscle forces. Extrinsic muscles have their origin outside of the hand and their insertion on the hand or carpus, whereas intrinsic muscles have both origin and insertion within the hand. Extrinsic muscles are either flexors or extensors, and intrinsic muscles contribute to both digital flexion and extension.

A. Extrinsic Extensor Muscles

The extrinsic extensors run through six different fibro-osseous retinacular compartments at the wrist level (Figure 10–8A). The first (most radial) compartment contains the abductor pollicis longus and the extensor pollicis brevis. The abductor pollicis longus inserts at the base of the thumb metacarpal and radially abducts the thumb, whereas the extensor pollicis brevis inserts on the dorsum of the proximal aspect of the proximal phalanx of the thumb and actively extends the metacarpophalangeal joint of the thumb.

The second extensor compartment contains the extensor carpi radialis longus and the extensor carpi radialis brevis. The extensor carpi radialis longus, inserting on the index metacarpal, dorsiflexes and radially deviates the wrist, and the extensor carpi radialis brevis, inserting into the base of the middle metacarpal, provides balanced wrist dorsiflexion.

The third compartment contains the extensor pollicis longus, which runs longitudinally down the forearm through the third compartment and turns abruptly radialward about Lister tubercle, a dorsal prominence on the distal radius. Because its insertion is on the distal phalanx, the extensor pollicis longus provides forceful extension of the thumb interphalangeal joint. The oblique course of the extensor pollicis longus tendon provides a significant adduction component to the pull of the extensor pollicis longus.

The fourth extensor compartment contains the extensor indicis proprius and the extensor digitorum communis, whereas the fifth compartment contains the extensor digiti quinti. These three muscles each have a role in digital extension at the metacarpophalangeal, proximal interphalangeal, and distal interphalangeal joints of the fingers. The principal bony insertion of the extrinsic digital extensors is on the dorsal proximal aspect of the middle phalanx. Metacarpophalangeal joint extension is provided by extrinsic extensor force transmitted through the sagittal bands. Distal interphalangeal joint extension is achieved through the conjoined lateral bands that are composed of tendinous slips from the extrinsic and intrinsic tendons.

The extensor indicis proprius inserts on the index finger ulnar to the extensor digitorum communis. The extensor digitorum communis inserts on the index, middle, ring, and, in some cases, little fingers. The extensor digiti quinti tendon inserts on the little finger ulnar to the extensor digitorum communis insertion.

The extensor carpi ulnaris tendon runs through the sixth compartment and inserts at the base of the little-finger metacarpal. It provides wrist extension and ulnar deviation.

The extensor digitorum communis tendons of the middle, ring, and little fingers are tethered together by juncturae tendinum over the dorsum of the hand proximal to the metacarpophalangeal joint (Figure 10–8B). The extensor indicis proprius tendon may be recognized at the wrist level as possessing the most distal muscle belly of any of the digital extensor tendons.

The digital extensor tendons are stabilized over the midline of the metacarpophalangeal joint by their attachment to sagittal band fibers (Figure 10–9). The sagittal band fibers insert onto the volar proximal phalanx and onto the lateral borders of the volar plate. The sagittal band fibers form a sling that allows proximal extrinsic extensor tension to be transmitted to the proximal phalanx, permitting metacarpophalangeal joint extension without a tendinous insertion onto the proximal phalanx. By holding the extrinsic extensor tendon balanced over the prominence of the metacarpal head, the sagittal bands normally keep the extrinsic extensor as far as possible away from the center of rotation of the metacarpophalangeal joint, thereby giving it the greatest mechanical efficiency. With rupture or attenuation of the sagittal band fibers, the extrinsic extensor tendon sublux to the ulnar side of the metacarpal head.

B. Extrinsic Flexor Muscles

The extrinsic finger flexors are the flexor digitorum profundus and the flexor digitorum superficialis. The flexor digitorum profundus inserts on the proximal volar aspect of the distal phalanx, flexing the distal interphalangeal joint as well as the proximal interphalangeal and metacarpophalangeal joints. The flexor digitorum superficialis acts as a flexor of the proximal interphalangeal and metacarpophalangeal joints. It lies palmar to the flexor digitorum profundus tendon in the palm, splits at the level of the metacarpophalangeal joint, and passes dorsal to the flexor digitorum profundus tendon before reattaching or inserting into the middle phalanx. Although the extrinsic flexors provide metacarpophalangeal joint flexion, this occurs only

contributes to metacarpophalangeal joint flexion and proximal and distal interphalangeal joint extension. The third dorsal interosseous usually has a single muscle belly, which inserts into the dorsal hood apparatus. The insertion of the volar interosseous muscles is also into the hood apparatus (see Figure 10–9).

All interosseous muscles course palmar to the axis of motion of the metacarpophalangeal joint and dorsal to the transverse intermetacarpal ligament. Their tendinous insertions are into the lateral band fibers, which pass dorsal to the axis of motion of the proximal and distal interphalangeal joints. When the metacarpophalangeal joint is flexed, the interossei are less effective in extending the interphalangeal joints than when the metacarpophalangeal joint is in extension or slight flexion.

The four lumbrical muscles insert into the radial lateral band of the dorsal hood aponeurosis of each finger. The lumbricals originate from the flexor digitorum profundus tendons of the corresponding finger. Their course is more volar than that of the dorsal or palmar interosseous muscles because they lie palmar to the transverse intermetacarpal ligament. The lumbrical muscles modulate flexor and extensor digital tone and may have a role in digital proprioception. Contraction of the profundus muscle belly draws the profundus tendon proximally and shifts the lumbrical origin proximally, thereby increasing tension on the dorsal hood fibers that extend the proximal and distal interphalangeal joints. Contraction of the lumbrical muscle draws the proximal profundus distally and reduces tension on the flexor digitorum profundus at the distal interphalangeal joint, so that distal interphalangeal joint extension is facilitated.

The abductor digiti quinti, like the first, second, and fourth interossei, has two tendons of insertion. One of these tendons inserts directly onto the bone of the abductor tubercle along the ulnar aspect of the little finger proximal phalanx, and the other insertion is into the dorsal hood apparatus. The flexor digiti quinti inserts onto the ulnar tubercle at the base of the proximal phalanx but does not insert into the dorsal hood apparatus. The primary function of the flexor digiti quinti is flexion of the metacarpophalangeal joint.

D. Dorsal Hood Apparatus

The dorsal hood apparatus, frequently referred to as the extensor mechanism, is the confluence of intrinsic and extrinsic tendon insertions on the dorsal aspect of the finger (see Figure 10–9). Through dorsal hood attachments, the extrinsic extensor muscles extend the metacarpophalangeal joint, the intrinsic muscles flex the metacarpophalangeal joint, and both the intrinsic and extrinsic muscles extend the proximal and distal interphalangeal joints.

Extension of the metacarpophalangeal joint is achieved through the action of the extrinsic extensor tendons pulling through the sagittal band sling mechanism, which lifts up the proximal phalanx. Flexion of the metacarpophalangeal joint is achieved both by the tendinous insertion of the intrinsics on the proximal phalanx and by a similar sling effect created by oblique fibers of the intrinsic mechanism blending into the hood, which flexes the metacarpophalangeal joint. Additionally, the flexor digitorum profundus and superficialis secondarily flex the metacarpophalangeal joint.

Extension of the proximal interphalangeal joint is achieved through the action of the central slip, which is the bony insertion of the extrinsic digital extensors on the middle phalanx. In addition, the intrinsic muscles contribute to proximal interphalangeal joint extension through medial slips from the lateral band, which run centrally to insert on the proximal dorsal aspect of the middle phalanx as part of the central slip.

Distal interphalangeal joint extension is achieved through both intrinsic and extrinsic forces pulling through the radial and ulnar conjoined lateral bands, which merge to form the terminal tendon insertion. The intrinsic contribution to the conjoined lateral band is through its insertion into the lateral band. The extrinsic contribution to distal interphalangeal joint extension occurs through lateral slip fibers that diverge from the central slip over the dorsum of the proximal phalanx and join the lateral band to form the conjoined lateral band. The conjoined lateral bands from the radial and ulnar side converge distally as the terminal tendon inserting on the distal phalanx.

DISRUPTION OF EXTENSOR MUSCLE INSERTIONS

1. Sagittal Band Disruption

Anatomy & Clinical Findings

The sagittal band fibers transmitting extrinsic extensor power may be disrupted by laceration or, more often, may become attenuated because of underlying synovitis of the metacarpophalangeal joint, as occurs in RA. When the sagittal band fibers along either the radial or ulnar aspect of the dorsal hood become attenuated, the extensor tendon may sublux into the valley between the adjacent metacarpal heads. Because the subluxed extrinsic extensors are mechanically less effective at extending the metacarpophalangeal joint, full active extension of this joint may be lost. This phenomenon occurs commonly in RA. It also may result from tearing of the sagittal band fibers with torquing activity such as occurs in the middle finger with pitching a baseball.

Treatment

An acute tear of the radial sagittal band may be treated by splinting. If this is ineffective, surgical repair may be indicated. Chronic injuries are treated by releasing the ulnar sagittal band and recentralizing the extensor tendon by placing a strip of the tendon around the radial collateral ligament.

2. Boutonnière Deformity

Anatomy & Clinical Findings

When the central slip is disrupted by laceration or closed rupture or elongated by synovitis of the proximal interphalangeal joint, the direct bony insertion of the extrinsic extensors on the middle phalanx is lost. When the insertion of the medial slips from the lateral band is also lost, active proximal interphalangeal joint extension is lacking. The finger is rapidly drawn into a position of proximal interphalangeal joint flexion as the unopposed motion of the flexor digitorum sublimis and profundus draws the finger into flexion (Figure 10–10). The lateral bands migrate apart as the finger is flexed and are drawn into a progressively more palmar position, eventually coming to lie palmar to the axis of flexion of the joint. In the subluxed position, the lateral bands become a deforming force contributing to the tendency of the finger to flex at the proximal interphalangeal joint.

With central slip disruption, the force normally transmitted through the central slip to the middle phalanx from both extrinsic extensor and intrinsic muscles bypasses the proximal interphalangeal joint and is refocused on the distal interphalangeal joint, amplifying the force of extension of this joint and hyperextending it. Because the distal interphalangeal joint is relatively resistant to active flexion, contraction of the flexor digitorum profundus muscle primarily flexes the proximal interphalangeal joint and is relatively ineffective in flexing the distal interphalangeal joint, unless the proximal interphalangeal joint is supported in maximal extension. The digit rapidly assumes the boutonnière deformity posture of proximal interphalangeal joint flexion and distal interphalangeal joint hyperextension.

Treatment

Because the proximal interphalangeal joint is at the center of the complex balance of the intrinsic and extrinsic forces, restoration of proper balance and tension on the central slip may be technically difficult. When the central slip is acutely lacerated, it should be directly repaired and the joint pinned in full extension for 3–6 weeks to protect the integrity of the repair. Closed ruptures of the central slip, if diagnosed acutely, should be treated with 6 weeks of splinting of the proximal interphalangeal joint in full extension. When diagnosis is delayed even a few weeks, a fixed flexion contracture of the proximal interphalangeal joint is usual.

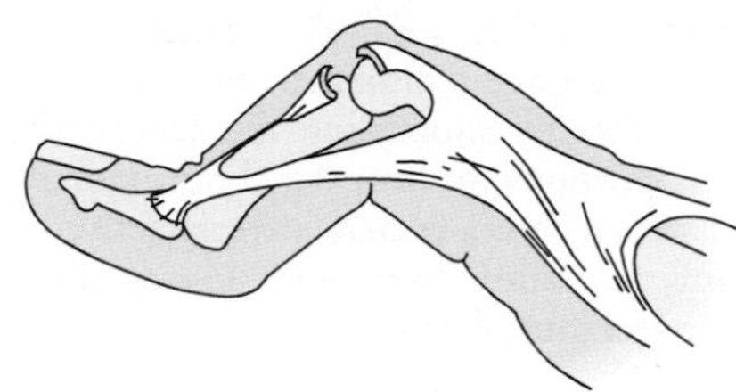

Figure 10–10. Boutonnière deformity caused by loss of active proximal interphalangeal extension secondary to loss of the central slip insertion on the proximal dorsal middle phalanx. (Reproduced, with permission, from Way LW, ed: *Current Surgical Diagnosis & Treatment,* 10th ed. Appleton & Lange, 1994.)

Surgical treatment of closed rupture of the central slip in a finger that develops a fixed flexion contracture is frequently disappointing because the surgical procedure must both release the contracture on the palmar aspect of the joint and augment proximal interphalangeal joint extension on the dorsal aspect. A better strategy employs prolonged splinting to diminish the extent of the fixed proximal interphalangeal joint flexion contracture. Among the variety of splints available for this, the Capener splint and the Joint Jack splint are particularly useful. Serial casting of the finger with a circumferential digital cast that is changed every few days may also be helpful in bringing the proximal interphalangeal joint into extension. During the period of splinting, the patient should be instructed to carry out active flexion of the distal interphalangeal joint, with the middle phalanx supported in extension. Care should be taken to assure that splints and casts allow distal interphalangeal joint flexion. Once full proximal interphalangeal joint extension is achieved, splinting should be continued full time for an additional 6–12 weeks. In many instances, this achieves sufficient tightening of the central slip to permit satisfactory active proximal interphalangeal joint extension.

If active extension cannot be restored with prolonged splinting, several operative interventions may be considered. The first, a Fowler type of tenotomy, obliquely divides the dorsal hood apparatus over the middle phalanx, proximal to the terminal tendon insertion. This diminishes distal interphalangeal joint hyperextension and may improve active proximal interphalangeal joint extension by refocusing intrinsic and extrinsic forces at the more proximal joint.

Alternatively, other surgical techniques attempt to more directly augment proximal interphalangeal joint extension, either by shortening the central slip or by mobilizing portions of one or both lateral bands. Although such techniques may increase active extension of the joint, they often do so at the loss of full proximal interphalangeal joint flexion.

3. Mallet Finger

Anatomy & Clinical Findings

The mallet finger deformity is characterized by a loss of full active distal interphalangeal joint extension with full passive ROM evident. The mallet finger reflects the loss of normal extensor force transmission via the terminal tendon insertion onto the distal phalanx. The unopposed flexor digitorum profundus pulls the distal joint into flexion (Figure 10–11). The usual mechanism of injury involves sudden passive flexion of the actively extended distal interphalangeal joint. Disruption of the terminal tendon may be entirely confined to the tendon or may involve an avulsed fracture fragment from the dorsal lip of the distal phalanx proximal articular surface.

Because the avulsed fragment includes the terminal tendon insertion, the clinical appearance of soft tissue and bony mallet fingers is similar. The distal joint rests in flexion, a posture that cannot be actively changed. Full passive extension of the distal interphalangeal joint is possible.

Treatment

A radiograph should be obtained to determine whether a fracture is present and, if the dorsal fragment is large, whether the distal phalanx is subluxed palmarward. If the joint is congruent, splinting is recommended even if a small articular surface fracture site gap persists. The distal interphalangeal joint should be splinted in extension continuously for 8 weeks, and the finger may then be tested. If residual drooping of the distal joint is noted, an additional 2–4 weeks of splinting is required.

Kalainov DM et al: Non-surgical treatment of closed mallet finger fractures. J Hand Surg Am 2005;30:580. [PMID: 15925171]

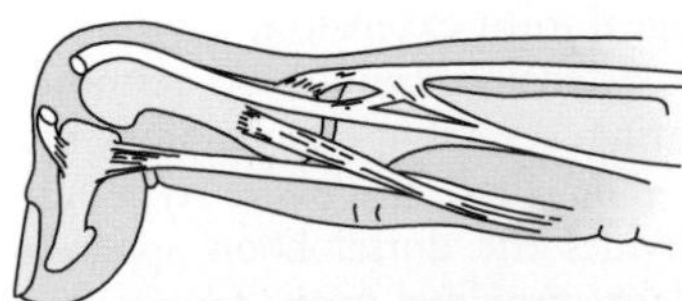

Figure 10–11. Mallet finger deformity is secondary to loss of terminal tendon insertion on the distal phalanx. (Reproduced, with permission, from Way LW, ed: *Current Surgical Diagnosis & Treatment,* 10th ed. Appleton & Lange, 1994.)

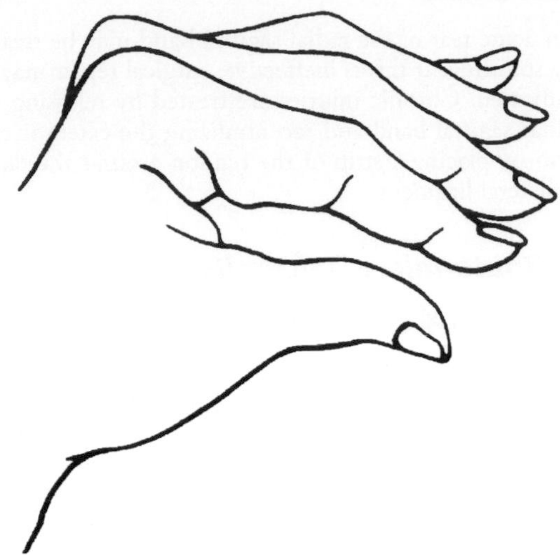

Figure 10–12. Intrinsic plus position.

INTRINSIC PLUS & INTRINSIC MINUS POSITIONS

Together, the interossei and lumbricals flex the metacarpophalangeal joints and extend the proximal and distal interphalangeal joints. Hence, the posture of the hand in which the metacarpophalangeal joints are flexed and the proximal and distal interphalangeal joints are extended is known as the intrinsic plus position (Figure 10–12). This is an ideal position for splinting the hand because the collateral ligaments of the metacarpophalangeal and interphalangeal joint are taut, and because it is also ideal for immobilization of most hand injuries, it is termed the *position of safety* or *position of advantage.*

The normal excursion of the intrinsic muscles is sufficient to allow simultaneous passive positioning of the metacarpophalangeal joints in extension while the proximal and distal interphalangeal joints are flexed. This posture, known as the intrinsic minus position, requires full excursion of the relaxed intrinsic muscles (see Figure 10–12, Figure 10–13). When the intrinsic muscles are paralyzed, the hand tends to assume the intrinsic minus posture, sometimes referred to as a clawhand. Although the extrinsic extensors have fibers that can provide proximal and distal interphalangeal joint extension in the hand with competent intrinsic muscles, in the intrinsic minus hand their excursion is expended in unopposed metacarpophalangeal joint hyperextension. Thus, the hand devoid of intrinsic power is unable to achieve active extension of the proximal and distal interphalangeal joints, unless the metacarpophalangeal joint is flexed by other means.

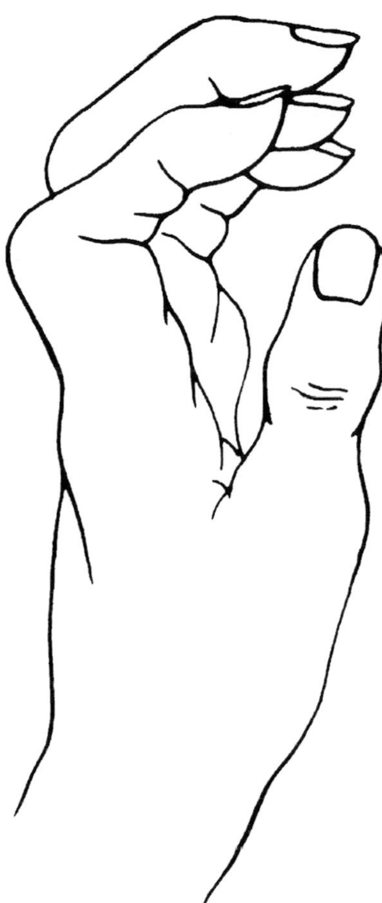

Figure 10–13. Intrinsic minus position secondary to low median and ulnar nerve palsies.

Treatment

Surgical correction of the intrinsic minus hand must either prevent passive hyperextension of the metacarpophalangeal joint or restore active control of metacarpophalangeal joint flexion. This may be achieved either by tenodesis or capsulodesis across the metacarpophalangeal joint or by an active tendon transfer. Once metacarpophalangeal joint hyperextension is prevented, the extrinsic extensors usually can effectively open the hand by extending the proximal and distal interphalangeal joints. If active proximal interphalangeal joint extension is not possible through the extrinsic extensors when the metacarpophalangeal joint is flexed, then tendon transfer for metacarpophalangeal joint flexion should be inserted into the digital lateral bands. This augments proximal interphalangeal joint extension and provides metacarpophalangeal joint flexion.

INTRINSIC MUSCLE TIGHTNESS

Anatomy & Clinical Findings

When the lumbricals and interossei become contracted and overly tight, the limitation of their excursion does not permit full simultaneous metacarpophalangeal joint extension and interphalangeal joint flexion. The intrinsic tightness test was originally described by Finochietto and later by Bunnell (Figure 10–14). It is accomplished by first determining that the metacarpophalangeal and interphalangeal joints each have a full range of passive joint motion in a reduced position. The metacarpophalangeal joint is then passively held in an extended position while the examiner attempts to flex the proximal and distal inter-

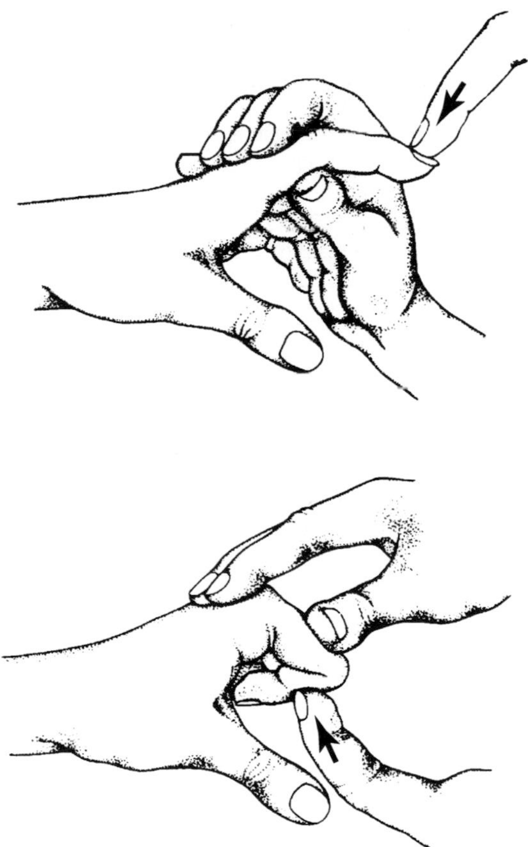

Figure 10–14. Intrinsic tightness test is performed by flexing the proximal interphalangeal joint with the metaphalangeal joint extended and flexed. Tightness to proximal interphalangeal flexion occurs with the metaphalangeal joint extended. (Reproduced, with permission, from Green DP, ed: *Operative Hand Surgery,* 2nd ed. Churchill Livingstone, 1988.)

phalangeal joints passively. If full passive flexion of the proximal and distal interphalangeal joints is not possible in this position, the intrinsic muscles are deemed tight.

Causes of intrinsic muscle tightness include conditions as diverse as RA, neurologic dysfunction secondary to closed head injury, and crush injury of the hand.

Treatment

Surgical treatment of intrinsic tightness may be carried out as an isolated procedure or in combination with metacarpophalangeal joint reconstruction. The intrinsic force is diminished either by intrinsic muscle tenotomy or by resection of a triangular segment of one or both lateral bands. The intrinsic tightness test may be used intraoperatively to judge the adequacy of intrinsic muscle release.

SWAN-NECK DEFORMITY

Anatomy & Clinical Findings

Swan-neck deformity is characterized by hyperextension of the proximal interphalangeal joint and flexion of the distal interphalangeal joint (Figure 10–15). The pathophysiology of swan-neck deformity involves either primary or secondary stretching or disruption of the volar plate's restraint on proximal interphalangeal joint hyperextension. Synovitis of the proximal interphalangeal joint secondary in patients with RA may distend the joint and thus render the volar plate ineffective in preventing proximal interphalangeal joint hyperextension. Overly forceful intrinsic muscle contraction (as occurs with an intrinsic plus deformity) transmits an abnormally high force through the central slip, hyperextending the proximal interphalangeal joint. When the proximal interphalangeal joint is hyperextended, the dorsal hood apparatus is relatively ineffective in extending the distal interphalangeal joint, allowing the distal interphalangeal joint to fall into flexion.

In some fingers, a fixed extension contracture or ankylosis of the proximal interphalangeal joint may occur as a consequence of swan-neck deformity. In other fingers, the proximal interphalangeal joint remains supple but the finger is locked in a hyperextended posture.

Treatment

Surgical treatment of swan-neck deformity secondary to intrinsic tightness requires diminishing intrinsic muscle force, usually through resection of a triangle of the proximal lateral band and dorsal hood. A new checkrein to proximal interphalangeal joint extension is created, either through tenodesis of one slip of the flexor digitorum superficialis or tenodesis in which one of the lateral bands is rerouted volar to the center of rotation of the proximal interphalangeal joint, recreating the sagittal oblique retinacular ligament.

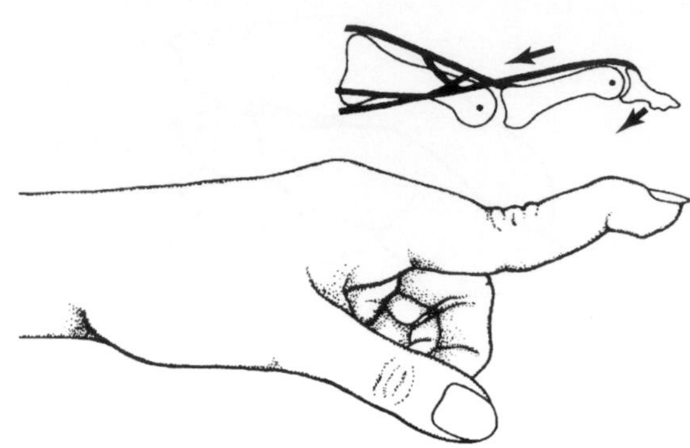

Figure 10–15. Swan-neck deformity. (Reproduced, with permission, from American Society for Surgery of the Hand: *The Hand: Examination and Diagnosis,* 2nd ed. Churchill Livingstone, 1983.)

Bruner S, Wittemann M, Jester A et al: Dynamic splinting after extensor tendon repair in zones V to VII. J Hand Surg. 2003B;28:224. [PMID: 12809652]

DISORDERS OF THE TENDONS OF THE HAND

FLEXOR TENDON INJURY

Anatomy

The extrinsic flexors of the finger consist of the flexor digitorum profundus and the flexor digitorum superficialis. The flexor digitorum profundus originates from the proximal ulna and the interosseous membrane. In the forearm, it divides into two muscle groups: the most radial component supplying the index finger and the ulnar component supplying the middle, ring, and little fingers. The flexor digitorum profundus and the flexor pollicis longus muscles form the deep compartment of the volar forearm. As the flexor digitorum profundus and flexor pollicis longus tendons travel through the carpal tunnel, they occupy the floor of the carpal tunnel.

The tenosynovial sheath of the flexor pollicis longus is continuous with the radial bursa; the tenosynovial sheath to the little finger is continuous with the ulnar digital bursa. In some patients, these two bursae communicate, allowing a so-called horseshoe abscess to spread between the thumb and little finger if infection occurs in the flexor tendon sheath of either one of these digits.

The lumbricals originate from the radial side of the index, middle, ring, and little fingers in the palm. The profundus tendon passes through the bifurcation of the flexor digitorum superficialis before inserting into the proximal palmar base of the distal phalanx. The innervation of the flexor digitorum profundus of the index and middle fingers is through the anterior interosseous branch of the median nerve, whereas the profundus of the ring and little fingers is innervated by the ulnar nerve. The flexor digitorum profundus provides digital flexion at both the proximal and distal interphalangeal joints.

The flexor digitorum superficialis has two heads: The radial head originates from the proximal shaft of the radius, and the humeral ulnar head originates from the medial humeral epicondyle and coronoid process of the ulna. Each digit has a corresponding independent superficialis muscle. As the superficialis tendons pass through the carpal tunnel, the tendons of the middle and ring fingers are more superficial and central than those of the index and little fingers. In the proximal aspect of the finger, the flexor digitorum superficialis tendon bifurcates around the flexor digitorum profundus at the beginning of the A2 pulley. The flexor digitorum superficialis tendon slips then reunite distally at the Camper chiasm, with approximately half of the fibers staying on the ipsilateral side and half crossing to the contralateral side of the finger. The tendon then inserts via radial and ulnar slips into the proximal metaphysis of the middle phalanx. The entire flexor digitorum superficialis muscle receives innervation from the median nerve. The primary function of the superficialis is digital flexion at the proximal interphalangeal joint.

The flexor pollicis longus originates from two heads: The radial head takes origin from the proximal radius and interosseous membrane, and an accessory head originates from the coronoid process of the ulna and from the medial epicondyle of the humerus. In the palm, the flexor pollicis longus tendon transverses between the abductor pollicis brevis and the flexor pollicis brevis. The flexor pollicis longus inserts into the proximal base of the thumb distal phalanx and is innervated by the anterior interosseous branch of the median nerve. The flexor pollicis longus flexes both the interphalangeal and metacarpophalangeal joints of the thumb.

As the flexor tendons pass distal to the metacarpal neck, they enter the fibroosseous tunnel, or digital flexor sheath. The fibroosseous tunnel extends distally to the proximal aspect of the distal phalanx. The tendinous sheath consists of annular pulleys, which provide mechanical stability, and cruciate pulleys, which provide flexibility (Figure 10–16). The first, third, and fifth annular pulleys (A1, A3, and A5) are located over the metacarpophalangeal, proximal interphalangeal, and distal interphalangeal joints, respectively, and the second and fourth pulleys (A2 and A4) are situated over the middle portion of the proximal and middle phalanges. The A2 and A4 pulleys are the most essential in maintaining the mechanical advantage of the flexor tendons.

The tenosynovium that lines the fibroosseous tunnel supplies both nutrition and lubrication to the poorly vascularized flexor tendons. Proximal to the sheath, the tendons are well vascularized by the peritenon. Within the sheath, tendon vascularity is supplied via the vincula system: the vinculum longus and brevis.

Following injury, the flexor tendon heals through both extrinsic and intrinsic mechanisms. Extrinsic tendon healing occurs via cells brought to the site of repair by ingrowth of capillaries and fibroblasts; formation of adhesions follows at the repair site. Intrinsic healing occurs from tenocyte within the tendon. The goal of flexor tendon repair and postoperative care is to encourage both intrinsic and extrinsic healing without the formation of thick adhesions, which would limit tendon excursion and ultimately result in restricted motion of the finger.

Clinical Findings

The time since injury as well as the mechanism of injury (sharp open injury versus closed avulsion injury) should be noted in the history.

A. Normal Cascade of Fingers

The resting posture of the fingers should be observed. Disruption of the normal cascade of increasing flexion in the relaxed fingers as one moves from the index finger to the little finger should arouse suspicion of tendon disruption (Figure 10–17).

B. Normal Tenodesis Phenomenon

Tendon integrity may also be evaluated by taking advantage of the normal tenodesis positioning of the

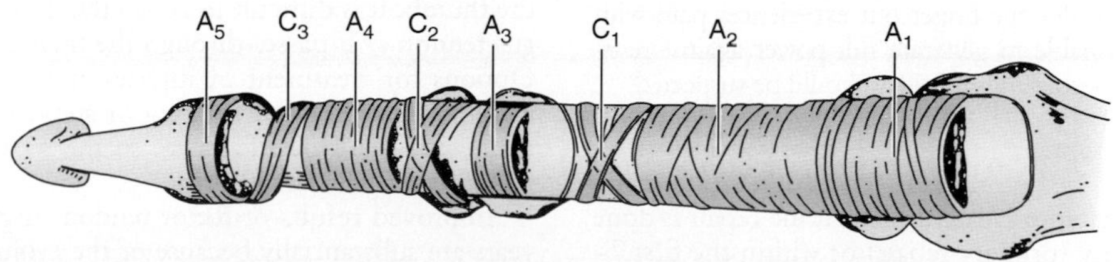

Figure 10–16. Annular (A) and cruciate (C) pulley locations.

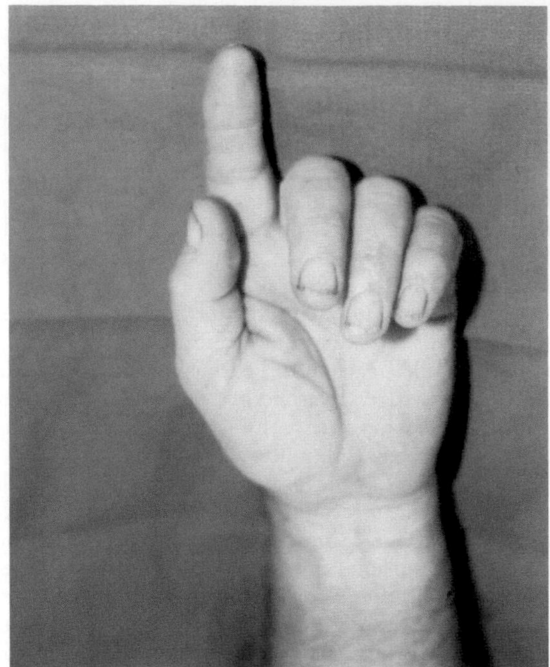

Figure 10–17. If the index finger remains extended when the hand is at rest, its flexor tendons are severed.

digits, which occurs as the wrist is passively brought through a ROM. Normally, as the wrist is dorsiflexed, the digital extensors relax and the finger flexors become taut, passively flexing the fingers in the normal cascade pattern. When the muscles of the proximal forearm are squeezed, the fingers normally flex involuntarily.

C. Testing of Individual Tendons

Isolated testing of the superficialis and profundus tendons is employed to determine the integrity of each tendon (see Figures 10–2 and 10–3). Because the flexor digitorum superficialis of the little finger is not independent of the ring finger in many individuals, either because of cross connections between the two tendons or because of congenital absence of the tendon, it may be impossible from clinical examination to detect injury to the flexor digitorum superficialis tendon of the little finger. The strength of flexion should be noted as each of the tendons is tested. If the patient is able to flex the finger but experiences pain with flexion and is unable to generate full power against resistance, a partial flexor tendon injury should be suspected.

Treatment

Functional outcomes are equivalent if the repair is done the day of injury (primary repair) or within the first 7–10 days after the injury (delayed primary repair).

Because repair requires proper visualization of both ends of the tendon, the wound may need to be electively extended. The tendon ends must be gently retrieved because trauma to the flexor tendon sheath creates adverse scarring. Tendons should not be grasped along their tenosynovial surfaces. The A2 and A4 pulleys should be preserved. A maximum of 1 cm may be debrided from the tendon ends without compromising eventual digital extension. A core suture of either 3-0 or 4-0 braided synthetic material is secured to coapt tendon ends (Figure 10–18).

The flexor tendon repair is strengthened by employing four strands of suture across the repair site rather than two. A running 6-0 nylon epitendinous suture completes the tendon repair. The role of flexor tendon sheath repair remains controversial.

Because the results and complications of flexor tendon repair vary by level of injury, five zones of injury are defined (Figure 10–19). Zone I extends from the insertion of the profundus on the distal phalanx to the insertion of the flexor digitorum superficialis on the middle phalanx. The tendon may be directly repaired if the distal stump is large enough, or it may be reinserted to bone. Care must be taken not to advance the tendon more than 1 cm.

Zone II, which extends from the proximal portion of the A1 pulley to the insertion of the superficialis tendon, is the most problematic region of injury because it contains both the profundus and superficialis tendons in a relatively avascular region. Care must be taken to preserve the vincular blood supply. When both the superficialis and profundus tendons are divided, it is preferable to repair both tendons because greater digital independence of motion may be achieved with a somewhat lower risk of tendon rupture during the rehabilitation period. Repair of the superficialis tendon as well as the profundus tendon also diminishes the likelihood of proximal interphalangeal joint hyperextension deformity.

Zone III injuries are located between the proximal edge of the A1 pulley and the distal edge of the transverse carpal ligament.

In zone IV injuries, the area beneath the transverse carpal ligament, a step-cut release and repair of the transverse carpal ligament should be performed to prevent flexor tendon bowstringing.

Zone I and II injuries of the thumb are handled similarly to those of analogous finger zones. In zone III of the thumb, it is difficult to access the flexor pollicis longus tendon as it passes through the thenar musculature. Options for treatment of injuries at this level include either primary tendon grafting or step-cut lengthening of the tendon in the forearm, so the repair is distal to the obscuring thenar muscles.

Improved results of flexor tendon surgery in recent years are substantially because of the evolution of postoperative therapy programs. Immobilization of the fin-

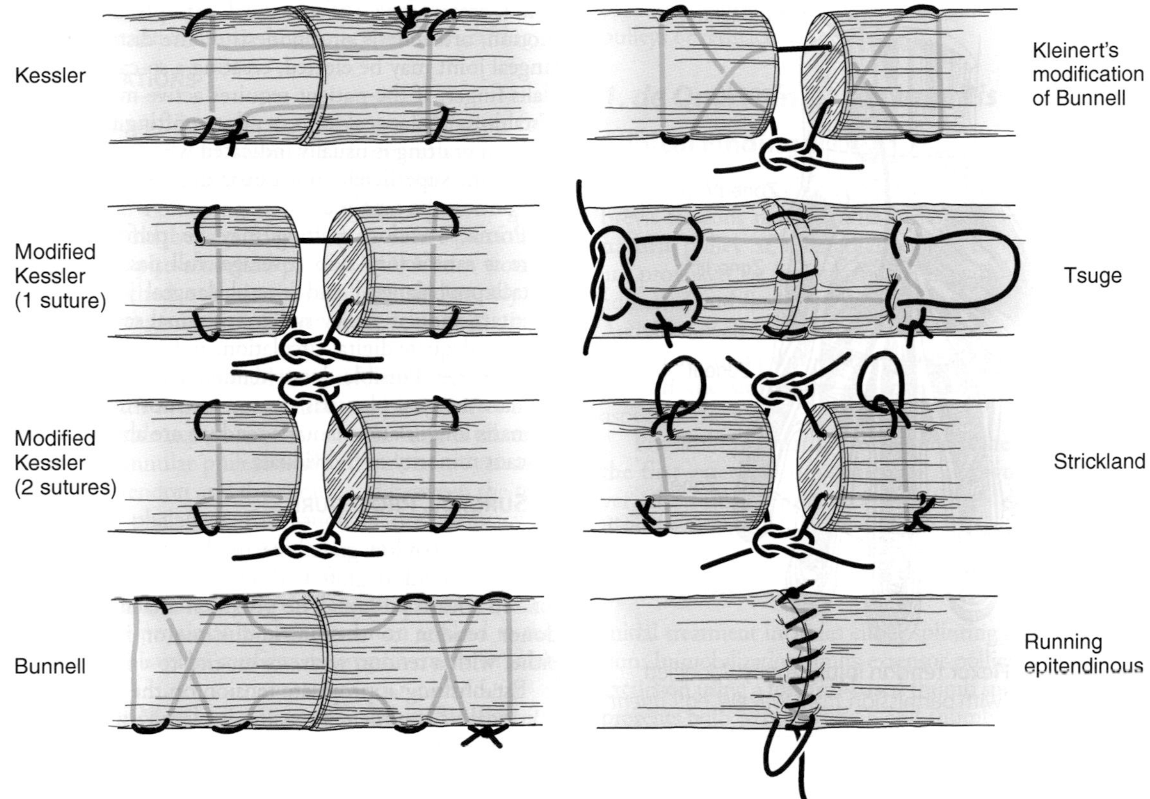

Figure 10–18. **Kessler sutures and other types of sutures for flexor tendon repair.** (Reproduced, with permission, from Green DP, ed. *Operative Hand Surgery*, 2nd ed. Churchill Livingstone, 1988.)

ger after tendon repair is appropriate only in very young or otherwise uncooperative patients. Following flexor tendon injury, the wrist should be immobilized at approximately 30 degrees of flexion, the metacarpophalangeal joints at approximately 45 degrees of flexion, and the interphalangeal joints at 0–15 degrees of flexion. A program of passive ROM exercises should be initiated that decreases the adhesions at the repair site and enhances intrinsic tendon repair. Passive motion may be achieved either through rubber band splinting to flex the finger passively or by having the patient move the finger passively. At 4–6 weeks following repair, active flexion and extension exercises are allowed as splinting is discontinued. At 6–8 weeks, passive extension exercises and isolated blocking is encouraged. After 8 weeks, the patient may begin flexion against resistance.

When a four-strand repair is performed, active assisted motion is begun within the first 2 weeks. In this program, the wrist is extended and the fingers are passively flexed. The patient is then asked to flex the fingers actively to hold this position.

With four-strand techniques for flexor tendon repair, active motion can begin earlier than with a two-strand repair. In properly motivated and cooperative patients, an active hold program is begun during the first week. The therapist passively brings the hand into flexion and the patient is asked to maintain the position.

Flexor Tendon Avulsion Injuries

The flexor tendon may be avulsed from its bony insertion, usually by forced extension of the finger while the finger is simultaneously actively flexed. An estimated 75% of flexor digitorum profundus avulsion injuries involve the ring finger. Such injuries commonly occur in football or rugby, when the athlete grabs an opponent's jersey and a finger is involuntarily extended as the opponent attempts to elude tackle.

Flexor digitorum profundus avulsion injuries may be classified according to the level of profundus tendon retraction. In type 1 injuries, the tendon retracts proximally from the sheath into the palm. Repair of these

lum may be elected. Because most patients with symptomatic disease have more than one abductor pollicis longus slip, the extensor pollicis brevis tendon must be identified and decompressed. In some cases, the first extensor compartment is divided by a septum, creating two separate tendon sheaths. In such cases, the more dorsal component sheaths must be opened to allow unconstrained extensor pollicis brevis tendon gliding.

Extreme caution must be exercised in carrying out the skin incision and subcutaneous dissection in this region because injury to the sensory branch of the radial nerve as it runs over the first compartment is a troublesome complication that may overshadow any benefit from tendon decompression.

2. Flexor Tenosynovitis (Trigger Finger & Trigger Thumb)

Clinical Findings

Flexor tenosynovitis or tenovaginitis is characterized by pain and tenderness in the palm at the proximal edge of the digital A1 pulley (Figure 10–21). Patients frequently note catching or triggering of the affected finger or thumb after forceful flexion. In more severe cases, the opposite hand must be used to force the finger or thumb passively into extension. In the most severe cases, the finger becomes locked in a flexed position. Triggering is often more pronounced in the morning than later in the day. Stenosing tenosynovitis is more common in diabetic patients than in nondiabetic patients. When multiple digits are involved, the possibility of diabetes should be considered.

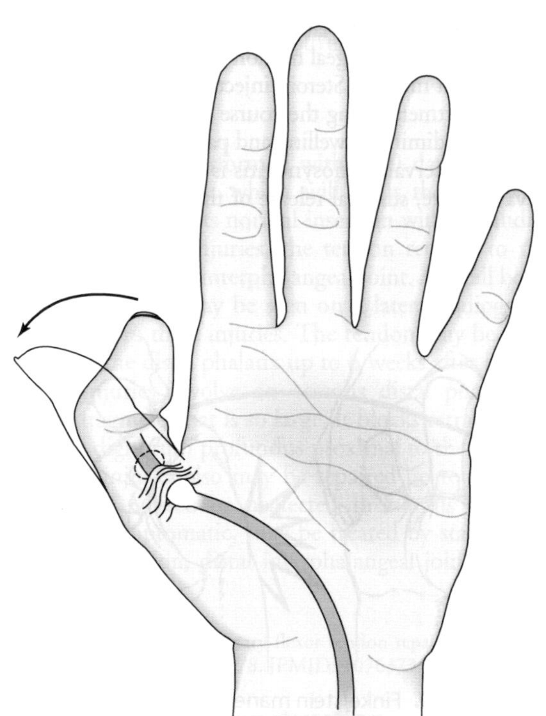

Figure 10–21. Trigger thumb. (Reproduced, with permission, from American Society for Surgery of the Hand: *The Hand: Examination and Diagnosis,* 2nd ed. Churchill Livingstone, 1983.)

Treatment

Most triggering digits may be successfully treated by long-acting steroid injection into the flexor sheath. To inject a trigger finger, the needle is inserted at the proximal palmar crease for the index finger and the distal palmar crease for the middle, ring, and small fingers. The needle enters the flexor tendon and pressure is applied to the plunger. The needle is slowly backed out until the needle is between the tendon and the tendon sheath, discerned by loss of plunger resistance. One milliliter of a combination of a short-acting anesthetic and steroid are given. The injection may be repeated if symptoms recur after an initially positive response to injection.

Surgical release of the A1 pulley is curative in digits refractory to steroid injection. Release is accomplished by directly exposing the pulley and incising its transversely oriented fibers longitudinally. The fibers of the A2 pulley must be spared to preserve effective digital flexion. Percutaneous release of the A1 pulley may be accomplished with a needle on the middle and ring fingers, especially if they actively lock. In patients with RA, the entire annular pulley system should be preserved to prevent further ulnar drift of the fingers. Triggering in these patients is treated by tenosynovectomy and excision of one slip of the flexor digitorum superficialis.

3. Flexor Carpi Radialis Tenosynovitis

Clinical Findings

Flexor carpi radialis tenosynovitis is characterized by pain with wrist motion, particularly active wrist flexion or passive wrist dorsiflexion. Marked tenderness is elicited on palpation of the skin overlying the tendon, particularly over the trapezium.

Treatment

Conservative care includes splinting the wrist in flexion and administration of oral antiinflammatory medication. If these measures are ineffective, a long-acting steroid may be injected about the tendon at the trapezial level.

Surgical decompression of the flexor carpi radialis is considered if conservative measures are ineffective. Decompression unroofs the tendon sheath in the distal forearm and across the wrist. The fibroosseous sheath is further decompressed by resection of the palmar ulnar ridge of the trapezium overlying the tendon.

Finsen V, Hagen S: Surgery for trigger finger. Hand Surg 2003; 8:201. [PMID: 15002098]

Hwang M et al: Referred pain pattern of the abductor pollicis longus muscle. Am J Phys Med Rehabil 2005;84:593. [PMID: 16034228]

Ragoowansi R, Acornley A, Khoo CT: Percutaneous trigger finger release: The "lift-cut" technique. Br J Plast Surg 2005;58:817. [PMID: 15936736]

Wilhelmi BJ et al: Trigger finger release with hand surface landmark ratios: An anatomic and clinical study. Plast Reconstr Surg 2001;108(4):908. [PMID: 11547146]

Zingas C et al: Injection accuracy and clinical relief of de Quervain's tendinitis. J Hand Surg Am 1998;22:89.

VASCULAR DISORDERS OF THE HAND

Anatomy

The blood supply to the hand is predominantly through the ulnar and radial arteries. The ulnar artery is larger than the radial artery and provides the primary arterial contribution to the hand. In most hands, the ulnar artery supplies the superficial palmar arch, which provides the principal blood supply to the common and proper digital arteries. The radial artery enters the hand by passing deep to the tendons of the first dorsal compartment across the anatomic snuffbox, dives palmarward between the bases of the first and second metacarpals, and forms the deep palmar arch. The median artery, a remnant of the embryologic vascular supply to the developing upper limb, contributes to the superficial palmar arch in 10% of patients.

The superficial palmar arch is located distal to the deep palmar arch. The arterial arch is complete, with total communication between the radial and ulnar arteries in 34% of hands and incomplete communication in 20%. The remaining hands have limited communication between the ulnar and radial arteries in varied configurations. The deep palmar arch runs alongside the motor branch of the ulnar nerve as it travels transversely just palmar to the proximal metacarpal shafts. The princeps pollicis artery is derived from the deep palmar arch in 98% of patients. The deep palmar arch also supplies the deep metacarpal arterial branches, which provide secondary blood flow to the digital arteries.

Clinical Findings

Patients with vascular insufficiency frequently complain of cold intolerance. When color changes occur, paleness or whiteness of the fingers is more suggestive of loss of inflow, whereas redness or bluish discoloration suggests inadequate venous return. Ulcerations of the tips of the fingers may denote ischemia.

The duration of vascular symptoms should be noted. If the abnormality is congenital in origin, changes in symptoms over time should be documented. The occupational history should record whether the patient uses vibrating tools or is subjected to repetitive blunt hand trauma during work. Occupations requiring outdoor work in all seasons (construction) or in a cold environment indoors (butchering) are noted. A history of trauma may suggest arterial or periarterial damage. Any sports activities that involve repeated trauma to the hand should be recorded; golfers, baseball catchers, and handball players are particularly at risk of closed vascular injury. Exposure to vasoconstrictive drugs, and particularly tobacco, should be noted. Other evidence of vascular disease should be sought, as well as diseases with vascular effects such as scleroderma or diabetes. Pulses are palpated, noting thrills or bruits.

A. Allen Test

The Allen test allows assessment of the extent of connection between the radial and ulnar arteries through the palmar arches. The examiner compresses both the radial and ulnar arteries at the wrist and then asks the patient to flex and extend the fingers repetitively. After the hand blanches, pressure is released from the radial artery while compression is maintained on the ulnar artery. The examiner observes how long it takes for each of the fingers to regain its pink color. The initial step is repeated with both vessels compressed, and the ulnar artery occlusion is then released while pressure is maintained on the radial artery. Again, examination of the reperfusion of the fingers reveals which digits are primarily supplied through the ulnar artery. In this fashion, the extent of interconnections between the radial and ulnar arteries may be assessed.

B. Diagnostic Studies

Noninvasive vascular diagnostic studies include Doppler scans, which detect the presence of flow; plethysmography, which determines the pulse volume difference between brachial and digital arteries; and cold stress testing, a technique that evaluates the effect of cold on arterial spasm. Invasive diagnostic procedures include arteriography, digital subtraction arteriography, and early-phase radionuclide scans.

ARTERIAL OCCLUSION

1. Arterial Trauma

Clinical Findings

Partial or complete division of an artery may occur as the result of lacerations, acute injection trauma, or cannulation injuries. Hemorrhage from arterial disruption should initially be treated with direct pressure. Total arterial division must be repaired if distal vascularity is inadequate. Partial arterial injuries may bleed profusely because the lacerated vessel ends are tethered to one another and are unable to retract, constrict, and occlude further flow. Partial arterial injury may require resection with or without reconstruction to prevent the formation of aneurysms or arteriovenous fistulas. Injection injury may produce either spasm or occlusion.

Treatment

The primary objective in treating arterial injuries is the restoration of adequate distal blood flow. Attempts may be made to remove distal clots with Fogarty catheters. If this is unsuccessful, clot-dissolving agents such as urokinase, local or systemic vasodilators, and stellate ganglion blocks may be employed to diminish vascular spasm. Care must be taken when using multiple agents to ensure they do not interfere with one another. For instance, use of urokinase after an axillary block may produce axillary artery hemorrhage, thereby compounding the problem.

2. Thrombosis

Clinical Findings

The ulnar artery is the most common site of upper extremity arterial thrombosis. This entity, also known as ulnar hammer syndrome hypothenar hammer syndrome, is most often the result of repetitive trauma to the hypothenar area of the hand. Patients may complain of a tender pulsatile mass on the ulnar side of the palm. In some instances, presenting symptoms reflect a low ulnar nerve palsy secondary to compression of the ulnar nerve by the aneurysm at the level of the Guyon canal. Distal vascular insufficiency may be evident in the ring and little fingers.

Treatment

If evaluation demonstrates that all the fingers are well perfused by the radial artery alone, excision of the segment of the ulnar artery containing the aneurysm or thrombosed segment and ligation of the vessel ends is curative. Simple division of the vessel may confer a modest sympathectomy effect to the residual ulnar artery because sympathetic fibers surrounding the ulnar artery are disrupted at the time of vessel division. If, however, digital perfusion is inadequate after a vessel segment is resected and the tourniquet deflated, a segmental vein graft is required to reconstitute the ulnar artery.

3. Aneurysm

A distinction should be made between true and false aneurysms. In a true aneurysm, all layers of the arterial wall are involved. These aneurysms are usually caused by blunt trauma but may also be secondary to degeneration or infection. False aneurysms are characterized by partial wall involvement, with periarterial tissues forming a false wall lined by endothelium. False aneurysms are most common following penetrating trauma, such as stab wounds.

Both true and false aneurysms should be treated with resection. As discussed in the section about ulnar hammer syndrome, the necessity of vascular reconstruction is dictated by the adequacy of distal perfusion after tourniquet release.

VASOSPASTIC CONDITIONS

Clinical Findings

Raynaud phenomenon, Raynaud disease, and Raynaud syndrome are often confused. Raynaud phenomenon is a condition in which pallor of the digits occurs with or without cyanosis on exposure to cold. Raynaud disease (primary Raynaud) is present when Raynaud phenomenon occurs without another associated or causative disease. Raynaud disease most commonly occurs in young (less than 40 years) women and is often bilateral, without demonstrable peripheral arterial occlusion. In severe cases, patients may develop gangrene or atrophic changes limited to the distal digital skin. Raynaud syndrome (secondary Raynaud) occurs when Raynaud phenomenon is associated with another disease, such as connective tissue disorders (systemic lupus erythematosus), neurologic disorders, arterial occlusive disorders, or blood dyscrasias.

Treatment

All patients with Raynaud phenomenon experience cyclic episodes of digital pallor alternating with episodes of cyanosis and hyperemia. Treatment includes protection of the hands from cold by the use of gloves or mittens. Patients should be strongly encouraged to cease all cigarette or cigar smoking. Drug treatment attempts to diminish occlusive phenomena. Alpha-receptor blocking agents, nitroglycerin ointment, nifedipine, and other calcium channel blockers are effective in decreasing spasm. Digital artery sympathectomy, the surgical stripping of the periarterial tissue of the common digital artery over a short segment at the distal palmar level, may improve circulation to ischemic digits.

Balogh B et al: Adventitial stripping of the radial and ulnar arteries in Raynaud's disease. J Hand Surg Am 2002;27:1073.

Ruch DS et al: Arterial reconstruction for radial artery occlusion. J Hand Surg [Am] 2000;25:282. [PMID: 10722820]

Ruch DS et al: Periarterial sympathectomy in scleroderma patients: Intermediate-term follow-up. J Hand Surg [Am] 2002;27(2): 258. [PMID: 11901385]

DISORDERS OF THE NERVES OF THE HAND

PERIPHERAL NERVE INJURY

Anatomy

Peripheral nerves consist of a mixture of myelinated and unmyelinated axons. Motor, sensory, and sympathetic fibers often travel together in a single nerve. Axons are grouped in bundles termed *fascicles,* which are surrounded by perineurium. The fine connective tissue between axons within a fascicle is called *endoneurium.* Fascicles are held together as a nerve by the epineurium. Nerves are considered monofascicular, oligofascicular, or polyfascicular, depending on the number of fascicles. The relationship between fascicles changes along the longitudinal course of the nerve. The degree of fascicular change decreases distally. The mesoneurium, which is the connective tissue surrounding the epineurium, facilitates longitudinal gliding of the nerve.

After a nerve is injured, a number of changes occur. The somatosensory cortex reorganizes so the area represented by the injured nerve diminishes. The cell body of the lacerated axon increases in size. The production of materials for repair of the cytoskeleton is increased, and the production of neurotransmitters decreases. At the proximal segment of the injured axon, further proximal degeneration occurs based on the severity of the injury. In the axon distal to the laceration, Schwann cells phagocytose the axon, allowing the surrounding myelin tube to collapse.

Within 24 hours of injury, axonal sprouting occurs from the proximal stump. Multiple axons in a fascicle form a regenerating unit. The number of axons in the unit decreases with time. Longitudinal growth of the regenerating nerve depends on the ability of the axons to adhere to trophic factors in the basal lamina of the Schwann cell. Changes also occur at the distal end of the nerve. At the motor endplate, the muscle fibers atrophy. The sensitivity and number of acetylcholine receptors increases as their location expands from pits to the entire length of the muscle fiber. If the muscle fiber is reinnervated, both old and new motor endplates become active. The recovery of strength is greatest after primary nerve repair, less vigorous after repair with nerve grafting, and weakest after direct implantation of the nerve end into muscle. Muscle reinnervation occurs only if the axon reaches the muscle within a year. In contrast, sensory receptors may be effectively reinnervated years after injury.

Nerve injures are classified into three types. (1) Neurapraxia is a conduction block that occurs without axonal disruption. Recovery is usually complete within days to a few months. (2) Axonotmesis describes an injury in which axonal disruption occurs, with the endoneurial tube remaining in continuity. The intact endoneurial tube provides the regenerating sprouting axons with a well-defined path to the end organs. Because axonal growth occurs at approximately 1 mm/day, recovery is good but slow. (3) Neurotmesis refers to transection of the nerve. Unless the nerve is repaired, the regenerating axons cannot find a suitable path and recovery does not occur. The frustrated sprouting axons form a neuroma at the distal end of the proximal segment of the lacerated nerve.

Diagnostic Studies

Preoperative and postoperative assessment of motor and sensory function include quantitative measurement of pinch and grip strength, static and moving two-point discrimination, and vibration and pressure measurements. Two-point discrimination reflects innervation density, whereas vibration and pressure measurements gauges innervation threshold.

Treatment

Nerve repair should be carried out with magnification and microsurgical technique. A tension-free repair provides the ideal environment for nerve regeneration. Tension at the repair site may be diminished by advancement of the nerve (ie, anterior transposition of the ulnar nerve for proximal forearm ulnar nerve laceration) or by limitation of joint motion. If a tension-free repair is impossible, nerve grafting is necessary to bridge the defect in the nerve. Frequently used donor nerves include the sural nerve, the anterior branch of the medial antebrachial cutaneous nerve, and the lateral antebrachial cutaneous nerve.

Primary repair is preferred to nerve grafting because the latter procedure requires two sites of nerve coaptation. Epineurial repair is usually performed under magnification, using 8-0 or 9-0 suture (Figure 10–22A). When a particular fascicular group (eg, motor branch of the median nerve) is recognized as mediating a specific function, it may be repaired separately (Figure 10–22B). Postoperative therapy may include motor and sensory reeducation to maximize the clinical result.

Primary nerve repair is indicated after a sharp nerve division occurs. After avulsion injuries, repair even by nerve grafting cannot be performed until the proximal and distal extent of injury is known. When closed nerve injury occurs, sensory and motor function is closely monitored. If no recovery is seen within 3 months, electrodiagnostic studies are carried out. If no electrical evidence of recovery is documented, the nerve is explored, and neurolysis, secondary nerve repair, or nerve grafting is accomplished.

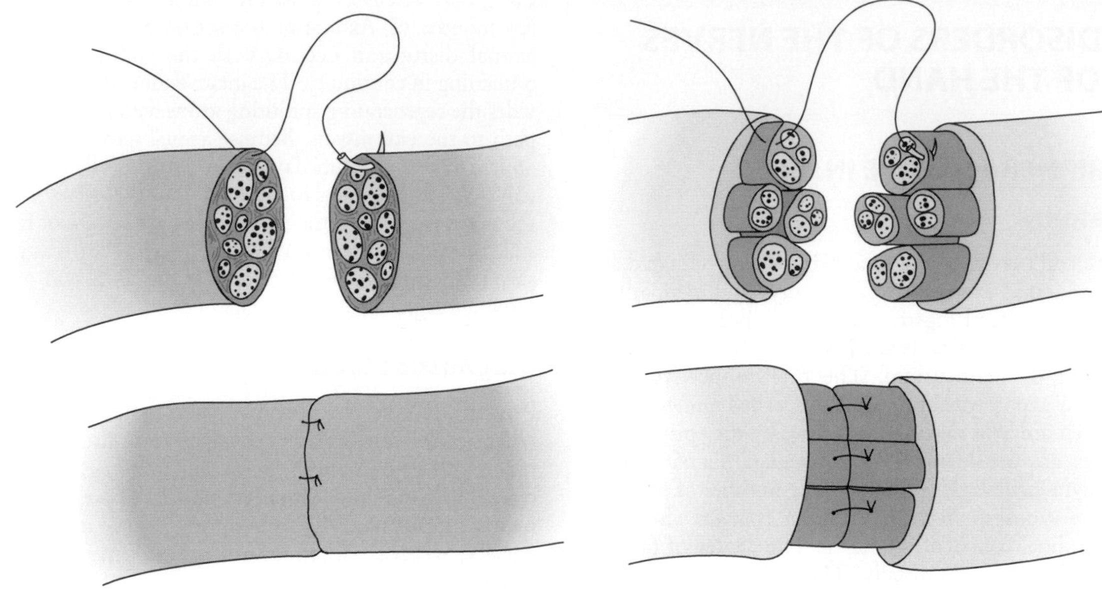

Figure 10–22. **A:** Schematic diagram of epineurial repair technique. **B:** Group fascicular repair technique. (Reproduced, with permission, from Mackinnon SE, Dellon AL: *Surgery of the Peripheral Nerve.* Thieme, 1988.)

COMPRESSIVE NEUROPATHIES

Compressive neuropathies are a group of nerve injuries that have common pathophysiology factors and occur at predictable sites of normal anatomic constraint. Nerve dysfunction is the result of neural ischemia in the compressed segment. Symptoms may resolve after release of the anatomic structures producing pressure on the nerve, particularly when compression is neither severe nor long standing.

1. Median Neuropathy

Carpal Tunnel Syndrome

A. Anatomy

Compression of the median nerve within the carpal tunnel is the most common upper extremity compressive neuropathy. The carpal tunnel is that space along the palmar aspect of the wrist anatomically bounded by the scaphoid tubercle and the trapezium radially, the hook of the hamate and the pisiform ulnarly, the capitate dorsally, and the transverse carpal ligament palmarly (Figure 10–23).

B. Clinical Findings

Carpal tunnel syndrome is often idiopathic. It is associated with pregnancy, amyloidosis, flexor tenosynovitis, overuse phenomenon, acute or chronic inflammatory conditions, traumatic disorders of the wrist, endocrine disorders (diabetes mellitus and hypothyroidism), and tumors within the carpal tunnel.

Differential diagnosis includes compression of the median nerve or cervical roots in other anatomic locations. Diabetic neuropathy may produce symptoms similar to those of carpal tunnel syndrome, and patients with diabetic neuropathy may develop concomitant carpal tunnel syndrome.

1. Symptoms and signs—Most patients complain of numbness in the thumb and index and middle fingers, though many note that the entire hand feels numb. Pain rarely prevents the affected individual from falling asleep but characteristically awakens the patient from sleep after a number of hours. After a period of moving the fingers, most patients are able to return to sleep. Many patients complain of finger stiffness upon arising in the morning.

Discomfort or numbness, or both, may be incited by activities in which the wrist is held in a flexed position for a sustained period of time (eg, holding a steering wheel, telephone receiver, book, or newspaper). Discomfort and pain may radiate from the hand up the arm to the shoulder or neck. The patient may complain of clumsiness when trying to perform tasks such as unscrewing a jar top and may experience difficulty in holding on to a glass or cup securely.

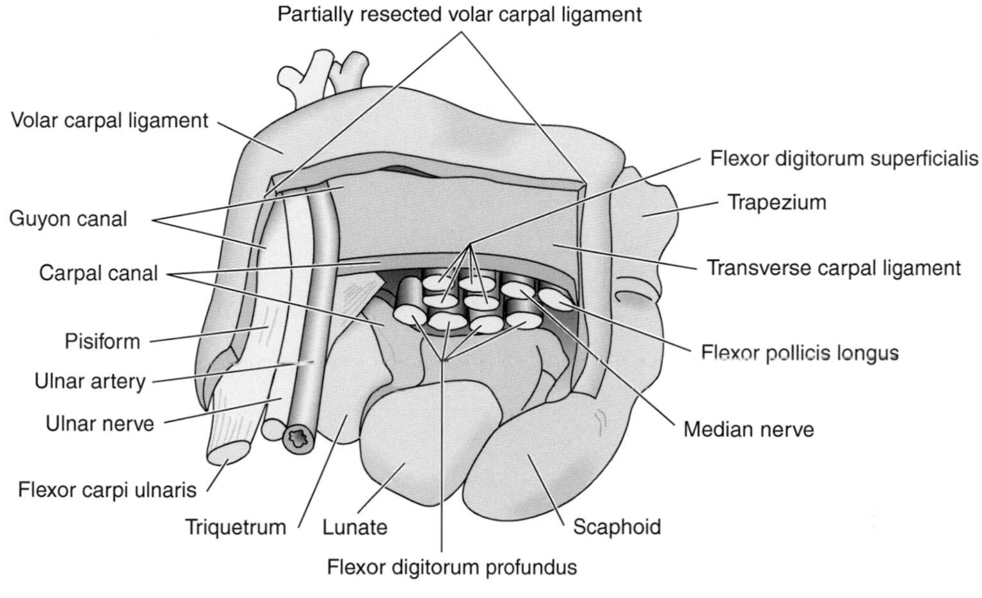

Figure 10–23. The Guyon canal and carpal tunnel and contents. (Cross section of supinated right wrist, viewed from proximal to distal.) Note the relationship between the transverse carpal ligament and the volar carpal ligament (partially resected). (Reproduced, with permission, from Reckling FW, Reckling JB, Mohn MP: *Orthopaedic Anatomy and Surgical Approaches.* Mosby-Year Book, 1990.)

Atrophy of muscles innervated by the median nerve is visible in severe long-standing cases but is uncommon in most cases of recent onset. Weakness of the abductor pollicis brevis muscle may be detected by careful manual muscle testing.

2. Provocative tests—Three provocative tests, the Phalen maneuver, the Tinel sign, and the wrist compression test, are helpful in establishing the diagnosis of carpal tunnel syndrome.

a. Tinel sign—The Tinel sign is elicited by percussing the skin over the median nerve just proximal to the carpal tunnel; when it is positive, the patient complains of an electric or tingling sensation radiating into the thumb, index, middle, or ring fingers.

b. Phalen maneuver—The Phalen wrist flexion sign, or Phalen maneuver, is usually positive in patients with carpal tunnel syndrome and is thought by many to be even more diagnostic than the Tinel sign. When this maneuver is performed, the elbow should be maintained in extension while the wrist is passively flexed (Figure 10–24). The time is then measured from initiation of wrist flexion to onset of symptoms; onset within 60 seconds is considered supportive of the diagnosis of carpal tunnel syndrome. Both the time to onset and the location of paresthesias should be recorded.

c. Wrist compression test—pressure over the median nerve proximal to the wrist provoke symptoms within 30 seconds. The test is confirmatory to other physical signs of median nerve compression.

3. Two-point discrimination test—Two-point discrimination is often diminished in the finger pulps of patients with carpal tunnel syndrome. Sensation in the radial aspect of the palm should be normal, however, because the palmar cutaneous branch of the median nerve does not pass through the carpal tunnel.

4. Imaging studies—The diagnostic evaluation may include a radiograph of the wrist, including a carpal tunnel view.

5. Electrodiagnostic studies—Nerve conduction velocities and electromyography help localize nerve compression to the wrist and evaluate residual neural and motor integrity. Nerve conduction velocity (NCV) and electromyogram (EMG) studies are indicated for patients who have failed conservative care and are considered candidates for surgery. A motor distal latency greater than 3.5–4.0 ms is the best indicator of carpal tunnel syndrome.

C. Treatment

1. Conservative measures—Because the pressure within the carpal tunnel increases if the wrist is held in sus-

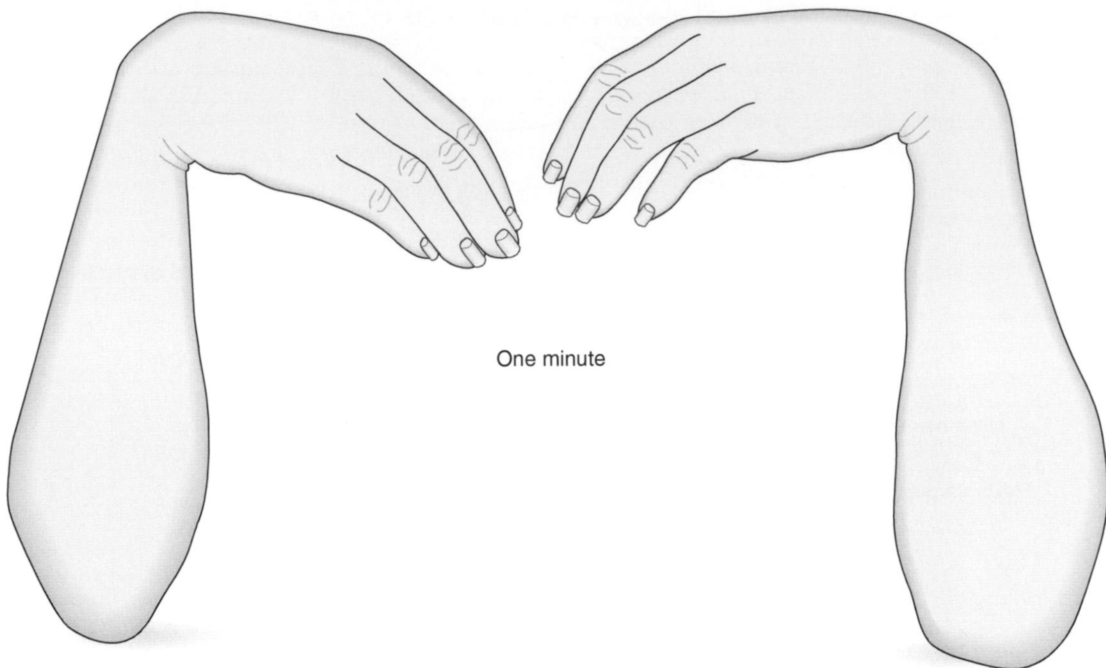

Figure 10–24. Phalen maneuver. (Reproduced, with permission, from American Society for Surgery of the Hand: *The Hand: Examination and Diagnosis,* 2nd ed. Churchill Livingstone, 1983.)

tained flexion (usual sleep posture) or sustained extension, the initial treatment of carpal tunnel syndrome should include a splint that maintains the wrist in a neutral position at night. Clinical improvement with this simple measure adds further support to the diagnosis of carpal tunnel syndrome. Activities that provoke symptoms may be modified with simple measures such as adjustment of keyboard height and rotation of repetitive job activities.

Injection of steroids into the carpal tunnel often decreases the inflammatory response around the flexor tendons and diminishes symptoms. To inject the carpal tunnel, a 25-gauge 1.5-inch needle is placed at the palmar wrist crease just ulnar to the palmaris longus tendon. If the palmaris longus is absent, a line along the radial border of the ring finger is drawn to the wrist crease. Before placing the needle, patients are told they may experience an electric shock sensation in the fingers. If this sensation occurs, the needle may be in the median nerve, and the injection should not be given. The needle is withdrawn and placed a few millimeters ulnar. When inserting the needle, first the skin is punctured, then a pop is felt as the needle passes through the transverse carpal ligament. A mixture of a short-acting anesthetic and steroid is injected. Transient relief of symptoms after injection suggests a greater likelihood of a favorable result after surgical decompression.

2. Surgical treatment—Patients unresponsive to conservative measures may benefit from surgical division of the transverse carpal ligament. This division may be accomplished through either direct open exposure or through an endoscopic approach. The open incision is made in the palm over the transverse carpal ligament, staying ulnar to the axis of the palmaris longus, along the longitudinal axis of the radial border of the ring finger. This incision avoids injury to the palmar cutaneous branch of the median nerve. After incising the palmar fascia longitudinally, the transverse carpal ligament is identified and sectioned longitudinally under direct observation. Endoscopic division of the transverse carpal ligament avoids a potentially tender palmar incision with either a single wrist portal proximal to the palm or with a combined proximal portal and short midpalmar portal along the axis of the open incision. Although some studies noted an earlier return to work activities after endoscopic release, the incidence of iatrogenic nerve and tendon injuries and late recurrence of symptoms form incomplete ligament division may be higher with endoscopic release than with open release. Both types of procedures are effective ways of treating carpal tunnel syndrome. The decision of which technique to use is based on the surgeon's experience. Endoscopic carpal tunnel release should not be used for treatment of recurrent carpal tunnel syndrome.

Patients are encouraged to actively move their fingers from the first postoperative day. Wrist motion is begun within the first week. Incisional tenderness often prevents patients from fully using their hands and returning to unrestricted work for the first 4–8 weeks. If patients have difficulty with hand function 3–4 weeks after surgery, a therapy program is prescribed consisting of desensitization, ROM, and strengthening.

Pronator Syndrome

A. Anatomy

The median nerve may be compressed in the proximal forearm by one or more of the following structures: ligament of Struthers, lacertus fibrosus, pronator teres muscle, or proximal fibrous arch on the undersurface of the flexor digitorum superficialis muscle.

B. Clinical Findings

Patients with pronator syndrome complain of pain that is usually more severe in the volar forearm than in the wrist or hand. Pain usually increases with activity. Complaints of numbness in the thumb, index, middle, and ring fingers may initially suggest the possibility of carpal tunnel syndrome. Night symptoms, however, are unusual in cases of isolated pronator syndrome.

Examination may reveal sensory and motor deficits similar to those seen in carpal tunnel syndrome, but significant differences may be detected on careful evaluation. Dysesthesia may include the distribution of the palmar cutaneous nerve. The Tinel sign is positive at the forearm level rather than at the wrist. The Phalen maneuver does not provoke symptoms. Patients may experience pain with resistance to contraction of the pronator teres or flexor digitorum superficialis muscles tested by resistance to forearm pronation or to isolated flexion of the proximal interphalangeal joints of the long and ring fingers.

C. Treatment

Evaluation of symptomatic patients should include electrodiagnostic studies if a 6-week course of immobilization fails to effect improvement. Surgical treatment requires generous decompression of all potentially constricting sites.

Anterior Interosseous Syndrome

A. Anatomy

The anterior interosseous nerve branch divides from the median nerve 4–6 cm below the elbow. This branch of the nerve innervates the flexor pollicis longus, flexor digitorum profundus of the index and middle fingers, and pronator quadratus muscles. The anterior interosseous nerve may be compressed by the deep head of the pronator teres, the origin of the flexor digitorum superficialis, a palmaris profundus, or the flexor carpi radialis. In addition, accessory muscles connecting the flexor digitorum superficialis to the flexor digitorum profundus proximally and Gantzer muscle (the accessory head of the flexor pollicis longus) may impinge on the anterior interosseous nerve.

B. Clinical Findings

Patients affected with anterior interosseous nerve syndrome complain of inability to flex either the thumb interphalangeal joint or the index-finger distal interphalangeal joint. In contrast to those with pronator syndrome, these patients do not complain of numbness or pain.

C. Treatment

Surgical decompression of the anterior interosseous nerve may be indicated when the syndrome does not spontaneously improve. All potentially compressing structures must be exposed and released.

2. Ulnar Neuropathy

Cubital Tunnel Syndrome

A. Anatomy

The ulnar nerve is most commonly compressed at the cubital tunnel, along the medial side of the elbow. Compression may occur between the ulnar and humeral origins of the flexor carpi ulnaris or at the proximal border of the cubital tunnel because the nerve is tethered anteriorly with elbow flexion (Figure 10–25).

B. Clinical Findings

Patients affected with cubital tunnel syndrome most often complain of paresthesia and numbness involving the ring and little fingers. Because symptoms may be aggravated or provoked by sustained elbow flexion, patients may complain of increased symptoms while talking on the telephone. Many patients complain of being awakened at night by the symptoms, most often when sleeping with the elbows flexed. Patients whose exam demonstrates weakness of muscles innervated by the ulnar nerve may note clumsiness and lack of dexterity.

1. Provocative tests—

a. Tinel sign—A positive Tinel sign is noted when percussion over the ulnar nerve at the elbow provokes paresthesias along the ulnar forearm and hand. The nerve may be noted to sublux over the medial epicondyle as the arm is brought into flexion.

b. Motor strength—Motor strength should be assessed both in intrinsic muscles innervated by the ulnar nerve (first dorsal interosseous muscle) and in extrinsic muscles innervated by the ulnar nerve (flexor digitorum profundus of the little finger).

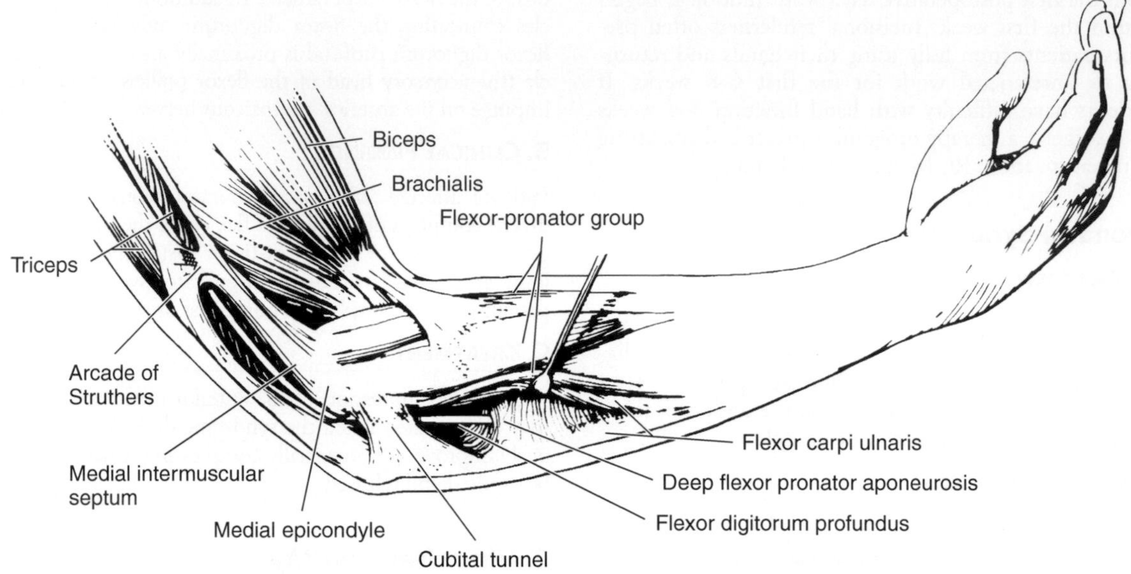

Figure 10–25. **Points of constriction of the ulnar nerve at the elbow.** (From Amadio PC: Anatomic basis for a technique of ulnar nerve transposition. Surg Radiol Anat 1986;8:155; used, with permission, from Mayo Foundation.)

c. Froment sign—With weakness of the ulnar nerve innervated adductor pollicis muscle, a positive Froment sign may be observed. As the patient tries to hold a piece of paper placed between the thumb and the index finger, the thumb interphalangeal joint flexes in an attempt to substitute flexor pollicis longus activity for inadequate adductor pollicis strength.

d. Elbow flexion test—The ulnar nerve may be rendered symptomatic by fully flexing the elbow with the wrist in the neutral position. The elbow flexion test, a provocative maneuver, is considered positive if paresthesia is elicited in the ring and little fingers within 60 seconds. The location of the paresthesia and the time between initiation of elbow flexion and the onset of symptoms should be recorded.

C. Treatment

1. Conservative treatment—Conservative treatment may include the use of an elbow pad to protect the nerve from trauma or a splint holding the elbow at approximately 45 degrees of flexion. The splint may be worn continuously or at night only, depending on the frequency and intensity of symptoms.

2. Surgical treatment—Electrodiagnostic studies should be obtained if conservative treatment does not alleviate the symptoms, particularly if motor weakness is evident. The reliability of nerve conduction studies at the elbow depends on the ability of the electromyographer to measure the length of the ulnar nerve accurately.

Numerous procedures are described to relieve ulnar nerve compression at the elbow. These include simple decompression of the ulnar nerve within the cubital tunnel or decompression with anterior transposition of the nerve subcutaneously, intramuscularly, or submuscularly into the flexor pronator mass. When the nerve is transposed, great care must be taken to excise the medial intermuscular septum proximally and to release the aponeurosis between the humeral and ulnar origins of the flexor carpi ulnaris distally, to avoid creating a new area of impingement.

An alternative surgical strategy involves decompression of the nerve and medial epicondylectomy. This technique removes the prominence against which the ulnar nerve is tethered with elbow flexion. After surgery, initial rehabilitation focuses on regaining elbow ROM. Strengthening begins at 4–6 weeks, and the patient is usually able to return to unrestricted work at 8–12 weeks.

Ulnar Tunnel Syndrome

A. Anatomy

The ulnar nerve passes from the forearm into the hand through the Guyon canal (see Figure 10–23). The anatomic borders of the Guyon canal are the pisiform and pisohamate ligament ulnarly, the hook of the hamate and insertion of the transverse carpal ligament radially, and the volar carpal ligament forming the roof of the tunnel.

B. Clinical Findings

Examination should document ulnar nerve sensory and motor integrity. In contrast to the findings in cubital tunnel syndrome, the Tinel sign is positive at the wrist rather than at the elbow. Extrinsic motor function is normal. The region of compression should be delineated by electrodiagnostic studies. In some cases MRI studies demonstrate a space-occupying lesion such as a ganglion compressing the nerve within the Guyon canal.

C. Treatment

When splinting is ineffective, surgical decompression should be considered. When symptoms exist in tandem with carpal tunnel syndrome, release of the transverse carpal ligament favorably alters the shape and size of the Guyon canal. Postoperative care is the same as following carpal tunnel release.

3. Radial Neuropathy

Radial Tunnel Syndrome

A. Anatomy

The radial nerve may be rendered symptomatic if compressed in the region of the radial tunnel. Points of impingement along the radial tunnel, located at the level of the proximal radius, include fibers spanning the radiocapitellar joint, the radial recurrent vessels, the extensor carpi radialis brevis, the tendinous origin of the supinator (arcade of Frohse), and the point at which the nerve emerges from beneath the distal edge of the supinator.

B. Clinical Findings

Because radial tunnel syndrome often occurs in combination with lateral epicondylitis, the two diagnoses are frequently confused. Patients with radial tunnel syndrome experience pain over the midportion of the mobile wad (brachioradialis, extensor carpi radialis longus, and extensor carpi radialis brevis muscles), whereas the pain experienced by patients with lateral epicondylitis is located at or just distal to the lateral epicondyle. Patients with radial tunnel syndrome experience pain when simultaneously extending the wrist and fingers while the long finger is passively flexed by the examiner (positive long-finger extension test). Patients with radial tunnel syndrome often also experience pain with resisted forearm supination.

C. Treatment

Conservative treatment of radial tunnel syndrome includes measures to avoid forceful extension of the wrist and fingers. The wrist is splinted in dorsiflexion while the forearm is immobilized in supination. Persistent symptoms in spite of splinting may be treated by surgical decompression of the radial nerve. Concomitant lateral epicondylitis should be treated surgically at the same time that the radial nerve is decompressed.

Posterior Interosseous Nerve Syndrome

A. Anatomy

The radial nerve splits into the posterior interosseous nerve and the superficial sensory branch of the radial nerve after passing anteriorly to the radiocapitellar joint. The posterior interosseous nerve then passes beneath the origin of the extensor carpi radialis brevis, radial recurrent artery, and arcade of Frohse. The posterior interosseous nerve is most commonly entrapped at the proximal edge of the supinator, although entrapment may also occur at either the middle or the distal edge of the supinator muscle.

B. Clinical Findings

In contrast to radial tunnel syndrome, patients with posterior interosseous nerve syndrome experience extrinsic extensor weakness. Pain may be less than that of patients with radial tunnel syndrome.

Paralysis may be either partial or complete. Because the brachioradialis, extensor carpi radialis longus, supinator, and often extensor carpi radialis brevis are innervated by the radial nerve proximal to the posterior interosseous nerve branch, these muscles are spared. Digital extension at the metacarpophalangeal joint is the principal deficit from loss of extensor digitorum communis, extensor indicis proprius, and extensor digit quinti function.

The differential diagnosis in a patient with spontaneous loss of digital extension should include the possibility of multiple tendon ruptures in addition to possible radial neuropathy, particularly in patients with RA. The tenodesis effect, in which the fingers extend as the wrist is passively flexed, is preserved in posterior interosseous nerve syndrome but absent if the extensor tendons are ruptured.

C. Treatment

Treatment of posterior interosseous nerve syndrome requires thorough decompression of the nerve. If motor recovery does not occur, tendon transfers restore digital extension.

4. Thoracic Outlet Syndrome

Anatomy

The brachial plexus exits the base of the neck and upper thorax through the thoracic outlet. Anatomic boundaries of the outlet are the scalenus anterior muscle anteriorly, the scalenus medius muscle posteriorly, and the first rib inferiorly. Thoracic outlet syndrome, usually resulting from irritation of the C8- and T1-derived nerves, may be caused by a cervical rib, a fiber spanning from a rudimentary cervical rib, tendinous bands from the scalenus anterior to the medius muscles, or hypertrophic clavicle fracture callus. Poor posture with slumping shoulders or prolonged military brace position are each implicated as a contributing factor.

Clinical Findings

The symptoms of thoracic outlet syndrome are often vague. Symptoms may include pain in the C8-T1 dermatome, with a variable degree of intrinsic muscle weakness. Patients may experience vascular symptoms if the axillary artery is simultaneously being compressed in the thoracic outlet region.

A. Provocative Tests

1. Elevated stress test—Physical examination of the patient with suspected thoracic outlet syndrome should include an elevated stress test, in which the patient's shoulders are kept extended and the arm is externally rotated 90 degrees at the shoulder. The patient is then asked to open and close the hands with the arms elevated for 3 minutes. Reproduction of symptoms is suggestive of thoracic outlet syndrome.

2. Other tests—The Adson sign and the Wright test may be helpful in detecting vascular compression. In a positive Adson test, the radial pulse is obliterated when the arm is dependent and the head is turned to the affected side. In the Wright test, the pulse is obliterated when the shoulder is abducted, externally rotated, and the head is turned away from the involved shoulder. In addition, this maneuver should reproduce the patient's symptoms. Physical examination should document C8-T1 sensation and intrinsic muscle strength.

B. Diagnostic Studies

Workup of the symptomatic patient should include radiographs of the cervical spine to rule out a cervical rib, electrodiagnostic studies to assess the function of the lower nerve roots, and Doppler studies of the arm in varied positions to assess compression of the axillary artery.

Treatment

Initial treatment includes postural exercises. Patients who are unresponsive to conservative treatment or have demonstrable weakness may benefit from surgical resection of a cervical rib, resection of the first rib, or scalenotomy.

5. Cervical Root Compression

Clinical Findings

Cervical spine root compression may result in complaints of hand pain or weakness. It is useful to inquire routinely about pain or limitation of motion of the cervical spine. If the patient was involved in an accident involving sudden neck flexion and extension, this should be noted. Cervical root compression may occur from a herniated cervical disk, cervical spondylosis, intervertebral foraminal osteophytes, or, rarely, a cervical cord tumor.

Patients with cervical root compression most often complain of pain in a radicular rather than a peripheral nerve distribution. In spite of symptoms involving the hand, most patients, when carefully questioned, are able to distinguish pain that begins in the neck and radiates to the hand from pain that begins in the hand and radiates proximally to the neck. Pain may be exacerbated with neck motion (flexion and extension, lateral bending, or rotation), coughing, or sneezing.

A. Spurling Test

Physical examination of the patient with cervical radiculopathy frequently demonstrates either a decreased range of neck motion or pain with neck motion. Symptoms may be reproduced with axial compression on the patient's head (positive Spurling test). Detailed sensory and motor examination may reveal deficits in the domain of one or more roots.

B. Double-Crush Syndrome

The occasional simultaneous presentation of cervical radiculopathy with peripheral entrapment neuropathy is termed the *double-crush syndrome.* Whether compression at one level renders a nerve more vulnerable to compressive forces at a second level or whether such cases simply represent two common entities in the same extremity remains the subject of debate.

Treatment

If a nerve is compressed at more than one location, the more symptomatic area is usually treated first. If both areas are equally symptomatic, the simpler of the two operations is chosen.

Lindley SG, Kleinert JM: Prevalence of anatomic variations encountered in elective carpal tunnel release. J Hand Surg Am 2003;28:849. [PMID: 14507518]

Morgenlander JC et al: Surgical treatment of carpal tunnel syndrome in patients with peripheral neuropathy. Neurology 1997;49:1159. [PMID: 9339710]

Naidu SH et al: Median nerve function in patients undergoing carpal tunnel release: Pre- and post-op nerve conductions. Electromyogr Clin Neurophysiol 2003;43:393. [PMID: 14626718]

Trumble TE et al: Single-portal endoscopic carpal tunnel release compared with open release: A prospective, randomized trial. J Bone Joint Surg Am 2002;84:1107. [PMID: 12107308]

Upton AR, McComas AJ: The double crush in nerve entrapment syndromes. Lancet 1973;2:359. [PMID: 4124532]

DISORDERS OF THE FASCIA OF THE HAND

DUPUYTREN DISEASE

Dupuytren disease is characterized by a nodular thickening on the palmar surface of the hand affecting the preexisting palmar fascia (Figure 10–26). It is a progressive condition, resulting from pathologic changes mediated by the myofibroblast. Dupuytren disease occurs most commonly in patients between 40 and 60 years of age. It is observed more often in men, in whom it appears earlier and is often more aggressive. Flexion contractures most frequently occur at the metacarpophalangeal joints but may also tether the proximal interphalangeal joint and, less commonly, the distal interphalangeal joint. The little and ring fingers and the thumb index web are the most commonly involved areas. Ectopic deposits may occur in the dorsum of the proximal interphalangeal joint (knuckle pads), the dorsum of the penis (Peyronie disease), and the plantar fascia of the foot (Ledderhose disease).

Epidemiologic Factors

A number of predisposing factors are identified. The disease most commonly appears in patients of northern European ancestry and is occasionally encountered in Asians; it is rarer in other racial groups. Dupuytren disease is associated with epilepsy medications taken for seizure disorders and with alcoholism, smoking, and diabetes. The relationship of work and trauma to the development of the disease remains controversial. The most aggressive disease occurs in patients who have a family history of disease and in those who have onset of disease prior to 40 years of age. More severely involved patients may have extensive bilateral involvement and ectopic deposits on the dorsum of the hands and the feet. Although these patients often undergo surgery at an early age, both extension and recurrence of the disease is common.

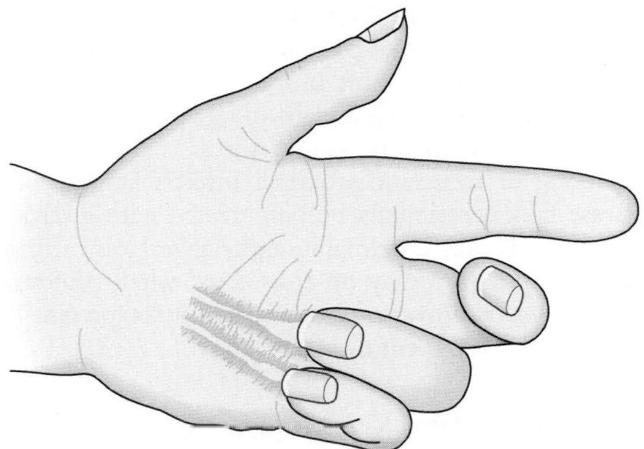

Figure 10–26. **Dupuytren contracture.** (Reproduced, with permission, from American Society for Surgery of the Hand: *The Hand: Examination and Diagnosis,* 2nd ed. Churchill Livingstone, 1983.)

Anatomy

Dupuytren contracture distorts the anatomy of the palmar fascia. Flexion contractures of the metacarpophalangeal joint are caused by pathologic contracture of pretendinous bands at a superficial level. Contracture of the natatory ligaments produces web space contractures and scissoring of the fingers. The transverse fibers of the palmar aponeurosis remain uninvolved, except at the base of the thumb. In the fingers, the superficial volar fascia, lateral digital sheath, spiral band, and Grayson ligaments may contract alone or in combination to produce flexion contracture of the proximal interphalangeal joint. When a spiral band contracts, the digital nerve is often displaced palmarly to the band from proximal lateral to distal central in the region of the proximal phalanx.

Treatment

Nonsurgical treatment is ineffective in reversing or halting Dupuytren disease. The primary indication for surgery is a fixed contracture of more than 30 degrees at the metacarpophalangeal or any degree of flexion contracture at the proximal interphalangeal joint.

Surgical exposure may be achieved through either transverse or longitudinal skin incisions. A transverse incision across the distal palmar skin crease is useful when extensive palmar involvement is anticipated. Transverse incisions are usually sutured; if there is excessive tension, the wound may be left open to heal by secondary intention. When longitudinal exposure of the finger is needed, Brunner zigzag incisions are useful. An alternative is a longitudinal incision that is modified for closure by a series of Z-plasty flap transpositions.

The goal of surgical release is to achieve a regional fasciectomy or subtotal palmar fasciectomy that allows maximal untethered joint motion. A local fasciotomy may occasionally be elected in older, more debilitated patients with severe joint contractures.

Severe or recurrent proximal interphalangeal joint disease may occasionally be best treated with a salvage procedure, usually proximal interphalangeal joint arthrodesis. Amputation may be considered when profound stiffness or neurovascular compromise is present in patients with recurrent disease.

Complications

The most common postoperative complication is hematoma, which may expand and compromise skin flaps and act as a nidus for infection. To diminish the possibility of postoperative hematoma, the tourniquet should be released and meticulous hemostasis obtained prior to wound closure. Tight skin closure should be avoided. If limited flap necrosis occurs, the affected regions should be treated by open dressing changes. If skin loss is extensive, skin graft application may be necessary to gain early wound closure.

Joint stiffness may occur, particularly after extensive surgical release of the long-standing fixed proximal interphalangeal joint. Extensive therapy is often necessary, consisting of both active and passive exercises and splinting.

Mild sympathetically mediated pain (reflex sympathetic dystrophy) is not uncommon. For patients who have a more severe form, hospitalization with elevation, sympathetic blocking agents, oral steroids, and intensive therapy may be necessary.

Prognosis

Contracture correction is usually maintained at the metacarpophalangeal joints. Recurrence is more common at the proximal interphalangeal joint, particularly when the extent of preoperative proximal interphalangeal joint contracture was more than 60 degrees. Long-term postoperative night splinting may diminish the extent of residual digital flexion contracture.

Forsman M et al: Dupuytren's contracture; increased cellularity—Proliferation, is there equality? Scand J Surg 2005;94:71. [PMID: 15865122]

Godtfredsen NS et al: A prospective study linked both alcohol and tobacco to Dupuytren's disease. J Clin Epidemiol 2004;57:858. [PMID: 15485739]

Ketchum LD, Donahue TK: The injection of nodules of Dupuytren's disease with triamcinolone acetonide. J Hand Surg Am 2000;25:1157. [PMID: 11119679]

McFarlane RM: On the origin and spread of Dupuytren's disease. J Hand Surg [Am] 2002;27(3):385. [PMID: 12015711]

COMPARTMENT SYNDROMES

Compartment syndromes are a group of conditions that result from increased pressure within a limited anatomic space, acutely compromising the microcirculation and threatening the viability of the tissue within that space.

Recurrent or chronic compartment syndrome results from increased pressure within the compartment with a specific activity, most commonly in athletes during exercise. Symptoms of muscle weakness may be severe enough to stop the exercise activity in spite of the patient being asymptomatic between recurrences.

The Volkmann ischemic contracture is the result of an acute compartment syndrome in which fibrous tissue has replaced dead muscle. Because nerve injury is not always associated with this condition, sensation and intrinsic muscle function may be normal distal to the involved compartment. Because there is often no associated nerve injury, no sensory deficit or loss of motor function may be detected in the nerve domain distal to the involved compartment.

Etiologic Factors

The most common causes of compartment syndrome are fractures, soft-tissue crush injuries, arterial injuries either caused by localized hemorrhage or postischemic swelling, drug overdose with prolonged limb compression, and burn injuries. In most cases, fractures are closed or, if open, are grade 1 injuries, with only limited disruption of the compartmental soft-tissue envelopes.

The pathophysiology of compartment syndrome is a consequence of closure of small vessels. Increased compartment pressure increases the pressure on the walls of arterioles within the compartment. Increased local pressure also occludes small veins, resulting in venous hypertension within the compartment. The arteriovenous gradient in the region of the pressurized tissue becomes insufficient to allow tissue perfusion. Because the elevated pressure within the compartment is not high enough to occlude major arteries completely as they pass through the compartment, distal pulses usually remain strong in spite of increasing tissue ischemia in the affected soft-tissue compartment.

Clinical Findings

The diagnosis of compartment syndrome is established predominantly on clinical findings. The clinician must have a high index of suspicion whenever a closed compartment has the potential for bleeding or swelling. Compartment syndromes are characterized by pain out of proportion to the initial injury. Pain is often persistent, progressive, and unrelieved by immobilization. Pain may be accentuated by passive stretching of involved muscles. Diminished sensation may be noted in the distribution of the nerve whose compartment is being compressed. This phenomenon is believed to be secondary to nerve ischemia. A third sign is weakness and paralysis of muscles within the compartment. A fourth sign is tenseness of the compartment on palpation. Of the preceding signs and symptoms, pain with passive muscle stretching is the most sensitive in detecting compartment syndrome.

If the diagnosis of compartment syndrome is in question, the clinician is obligated to ascertain the pressure within the potential affected compartments. Various methods are available, including a portable handheld pressure monitor or a simple modification of a mercury manometer connected to tubing and a three-way stopcock. Although the exact pressure threshold for requiring fasciotomy is controversial, fasciotomy should be strongly considered whenever the compartment pressure is greater than 30 mm Hg in the forearm. Pressure measurements of the compartments of the hand are difficult to interpret. The decision to perform a fasciotomy of the hand or finger is based solely on clinical judgment.

Treatment

Once the diagnosis of compartment syndrome is established, fasciotomy of the involved compartment should be performed as soon as possible because elevation of compartment pressure of more than 30 mm Hg for more than 8 hours is associated with irreversible tissue death. Prophylactic fasciotomy should also be considered in patients in whom ischemia is present for more than 4 hours. All patients undergoing forearm or arm replantation should have a fasciotomy performed at the time of the initial surgical procedure.

The volar compartment of the forearm is the upper extremity compartment most often requiring release (Figure 10–27A). The skin incision should extend from the elbow to the carpal tunnel. The preferred skin incision extends from the medial side of the biceps and swings ulnarly toward the medial epicondyle. Care must be taken to incise the lacertus fibrosus at the elbow

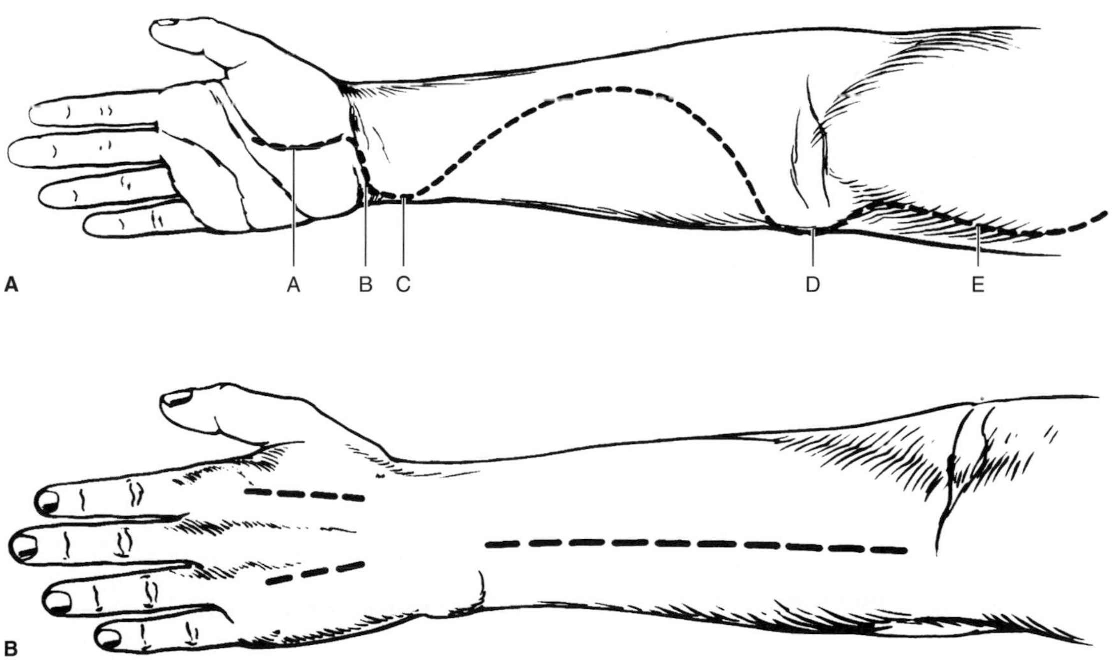

Figure 10–27. **A:** Various skin incisions used for performing a volar arm fasciotomy. **B:** To decompress the dorsal and mobile wad compartments, straight incisions are preferred because fewer veins are damaged. (Reproduced, with permission, from Green DP, ed: *Operative Hand Surgery*, 2nd ed. Churchill Livingstone, 1988.)

level. The incision may be extended in a radial direction to allow decompression of the mobile wad. In the distal half of the forearm, the incision runs along the ulnar border. The flap is designed to allow coverage of the median nerve in the distal forearm when the wounds are left open at the conclusion of the procedure. The incision is extended obliquely across the wrist to provide exposure of the carpal tunnel in the proximal palm.

An epimysiotomy of the individual superficial and deep compartment muscle bellies should be performed as needed. Care should be taken to ensure that the deep compartment musculature (the flexor pollicis longus and flexor digitorum profundus muscles) is completely decompressed. The skin incision should be partially closed over the median nerve in the hand and distal forearm. The proximal wound over muscle should be left open. The patient should be returned to the operating room within 48 hours for reevaluation. At the second surgery, dressings are changed and secondary debridement is accomplished if nonviable muscle remains. In some instances, it is possible to close the wound secondarily; in most cases, split-thickness skin grafting of the residual skin defect is a safer alternative. Decompression of the dorsal forearm when necessary may be accomplished with a dorsal longitudinal incision (Figure 10–27B).

In the hand, the connections between compartments are limited; therefore, each compartment should be released individually. This may be accomplished by two longitudinal dorsal incisions over the index and ring metacarpals. Through these incisions, each of the interosseous compartments can be entered on both the radial and ulnar sides of each metacarpal. Separate volar incisions are needed when decompression of the thenar and hypothenar compartments is necessary on the palm of the hand.

In the finger, fasciotomy may be required for treatment of either severe trauma or snakebite injuries. Because compartment pressures in the finger are impossible to measure accurately, the indications for finger fasciotomy are based on the degree of swelling. Midaxial incisions along the ulnar side of the index, middle, and ring fingers and the radial side of the little finger and thumb allow satisfactory digital decompression. Care is taken to retract the neurovascular bundle palmarward, and the fascia between the neurovascular bundle and the flexor tendon sheath are then incised. Digital wounds are left open postoperatively, and wound closure is achieved either secondarily or with a split-thickness skin graft.

Botte MJ, Keenan MA, Gelberman RH: Volkmann's ischemic contracture of the upper extremity. Hand Clin 1998;14:483. [PMID: 9742427]

Dente CJ et al: A review of upper extremity fasciotomies in a level I trauma center. Am Surg 2002;70:188. [PMID: 15663051]

Hovius SE, Ultee J: Volkmann's ischemic contracture. Prevention and treatment. Hand Clin 2000;16:647. [PMID: 11117054]

Ultee J, Hovius SE: Functional results after treatment of Volkmann's ischemic contracture: A long-term followup study. Clin Orthop 2005;431:42. [PMID: 15685054]

FRACTURES & DISLOCATIONS OF THE HAND

FRACTURES & DISLOCATIONS OF THE METACARPALS & PHALANGES

Fractures of the metacarpals and phalanges account for approximately 10% of all fractures. More than half of all hand fractures are work related. Fractures of the border digits, thumb, and little finger are most common. The most commonly fractured bone is the distal phalanx, accounting for 45–50% of all hand fractures.

Clinical Findings

Description of a phalangeal or metacarpal fracture should include notation of the bone involved, the location within the bone (base, shaft, or neck), and whether the fracture is open or closed. Further determination should be made as to whether the fracture is displaced or nondisplaced, if it has an intraarticular component, and whether rotational or angular deformity is present.

Because rotational malalignment of a metacarpal or phalangeal fracture is difficult to evaluate from a radiograph, physical examination is essential. The patient is asked to flex actively the fingers individually and together. Nail rotation, finger orientation, and overlapping of the fingers is assessed. Associated vascular, nerve, and tendon injuries, as well as the adequacy of soft-tissue coverage, also should be evaluated.

Treatment

Treatment of metacarpal and phalangeal fractures requires accurate diagnosis, reduction, sufficient immobilization to maintain the fracture reduction, with early motion of the uninvolved fingers to prevent stiffness. Immobilization should usually place the hand in an intrinsic plus, or safe, position to avoid secondary joint contracture (see Figure 10–12). Immobilization should rarely exceed 3 weeks for phalangeal fractures or 4 weeks for metacarpal fractures. Because radiologic union usually lags behind clinical union in the hand, initiation of digital motion should not be delayed until radiologic union is visible. Prolonged immobilization increases the likelihood of residual stiffness.

The fixation required to maintain fracture reduction depends on the fracture characteristics. Stable fractures may be treated by either buddy taping the affected finger to an adjacent finger and allowing early motion or with a brief period of splint immobilization. Repeat radiographs at 7–10 days document maintenance of fracture reduction. Initially displaced unstable fractures that require closed reduction to achieve proper alignment require external immobilization with a cast or splint.

When external immobilization is impossible or unlikely to maintain fracture reduction, internal fixation is required. Internal fixation techniques useful in the management of hand fractures include Kirschner (K)-wire fixation, interosseous wiring, tension band wiring, interfragmentary screw fixation, or fixation with plates and screws. K-wire fixation is versatile but lacks the rigidity of other techniques. Additional stability may be achieved by combining K-wire fixation with tension band wires. Interfragmentary screws provide ideal fixation for long oblique fractures, in which the obliquity of the fracture is more than two times the diameter of the fractured bone. Plates and screws in the hand are particularly helpful in open metacarpal fractures with bone loss. When segmental bone loss occurs, initial treatment includes debridement of an associated open wound and maintenance of skeletal length with either internal or external fixation. After the soft-tissue coverage is established, bony graft reconstruction may be coupled with definitive internal fixation.

1. Physeal Fractures

Approximately a third of all fractures of the immature skeleton involve the epiphysis. Salter-Harris physeal fractures are divided into five types. Type 1 fractures, which shear through the growth plate without extension into the epiphysis or metaphysis, may be effectively treated with simple immobilization. Type 2 fractures, in which a metaphyseal fracture fragment is attached to the epiphysis, can usually be reduced in a closed fashion and immobilized with a splint. One of the more common type 2 fractures is the so-called extraoctave fracture at the base of the proximal phalanx of the little finger, caused by forceful ulnar deviation of the finger. Reduction may be accomplished by metacarpophalangeal joint flexion and little-finger radial deviation. Type 3 and 4 fractures are intraarticular injuries. When displaced, these fractures require open reduction to achieve restoration of the articular surface and physis. Type 5 fractures are uncommon in the phalanges, occurring most often in the finger metacarpals as a result of axial compression. Type 5 crush injuries to the growth plate may provoke either partial or complete fusion of the physis and thereby result in late angular deformity or digital shortening.

2. Distal Phalanx Fractures

Distal phalangeal fractures occur most often in the middle finger and the thumb. These fractures usually result from a crushing injury, such as occurs with a misdirected hammer striking a thumb holding a nail or a protruding middle-finger distal phalanx caught in a closing door.

Precise reduction of distal phalangeal fracture fragments is not required in closed injuries, unless the articular surface is involved. Treatment consists of splinting the bone and distal interphalangeal joint for protection and pain relief. While the distal interphalangeal joint is splinted, motion should be encouraged at the metacarpophalangeal and proximal interphalangeal joints. Splint protection may be discontinued at 3 weeks.

Nail matrix injuries are often associated with open distal phalanx fractures. Proper treatment of these fractures requires removal of the nail, irrigation of the fracture and nail bed, and nail bed repair with fine absorbable sutures. Fracture reduction is usually accomplished by nail matrix repair and replacement of the nail. In rare cases, pin fixation of markedly displaced distal phalanx fractures may be required. After nail bed repair, either the original nail, a nail prosthesis, a piece of aluminum suture package, or a piece of gauze should be interposed between the nail roof and the nail bed to prevent synechia (adhesion) formation.

Displaced open distal phalangeal epiphyseal injuries are most often caused by flexion of the distal phalanx with the apex at the dorsal physis. The nail is often avulsed dorsal to the eponychia. Treatment requires nail removal, irrigation, reduction of the fracture, and nail bed repair. Failure to appreciate the open nature of a displaced type 1 fracture of the distal phalanx may result in osteomyelitis with growth arrest of the distal phalanx.

3. Proximal & Middle Phalanx Fractures

Angulation of fractures of the proximal and middle phalanges reflects the tendon forces inserting on the bone. The middle phalanx has an extensor force transmitted to it by the central slip attaching dorsally and proximally. The terminal extensor tendon inserts dorsally and distally into the terminal phalanx, providing a secondary dorsiflexion force. The flexor digitorum superficialis inserts volarly over the middle three fifths of the middle phalanx. Therefore, middle phalanx fractures that occur proximal to the flexor digitorum superficialis insertion angulate with the fracture apex dorsally; fractures that occur distal to the superficialis insertion angulate with the apex palmarly. Proximal phalangeal fractures tend to angulate with the apex palmarly because of the force of lateral bands that pass palmarward to the axis of the metacarpophalangeal joint and dorsalward to the axis of the proximal interphalangeal joint.

Adhesions involving the flexor or extensor tendons are a major complication of proximal and middle phalangeal fractures. Fracture displacement increases the likelihood of tendon adherence and limitation of joint motion. Malunion or malrotation of the fractures may require secondary correction.

Early appropriate treatment of these fractures attempts to prevent complications. In a stable nondisplaced or impacted fracture, only temporary splint protection is required, followed by dynamic splinting such as buddy taping to an adjacent finger. Radiographic follow-up is needed to document maintenance of the reduction. Patients who require closed reduction and immobilization should have the forearm, wrist, and injured digits as well as an adjacent digit immobilized in a plaster cast or gutter splint.

4. Metacarpal Fractures

Metacarpal Head Fractures

Intraarticular fractures of the metacarpal head require open reduction and internal fixation if more than 20–30% of the joint surface is involved. Realigned articular fracture fragments may be held in place with either a K-wire or small screw. Fractures with marked comminution of the metacarpal head distal to the ligament origin may not be amenable to precise internal fixation and may be treated with early mobilization with distraction traction.

Metacarpal Neck Fractures

Metacarpal neck fractures are most frequent in the little finger, although they may occur in any metacarpal. Metacarpal neck fractures result from a direct blow, either delivered to the hand or by the hand striking a solid object (animate or inanimate). Comminution of the volar cortex results in collapse deformity with apex dorsal angulation (Figure 10–28). Greater residual fracture angulation may be accepted in the ring and little fingers because the greater mobility in the ulnar carpometacarpal joints allows greater compensatory motion. The flexion and extension arc is 15 degrees in the ring-finger carpometacarpal joint and 30 degrees in the little finger.

Fracture site angulation of more than 10 degrees should not be accepted in the index and middle fingers. Fractures of the ring and little fingers with initial angulation of less than 15 degrees should be immobilized in a gutter splint for 10–14 days. When angulation is 15–40 degrees, reduction should be accomplished before an ulnar gutter splint immobilization is employed for 3 weeks. With angulation of more than 40 degrees, extensor lag may be noted at the proximal interphalangeal joint, and the patient may complain of a "marble" in the palm when making a fist. If closed reduction cannot be maintained, internal fixation may be employed.

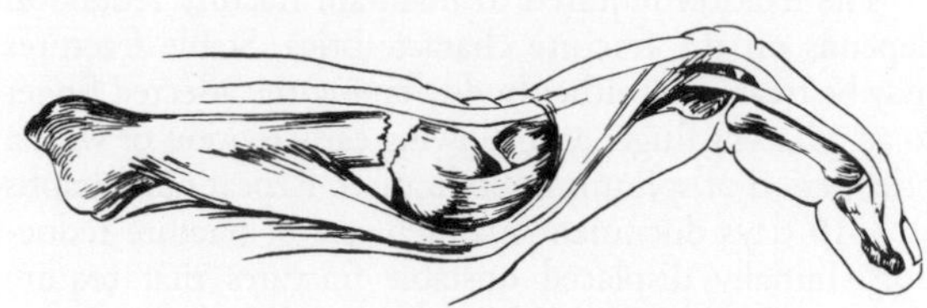

Figure 10–28. **Boxer's fracture. If the angulation in a metacarpal neck fracture is severe, clawing may result when the patient attempts to extend the finger. This is a good clinical test to supplement the evaluation of the severity of the angulation as seen radiographically.** (Reproduced, with permission, from Rockwood CA Jr et al, ed: *Fractures in Adults,* 3rd ed. Lippincott, 1991.)

Metacarpal Shaft Fractures

Metacarpal shaft fractures result from a direct blow or crushing injury. Dorsal angulation of the fracture fragments is secondary to the interosseous muscle forces. The closer the fracture is to the carpometacarpal joints, the greater the lever arm and, hence, the less angulation can be tolerated. Less shortening occurs in isolated fractures of the middle and ring metacarpals than in the index or little fingers because the deep intermetacarpal ligaments of two adjacent rays tether the fractured metacarpal distally. Isolated metacarpal fractures may be treated with cast or splint immobilization for 4–6 weeks. Displaced metacarpal shaft fractures may be fixed percutaneously with a longitudinal pin or by percutaneously pinning the fractured metacarpal to an adjacent metacarpal. Skeletal fixation is essential if metacarpal rotational deformity cannot be corrected with closed means because modest metacarpal malrotation results in substantial digital overlap. Dorsal angulation of more than 10 degrees in index and middle metacarpals and more than 20 degrees in ring and little metacarpals, shortening of more than 3 mm, or multiple displaced metacarpal fractures should be treated with operative intervention. Long spiral fractures may be effectively fixed with multiple screws, and transverse fractures are usually most securely fixed with dorsally applied plates. When two or more metacarpals are simultaneously fractured, the splinting effect of the intact adjacent metacarpals is lost. Secure fixation with screws or plates should be employed in at least one of the multiple injured metacarpals.

5. Joint Injuries

Distal Interphalangeal Joint

The most common intraarticular fracture of the distal interphalangeal joint is a bony mallet finger, in which a portion of the articular surface is avulsed by the extensor tendon. Most bony mallet injuries can be treated with splinting in extension for 6 weeks. Indications for fixation of these fractures are controversial. Internal fixation should be considered in fractures that include articular surface loss greater than 30% and subluxation of the joint.

Dislocation of the distal interphalangeal joint is uncommon without an associated fracture. Closed reduction with temporary splint protection allows early mobilization to begin within 7–10 days.

Condylar Fractures

Condylar fractures may occur in either the proximal or middle phalanges. These fractures are most often athletic injuries. Anteroposterior, lateral, and oblique radiographs are necessary to identify the fracture fragments. If the injury is inadequately appreciated, angulation of the finger and joint incongruity may lead to stiffness, deformity and early degenerative arthritis. Displaced fracture should be openly reduced and internally fixed if the condylar fracture is displaced by more than 2 mm. If both condyles are fractured, they must be precisely secured together and then secured to the phalangeal shaft. The collateral ligament insertion to the condyle must be preserved because it is the only blood supply to the fragment. Permanent stiffness may be anticipated in complex condylar fractures.

Proximal Interphalangeal Joint Dislocation & Fracture-Dislocation

Dorsal dislocations of the proximal interphalangeal joint are more common than palmar or lateral dislocations. Dorsal dislocations may be separated into three types (Figure 10–29). In type 1 dislocations, a hyperextension injury avulses the volar plate from the base of the middle phalanx, and the collateral ligaments partially split from the middle phalanx and the joint surface remain intact. Type 2 dislocations are dorsal dislocations similar to type 1 injuries, except that a larger portion of the collateral ligament is torn. In type 3 injuries, dorsal dislocation occurs with proximal retraction of the middle phalanx. A portion of the middle phalangeal palmar base may be sheared away. Stable fracture-dislocations are associated with fractures in which less than 40% of the middle phalanx base is fractured. Unstable fracture-dislocations have more than 40% bone fracture involvement and are associated with complete loss of collateral ligament stability.

Treatment of proximal interphalangeal joint dislocations depends on the dislocation type. Stable type 1 and 2 injuries should be treated by closed reduction and immobilization in a dorsal splint in 30 degrees of flexion for 1–2 weeks. After reduction and splinting, a radiograph should document the reduction. While in the splint, patients are encouraged to flex the proximal interphalangeal joint actively. After 2–3 weeks, the splint is removed. The finger may be buddy taped to an adjacent finger during sports for the next month.

Unstable fracture-dislocations should be treated with closed reduction. Considerable flexion (more than 75 degrees) may be necessary to achieve reduction. Again,

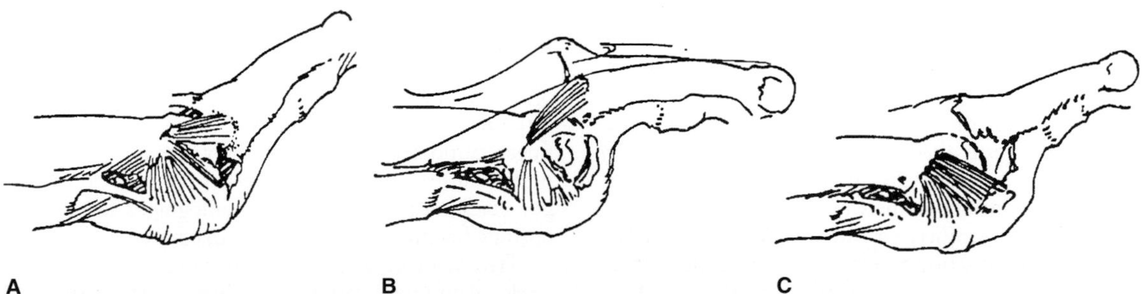

Figure 10–29. Various dorsal dislocations of the proximal interphalangeal joint. **A:** Type 1 (hyperextension). The volar plate is avulsed, and an incomplete longitudinal split occurs in the collateral ligaments. The articular surfaces maintain congruous contact. **B:** Type 2 (dorsal dislocation). There is complete rupture of the volar plate and a complete split in the collateral ligaments, with the middle phalanx resting on the dorsum of the proximal phalanx. The proximal and middle phalanges lie in almost parallel alignment. **C:** Type 3 (fracture-dislocation). The insertion of the volar plate, including a portion of the volar base of the middle phalanx, is disrupted. The major portion of the collateral ligaments remains with the volar plate and flexor sheath. A major articular defect may be present.

radiographs must document congruent joint reduction. An extension block splint allows active proximal interphalangeal joint flexion while constraining extension. The splint is straightened by 10-degree increments each week until approximately 6 weeks after reduction, when splinting may be discontinued. If closed reduction cannot be achieved, open reduction is required. When a single large palmar articular fragment is present, internal fixation may be attempted. If the fracture is comminuted, however, either volar plate arthroplasty or an axial traction technique that allows early controlled passive joint motion is necessary.

Radial lateral proximal interphalangeal dislocation is six times more common than ulnar lateral interphalangeal dislocation. These dislocations are associated with avulsion of the volar plate, extensor mechanism, or a portion of the phalangeal base. After the joint is reduced, the residual joint stability should be assessed by observing the active ROM. Stable fracture-dislocations are immobilized at 5–10 degrees of flexion for 3 weeks, and then active ROM activities are allowed.

Palmar proximal interphalangeal dislocations are unusual. The condyle of the proximal phalanx may buttonhole between the central slip and the lateral bands. Closed reduction may be attempted by applying traction to the fingers after flexing both the metacarpophalangeal and proximal interphalangeal joints. If closed reduction is successful, the digit should be splinted in extension for 3–6 weeks to allow healing of the extensor rent. If closed reduction is unsuccessful, open reduction is necessary to free the condyle from the rent in the extensor mechanism.

Metacarpophalangeal Joint

Dorsal metacarpophalangeal dislocations most commonly involve either the index or little finger. The volar plate is ruptured proximally from the metacarpal by hyperextension injury. If the joint is subluxed and the volar plate has not yet become interposed in the joint, closed reduction may be achieved by flexion of the joint. Traction across the subluxated metacarpophalangeal joint can transform a reducible joint into an irreducible, dislocated joint. Once the joint dislocates, the volar plate becomes interposed between the dislocated articular surfaces. This injury, termed *complex* or *irreducible,* requires open reduction to extract the volar plate from between the articular surfaces (Figure 10–30). Open reduction may be accomplished through either a palmar or dorsal approach. If the palmar approach is used, care should be taken to avoid injury to the radial digital nerve of the index finger or the ulnar digital nerve of the small finger. The A1 pulley is incised to release the tension of the flexor tendons on the volar plate. If the dorsal approach is used, the volar plate is incised longitudinally to facilitate reduction.

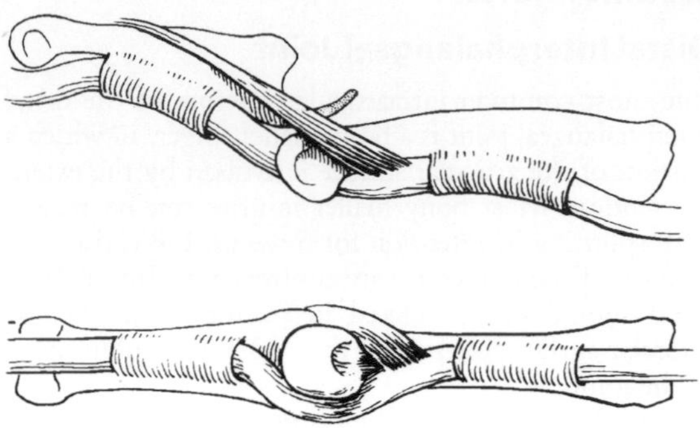

Figure 10–30. Complex dislocation of the metacarpophalangeal joint. In the upper lateral diagram, the palmar plate is locked between the head of the metacarpal and the base of the proximal phalanx. In the lower diagram, an anterior view, the head of the metacarpal can be seen trapped between the flexor digitorum profundus on one aspect and the lumbrical on the other. (Reproduced, with permission, from Lister G: *The Hand: Diagnosis and Indications,* 3rd ed. Churchill Livingstone, 1993.)

Postoperatively, the metacarpophalangeal joint is immobilized in approximately 30 degrees of flexion for 3–5 days. Splinting that allows active motion is maintained for 3 weeks.

Although lateral dislocations of the metacarpophalangeal joint are rare, isolated radial collateral ligament ruptures may occur. These injuries should also be immobilized in approximately 30 degrees of flexion for 3 weeks. The fingers should be protected from ulnar stress for an additional 3 weeks. Unstable index- and middle-finger radial collateral ligament tears may be surgically repaired.

Finger Carpometacarpal Joints

Sprains and fracture-dislocations may involve any of the carpometacarpal joints. Sprains of the index- and middle-finger carpometacarpal joints may occur with palmar flexion and torsion. If tenderness is localized to the carpometacarpal joint and careful radiographs fail to demonstrate fracture, a sprain may be diagnosed.

Treatment of acute sprain injuries consists of 3–6 weeks of immobilization. If localized pain persists, steroid injection may be considered. Chronic pain at the index middle trapezoid capitate joint may be treated with either carpal boss excision or arthrodesis of the carponmetacarpal joint. Carpometacarpal fracture-dislocations of the ring and little fingers are usually secondary to direct or longitudinal blows. Dorsal dislocations are more common than volar dislocations. Oblique views with partial pronation and supination may be required to visualize the carpometacarpal joint clearly. Closed reduction may be achieved with longitudinal distraction. The reduction may be maintained by percutaneous K-wire fixation. When fracture-dislocation of the little-finger metacarpal articular surface shears off a fragment of the hamate, displacement of the metacarpal shaft is likely. Because of forces of the extensor carpi ulnaris and the hypothenar muscles, the metacarpal shaft tends to displace proximally and angulate palmarly. Longitudinal traction and percutaneous K-wire fixation of the ring- and little-finger metacarpals stabilize these fractures. Open reduction is necessary for an irreducible dislocation or for chronic fracture-dislocations. If the patient develops degenerative arthritis of the hamate metacarpal joint, arthrodesis of the ring- or small-finger carpometacarpal joint (or both) is well tolerated.

Thumb Metacarpophalangeal Joint

The most common injury to the metacarpophalangeal joint is sprain of the ulnar collateral ligament of the thumb (gamekeeper's thumb, skier's thumb). This injury occurs when the thumb is forced into radial deviation, stressing the ulnar collateral ligament. When the ulnar collateral ligament tears from its phalangeal insertion, the adductor aponeurosis may become interposed between the retracted ligament, preventing healing of the ligament to the proximal phalanx with closed treatment (Stener lesion). Evaluation of the integrity of the ligament may be made by radially stressing the flexed metacarpophalangeal joint under local anesthesia. Radial deviation that is more than 30 degrees from that of the opposite thumb is diagnostic of a totally disrupted, incompetent ligament.

Closed treatment of a partial ligament tear may be accomplished with a thumb spica splint for 3–4 weeks. Complete disruption of the ligament requires surgical exploration and reattachment to the bone. Avulsion of the ulnar collateral ligament may also occur with a bony fragment. If the fragment is greater than 15% of the articular surface or if the avulsed fragment is displaced more than 5 mm, open repair of the ligament is recommended.

Chronic symptomatic ulnar collateral ligament injuries may be repaired if the residual ligament is of sufficient quality. Supplementation of the repair with either tendon transfer or tendon grafting may be useful. In patients who develop traumatic arthritis or if ligament reconstruction is not deemed feasible, arthrodesis of the metacarpophalangeal joint is preferred.

Thumb Carpometacarpal Joint

Four patterns of thumb metacarpal fracture are most commonly encountered.

A. Bennett Fracture

Bennett fracture is an intraarticular fracture in which the small volar radial fragment of the metacarpal articular surface remains attached to the anterior oblique ligament, and the remainder of the metacarpal articular surface and shaft is displaced proximally, radially, and into adduction in response to the force of the adductor pollicis and abductor pollicis longus muscles insertion on the metacarpal (Figure 10–31). Acute Bennett fractures may often be reduced by traction and pressure on the proximal metacarpal, with slight pronation. The reduction may then be stabilized by percutaneous pin fixation through the metacarpal shaft into either the fragment or the trapezium. If satisfactory reduction cannot be achieved by closed means, open reduction and internal fixation is required.

B. Rolando Fracture

The Rolando fracture is a comminuted T or Y intraarticular fracture of the base of the thumb metacarpal. When large fragments are present, open reduction and internal fixation is possible. When the joint is highly comminuted, cast immobilization, traction, or limited open reduction and internal fixation with cast immobilization may be employed.

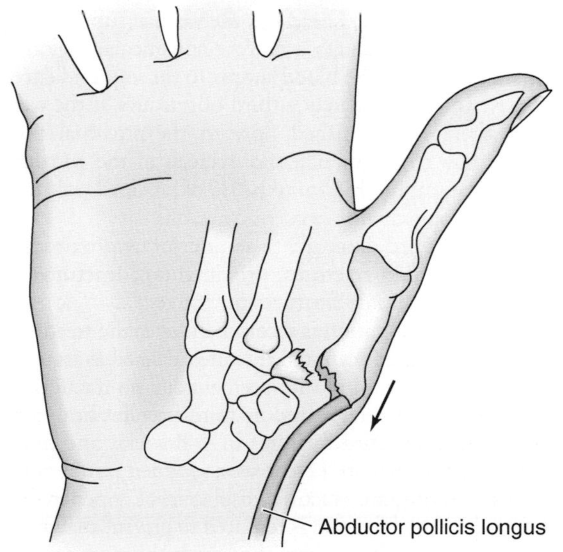

Figure 10–31. Bennett fracture. The first metacarpal shaft is displaced by the pull of the muscle. (Reproduced, with permission, from American Society for Surgery of the Hand: *The Hand: Examination and Diagnosis,* 2nd ed. Churchill Livingstone, 1983.)

C. Extraarticular Fracture

Extraarticular fractures are less likely to develop traumatic arthritis than intraarticular fractures. Because of the mobility of the carpometacarpal joint of the thumb, up to 30 degrees of angulation can be accepted without functional loss.

D. Epiphyseal Fracture

Epiphyseal fractures of the thumb metacarpal are treated in a fashion similar to other Salter-Harris fractures.

Freeland AE, Lineaweaver WC, Lindley SG: Fracture fixation in the mutilated hand. Hand Clin 2003;19:51.

Kiefhaber TR, Stern PJ: Fractures dislocations of the proximal interphalangeal joint. J Hand Surg Am 1998;23:368.

Page SM, Stern PJ: Complications and range of motion following plate fixation of metacarpal and phalangeal fractures. J Hand Surg Am 1998;23:827.

WRIST INJURIES

Scaphoid Injuries

The scaphoid is the most commonly fractured bone in the carpus. Anatomically, the scaphoid may be divided into proximal, middle, and distal thirds. The middle third is termed the *waist.* The scaphoid tubercle forms a distal volar prominence. Because the scaphoid articulates with four carpal bones and the radius, most of its surface is composed of articular cartilage, leaving little room for vascular perforation. Therefore, the vascular supply to the scaphoid comes through a narrow nonarticular region in the waist. Most of the blood supply to the scaphoid enters distally. In approximately a third of fractures at the waist level, there is diminished flow to the proximal pole, which may result in ischemic necrosis of the proximal pole of the scaphoid. Almost 100% of proximal pole fractures develop ischemic or aseptic necrosis.

Middle third fractures account for approximately 70% of scaphoid fractures, proximal pole fractures for 20%, and distal pole fractures for the rest.

Cast immobilization is recommended in the treatment of all nondisplaced scaphoid fractures, defined as fractures with less than 2 mm of displacement and no fracture site angulation. On average, middle third fractures heal in 6–12 weeks, distal third fractures in 4–8 weeks, and proximal third fractures in 12–20 weeks. When initial radiographs demonstrate fracture displacement, open reduction and internal fixation is required to prevent malunion. Internal fixation is accomplished with either smooth K-wires or a buried compression screw. Because of the time to union in scaphoid fractures, some surgeons recommend primary fixation of these fractures even when nondisplaced. Newer studies demonstrate that percutaneous fixation of nondisplaced waist fractures decreases or eliminates the period of cast immobilization.

Delayed union may be treated with either prolonged casting or open reduction, curettage, and bone grafting. Nondisplaced ununited fractures may be treated by percutaneous screw fixation. If fracture site angulation or collapse is present, a cortical cancellous volar graft is employed to correct the deformity. The graft must be stabilized with either a buried compression screw or K-wires. If the proximal pole is avascular and no radiocarpal arthritis is present, revascularization of the scaphoid with a vascularized bone graft from the dorsal radius should be performed.

Once degenerative arthritis is evident at the radiocarpal joint, salvage procedures include proximal row carpectomy, scaphoid excision and midcarpal arthrodesis, or total wrist arthrodesis.

Lunate & Perilunate Dislocations

Lunate and perilunate dislocations are the result of a powerful force causing disruption of the ligamentous support about the lunate. The mechanism of these injuries is usually dorsiflexion, ulnar deviation, and intercarpal supination. Mayfield defined four stages of disruption. Stage 1 injuries demonstrate disruptions of the scapholunate ligament. Stage 2 injuries also include tears of the ligaments dorsal to the lunate. In stage 3 injuries, the arc of disruption extends across the lunotriquetral ligament. Stage 4 injuries have total disruption of the entire lunate ligamentous support. The sequence of injuries is paralleled by a progression of clinical entities from scapholunate dissociation to perilunate dislocation to lunate dislocation.

When the entire carpus except the lunate dislocates and the lunate remains normally seated in the lunate fossa of the radius, the abnormality is termed *perilunate dislocation* (Figure 10–32). When the relationship between the carpus and the radius is maintained but the lunate is dislocated palmarward into the carpal tunnel, the condition is termed *lunate dislocation.* Both lunate and perilunate dislocations imply disruption of ligamentous connections between the scaphoid and the lunate, between the capitate and the lunate, and between the lunate and the triquetrum. Although the lunate is bound to the scaphoid by the scapholunate ligament and to the triquetrum through the lunotriquetral ligament, the interval between the lunate and the capitate, known as the space of Poirier, lacks direct ligamentous connection.

A variant of perilunate dislocation is transscaphoid perilunate dislocation. With this injury, the arc of disruption passes through the scaphoid rather than the scapholunate ligament. The disruption then passes between the proximal scaphoid and the capitate, between the capitate and the lunate, and between the lunate and the triquetrum.

Intercarpal ligamentous disruptions heal if the normally connected bones are maintained in an anatomic

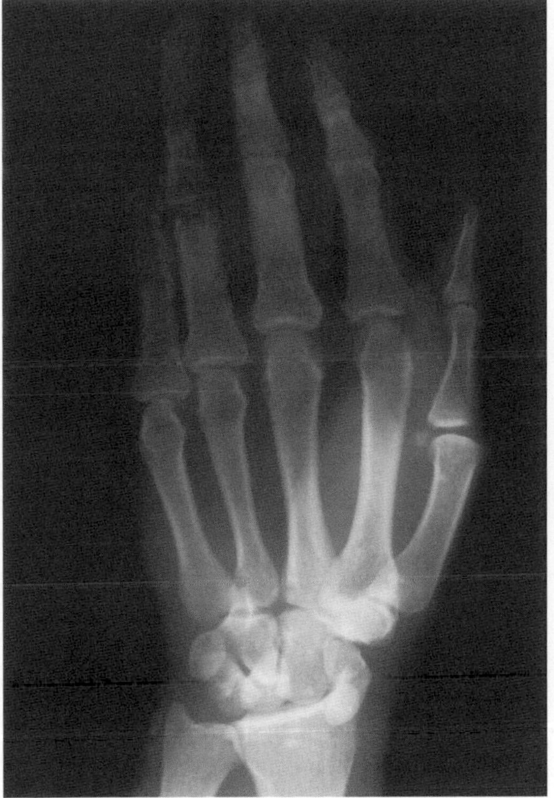
A

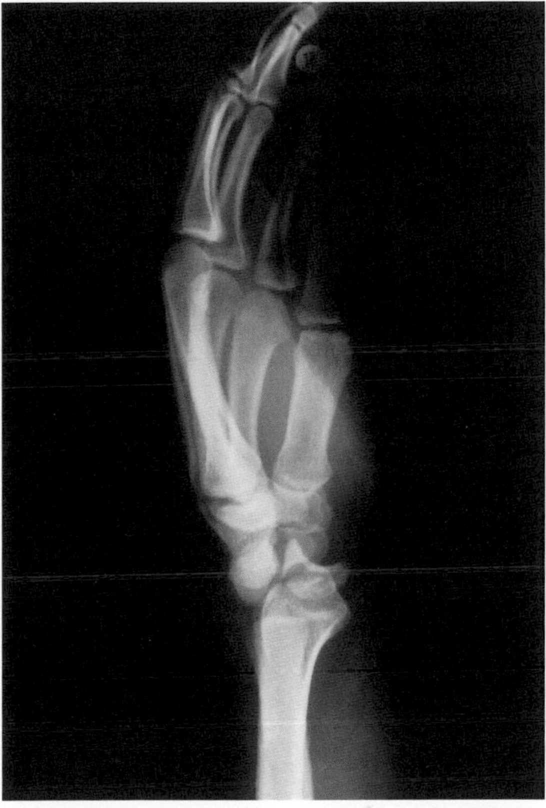
B

Figure 10–32. Perilunate dislocation: Anteroposterior view (**A**); lateral view (**B**).

relationship. Intercarpal dislocations should be reduced initially in a closed fashion. Reduction is usually achieved by longitudinal traction and direct pressure on the dislocated carpal bone or bones. Occasionally, anatomic alignment of the carpus can be achieved and maintained with closed reduction and cast application. In most instances, however, open reduction, pin fixation, and direct ligamentous repair is necessary to secure anatomic reduction. Surgical treatment of perilunate and lunate dislocations often requires both palmar and dorsal approaches. Through the dorsal approach, intercarpal alignment is visualized, adjusted, and stabilized. The palmar approach is employed to release the median nerve at the carpal tunnel and to repair the rent in the space of Poirier.

Kienböck Disease

Kienböck disease results from ischemic necrosis of the lunate. The cause of the condition is the subject of extensive debate. The condition is more common in patients with a negative ulnar variance, in which the ulna is shorter than the radius. It is unclear whether the relatively shorter ulna alters and increases the force transmitted to the lunate through the lunate fossa of the radius or whether the altered stress causes the lunate to be shaped in a more triangular and less cuboid or trapezoidal configuration.

Kienböck disease may be classified based on the extent of collapse (Figure 10–33). Stage I disease demonstrates a linear compression fracture but an otherwise normal-appearing architecture and density. MRI studies show poor vascularity of the lunate in stage I (Figure 10–34). In stage II disease, the density is abnormal on plain films. By stage III, lunate collapse is present. Stage III disease is subdivided into stage IIIA, in which the lunate is collapsed but carpal height remains normal, and stage IIIB, in which the lunate is collapsed and carpal height is also abnormal. In stage IV wrists, extensive osteoarthritic changes are present.

The current recommendations for the treatment of Kienböck disease include radial shortening osteotomy for ulnar-negative or neutral variance when no carpal collapse is present. If the patient initially demonstrates a

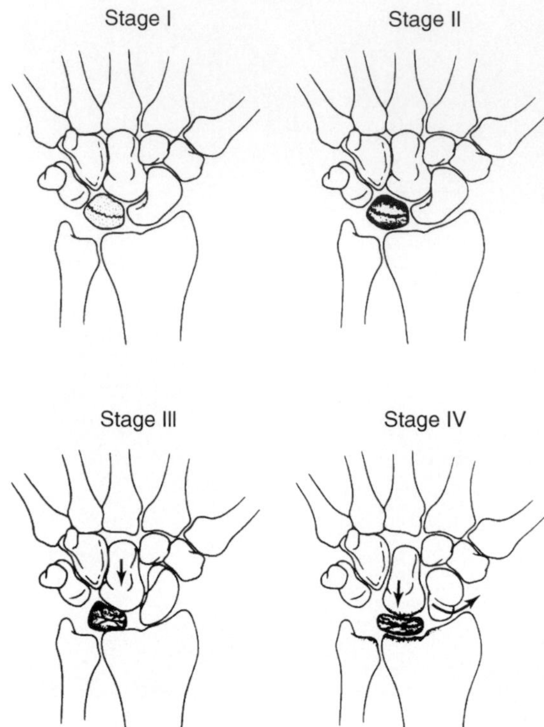

Figure 10–33. Staging of Kienböck disease (after Lichtman). Stage I: Routine radiographs (posteroanterior, lateral) are normal, but tomography may show a linear fracture, usually transverse through the body of the lunate. MRI confirms avascular changes. Stage II: Bone density increase (sclerosis) and a fracture line are usually evident on the posteroanterior radiograph. Posteroanterior and lateral tomograms demonstrate sclerosis, cystic changes, and often a clear fracture. There is no collapse deformity. Stage III: Advanced bone density changes are present, with fragmentation, cystic resorption, and collapse. The diagnosis is evident from posteroanterior radiograph. Tomograms (posteroanterior and lateral) show the degree of lunate infractionation and amount of fracture displacement. Proximal migration of the capitate is present, and there is mild to moderate rotary alignment of the scaphoid. Stage IV: Perilunate arthritic changes are present, with complete collapse and fragmentation of the lunate. Carpal instability is evident, with scaphoid malalignment and capitate displacement into the lunate space. (Reproduced, with permission, from Rockwood CA Jr et al, eds: *Fractures in Adults,* 3rd ed. Lippincott, 1991.)

positive ulnar variance, recommendations include either a capitate shortening osteotomy or an intercarpal arthrodesis of the scaphoid, trapezium, and trapezoid. A new technique restores the anatomic height of the lunate with a vascularized bone graft and additional cancellous bone. In stage IIIB and IV wrists, consideration is given to either proximal row carpectomy or wrist arthrodesis. Silicone replacement of the lunate is no longer advised for Kienböck disease.

Carpal Instability

To evaluate the orientation of the carpus properly, true anteroposterior and lateral radiographs are required. The anteroposterior view should be obtained with the forearm positioned in neutral rotation to allow a precise standardized evaluation of the relationship between the distal radius and the distal ulna. When the ulna is shorter than the radius, the term *negative ulnar variance* is used, and when the ulna extends further distally than the radius, the term *positive ulnar variance* is used.

The anteroposterior radiograph should demonstrate the close relationship of the scaphoid and the lunate. Normally, the ossified portions of these two bones are separated by their abutting respective articular cartilage shells, creating a radiographic gap of 3 mm or less. In an adult a gap of more than 3 mm is considered abnormal and indicates separation of these two bones secondary to ligamentous disruption. When the scapholunate gap is abnormally wide on a standard radiograph, the abnormality is referred to as static scapholunate dissociation (Figure 10–35). When the standard anteroposterior radiograph is normal but an anteroposterior radio-

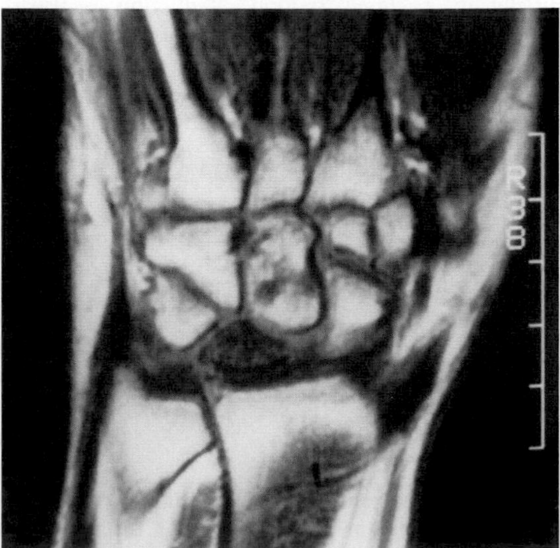

Figure 10–34. MRI showing Kienböck disease.

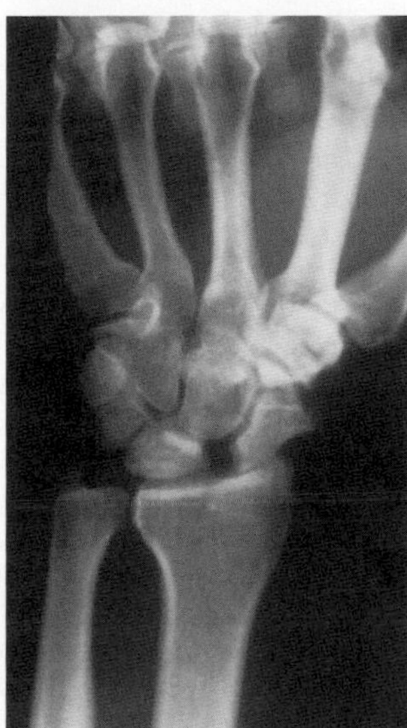

Figure 10–35. Anteroposterior view of static scapholunate dissociation.

graph taken with the fingers squeezing tightly to form a fist reveals an abnormal gap, the condition is referred to as dynamic scapholunate dissociation.

The lateral radiograph should be obtained with the wrist in a neutral position, neither flexed nor extended. The lateral radiograph is often overlooked because of the projected superimposition of shadows. This normal overlapping allows measurement of a number of angles between bones. Normally, the middle metacarpal, capitate, lunate, and radius are collinear. The long axis of the radius is readily defined. Establishing the relationship of the scaphoid to the radius requires defining a line drawn along the most palmar portions of the distal and proximal poles of the scaphoid. The axes of the radius and the scaphoid intersect, forming the radioscaphoid angle (Figure 10–36). This angle is usually between 40 and 60 degrees. When the angle is greater than 60 degrees, the scaphoid is abnormally flexed.

The orientation of the lunate viewed on the lateral radiograph is derived by first establishing a line between the most distal palmar and dorsal lips of the lunate. A second line is then drawn perpendicular to the first line, establishing the axis of the lunate. The angle between the radial and lunate axes (radiolunate angle) is normally less than 15 degrees.

The orientation of the lunate seen on the lateral radiograph normally reflects a ligamentous balancing of the influences of the adjacent scaphoid and triquetrum. The scaphoid tends to tether the lunate into flexion through the scapholunate ligament, whereas the triquetrum tends to tether the lunate into extension (dorsiflexion) through the lunotriquetral ligament. When the scapholunate ligament is disrupted, the scaphoid tends to flex excessively, and the lunate, under the unopposed influence of the triquetrum, dorsiflexes (dorsal intercalated segment instability [DISI]) (Figure 10–37). When the lunotriquetral ligament is disrupted, the lunate, under the unopposed influence of the scaphoid, is flexed

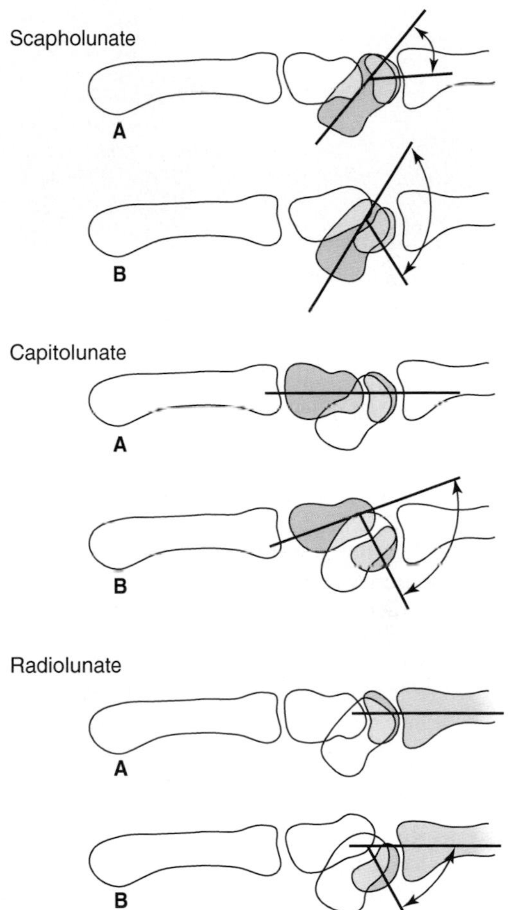

Figure 10–36. Carpal angle measurements are of considerable aid in identifying carpal instability patterns. A = normal angle; B = abnormal angle seen in dorsiflexion instability. The capitolunate angle should theoretically be 0 degrees with the wrist in neutral position, but the range of normal probably extends to as much as 15 degrees. The scapholunate angle may be the most helpful; an angle of greater than 80 degrees is definite evidence of dorsiflexion instability. The radiolunate angle is abnormal if it exceeds 15 degrees. (Reproduced, with permission, from Green DP, ed: *Operative Hand Surgery*, 2nd ed. Churchill Livingstone, 1988.)

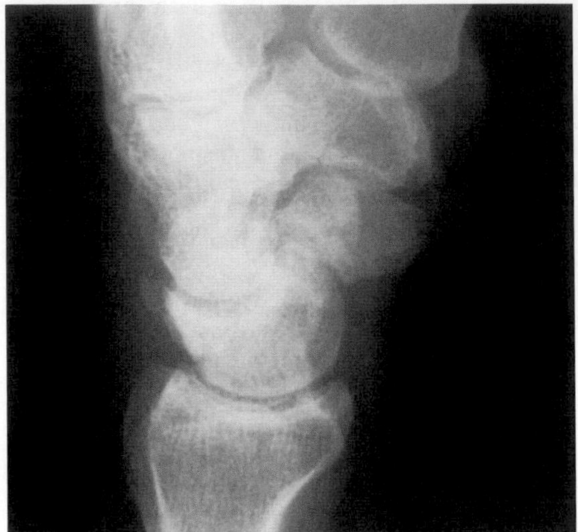

Figure 10–37. Lateral radiograph of dorsal intercalated segment instability.

(volar intercalated segment instability [VISI]). The optimal treatment for DISI is currently an area of intense interest. Acute ligamentous disruption is usually treated with direct ligamentous reapproximation and repair. When ligamentous repair is not possible and articular surfaces are free of degenerative change, ligamentous reconstruction, dorsal capsular ligamentodesis, or intercarpal fusions may be considered.

Degenerative arthritis occurs in wrists subjected over time to loads applied to noncongruently articulating carpal bones. The scapholunate advanced collapse (SLAC) wrist pattern describes the evolution of degenerative arthritis resulting from disruption of the scapholunate ligament (Figure 10–38). The earliest evidence of degenerative change is seen at the radioscaphoid joint, and, with time, degenerative change progresses to include the capitate lunate articulation. When radioscaphoid change is present but the articular surface of the capitate retains its normal articular cartilage, proximal row carpectomy (removal of the scaphoid, lunate, and triquetrum) allows preservation of wrist motion as the capitate head shifts proximally to articulate within the lunate fossa of the distal radius. When degenerative change is present at the capitate lunate portion of the midcarpal joints in addition to radioscaphoid change, the scaphoid may be excised and intercarpal fusion of the capitate, lunate, triquetrum, and hamate is accomplished. This selective intercarpal fusion procedure provides motion through the residual radiolunate articulation. The ultimate salvage procedure, complete wrist fusion, provides reliable pain relief while permanently sacrificing wrist motion.

Distal Radioulnar Joint

The distal radioulnar joint (DRUJ) is composed of two joints. The proximal and distal articulations of the ulna and radius allow forearm rotation. The ulna also articulates with the ulnar carpus through the triangular fibrocartilage complex (TFCC). Approximately 20% of the load from the hand to the forearm passes through the ulnocarpal joint. Problems at the DRUJ are related to one or both of these joints.

When the ulnar variance is positive, the patient may develop an ulnocarpal impaction syndrome. This often presents with pain on the ulnar side of the wrist, particularly with ulnar deviation. Radiographs may demonstrate degenerative changes of the distal ulna and ulnar lunate. Treatment consists of shortening the ulna, accomplished by removing 2–3 mm of the ulnar head (wafer procedure) either by open method, by arthroscope, or by an ulnar-shortening osteotomy, performed in the diaphyseal ulna, and fixed with a plate and screws. After the wafer procedure, patients often complain of ulnar pain for a prolonged (3–6 month) period. Approximately 50% of patients who have an ulnar shortening osteotomy require plate removal after osteotomy healing.

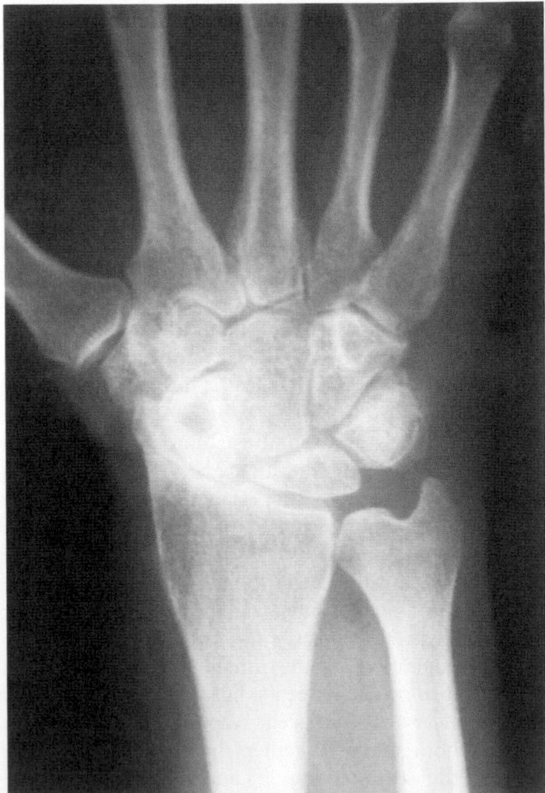

Figure 10–38. Scapholunate advanced collapse pattern.

Another source of ulnar-sided wrist pain is a tear of the TFCC. Tears are divided into degenerative and traumatic types. Degenerative tears are usually related to ulnocarpal impaction. Traumatic tears usually occur after a twisting injury of the wrist. Central tears and tears near the attachment of the TFCC to the radius are usually treated with an arthroscopic debridement. Tears in the well-vascularized periphery of the TFCC are treated with either arthroscopic or open repair. After repair, patients are maintained in a long arm cast for 6 weeks to allow fibrocartilage healing.

Arthritis between the distal radius and ulna can be caused by traumatic, degenerative, or inflammatory arthritis. Treatment consists of hemiresection or complete excision of the ulnar head (Darrach procedure). An alternative treatment, the Suave-Kapandji procedure, fuses the DRUJ and creates a pseudarthrosis of the distal ulna. This is particularly useful in the presence of ulnar translocation of the carpus.

Instability of the DRUJ is difficult to treat. Instability is usually the result of trauma, but it may occur after an excessive distal ulna resection. Treatment requires detection and correction of any degree of malunions in the radius or ulna. A number of soft-tissue operations are designed to stabilize the distal ulna, all with varying degrees of success.

Adams BD, Berger RA: An anatomic reconstruction of the distal radioulnar ligaments for posttraumatic distal radioulnar joint instability. J Hand Surg [Am] 2002;27(2):243. [PMID: 11901383]

Aldridge JM III, Mallon WJ: Hook of the hamate fractures in competitive golfers: Results of treatment by excision of the fractured hook of the hamate. Orthopedics 2003;26:717. [PMID: 12875568]

Berger RA: The anatomy of the ligaments of the wrist and distal radioulnar joints. Clin Orthop 2001;(383):32. Review. [PMID: 11210966]

Cohen MS, Kozin SH: Degenerative arthritis of the wrist: Proximal row carpectomy versus scaphoid excision and four-corner arthrodesis. J Hand Surg [Am] 2001;26:94. [PMID: 11172374]

Gelberman RH et al: Ulnar variance with Kienböck's disease. J Bone Joint Surg Am 1975;57:674. [PMID: 1150712]

Rettig ME et al: Open reduction and internal fixation of acute displaced scaphoid waist fractures. J Hand Surg [Am] 2001;26(2): 271. [PMID: 11279573]

Shin AY et al: Treatment of isolated injuries of the lunotriquetral ligament. A comparison of arthrodesis, ligament reconstruction and ligament repair. J Bone Joint Surg Br 2001;83(7):1023. [PMID: 11603516]

Shin AY, Bishop AT: Pedicled vascularized bone grafts for disorders of the carpus: Scaphoid nonunion and Kienböck's disease. J Am Acad Orthop Surg 2002;10:210. [PMID: 12041942]

Slade JF III et al: Percutaneous internal fixation of selected scaphoid nonunions with an arthroscopically assisted dorsal approach. J Bone Joint Surg Am 2003:85:20. [PMID: 14652390]

Steinmann SP et al: Use of the 1,2 intercompartmental supraretinacular artery as a vascularized pedicle bone graft for difficult scaphoid nonunion. J Hand Surg [Am] 2002;27(3):391. [PMID: 12015712]

Szabo RM et al: Dorsal intercarpal ligament capsulodesis for chronic, static scapholunate dissociation: Clinical results. J Hand Surg Am 2002;27A:978. [PMID: 12457347]

FINGERTIP INJURIES

SOFT-TISSUE INJURIES

Because of the importance of the fingertip in providing a contact surface for sensate prehension, injuries to the fingertip may result in troublesome disability. The pulp of the fingertip is normally covered by tough, highly innervated skin, anchored to the phalanx by fibrous septa. The dorsum of the fingertip is composed of the nail and nail bed.

Treatment

The goals in treatment of fingertip injuries are to provide adequate sensation, minimal tenderness, satisfactory appearance, and full joint motion. Preservation of length should be balanced with the other goals.

The choice of treatment depends on the size and location of the defect. The mechanism of injury (sharp, crushing, or avulsion), the presence of exposed bone, and the angle of soft-tissue loss are considered in planning treatment.

A. Open Wound Care

The simplest treatment is open wound care, which is indicated in most injuries in children and in defects of 1 cm^2 or less in adults. The wound is thoroughly cleansed. Bone is shortened so it is covered by soft tissue and the length of the bone is the same as the length of the nail bed. Dressings are changed until the wound is healed. The disadvantages of the open method are the possibility of stump tenderness and prolonged healing time. Advantages include the ability to initiate movement immediately and to thus preserve full digital motion.

B. Composite Grafting

Replacement of the amputated part as a composite graft (skin and subcutaneous tissue) is indicated in children and selected adults with sharp distal amputations. When successful, this treatment gives the best appearance. The disadvantage, the unpredictable viability of the part, may result in recovery delayed by failure and secondary procedures.

C. Microvascular Replantation

Microvascular replantation is possible in selected sharp amputations distal to the distal interphalangeal joint. Disadvantages include the expense of complex surgery and the time lost from work.

D. Primary Shortening and Closure

Primary bone shortening and closure is indicated when more than 50% of the distal phalanx is lost or the nail matrix is irreparably damaged. This one-stage procedure allows for immediate mobilization. In performing the procedure, the end of the distal phalanx bone should be trimmed to provide a tension-free soft-tissue closure. The nail bed should be trimmed as far proximal as the bone. If the nail bed is pulled over the end of the shortened bone, a hook-shaped nail results. Neurectomy of digital nerves under traction allows the nerve ends to retract into soft tissue proximal to the ultimate scar.

E. Skin Grafting

Skin grafting may also be employed to obtain closure if no bone is exposed. Split-thickness grafts may be placed on a less well vascularized bed. Split-thickness grafts contract more than full-thickness grafts. As the graft shrinks, the area of sensory loss also shrinks. The appearance and durability of scar tissue may be less than ideal, however.

Full-thickness skin grafts provide more durable coverage and better appearance. Care should be taken to match the pigmentation of the skin at the donor and recipient sites. The ulnar border of the hand provides an ideal donor source. Full-thickness grafts require a better vascularized bed to assure survival.

F. Skin Flaps

Local advancement skin flaps are useful in the treatment of fingertip injuries.

1. V-Y advancement skin flaps—V-Y advancement skin flaps may advance palmar tissue or unite two lateral skin flaps. These skin flaps are helpful in the management of transverse or dorsal oblique amputations in which soft-tissue tip coverage is needed and further skeletal shortening deemed undesirable. Complete separation of the vertical septa between the skin and the bone is required to mobilize skin flaps for advancement. The septa between the flap and the proximal skin must then be divided. Traction on the flap helps differentiate the septa from vessels and nerves.

2. Moberg palmar advancement flap—Defects of up to 1.5 cm on the thumb may be covered by a palmar advancement flap, first described by Moberg. Bilateral midlateral incisions dorsal to the neurovascular bundles of the thumb allow mobilization of the flap from the flexor tendon sheath. The flap may be maximally advanced by flexion of the thumb interphalangeal joint. When additional coverage is required, the skin of the flap may be transversely divided at the metacarpophalangeal crease while the neurovascular bundles are preserved, the distal portion of the flap may be advanced further, and a skin graft may be placed between the distal flap and the proximal flap. Disadvantages of this flap include the possibility of interphalangeal joint flexion contracture and the potential for dorsal tip necrosis if dorsal vascular branches to the digit are injured.

3. Regional skin flaps—Regional skin flaps are considered when fingertip skin is lost but nail and bone are preserved.

a. Cross-finger flap—The cross-finger flap is the most commonly used distant flap. Skin is elevated from the dorsum of the adjacent finger, with care taken not to incise the extensor paratenon. The skin is then rotated palmarward and sewn to the palmar defect of the involved finger. The donor region on the donor finger is skin grafted. The transposed flap is divided from the donor finger after 2 weeks. Joint stiffness is a potential complication in both the donor and recipient digits. The creation of a defect on a normal digit is another disadvantage.

b. Thenar flap—The thenar flap may be used in children and young (less than 25 years) adults in whom the potential for joint stiffness is less. More subcutaneous fat is transferred with a thenar flap than with a cross-finger flap. Thenar skin flaps usually result in good matching of color and texture with the pulp.

NAIL BED INJURIES

Clinical Findings

Nail bed injuries, often neglected, should be carefully attended to because the nail enhances sensibility, provides protection and fine manipulation of the finger, and gives the finger a normal appearance. The nail bed may be injured by subungual hematoma, nail matrix laceration, avulsion of the nail matrix from the nail fold, or complete loss of the nail matrix.

Treatment

When a subungual hematoma involves more than 50% of the subungual area, the nail should be removed and the nail bed laceration repaired with fine absorbable suture. Either the nail is replaced or a dressing is placed under the nail fold to prevent synechia formation with resultant splitting of the nail. Nail bed defects are treated with split-thickness nail bed grafts taken from either an adjacent uninjured fingernail or a toenail.

When nail bed injuries occur with an open distal phalangeal fracture, pin fixation of the fracture may be considered because it stabilizes the nail bed repair.

Caution is required in the treatment of nail bed injuries in children, who often suffer injury from having a fingertip slammed in a door. The nail often lies dorsal to the nail fold, and a small subungual hematoma is noted. If a radiograph is obtained, usually a physeal fracture of the distal phalanx is observed. Because the nail bed laceration communicates with the physeal fracture, this injury represents an open fracture and must be treated appropriately. The nail should be removed and the fracture site irrigated. An interposed portion of the nail bed often must be extracted from between the fragments of the physeal fracture. If the fracture is unstable, pin fixation facilitates nail bed repair. Failure to appreciate the open nature of this pediatric injury may result in osteomyelitis and physeal arrest of the distal phalanx.

Heistein JB, Cook PA: Factors affecting composite graft survival in digital tip amputations. Ann Plast Surg 2003;50:299. [PMID: 12800909]

THERMAL INJURY

ACUTE BURN INJURY

Degree of Injury

A. First-Degree Burns

Burns are characterized by the depth of skin injury. First-degree burns involve only the epidermis. Patients usually present with swollen red areas, and care is symptomatic.

B. Second-Degree Burns

Second-degree burns involve both the epidermis and the superficial portion of the dermis. These burns may be identified by skin blistering and blanching of the skin when pressure is applied. Second-degree burns are subdivided into superficial and deep burns. Superficial second-degree burns are treated with topical antibiotics such as silver sulfadiazine. The extremity is elevated and the hand splinted in the intrinsic plus position. With the wrist in 30 degrees of extension, the metacarpophalangeal joint is flexed and the interphalangeal joints are extended. The thumb should be maintained in an abducted position to prevent contracture of the first web space. The patient should begin a vigorous therapy program emphasizing active ROM as soon as it is tolerated. Compression garments may deduce swelling and scar hypertrophy after reepithelialization.

In deep second-degree burns, excision of the remaining portion of the skin and application of a skin graft does not produce long-term results superior to those achieved with spontaneous healing. Therefore, the treatment of deep second-degree burns should be similar to that of superficial second-degree burns.

C. Third-Degree Burns

Third-degree burns involve the entire epidermis, dermis, and a portion of the subcutaneous region. These burns result in waxy dry regions often having a nontender central area, caused by burning of the neural tissue. Third-degree burns should be treated with excision within the first 3–7 days and a split-thickness skin graft applied to the involved areas.

D. Fourth-Degree Burns

In addition to involvement of the skin, fourth-degree burns involve deep tissues, including muscle, tendon, and bone. Often, the only effective treatment for these burns is amputation of the involved part, with appropriate soft-tissue coverage of the residual stump.

Complications

A. Neurovascular Complications

The neurovascular status of the burned hand should be carefully monitored. Massive swelling necessitates release of compartments of the hand and forearm. Digital releases are best performed by longitudinal releases along the ulnar border of the index, middle, and ring fingers and along the radial border of the thumb and little finger. Longitudinal incisions on the dorsal hand allow decompression of interosseous muscle compartments. Incisions are made along the medial and lateral aspects of the arm and forearm.

B. Late Complications

1. Joint contractures—Joint contractures are the most common complications of upper extremity burns. At the elbow, these are most often flexion contractures. Treatment consists of soft-tissue release and either skin grafting of open regions or rotation of local skin flaps. Elbow motion may also be limited by the development of heterotopic ossifications. Excision of the ossification may be successful if delayed until the area of ossification has matured, often 1.5–2 years after the burn injury. Because the area of most intense heterotopic ossification is posteromedially, care must be taken to define and protect the ulnar nerve during elbow release surgery.

2. Wrist and hand contractures—Wrist contracture may tether the hand into either a flexed or extended position, depending on the region of the burn. In the fingers, burns usually involve the thin skin on the dorsum of the finger, often disrupting the central slip insertion onto the middle phalanx. The loss of active proximal interphalangeal joint extension combined with dorsal hand burns may result in development of a clawlike deformity, with flexion contractures of the proximal interphalangeal joints and hyperextension contracture at the metacarpophalangeal joint.

Treatment of metacarpophalangeal joint extension contracture usually requires release of the dorsal scar, addition of a dorsal skin graft, and dorsal metatarsophalangeal joint capsular release. Proximal interphalangeal flexion contractures may also occur secondary to scarred volar skin. In such cases, soft tissue release may be accomplished with either Z-plasty flap transposition or by palmar scar excision and full-thickness skin graft application. The most predictable treatment of severe proximal interphalangeal joint contracture in the burn patient is arthrodesis of the proximal interphalangeal joint.

Adduction contracture, the most common thumb deformity in the burned hand, may be difficult to resolve fully. The extent of release required depends on the degree of contracture. A modest adduction contracture may be effectively treated with Z-plasty of the thenar skin to regain adequate abduction in the first web space. With more severe contracture, release of the adductor pollicis from its origin or at its insertion and release of the first dorsal interosseous muscle origin from the thumb metacarpal may be required. If web space skin coverage is inadequate after muscle release, full-thickness skin grafting or local or distant skin flaps may be needed.

Ideally, first web space contracture should be avoided by carefully maintaining the first web space during the initial phases of burn treatment. When the extent of web space burn is severe and the normal first web cannot be maintained with dressings, an external fixator should be placed, spanning the thumb and index-finger metacarpals.

ELECTRICAL BURNS

The extent of injury in electrical burns is proportional to the amount of current that passes through the involved portion of the body. The Ohm law states that the amount of current is equal to the voltage divided by the resistance. Therefore, for a given voltage, those structures that have a lower resistance conduct a greater amount of current. The relative resistance of structures in the arm from least resistance to greatest resistance is as follows: nerve, vessel, muscle, skin, tendon, fat, and bone. Alternating current is more injurious than direct current. Because of its frequency, alternating current produces muscle tetany in the finger flexors, which may prevent the patient from releasing the grasped current source. The duration of contact plays a direct role in the severity of injury because a longer contact period results in more electrical energy passing through the body.

Clinical Findings

The greatest current density occurs at the entrance and exit wounds, usually apparent as charred areas that are blackened and surrounded by a gray-white zone, an area of tissue necrosis in which the tissue is still intact but will die. These areas are surrounded by a red zone, in which there is a variable extent of vessel thrombosis, coagulation, and necrosis.

High-voltage, or arc, burns produce a greater thermal than electric injury. Arc burns may extend across flexor surfaces from the hand to the wrist or from the forearm to the arm. Arc burns are usually associated with a high temperature of 3000–5000°C.

It is difficult to assess precisely the extent of tissue necrosis in burn wounds at the time of initial presentation. All burn patients should be examined for fractures, particularly cervical spine fractures, because electrical burn patients were possibly thrown a distance by the current. The possibility of either compartment syndrome or concomitant peripheral nerve injury must also be considered. Patients should be admitted to an intensive care unit and monitored for cardiac arrhythmia, renal failure, sepsis, secondary hemorrhage, and neurologic complications to the brain, spinal cord, or peripheral nerves.

Treatment

Treatment for upper extremity burns consists of initially debriding clearly nonviable tissue. The decision to carry out fasciotomy and nerve decompression should be guided by examination. A second debridement is performed 48–72 hours later, for tissue in the gray-white zones. Debridement should be continued every 48–72 hours until a stable wound is achieved. The extent of necrosis often appears to increase with each successive debridement. This phenomenon reflects both an underestimation of the extent of initial injury and progressive vascular thrombosis. After all necrotic tissue is debrided, reconstruction is accomplished with either local or distant skin flaps or amputation.

CHEMICAL BURNS

The severity of chemical burns is directly proportional to the concentration and penetrability of the offending agent, the duration of skin exposure, and the mechanism of contact. Tissue destruction continues until either the chemical combines with tissue or the agent is neutralized by an applied secondary agent or washed from the skin surface. The mainstay of treatment of chemical burns of the skin is irrigation with water.

Two notable exceptions are burns resulting from hydrofluoric acid and from white phosphorous. Because hydrofluoric acid cannot be removed with water, calcium gluconate 10%, either applied to the skin as a gel or injected subcutaneously, is required to neutralize the acid. Patients with hydrofluoride burns experience severe pain seemingly out of proportion to the injury. White phosphorus burns, also refractory to water irrigation, are treated with 1% copper sulfate solution.

Iatrogenic chemical burns may occur with extravasation of chemotherapeutic agents administered intravenously. Chemotherapeutic agents are classified as vesicants, which include doxorubicin and vincristine and have a high probability of causing skin necrosis, and nonvesicants, which include cyclophosphamide. Management of both types of injury requires early surgical debridement of the region of extravasation. Secondary wound coverage may be obtained by either split-thickness skin grafting or skin flap coverage.

COLD INJURY (FROSTBITE)

Clinical Findings

Frostbite occurs as the result of cellular injury when the cell membrane is punctured by ice crystals formed in the extracellular space. With the formation of ice crystals, osmotic gradients develop, leading to cell dehydration and electrolyte disturbances. Patients may develop severe vasoconstriction as a result of increased sympathetic tone. Vessel endothelial injury may cause thrombosis. With capillary endothelial damage, leakage occurs into the extracellular space, resulting in hemoconcentration and sludging within the capillary system.

Frostbite injuries may be classified as either superficial or deep. Superficial frostbite involves only the skin and usually heals spontaneously, whereas deep frostbite damages both the skin and subcutaneous structures (Figure 10–39). As with burn injuries, the depth of the area of necrosis is difficult to determine initially.

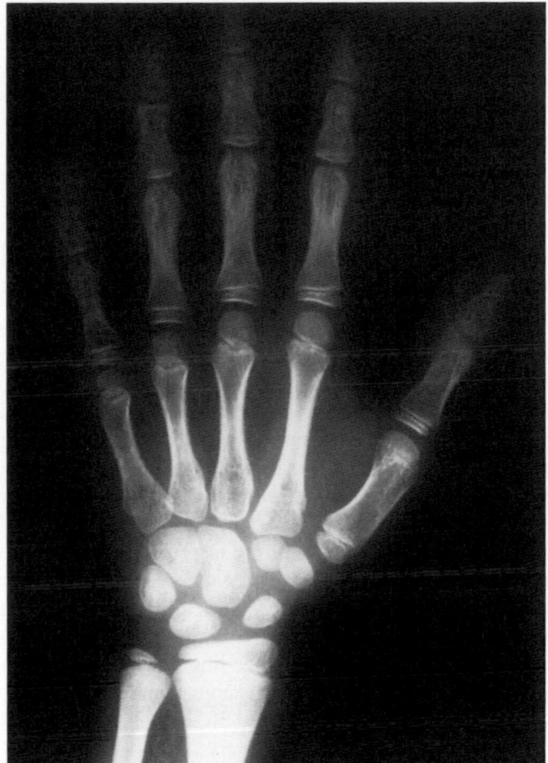

Figure 10–39. Radiograph of deformities of the fingers of the left hand in a 12-year-old girl caused by frostbite incurred at 2 years of age. Note destruction of epiphyses of middle and distal phalanges of all fingers and deformity of epiphysis of proximal phalanx of little finger. Osseous changes in right hand were similar.

Treatment

The initial treatment of frostbite consists of rewarming the part and providing pain relief. The core body temperature should be restored and the frozen extremity rapidly rewarmed in a water bath at 38–42°C. Because rapid rewarming induces considerable pain, it should be delayed until adequate analgesia can be administered. After rewarming, treatment should include elevation of the hand, local wound care, and dressing changes. Frequent whirlpool debridement and active ROM exercises should be instituted. The role of anticoagulants and sympathectomy in increasing blood flow is controversial.

Long-Term Sequelae

Long-term sequelae depend on the extent of initial injury. Adult patients may develop osteoarthritis of the interphalangeal joints. Skeletally immature patients may develop epiphyseal destruction, with digital shortening, nail dysplasia, and joint destruction. Severe injuries may produce intrinsic muscle atrophy or vasospastic syndrome secondary to increased sympathetic tone. Vasospasm may lead to severe pain, coldness, or edema of the finger; trophic changes leading to decreased nail or hair growth; or Raynaud phenomenon. In severe injuries, mummification of nonviable portions of the fingers may become apparent. Amputation or surgical debridement of these mummified parts should usually be delayed 60–90 days, unless local infection develops. This delay allows maximal reepithelialization beneath the nonviable tissue.

Woo SH, Seul JH: Optimizing the correction of severe postburn hand deformities by using aggressive contracture releases and fasciocutaneous free-tissue transfers. Plast Reconstr Surg 2001;107(1):1. [PMID: 11176593]

HIGH-PRESSURE INJECTION INJURY

Injection machinery used in industry may create pressures of 3000–10,000 psi. The amount of pressure reflects both the design of the nozzle aperture and the distance between the nozzle and the finger. Virtually all patients who sustain injuries with pressures of over 7000 psi require amputation.

Clinical Findings

Injection injuries usually puncture the palmar digital pulp, track to the flexor tendon sheath, and fill the tendon sheath with the injected material. These injuries have a poor prognosis. Injections into the palm have a somewhat better prognosis because the site of the material is unconfined by fascial planes. Prognostic factors include the time interval from injury to treatment, as well as the amount and type of material injected. Whereas paint injection may cause more necrosis of the finger, grease injection more often leads to fibrosis of the finger. The amputation rate for paint injection injuries is approximately 60%; the rate for grease injection injuries is 20%.

The examiner must be wary of an innocuous-appearing entrance wound at the time of presentation. Initial pain may be modest but increases with time as more distal swelling and early necrosis occur.

Treatment

The effectiveness of corticosteroids administered every 6 hours remains controversial in the treatment of injection injuries. Patients should be operatively treated soon after the injury occurs. Thorough debridement of all injected material is easier when the injected material is pigmented. Nonpigmented materials such as kerosene or turpentine are considerably more difficult to remove thoroughly. The hand should be splinted in the safe position. Sympathetic blocks may be helpful in managing pain. Repeat debridement should be done if there is doubt about the adequacy of the initial procedure.

Although injection injuries may appear simple, these severe injuries compromise function and result in amputation. The seriousness of these injuries should be recognized at the time of presentation.

Christodoulou L et al: Functional outcome of high-pressure injection injuries of the hand. J Trauma 2001;50:717. [PMID: 11303170]

Gutowski KA et al: High-pressure hand injuries caused by dry cleaning solvents: Case reports, review of the literature, and treatment guidelines. Plast Reconstr Surg 2003;111:174. [PMID: 12496578]

Luber KT, Rehm JP, Freeland AE: High-pressure injection injuries of the hand. Orthopedics 2005;28:129. [PMID: 15751366]

INFECTIONS OF THE HAND

Felon

A felon is an abscess of the pulp space of the distal phalanx. Vertical septa between the skin and the bone create small closed compartments within the pulp space. Infection in this region produces localized erythema, swelling, and throbbing pain.

Treatment of these infections requires incision and drainage, with release of the vertical septa to decompress the pulp space completely (Figure 10–40). A drain is placed in the wound, the hand is elevated, and intravenous antibiotics are administered.

Paronychia

Paronychia is the most common digital infection. The paronychia is the gutter along both the radial and ulnar borders of the fingernail. The eponychium is the roof of the nail over the nail lunula. Paronychial infections may be classified as acute or chronic.

A. Acute Infection

Acute infections are most often caused by *Staphylococcus aureus.* These infections begin as a localized cellulitis, with erythema around the nail. Untreated, this cellulitis may progress to an abscess at the nail margin.

Treatment of early infection includes warm soaks and oral antibiotics. Once an abscess forms, incision and drainage is required. To debride the region adequately, either an incision is made in the abscess and the abscess packed, or a portion of the lateral nail is removed and the abscess decompressed.

B. Chronic Infection

Chronic paronychial infections are most often caused by *Candida* species. These occur commonly in patients who work with their hands in water, such as bartenders or dishwashers. Patients may have repeated episodes of acute infection in addition to chronic infection.

Treatment of chronic infection may be accomplished by eponychial marsupialization, excision of a segment of the eponychia without incision of the nail roof. Simultaneous nail removal may increase the effectiveness of marsupialization.

Web Space Abscess

Web space abscesses most often occur after palmar puncture wounds. The infection spreads from the palm along the path of least resistance to the dorsal web space. Treatment requires dorsal and palmar incision, drain placement, open wound care, and appropriate antibiotic coverage.

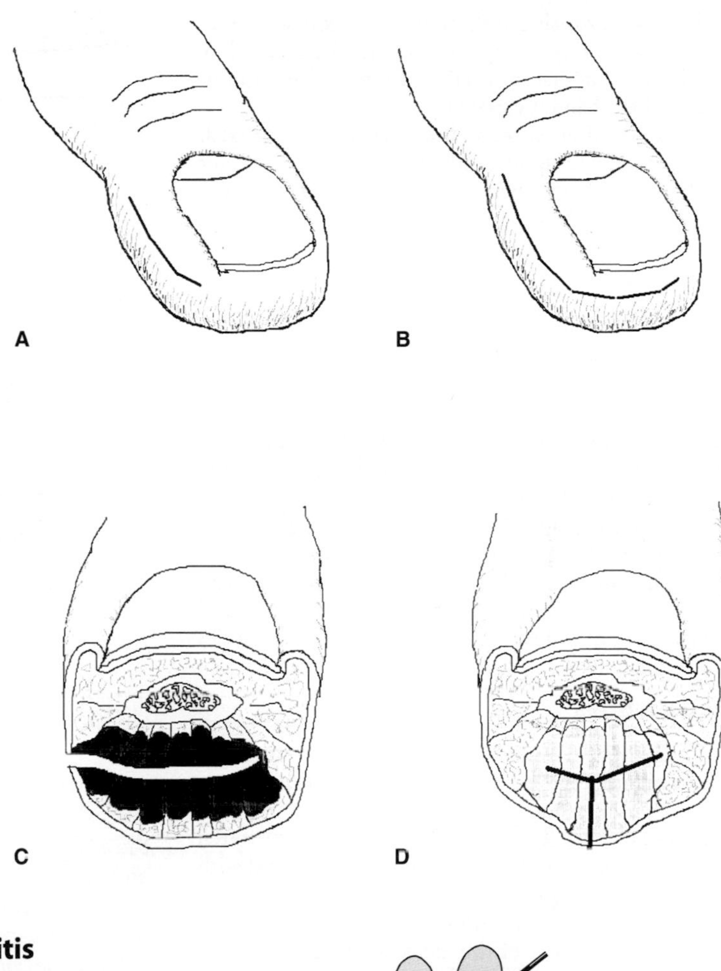

Figure 10–40. Incisions for drainage of felons. **A:** Unilateral longitudinal approach that should be used for most felons. It is generally made on the ulnar side of the finger, unless it is the little finger, to preserve sensation. **B:** The hockey stick, or J, incision should be reserved for extensive or severe abscess or felon. **C:** The incision must decompress the longitudinal septa but should not go through and through. **D:** The felon that points volarly may be decompressed through a longitudinal midline incision, which is preferable because of less risk to sensory nerves. A transverse incision may also be made, but there is risk of damage to the digital nerves. (Courtesy of HB Skinner, ©copyright 2002.)

Flexor Suppurative Tenosynovitis

Kanavel described four cardinal signs of acute suppurative tenosynovitis: (1) pain on passive digital extension; (2) flexed position of the digit; (3) symmetric swelling of the digit, which may include the palm; and (4) tenderness with palpation along the flexor tendon sheath. Acute suppurative tenosynovitis of the flexor pollicis longus sheath may extend into the thenar space. Likewise, infections in the flexor sheath of the little finger may extend into the ulnar bursa. In some patients, coalescence between the radial and ulnar bursas may allow infection to track in a horseshoe pattern, extending from the thumb to the little finger.

Treatment of acute suppurative tenosynovitis requires incision, irrigation, and drainage. Although an extensive midlateral incision may be used, limited incisions are preferred. Short incisions over the proximal (metacarpophalangeal joint region) and distal (distal interphalangeal region) margins of the flexor tendon sheath allow thorough sheath irrigation (Figure 10–41). The sheath is opened distally and a small tube (16-gauge catheter or number 8 pediatric feeding tube) is inserted. A drain is

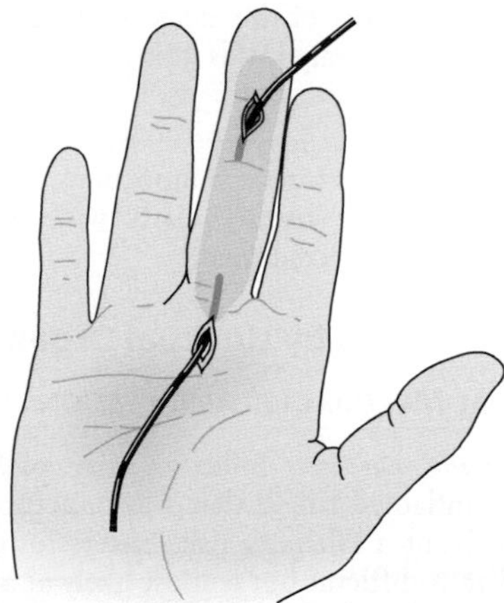

Figure 10–41. Drainage and closed irrigation for flexor sheath infection. The antibiotic solution drips in through the distal catheter and drains out through the proximal one. (Reproduced, with permission, from Way LW, ed: *Current Surgical Diagnosis and Treatment,* 10th ed. Appleton & Lange, 1994.)

placed in the flexor sheath through the proximal wound. Irrigation of the finger is performed with 5 mL of saline injected every 2 hours. Intravenous antibiotics are administered, and the hand is elevated.

Two days after surgery the dressing is changed. Swelling should be significantly decreased. The catheter is removed, and the patient is encouraged to begin active ROM exercises.

Bite Injuries

Although bite wounds may initially appear harmless, a bite may inoculate deep tissues with virulent organisms.

A. Cat and Dog Bites

Because the small puncture wounds of cat bites are more likely to be disregarded than the large tearing wounds of dog bites, late sequelae are more common after cat bites. Cat and dog bites frequently harbor *Pasteurella multocida,* an organism best treated with ampicillin, penicillin, or a first-generation cephalosporin. Acute animal bites may be treated with incision and drainage and an initial course of intravenous antibiotics in the emergency room followed by oral antibiotics.

B. Human Bites

Most human bite wounds result from a fist striking a tooth, which readily penetrates the skin, subcutaneous tissue, extensor tendon, and capsule of the metacarpophalangeal joint (Figure 10–42). Human bites often contain *Eikenella corrodens,* an organism best treated with penicillin or ampicillin. Human bite wounds should be excised and drained, and intravenous antibiotic therapy instituted. Arthrotomy of the metacarpophalangeal joint and irrigation is necessary if this injury is suspected.

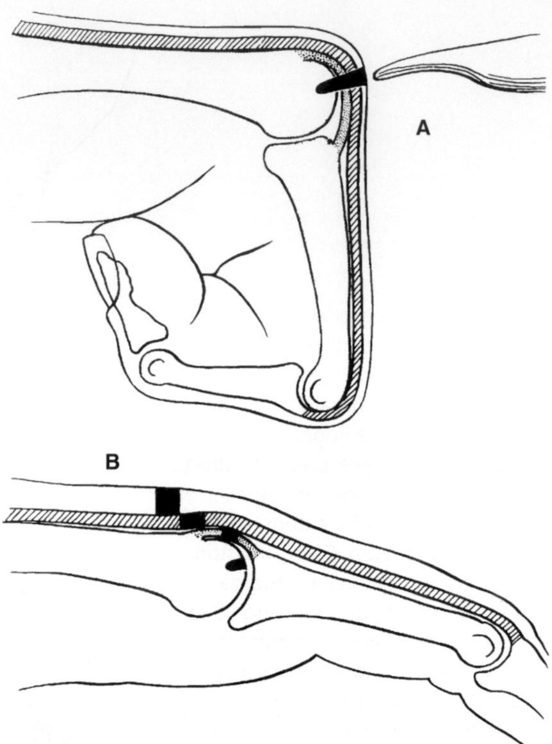

Figure 10–42. Human bite wound of metacarpophalangeal joint. **A:** The tooth pierces the clenched fist of the attacker, penetrating skin, tendon, joint capsule, and metacarpal head. **B:** When the finger is extended by swelling and at surgery, the four puncture wounds do not correspond. (Reproduced, with permission, from Lister G: *The Hand: Diagnosis and Indications,* 3rd ed. Churchill Livingstone, 1993.)

C. Spider Bites

Although most spider bites are innocuous, the bite of a brown recluse spider requires early wide excision to control the locally injected toxin.

Infection Caused by Unusual Organisms

A. Atypical Mycobacterial Infection

Mycobacterium marinum infection may present as a chronically inflamed finger that was punctured by the spine or a fin of a saltwater fish. Successful culture of the organism is difficult but is most likely at a temperature of 30–32°C. Antitubercular drug therapy is effective in treating and eradicating these infections.

B. Gram-Negative Infection

Because of the risk of a gram-negative infection following mutilating farm injuries or injuries with possible fecal contamination, these patients should be treated with broad-spectrum antibiotics.

C. Anaerobic Infection

When *Clostridium perfringens* infection occurs after hand injury, immediate wide fasciotomy and intravenous penicillin should be instituted. Hyperbaric oxygen therapy may be helpful. If infection cannot be adequately controlled, amputation may be necessary to avoid death.

The possibility of *Clostridium tetani* contamination must be remembered with any puncture wound. Initial evaluation of all patients with penetrating wounds must include questioning about tetanus inoculation. If inoculation is not up to date, antitoxin should be administered.

D. Gonorrhea

A patient who presents with an isolated septic joint or tenosynovitis without a history of puncture wound may have a hematogenous gonorrheal infection. Treatment consists of culturing the involved organism on the appropriate media and treatment with penicillin or tetracycline.

E. Necrotizing Fasciitis

The causative agent in necrotizing fasciitis is most commonly hemolytic *Staphylococcus*. Treatment consists of wide surgical debridement to the fascia and appropriate antibiotics.

F. Herpetic Whitlow

Herpes simplex infections may involve the fingertips. They are most common in medical or dental personnel who care for the oral tracheal area and are also seen in small children. It may be difficult to distinguish herpetic lesions from acute bacterial infections of the fingers. Close examination reveals the presence of groups (crops) of vesicles, with surrounding erythema. Aspiration of a vesicle yields clear fluid. Serial viral titers confirm the diagnosis. Unlike bacterial infections, herpetic whitlow should not be incised but simply treated with splinting and elevation.

Connor RW, Kimbrough RC, Dabezies MJ: Hand Infections in patients with diabetes. Orthopedics 2001;24:1057. [PMID: 11727802]

Huish SB et al: Pyoderma gangrenosum of the hand: A case series and review of the literature. J Hand Surg 2001;26A:679. [PMID: 11466644.]

Karanas YL, Bogdan MA, Chang J: Community acquired methicillin-resistant *Staphylococcus aureus* hand infections: Case reports and clinical implications. J Hand Surg Am 2000;25: 760. [PMID: 1093220]

Perron AD, Miller MD, Brady WJ: Orthopedic pitfalls in the ED: Fight bites. Am J Emerg Med 2002;20:114. [PMID: 11880877]

ARTHRITIS OF THE HAND

OSTEOARTHRITIS

Osteoarthritis is a slowly progressive polyarticular disorder of unknown cause, predominantly affecting the hands and large weight-bearing joints. Clinically, osteoarthritis is characterized by pain, deformity, and limitation of motion. Focal erosions, articular cartilage space loss, subchondral sclerosis, cyst formation, and peripheral joint osteophytes are evident on radiographic examination.

Epidemiologic Factors

The disease occurs commonly in older individuals, with approximately 80–90% of adults older than 75 years showing radiographic evidence of osteoarthritis. The strongest predictors of developing osteoarthritis of the hand are female gender, increasing age, and positive family history.

The most frequently involved joints in the hand are the distal interphalangeal joints, carpometacarpal joint of the thumb (Figure 10–43), and proximal interphalangeal joints. The bony enlargements commonly seen in the osteoarthritic distal interphalangeal joint are referred to as Heberden nodes, whereas osteoarthritic enlargements at the proximal interphalangeal joint are known as Bouchard nodes.

Secondary osteoarthritis may develop in the hand as the result of trauma, avascular necrosis, prior inflammatory arthritis, or metabolic disorders.

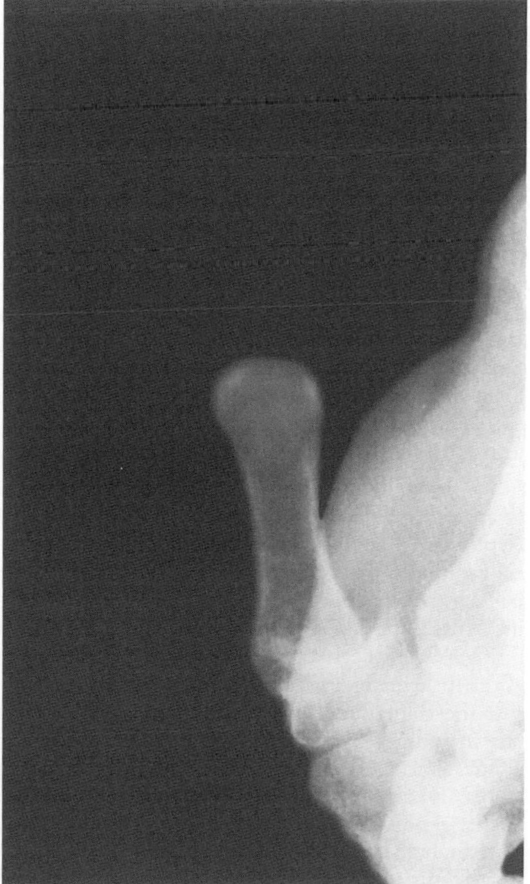

Figure 10–43. Osteoarthritis of the carpometacarpal joint of the thumb.

Clinical Findings

Patients with osteoarthritis of the hand often complain of activity-induced or work-related pain. Most patients experience periods of exacerbation and remission. Functional limitations result from pain, weakness, loss of motion, and deformity. Tenderness and enlargement of the distal and proximal interphalangeal joints are noted on examination. Axial compression of the thumb trapeziometacarpal with a circumduction motion (grind test) reproduces pain. As the disease progresses, radial subluxation of the thumb metacarpal on the trapezium may develop, leading to adduction deformity of the metacarpal.

Treatment

Nonoperative treatment includes oral nonsteroidal anti-inflammatory medication (NSAIDs), long-acting intraarticular steroid injection, and splint immobilization.

The primary indication for surgery is pain unresponsive to oral medication and splinting. Distal interphalangeal joint arthrodesis relieves pain, corrects deformity, and resolves joint instability. Because the severely arthritic distal interphalangeal joint is often stiff, the additional loss of motion occasioned by arthrodesis is usually well tolerated. The distal interphalangeal joint is fused in 10–15 degrees of flexion, a position in which the fingernail is parallel with the axis of the middle phalanx.

At the proximal interphalangeal joint, pain is the primary indication for surgery. Implant arthroplasty may be helpful in relieving pain and retaining motion in the ring and little fingers. The motion attained from implant arthroplasty is less in the proximal interphalangeal joints than in the metacarpophalangeal joints. Implant arthroplasty is usually avoided in the index- or middle-finger proximal interphalangeal joint because of residual instability to lateral or key pinch.

Arthrodesis effectively relieves pain at the proximal interphalangeal joint and provides pinch stability. The ideal position of arthrodesis varies from the radial to the ulnar digits. The index-finger proximal interphalangeal joint is usually fused at 40 degrees of flexion, the middle finger at 45 degrees, the ring finger at 50 degrees, and the little finger at 55 degrees.

At the trapeziometacarpal joint, conservative treatment includes a hand-based thumb spica splint with the interphalangeal joint left free, cortisone injections, and NSAIDs. Many patients with advanced degenerative changes on radiograph obtain good pain relief with conservative therapy.

The primary indication for surgery is persistent pain. Trapezium resection arthroplasty relieves pain at the trapeziometacarpal joint and allows retention of full metacarpal base motion. Either the distal half of the trapezium or the entire trapezium may be resected. A tendon interposition is created using either the flexor carpi radialis or a slip of the abductor pollicis longus. The tendon may be threaded through a drill hole in the articular surface of the thumb metacarpal to suspend the thumb. The remaining tendon is rolled into a so-called anchovy and placed in the space of the excised trapezium. This reconstruction prevents impingement of the metacarpal on the scaphoid. After surgery, the thumb is immobilized in a cast or splint for 6 weeks.

Arthrodesis of the thumb carpometacarpal joint is an alternative to trapeziectomy. With the joint fused, patients are unable to lay their hand flat on a table. However, pain relief is excellent, and it may be the procedure of choice for a young laborer.

RHEUMATOID ARTHRITIS

RA is a chronic inflammatory disease of unknown cause. The combined effect of tenosynovitis and synovitis on joints and periarticular tissues results in progressive joint destruction and deformity. RA affects 0.3–1.5% of the population. Women are two to three times more commonly affected than men.

Clinical Findings

Evaluation of the hand affected by RA requires care. The goal is to determine which of the patient's many problems—pain, weakness, or mechanical dysfunction—is most problematic. Evaluation detects tendon rupture, adherence, or triggering as well as nerve compression symptoms. The most common nerve compression syndromes involve compression of the median nerve at the wrist and compression of the radial nerve at the elbow. The appearance of rheumatoid nodules and ulnar drift deformity at the metacarpophalangeal joint may be disturbing aesthetically. Rheumatoid nodules, occurring in 20–25% of patients with RA, are not treated unless associated with erosion, pain, or infection.

Treatment

The shoulder, elbow, forearm, wrist, and hand should be examined individually. The goal of surgical reconstruction is restoration of a functional upper extremity, not just a functional hand. Indications for surgical intervention include relieving pain, slowing the progression of disease, improving function, and improving appearance.

Surgical treatment may be classified as either preventive or corrective. Preventive options include tenosynovectomy and synovectomy. Corrective procedures include tendon transfers, nerve decompression, soft-tissue reconstruction, and arthrodesis.

Synovectomy is considered in patients who have pauciarticular persistent synovitis while under good medical control. Contraindications to synovectomy include rapidly progressive disease, multiple joint involvement, and underlying joint destruction.

A. Elbow Reconstruction

Synovitis of the elbow joint may cause pain, joint destruction, and radial nerve compression. Nodules or bursas are common over the olecranon. Surgical treatment of the rheumatoid elbow includes radial head excision and synovectomy. As the disease progresses, consideration may be given to total elbow arthroplasty.

B. Wrist Reconstruction

RA frequently involves the wrist and occurs in a predictable pattern. On the radial side of the wrist, the radioscaphocapitate and the radiolunototriquetral ligaments are attenuated, permitting rotatory displacement of the scaphoid. Scapholunate dissociation is followed by radiocarpal collapse.

On the ulnar side of the wrist, the ulnar carpal ligaments become attenuated, allowing the carpus to drift radially as the carpus translates ulnarward. Attenuation of the distal radioulnar joint allows the head of the ulna to displace dorsally, producing caput-ulnae syndrome. The extensor carpi ulnaris tendon displaces volarly. These changes lead to supination of the carpus on the radius, ulnar translocation of the carpus, and a concomitant radialward displacement of the metacarpals (Figure 10–44). The carpus may also dislocate volarly beneath the radius.

Surgical treatment consists of extensor tenosynovectomy, with transposition of the dorsal retinaculum over the wrist joint to reinforce the capsule, and wrist synovectomy. The extensor carpi ulnaris tendon can be relocated from a volar to a dorsal position.

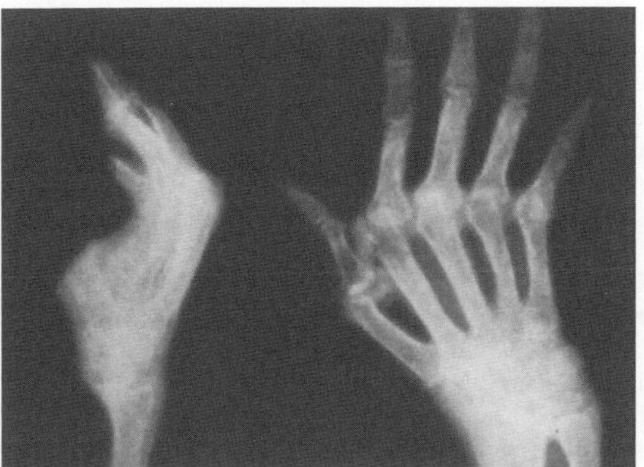

Figure 10–44. Radialward displacement of the metacarpals in rheumatoid arthritis.

If pain is present over the distal ulna or if rupture of the little- or ring-finger extensor tendon results from a sharp prominence of the distal ulna, then resection of the distal ulna is performed. Fusion of the rheumatoid wrist provides stability and may increase function. Either a total wrist arthrodesis or a radiolunate arthrodesis may be elected, depending on the extent of midcarpal joint involvement.

C. Hand Reconstruction

Triggering of the digits is a common problem caused by flexor tenosynovitis. The A1 pulley should not be incised in the treatment of rheumatoid trigger digits. Loss of the A1 pulley increases the tendency of the fingers to drift ulnarward. Instead, tenosynovectomy and excision of the ulnar slip of the sublimis tendon should be considered.

If flexor tendon rupture occurs, treatment may include tendon transfer, bridge grafting, or joint fusion. The flexor tendon that most commonly ruptures is the flexor pollicis longus because it rubs over an osteophyte on the volar aspect of the scaphotrapezial joint (Mannerfelt lesion). Extensor tendon ruptures are caused by attrition of the common extensor tendon of the ring and little fingers over the distal ulna (Vaughn-Johnson syndrome).

Treatment of the arthritic hand depends on the joints involved. The distal interphalangeal joint is usually best treated by arthrodesis. At the proximal interphalangeal joint, synovectomy may be performed if synovitis is isolated to the proximal interphalangeal joint without multiple joint involvement. Alternatives for the more involved joint are arthroplasty or arthrodesis.

At the metacarpophalangeal joint, inflammation of the synovium may cause the extensor mechanism to sublux ulnarly because of attenuation of the radial sagittal band. The mechanism may be relocated to improve function of the joint. For isolated joints without significant destruction, synovectomy may be performed. With more severe joint destruction, resection implant arthroplasty is required (Figure 10–45). Subluxation and ulnar drift alone are not absolute indications for arthroplasty if satisfactory function of the hand remains. Arthroplasty does not increase the ROM of the metaphalangeal joints, but it changes its arc. Because most patients have severe flexion and ulnar deviation of the joints, arthroplasty provides a more functional ROM, especially for grasping large objects. Because the implants fracture with extensive use, silicone arthroplasty is indicated only in the low-demand hand and is therefore better suited to rheumatoid than osteoarthritic patients.

1. Boutonnière deformity—In addition to arthritis, various finger deformities occur related to soft-tissue damage. At the proximal interphalangeal joints, the most common is boutonnière deformity. Because of proximal interphalangeal joint synovitis, the central slip is either elongated or ruptured, which allows the proximal interphalangeal joint to flex and the lateral bands to

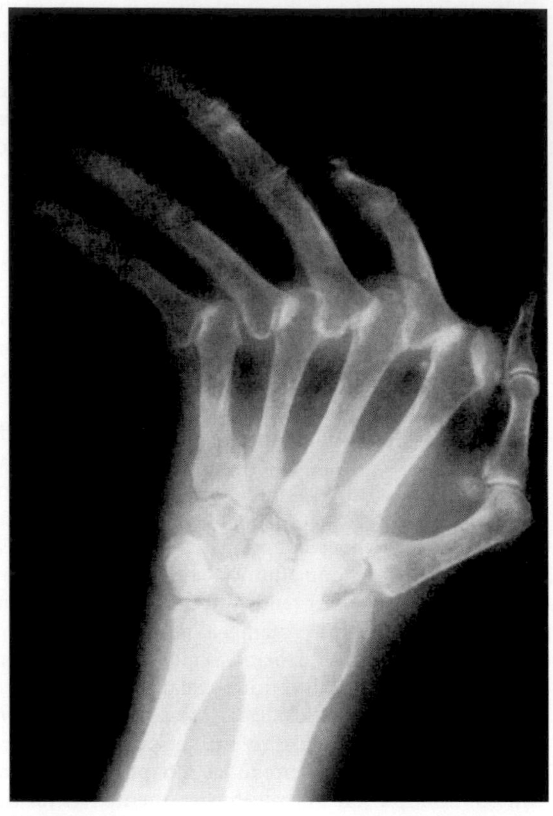

A

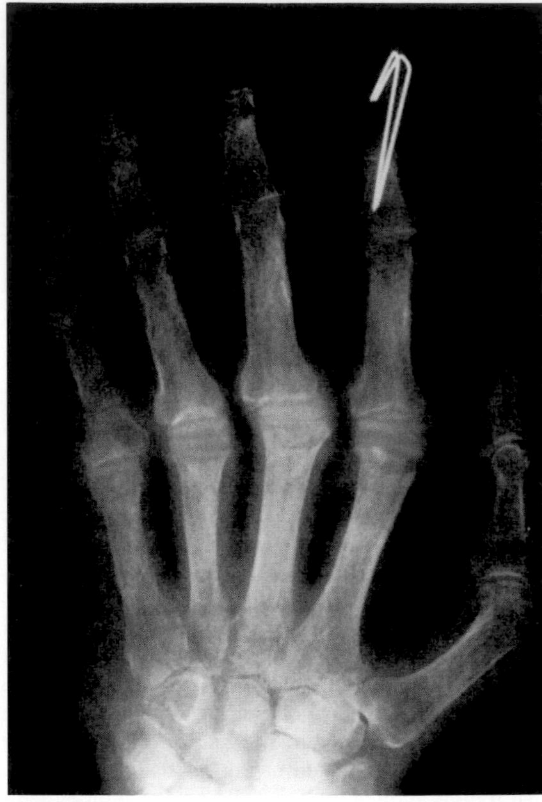

B

Figure 10–45. **A:** Preoperative view of metacarpophalangeal joint in rheumatoid arthritis. **B:** Following resection arthroplasty.

sublux volarly. As the lateral bands migrate below the proximal interphalangeal joint axis, they become active proximal interphalangeal flexors rather than extensors. In addition to increasing the proximal interphalangeal joint deformity, the relative shortening of the extensor mechanism leads to distal interphalangeal joint hyperextension. Treatment of mild boutonnière deformities, which are passively correctable, consists of synovectomy and splinting. Lateral band reconstruction may be considered to relocate the bands dorsal to the axis of rotation. Alternatively, tenotomy of the terminal slip may be done to allow relaxation of the extensor mechanism and prevent hyperextension of the distal interphalangeal joint. Once moderate deformity of the proximal interphalangeal joint occurs (30- to 40-degree flexion deformity, with a flexible joint and preservation of the joint space), consideration may be given to reconstruction of the central slip as well as lateral band reconstruction and terminal tendon tenotomy. In the final stage of boutonnière deformity, the joint deformity becomes fixed, and the best form of treatment is arthroplasty or fusion.

2. Swan-neck deformity—Swan-neck deformities consist of hyperextension at the proximal interphalangeal joint and flexion at the distal interphalangeal joint. The mechanism of swan-neck deformity is terminal tendon rupture or attenuation, with secondary hyperextension of the proximal interphalangeal joint resulting from overpulling of the central slip or proximal interphalangeal joint hyperextension caused by laxity of the volar plate, rupture of the flexor digitorum superficialis, or intrinsic tightness. The most common of these mechanisms is intrinsic tightness secondary to metacarpophalangeal joint synovitis.

Swan-neck deformities are divided into four stages. In stage 1, the joints are supple in all positions. Treatment consists of splinting, distal interphalangeal joint fusion, or soft-tissue reconstruction to limit proximal interphalangeal joint hyperextension. In stage 2, proximal interphalangeal flexion is limited because of intrinsic tightness. Intrinsic release with or without reconstruction of the metacarpophalangeal joint may be of benefit. In stage 3, proximal interphalangeal joint motion is limited in all positions, yet the joint is still preserved. Mobilization of the lateral bands may help relieve this deformity. Finally, in stage 4, the proximal interphalangeal joint is arthritic. Either proximal interphalangeal arthrodesis or arthroplasty should be considered for stage 4 joint destruction.

3. Synovitic metacarpophalangeal joint deformity— The metacarpophalangeal joints subluxes volarly and ulnarly in RA. This deformity results from synovial invasion of the collateral ligaments with secondary laxity, volar and ulnar forces that are normally present on the joint, augmentation of these forces by radial deviation of the wrist, attenuation of the radial sagittal band (allowing ulnar subluxation of the extensor tendon), and contracture of the intrinsic muscles. Treatment of the synovitic metacarpophalangeal joint consists of medical management and splinting. When the joint space is preserved, surgical synovectomy may provide symptomatic relief. Once moderate joint destruction or volar subluxation and ulnar deviation occurs, the decision about surgery is based on the function of the hand. When the patient is still able to use the hand for activities of daily living, splinting and other assistive aids are provided. Once loss of function is noted, metacarpophalangeal arthroplasty is considered. In performing metacarpophalangeal arthroplasty, the wrist deformity should first be corrected, and all soft-tissue releases required to relieve the subluxing forces should be performed. The radial collateral ligament of the index finger should be reconstructed, and the extensor tendon should be relocated. Postoperatively, extensive splinting and therapy are required to hold the hand in proper position. Therapy utilizes an outrigger splint holding the wrist in dorsiflexion and the metaphalangeal joints in full extension and neutral radial-ulnar alignment. The splint is worn full time for 6 weeks and part time for 3 months. The patient wears a resting pan splint at night for 1 year.

D. Thumb Reconstruction

Three patterns of rheumatoid thumb deformities are defined. In type 1 deformity, the metacarpophalangeal joint is flexed while the interphalangeal joint is hyperextended and the thumb metacarpal is secondarily abducted. In type 2 and 3 deformities, carpometacarpal subluxation leads to metacarpal adduction. In type 2 deformities, interphalangeal joint hyperextension develops with metacarpophalangeal flexion, and in type 3 deformities, the metacarpophalangeal joint is hyperextended and the interphalangeal joint is flexed. Type 2 deformities are unusual. Type 1 deformities are usually initiated by synovitis of the metacarpophalangeal joint, leading to attenuation of the extensor pollicis brevis tendon, intrinsic muscle tightness, and ulnar and volar displacement of the extensor pollicis longus.

Treatment is based on the degree of progression. In type 1 deformities, if the metacarpophalangeal and interphalangeal joints are passively correctable, synovectomy and extensor reconstruction may be performed. If the metacarpophalangeal joint flexion deformity is fixed, arthrodesis or arthroplasty of the joint is considered. When fixed metacarpophalangeal flexion and interphalangeal extension deformities are present simultaneously, the interphalangeal joint is fused and the metacarpophalangeal joint is replaced with an arthroplasty or also undergoes arthrodesis.

Type 3 deformities are analogous to swan-neck deformities of the fingers. The carpometacarpal joint disease allows dorsal and radial subluxation of the joint, with secondary adduction contraction of the metacarpal and hyperextension of the metacarpophalangeal joint. Treatment with minimal metacarpophalangeal deformity (stage 1) or passively correctable metacarpophalangeal deformity (stage 2) consists of splinting and carpometacarpal arthroplasty or fusion. Once the metacarpophalangeal deformity becomes fixed (stage 3), first web release and carpometacarpal arthroplasty are required.

E. Surgical Priorities

When multilevel deformity is present, consideration should be given to combined procedures. If wrist and metacarpophalangeal deformities are both present, the wrist should be fused prior to or simultaneously with metacarpophalangeal joint reconstruction. When both metacarpophalangeal and proximal interphalangeal joint deformities are present, motion-preserving procedures such as arthroplasty should be carried out at the metacarpophalangeal joint. Treatment of concomitant proximal interphalangeal joint involvement depends on the stage of deformity. Mild to moderate proximal interphalangeal joint deformities can either be ignored or treated by closed manipulation and pin fixation. With severe deformity, arthrodesis of the proximal interphalangeal joint should be performed.

In all cases, attempts should be made to perform multiple procedures under a single anesthetic. These patients often require numerous operations for multiple joints of the upper and lower extremities, and surgical and rehabilitation time must be used judiciously.

Other Inflammatory Arthritides

Other inflammatory conditions related to RA may affect the hand, producing joint destruction and deformity.

A. Juvenile Rheumatoid Arthritis

In juvenile rheumatoid arthritis (JRA), early epiphyseal closure occurs as a result of synovitis and increased periarticular blood flow. Narrowing of phalangeal and metacarpal medullary canals makes implant arthroplasty difficult. The metacarpophalangeal joints may deviate radially rather than ulnarly.

B. Arthritis Mutilans

In arthritis mutilans, axial shortening because of marked bone loss occurs while the soft-tissue envelope is preserved. Early joint fusion is required to avoid progressive bone loss.

C. Systemic Lupus Erythematosus

Systemic lupus erythematosus (SLE) affects periarticular soft tissue, resulting in joint laxity with secondary dysfunction. Synovitis is minimal in lupus, and therefore the articular cartilage is preserved. Soft-tissue reconstruction is ineffective, and joint fusions are preferable to restore stability and function. The exception to this is the metacarpophalangeal joints, where implant arthroplasty may be appropriate, even though normal articular cartilage is sacrificed.

D. Psoriatic Arthritis

Psoriatic arthritis presents deformities similar to that of RA. The hand has a marked tendency to become stiff. In psoriatic arthritis, the metacarpophalangeal joints become stiff in extension, whereas in RA, these joints tend to become stiff in flexion.

Davis TR, Brady O, Dias JJ: Excision of the trapezium for osteoarthritis of the trapeziometacarpal joint: A study of the benefit of ligament reconstruction or tendon interposition. J Hand Surg Am 2004;29:1069. [PMID: 15576217]

Day CS et al: Basal joint osteoarthritis of the thumb: A prospective trial of steroid injection and splinting J Hand Surg Am 2004;29:247. [PMID: 15043897]

Fulton DB, Stern PJ: Trapeziometacarpal arthrodesis in primary osteoarthritis: A minimum two-year follow-up study. J Hand Surg Am 2001;26:109. [PMID: 11172376.]

Jain A et al: Influence of steroids and methotrexate on wound complications after elective rheumatoid hand and wrist surgery. J Hand Surg Am 2002;27:449. [PMID: 12015719]

HAND TUMORS

Nearly all mass lesions in the hand or wrist are benign conditions. Foreign body granulomas, epidermoid inclusion cysts, and neuromas are usually related to prior trauma. Ganglions and fibroxanthomas arise adjacent to joints or tendon sheaths.

Ganglion

Ganglions are the most common soft-tissue tumors of the hand and wrist. They are cystic structures filled with a mucinous fluid but without a synovial or epithelial lining. In most cases, a stalk can be identified communicating between the cyst and an adjacent joint or tendon sheath. The most common locations for ganglions are the wrist, digital flexor sheath, and distal interphalangeal joint (Figure 10–46).

A. Dorsal Wrist Ganglion

Dorsal wrist ganglions arise from the dorsal capsule of the scapholunate joint. Small firm dorsal ganglions may be barely palpable but highly symptomatic, whereas large ganglions are often soft and only mildly symptomatic. Aspiration and steroid injection may provide transient symptomatic relief, but recurrence is frequent. Symptomatic lesions can be surgically excised, with expectation of cure if care is taken to excise the stalk of the lesion with a capsular base from the lesion's origin. Because these lesions arise from the dorsal portion of the scapholunate ligament, care must be taken to preserve the ligament's integrity to avoid an iatrogenic scapholunate dissociation.

B. Palmar Wrist Ganglion

Palmar wrist ganglions present as swellings on the palmar radial aspect of the wrist, adjacent to the radial artery. These lesions arise from either the palmar radios-

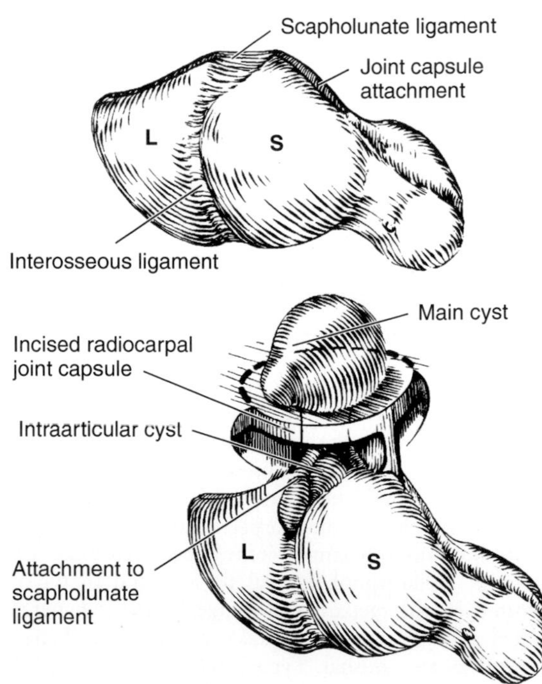

Figure 10–46. **The ganglion and scapholunate attachments are isolated from the remaining uninvolved joint capsule (not shown).** (Reproduced, with permission, from Green DP, ed: *Operative Hand Surgery*, 2nd ed. Churchill Livingstone, 1988.)

caphoid or palmar scaphotrapezial joint. Surgical resection of the palmar radial ganglion requires mobilization and protection of the adjacent radial artery.

C. Flexor Sheath Ganglion

Flexor sheath ganglions present as firm mass lesions over the palmar aspect of the flexor sheath. The mass is usually between 3 and 8 mm in diameter and often so firm that it is presumed to be a bone exostosis. Treatment of symptomatic lesions is accomplished with aspiration or excision.

D. Mucous Cyst

Mucous cysts are ganglions arising from the distal interphalangeal joint. The neck of the ganglion arises either the radial or ulnar side of the extensor terminal tendon. Surgical excision requires debridement of the joint osteophyte. If the skin is thinned, a local rotation flap is required for soft-tissue coverage after excision.

E. Fibroxanthoma

Fibroxanthomas are also known as giant cell tumors of tendon sheath or tendon sheath xanthomas. These slowly enlarging, firm lesions are usually painless, often arising from an interphalangeal joint. They lesion are usually fixed to deep tissues, more often on the palmar aspect of the hand or finger. Surgical resection requires delineation of adjacent nerves that may be displaced, compressed, or encircled by a fibroxanthoma.

F. Epidermoid Inclusion Cyst

Epidermoid inclusion cysts are usually the result of previous trauma, such as a puncture wound, stab wound, or laceration. Epidermal cells become embedded in the subcutaneous tissue, gradually into an enlarging pearlike mass. Eventually, the mass becomes noticeable, particularly when it is located over the palmar aspect of the pulp. Surgical treatment is excision of the mass without rupture.

G. Foreign Bodies

Foreign bodies may act as a nidus, inciting the development of a surrounding granuloma. This situation may be associated with a local inflammatory reaction or frank infection. Treatment consists of excision.

H. Neuromas

Neuromas, the bulbous enlargement of the distal end of a severed nerve, are a normal response to nerve transection. Neuromas are inevitable in all amputations of the hand. If the neuroma enlargement of the distal end of the proximal segment of the transected nerve is in an area of palmar pulp contact, the lesion may be highly symptomatic. Treatment alternatives include neuroma revision or transposition of the neuroma to a location away from contact stress.

CONGENITAL DIFFERENCES

Congenital hand differences occur in approximately 1 in 1500 live births. The term *differences* is favored over the traditional terms *abnormality, anomaly,* or *malformation.* Many congenital hand differences are part of a well-delineated association or syndrome. The abnormality may suggest that other regions of the body or organ systems be evaluated. When an infant is seen with bilateral total absence of the radius and normal or very mildly hypoplastic thumbs, the possibility of thrombocytopenia with absent radius (TAR) syndrome should be considered and a platelet count obtained. Radial absence may also be associated with the VATER association, children with abnormalities that may include *v*ertebral, *a*nal, *t*racheal, *e*sophageal, and *r*enal defects.

A number of frequently encountered conditions such as cleft hand are inherited as autosomal-dominant traits. The expertise of an experienced geneticist is invaluable in providing counsel to families considering additional children and to patients wishing to know the likelihood that their offspring would be affected by the disorder.

The two most commonly encountered conditions are syndactyly and polydactyly. In white populations, syndactyly is more common, and in African American populations, polydactyly is the most commonly encountered congenital hand anomaly.

Syndactyly

Syndactyly, the webbing together of digits, is simple if soft tissue alone is involved and complex if bone or nails are joined (Figure 10–47). Surgical release of syndactyly requires the use of local flaps to create a floor for the interdigital web space and to partially surface the adjacent sides of the separated digits. Residual defects along

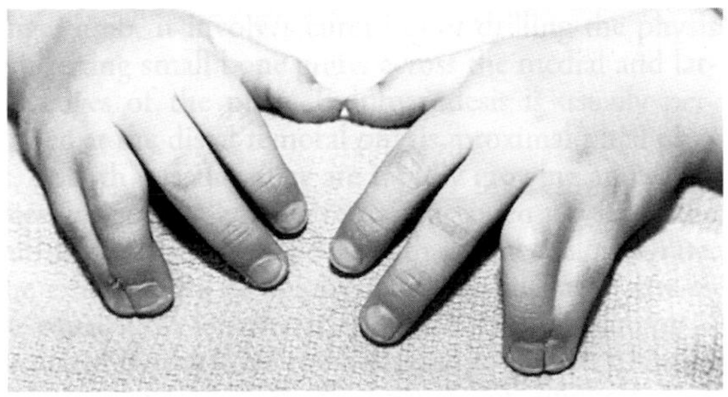

Figure 10–47. Bilateral complex syndactyly of the ring and little fingers.

Table 11–1. Causes of limb-length inequality.

Infectious causes
Osteomyelitis
Septic arthritis
Neoplastic causes
Arteriovenous malformations
Hemangioma
Neuromuscular causes
Cerebral palsy
Isolated limb paralysis
Poliomyelitis
Traumatic causes
Malunion of long bones
Physeal injury
Other causes
Avascular necrosis of femoral head (and physis)
Congenital amputations
Legg-Calvé-Perthes disease

data be collected on this growth for several years (ie, scanograms for leg-length measurement, skeletal age).

2. Femoral shortening—If a child reaches the age when bone growth is insufficient to make epiphysiodesis practical, the long leg may be shortened at skeletal maturity by femoral shortening. This may be performed as an open procedure by removing a segment of femur and fixing the bone with a plate and screws. It may also be done as a closed procedure, using an intramedullary femoral rod introduced through a buttock incision for fixation. A cylindrical segment of femur is cut out of the bone using intramedullary saws, and the bone is pushed aside to allow the femur to shorten over the rod. The excised bone segment eventually resorbs.

3. Other techniques—Leg-length inequalities projected to be 6 cm or more generally do not respond well to the previously described treatments, which in these cases may lead to unacceptably short stature or limb segments. Although some discrepancies are so severe that amputation of the foot and prosthetic fitting are required, techniques of bone lengthening are successful in treating these children (see Chapter 1).

Anderson M et al: Growth and predictions of growth in the lower extremities. J Bone Joint Surg Am 1963;45:1.

Birch JG, Samchukov ML: Use of the Ilizarov method to correct lower limb deformities in children and adolescents. J Am Acad Orthop Surg 2004:12:144. [PMID: 15161167]

Little DG et al: A simple calculation for the timing of epiphysiodesis. J Pediatr Orthop 1996;16:173.

Moseley CF: Assessment and prediction in leg-length discrepancy. Instr Course Lect 1989;38:325.

Surdam JW, Morris CD, DeWeese JD et al: Leg length inequality and epiphysiodesis: Review of 96 cases. J Pediatr Orthop 2003; 23:381. [PMID: 12724605]

2. Dwarfism & Other Disorders of Growth

Orthopedic disorders (achondroplasia, multiple epiphyseal dysplasia) or other syndromes (Down syndrome, Marfan syndrome) often accompany dwarfism. The classification of skeletal syndromes and dysplasias is undergoing rapid change as knowledge is gained using molecular, biologic, and genetic techniques. A detailed review is outside the scope of this text; Table 11–2 lists

Table 11–2. Orthopedic involvement in selected syndromes and dwarfing conditions.

Achondroplasia
Short limbs; genu varum; exaggerated lumbar lordosis; spinal stenosis; ligamentous laxity
Apert syndrome
Foot deformities; hand and foot polydactyly
Arthrogyposis
Severe joint stiffness, contractures, and dislocations; resistant clubfoot
Cleidocranial dysplasia
Absent clavicles; coxa vara
Diastrophic dysplasia
Severe clubfoot; joint dislocations; joint stiffness; cervical kyphosis; scoliosis
Down syndrome
Cervical (C1–C2) instability; hip dislocation; ankle valgus; ligamentous laxity
Enchondromatosis
Asymmetric multiple enchondromas in long bones; limb-length inequality; angulation of long bones
Fibrous dysplasia
Multiple fibrous lesions in bone; limb bowing or shortening; occasional endocrine disorders
Larsen syndrome
Hip, knee, and radial head dislocations; severe cervical kyphosis and instability; scoliosis
Marfan syndrome
Scoliosis
Metaphyseal chondrodysplasia
Moderate dwarfing; genu varum; ligamentous laxity; cervical instability
Multiple epiphyseal dysplasia
Mild dwarfism; joint surface deformities with premature osteoarthritis; angular limb deformities
Multiple hereditary exostoses
Mild dwarfing; osteochondroma (external enlargements) at all long bone ends
Osteogenesis imperfecta
Bone fragility and multiple fractures; bowing of bones; scoliosis; mild to moderate dwarfing
Spondyloepiphyseal dysplasia
Severe dwarfing; coxa vara; genu valgum; scoliosis; odontoid hypoplasia, instability, and deformity

some of these conditions and the major orthopedic problems associated with them.

INFECTIOUS PROCESSES

1. Hematogenous Osteomyelitis

Osteomyelitis, an infection of bone tissue, usually occurs in the marrow cavity but sometimes affects the cortex as well. In children, it is most commonly the result of hematogenous spread, frequently following an upper respiratory infection or partially treated distant infection. Direct inoculation of bacteria into an open fracture or penetrating wound can also lead to infection and may resemble other serious bacterial infections in children (Table 11–3).

Clinical Findings

Acute bacterial hematogenous osteomyelitis usually occurs in the metaphysis following sludging of bacteria-laden blood in the venous sinusoids. The majority of cases are caused by *Staphylococcus aureus*. As the infection progresses, edema fluid and infected purulent tissue invade the porous cortex and elevate the periosteum, which is highly resistant to infection because of its extreme vascularity. The pressure of the pus beneath the richly innervated periosteum causes localized pain. Eventually, if the infection is untreated, the periosteum itself ruptures, and infected tissue spills into the surrounding soft tissue or ruptures the skin (Figure 11–1).

Table 11–3. Common pathogens in pediatric bone and joint infections.

Osteomyelitis
Group A *Streptococcus*
Salmonella (with sickle cell)
Staphylococcus aureus
Septic joint
Escherichia coli (neonatal)
Group A *Streptococcus*
Haemophilus influenzae (age 6–24 months) in non-HIB immunized patients
Neisseria gonorrhoeae (adolescent)
Pneumococcus
Proteus (neonatal)
Staphylococcus aureus
Streptococcus fecalis (neonatal)
Soft-tissue infection
Escherichia coli (neonatal)
Group A *Streptococcus*
Proteus
Pseudomonas
Staphylococcus aureus
Streptococcus fecalis (neonatal)

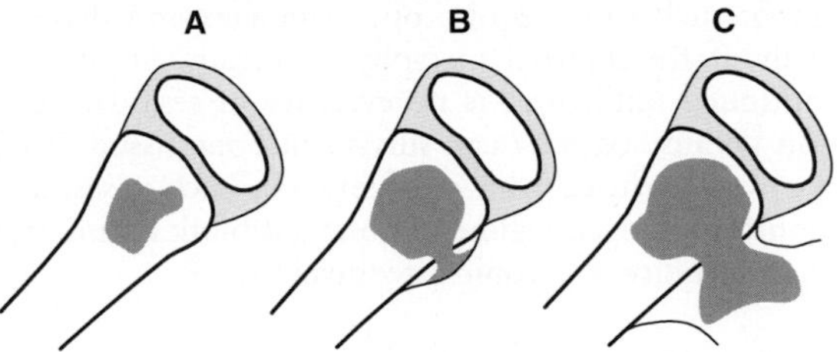

Figure 11–1. Hematogenous osteomyelitis in children. Cellulitic phase (**A**) can exude through the cortex, raising periosteum (**B**). Late rupture into soft tissues (**C**) is rare, unless infection is untreated.

The accumulated purulence in the marrow cavity and under the periosteum creates an efficient avascular culture medium in the cortex between them. This dead cortex is called sequestrum, and, if it is large, surgical removal may be required to control the infection.

The elevated periosteum responds to infection by producing a shell of periosteal new bone called involucrum, which provides some stability to the infected bone and rarely becomes infected itself.

Pain and tenderness at the infection site are universal signs, limping is common, and frequently the child is irritable. Fever and leukocytosis are common but not universal, and the erythrocyte sedimentation rate (ESR) is almost always elevated, usually to 50 mm/hour or more. C-reactive protein (CRP) is elevated. Clinical examination is usually sufficient to make the diagnosis; occasionally bone scans or MRI may be required to help localize lesions. Although the diagnosis is usually clear, osteomyelitis should be suspected if a child has bone pain in the absence of other systemic signs but has recently received antibiotic treatment for other conditions.

Treatment

A. Early Treatment

Treatment depends on the duration of symptoms and findings on radiograph. If the infection is detected early, no visible radiograph changes usually are apparent except for soft-tissue swelling. In that case, intravenous and, later, oral antibiotics may resolve the infection. Aspiration of the metaphysis should be done for culture before beginning antibiotic therapy. Up to 30–40% of cultures may be negative despite other clear evidence of bacterial infection; in that case, empirical treatment (usually with antistaphylococcal antibiotics) is appropriate.

B. Treatment for Advanced Infection

In advanced cases, lytic defects or osteoporosis may be present, and periosteal reaction may be visible on radiograph; such cases require open drainage and debridement of the infected metaphysis. Treatment must be continued until there is no evidence of residual infection because bacteria can survive in bone tissue that is not well perfused with antibiotic. In such cases, a 3-month prolonged regimen of oral antibiotics minimizes the possibility of chronic osteomyelitis.

Hamdy RC et al: Subacute hematogenous osteomyelitis: Are biopsy and surgery always necessary? J Pediatr Orthop 1996; 16:220.

Scott RJ et al: Acute osteomyelitis in children: A review of 116 cases. J Pediatr Orthop 1990;5:649.

2. Septic Joint

Septic arthritis in children, like osteomyelitis, usually is hematogenous in origin. The bacterial complications are similar to those seen in bone infections (see Table 11–3). Septic joints frequently follow upper respiratory infections; they may be delayed in onset by a week or more and may present in an attenuated form when a previous infection was partially treated.

Clinical Findings

The classic septic joint in a child presents a dramatic picture: The joint is splinted by muscle spasm, and motion of even a few degrees causes extreme pain. There may be effusion, but findings may be less striking if antibiotics were used in the recent past. During this acute inflammatory phase, children are more comfortable if the involved joint is immobilized.

Although white blood cell counts and the ESR are usually elevated, the definitive diagnosis of septic joint requires aspiration and synovial fluid analysis. Sterile aspiration does not harm the joint and should be done immediately when the diagnosis is suspected. Aspiration of deep joints such as the hip may require radiographic control.

Synovial white blood cell counts range from 50,000/μL (in nonpyogenic infections such as *Neisseria gonorrhoeae*) to over 250,000/μL (*S. aureus*). This white cell response, with the concomitant high level of lysosomal enzyme release, is most destructive of articular cartilage in septic joints. Although synovial fluid cultures give definitive guidance for therapy, antibiotic treatment can initially be based on results of Gram staining. In addition, immunochemical tests may offer rapid identification of certain pathogens.

Treatment

Treatment always includes drainage of the joint. In easily accessible joints, such as the finger or knee, certain low-grade infections may respond well to repeated aspirations. In most cases, however, surgical drainage by arthrotomy or arthroscopy is preferable.

Antibiotics easily cross the synovial membrane and are continued until the joint inflammation is resolved, usually for at least 3 weeks. Intravenous administration is used initially but may often be followed by oral medication once the temperature, sedimentation rate, and leukocyte count return to normal.

Darville T, Jacobs RF: Management of acute hematogenous osteomyelitis in children. Pediatr Infect Dis J 2004;23:255. [PMID: 15014303]

Kim HKW et al: A shortened course of parenteral antibiotic therapy in the management of acute septic arthritis of the hip. J Pediatr Orthop 2000;20:44. [PMID: 10641687]

3. Septic Hip

Septic hip is one of the true surgical emergencies in pediatric orthopedics. It must be differentiated from transient synovitis of the hip, which is a benign condition (see the section on transient synovitis of the hip).

Because of the unique structure and blood supply of this joint (Figure 11–2), purulence within the joint cap-

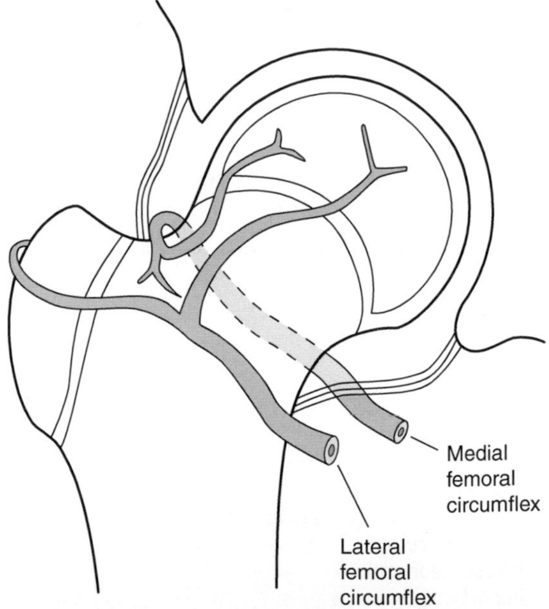

Figure 11–2. The blood supply of the proximal femur is unusual because the capsule interferes with the direct routing of blood vessels. The epiphyseal vessels emerge distal to the capsule and course up the surface of the femoral neck, rendering them susceptible to injury, thrombosis, or blockage by increased intraarticular pressure.

sule can cause thrombosis of epiphyseal vessels and necrosis of the proximal femoral epiphysis. Neglected septic hips may subluxate or dislocate because of effusion and laxity caused by hyperemia. For these reasons, septic hip (or osteomyelitis of the proximal femur) always requires surgical drainage. Delay of even 4–6 hours may compromise the vascularity of the hip. An anterior approach is preferred to reduce the risk of vascular injury and subluxation.

Septic hip in a growing child is also a special orthopedic case because the femoral neck (which is intraarticular) is actually the anatomic metaphysis of the proximal femur. It is thus susceptible to hematogenous osteomyelitis, which may rupture into the hip joint and cause sepsis.

A common clinical problem is the differentiation between septic and hip and transient synovitis of the hip. Juvenile arthritis may occasionally be included in the differential. Table 11–4 highlights differences in the conditions.

Kocher MS, Mandiga R, Zurakowski D et al: Validation of a clinical prediction rule for the differentiation between septic arthritis and transient synovitis of the hip in children. J Bone Joint Surg Am 2004;86-A:1629. [PMID: 15292409]

4. Puncture Wounds of the Foot

Sneakers and tennis shoes offer little protection from nail punctures of the plantar surface of the foot. The penetrating nail may carry *Pseudomonas* bacteria (which contaminates the soles of tennis shoes) into the plantar fascia, although one series found *S. aureus* or Group A *Streptococcus* to be most common.

The symptoms of infection include redness, swelling, and pain that persist longer than 1 week. Surgical incision and drainage of the abscess and foreign body excision, when present (approximately one sixth of cases), are usually curative. Interestingly, prophylactic use of antibiotics does not seem to lessen the chance of developing late abscess. Late presentation is a marker for deep infection.

Eidelman M et al: Plantar puncture wounds in children: Analysis of 80 hospitalized patients and late sequelae. Isr Med Assoc J 2003;5:268. [PMID: 14509132]

5. Skeletal Tuberculosis

As in the adult, *Mycobacteria* organisms may invade the pediatric skeleton by hematogenous spread to bone or synovium while the initial pulmonary infection goes undetected. The most common sites of invasion are the hip and spine. Tuberculosis should be considered, and skin tests performed, in children suffering from chronic atypical musculoskeletal infections, particularly if the child is immunosuppressed.

Clinical Findings

Hip involvement is characterized by a chronic limp associated with a flexion contracture. In addition, muscle atrophy of the thigh may be striking. Radiographic examination discloses osteoporosis, joint narrowing, and irregular erosions.

Spine involvement may include paraspinal abscess (best visualized by CT scan or MRI), vertebral destruction, or kyphosis, which may be severe and lead to paralysis.

Treatment

Treatment of skeletal tuberculosis consists of combination chemotherapy, with surgical debridement in resistant cases. Occasionally, surgical fusion of joints or spine may be required.

Teo HE, Peh WC: Skeletal tuberculosis in children. Pediatr Radiol 2004;34:853. [PMID: 15278319]

Table 11–4. Clinical differential diagnosis of inflammatory hip conditions.

	Septic Hip	Transient Synovitis of Hip	Juvenile Arthritis of Hip
Pain	Severe	Moderate–severe	Moderate
Gait	Cannot walk	Limp or cannot walk	Limp
Fever	Common	No	No or low grade
Radiograph	Negative	Negative	Joint narrowing
WBC	Elevated	Normal	Normal–elevated
Aspirate	Turbid; 5000–250,000 WBC; bacteria present	Normal	25,000–50,000 WBC with monocytes
Treatment	Urgent surgical drainage; antibiotics	Symptomatic	Salicylates, rest, physical therapy

WBC = white blood cells.

6. *Diskitis in Children*

Diskitis is a low-grade inflammatory process involving the intervertebral disk, usually in the lumbar spine. It affects children at any age, although it is most frequent between 2 and 6 years of age. The disorder is caused by hematogenous bacterial seeding, with the most common cultures growing *S. aureus* from the disk aspirate. The classic presentation in a toddler is refusal to walk; pain is not a prominent symptom in this age group. Older children (up to early teen years) may have either back or abdominal pain.

Clinical Findings

Small children may have limitation of passive hyperextension of the spine (in the prone position) with no other findings. Older children have splinting of the paraspinous muscles and pain with percussion. The ESR may be normal or elevated; those patients with an elevated ESR are more likely to have bacterial growth if cultures are done. Aspirate cultures may be negative in up to 40% of patients. Radiographs at first are normal but eventually demonstrate disk space narrowing with sclerosis of adjoining endplates, best visualized on spot lateral views. Bone scan is positive in those children with negative radiographs.

Treatment

Management depends on the severity of clinical findings because a large number of diskitis patients have self-limited disease and improve spontaneously. Children with sepsis or elevated ESR may benefit from disk aspiration and culture. Less ill children are usually treated with empirical antistaphylococcal oral antibiotics for 6 weeks. Pantaloon spica cast may occasionally be required for symptom relief. Long-term outcome is universally favorable, although occasional spontaneous fusion of the disk space occurs.

Early SD, Kay RM, Tolo VT: Childhood diskitis. J Am Acad Orthop Surg 2003;11:413. [PMID: 14686826]

METABOLIC DISORDERS

1. *Rickets & Rickets-Like Conditions*

Nutritional rickets is a dietary deficiency of vitamin D that interferes with skeletal ossification. In the United States, vitamin supplementation of food and milk has virtually eliminated the dietary form of rickets. Numerous rickets-like metabolic conditions persist with orthopedic consequences, however.

Renal Osteodystrophy

Renal osteodystrophy, a disorder of calcium, phosphorus, vitamin D, and parathyroid function in children with chronic renal disease, has potentially serious skeletal manifestations. In transplantation patients, the condition can be aggravated by chronic illness and antimetabolite or steroid usage.

Osteoporosis, leading to compression fractures of the spine, is a common complication. Delayed healing of fractures is also common. Inadequate metaphyseal ossification during skeletal growth results in wide, irregular cartilaginous growth plates, which tend to slip slowly, sometimes producing grotesque hip, knee, and ankle deformities. Such deformities are usually best treated only after transplantation or other improvement in renal status. Occasionally, severe functional disabilities may require osteotomy to correct deformity before renal transplantation. Healing may be delayed, however, and the condition may recur.

Hypophosphatemic Rickets

Hypophosphatemic rickets (vitamin D–resistant rickets) is an dominant X-linked condition in which vitamin D production and metabolism are normal but renal tubular loss of phosphate interferes with skeletal ossification. The major manifestations are a mild-to-moderate decrease in stature and bowing of the lower extremities.

The medical history usually discloses a parent or sibling with short stature and bowlegs. In addition, serum phosphorus is reduced, and serum calcium is normal. Radiographic examination discloses characteristic widening of growth plates, funnel-like beaking of the metaphyses, and curvature of the femoral and tibial shafts, which are normally straight (Figure 11–3).

Medical treatment with megadoses of vitamin D and phosphorus supplementation may not be curative. Functionally disabling deformities can be corrected by multiple-level osteotomies, which usually require bilateral surgery. Because postosteotomy healing is delayed and recurrence of deformity is common until maturity, surgery should be postponed until adolescence, if possible.

Saland JM: Osseous complications of pediatric transplantation. Pediatr Transplant 2004;8:400. [PMID: 15265169]

Santos F et al: Alterations of the growth plate in chronic renal failure. Pediatr Nephrol 2004;20:330. [PMID: 15549411]

HIP DISORDERS

1. *Transient Synovitis of the Hip*

Transient synovitis of the hip is a benign, nontraumatic, self-limited disorder that mimics septic hip in clinical presentation. The physician confronting this condition must exclude septic hip, which is a surgical emergency.

Although the cause of transient synovitis is unclear, evidence suggests it is associated with immune responses to viral or bacterial antigens, mediated through the synovial membrane. Synovial fluid rapidly accumulates under pressure in the hip joint, and there may be severe pain from capsular distension. The fluid is resorbed within 3–7 days, with no long-term sequelae.

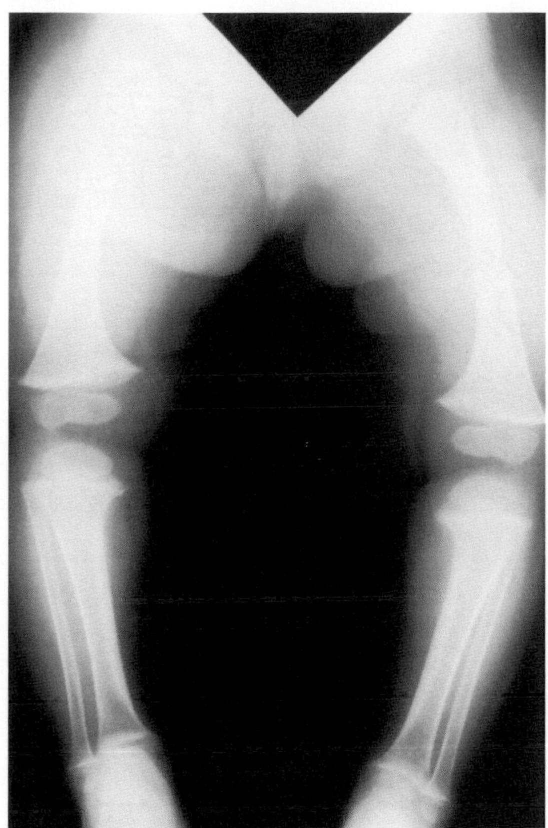

Figure 11–3. Hypophosphatemic rickets. Radiographs demonstrate bowing of long bones and flared, irregular physes (see text).

Clinical Findings

As with septic hip, upper respiratory tract infections often precede transient synovitis by a few days to 2 weeks. The hip contains excess synovial fluid and is held in flexion, abduction, and external rotation because this is the joint's position of maximum capacity. The joint may be sore and resistant to movement, but subluxation does not occur. Usually, the patient allows careful passive movement.

Radiographs reveal only capsular swelling, and effusion may be detected on ultrasound. Leukocytosis is absent, and ESR and CRP are not elevated.

Although experienced physicians frequently suspect transient synovitis based only on clinical examination, aspiration of the hip following confirmation of needle position by radiograph is the safest approach. Synovial fluid does not show elevation of the white blood cell count, and bacterial cultures are negative.

Treatment

Treatment of transient synovitis includes simple analgesics and splintage, usually by bed rest, until symptoms resolve.

The early stages of Legg-Calvé-Perthes disease (see section on Legg-Calvé-Perthes disease) may include a synovitic stage that, until the development of characteristic radiograph findings, is indistinguishable from transient synovitis. No evidence indicates that transient synovitis leads to Legg-Calvé-Perthes disease itself. Typically, the pain is less severe than in transient synovitis, the children are a bit older (older than 4–5 years), and there is no history of recent illness.

Luhmann SJ et al: Differentiation between septic arthritis and transient synovitis of the hip in children with clinical prediction algorithms. J Bone Joint Surg Am 2004;86:956. [PMID: 15118038]

2. Developmental Dysplasia of the Hip

Developmental dysplasia of the hip is one of the most serious problems in pediatric orthopedics. The neonatal hip is a relatively unstable joint because the muscle is undeveloped, the soft cartilaginous surfaces are easily deformed, and the ligaments are lax. Exaggerated positioning in acute flexion and adduction in utero may occur, especially in breech presentation. This situation may cause excess stretching of the posterior hip capsule, which renders the joint unstable after delivery. Laxity may reflect family history or the presence of maternal relaxin hormone in the fetal circulatory system.

This relative instability may lead to asymptomatic subluxation (partial displacement) or dislocation (complete displacement) of the hip joint. Displacement of the femoral head in the infant is proximal (posterior and superior) because of the pull of the gluteal and hip flexor muscles. In the subluxated hip, asymmetric pressure causes progressive flattening of the posterior and superior acetabular rim and medial femoral head (*dysplasia* is the term to describe these structural deviations from normal).

In the completely dislocated hip, dysplasia also occurs because normal joint development requires concentric motion with normally mated joint surfaces. The shallow, deformed dysplastic joint surfaces predispose to further mechanical instability and the inexorable progression of undetected, and therefore untreated, developmental dysplasia of the hip.

Developmental dysplasia of the hip (DDH) occurs in approximately 1 in 1000 live births in whites, is less common in blacks, and may be more common in certain ethnic groups such as North American Indians. In all groups, this disorder is more likely if certain risk factors are present, such as positive family history, ligamentous laxity, breech presentation (and, by association, cesarean delivery), female gender, large fetal size, and first-born status. Dislocations may be bilateral but are more often unilateral and on the left side.

Clinical Findings

Reversal of dysplasia and subsequent normal hip development depend on early detection of DDH. Early detection is made more challenging by lack of a definitive test or finding on examination. Moreover, because this disorder is painless, there are no symptoms in the infant. Detection of bilateral dislocations may be particularly difficult.

Radiographs are usually not useful in newborn infants because the femoral head is composed of radiolucent cartilage. Ultrasound examination is helpful, but false-positive results are common before 8–10 weeks of age. The test is expensive, and interpretation requires comprehensive training. Thus, the best test for this disorder is careful physical examination at birth, repeated at each well-infant check until the child is walking normally. A high index of suspicion is mandatory, especially if risk factors are present.

A. Tests for Dysplasia

Several examination maneuvers require a quiet, relaxed infant and commonly produce false-negative findings. Although it is imperative to detect subluxated or dislocated hips, it is also helpful to identify the very lax (unstable) but still located hip. This type of joint may either dislocate later or exhibit subtle dysplasia during growth that can cause premature osteoarthritis.

1. Asymmetric skin folds—A dislocated hip displaces proximally, causing the leg to be marginally shorter. This occasionally leads to the accordion phenomenon, with wrinkling of thigh skin folds. The most significant fold is between the genitals and gluteus maximus region. This test is not very reliable, frequently producing false-positive and false-negative results (Figure 11–4A).

2. Galeazzi test—With the child lying on a flat surface, flex the hips and knees so the heels rest flat on the table, just distal to the buttock (Figure 11–4B). A dislocated hip is signaled by relative shortening of the thigh compared with the normal leg, as shown by the difference in knee height level. This test is almost always useless in children younger than 1 year and is negative if dislocation is bilateral.

3. Passive hip abduction—The flexed hips are gently abducted as far as possible (Figure 11–4C). If one or both hips are dislocated, the femoral head (the pivot point during abduction) is posterior, causing relative tightness of the adductor muscles. Asymmetric abduction or limited abduction (usually less than 70 degrees from the midline) is a positive finding. When the hip is lax (dislocatable but not dislocated), the abduction test is normal despite the presence of subluxation or dislocation.

4. Barlow test—A provocative test that picks up an unstable but located hip, the Barlow test is unsuitable for a dislocated hip. The flexed calf and knee are gently grasped in the hand, with the thumb at the lesser trochanter and fingers at the greater trochanter (knee flexion relaxes the hamstrings). The hip is adducted slightly and gently pushed posteriorly and laterally with the palm (Figure 11–4D, F). Detection of so-called pistoning, or the sensation of the femoral head subluxating over the posterior rim of the acetabulum, is a positive finding.

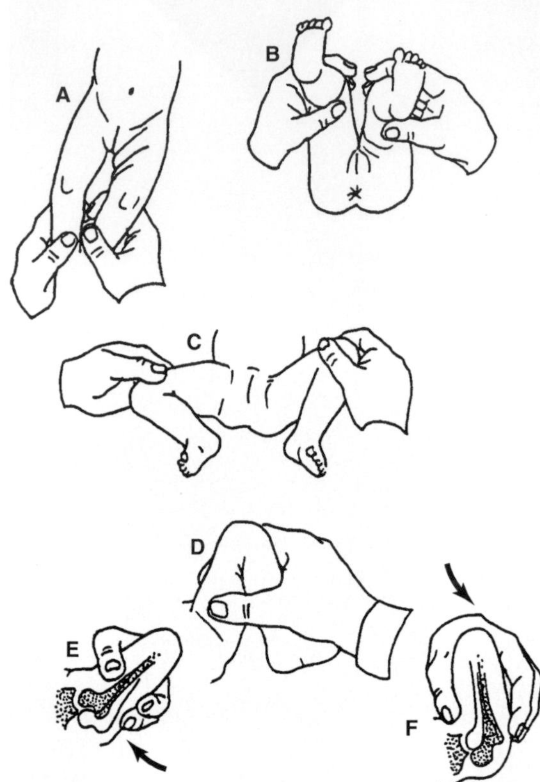

Figure 11–4. Clinical examination of developmental dislocation of the hip. In all pictures, the child's left hip is the abnormal side. **A:** Asymmetric skin folds. **B:** Galeazzi test. **C:** Limitation of abduction. **D, E, F:** Ortolani and Barlow tests (see text).

5. Ortolani test—This test detects hips that are already dislocated. The flexed limb is grasped as in the Barlow test. The hip is abducted while the femur is gently lifted with the fingers at the greater trochanter (Figure 11–4D, E). In a positive test, there is a sensation of the hip reducing back into the acetabulum. Reduction is felt but not heard: The old concept of a so-called hip click is incorrect. The Ortolani test may be negative at 2–3 months of age, even when the hip is dislocated, because of the development of soft-tissue contracture.

B. Imaging Studies

In the infant, diagnosis is made by physical examination alone, and radiographs are generally unnecessary. Dysplasia, instability, and dislocation may appear on ultrasound studies, which can allow visualization of hip contour and stability before ossification is present. Sonography is a dynamic examination that requires an experienced interpreter, and there can be false positives prior to 6–10 weeks of age. Radiographs may be used at any age, but the absence of ossified structures renders them inaccurate in the newborn. After 4–6 months, when the ossific nucleus appears in the femoral head, radiographs are more helpful. Because much of the skeleton is cartilaginous at this age, certain lines and angles may be drawn on radiographs to allow estimates of geometric parameters (Figure 11–5). These may suggest evidence of acetabular dysplasia (a more vertical slope of the acetabular roof, measured as the acetabular index); femoral dysplasia (small or absent ossification center in the femoral head); or lateral superior displacement of the femoral head.

Increased femoral anteversion (external rotation of the femoral head and neck) is often present in DDH but not visible. Increased anteversion may be seen as an increase in relative femoral neck valgus in the older child.

C. Detection of Dysplasia in the Older Child

As the infant grows older, many diagnostic maneuvers that are positive in a young infant become negative because soft-tissue changes accommodate the displaced structures. Thus, the Ortolani and Barlow signs can be negative, even in the face of grossly abnormal hip development, making detection particularly difficult (especially between 4 and 15 months of age). The first signs of developmental dysplasia may then not be recognized until the child begins to walk and demonstrates a waddling gait with excessive lumbar lordosis. Radiographs at this age are diagnostic.

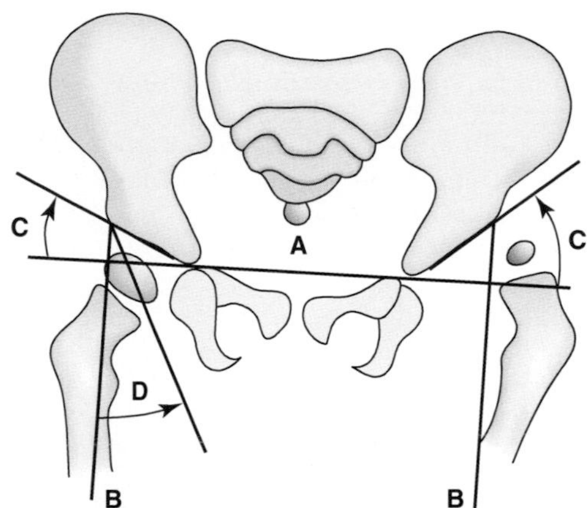

Figure 11–5. Lines drawn for measurement in developmental dysplasia of the hip. In the figure, the patient's left hip (on the right of the figure) is the subluxated one. **A:** Hilgenreiner line is a horizontal line of the pelvis, drawn between the triradiate cartilages. The proximal femoral ossification center should be below this line. **B:** Perkins line is a vertical line (perpendicular to Hilgenreiner line) drawn down from the lateral edge of the acetabulum. The femoral head ossification center, as well as the medial beak of the proximal metaphysis, should fall medial to this line. **C:** The acetabular index is the angle between Hilgenreiner line and a line joining the acetabular center (triradiate) with the acetabular edge as it intersects Perkins line. It measures acetabular depth and should be below 30 degrees by 1 year of age and below 25 degrees by 2 years of age. **D:** The center-edge angle is the angle between Perkins line and a line joining the lateral edge of the acetabulum with the center of the femoral head. It is a measure of lateral subluxation that becomes smaller as the hip subluxates laterally. Normal is 20 degrees or greater.

Treatment

Treatment of DDH should be initiated as soon as the diagnosis is suspected. Early treatment is generally successful, whereas a delay in treatment may result in permanent dysplastic changes. Exact treatment depends on patient age at presentation and degree of involvement. Regardless of age, treatment may fail, and the physician may need to institute a more complex treatment plan. The current recommendations described next.

A. Age 0–6 Months

A dislocated hip at this age may spontaneously reduce over 2–3 weeks if the hip is held in a position of flexion. This is best accomplished with the Pavlik harness (Figure 11–6), a canvas device that holds the hips flexed at 100 degrees and prevents adduction but does not limit further flexion. Movement in the harness is beneficial for the joint and helps achieve gradual spontaneous reduction and stabilization of the hip. The Pavlik harness presents a low risk of avascular necrosis (see section on avascular necrosis of the hip). This treatment should not be continued beyond 3–4 weeks if there is no improvement. The failure rate of the Pavlik harness is approximately 10%, necessitating more invasive treatment, such as closed or open reduction.

B. Age 6–15 Months (Before Walking)

Gentle manipulative reduction of the dislocation under a general anesthetic and maintenance of a located position for 2–3 months in a spica cast usually stabilizes the joint. Even after the hip is stable, any residual dysplasia

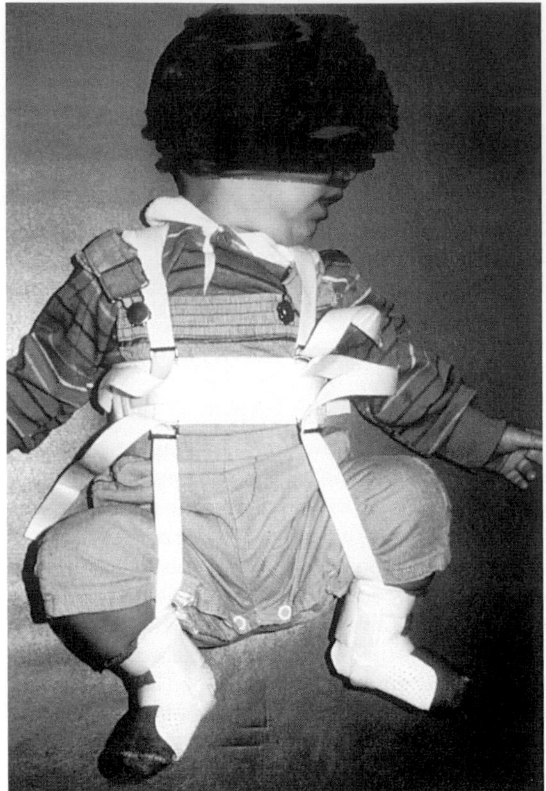

Figure 11–6. The Pavlik harness, a device used for treatment of hip dislocation, subluxation, and dysplasia.

must be treated by bracing or surgery. In the past, prereduction skin traction was thought to reduce the risk of avascular necrosis. It is now believed that adequate hip flexion and limited abduction in the spica cast is the most important safety factor, and most surgeons no longer use traction.

C. Age 15 Months to 2 Years

In toddlers or young children in whom closed reduction failed, open reduction of the hip is required. Severe flattening of the acetabulum with distortion of the normal spherical femoral head shape is found on opening the hip. The limbus (acetabular rim) may be flattened and inverted, and the ligamentum teres is always hypertrophic. Fibrofatty tissue occupying the center of the acetabulum must be removed. Femoral shortening osteotomy may be required at the time of open reduction to reduce soft-tissue tension and minimize the risk of avascular necrosis. After reduction, the position is maintained by capsular repair (capsulorrhaphy) and a cast, until stability is achieved. Prolonged bracing or surgery is often required to resolve the residual dysplasia that accompanies untreated dysplasia in this group of children.

D. Age Older Than 2 Years

Significant residual dysplasia is present in children with DDH who are untreated at this age. Dysplasia may also persist despite successful reduction performed by any method at an earlier age. The dysplasia may be accompanied by a limp, and radiographs show a high acetabular index (more vertical acetabular roof), increased valgus of the femoral neck, and subluxation of the femoral head.

Surgical correction of dysplasia creates a stable mechanical environment that permits remodeling to a more normal joint during growth. Treatment requires bony procedures, either on the acetabular or femoral sides of the joint, or on both sides. Acetabular procedures, such as the Salter or Pemberton osteotomies, improve the acetabular index and increase the mechanical stability of the joint.

Femoral osteotomy corrects the anteversion and femoral neck valgus that characterize femoral dysplasia. The exact selection of osteotomy site may be based on maximum radiographic dysplasia or on the individual surgeon's preference. All of the osteotomies require that the femoral head be spherical and the hip joint concentrically reduced before an attempt can be made to correct the dysplasia. In general, the osteotomy should address the site of dysplasia, that is, acetabular dysplasia is not ideally treated with femoral osteotomy. Nevertheless, femoral osteotomy, if performed before 4 years of age, stimulates a dysplastic shallow acetabulum to remodel into a more normal shape. This occurs because the femoral osteotomy renders the hip joint more stable, thus allowing the normal mechanisms of growth to take over. Similarly, patients exhibit a progressive decrease in femoral dysplasia following successful acetabular osteotomy.

1. Salter osteotomy—Salter osteotomy is a surgical procedure to redirect the acetabulum in DDH (Figure 11–7). Animal models demonstrate that residual hip dysplasia is accompanied by acetabular malrotation and deficiency in the anterolateral acetabular rim. Salter osteotomy corrects this deficiency by rotating the acetabular region anteriorly and laterally.

The procedure is indicated in children 18 months to 10 years of age in whom concentric reduction of the hip was achieved. It is used to correct moderate acetabular dysplasia and can improve the acetabular index by 15 degrees. It may also be used to stabilize the hip at the time of open reduction. The pelvis above the hip joint is exposed subperiosteally. A transverse cut is made, using a wire saw, from the sciatic notch to the anteroinferior iliac spine, and the entire distal fragment (including the acetabulum) is spun on the pivot points

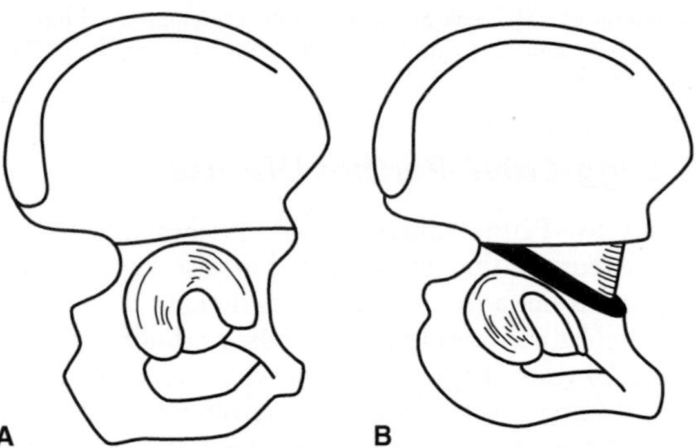

Figure 11–7. Salter innominate osteotomy, used for managing acetabular dysplasia. After a transverse cut is made above the acetabulum (**A**), the acetabular fragment is rotated forward and outward (**B**) to improve acetabular coverage.

of the notch and the pubic symphysis. This redirects the entire dysplastic acetabulum to a more horizontal stable position. A bone graft and pins hold the osteotomy open until it heals. A spica cast is used for 6 weeks to protect the graft during healing.

Salter osteotomy requires a second operation to remove the fixation pins. Because the geometric reorientation afforded is limited, there may be residual dysplasia. In addition, failure to achieve a concentric reduction before pelvic osteotomy usually renders the procedure ineffective.

2. Pemberton osteotomy Indications for the Pemberton osteotomy (Figure 11–8) are similar to those of the Salter osteotomy, and frequently one or the other is selected according to the surgeon's experience or preference. The Pemberton procedure is particularly suited for correction of the long stretched-out dysplastic acetabulum because it reduces the capacity of an overly spacious acetabulum. This is done by cutting above the acetabular roof, down to the flexible triradiate cartilage (the growth plate of the center of the acetabulum). The roof fragment is then pried down to a more horizontal position and held in place by wedging a bone graft into the resulting defect. The fold thus produced in the center of the acetabulum may cause temporary stiffness. In younger children, this quickly remodels, but it is the major reason many surgeons do not perform this procedure on children older than 7–8 years.

Like the Salter procedure, Pemberton osteotomy requires concentric reduction before it is performed. For the Pemberton osteotomy, the pelvis is exposed above the joint. Under radiographic guidance, a curved osteotome is used to cut the pelvic bone from the acetabular roof down to the triradiate cartilage (the central growth plate of the acetabulum). The flexible cartilage allows the fragment to be hinged down over the femoral head, producing a more horizontal acetabular roof. A bone graft from the upper ilium wedges into the osteotomy site to maintain correction, and a spica cast is used until healing, which takes approximately 6 weeks.

Rarely, early extrusion or graft collapse occurs, and transient stiffness may be seen in older children. Because there is no internal fixation, a second procedure is unnecessary.

3. Femoral osteotomy—Femoral osteotomy (Figure 11–9) may be used to correct severe increased femoral anteversion or coxa valga (a high neck-shaft angle), conditions that are sometimes seen in residual DDH.

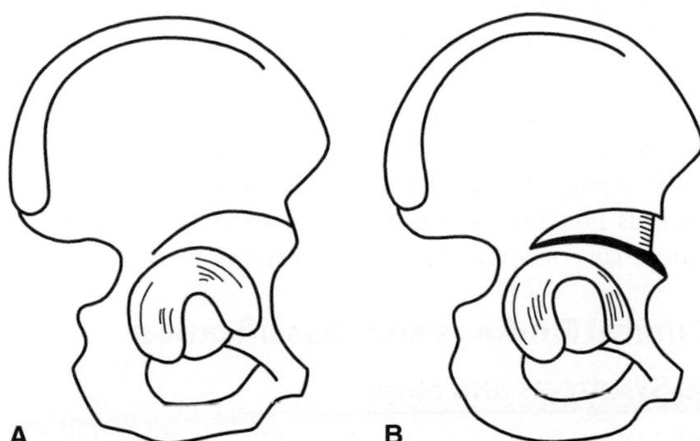

Figure 11–8. Pemberton pericapsular iliac osteotomy. An osteotomy cut is made above the acetabulum down to the flexible triradiate cartilage (**A**). The fragment is pried down to improve acetabular coverage and held with a bone graft (**B**).

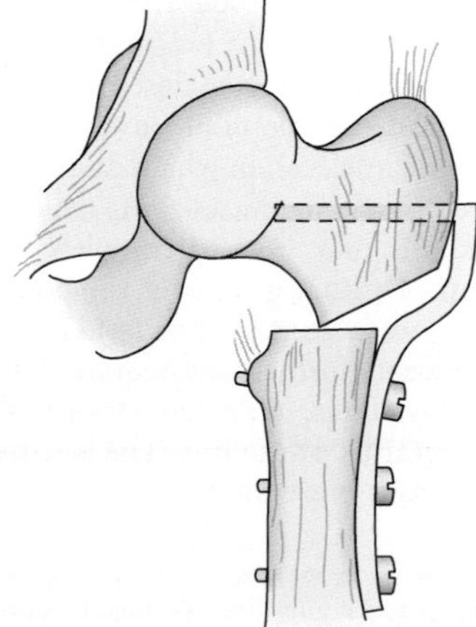

Figure 11–9. Femoral osteotomy is performed at the intertrochanteric level and fixed with a plate and screws.

The procedure is particularly indicated when radiographs taken with the hip in abduction and external rotation show improvement in the overall congruency of the hip. Redirection of an anteverted proximal femur in valgus angulation stimulates spontaneous improvement in dysplastic acetabula in children younger than 4 years.

Femoral osteotomy is performed using a lateral approach, with the cut made across the intertrochanteric region of the femur. This site is chosen both because it is distal to the blood supply of the femoral head and because the cancellous bone heals easily. A metal bladeplate is placed in the proximal (femoral neck) fragment, usually after positioning with a provisional guidewire. The femoral neck fragment is rotated into a more horizontal position (varus) and is then internally rotated to correct excessive anteversion. The exact degree of correction is determined by preoperative radiograph positioning to achieve maximum congruence and correction of radiographic dysplasia. The plate portion is then clamped to the shaft of the bone and fixed with screws. A spica cast is usually used to supplement fixation.

After healing (6 weeks), the patient may resume walking. A Trendelenburg limp is common for 1–2 years after femoral osteotomy because of the geometric distortion of the relationship between the joint and insertion of the abductor muscles. This resolves as the femur remodels with growth and does not present a long-term problem.

Avascular Necrosis of the Hip

If a reduction maneuver for DDH was forceful or if there is tension in the soft tissues around the hip, the resulting compression of the joint may cause transient blockage of the blood supply to the femoral head. The subsequent death of the ossific nucleus and proximal growth plate of the femur (avascular necrosis) is a complication of treatment rather than of the disorder itself. A well-recognized cause of avascular necrosis is exaggerated forced abduction in the spica cast used after closed or open reduction. Avascular necrosis may be mild (involving a small fraction of the ossific nucleus), in which case it may go undetected and be of little significance. At the other extreme, avascular necrosis may lead to complete femoral head death and loss of future growth at the proximal physis. As it revascularizes, a dead femoral head may deform significantly, subluxate further, and require abduction bracing or osteotomy. Thus, it can cause leg-length inequality or early osteoarthritis of the hip. The best treatment for avascular necrosis is prevention.

Lehmann HP, Hinton R, Morello P et al: Developmental dysplasia of the hip practice guideline: Technical report. Committee on Quality Improvement, and Subcommittee on Developmental Dysplasia of the Hip. Pediatrics 2000;105(4):E57. [PMID: 10742378]

Weinstein SL, Mubarak SJ, Wenger DR: Developmental hip dysplasia and dislocation: Part II. Instr Course Lect 2004; 53:531. [PMID: 15116642]

3. Legg-Calvé-Perthes Disease

Legg-Calvé-Perthes disease (LCP, Perthes disease) is a serious but self-limited pediatric hip disorder. Although its cause is unknown, the disease is thought to be related to avascular necrosis of the hip. It affects children between 4 and 10 years of age and is somewhat more common in boys. Children with the disease are often small for their age and have retarded bone age. The disease is generally unilateral. If it is bilateral, other conditions, such as Gaucher disease or multiple epiphyseal dysplasia, must be considered. Newer investigations suggest that some cases of LCP might be related to a variety of transient or permanent hypercoagulation states. This research is not yet been confirmed in multiple centers. Surprisingly, trauma is not considered a causative factor in LCP.

Although early radiographs may be negative, they eventually show fragmentation, irregularity, and collapse of part or all of the femoral head ossification center (Figure 11–10). The few pathologic specimens that were examined suggest that multiple rather than single episodes of avascular necrosis occur over a period of months. Early bone scans may show a filling defect corresponding to areas of necrosis, and MRI is typical of avascular necrosis. The disease has a characteristic course (see Figure 11–10). Initially, the avascular episodes are silent and the child is asymptomatic. As the disease progresses, the necrotic femoral epiphysis is revascularized. Osteoclasts remove dead bone while osteoblasts simultaneously lay down new bone on the dead trabeculae (a process known as creeping substitution). During this phase, the femoral head is mechanically weak. Fragmentation and collapse of the bony structure may then occur, causing geometric flattening and deformity of the ossific nucleus and femoral head. The newly replaced bone takes the shape of the collapsed head.

At this point, continued growth may allow gradual remodeling and improvement of the femoral head shape until maturity. The symptomatic collapse phase rarely exceeds 1–1.5 years, but full revascularization and remodeling may continue silently for several years thereafter.

Clinical Findings and Classification

A. Symptoms and Signs

The clinical presentation of LCP in a child 4–10 years of age is usually a painless limp. If pain is present, it may be mild and referred to the thigh or knee. Physical examination discloses atrophy of the thigh on the affected side and, usually, limited hip motion. The typical patient has a flexion contracture of 0–30 degrees,

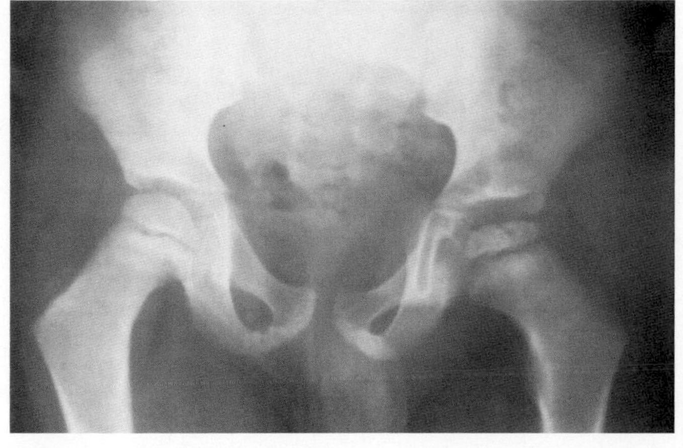

A

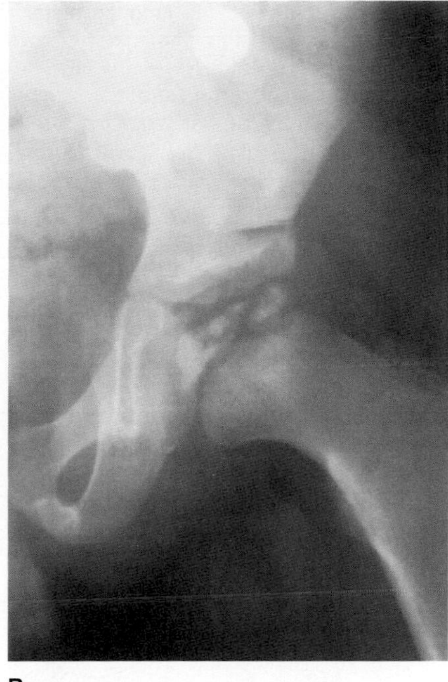

B

Figure 11–10. Legg-Calvé-Perthes disease. **A:** Central necrotic fragment with collapse. **B:** Same patient after healing and partial remodeling.

loss of abduction compared with the opposite side (in severe cases, no abduction beyond 0 degrees), and loss of internal rotation of the hip.

B. Imaging Studies

Radiographs may be negative at first, probably because the initial softening of the femoral head is sufficient to cause symptoms but insufficient to change the radiographic appearance of the femoral head. The eventual characteristic collapse of portions of the femoral head is diagnostic of the disease, however.

The exact extent of necrosis, which is usually estimated in fourths of the head using the Catterall classification (Figure 11–11), is helpful in determining whom to treat. It may require additional radiographs.

An alternative radiograph classification uses the lateral third of the femoral epiphysis (the so-called lateral pillar). Collapse of this structure suggests a poor prognosis for late deformity, whereas maintenance of pillar height correlates with good long-term results. Partial collapse suggests an intermediate prognosis. The difficulty with all classification systems is their reproducibility and the need to delay until the collapse phase before the exact extent of involvement is clear.

There is little value in bone scans or MRI in the clinical management of LCP.

Treatment Options

A. No Treatment

Children with bone age less than 5 years and children who exhibit relatively minor involvement (less than half of the femoral head) rarely need treatment. In these children, so much of the femoral head is cartilage, and therefore unaffected by necrosis, that mechanical collapse does not markedly decrease sphericity. Also, younger children have tremendous remodeling potential, and minor collapse can be outgrown before maturity. Older children who exhibit some radiograph changes but have excellent range of motion (ROM) may require only observation and serial reexamination.

B. Nonoperative and Operative Treatment

The issues surrounding selection of patients with LCP who need treatment are as highly controversial as the treatment itself. Most experts agree that children who maintain excellent motion (particularly abduction greater than 30 degrees in the absence of flexion contracture) may not require intervention. In children older than 4–5 years with significant collapse or progressive loss of abduction, treatment is frequently recommended.

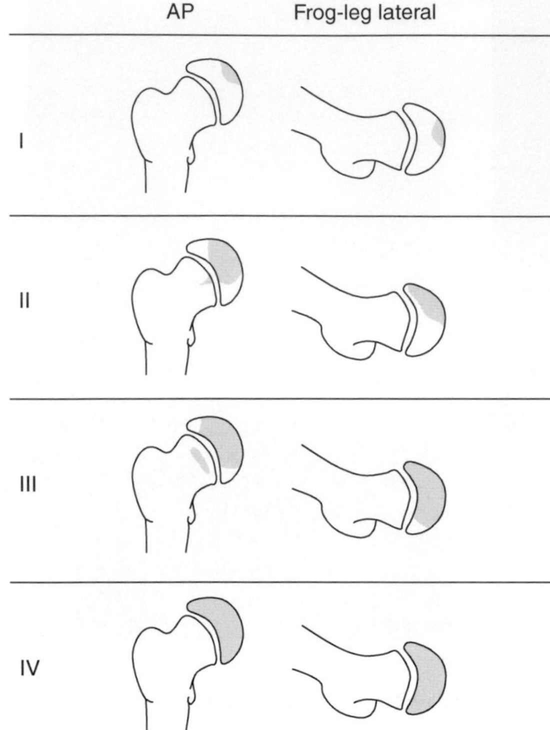

Figure 11–11. The Catterall classification is used to determine probable course and prognosis of Legg-Calvé-Perthes disease. It is based on progressive involvement of approximate fourths of the femoral head.

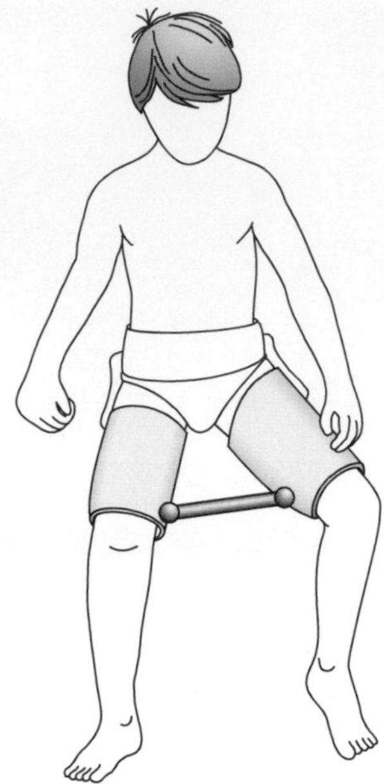

Figure 11–12. Abduction bracing is one method used for ambulatory treatment of Legg-Calvé-Perthes disease.

No evidence indicates that use of crutches or relief of weight bearing has any effect on femoral head collapse in this disease. For those children requiring it, however, treatment should minimize the effects of collapse and subluxation that often occur when the femoral head deforms. This is best achieved by abduction of the hip until subluxation resolves. The molding action of the acetabular shape is thought to help improve the contour of the collapsing femoral head. Abduction can be accomplished nonoperatively by holding the legs in abduction (Petrie) casts or using an ambulatory brace (Figure 11–12).

Operative procedures are advocated by some and include varus femoral osteotomy and Salter osteotomy, which were adapted from hip dysplasia treatment to control the subluxation seen in some cases of LCP. Healing usually occurs within 18 months.

Despite many studies, there is still no consensus for the best method of treatment; some patients do well without treatment, whereas others have a poor result after aggressive treatment. Prognosis can often be predicted from the knowledge of certain factors (Table 11–5).

Balasa VV, Gruppo RA, Glueck CJ et al: Legg-Calve-Perthes disease and thrombophilia. J Bone Joint Surg Am 2004;86-A:264. [PMID: 15590848]

Herring JA, Kim HT, Browne R: Legg-Calve-Perthes disease. Part II: Prospective multicenter study of the effect of treatment on outcome. J Bone Joint Surg Am 2004;86-A:2121. [PMID: 15466720]

Table 11–5. Factors in long-term prognosis for patients with Legg-Calvé-Perthes disease.

Relative Prognosis	Good	Poor
Age at diagnosis	< 5 years	> 8–9 years
Hip motion[a]	Maintained (abduction > 30°)	Stiff (abduction < 15°)
Extent of involvement	< 50% of femoral head	> 50% or total femoral head
Radiograph features	Little or no subluxation	Subluxation, lateral calcification

[a]During first year of treatment.

4. Slipped Capital Femoral Epiphysis

Slipped capital femoral epiphysis is an adolescent hip disorder characterized by displacement of the femoral head on the femoral neck. Displacement changes the geometry of the upper end of the femur and hinders hip function (Figure 11–13). This disorder is one of the main causes of premature osteoarthritis in young adults.

Slipped capital femoral epiphysis usually affects both male and female adolescents 11–13 years of age. In 30% of patients, the condition is bilateral, although both legs are not always affected simultaneously. The typical patient is overweight—often markedly so—and is in either late prepuberty or early puberty. Rarely, the patient is tall, asthenic, and rapidly growing.

This disorder occurs at a time when the cartilage physis of the proximal femur is thickening rapidly under the influence of growth hormone. The vigorous secretion of sex hormone has not yet begun, however, so the mechanical effect of sex hormones on closure and stabilization of the growth plate is absent. This combination of thick growth plate cartilage (weaker than bone and subject to shear), lack of sexual maturity (which would stabilize the physis), mechanical stress (caused by obesity), and the peculiar anatomic mechanics of the hip joint renders the growth plate susceptible to slippage.

The direction of the slip is always posterior and often medial, and the mechanical bases of chronic and acute disorders are the same. In chronic slipped capital femoral epiphysis, the most common form (90% of patients), the femoral head slips insidiously at the growth plate over the course of several months. In the acute form, the femoral head is suddenly displaced, a condition that can be superimposed on chronic changes. Displacement may occur during normal activity or following minor trauma.

Because slipped capital femoral epiphysis is a progressive disorder and the prognosis depends on the severity of the slippage, early detection and prompt treatment are imperative.

Clinical Findings

A. Symptoms and Signs

The onset of chronic slipped capital femoral epiphysis is usually insidious, with a history of a painful limp for 1 to several months prior. The pain is characteristically aching and located in the thigh or knee rather than the hip. This referred pain to the knee is responsible for many misdiagnoses. Patients may be seen for knee pain and dismissed as normal after a negative knee examination and radiographs. A high index of suspicion is required to detect slipped capital femoral epiphysis in the obese limping adolescent complaining of knee pain. The change in hip ROM is usually diagnostic. Loss of abduction and internal rotation of the hip are evident, although these may be difficult to identify in the grossly overweight child. There is almost always a characteristic obligatory external rotation of the hip when it is flexed because of the distorted hip anatomy caused by the disorder. The femoral head is posterior to its normal position, so the flexed hip must externally rotate to keep the head within the acetabulum.

Acute slipped capital femoral epiphysis is accompanied by severe pain and limping, which may render the patient immobile. The onset is sudden, following little or no trauma, and examination discloses a painful, guarded, restricted range of hip motion. An acute slip is analogous to an epiphyseal fracture. In its unstable form, the patient is unable to bear weight, and there is a high rate of avascular necrosis. In its stable form, the sudden increase in displacement is painful, but limited weight bearing is possible and the risk of avascular necrosis appears to be lower.

B. Imaging Studies

Slipped capital femoral epiphysis can be difficult to detect on standard anteroposterior (AP) radiographs (Figure 11–14). A frog-leg lateral view is the best for detecting mild forms because slippage is always poste-

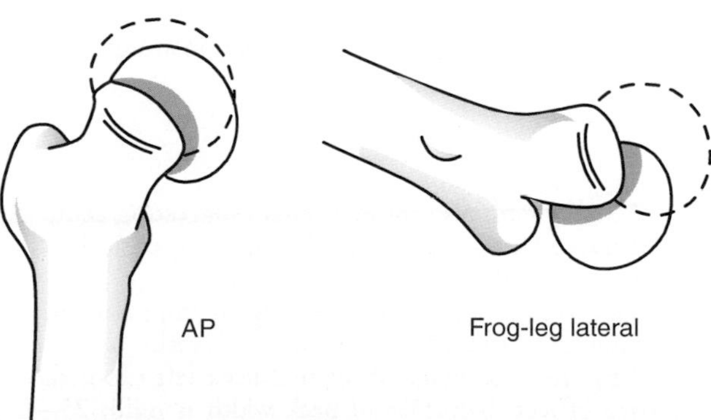

Figure 11–13. Anteroposterior (AP) and frog-leg views of a slipped epiphysis. The dotted lines show the normal position of the femoral head.

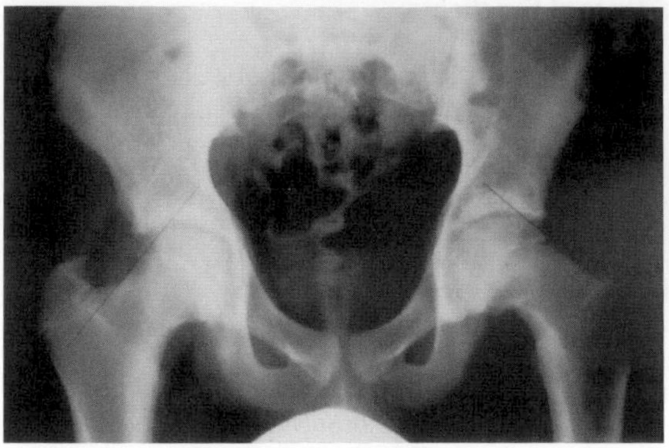

A

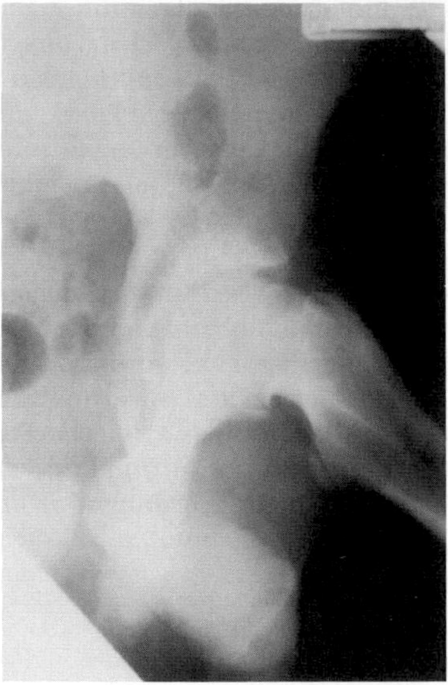

B

Figure 11–14. Radiograph diagnosis of left slipped capital femoral epiphysis. **A:** Anteroposterior film shows subtle medial displacement of left epiphysis, best appreciated by drawing a line (Klein line) along the lateral side of the normal and abnormal femoral neck. The slipped epiphysis does not protrude lateral to this line. **B:** Frog-leg lateral radiograph clearly demonstrates posterior displacement.

rior. A radiograph also shows changes suggesting acute or chronic forms, information that may be critical to management of the disorder.

Establishing the severity of slippage is important in determining treatment and prognosis. Severity is estimated by the percentage of femoral neck left exposed. Slippage of less than 25% of neck width is mild; 25–50% is moderate; and more than 50% is severe.

Treatment

Slipped capital femoral epiphysis is usually a progressive disease that requires prompt surgical treatment. Because the changes in the chronic form occur so slowly, it is impossible to manipulate the femoral head into a better position. Treatment consists of fixing the slip in its current position and preventing progression. This is done by inserting one or more screws or pins across the growth plate, regardless of the severity of the slip (pinning in situ).

Following surgery, aching rapidly resolves, and during the remaining 2–3 years of skeletal growth, the extent of remodeling of the distorted proximal femur may be considerable, leading to an improved ROM.

Acute slips, if unstable, may be gently reduced before fixation, but the risk of further damage to the tenuous blood supply of the proximal femur and subsequent avascular necrosis is always significant. For this reason, many surgeons accept the position of an acute slip and pin it in situ.

In some cases, high-grade slipped capital femoral epiphysis does not remodel sufficiently with growth, despite treatment. In these cases, a residual, chronically painful limp is present, requiring correction by proximal femoral osteotomy. The osteotomy site may be at the level of the slip, which is mechanically effective but relatively risky for the blood supply. Alternatively, osteotomy can be performed at the trochanteric level; this is a safer procedure for correction of the functional deformity but does not resolve the exact anatomic deformity.

Complications

A. Chondrolysis

In addition to the problems of impingement of the anterior metaphyseal prominence, which can impede motion, some patients with slipped capital femoral epiphysis develop chondrolysis, a poorly understood degeneration of the hip articular cartilage. It may be painful and may progress to severe joint narrowing and degenerative changes within 6 months.

During chondrolysis, cartilage is replaced by fibrous tissue, the joint capsule thickens and contracts, and joint motion is lost. Typically, the joint stiffens in flexion, abduction, and external rotation. Radiographs disclose joint narrowing, irregularity, and subchondral sclerosis, as well as regional osteoporosis from disuse.

Chondrolysis can result from iatrogenic malposition (permanent penetration) of pins or screws used for fixation of slipped capital femoral epiphysis. Although brief penetrations during surgery are probably common and cause no complications, unrecognized permanent pin penetration is disastrous. Chondrolysis also appears without obvious penetration and occasionally is detected in patients before treatment begins.

Chondrolysis is treated by nonsteroidal antiinflammatory medications (NSAIDs), aggressive physical therapy and ROM exercises, and observation. Capsular release is sometimes useful in resistant cases. Approximately half of patients eventually recover satisfactory painless motion. The other half may require hip fusion for symptomatic relief.

B. Avascular Necrosis

Patients with an acutely slipped capital femoral epiphysis can develop avascular necrosis of the femoral head (see section on developmental dysplasia of the hip). Because such patients are teenagers, the prognosis is poor, although some patients with partial head involvement regain a painless hip after a 1–2 years of symptoms. Some patients with painless but abnormal ROM may be treatable by intertrochanteric osteotomy to reorient the arc of motion. Long-term pain following avascular necrosis is treated by hip fusion.

C. Prognosis

A slipped epiphysis is a major cause of early osteoarthritis. In general, the higher the degree of slip, the earlier the degenerative changes begin. In fact, a statistical increase in degenerative arthritis is evident even in the radiographically normal hip of patients with a contralateral slipped epiphysis. This suggests that subclinical bilateral involvement is more common than recognized.

Loder RT, Greenfield ML: Clinical characteristics of children with atypical and idiopathic slipped capital femoral epiphysis: Description of the age-weight test and implications for further diagnostic investigation. J Pediatr Orthop 2001;21:481. [PMID: 11433161]

Perron AD, Miller MD, Brady WJ: Orthopedic pitfalls in the ED: Slipped capital femoral epiphysis. Am J Emerg Med 2002;20:484. [PMID: 12216050]

Tokmakova KP, Stanton RP, Mason DE: Factors influencing the development of osteonecrosis in patients treated for slipped capital femoral epiphysis. J Bone Joint Surg Am 2003;85-A:798. [PMID: 12728027]

FOOT DISORDERS

1. Metatarsus Adductus

Metatarsus adductus (metatarsus varus) is the most common foot deformity in the newborn infant, occurring in 5 in 1000 live births, frequently bilaterally. Although it is usually isolated, several apparently unrelated deformities (such as DDH) are statistically more likely to occur in the presence of this disorder. The cause is unknown but might be related to so-called uterine packing.

Clinical Findings

The hallmark of metatarsus adductus is medial deviation of the forefoot, with the apex of the deformity at the midtarsal region. The hindfoot is normal. A deep skin crease frequently is evident at the medial border of the foot, suggesting the deformity has been present for some time. The adducted forefoot usually can be passively corrected to a neutral position but occasionally is fairly rigid. When the examining physician places a hand on the forefoot so as to hide it, the ankle has full movement.

Treatment

Metatarsus adductus tends to be self-correcting. Even severe cases generally resolve by 12–18 months of age without treatment. Nevertheless, many orthopedists use passive stretching to reassure parents the child is being treated. Indeed, some evidence indicates that passive correction and serial plaster casting can speed resolution of the disorder. Recurrence after brief casting is frequent in young children, however, and treatment for metatarsus adductus is usually not recommended.

2. Congenital Clubfoot

Congenital clubfoot (equinovarus foot; talipes equinovarus) is a severe fixed deformity of the foot (Figure 11–15). It is characterized by fixed ankle plantar flexion

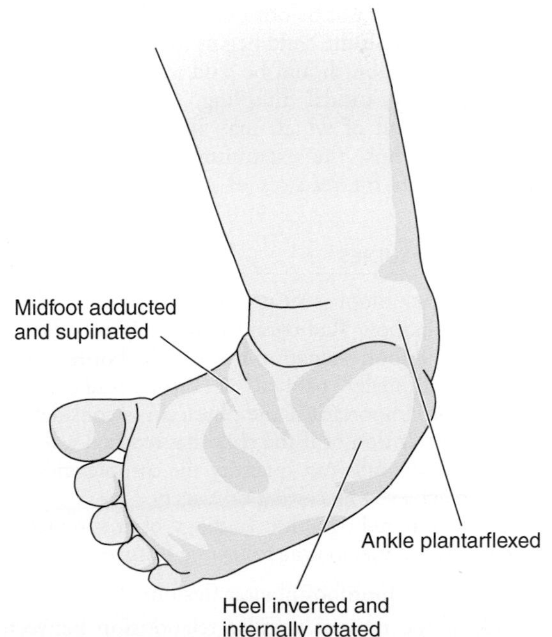

Figure 11–15. Clinical appearance of congenital right clubfoot.

(equinus), inversion and axial internal rotation of the subtalar (talocalcaneal) joint (varus), and medial subluxation of the talonavicular and calcaneocuboid joints (adductus). Severe cavus may be present, with a medial and plantar midfoot crease. Whether unilateral or bilateral, the deformity is more common in males, although when it occurs in females, it tends to be more severe.

The incidence in the newborn population is 1 in 1000, with increased risk for families in which even distant members have the deformity. There is considerable evidence that clubfoot is an inherited trait, but the disorder appears to reflect polygenetic expression, and exact inheritance patterns are unclear. Although most are isolated deformities and considered idiopathic, clubfoot may frequently be present in association with a wide variety of syndromes that affect the musculoskeletal system.

Clinical Findings

A. Symptoms and Signs

Clinical diagnosis of clubfoot is uncomplicated. Because it is a rigid deformity, clubfoot cannot be passively corrected the way metatarsus adductus can. Frequently, the foot is so severely internally rotated and inverted that the sole faces superiorly. Occasionally, the plantar flexion of the ankle is not obvious because the posterior tip of the calcaneus is small, high, and difficult to palpate. Clubfoot is always associated with a permanent decrease in calf circumference related to fibrosis of the calf musculature. This may not be obvious at birth but becomes more apparent after the child begins to walk.

Special attention should be paid to the presence of spine deformity, caudal dimpling, or midline spinal hairy patches, all of which may imply a neurogenic component. Thus, the examining physician should carefully search for features of other deformities or syndromes.

B. Imaging Studies

Increasingly, clubfoot is suspected from prenatal ultrasound examination. Radiographs are rarely of value in the initial clubfoot evaluation because the bones of the foot are minimally ossified at birth. Radiographs become more important if the physician is considering surgical intervention or if the child has reached walking age, and radiographs can quantify the completeness of correction achieved by casting or surgery.

The typical radiographic findings of incompletely treated clubfoot include the following features:

1. presence of hindfoot plantar flexion;
2. lack of the normal angular relationship between the talus and calcaneus (so-called parallelism of talus and calcaneus); and
3. residual medial subluxation or displacement of the navicular on the talus and the cuboid on the calcaneus (Figure 11–16).

Treatment

A. Conservative Treatment

Clubfoot always requires treatment, which should begin at birth. The initial approach is passive manipulation and positioning to the corrected position. In the United States, the majority of orthopedists use serial manipulation and casting, usually at 1-week intervals in the first month of life, and at 1- to 2-week intervals thereafter. In other parts of the world, strapping (with adhesive tape) or splinting with a variety of braces are popular methods (in addition to serial casting) for maintaining the manipulated correction. When casting is performed, there is agreement that specific techniques are more likely to be successful (Ponseti method). Even when the deformity responds to casting, there is usually sufficient Achilles tightness that a heel cord lengthening needs to be done at 4 weeks or later to facilitate cast correction.

The combination of careful casting and limited release allows most clubfeet to be corrected adequately, and long-term bracing for a year or more maintains the correction until the child is walking well. When satisfactory correction is not obtained, more extensive surgery is necessary. Although nonoperative treatment may be conceptually similar to training a bonsai tree, in that the joints are carefully held in a corrected position during growth, the analogy is limited. In clubfoot, the ligaments and joint capsules are severely contracted and thickened and, unlike supple tree limbs, may not stretch despite carefully executed manipulation and casting. In addition, the manipulation that encourages tension in these shortened ligaments may produce damaging compressive forces on delicate cartilaginous anlages of future tarsal bones. For these reasons, many surgeons limit nonoperative treatment to 12 weeks and then reassess the degree of correction attained. If clinical and radio-

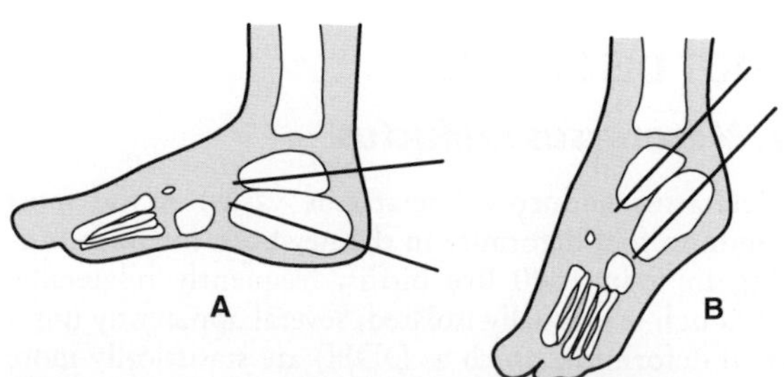

Figure 11–16. Diagrammatic appearance of radiograph in clubfoot. **A:** Normal foot. **B:** Clubfoot.

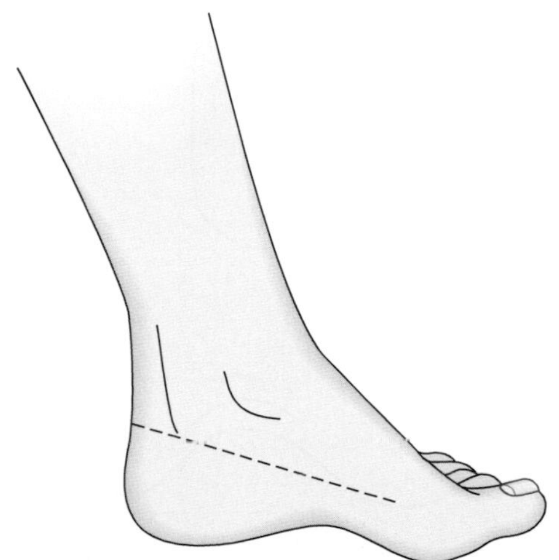

Figure 11–17. Cincinnati incision used for surgical correction of clubfoot.

logic evidence indicates significant correction, casting continues. Otherwise, surgery is required. Failure of nonoperative treatment is common, particularly in girls (where the deformity is often more severe) and in bilateral cases.

B. Surgical Treatment

Surgical correction of all clubfoot deformities is generally performed in one stage. At times, the casting corrects most of the midfoot deformity, and simple posterior release (ankle capsulotomy and Achilles tendon lengthening) are all that is required. Frequently, the surgeon must consider correction of the entire group of deformities through a comprehensive, extensive surgical approach.

One common approach uses the so-called Cincinnati incision, which extends from the navicular bone medially, around the superior portion of the heel, to the cuboid bone laterally (Figure 11–17). During surgery, the medial posterior tibial neurovascular bundle must be identified and protected. The tendons of the posterior tibialis, flexor digitorum longus, flexor hallucis longus, and Achilles tendon are Z-lengthened. The capsules of the talonavicular joint, subtalar (talocalcaneal) joint, and posterior ankle joint are released to allow repositioning of the bones of the hindfoot and midfoot.

The navicular is usually subluxated medially on the head of the talus and must be repositioned onto its normal location. The calcaneus is both inverted and internally rotated on the talus. This is corrected by manually derotating the subtalar joint and tilting the calcaneus back into a neutral position. These corrections are usually held in place after reduction by inserting small K-wires, which are removed after 4–6 weeks.

The ankle is repositioned by dorsiflexion to neutral prior to repair of the lengthened Achilles tendon. Postoperative casting allows the gaping capsule to reform with the bones of the clubfoot in their appropriate, corrected position.

C. Complications

Early complications of clubfoot surgery are rare, but the rate of recurrence within 3 years is 5–10%. Mild recurrence of deformity is fairly common, and even when deformity is permanently corrected, the foot always remains smaller and stiffer than normal and calf circumference is reduced. Families must be informed of this possibility early in treatment so they have realistic expectations about the outcome.

If surgical release is too aggressive, overcorrection with late heel valgus and an overlengthened heel cord can occur. There is broad agreement that a slightly underreleased clubfoot is much more functional that an overreleased one, and the trend to less surgery and more conservative treatment is currently strong.

Dobbs MB, Morcuende JA, Gurnett CA et al: Treatment of idiopathic clubfoot: An historical review. Iowa Orthop J 2000;20:59. [PMID: 10934626]

Herzenberg JE, Radler C, Bor N: Ponseti versus traditional methods of casting for idiopathic clubfoot. J Pediatr Orthop 2002;22:517. [PMID: 12131451]

3. Calcaneovalgus Foot

Calcaneovalgus foot is generally considered a uterine-packing problem in which the foot is markedly dorsiflexed at birth so the dorsum of the foot sits against the anterior surface of the tibia (Figure 11–18). The hind-

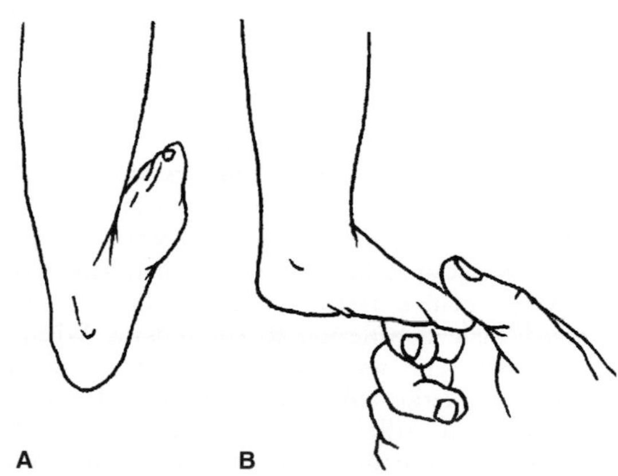

Figure 11–18. Calcaneovalgus foot as it appears in relaxed position (**A**) and maximally plantar flexed (**B**).

foot is usually in moderate eversion (valgus) as well. Although some flexibility is present with the deformity, there is resistance to full motion, and most cases do not allow ankle plantar flexion beyond a right angle.

Despite its dramatic appearance, calcaneovalgus foot corrects spontaneously within 2–3 months. Although some orthopedists brace or apply serial casts and many recommend stretching exercises, all true calcaneovalgus feet resolve without treatment.

Congenital Vertical Talus

Calcaneovalgus foot must be differentiated from a much rarer condition known as congenital vertical talus (congenital rocker-bottom foot, congenital complex pes valgus). In this deformity, although the foot appears to lie against the anterior tibia, the hindfoot is actually plantar flexed because of contracture of the posterior calf muscles. To accommodate plantarflexion of the hindfoot and dorsiflexion of the forefoot, the midfoot joints (talonavicular and calcaneocuboid joints) must subluxate or dislocate dorsally.

Congenital vertical talus often accompanies genetic disorders, syndromes such as arthrogryposis, or neuromuscular disorders such as spina bifida. It is occasionally found in otherwise normal infants, however. Treatment is usually surgical, and casting does not resolve the disorder.

4. Cavus Foot

Cavus foot is a foot with an abnormally high arch. Although it is difficult to ascribe a particular threshold of arching beyond which treatment is necessary, most deformities are dramatic enough to make diagnosis straightforward (Figure 11–19).

Cavus foot frequently accompanies hindfoot varus deformity (cavovarus foot), and there may be clawing of the toes and demonstrable weakness of ankle or foot muscles. In addition, calluses beneath the metatarsal heads and heel skin are common.

Clinical Findings

One of the most common symptoms of cavus foot is anterior ankle pain, sometimes associated with toe walking. This paradoxical situation occurs because of the pathologic anatomy of the cavus foot. The forefoot is severely plantar flexed on the hindfoot, requiring marked ankle dorsiflexion to compensate. When the cavus becomes too severe, ankle dorsiflexion is blocked, leading to anterior ankle impingement and pain. The inability to dorsiflex further compromises forefoot clearance, and, eventually, only the metatarsals can contact the floor. This can be misinterpreted as ankle plantarflexion contracture, leading to unnecessary (and possibly harmful) heel cord release.

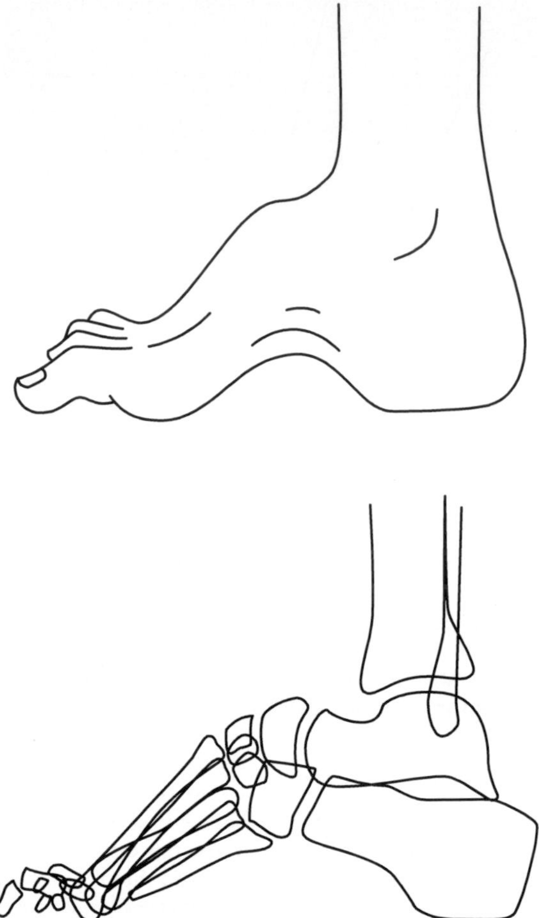

Figure 11–19. Cavus foot: clinical appearance and radiographic appearance.

The cause of cavus foot is usually muscle imbalance in a growing foot. Thus, cavus is rarely found in early childhood but is fairly frequent after 8–10 years of age. Although intrinsic muscle weakness is a major cause of cavus foot, weakness of the peroneal or anterior tibialis muscles is also implicated. Cavus foot is rarely found in the absence of an underlying neuromuscular condition.

Cavus foot is a marker for neuromuscular disease. Diagnosis requires a thorough search for the underlying cause and may require neurologic consultation, spinal MRI, and electromyographic (EMG) studies. Table 11–6 lists common neuromuscular causes of cavus foot.

Treatment

Conservative treatment of cavus foot includes accommodation by shoe modifications or inserts. These modalities

Table 11–6. Common neuromuscular causes of cavus foot.

Cerebral palsy
Charcot-Marie-Tooth disease
Compartment syndrome
Diastematomyelia
Friedrich ataxia
Muscular dystrophy
Spinal cord tumor
Spinal dysraphism (spina bifida)

do not actually correct the condition; severe deformity requires surgical correction by tendon transfers to restore muscle balance, by midfoot osteotomy to correct bony deformity, or by triple arthrodesis (hindfoot fusion in a corrected position).

Schwend RM, Drennan JC: Cavus foot deformity in children. J Am Acad Orthop Surg 2003;11:201. [PMID: 12828450]

5. Pes Planus (Flatfoot)

Flatfoot refers to loss of the normal longitudinal arch of the medial foot. Many cases of flatfoot are inherited, and a careful family history may uncover other persons with the condition. The foot is usually flexible, so the arch appears when the foot is not bearing weight. Hindfoot valgus (heel eversion) is often present. In severe cases, flatfoot may be painful, but this aspect of the deformity is often overemphasized.

Clinical Findings

Physical determination of the flexibility of the flatfoot requires careful examination. Subtalar motion is usually normal. In feet that exhibit a flat arch and valgus heel while standing, examination from the posterior aspect frequently discloses a normal arch and varus heel by muscle action when the patient stands on tiptoe. If these signs of a flexible flatfoot are not present, alternative diagnoses such as tarsal coalition (see section on tarsal coalition) should be considered. The physician should also look for painful plantar calluses.

Standing radiographs disclose loss of the normal medial longitudinal arch and may show mild lateral subluxation of the talonavicular joint as well. In severe chronic cases, degenerative talonavicular spurring may be present.

Treatment

Symptomatic treatment (shoe modifications, arch supports, and plantar inserts) is appropriate because no long-term treatment can alter the anatomic features of the disorder. Posterior tibial advancement, subtalar joint elevation or fusion, and elongation osteotomy of the lateral calcaneal neck may not provide reproducible, predictable resolution of the problem.

6. Tarsal Coalition

Tarsal coalition is a congenital connection between two or more tarsal bones. Coalitions may be fibrous, cartilaginous, or bony. Coalitions usually occur between two bones and are cartilaginous in early life but eventually ossify (or nearly ossify) as the foot matures. Frequently bilateral, coalitions often follow an autosomal-dominant inheritance pattern.

The most common sites for tarsal coalition are between the calcaneus and the navicular laterally (Figure 11–20) and between the talus and the calcaneus medially.

Clinical Findings

Symptoms of tarsal coalition may include foot pain and stiffness as the lesion begins to ossify during early adolescence. The resulting stiffness and abnormal intertarsal movement patterns in the hindfoot lead to progressive loss of subtalar motion and fixed valgus (eversion) of the heel. Tarsal coalition is often called peroneal spastic flatfoot because the peroneals appear to be protectively overactive. As the lesion matures, pain may diminish but stiffness increases, and the abnormal valgus posture persists.

This diagnosis should be suspected in adolescents with foot pain, valgus heel, and decreased subtalar motion. Lateral anteroposterior and oblique radiographs of the foot confirm the diagnosis of calcaneonavicular coalition, but special subtalar radiographs (Harris views), CT scan, or MRI may be necessary to delineate medial talocalcaneal lesions.

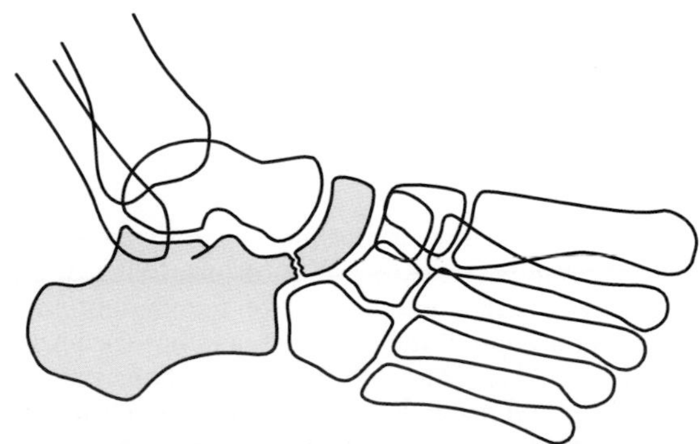

Figure 11–20. Calcaneonavicular tarsal coalition is best seen on oblique radiograph projection.

Treatment

Not all coalitions require treatment. The decision to initiate treatment depends on the severity of pain, stiffness, and fixed valgus. Conservative treatment consists of casting to reduce pain and peroneal spasm. If this fails, the coalition can be surgically resected and the resultant space filled with autologous fat or muscle to prevent recurrence. In late or neglected cases with pain or deformity, hindfoot fusion by triple arthrodesis is effective treatment for both symptoms.

Harris EJ, Vanore JV, Thomas JL et al: Clinical Practice Guideline Pediatric Flatfoot Panel. Diagnosis and treatment of pediatric flatfoot. J Foot Ankle Surg 2004;43:341. [PMID: 15605048]

7. Toe Deformities

Toe deformities occur as isolated conditions, in association with similar hand deformities, and as part of other syndromes. The more commonly found deformities are presented here, with mention of associated hand problems.

Simple Syndactyly

Simple syndactyly, a connection of two or more toes, is the most common toe deformity. The webbing is complete, or a proximal fraction of the web is absent. This disorder demonstrates a strongly familial inheritance pattern and causes no symptoms. It is rarely treated in the foot. In the hand, however, surgical separation is required to restore normal finger function.

Acrosyndactyly

Acrosyndactyly is joining of the tip of two or more toes distally with an open web. It is most commonly seen in conjunction with oligohydramnios, congenital soft-tissue constriction bands, and congenital amputations (Streeter dysplasia).

In the hand, acrosyndactyly interferes with independent finger function and should be treated surgically (usually at approximately 6–12 months of age). In the foot, it is usually asymptomatic and may be left untreated.

Polydactyly

Polydactyly is the presence of more than five digits on either the hands or the feet. It is frequently hereditary and often bilateral. Duplication of the thumbs may mirror duplication of the great toes, and both generally require surgical treatment. Both preaxial (duplication of medial toes and radial digits) and postaxial polydactyly (duplication of the lateral toes or ulnar digits) often accompany genetic syndromes and should prompt the physician to look for other symptoms.

8. Constriction Bands (Amniotic Bands)

During gestation, protein-laden amniotic material can condense around limb segments. These amniotic bands may indent delicate embryonic tissues, causing constriction rings or even necrosis and resorption of the distal segment (congenital amputation). Constriction bands may be isolated or associated with Streeter dysplasia. The syndactyly of Streeter dysplasia differs from simple syndactyly in that the distal, rather than proximal, web is obliterated (acrosyndactyly). It is thought to be an acquired, rather than hereditary, condition, caused by shearing of the delicate tips of the embryonic digits, followed by conjoined healing of distal digits.

Constriction bands may be very deep and circumferential and occasionally must be released surgically by Z-plasty immediately after birth to avoid postnatal necrosis. Usually, only half of the circumference of a band is released at one time, to protect any remaining blood supply in the other half. Reports of successful one-stage resection and Z-plasty of constriction bands suggest that the remaining blood supply is probably subfascial and interosseous.

9. Adolescent Bunions (Hallux Valgus)

Although bunion (prominence of the medial metatarsophalangeal joint of the great toe) is rare in children, this troublesome deformity often requires treatment. It is frequently hereditary, usually seen in early adolescence, and almost always found in conjunction with a wide forefoot caused by varus (medial deviation) of the first metatarsal shaft (metatarsus primus varus). The wide forefoot allows severe lateral deviation of the great toe (hallux valgus), causing the prominent base of the great toe to rub against the inside of the shoe and create a painful bunion (Figure 11–21).

Although conservative measures may relieve discomfort, many adolescent bunions are progressive and require surgical management. Surgery must address each aspect of the deformity. The surgeon must trim the bunion, correct the varus angulation of the first metatarsal by osteotomy, and centralize and balance the hallux valgus by lengthening the adductor hallucis muscle. There is a fairly high incidence of recurrence of the deformity following surgery.

Johnson AE et al: Treatment of adolescent hallux valgus with the first metatarsal double osteotomy: The Denver experience. J Pediatr Orthop 2004;24:358. [PMID: 15205615]

TORSIONAL & ANGULAR DEFORMITIES OF THE KNEE & LEG

Torsional (rotational) and angular deformities are a major source of referrals to pediatric orthopedic surgeons (Figure 11–22). Most of these patients are young

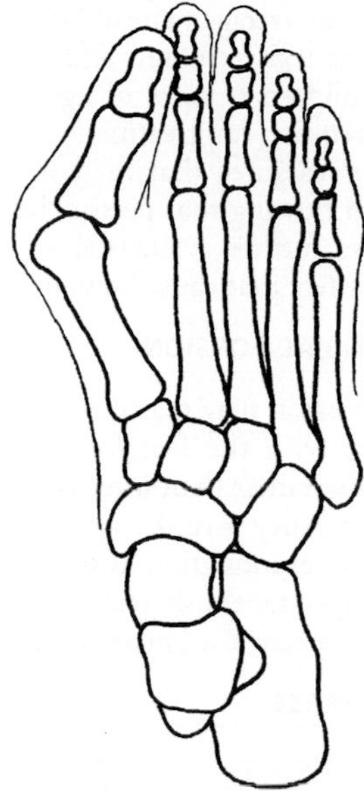

Figure 11–21. Adolescent bunion (hallux valgus) is generally accompanied by a wide forefoot with splaying of the first metatarsal (metatarsus primus varus).

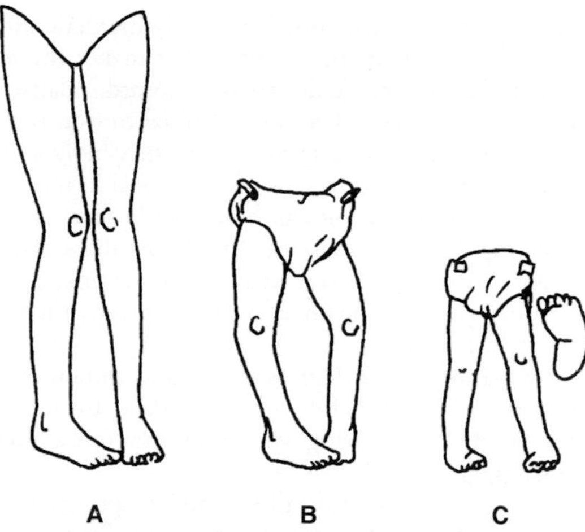

Figure 11–22. The major causes of clinical in-toeing include increased femoral anteversion (**A**), internal tibial torsion (**B**), and metatarsus adductus (**C**).

(less than 5 years) and have internal rotational deformities resulting in a so-called pigeon-toed gait.

The internal rotation, which can occur at the level of the thigh, leg (shin), or foot, is a cosmetic problem. Little evidence indicates that any of the so-called torsional deformities are harmful to the child or cause significant disability in the adult. Angular deformities (usually varus or valgus at the knee) are also usually benign, although careful evaluation and workup, including radiograph or other imaging modalities, occasionally disclose conditions requiring treatment. Nevertheless, most torsional and angular deformities are physiologic variations of normal anatomy, and they correct spontaneously over time.

Increased Femoral Anteversion

The normal femoral neck does not lie exactly in the frontal (coronal) plane but rather projects anteriorly from the plane at an angle called the angle of anteversion (Figure 11–23). Infants have anteversion of as much as 40 degrees, but this angle gradually reduces with growth, so normal adult femurs exhibit anteversion of 15 degrees. In some children, this gradual regression is slow or incomplete, causing the child to have excessive anteversion compared with an average child of the same age. This excessive anteversion produces a relative increase in internal femoral rotation. The clinical manifestation of this increased internal rotation and decreased external rotation of the hip is in-toeing during walking.

Observation of the walking child discloses internal rotation of the entire femur by the medial position of the patella. Although parents may consider this pigeon-toed gait unsightly, increased femoral anteversion is a normal variant that has no effect on function.

Increased femoral anteversion gradually decreases, with improvement in in-toeing, until 9 years of age. Subsequently, persistent in-toeing in the adult becomes more likely. Increased femoral anteversion requires no treatment.

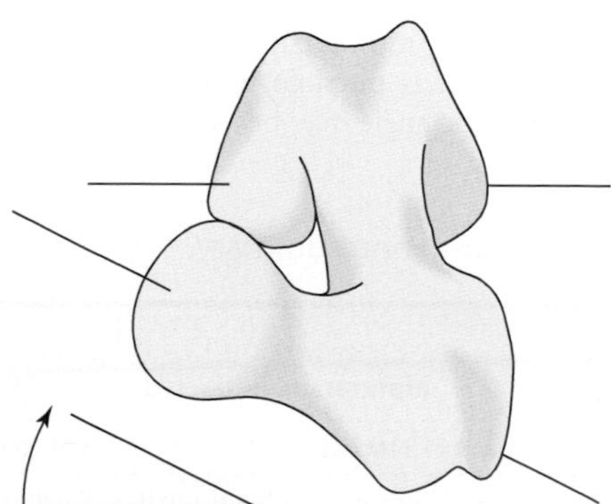

Figure 11–23. The angle of anteversion describes the inclination of the femoral neck forward of (anterior to) the frontal plane.

Internal Tibial Torsion

Some infants are born with a relatively dramatic internal twisting (torsion) of the tibia that makes the foot and ankle appear markedly rotated inward, relative to the axis of the knee. This internal tibial torsion is usually bilateral, frequently familial, and inevitably a normal variant in the wide torsional range seen in infants.

Internal tibial torsion can be clinically measured by comparing the bimalleolar axis (imaginary line connecting the medial and lateral malleoli of the ankle) with the frontal plane of the knee as determined by the position of the patella.

Torsion of 30–40 degrees is not uncommon in the newborn. When the child starts to walk, torsion can cause significant in-toeing, which, in turn, causes excessive tripping.

With growth, internal tibial torsion spontaneously resolves, and normal foot position and walking eventually occur. Some children improve by 24 months of age but may require up to 4 years for full resolution of the torsion. Internal tibial torsion requires no treatment. There is no scientific evidence that braces or shoe modifications alter the natural correction of the deformity.

Metatarsus Adductus

Metatarsus adductus may cause apparent in-toeing in the young child, leading to its inclusion as a torsional deformity. It is described in the previous section on the foot (Table 11–7).

Staheli LT et al: Lower extremity rotational problems in children. Normal values to guide management. J Bone Joint Surg AM 1985;67:39.

Bowlegs, Knock-Knee, & Genu Varum

Many infants have bilateral symmetric bowing of the legs, which may persist in the first 1–2 years of walking before developing into an exaggerated knock-kneed condition. The knock-knee is most dramatic at 3–6 years of age when it is known as physiologic genu valgum. At this time, the anatomic angle may be as high as 15 degrees of valgus. The genu valgum then gradually remodels spontaneously to the adult average value of 5–7 degrees of valgus.

Bowing of the legs in infants and excessive valgus of the knees in children 6 years of age are normal phenomena that require no treatment, although parents may have to be reassured that the condition is benign. The rare case of bowing that persists beyond 3 years of age may require further evaluation or treatment. Following are disorders that cause bowing.

A. Internal Tibial Torsion

Internal tibial torsion may masquerade as bowing when the child walks with the feet forward and the knees rotated externally rather than internally. As the laterally facing knees flex, they give the appearance of bowlegs. Careful physical examination discloses internal tibial torsion, which spontaneously resolves by 4 years of age. As the torsion corrects, the apparent bowlegs disappear.

B. Blount Disease

Also known as tibia vara, Blount disease is a poorly understood loss of medial tibial physeal growth that causes progressive bowing of the leg (Figure 11–24). It may occur as early as 3 years of age and can be bilateral or unilateral. If unilateral, the condition may be suspected earlier because it is obvious by comparison with the other leg. Excessive loading of the knee by early walking in heavy children with physiologic bowing of the legs may contribute to the development of Blount disease, but this is not proven. It occurs in all racial groups but is particularly common in blacks and Hispanic children.

Diagnosis of Blount disease is based on radiographic evidence of decreased medial tibial physeal growth. Later, the medial articular surface is distorted and the medial physis fuses. This allows progressive angular deformity to develop as the lateral growth plate continues elongating while the medial side is tethered.

Mild cases of Blount disease may improve spontaneously. Although some orthopedists recommend bracing to assist the process, there is no consensus that this is necessary or effective.

Table 11–7. In-toeing summary.

	Metatarsus Adductus	Internal Tibial Torsion	Internal Femoral Torsion (Increased Femoral Anteversion)
Age at resolution	12 months	3–4 years	9–10 years
Leg position	Femur and tibia normal	Patella forward; foot/ankle internally rotated	Patella internally rotated
Hip examination	Normal	Normal	Internal rotation exceeds external rotation

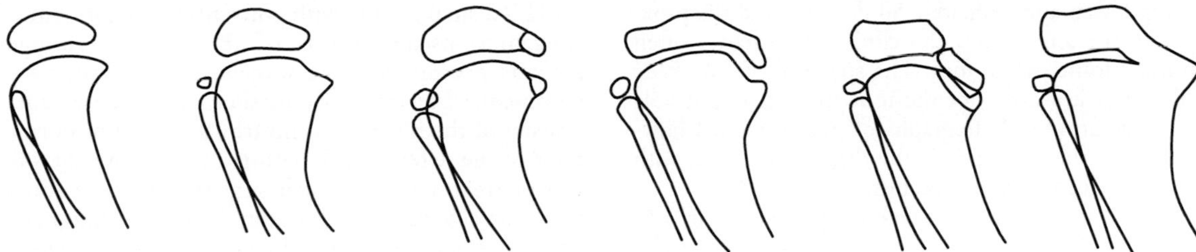

Figure 11–24. The Langenskiöld diagrammatic classification of radiographic changes in Blount disease (infantile tibia vara). The higher grades are associated with permanent closure of the medial tibial physis, which leads to progressive varus and internal rotation deformity with growth.

Severe or progressive cases of Blount disease require surgical correction by tibial osteotomy to regain the normal physiologic valgus angle of the knee. Surgery reduces the physiologic load on the medial tibial plateau and may allow normal growth. Slight overcorrection of the bowing often ensures load reduction, and the resulting valgus slowly resolves as the child grows.

Surgical treatment early in life is now popular, and many orthopedists recommend osteotomy after 3–4 years of age if radiographic changes are present. In early cases, surgical correction may cause reversal of the radiographic findings. Once physeal bridging occurs, however, there is no alternative to repeated surgical correction of angular deformity and leg-length inequality until growth ceases at maturity. Controlled studies of the issues involved in treatment of Blount disease by bracing and surgery are not available.

C. Rickets

Metabolic disorders of calcium intake can decrease the rate of calcification and ossification of physeal cartilage, causing the development of softer bones, so to speak, that are prone to bowing. Vitamin and calcium dietary supplements have virtually eliminated nutritional rickets in the United States. Hypophosphatemic rickets was discussed earlier in the section on metabolic bone disease.

Accadbled F, Laville JM, Harper L: One-step treatment for evolved Blount's disease: Four cases and review of the literature. J Pediatr Orthop 2003;23:747. [PMID: 14581778]

Ferrick MR, Birch JG, Albright M: Correction of non-Blount's angular knee deformity by permanent hemiepiphysiodesis. J Pediatr Orthop 2004;24:397. [PMID: 15205622]

Fraser RK et al: Medial physeal stapling for primary and secondary genu valgum in late childhood and adolescence. J Bone Joint Surg BR 1995;77:733.

Heath CH, Staheli LT: Normal limits of knee angle in white children—genu varum and genu valgum. J Pediatr Orthop 1993;13:259.

Langenskild A, Riska EB: Tibia vara (osteochondrosis deformans tibiae): A survey of seventy-one cases. J Bone Joint Surg Am 1964;46:1405.

Tibial Bowing & Pseudarthrosis

The tibia has a propensity to exhibit congenital angular deformities (bowing of the tibial shaft), which, although rare, are significant. The direction of the bowing is important in both diagnosis and prognosis and usually detectable at birth. Bowing direction is described by the apex of the bow, not the direction of displacement of the distal part (Figure 11–25).

A. Congenital Posteromedial Bowing of Tibia

Congenital posteromedial bowing of the tibia is a unilateral birth deformity of the distal fourth of the tibia. The apex of the bow is posteromedial, and often a skin dimple is present over the area. Because of the angle of

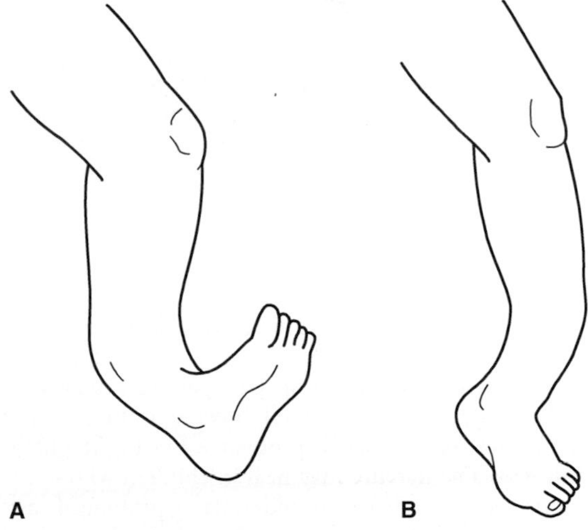

Figure 11–25. The major types of tibial bowing. **A:** Posteromedial bowing. The angulation spontaneously corrects, but with limb-length inequality. **B:** Anterolateral bowing. This disorder eventually progresses to spontaneous tibial fracture with resistant pseudarthrosis (see text).

bowing (often approximately 50 degrees) and the proximity to the ankle joint, the clinical appearance often mimics calcaneovalgus foot. The spatial position of the ankle joint, however, not the foot itself, is responsible for the deformity. Radiographs of posteromedial bowing disclose the curvature of the distal tibia, often with sclerosis in the underlying section of bone.

Despite its dramatic appearance, posteromedial tibial bowing corrects spontaneously in all cases. Some authors recommend casting to bring the dorsiflexed foot down to plantigrade position, but because the actual deformity is not related to the foot, this advice is not logical: Patients who are never casted resolve as quickly as those who are.

The tibial curvature remodels enough by 3 years of age that the limb appears cosmetically straight, although some bowing may be evident on radiograph for 5–8 years. All patients with posteromedial bowing are left with a leg-length discrepancy. At maturity, the involved limb is relatively as much shorter than the longer limb as it was at birth. Therefore, although the angular deformity needs no treatment, long-term follow-up and treatment of limb inequality is necessary in all cases.

Pseudarthrosis of Tibia

B. Congenital Anterolateral Bowing of Tibia and Congenital Pseudoarthrosis of the Tibia

Congenital anterolateral bowing of the tibia and congenital pseudoarthrosis of the tibia represent the other extreme of tibial bowing. For reasons not understood, anterolateral bowing in the distal third of the tibia and fibula is associated with inevitable progressive sclerosis and atrophy of the tibial shaft underlying the deformity. The ultimate fate of this atrophic abnormal bone is spontaneous fracture, which does not heal as readily as most fractures in children do (ie, pseudoarthrosis). Some children with this condition are born with a tibial fracture, whereas others simply have anterolateral bowing and sclerosis at birth, with fractures occurring up to 8–10 years of age. In approximately 30% of cases, coexisting neurofibromatosis is present.

All children with variations of this disorder require treatment. Because the prognosis is worse for those whose fracture occurs at a younger age, treatment methods vary. If anterolateral bowing is present but fracture has not occurred, protective bracing might be indicated. The fracture may heal in children whose first fracture occurs at 8 years or older, using prolonged casting or surgical bone grafting (with or without internal fixation).

Bone grafting in children whose fracture occurs before 3 years of age almost always fails, although repeated attempts to graft show some success.

The dismal results with conventional treatment of congenital pseudarthrosis of the tibia in younger patients prompted some surgeons to try innovative treatments. Electrical stimulation, free microvascular transfer of the fibula, and Ilizarov transport of normal bone to the defect are all reported to improve the success of treatment. So much surgery may be required to achieve a functional result, however, that many patients eventually undergo amputation to achieve rapid return to the normal functional activities of childhood.

Johnston CE: Congenital pseudarthrosis of the tibia: Results of technical variations in the Charnley-Williams procedure. J Bone Joint Surg Am 2002;84:1799. [PMID: 12377911]

Kim HW, Weinstein SL: Intramedullary fixation and bone grafting for congenital pseudarthrosis of the tibia. Clin Orthop 2002;405:250. [PMID: 12461381]

Morrissey RT: Congenital pseudarthrosis of the tibia: Factors that affect results. Clin Orthop 1982;166:21.

Ohnishi I et al: Treatment of congenital pseudarthrosis of the tibia: A multicenter study in Japan. J Pediatr Orthop 2005;25:219. [PMID: 15718906]

Tudisco C et al: Functional results at the end of skeletal growth in 30 patients affected by congenital pseudarthrosis of the tibia. J Pediatr Orthop B; 2000,9:94.

KNEE DISORDERS

1. Discoid Meniscus

The normal menisci of the knee are semilunar in shape and wedge shaped in cross section. They deepen the flat tibial articular surface to allow cupping of the rounded femoral condyles. The medial meniscus is longer and narrower than the lateral meniscus.

Rarely, the lateral meniscus remains congenitally round (or discoid) instead of acquiring its normal semilunar shape (Figure 11–26). This reduces its cupping function and may cause some instability of either the lateral compartment of the knee or hypermobility of the lateral meniscus itself.

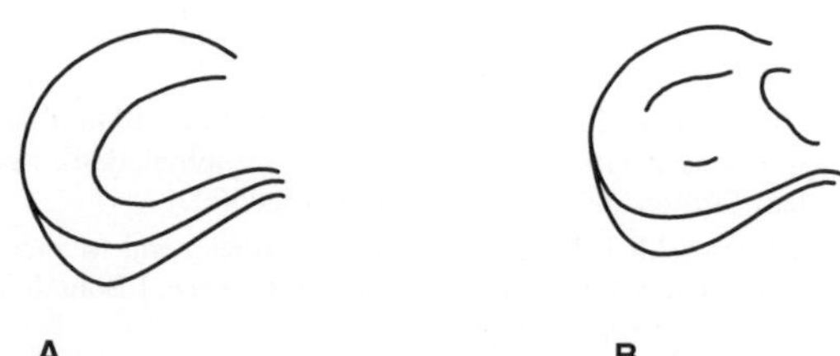

Figure 11–26. **A:** Normal lateral meniscus. **B:** Discoid lateral meniscus, which may cause clicking, effusion, or pain.

Clinical Findings

The classic physical finding of discoid meniscus is loud clicking over the lateral meniscus during flexion and extension of the knee. This clicking is usually painless but may be accompanied by aching or effusion. Physical exam may demonstrate an extension block. Discoid meniscus may be suspected on radiograph by widening of the lateral knee compartment, a subtle increase in subchondral sclerosis laterally, and convexity of the lateral tibial articular surface. Confirmation is attained on arthrography or MRI. The abnormal mechanical function of discoid lateral meniscus makes it susceptible to tears, particularly in children older than 10 years.

Treatment

In the past, symptomatic discoid menisci were treated by total lateral meniscectomy, but the resultant late degenerative knee changes dictate a far more conservative course. Current practice is to avoid treatment unless symptoms are significant and disabling. If treatment is required, the safest approach appears to be arthroscopic removal of the central portion of the discoid shape, thus sculpting the lateral meniscus into a roughly semilunar form.

Ahn JH et al: Discoid lateral meniscus in children: Clinical manifestations and morphology. J Pediatr Orthop 2001;21:812. [PMID: 11675561]

Kelly BT, Green DW. Discoid lateral meniscus in children. Current Opin Pediatr 2002;14:54. [PMID: 11880735]

Washington ER III et al: Discoid lateral meniscus in children. Long-term follow-up after excision. J Bone Joint Surg AM 1995;77:1357. [PMID: 7673286]

2. Chondromalacia and Internal Derangements of the Knee

Patellar chondromalacia and patellar subluxation are common in active adolescents, particularly in females who have small patellas and a slight exaggeration of knee valgus and quadriceps (Q) angle. Meniscal and ligament injuries are managed as in the adult, although these injuries are not as common in children.

A somewhat more conservative approach to suspect internal knee derangements is warranted in most children. The diagnostic accuracy of both physical exam and complex imaging studies (such as MRI) is surprisingly low in children. False-positive MRIs are particularly typical in children.

These disorders are described in Chapter 3, Musculoskeletal Trauma Surgery, and Chapter 4, Sports Medicine.

3. Osteochondritis Dissecans

Osteochondritis dissecans is a poorly understood disorder usually of the distal femoral condyle ossification center, although other joints (talus, elbow) can be affected. A portion of the joint surface softens, shears, or separates through the articular cartilage and underlying bone (Figure 11–27). This disorder is common, but not exclusive, in children 8–14 years of age; however, it is an infrequent problem in the adult.

The disease appears to be caused by a combination of two factors: (1) mechanical shearing or injury from activity and (2) femoral condyle susceptibility (fragility) resulting from immature ossification of the femoral condyle (which can be quite irregular in children). The importance of each factor depends on age. Athletic trauma seems more important in older children and adults, whereas in younger children, ossification defects render the femoral condyle more susceptible to minor repetitive injury.

Clinical Findings

A. Symptoms and Signs

Symptoms and physical findings can be highly variable. Younger children may have an asymptomatic radiographic abnormality of condylar fragmentation or may simply have a vague aching after strenuous activity. Older children and adults may have pain, effusion, and locking or catching if the affected fragment actually separates and becomes a loose body in the knee joint.

B. Imaging Studies

Plain radiographs show an irregular fragment of the surface that is usually sclerotic but may be osteopenic, and is usually on the lateral side of the medial condyle. It is often necessary to obtain tangential views of the condyle such as notch views. Occasionally, the defect is visible only on lateral projection. Contralateral comparison views should

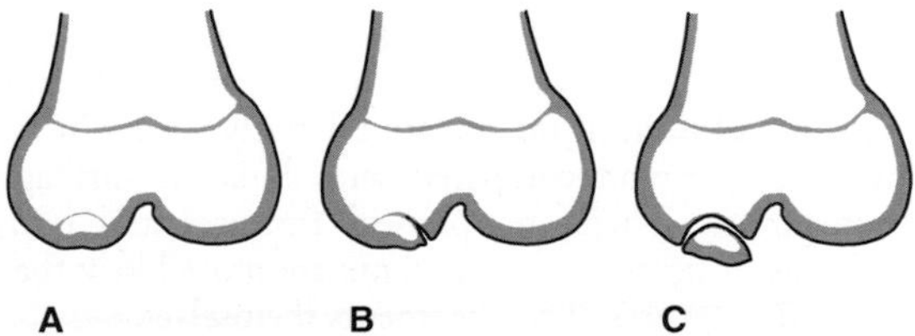

Figure 11–27. Various forms of the osteochondritis dissecans lesion found in children. **A:** Defect in ossification center without cartilage defect. **B:** Lesion with a hinged flap. **C:** Complete separation of bone and cartilage, which can lead to loose body in the knee joint.

always be obtained. So-called ossification defects that mimic osteochondritis dissecans may be normal ossification fronts, seen to be bilateral and symmetric.

In children older than 11–12 years, MRI or arthrography is used to determine whether the underlying bone alone is involved or whether there is an actual separation of overlying cartilage. Although these studies are helpful in refining treatment strategy in this age group, they are seldom useful in younger children.

Treatment

Young children with asymptomatic osteochondritis dissecans need not be treated because most of these lesions heal spontaneously. In preadolescents with symptoms or with large lesions seen on radiographs, simple immobilization with either a knee immobilizer or cylinder cast for 6 weeks frequently heals the defect and eliminates symptoms.

Sometimes immobilization is not effective, though. If the lesion is large and accompanied by cartilage separation or displacement, or if the skeleton has reached maturity, treatment may be the same as in the adult. This includes arthroscopic debridement and stabilization of the loose fragment using pins for internal fixation. Excision is less likely to result in a good result. The presence of open physes may necessitate modifications of standard adult techniques.

Hefti F et al: Osteochondritis dissecans: A multicenter study of the European Pediatric Orthopedic Society. J Pediatr Orthop B 1999;8:231.

Letts M, Davidson D, Ahmer A: Osteochondritis of the talus in children. J Pediatr Orthop 2003;23:617. [PMID: 12960624]

Wright RW et al: Osteochondritis of the knee: Long-term results of the excision of the fragment. Clin Orthop 2004;424:239. [PMID: 15241178]

4. Ligament & Epiphyseal Injury

Children who have not reached skeletal maturity have far fewer major ligament injuries of the knee than do older children and adults. Smaller children tend to participate in lower impact activities and sports, and their lack of muscle bulk (which increases during adolescence) limits body acceleration and the force of collision. In addition, ligaments are relatively strong in the immature skeleton compared with bone or cartilaginous physes. Therefore, physeal fractures and bony avulsions of ligament attachments are more likely than traumatic ruptures of the ligaments themselves.

Residual instability may occur in the child's knee after varus or valgus injury. In the adult, such instability is considered clinical evidence of ligament injury. In children, however, the physis rather than the ligament may be the site of failure. Instability can be caused by a physeal fracture that hinges open rather than the joint opening (Figure 11–28). It is usually clinically obvious that fracture is present, although stress radiographs may help in questionable cases.

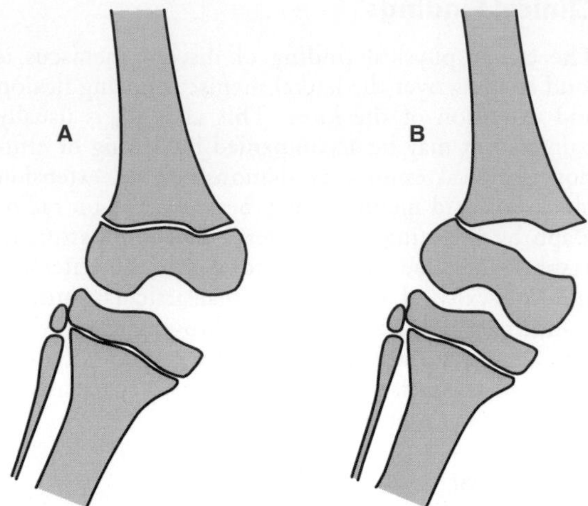

Figure 11–28. Stress radiograph of the unstable knee in an immature patient may reveal ligament rupture (**A**) or separation of the femoral physis (**B**).

Major intraarticular disruptions of the knee joint (meniscal tear or cruciate ligament injury) are rare in children. Detection may be delayed because symptoms may be less severe than in the adult and their presence not given as much weight in the differential diagnosis. Meniscus injury, particularly when peripheral, may lend itself to arthroscopic repair because of the excellent blood supply in children. Anterior cruciate rupture can be difficult to manage surgically in children because the anatomic sites of the tibial or femoral physes limit the options for reattachment. With the exception of cruciate injuries, most childhood knee ligament injuries are treatable by 2–4 weeks of splinting and return to function, as tolerated by pain. Physical therapy is rarely necessary in children younger than 15 years. A review of the major signs, symptoms, diagnostic procedures, and treatment options can be found in Chapter 4, Sports Medicine.

Not all effusions in the knee are traumatic, particularly in younger children. Because children at play are always suffering minor injuries, a history of injury may be inaccurate. The physician must remember to consider septic arthritis and pauciarticular juvenile rheumatoid arthritis in the differential diagnosis of effusion.

Beasley LS, Chudik SC: Anterior cruciate ligament injury in children: Update of current treatment options. Curr Opin Pediatr 2003;15:45. [PMID: 12544271]

Luhmann SJ: Acute traumatic knee effusions in children and adolescents. J Pediatr Orthop 2003;23:199. [PMID: 12649021]

OSGOOD-SCHLATTER DISEASE

The proximal tibial physis contains a transverse component that contributes to longitudinal growth and an anterior tongue that contains the attachment of the patellar tendon. In preadolescent and adolescent children (usually boys), the distal tip of this tongue may undergo fragmentation from chronic tensile stress, and enlargement from the resultant hyperemic response, which is known as Osgood-Schlatter disease. As the tibial tubercle becomes increasingly prominent, a painful bursa can form over it.

Clinical Findings

Symptoms vary from mild aching at the tubercle to severe pain with patellar function and exaggerated bursal tenderness. Radiographs of the lateral proximal tibia show the characteristic fragmentation (Figure 11–29).

Treatment

Treatment is symptomatic, including analgesics, knee pads to avert direct pressure, quadriceps stretching, avoidance of sports activities, and brief casting or splinting for painful cases. The disorder resolves spontaneously when the physis closes at skeletal maturity. No evidence indicates that physical activity within the limits of pain is harmful to the child with Osgood-Schlatter disease.

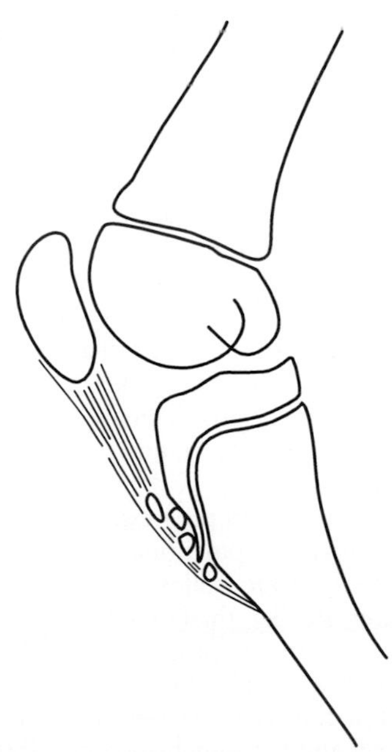

Figure 11–29. Osgood-Schlatter disease. The radiographs would show characteristic fragmentation of the tibial tubercle apophysis, similar to diagram.

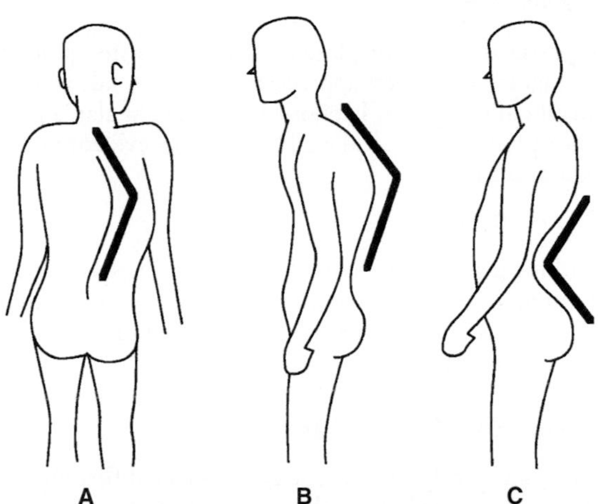

Figure 11–30. Definitions of spinal deformities. **A:** Scoliosis. **B:** Kyphosis. **C:** Lordosis. Frequently, a combination of deformities occur in individual patients (ie, kyphoscoliosis).

Krause BL et al: Natural history of Osgood-Schlatter disease. J Pediatr Orthop 1990;10:65.

SPINAL CURVATURE

Spinal curvature may occur in any age group and present with variable findings. Curvatures may be idiopathic, congenital, or accompany a wide variety of neuromuscular disorders, tumors, and infections. Curvatures may be small and nonprogressive or may worsen and require aggressive treatment. Sometimes, spinal curvature is the first clue to important underlying disease. Figure 11–30 shows the different types of spinal deformities.

Types of Curvatures

A. Scoliosis

Scoliosis is a lateral spinal curvature in the frontal plane, best appreciated by physical examination from the patient's back and by anteroposterior radiographs. Curvatures, which may be single or multiple, are described by the direction of their convexity. In a flexible spine, the presence of a single (more rigid) curvature can lead to physiologic compensatory curvatures in the opposite direction, above and below the primary curvature. True scoliosis always includes a rotational component that may not be fully appreciated on radiograph and generally includes a lordotic component as well (see section on lordosis). Surprisingly, lateral curvature is often undetected externally. The rotation of vertebrae that accompanies scoliosis is the physical feature that allows clinical detection.

B. Kyphosis

Kyphosis is a forward (flexed) curvature of the spine in the sagittal plane, best appreciated from the side and by lateral radiographs. If kyphosis is acutely angular, a posterior prominence called a gibbus may be evident in the sagittal plane.

C. Lordosis

Lordosis is a hyperextension deformity of the spine, most common in the lumbar spine but also often accompanying scoliosis. Lumbar lordosis may be secondary to flexion contracture of the hip.

Detection of Curvature

Although spinal curvatures may be detected first during routine radiograph, most lesions are best diagnosed by physical examination. Spinal examination should proceed according to the following specific protocol:

1. Place the patient in the standing position (Figure 11–31).
2. Check the level of the pelvis and look for obvious asymmetry of the rib, scapula, neck, and shoulder height (leg-length inequality can cause apparent scoliosis, which disappears when the short leg is elevated on blocks).
3. Level the pelvis by seating the child on a firm surface if the pelvis cannot be leveled while standing. This is the case in children with hip contracture from neuromuscular disease.
4. Have the child bend forward, carefully noting any asymmetric prominence of the lumbar paraspinous muscle, rib cage, or scapula, which suggests the rotational portion of scoliosis. The magnitude of asymmetry corresponds to the severity of the curvature, with convexity of the curvature directed toward the most prominent side.
5. From the side, check for prominence of the spine that might indicate kyphosis, both in the upright and forward-bending position.
6. Perform a careful neurological exam, including upper extremity reflexes and abdominal reflexes in addition to thorough lower extremity neurological examination.
7. Use radiographs to assess type, severity, and location of the curvature and to look for underlying lesions. Because primary scoliosis and kyphosis curvatures are always stiffer than uninvolved spine segments, bending radiographs may reveal which curvatures are "structural" and which are more flexible compensations (secondary curvature). The Cobb method is usually used to measure curvatures (Figure 11–32). The degree of tilt between the most affected vertebral end plates describes curvature magnitude.

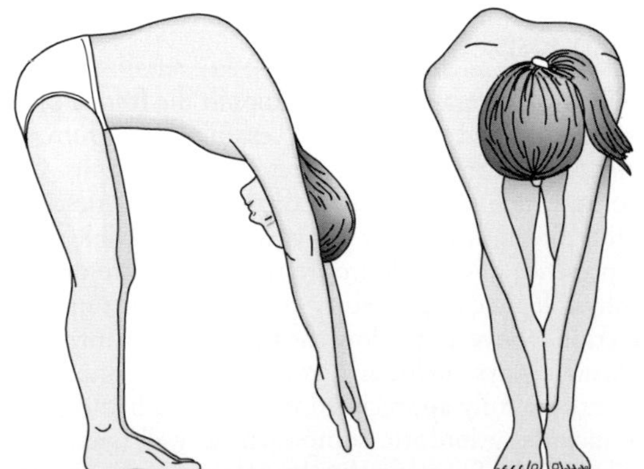

Figure 11–31. Examination of the spine for deformity is best carried out by observing for asymmetry and deformity as the patient bends forward (see text).

Scoliosis

A. Idiopathic Scoliosis

Idiopathic scoliosis has no apparent underlying cause. It is most common in early adolescent girls, although it can be found in either gender at any age. Adolescent idiopathic scoliosis typically is a convex curvature to the right in the thoracic portion of the spine (right thoracic curvature pattern). Patients with atypical curvature patterns and idiopathic curvature in younger children may require more extensive testing (eg, EMG, MRI) before the cause can be definitively designated idiopathic.

Many idiopathic curvatures progress in magnitude with growth and continue to do so until skeletal maturity. Therefore, the clinician must determine if the curvature is progressing and if the spine is still growing. Radiographs document progression, and observations of the ossification pattern of the iliac crest apophysis (Risser sign) are used to estimate skeletal maturity. This ossification pattern begins laterally at puberty and spreads medially across the ilium, capping and fusing with the bone at maturity.

Growing children with progressive curvatures should be treated. A variety of spinal braces is available to treat progression of idiopathic scoliosis. Children who mature with curvatures smaller than 35–40 degrees generally have no symptoms and no progression in adulthood. If a curvature progresses despite adequate bracing, surgery is the treatment of choice. Some curvatures are too rigid to brace effectively and can only be observed if they are relatively small. If curve magnitude exceeds 40 degrees, bracing is generally ineffective and surgical correction is the treatment of choice.

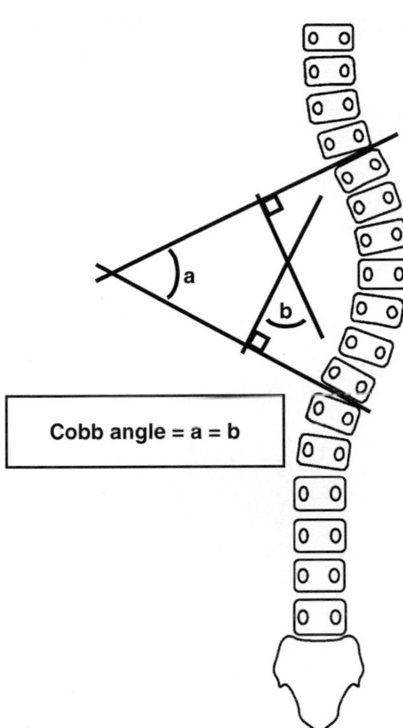

Figure 11–32. The Cobb method of measurement is commonly used to assess spinal curvature. It measures the angle between the far (top and bottom) endplates of the most inclined vertebrae. To allow the measurement lines to fit on the radiograph, lines at 90-degree angles to the endplates are often drawn, and their relative angles measured. Geometrically, these angles are the same.

Surgery for scoliosis corrects the deformity using metal rods that can be configured to push, pull, distract, or compress portions of the spine with curvature. The involved spinal segments are then fused together using iliac or allograft bone. Typically, a posterior fusion of the laminas and facets is sufficient for many cases of idiopathic scoliosis. Severe cases may also require anterior fusion through the thorax or retroperitoneal space.

B. Congenital Scoliosis

Congenital scoliosis is caused by malformations of vertebral shape. It does not refer to the age of the patient: Newborns can have idiopathic scoliosis, despite being born with spinal curvatures. Congenital vertebral malformations generally occur in early embryonic life (before 7 weeks) and are thought to represent errors in formation or segmentation of the spinal segments that originate from primitive mesenchymal condensations of embryonic cells (Figure 11–33).

Curvatures can originate when vertebral parts fail to form (eg, hemivertebrae, wedge vertebrae, butterfly vertebrae) or when embryonic somites fail to segment properly into individual vertebrae (eg, block vertebrae, unilateral unsegmented bar). Because of the embryonic timing of this process, children with congenital scoliosis frequently have abnormalities of other organ systems that form during the same embryonic period (eg, cardiac and renal systems).

Diagnosis of congenital scoliosis must be followed by a careful cardiac examination and by ultrasound or intravenous pyelography evaluation of the kidneys. Although neural tube damage is relatively rare, careful imaging of the spinal canal (MRI, EMG) may be required, especially if surgery is contemplated.

Congenital scoliosis may encompass one or many deformed vertebrae, and different types of vertebral abnormalities are often seen in the same patient. Sometimes, two deforming vertebrae cancel each other out, as it were, and no curvature is visible. For this reason, prediction of progression of the scoliosis depends on serial radiographs. If progression occurs, bracing is usually the first treatment, although surgery is indicated if progression is not halted by external means. Curvatures caused by unilateral unsegmented bars have such a strong tendency to progress that they should be treated by surgery as soon as they are detected.

C. Neuromuscular Scoliosis

Neuromuscular scoliosis includes a diverse group of curvature patterns that occur in association with various neuromuscular diseases. The cause varies with the disease. For example, scoliosis in children with cerebral palsy is usually caused by a combination of spasticity (overactivity of muscle) and weakness. Scoliosis in children with muscular dystrophy is the result of severe progressive muscle weakness that eliminates the paraspinous stability of the spinal column. Scoliosis in infants with spina

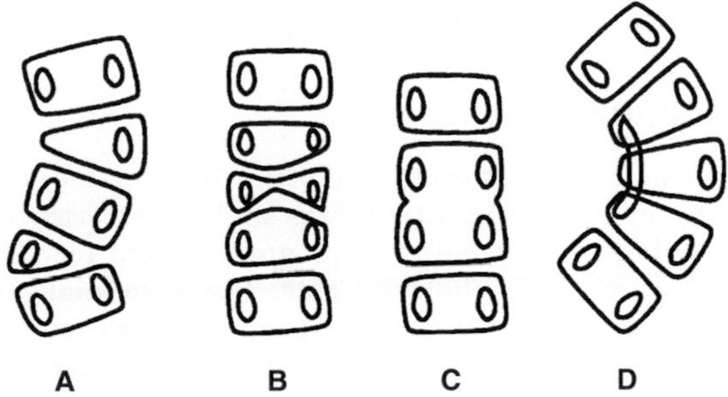

Figure 11–33. Vertebral anomalies of congenital scoliosis. **A:** Hemivertebra. **B:** Butterfly vertebra. **C:** Block vertebra. **D:** Unilateral unsegmented bar.

bifida (myelomeningocele) is frequently congenital (see previous discussion), related to loss of posterior elements, or associated with the development of a syrinx (central cystic fluid collection) in the spinal cord, a process similar to hydrocephalus.

Patients with neuromuscular scoliosis often develop curvatures at an early age, when surgical treatment is either impossible or would result in severe stunting of spinal growth. It is common to treat such children by daytime bracing, despite the fact that bracing alone is rarely sufficient to eliminate progression or the need for later surgery. In such cases, some surgeons feel that bracing may slow progression enough to allow additional skeletal growth, and spinal correction and fusion is postponed until puberty.

D. Other Scolioses

Childhood scoliosis can be associated with benign tumors of the spine, usually osteoid osteoma and osteoblastoma. Treatment of the tumor is usually curative, although long-standing lesions may require fusion as well.

Neurofibromatosis is associated with both scoliosis and kyphosis and characteristically leads to short high-grade curvatures requiring surgical treatment.

Dobbs MB et al: Prevalence of neural axis abnormalities in patients with infantile idiopathic scoliosis. J Bone Joint Surg Am 2002; 84:2230. [PMID: 12473713]

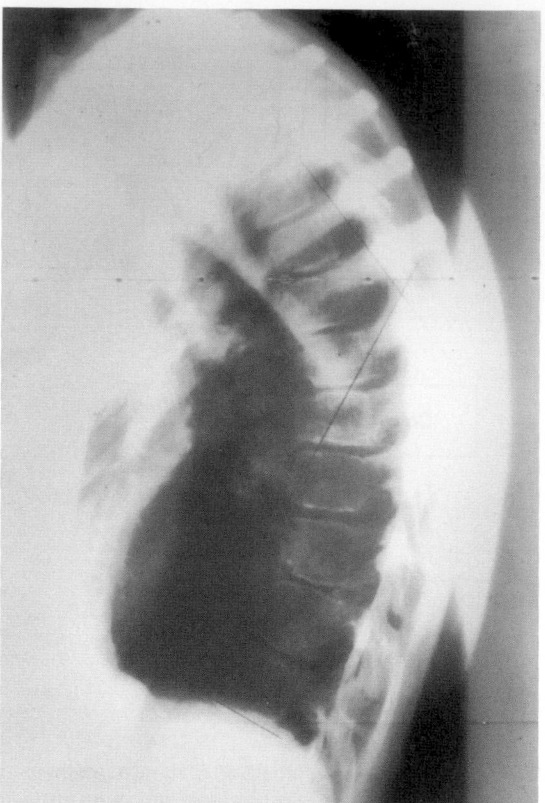

Figure 11–34. Scheuermann kyphosis is characterized by vertebral wedging, endplate changes, and kyphosis.

Kyphosis

Kyphosis may be congenital, traumatic, or acquired. Some patients with kyphosis need no treatment, whereas others require immediate surgical attention.

A. Postural Kyphosis (Postural Roundback)

Postural kyphosis, a variation of normal posture, is a cosmetic problem. There is no associated underlying disease, and the spine is flexible and capable of hyperextension. Although it may be worrisome to parents, little scientific evidence indicates that it requires, or responds to, treatment.

B. Scheuermann Kyphosis

Scheuermann kyphosis is a disorder of growth of the vertebral end plates that affects adolescents, particularly boys, and produces a progressive rigid forward curvature of the thoracic spine. Less commonly, it involves the lumbar spine, causing decreased lumbar lordosis (relative kyphosis). It is often moderately painful. Radiographs show wedging of vertebral bodies, irregularity of the endplates with radiographic lucent pits known as Schmorl nodules, and kyphosis (Figure 11–34).

Lumbar Scheuermann kyphosis responds to symptomatic treatment with nonnarcotic pain medications or a supportive lumbar corset. Thoracic involvement with pain or kyphosis of 15–20 degrees greater than normal can be managed with a Milwaukee brace. Brace treatment is usually effective in controlling pain and producing structural correction of the kyphosis. It can sometimes be used at night only so it will not have to be worn during school hours.

Scheuermann disease is the exception to the general rule that spinal bracing must be done during the growth phase to improve deformity. Patients as old as 18 years of age show improvement with the Milwaukee brace. Severe cases (40 degrees excessive kyphosis) may require surgical correction by spinal instrumentation and fusion.

C. Congenital Kyphosis

Congenital kyphosis is a rare but important group of diseases, which, like congenital scoliosis, may be caused by failure of formation of vertebrae (hemivertebrae) or failure of embryonic segmentation (anterior unsegmented bar). In most cases, the lesion tends to cause uneven growth, so kyphosis gradually increases as the spine elongates. This can produce bowstringing of the spinal cord over the kyphotic prominence and eventually cause paraplegia. For this reason, any progressive congenital kyphosis must be fused to prevent neurologic complications, regardless of the child's age.

D. Traumatic Kyphosis

Traumatic kyphosis is a traumatic compression of vertebrae that may lead to either cosmetic or symptomatic kyphosis. This may be prevented by early surgical stabilization of high-grade unstable traumatic spinal injuries.

E. Infectious Kyphosis

Infectious kyphosis refers to septic destruction of vertebral bodies, which can lead to severe kyphosis. In particular, tuberculous vertebral osteomyelitis can produce soft-tissue abscess, high-grade kyphosis, a sharp gibbus, and paraplegia. Bacterial infection can mimic this, although dramatic deformities are far more unusual.

Treatment includes chemotherapy, surgical debridement and drainage, decompression of the spinal cord, and spinal fusion to prevent further deformity.

Treatment

A. Bracing

Bracing can be used to slow progression of spinal curvatures, prevent progression, or improve underlying structural deformities. Many different types of braces are available, each with its own advocates and specific applications (Figure 11–35). When the goal is to provide postural support, slow progression, or postpone (but not prevent) surgery, a polypropylene body jacket, or so-called clamshell brace, may suffice for waking or sitting hours.

Long-term braces designed to arrest progression must be custom molded for the patient, with pads placed to exert appropriate pressure to reduce deformity. Depending on the anatomic level of the curvature, they may be positioned under the arm or may extend to the neck (Milwaukee brace). This type of brace is usually worn 24 hours a day.

All braces must be modified or replaced to accommodate growth. In general, bracing is only effective with flexible curvatures in growing children.

B. Surgical Treatment

Surgical intervention is indicated for curvatures that progress despite adequate conservative treatment (usually bracing). It is also required when spinal compression is imminent (tuberculous kyphosis, congenital kyphosis) or when a curvature is so severe that bracing is impossible and future progression likely.

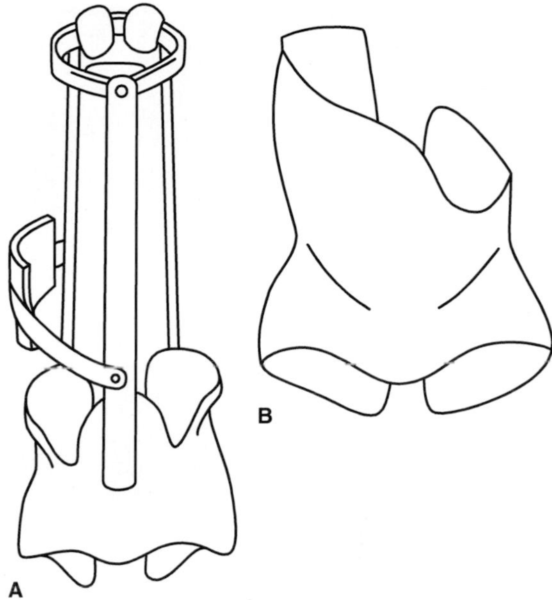

Figure 11–35. Two popular brace styles used for the treatment of spinal deformity are the Milwaukee brace (**A**) and the low-profile (Boston-type) brace (**B**).

1. Surgical stages—Surgery involves two separate stages: correction and stabilization. After posterior exposure of the spine, correction is achieved with a variety of mechanical internal fixation devices. These are usually rods with hooks, screws, wires, or other mechanisms to distract, compress, or bend spinal segments. Correction is rarely complete because mechanical and safety considerations limit the force that can be applied. Once correction is obtained, the cortex of spine is removed and bone graft is placed over the raw bone. Subsequently, solid fusion occurs within 6 months, permanently stabilizing the spine (Figure 11–36).

2. Treatment of severe curvatures—For small curvatures, posterior instrumentation and fusion are sufficient. Some large idiopathic curves and neuromuscular curves require anterior release and bone grafting to render enough acute flexibility for curvature correction and enough late stability for dependable fusion. Occasionally, fusion may fail, causing a pseudarthrosis that may be painful or may allow progression of a previously corrected curvature. In this case, fusion must be repeated.

Lonstein JE: Adolescent idiopathic scoliosis: Screening and diagnosis. Instr Course Lect 1989;38:105. [PMID: 2649563]

Danielsson AJ, Nachemson AL: Radiologic findings and curve progression 22 years after treatment for adolescent idiopathic scoliosis: Comparison of brace and surgical treatment with

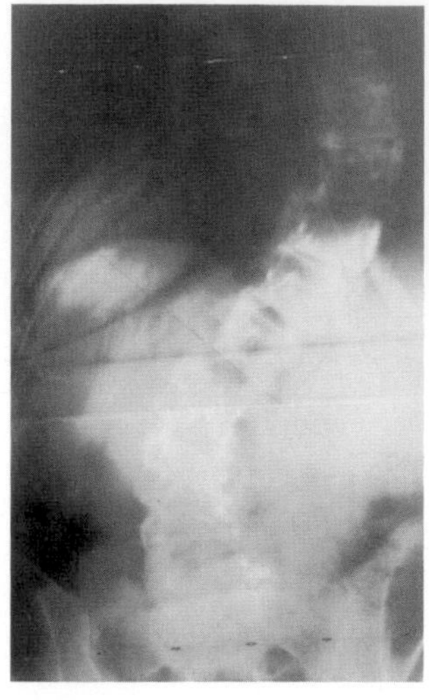

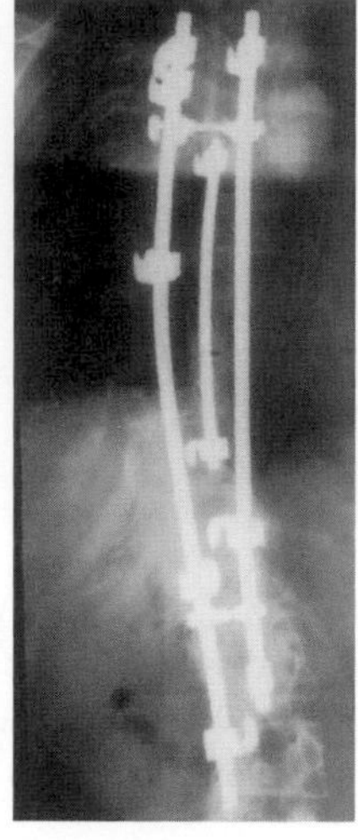

A B

Figure 11–36. Treatment of a scoliotic curve by instrumentation and fusion. Preoperative view (**A**) and postoperative view (**B**).

matching control group of straight individuals. Spine 2001;26:516. [PMID: 11242379]

Weinstein SL, Ponseti IV: Curve progression in idiopathic scoliosis. J Bone Joint Surg Am 1983;65:455. [PMID: 6833318]

NEUROMUSCULAR DISORDERS

Because muscle weakness or imbalance changes the underlying structure of a growing skeleton, neuromuscular diseases of children often require orthopedic evaluation. Treatment may be required to reverse skeletal deformity and contracture or to effect functional improvement.

Many childhood neuromuscular diseases require coordinating the services of the pediatrician, neurologist, physiatrist, therapist, educator, social worker, nurse, and parent.

1. Cerebral Palsy

Cerebral palsy is a static encephalopathy in a growing child. Although it is often birth related, the term also includes childhood head injury, stroke, metabolic brain conditions, and degenerative neurologic conditions.

The challenges to physicians evaluating cerebral palsy are making an accurate diagnosis and detecting correctable conditions. It is essential that functional evaluation of the child's condition take into account the need for education, communication, socialization, and mobility.

Types of Cerebral Palsy

The hallmark of most cases of cerebral palsy is alteration in motor tone (spasticity or dystonia). Spasticity is increased tone associated with stretching of muscle; dystonia is present without changing muscle length. Diagnosis of spasticity can be direct (increased tone, increased deep tendon reflexes, clasp-knife rigidity, and clonus) or inferred (shortening of muscles, contractures of joints, joint dislocations, and scoliosis). Dystonia can be confused with spasticity, but it does not generally lead to contractures.

A. Hemiplegia

Hemiplegia is spasticity involving only one side of the body. Most hemiplegia involves the pyramidal tract, especially at the cerebral cortex. It may be mild or severe and typically is more pronounced in the distal skeleton (hand and foot-ankle). Hemiplegia is usually caused by congenital loss of portions of the parietal, contralateral cerebral cortex. This loss may reflect vascular insufficiency, trauma, or porencephalic cysts.

Many patients with hemiplegia have normal development and intelligence. Children with hemiplegia frequently walk at a normal age, although sometimes with marked posturing of the involved side. Right hemiplegia (left cerebral cortex) may involve the Broca area and thus cause speech deficits. Because sensory and motor cortex areas are contiguous, hemiplegia is strongly associated with abnormalities of sensation and proprioception in the affected limbs. This may prove more disabling than the spasticity because a child may not appreciate an insensate limb as part of overall body image.

B. Diplegia

Diplegia, or diplegic cerebral palsy, is an encephalopathy usually associated with prematurity. It is characterized by relatively symmetric involvement of the lower extremities and lesser involvement of the upper extremities. Prematurity is often accompanied by intracerebral hemorrhage and periventricular leukomalacia, which lead to edema and necrosis in the region of the trigone. This involvement of the pyramidal tract and associated basal ganglia is the main cause of diplegia.

Most diplegic children exhibit mixed patterns of spasticity with a variety of less obvious neurologic symptoms, including ataxia, rigidity, and athetosis (dystonia). Many have normal intelligence (if the cortex is spared) but may suffer developmental delays caused by damage to associative fibers in the brain. Although they may initially be hypotonic ("floppy"), most diplegic patients develop high tone (dystonic rigidity) and spasticity by 12–18 months of age.

Diplegia, usually more severe in the lower extremities, is relatively symmetric. Many children with diplegia eventually walk, exhibiting a crouching gait characterized by flexed, internally rotated hips, flexed knees, and plantar-flexed ankles.

C. Quadriplegia

Quadriplegia (total body involvement) often occurs in children who suffer birth asphyxia, metabolic encephalopathy, or encephalitis. Severe spasticity, seizures, mental retardation, joint contractures, and scoliosis are typical but not always individually present in this type of cerebral palsy. Children with quadriplegia are particularly susceptible to spontaneous hip dislocations (because of hip muscle imbalance) and high-grade scoliosis. Both of these conditions interfere with sitting and may require surgery. Most quadriplegic patients require wheelchair assistance and do not walk.

D. Mixed Neurologic Involvement

Mixed neurologic involvement of extrapyramidal portions of the brain can cause athetosis, dystonia, ballismus, and ataxia. Many children with cerebral palsy exhibit subtle signs of some of these disorders, in addition to spasticity. In some children, one of these signs may predominate, but spasticity is absent. In general, prognosis varies with the anatomy of involvement.

Treatment

Before treating cerebral palsy, specific goals should be set for the patient. Although many important goals are not orthopedic, the surgeon may help the patient achieve them. Increased mobility, for instance, may facilitate achieving a variety of nonorthopedic goals. Especially urgent are the patient's ability to communicate, move independently, and socialize. Orthopedic treatment may improve sitting position in the wheelchair or improve walking by releasing muscles or joints.

Many children benefit from physical or occupational therapy during the first few years of life. Although the exact role of such therapy in cerebral palsy remains undefined, therapists often help parents and children deal more effectively with the complex problems presented by the disease. Therapists also help parents and children set optimistic and realistic goals for the future.

Bracing or surgery may be required to control effects of spasticity on individual joints and to decrease spasticity, correct dislocation or contracture, or control scoliosis. Surgery is ineffective in the case of extrapyramidal neurologic symptoms. A variety of nonorthopedic treatments are also used for cerebral palsy. Selective dorsal rhizotomy, a neurosurgical procedure to cut a portion of the posterior roots of the lumbar spinal cord, may reduce spasticity in selected patients by interrupting the reflex arc. Botulinum toxin injection (or phenol injection) into the motor endplate region of a muscle temporarily interrupts the nerve supply, relaxing a spastic muscle for several months and allowing therapy or other evaluation. Oral baclofen can reduce overall spasticity. Intrathecal baclofen, delivered by a subcutaneous pump, may offer relaxation of troublesome lower extremity muscle tension in both dystonic and spastic patients.

Hip subluxation is common in quadriplegia, and pelvic radiographs in young quadriplegic patients are needed to detect early, reversible involvement. Subluxation may be treated in children younger than 3–4 years by adductor muscle release, which improves abduction. Rarely, the anterior obturator nerve (which innervates the adductor longus muscle) is resected to weaken the adductors. In older children, bony reconstruction by varus-derotation osteotomy and acetabular reorientation or supplementation may be necessary to correct the bone malformation that results from the force of spastic muscles on the growing skeleton. Children who develop hip subluxation often develop scoliosis as well (see section on scoliosis).

A. Adductor Release

Adductor release may be done as an open procedure (usually by myotomy or transverse sectioning of the adductor longus and a portion of the adductor brevis) or by percutaneous adductor tenotomy (section of the tendon origin of the adductor longus at the pelvis). The exact technique and amount of release is dictated by the severity of contracture and other factors. When done for hip subluxation, adductor release is most effective before 3–4 years of age. It should be sufficient to allow hip abduction of 70–80 degrees on the operating table. When frank subluxation is present, some surgeons perform an anterior obturator neurectomy in addition to the adductor myotomy. This open procedure removes a segment of the obturator nerve that supplies the released adductor longus muscle, so the muscle remains loose after spontaneously reattaching after surgery.

Obturator neurectomy must be used carefully because it can cause excessive weakening of the adductors and, subsequently, late hip abduction contracture. After each of these procedures, the patient is casted in abduction for 3–4 weeks to allow muscle healing in the new elongated position.

Dynamic spasticity or joint contracture (the result of chronic spasticity) can interfere with walking in children with hemiplegia or diplegia. This may be treated by bracing involved joints in a functional position or by surgical lengthening of the muscle–tendon unit. Such muscle releases can be done by complete tenotomy, tendon Z-lengthening (common at the Achilles tendon), or lengthening of the aponeurosis of a muscle, which is often done for the iliopsoas or hamstrings (Figure 11–37).

It is convenient to combine multiple procedures for children with cerebral palsy. For example, a typical hemiplegic with a tiptoe (equinus) gait may benefit from lengthening the Achillis tendon to make the foot plantargrade. A typical diplegic patient with a crouching gait may benefit from hip flexor, hamstring, and Achilles tendon lengthenings performed bilaterally during a single operation. The exact timing and extent of surgery

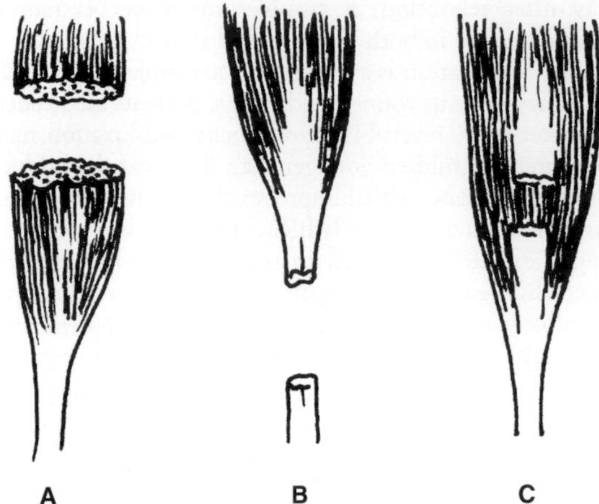

Figure 11–37. Schematic representation of surgical options for muscle release or lengthening in cerebral palsy. **A:** Myotomy; **B:** tenotomy; **C:** aponeurotomy.

are controversial among experts in cerebral palsy. Three-dimensional computerized gait analysis, performed in motion laboratories, can guide the surgeon.

B. Muscle Release for Dynamic Deformity

Muscle releases for dynamic deformity may be done in several ways, depending on the specific muscle, the presence of contracture, and the surgeon's preference. The goal is to weaken spastic muscles to reduce their abnormal influence while not lengthening them so much that the opposite deformity occurs. The more common procedures are described here.

1. Achilles tendon lengthening—Achilles tendon lengthening is usually done by Z-lengthening of the distal tendon. Cuts for Z-lengthening can be either open or percutaneous. The ankle is carefully dorsiflexed just beyond neutral to allow the tendon fibers to slide into an elongated position. The surgeon must avoid overlengthening (a matter of judgment) because an excessively weakened gastrocnemius-soleus group hinders walking and can actually encourage a deeper crouching gait.

2. Gastrocnemius lengthening—Gastrocnemius lengthening is required in patients whose gastrocnemius is considerably more spastic than the soleus. In such cases, ankle dorsiflexion is limited and ankle clonus occurs when the knee is extended, but free dorsiflexion occurs when the knee is flexed. In such patients, the gastrocnemius alone may be released by approaching the musculotendinous junction in the calf and sectioning the aponeurosis or by release of the insertion of the gastrocnemius where it attaches to the soleus and Achilles tendon. This effectively recesses the muscle, selectively weakening it while retaining soleus strength for pushoff during walking.

3. Hamstring lengthening—Hamstring lengthening is indicated when the hamstrings are tight (limited straight-leg raising) and knee flexion is persistent during the stance phase of gait (crouching gait). Usually, the distal medial and lateral hamstrings are released, but procedures vary widely among surgeons. On the medial side, the gracilis and semitendinosus tendons are usually Z-lengthened or tenotomized (transversely released). The semimembranosus is lengthened by transverse incision of its aponeurosis, which allows the interior muscle fibers to stretch and lengthen. Laterally, both heads of the biceps femoris can be managed by aponeurotic lengthening as well. The procedure must be done carefully to avoid cutting or stretching the sciatic or peroneal nerves. The leg is splinted or casted in extension for 3–4 weeks to allow soft-tissue healing.

4. Iliopsoas lengthening—The hip flexors (psoas and iliacus) may be released at the insertion of the conjoined tendon into the lesser trochanter, usually done in sitters also undergoing adductor release for spastic hip subluxation. If the child is walking and less weakening of hip flexion is desired, the psoas tendon alone can be sectioned at the level of the pelvic brim, retaining the iliacus portion of the muscle for strength.

DeLuca PA: The musculoskeletal management of children with cerebral palsy. Pediatr Clin North Am 1996;43:1135.

2. Myelomeningocele (Spina Bifida)

Myelomeningocele is a complex birth defect affecting the spinal cord and central nervous system. Although the cause is not fully understood, there is a hereditary component. Lack of maternal folic acid is identified as a causative factor in an estimated 50–70% of cases.

Embryologic Defect

The basic embryologic defect is a failure of complete tubulation and dorsal closure of the embryonic neural tube and placode, including incomplete closure of the skin over the spinal cord, resulting from lack of induction. In its mildest form, this spinal dysraphism consists of a simple spina bifida occulta or isolated meningocele (protrusion of spinal membranes, but not nerve, outside of the spinal canal, without neurologic deficit). The more severe varieties include herniation of membranes and nervous tissue through large dorsal bony and skin defects at birth and hydrocephalus with cerebral malformations (Figure 11–38).

Myelomeningocele can occur at any spinal level but usually is seen between levels T12 and S2. Because neural tissue fails to form properly, the child is paraplegic and insensate below the level of the dysraphism. The clinical determination of neurologic level is most easily accomplished by describing the last muscles contracting under active voluntary motor control (Table 11–8). This may

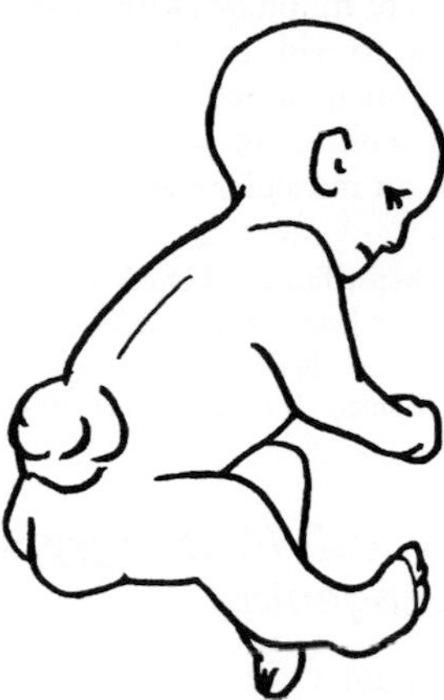

Figure 11–38. Spina bifida (myelomeningocele). The sac includes dysplastic spinal cord and membrane elements, and it must be surgically closed in the first days of life. Hydrocephalus and congenital scoliosis are commonly associated.

be difficult because of anatomic variability, the age of the child, and other central nervous system involvement.

Treatment of Orthopedic Problems

Orthopedic problems associated with myelomeningocele include clubfoot or congenital vertical talus, torsional deformities of the legs, contractures, hip dislocations, and scoliosis. The lack of sensation may allow extensive pressure sores to develop, or painless fractures may go undetected by patients. The health defects of children with spina bifida, in addition to their paralysis, usually include nonmusculoskeletal organ system problems such as hydrocephalus or Arnold-Chiari malformation (brain), syrinx formation or tethering (spinal cord), and neurogenic bladder or hydronephrosis (renal system). Early in life, most of these are more important than the orthopedic manifestations, and a team approach is needed to decide when and how best to coordinate management. The most pressing needs of the infant born with spina bifida are usually neural defect closure and ventricular shunting.

Orthopedic management depends on the deformities and the long-term mobility goals for the child. The level of paralysis often is helpful in determining whether the child will ultimately be able to walk (L5 or S1 function usually required) or will require a wheelchair (because of function only proximal to L4 or L5). Foot deformities such as clubfoot or congenital vertical talus usually require surgery. If foot deformities recur or progress, tethered cord should be suspected.

Spina bifida is theoretically a static neurologic disease, but many children exhibit a drifting deterioration of neurologic function as they grow; progression of foot deformities, especially during growth spurts, suggests tethering (and therefore stretching) of the cord. Hip dislocations, although dramatic on radiograph, frequently require no treatment; they are painless and tend to occur in children with neurologic involvement at L2 to L4, which precludes long-term walking.

A young child with scoliosis may require bracing until the thorax is long enough for spinal fusion. Scoliosis surgery is complicated by absent posterior neural arches. Some scoliosis seen with spina bifida is congenital (see section on scoliosis). If rapidly progressive scoliosis occurs, the physician should suspect a neurologic cause such as syrinx. Because of chronic exposure to latex materials in contact with mucous membranes and internal tissues (shunts, catheters), children with spina bifida are exceedingly susceptible to latex allergy, which can be fatal. Steps to limit latex exposure are essential in this population and must be observed by medical personnel working with them.

Bunch WH: Myelomeningocele: Part I. General concepts. Instr Course Lect 1976;xxv:61–64.

CDC (Centers for Disease Control and Prevention): Spina bifida and anencephaly before and after folic acid mandate—United States, 1995–1996 and 1999–2000. MMWR Morb Mortal Wkly Rep 2004;53:362. [PMID: 15129193]

Mazur JM, Menelaus MB: Neurologic status of spina bifida patients and the orthopedic surgeon. Clin Orthop 1991;264:54.

Oakshott P, Hunt GM: Long-term outcome in open spina bifida. Br J Gen Pract 2003;53:632. [PMID: 14601340]

Wehby MC et al: Occult tight filum terminale syndrome; Results of surgical untethering. Pediatr Neurosurg 2004;40:51. [PMID: 15292632]

Table 11–8. Muscle function at neurologic levels in myelomeningocoele (spina bifida).

Neurologic Level	Functions	Muscles Active
T12	Hip flexion (weak)	Iliopsoas (weak)
L1	Hip flexion	Iliopsoas
L2	Hip adduction (weak)	Adductor longus, brevis (weak)
L3	Hip adduction Knee extension (weak)	Adductors Quadriceps (weak)
L4	Knee extension Ankle dorsiflexion	Quadriceps Anterior tibialis (variable)
L5	Knee flexion Hip abduction	Medial hamstring Tensor fascia lata
S1	Knee flexion Ankle plantar flexion	All hamstrings Gastrocnemius-soleus
S2	Toe flexion	Flexor digitorum longus

3. Muscular Dystrophy

Duchenne muscular dystrophy is an X-linked disorder that presents orthopedic features in boys 6–9 years of age. The disorder is one of progressive muscle weakness, usually first involving more proximal muscles of the limb girdles. Pseudohypertrophy caused by replacement of gastrocnemius muscles (or other muscles) with fat is a classic finding, as is Gower sign (an inability to rise from the floor without using the hands to walk up the body and legs). As the muscles weaken, imbalance can cause fixed flexion contractures of the hip, knee, and ankle plantar flexors, which limits walking ability. Because weakness eventually forces patients into a wheelchair, a decision to brace or correct these contractures surgically depends on estimates of remaining strength and likely duration of ambulation after treatment. Most often, progressive foot deformities (usually equinovarus) require muscle release and correction (including bracing) because use of the wheelchair also requires relatively well-positioned feet.

As weakness progresses, the child requires an electric wheelchair for mobility. At this point, scoliosis begins to appear and is usually relentlessly progressive. Attempts to control the scoliosis of muscular dystrophy by wheelchair inserts and braces are ineffective. Early surgery (before cardiorespiratory status deteriorates) is often the best answer. Chapter 13, Rehabilitation, provides more information.

4. Myotonic Dystrophy

Myotonic dystrophy is a genetic muscle disease whose name reflects the hallmark of the disease: myotonic EMG potentials. The disease is often associated with mild-to-moderate retardation, obesity, and foot deformities. Initial diagnosis is made by identifying the characteristic myotonic face (weak perioral muscles with a distinctive pyramidal mouth), confirmed by EMG. Myotonic dystrophy worsens with each succeeding generation; genetic markers are available for diagnosis.

The most frequent foot deformity is equinovarus, often with weakness of the anterior tibialis and overactivity of the posterior tibialis. Surgery is often required, and recurrence requiring additional surgery is common. Surgical treatment of myotonic dystrophy foot deformities includes joint release (for passive correction of the deformity) and muscle transfers (for rebalancing muscle forces).

5. Spinal Muscular Atrophy

This heterogeneous group of disorders includes static and degenerative lesions of the anterior horn cell population in the spinal cord. These disorders all involve muscle weakness caused by a lower motor neuron lesion, that is, flaccid paralysis. Sensation is intact, and the major goals are mobility (with electric wheelchair), adaptive devices to aid in daily living (eg, feeding devices), and control of scoliosis, which is similar to management of scoliosis in advanced muscular dystrophy (see section on muscular dystrophy).

Green NE: The orthopaedic care of children with muscular dystrophy. Instr Course Lect 1987;36:267.

Voisin V, de la Porte S: Therapeutic strategies for Duchenne and Becker dystrophies. Int Rev Cytol 2004;240:1. [PMID: 15548414]

6. Arthrogryposis (Arthrogryposis Multiplex Congenita)

Arthrogryposis is not a disease per se but rather a symptom complex that includes joint contractures or dislocations, rigid skeletal deformities (especially clubfoot), shiny skin with decreased wrinkling and subcutaneous tissue, weakness, and muscle wasting. Although many factors contribute to arthrogryposis, the common link among the symptoms appears to be decreased fetal movement during a critical period in limb development. This can be caused by neurologic lesions (congenital absence of anterior horn cells, Werdnig-Hoffman spinal muscular atrophy, myelomeningocele), myopathic lesions (myotonic dystrophy, congenital myopathies), various syndromes (Moebius syndrome), or physical restriction associated with oligohydramnios.

Arthrogrypotic infants frequently have extension or flexion contractures of knees and elbows, dislocated hips, and severe clubfeet. The contractures may partially resolve with passive ROM therapy in the first 6–12 months of life; however, they must be released surgically after that if they interfere with walking or arm use. Hip dislocations may not limit function and often are not treated. Clubfeet require surgery, which is often of limited success; multiple operations are frequently necessary. Arthrogrypotic children are generally highly resourceful in achieving mobility, and they care for themselves completely independently, despite seemingly overwhelming skeletal problems.

TUMORS

Skeletal neoplasms, particularly benign ones, are fairly common in children. Common benign bone lesions of childhood include osteochondroma, osteoid osteoma, unicameral (simple) bone cysts, chondroblastoma, hemangioma, histiocytosis X (eosinophilic granuloma), and fibrous dysplasia. Malignant tumors, which are usually seen after 10 years of age, include Ewing sarcoma and osteosarcoma. Certain systemic diseases can be manifested in childhood as apparent bone tumors (hyperparathyroidism, renal disease, leukemia). Chapter 6 offers a detailed discussion of bone tumors.

AMPUTATIONS

Congenital Amputations & Absence of Segments

Congenital absence of limb segments at birth can occur sporadically, as part of a syndrome (Streeter dysplasia) or as a result of mutagens (eg, thalidomide). Absence may be terminal (eg, congenital below-knee amputation) or intercalary (eg, congenital shortening or absence of the humerus).

Although congenital amputations can be dramatic in appearance, the missing limb is not part of the child's body image. Thus, the child has a natural instinct to be mobile. Children with severe limb deficiencies at birth are almost always able to be completely independent and functional. They accept prostheses quite readily but only if the device truly improves their efficiency. For example, nearly all congenital above-elbow amputees reject artificial limbs, opting for function over appearance. Parents may harbor strong feelings of guilt over the child's condition, so the psychological issues associated with the condition are more those of the adults than the child.

It is not unusual for congenital amputations to require conversion to a level more easily fitted with a prosthesis. For example, fibular hemimelia (severe shortening of the tibia with absent fibula and foot deformity) sometimes can be most effectively treated by removing the foot and converting the limb to an ankle disarticulation level. This facilitates prosthetic fitting and simplifies management of the leg-length discrepancy, thus permitting normal function.

Boostra AM et al: Children with congenital deficiencies or acquired amputations of the lower limbs: Functional aspects. Prosthet Orthot Int 2000;24:19. [PMID: 10855435]

Ephraim PL et al: Epidemiology of limb loss and congenital limb deficiency: A review of the literature. Arch Phys Med Rehabil 2003;84:747. [PMID: 12736892]

Fixsen JA: Major lower limb congenital shortening: A mini review. J Pediatr Orthop B 2003;12:1. [PMID: 12488764]

Krebs DE, Fishman S: Characteristics of the child amputee population. J Pediatr Orthop 1984;4:8. [PMID: 6693574]

Rijnders LJ et al: Lower limb deficient children in the Netherlands: Epidemiological aspects. Prosthet Orthot Int 2000;24:13. [PMID: 10855434]

Traumatic Amputation

In contrast to the congenital amputee, the child with a traumatic amputation is particularly likely to be male, adolescent, rebellious, and troubled. Although pediatric traumatic amputations are often caused by inadvertent incidents, many result from high-risk behavior. These factors must be taken into account when dealing with the psychological issues of the patient and family; social, as well as medical, intervention is often appropriate.

The orthopedic management of traumatic amputees is modified in children by the presence of growth plates and the remarkable healing and rehabilitation powers of children. This must be considered during surgical completion of amputations because injury to the physis may cause severe shortening or angulation of a stump, rendering the amputation far less satisfactory than a similar amputation in the adult. The child amputee rarely has vascular problems, however, and the use of split-thickness skin grafting may allow preservation of length that would be impossible in most adults.

Overgrowth of Amputation Stump

Amputations through the long bones of children exhibit the unique phenomenon of terminal overgrowth. Eventually, the distal end of the stump may develop a long, thin, sometimes painful bony prominence. Overgrowth is not physeal in origin (ie, closure of the physis by epiphysiodesis does not eliminate its formation), and it appears to be related to aggressive bone formation associated with the periosteal membrane.

Although overgrowth can occur in any bone, it is most troublesome in the tibia, fibula, and humerus. When symptomatic, overgrowth is treated by resecting the spike of bone (revision of the amputation), but the process does continue, and recurrence is common. Some pediatric amputees require two or more surgical revisions during growth. Overgrowth ceases at skeletal maturity. Various attempts at capping the overgrowing bone end (using foreign materials or free epiphyseal grafts) have met with inconsistent success.

Tenholder M et al: Surgical management of juvenile amputation overgrowth with a synthetic cap. J Pediatr Orthop 2004;24:218. [PMID: 15076611]

FRACTURES

Common Pediatric Fracture Patterns

Many fractures in children are similar to their counterparts in adults. However, the added factor of growth contributes to the unique issues of fracture care in children. Pediatric bone is softer and more easily broken than adult cortical bone. Thus, the amount of energy required to produce a fracture is less in the child, even as soft-tissue injury is frequently less severe in the child than in the adult. In addition, the periosteal membrane in children is far thicker and more osteogenic than in adults. The periosteum is so leathery in immature humans that it frequently holds bone ends together, contributing greatly to stability and ease of manipulative reduction. The excellent osteogenic potential of pediatric periosteum permits rapid, aggressive fracture healing, so nonunions are extremely rare in children.

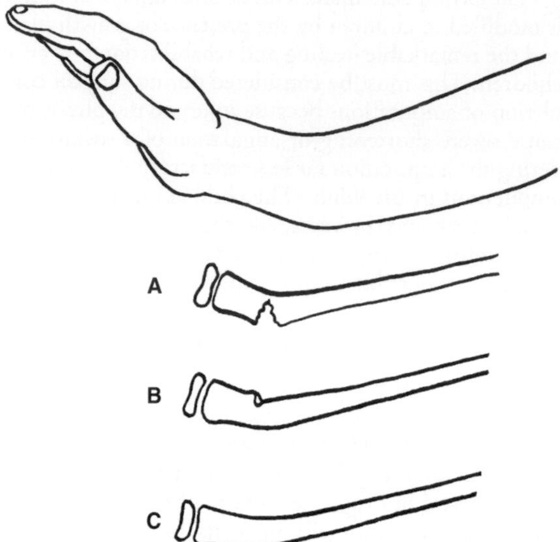

Figure 11–39. Softer bone in children can lead to unique fracture behavior (in addition to the fracture patterns seen in adults). **A:** Greenstick fracture; **B:** torus fracture; **C:** plastic deformation.

Less brittle pediatric bone is subject to fracture patterns unique to children (Figure 11–39). A greenstick fracture is a transverse crack that retains its continuity, just as a small moist twig breaks without actually snapping apart.

A torus fracture is a small buckle or impaction of one cortex with a slight bend on the opposite cortex. Plastic deformation is a change in the natural shape of a bone without a detectable fracture line.

Remodeling (gradual correction in alignment or size of a fractured bone back to normal) is generally far more rapid in children than in adults. Remodeling of angular deformities is particularly rapid when the deformity is in the same plane of motion as the nearest joint (Figure 11–40) or when the deformity is near a rapidly growing physis. Remodeling of rotational deformities is less reliable. Overgrowth is a singular feature of remodeling that occurs in certain fractures of the long bones, particularly the femur. It is a product of physeal stimulation by the hyperemic response to fracture and healing and may increase the length of a bone by 2 cm or more over the course of a year.

The combination of low-energy injury, rapid bone healing, and dependable remodeling of angular deformity makes it possible to treat many pediatric fractures by simple closed reduction (often incomplete) and casting. Surgical management of children's fractures is rarely required. The surgeon may accept a less-than-perfect reduction if the fracture is known to remodel into satisfactory alignment.

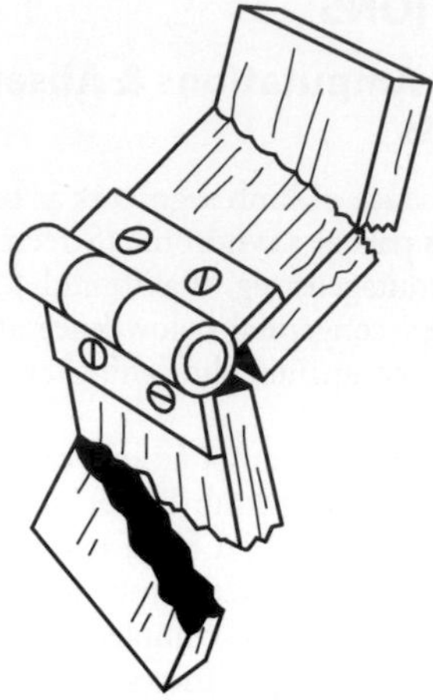

Figure 11–40. Remodeling of bone after fracture is most rapid when it is in the plane of a nearby joint. Schematically, if the joint is thought of as a hinge, the fracture above (in the plane of the hinge) is likely to remodel faster than the fracture below the hinge (out of plane).

1. Epiphyseal Fracture

The cartilage physeal plates are a region of low strength relative to the surrounding bone and are susceptible to fracture in the child. They are analogous to a scratch on a pane of glass, in which concentrated force facilitates damage. Once injury occurs, the physis usually is able to recover and resume growth. But if an offset occurs in the physeal substance, bone may grow across it (from epiphyseal bone to metaphyseal bone), forming a bridge that anchors further growth and leads to either progressive shortening or a worsening angulation (Figure 11–41).

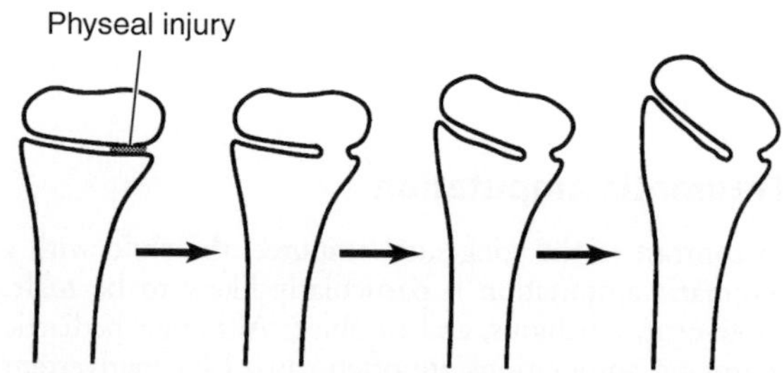

Figure 11–41. Progressive angular deformity can occur if there is asymmetric closure of the physis after fracture.

Because physes are near joints and physeal fractures are common, children may suffer injuries to joint surfaces that require careful surgical repair and realignment. Thus, open reduction is more likely in fractures involving physes and joints than in other pediatric fractures.

Most physeal fractures propagate through the weakest region of the cartilage. Physeal cartilage begins in a dense resting zone on the epiphyseal side, and chondrocytes gradually multiply, elongate, and arrange into longitudinal columns that produce longitudinal growth. Hypertrophic, balloonlike chondrocyte columns then undergo cell death, and the remaining cell walls are calcified and eventually ossify to form metaphyseal bone.

The weakest spot is usually the interface between hypertrophic dying columns of cells and the stiff calcified cell walls beneath them; this area is highly susceptible to shearing forces. Fortunately, the region also represents the boundary between the process of epiphyseal elongation (supported by the epiphyseal blood supply) and metaphyseal ossification (supported by the metaphyseal blood supply). Thus, physeal fractures do not often damage the growth potential of the physis because they do not interrupt its critical blood supply.

Although physeal fractures can occur in a wide variety of configurations, certain patterns are seen frequently enough that a descriptive classification aids in understanding physeal injury (Figure 11–42). Fractures that either cross the joint or result in spatial malalignment of portions of the physis have the worst prognosis.

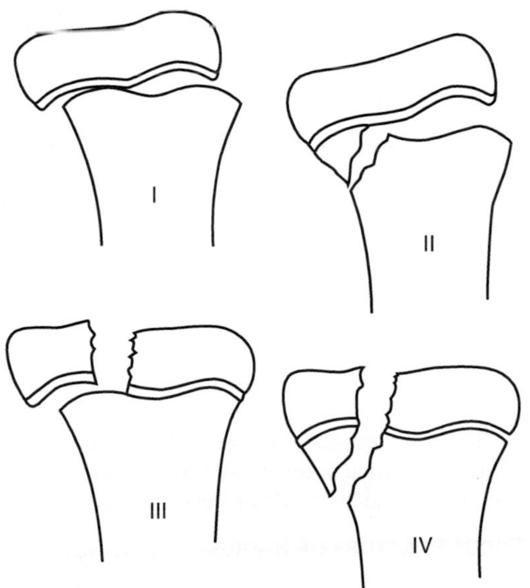

Figure 11–42. The Salter-Harris classification of physeal fractures is widely used to describe such injuries. With some exceptions, the potential for problems with growth arrest is greater in the higher numbered patterns.

Physeal fractures heal rapidly, usually within 4 weeks. Careful monitoring is required to detect early posttraumatic closure of the growth plate. Occasionally, an epiphyseal–metaphyseal bony bridge forms and tethers growth. If this growth is minor, surgical removal of the bridge (epiphyseal bar resection) may successfully restore physeal growth. Otherwise, the procedures for evaluation and treatment of limb-length inequality should be followed (see section 1. Limb-length inequality).

Salter RB, Harris WR: Injuries involving the growth plate. J Bone Joint Surg Am 1963;45:587.

2. Upper Extremity Fractures

Clavicle Fracture

Clavicle fractures are among the most common injuries in children. They are usually closed and may be treated with a simple sling. Healing occurs rapidly with abundant callus, which leaves a lump that may concern parents. This enlargement remodels over several years of growth.

An extremely rare condition, atraumatic congenital pseudarthrosis of the clavicle, can mimic the radiographic appearance of fracture. It may be right sided or bilateral, with little or no pain and no history of trauma. Treatment is generally unnecessary.

Proximal Humerus Fracture

Proximal humerus fractures are usually epiphyseal injuries (usually Salter-Harris type II injuries) that may progress into significant varus angulation (medial deviation). Fortunately, the proximal humerus is a rapidly growing physis and shoulder motion is full in all planes, so remodeling is rapid. These fractures generally require only a sling or shoulder immobilization for 3–4 weeks, without reduction. Rarely, fractures with extreme angulation (more than 90 degrees) may require surgical reduction and fixation.

Elbow Region Fracture

Most elbow region fractures are indirect injuries caused by a fall on the outstretched hand. Both diagnosis and treatment can be difficult in this serious group of injuries. Epiphyseal ossification is incomplete in the group that is susceptible to falls (2–10 years of age), making radiographs difficult to interpret (Figure 11–43). Swelling, if severe, can block venous or arterial structures and lead to forearm compartment syndromes. Reductions are often unstable, and operative intervention may be required. Most surgeons immobilize pediatric elbow fractures for 4 weeks after treatment. The most important fractures are listed next.

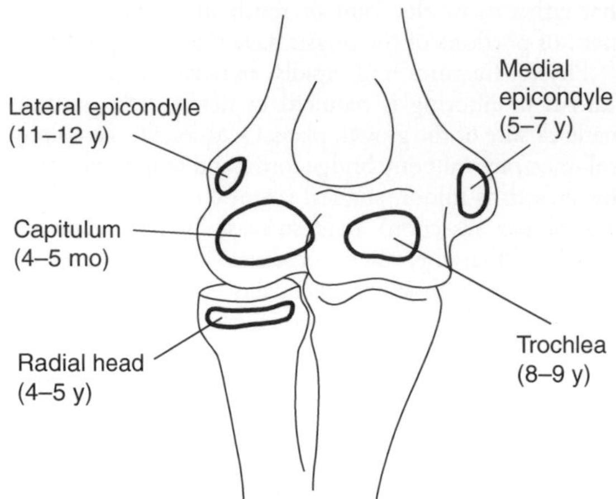

Figure 11–43. Ages of appearance of ossification centers. The ossification centers of the elbow region emerge at different ages as indicated and can complicate the interpretation of radiographs. It is often advisable to obtain comparison radiographs of the opposite elbow if injury is suspected.

A. Supracondylar Fracture of Humerus

Supracondylar fracture of the humerus occurs at the metaphyseal bone, proximal to the elbow joint, and does not involve the growth plate (Figure 11–44). Displacement may be severe, and nerve injury, usually caused by stretching, is common. If swelling is marked, there may be interruption of the blood supply; it is not uncommon for such a distal extremity to lack a pulse.

The most appropriate treatment is rapid anatomic reduction under general anesthesia. Because the reduction is highly unstable, many surgeons prefer to fix the fracture after reduction with percutaneous wires. Once the fracture is reduced, the swelling recedes rapidly and the pulse returns. On rare occasions, the surgeon must perform vascular or nerve exploration or repair.

Some displaced supracondylar humerus fractures are incompletely reduced or lose position because of fracture instability after apparently adequate initial reduction. These progress to a characteristic malunion with an apex-lateral angular deformity of the elbow (known as cubitus varus or so-called gunstock deformity). Although cosmetically unsightly, cubitus varus rarely has any significant functional consequences. If desired, it may be corrected by valgus osteotomy at the old fracture site.

B. Lateral Condyle Fracture

The lateral condyle fracture is an oblique shearing fracture of the lateral portion of the joint surface that occurs when the radial head drives into the capitulum of the humerus during a fall. The lack of significant ossification may obscure the fracture or give the false appearance of a benign Salter-Harris II fracture pattern, but most lateral condyle fractures are highly unstable Salter-Harris IV fractures (Figure 11–45). Because both the joint surface and the physis are displaced, they usually require open reduction and fixation using pins.

C. Radial Neck Fracture

Fracture of the radial neck is similar to a lateral condyle fracture. The radial neck just distal to the joint may angulate up to 70–80 degrees, although lesser angulation is more common (Figure 11–46). It is important to determine the location of the radial head despite traumatic angulation of the radial neck. Surprisingly, angulation of 45 degrees or less usually remodels spontaneously and requires only symptomatic treatment that permits early return to activity. Larger degrees of angulation can often respond to closed manipulation.

D. Forearm Fracture

Forearm fractures are a common result of falls. If they involve both bones, one bone may be completely displaced while the other only bends or suffers a greenstick fracture. In children, most forearm fractures that involve both bones can be treated successfully by closed reduction and casting; minor angular malalignment can easily be tolerated if rotational alignment of the bone ends is accurate. In addition, the ends of fractured bones often overlap. This is not necessarily of concern if alignment is satisfactory because side-to-side bone healing and remodeling are rapid in children.

E. Monteggia Fracture

Monteggia fracture is fracture of the ulna only, with the radius remaining intact. Because two-bone systems generally must fail in two spots if they break at all, the radial head dislocates from the capitulum. In such cases, reduction must include the elbow component. As with other pediatric forearm fractures, closed reduction is usually successful, although some Monteggia fractures require open reduction. The physician should be alert to the possibility of Monteggia fracture because the fracture can lead to chronic loss of elbow motion if it is not properly reduced.

In children, Galeazzi fracture of the radius, in which the distal radioulnar joint is dislocated, is far less common than the analogous Monteggia fracture.

F. Torus Fracture of Radius

Torus fracture of the radius is a minor buckle of the dorsal cortex of the distal radius, usually 1–2 cm proximal to the distal radial physis. It occurs after a minor fall on the hand. Many torus fractures are mistaken for wrist sprains because they are stable and not as painful

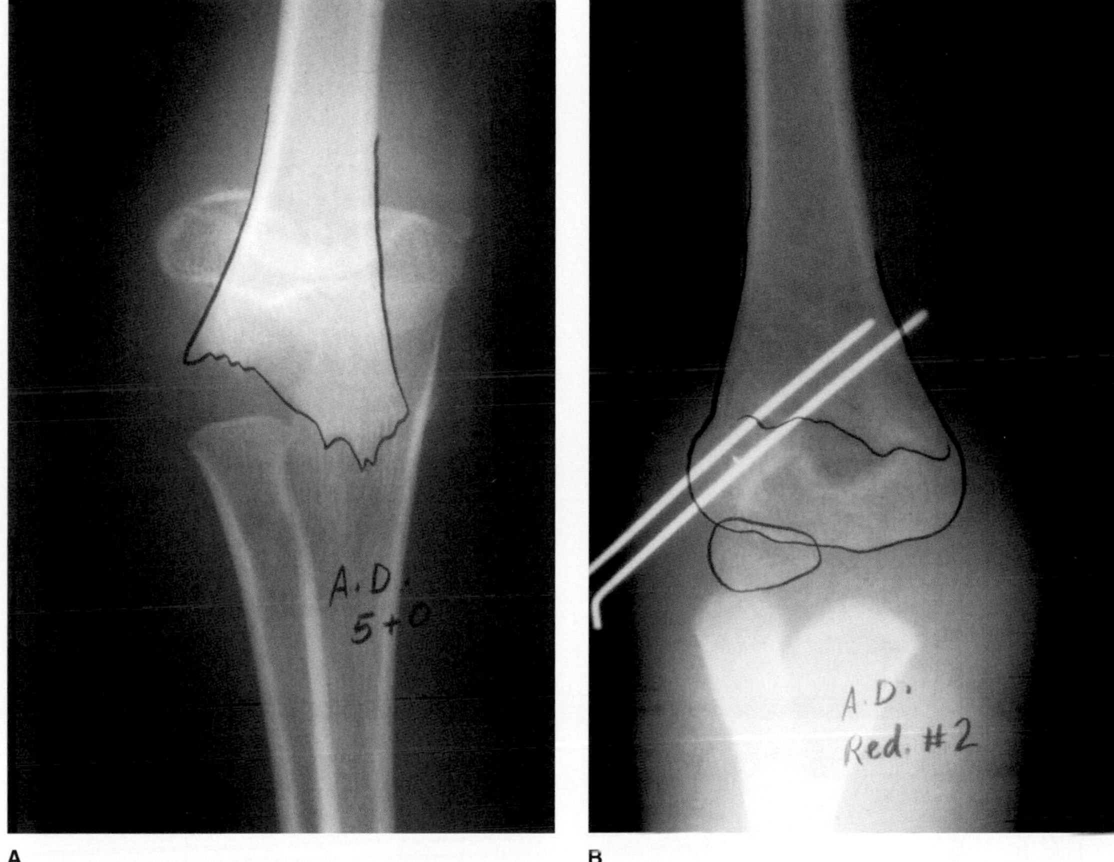

Figure 11–44. Displaced supracondylar fracture of the humerus. Injury film (**A**); after closed reduction and internal fixation using percutaneous pins (**B**).

as unstable fractures. They heal uneventfully in 3–4 weeks, with excellent long-term results.

Laumay F et al: Lateral humeral condyle fractures in children: A comparison of two approaches to treatment. J Pediatr Orthop 2004;24:385. [PMID: 15205620]

Mirsky EC et al: Lateral condyle fractures in children: Evaluation of classification and treatment. J Orthop Trauma 1997;11:117. [PMID: 9057147]

Wattenbarger JM, Gerardi J, Johnston CE: Late open reduction internal fixation of lateral condyle fractures. J Pediatr Orthop 2002;22:394. [PMID: 11961463]

Metacarpal & Phalangeal Fractures

Fractures of the metacarpals and phalanges commonly occur from crush injuries in children (eg, catching a hand or finger in a door) and are generally quite stable because the periosteum remains intact. Rarely severely angulated or rotationally malaligned, they can usually be managed by immobilization for 2–3 weeks.

3. Lower Extremity Fractures

Pelvic Fracture

Pelvic fractures in children are usually seen in conjunction with major blunt trauma. Gross displacement is fairly uncommon and usually can be treated symptomatically because the intact periosteum stabilizes the large flat bones. The patient should be carefully evaluated for intraabdominal and other injuries. Properly treated pelvic fractures in an immature skeleton resolve satisfactorily.

Adolescents exhibit a special type of avulsion fracture of apophyses because aggressive pulling of muscles during sports can detach an apophysis from its parent bone. These avulsion fractures are sometimes called transitional fractures because the physes are in transition within 2 years of skeletal maturity. During this time, relatively weak cartilage physes may not be strong enough to withstand the pull of growing muscles sud-

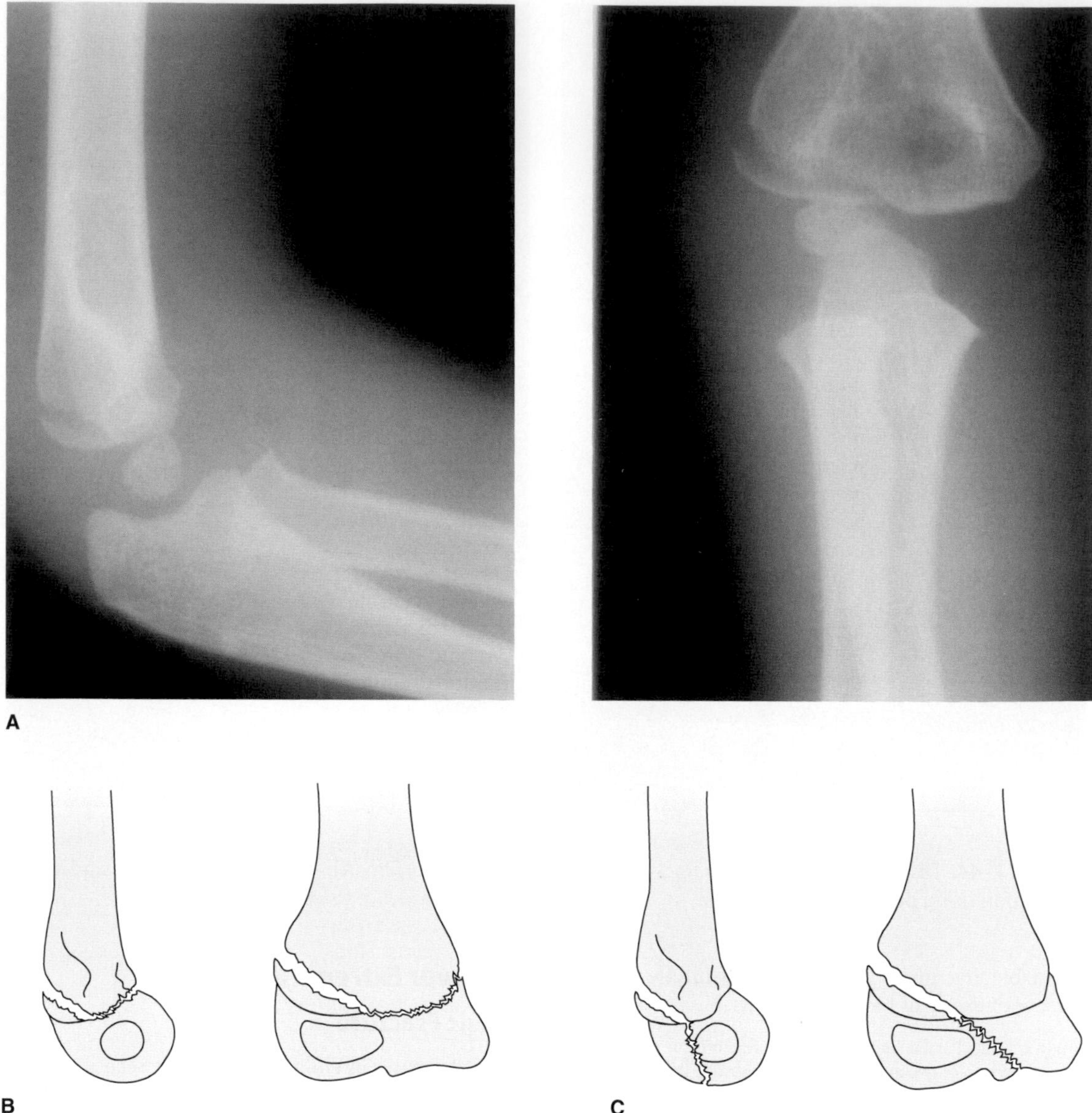

Figure 11–45. Lateral condyle fracture of the humerus (**A**) can easily be mistaken for a relatively simple Salter-Harris type II injury, which carries a good prognosis (**B**). In reality, however, it is almost always a Salter-Harris type IV injury, with a fracture pattern crossing both the joint surface and the physis (**C**); unless it is not displaced, it requires open reduction.

denly grown powerful under the influence of hormones. Transitional avulsion fractures may occur at the iliac crest (abdominal muscles), lesser trochanter of the femur (iliopsoas muscle), or ischial tuberosity (hamstring muscle). Transitional fractures of the pelvis and femur are treated symptomatically. Although these fractures do not require reduction, they may heal with a significant bump that requires excision later.

Tsirikos AI et al: Transepiphyseal fracture-dislocation of the femoral neck: A case report and review of the literature. J Orthop Trauma 2003;17:648. [PMID: 14574194]

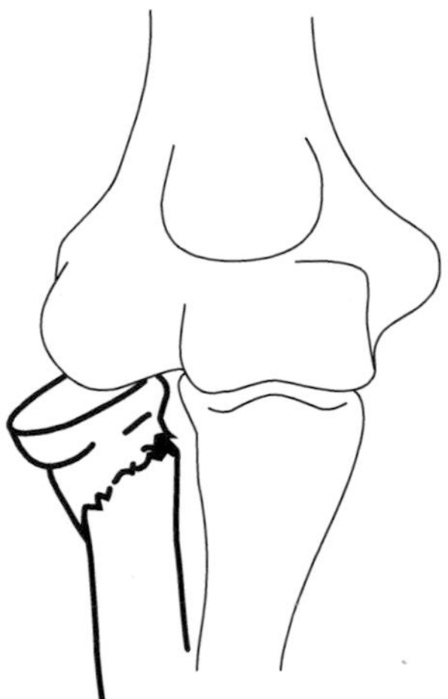

Figure 11–46. Fracture of the radial neck may angulate greatly yet still remodel spontaneously in the younger child.

Hip Fracture

Pediatric hip fractures are rare but may be serious because trauma to this area may produce significant injury. As in the adult, the fracture pattern may disrupt the blood supply of the proximal femoral head and lead to avascular necrosis of the proximal femoral epiphysis, femoral neck, or both. In older children, this can be a devastating complication; it is treated like LCP but may result in such severe collapse that hip fusion is required.

Femoral neck fractures in children are highly unstable and treated by reduction and internal fixation. The mechanical fixation may be imperfect because the surgeon must avoid injury to the proximal femoral physis. For this reason, a spica cast (body and legs) is generally used as well.

Odent T et al: Traumatic dislocation of the hip with separation of the capital epiphysis: 5 adolescent patients with 3–9 years of follow-up. Acta Orthop Scand 2003;74:49. [PMID: 12635793]

Femoral Shaft Fracture

Fractures of the femoral shaft are common injuries caused by falls as well as bicycle and motor vehicle accidents. In young children, they may be the result of child abuse. Although most are closed injuries, blood loss can be significant because of bleeding into the soft tissues of the thigh. Nerve injury is rare, and the fact that the fracture is surrounded by richly nourished muscle ensures rapid solid union (usually within 6 weeks).

Longitudinal muscle pull and spasm cause femoral shaft fractures to shorten and angulate. Initial treatment requires longitudinal traction (skin traction in younger children, skeletal traction in older children) to restore length and alignment. At this point, treatment largely depends on the patient's age.

Femur fractures in children 2–10 years of age have a strong tendency to exhibit overgrowth of 1–2.5 cm because of fracture hyperemia. In this age group, therefore, it may be desirable to use a cast and allow some shortening to occur. Rapid remodeling of the bone makes perfect reduction unnecessary. Most surgeons apply a spica cast immediately or within the first week.

Femoral overgrowth following fracture becomes unlikely in children older than 10 years. In these older children, the bone either must be kept to anatomic length by traction for 3–4 weeks (until sufficient callus has formed to stabilize length) or treated by intramedullary nails or other operative measures, as in the adult. Currently, flexible intramedullary nails are popular because they do not require reaming prior to insertion, and they are less likely to disrupt the precarious blood supply of the proximal femur. There is now a tendency at many centers to fix femur fractures using flexible nails in children 6 years and older.

After healing or cast removal, the child may begin walking. Limping is common in the first month after fracture because the hip girdle musculature regains its strength only slowly. No physical therapy is required, however, because normal walking permits spontaneous recovery, and long-term results of pediatric femur fractures are excellent.

Epiphyseal Separation

Epiphyseal separations (fracture) of the distal femoral physis are usually Salter-Harris type I or II injuries. All are caused by significant trauma, and injury to the growth mechanism of the plate is common. As many as 50% of cases exhibit subsequent growth arrest. Major neurovascular injury can occur, as with knee dislocations. Displaced epiphyseal separations require gentle reduction under general anesthesia. Some are so unstable, however, that they require percutaneous pin fixation for several weeks until the fracture is sticky, as it were, or healed enough so displacement does not occur. If physeal closure occurs, the treatment depends on age and remaining growth potential. (See discussion of limb-length inequality.)

Tibial Eminence Injury

The tibial eminence (spine), located entirely on the proximal tibial epiphysis, is the site of attachment of the anterior cruciate ligament. Twisting injuries of the knee can shear off the eminence and may displace it within the joint. Usually, the fragment reduces with full

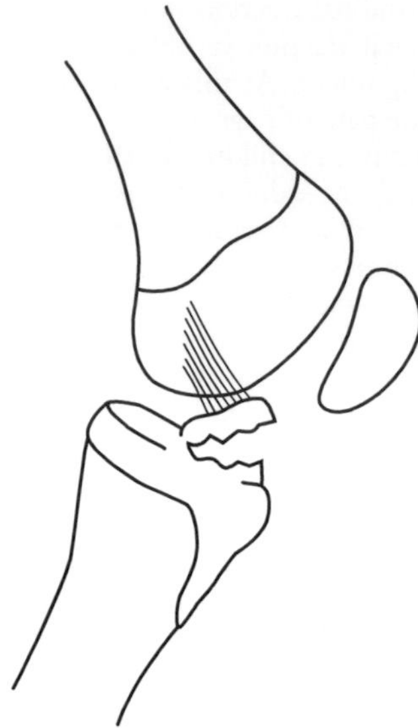

Figure 11–47. Tibial eminence fracture usually includes an anterior cruciate avulsion component. It can be treated nonoperatively if the fragment reduces with extension of the knee.

extension of the knee, but open reduction can be performed if necessary. Casting in extension is used for 6 weeks, until the bone heals (Figure 11–47). Unlike many other pediatric fractures, tibial eminence injuries often lead to mild long-term knee symptoms, especially during athletic activities.

Tibial Tubercle Avulsion Fracture

Tibial tubercle avulsion fractures are most often seen in adolescent males (13–14 years of age) who suffer sports-related injuries. The anterior tongue of the proximal tibial epiphysis is the site of attachment of the patellar tendon. During strenuous jumping, as in basketball, the tongue may avulse and displace. Sometimes the fracture extends into the joint and across the tibial joint surface. Tibial tubercle avulsions are transitional fractures in that they occur immediately before physeal closure and are not seen in younger children. Nearly all these fractures require open reduction and internal fixation, although the surgeon need not take the usual precautions when operating near the physis because maturity follows too rapidly to permit deformity.

Proximal Tibial Metaphyseal Fracture

Proximal tibial metaphyseal fractures are usually undisplaced or minimally displaced. In the absence of fibular overgrowth (Figure 11–48), they can exhibit troublesome late angular deformity (valgus) caused by tibial overgrowth after fracture. The phenomenon is most pronounced at the age of maximum physiologic valgus (3–6 years). Over a number of years, the valgus has a tendency to remodel, so the best approach is observation.

Tibial Shaft Fracture

Tibial shaft fractures, which are usually accompanied by fibula fractures, generally result from major trauma. An exception is the nondisplaced, isolated spiral tibial fracture often seen after minor trauma in children just learning to walk (toddler's fracture). In the pediatric population, open tibia fractures are fairly common. As

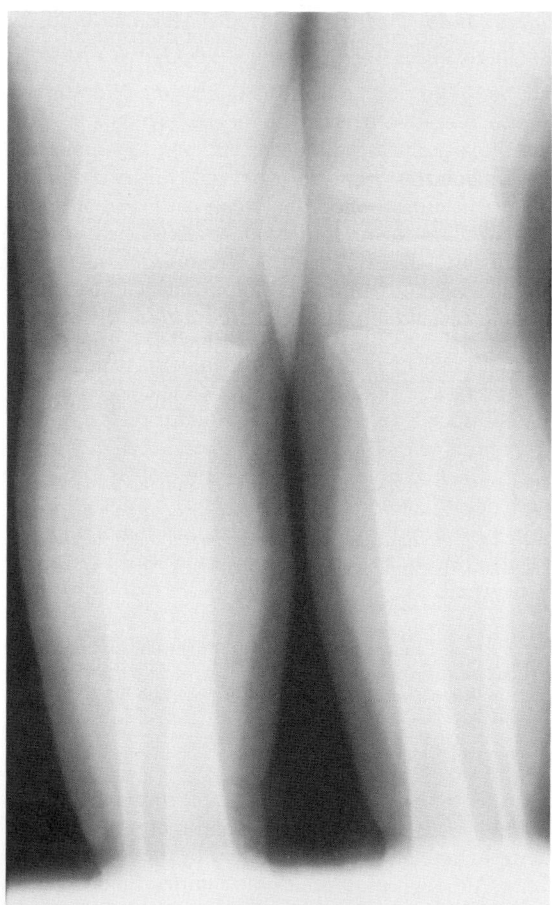

Figure 11–48. Even when not displaced, fracture of the proximal tibial metaphysis can stimulate the tibial physis and cause progressive valgus deformity, especially in patients younger than 6 years. Long-term observation indicates that slow remodeling eventually occurs.

in the adult, injury to neurovascular structures and compartment syndromes are major risks (see Chapter 3, Musculoskeletal Trauma Surgery). Open fractures of the tibia and fibula require surgical debridement, but because skin loss is less likely than in the adult, they can often be managed the same way as closed fractures, following lavage.

Most tibial fractures in children can be adequately aligned and immobilized in above-knee casts. Rare, unstable cases, some open fractures, or fractures in older children also may require external fixation or other devices to maintain reduction and alignment. As in the adult, pediatric tibia fractures are relatively slow to heal, frequently requiring 10–12 weeks; nonunion is rare, however.

Ankle Fracture & Distal Tibial Fracture

Ankle fractures and distal tibial fractures in younger children are often either metaphyseal or Salter-Harris type II distal tibial physeal injuries that heal rapidly. These fractures have very little tendency to suffer growth arrest or other serious consequences (Figure 11–49). In children 8–11 years of age, inversion injuries can push off the medial malleolus, causing an oblique Salter-Harris type IV fracture that disrupts both the joint and the growth plate. These fractures generally require open reduction for accurate realignment of the physis and articular surface. Subsequent growth arrest can cause a medial physeal bridge and produce a progressive varus deformity of the distal tibial articular surface as the lateral physis continues untethered elongation. If this occurs, either epiphyseal bar resection or corrective tibial osteotomy should be considered.

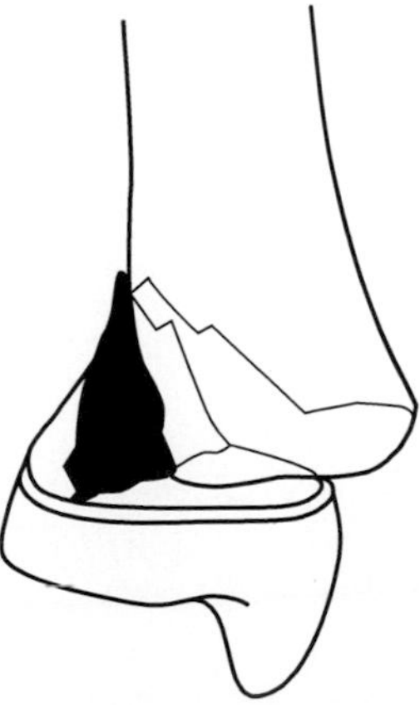

Figure 11–49. Simple fracture of the distal tibia (and fibula) at the ankle is usually a Salter-Harris type II pattern in patients younger than 10 years.

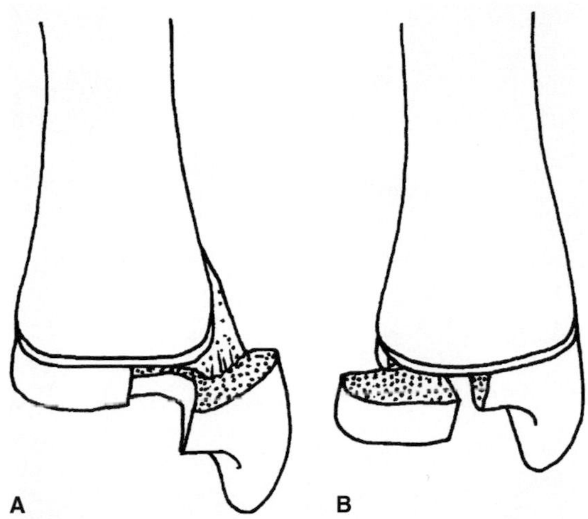

Figure 11–50. The triplane (**A**) and juvenile Tillaux (**B**) fractures are variations of ankle fracture that occur in the adolescent shortly before physeal closure. Because they involve the joint surface, such fractures may require open reduction.

The distal tibia is the site of several distinct transitional fracture patterns. These physeal injuries occur only at the end of growth, shortly before complete distal tibial physeal closure at maturity. The distal physis begins early closure medially, with gradual lateral closure over the next year. The exact fracture pattern depends on how much of the plate is still open and on the force applied (ie, mechanism of injury). When just the medial physis is closed, a triplane fracture (ie, sagittal, transverse, and frontal) of the distal tibia occurs (Figure 11–50). This fracture contains a complex of fracture lines and crosses the growth plate. Triplane fractures usually require open reduction, although minimally displaced injuries can be managed nonoperatively. CT scans may be necessary to define the exact fracture configuration for accurate treatment.

In slightly older patients, when only a small anterolateral segment of the physis remains open, this anterolateral fragment can be avulsed by fibers of the distal tibiofibular syndesmosis (juvenile Tillaux fracture). This is a Salter-Harris type III fracture involving the articular surface and frequently requires open reduction to restore perfect joint anatomy.

Spiegel PG et al: Epiphyseal fractures of the distal ends of the tibia and fibula: A retrospective study of two hundred and thirty-seven cases in children. J Bone Joint Surg Am 1978; 60:1046.

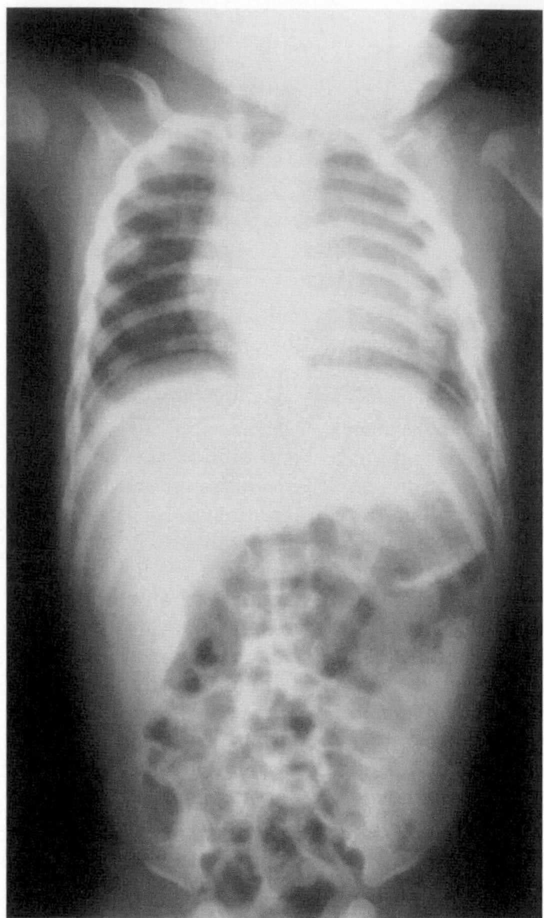

Figure 11–51. The presence of multiple fractures of various ages as well as unexplained long-bone fracture in a young child should suggest the diagnosis of child abuse.

INJURIES RELATED TO CHILD ABUSE

Child abuse crosses all socioeconomic boundaries and takes many forms. The musculoskeletal system is frequently the site of abuse-related injuries, but findings may be subtle or misleading. The most critical issue to consider in suspected abuse is whether the history can explain the injury adequately and believably.

The classic radiographic picture of abuse is the presence of multiple healing fractures of various ages; in the absence of a bone fragility syndrome, the diagnosis may thus be obvious (Figure 11–51). Soft-tissue injuries were found in 92% of children suspected of having been physically abused, with ecchymosis as the most common finding, increasing in incidence with age. Long bones (femur or humerus) are the bones most commonly fractured during child abuse. These fractures are transverse or oblique shaft injuries, a common pattern that is not by itself diagnostic. The history is often one of a minor fall or a limb "catching" in the side of the crib. But studies of fractures in young children disclosed that injury mechanisms of this type are almost never the cause of serious skeletal injury, and the dichotomy between story and findings is highly suggestive of abuse. A good rule of thumb is to consider any long bone fracture in a child younger than 3 years as abuse until proved otherwise.

The orthopedic management of abuse fractures is rarely complex, and simple closed methods usually suffice. Nearly all such fractures carry an excellent prognosis and heal or remodel rapidly. It is the detection of the abuse, and its subsequent social management, that are the main determinant of outcome.

McMahon P et al: Soft-tissue injury as an indication of child abuse. J Bone Joint Surg AM 1995;77:1179.

Oral R, Blum KL, Johnson C: Fractures in young children: Are physicians in the emergency department and orthopedic clinics adequately screening for possible abuse? Pediatr Emerg Care 2003;19:148. [PMID: 12813297]

Amputations

12

Douglas G. Smith, MD

Amputations are performed to remove extremities that are severely diseased, injured, or no longer functional. Although medical advances in antibiotics, trauma care, vascular surgery, and the treatment of neoplasms have improved the prospects for limb salvage, in many cases prolonged attempts to save a limb that should be amputated lead to excessive morbidity or even death. To counsel a patient regarding amputation versus limb salvage adequately, the physician must provide sufficient information about the surgical and rehabilitative steps involved with each procedure and must also appraise the probable outcome for function realistically with each alternative. Attempting to salvage a limb is not always in the best interest of the patient.

The decision to amputate is an emotional process for the patient, the patient's family, and the surgeon. The value of taking a positive approach to amputation cannot be overemphasized. It is not a failure and should never be viewed as such. The amputation is a reconstructive procedure designed to help the patient create a new interface with the world and to resume his or her life. The residual limb must be surgically constructed with care to maintain muscle balance, transfer weight loads appropriately, and assume its new role of replacing the original limb.

For patients to achieve maximal function of the residual limb, they also need a clear understanding of what to expect for an early postoperative prosthetic fitting, a rehabilitation program, and for long-term medical and prosthetic needs. For these discussions, the team approach to meeting the patient's needs can be especially rewarding. Nurses, prosthetists, physical and occupational therapists, and amputee support groups can be invaluable in providing the physical, psychologic, emotional, and educational support needed in returning patients to a full and active life. Many new amputees state that a peer visitor program was one of the most helpful events during their hospitalization and rehabilitation. The Amputee Coalition of America, a not-for-profit organization, supports this peer visitor training and can help locate programs that are available throughout the country.

SPECIAL CONSIDERATIONS IN THE TREATMENT OF PEDIATRIC PATIENTS

In infants and children, amputations are frequently associated with congenital limb deficiencies, trauma, and tumors. Congenital limb deficiencies are commonly described using the Birch revision of the Frantz and O'Rahilly classification system. Amelia is the complete absence of a limb; hemimelia is the absence of a major portion of a limb; and phocomelia is the attachment of the terminal limb at or near the trunk. Hemimelias can be further classified as terminal or intercalary. A terminal hemimelia is a complete transverse deficit at the end of the limb. An intercalary hemimelia is an internal segmental deficit with variable distal formation. In discussions of limb deficiencies, preaxial refers to the radial or tibial side of a limb, and postaxial refers to the ulnar or fibular side. The International Organization for Standardization (ISO) published a recommended classification for limb deficiencies in 1989 based on standard anatomic and radiologic characteristics and terminology. Although the ISO intentionally avoided the use of the terminology in the Frantz and O'Rahilly system, the older system is widely used, and the definitions and unusual language must still be understood by those caring for children with limb deficiency.

Reamputation of a congenital upper limb deficiency is rarely indicated, and even rudimentary appendages can often be functionally useful. In the lower limb, however, the ability to bear weight and the relative equality of leg lengths are mandatory for maximal function. Reamputation may be indicated in proximal femoral focal deficiency and congenital absence of the fibula or tibia to produce a more functional residual limb and improve prosthetic placement.

In the growing child, proportional change occurs in residual limb length from childhood to adulthood—an important concept to keep in mind when determining the surgical approach. A diaphyseal amputation in an infant or young child removes one of the epiphyseal growth centers, and the involved bone therefore does not keep proportional growth with the rest of the body. What initially appears to be a long transfemoral amputation in a small child can turn out to be a short and troublesome residual limb when the child reaches skeletal maturity. All attempts should be made to save the distal-most epiphysis by disarticulation. If this is not technically possible, the greatest amount of bone length should be saved.

Terminal overgrowth occurs in 8–12% of pediatric patients who had a surgical amputation. The growth of appositional bone at the transected end of a long bone exceeds the growth of the surrounding soft tissues. If left untreated, the appositional bone can penetrate through the skin (Figure 12–1). Terminal overgrowth of the transected bone does not occur as a result of the normal growth from the proximal physis pushing the distal end of the bone through the soft tissues, nor does it occur in limb disarticulations. Terminal overgrowth occurs most commonly in the humerus, fibula, tibia, and femur, in that order. Although numerous surgical procedures are used to manage this problem, the best approach consists of stump revision with adequate bone resection or autogenous osteochondral stump capping as originally described by Marquardt (Figure 12–2). If the stump-capping procedure is done at the time of original amputation, the graft material can be obtained from part of the amputated limb, such as the distal tibia, talus, or calcaneus. If a procedure is done later, the graft material can be obtained from the posterior iliac crest. Although techniques with nonautologous material are used, significant complications are reported. A report of using a modified Ertl osteomyoplasty to prevent terminal overgrowth in childhood limb deficiencies was not successful.

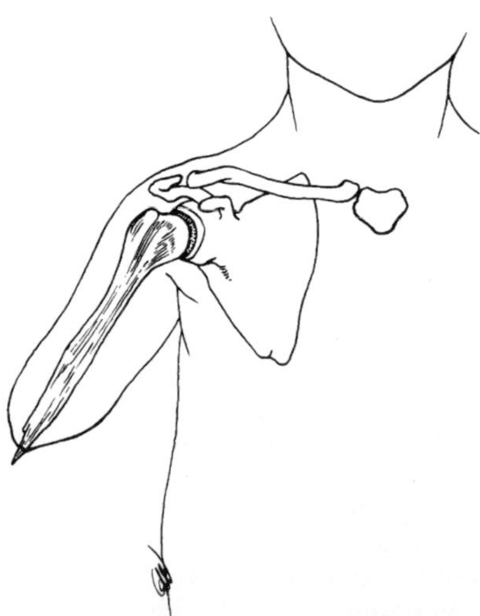

Figure 12–1. Terminal overgrowth of the transected bone in a pediatric amputee.

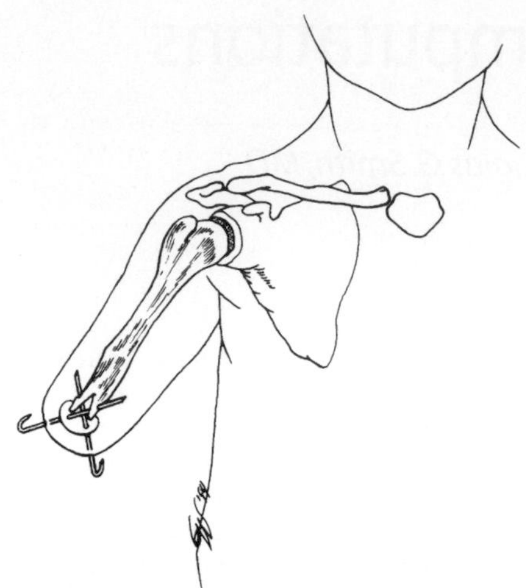

Figure 12–2. Stump-capping procedure. The bone end was split longitudinally and the osteochondral graft fixed temporarily with K-wires.

In a growing child, the fitting of a prosthesis can be challenging and requires frequent adjustments. Specialty pediatric amputee clinics can ease this process, provide family support, and make care more cost effective. The timing of prosthetic fitting should be initiated to coincide closely with normal motor skill development.

Prosthetic fitting for the upper limb should begin near the time the child gains sitting balance, usually around 4–6 months of age. A passive terminal device with blunt rounded edges is used initially. Active cable control and a voluntary opening terminal device are added when the child exhibits initiative in placing objects in the terminal device, usually in the second year of life. Myoelectric devices are usually not prescribed until the child masters traditional body-powered devices. The physical demand placed on prosthetic devices by children can often exceed the durability of current myoelectric designs, so maintenance and repair costs must be considered. The decision to prescribe a myoelectric device for a child is individual and depends on many factors, including the physical characteristics of the residual limb, the desires of the child, the training available, the proximity of prosthetic facilities for fitting and maintenance, and issues about funding.

Prosthetic fitting for the lower limb commonly begins when the child develops the ability to crawl and pull to a standing position, which is usually at 8–12 months. A child with a Syme amputation or a transtibial amputation generally adapts to a prosthesis with surprising ease, and although formal gait training is not required, educational efforts are focused on teaching the parents about the prosthesis. For a child with a transfemoral amputation, control of a knee unit should not be expected immediately. The knee unit should be eliminated or locked in extension until the child is ambulating well and demonstrates proficient use of the prosthesis. The initial gait pattern used by a child with a transfemoral amputation is not a normal heel strike, midstance, toe-off gait pattern but is instead a more circumducted gait pattern with a prolonged foot flat phase. Formal gait training is seldom warranted until the child reaches 5 or 6 years of age. Attempts to force gait training too early can be frustrating for all involved. When pediatric patients are allowed to develop their own gait patterns as they grow and gain improved motor coordination, they are surprisingly adept at discovering the most efficient gait pattern without formal training.

Bernd L et al: The autologous stump plasty: Treatment for bony overgrowth in juvenile amputees. J Bone Joint Surg Br 1991; 73:203. [PMID: 2005139]

Birch JG et al: Syme amputation for the treatment of fibular deficiency. An evaluation of long-term physical and psychological functional status. J Bone Joint Surg Am 1999;81(11):1511. [PMID: 10565642]

Drvaric DM, Kruger LM: Modified Ertl osteomyoplasty for terminal overgrowth in childhood limb deficiencies. J Pediatr Orthop 2001;21(3):392. [PMID 1137827]

Fixsen JA: Major lower limb congenital shortening: A mini review. J Pediatr Orthop B 2003;12:1. [PMID: 124887464]

Greene WG, Cary JM: Partial foot amputation in children: A comparison of the several types with the Syme's amputation. J Bone Joint Surg Am 1982;64:438. [PMID: 7061561]

International Organization for Standardization: ISO 8548-1: Prosthetics and orthotics—Limb deficiencies, Part 1: Method of describing limb deficiencies present at birth. International Organization for Standardization, 1989.

Pfeil J et al: The stump-capping procedure to prevent or treat terminal osseous overgrowth. Prosthet Orthot Int 1991;15:96.

Weber M: Neurovascular calcaneo-cutaneus pedicle graft for stump capping in congenital pseudarthrosis of the tibia: Preliminary report of a new technique. J Pediatr Orthop B 2002;11(1): 47. [PMID: 11866081]

GENERAL PRINCIPLES OF AMPUTATION

Epidemiology

Epidemiologic data on the incidence of amputation in the United States from 1993 to 2001 show the number of lower extremity amputations increased 14% from 99,522 to 113,379, and the average hospital charge for this procedure increased 38% from $24,332 to $33,562. Nearly two thirds of amputations are performed in individuals with diabetes, even though people with diabetes represent only 6% of the population.

Preoperative Evaluation & Decision Making

The decision to amputate a limb and the choice of amputation level can be difficult and are often subject to differences in opinion. Advances in the treatment of infection, peripheral vascular disease, replantation, and limb salvage complicate the decision-making process. The goals are to optimize a patient's function and reduce the level of morbidity.

A. Vascular Disease and Diabetes

Ischemia resulting from peripheral vascular disease remains the most frequent reason for amputation in the United States. Nearly two thirds of patients with ischemia also have diabetes. The preoperative assessment of these patients includes a physical examination and an evaluation of perfusion, nutrition, and immunocompetence. Preoperative screening tests can be helpful, but no single test is 100% accurate in predicting successful healing. Clinical judgment based on experience in examining and following many patients with vascular disease and diabetes is still the most important factor in preoperative assessment.

1. Doppler ultrasound studies—The most readily available objective measurement of limb blood flow and perfusion is by Doppler ultrasound. Arterial wall calcification increases the pressure needed to compress the vessels of patients with vascular disease, and this often gives an artificially elevated reading. Low-pressure levels are indicative of poor perfusion, but normal and high levels can be confusing because of vessel wall calcification and are not predictive of normal perfusion or of wound healing. Digital vessels are not usually calcified, and blood pressure levels in the toes appear to be more predictive of healing than do those in the ankles.

2. Transcutaneous oxygen tension measurements—Tests to measure transcutaneous partial pressure of oxygen (PO_2) are noninvasive and becoming more readily available in many vascular laboratories. These tests use a special temperature-controlled oxygen electrode to measure the PO_2 diffusing through the skin. The ultimate reading is based on several factors: the delivery of oxygen to the tissue, the utilization of oxygen by the tissue, and the diffusion of oxygen through the tissue and skin. Caution in interpreting the transcutaneous PO_2 measurements during acute cellulitis or edema is warranted because the presence of either of these disorders can increase oxygen utilization and decrease oxygen diffusion, thereby resulting in lower measurements of PO_2. Paradoxical measurements are also reported on the plantar skin of the foot. In spite of these limitations, transcutaneous PO_2 and transcutaneous partial pressure of carbon dioxide (PCO_2) are both statistically accurate in predicting amputation healing, but this does not rule out false-negative results.

3. Xenon studies—Xenon-133 (^{133}Xe) skin clearance studies are used successfully to predict healing of amputations, but the preparation of the mixture containing xenon-133 gas and saline solution and the administration of the test are time consuming, highly technician dependent, and expensive. A small amount of the xenon and saline solution is injected intradermally at various sites, and the rate of washout is monitored by gamma camera. Xenon-133 is almost never used today and is primarily of historical interest.

4. Fluorescence studies—Skin fluorescence studies use intravenous injection of fluorescein dye and subjective observation or digital fluorometers to assess skin blood flow and correlate this with the likelihood of successful wound healing. The technique is not commonly used, and studies to assess its accuracy yielded conflicting results.

5. Arteriography—Arteriography is not helpful in predicting successful healing of amputations, and this invasive test is probably not indicated solely for the purpose of selecting the proper level of amputation. Arteriography is indicated if the patient is truly a candidate for arterial reconstruction or angioplasty.

6. Nutrition and immunocompetence studies—Both nutrition and immunocompetence correlate directly with amputation wound healing. Many laboratory tests are available to assess nutrition and immunocompetence, but some are quite expensive. Screening tests for albumin level and total lymphocyte count are readily available and inexpensive. Several studies show increased healing of amputations in patients who have vascular disorders but have a serum albumin level of at least 3 g/dL and a total lymphocyte count exceeding 1500/mL. Nutritional screening is recommended to allow for nutritional improvement preoperatively and to help determine whether a higher level of amputation is needed.

7. Other issues—Activity level, ambulatory potential, cognitive skills, and overall medical condition must be evaluated to determine if the distal-most level of amputation is really appropriate for the patient.

For patients who are likely to remain ambulatory, the goals are to achieve healing at the distal-most level that can be fit with a prosthesis and to make successful rehabilitation possible. Newer studies of patients with vascular insufficiency and diabetes demonstrate that successful wound healing can be achieved in 70–80% of these patients at the transtibial or more distal amputation level. This is in sharp contrast to 25 years ago, when because of a fear of wound failure, surgeons elected to perform 80% of all lower extremity amputations at the transfemoral level.

For nonambulatory patients, the goals are not simply to obtain wound healing but also to minimize complications, improve sitting balance, and facilitate position transfers. Occasionally, a more proximal amputation more successfully meets these goals. For example, a bedridden patient with a knee flexion contracture might be better served with a knee disarticulation than a transtibial amputation, even if the biologic factors are present to heal the more distal amputation. Preoperative assessment of the patient's potential ability to use a prosthesis, the patient's specific needs for maintaining independent transfers, and the best weight distribution for seating can help in making wise decisions concerning the appropriate level of amputation and the most successful type of postoperative rehabilitation program.

Some nonambulatory patients do benefit from a partial foot amputation, or even transtibial amputation with prosthetic fitting, not with the goal of walking but to use that leg as a standing pivot for independent transfers. In these cases, prosthetic fitting is justified.

B. Trauma

As vascular reconstruction techniques improved, more attempts to salvage limbs were initially made, often with the result that multiple surgical procedures were subsequently required. In many cases, amputation was ultimately performed after a substantial investment of time, money, and emotional energy. Current studies offer guidelines for immediate or early amputation and show the value of amputation not only in saving lives but also in preventing the emotional, marital, and financial disasters that can follow unwise and desperate limb salvage attempts. Although several scoring systems for mangled limbs are published, none can perfectly predict when an amputation should be performed. These scores can help in the decision-making process, but good clinical experience and judgment are still required.

The absolute indication for amputation in trauma remains an ischemic limb with unreconstructable vascular injury. Massively crushed muscle and ischemic tissue release myoglobin and cell toxins, which can lead to renal failure, adult respiratory distress syndrome, and even death. In two groups of high-risk patients (multiply injured patients and elderly patients with a mangled extremity), limb salvage, even though technically possible, can become life-threatening and generally should be avoided. In all patients, the decision about whether to undertake immediate or early amputation of a mangled limb must also depend on whether it is an upper extremity or lower extremity.

An upper extremity can function with minimal or protective sensation, and even a severely compromised arm can serve as an assistive limb. An assistive upper extremity often functions better than the currently available prosthetic replacements. The decision of salvage versus amputation in the upper limb should be based on the chance of maintaining some useful function, even if that function is limited.

In the lower extremity, weight bearing is mandatory. A lower limb functions poorly without sensation, and an assistive limb is not useful. A salvaged lower limb often functions worse than a modern prosthetic replacement unless the limb can tolerate full weight bearing, is relatively pain free, has enough sensation to provide protective feedback, and has durable skin and soft-tissue coverage that does not break down whenever walking is attempted. The decision to salvage a mangled lower extremity should be based on providing a limb that can tolerate the demands of walking.

C. Frostbite

Exposure to cold temperatures can directly damage the tissue and cause a related vascular impairment from endothelial vessel injury and increased sympathetic tone. If the foot or hand is wet or directly exposed to the wind, cold injury can result even in temperatures above freezing. The immediate treatment involves restoring the core body temperature and then rewarming the injured body part in a water bath at a temperature of 40–44°C for 20–30 minutes. Rewarming can be painful, and the patient often requires opiate analgesia. After rewarming, the involved part should be kept dry, blisters left intact, and dry gauze dressings used. The goals are to keep the injured extremity clean and dry and to prevent maceration, especially between the digits.

The temptation to perform early amputation should be avoided because the amount of recovery can be dramatic. As the extremity recovers from frostbite, a zone of mummification (dry gangrene) develops distally, and a zone of intermediate tissue injury forms just proximal to this. Even at the time of clear demarcation, the tissue just proximal to the zone of mummification continues to heal from the cold insult, and although the outward appearance is often pink and healthy, this tissue is not totally normal. Delaying amputation can improve the chance of primary wound healing. It is not unusual to wait 2–6 months for definitive surgery. In spite of having mummified tissue, infection is rare if the tissue is kept clean and dry.

D. Tumors

Patients with musculoskeletal neoplasms face new choices in treatment with the development of limb salvage techniques and adjuvant chemotherapy and radiation therapy. If an amputation is chosen, the amputation incisions must be carefully planned to achieve the appropriate surgical margin.

Surgical margins (Figure 12–3) are characterized by the relationship of the surgical incision to the lesion, to the inflammatory zone surrounding the lesion, and to the anatomic compartment in which the lesion is located. The four types of margins are the intralesional margin, in which the surgical incision enters the lesion; the marginal margin, in which the incision enters the inflammatory zone but not the lesion; the wide margin, in which the incision enters the same anatomic compartment as the lesion but is outside of the inflammatory zone; and the radical margin, in which the incision remains outside of the involved anatomic compartment. Biopsy incisions and amputation incisions must be planned with careful consideration as to the tumor margin required.

Newer studies continue to evaluate the complex issues and outcomes of amputation versus limb-sparing procedures for patients with extremity sarcomas. Studies still suggest that functional outcomes in terms of kinesiologic parameters are comparable with either limb salvage or amputation. Both treatment groups report quality of life problems involving employment, health insurance, social isolation, and poor self-esteem. Overall survival remains comparable with either treatment. In some tumors, amputation may achieve better local disease control. These results confirm that the decision about treatment must be made on an individual basis, according to the specific lifestyle and needs of the patient.

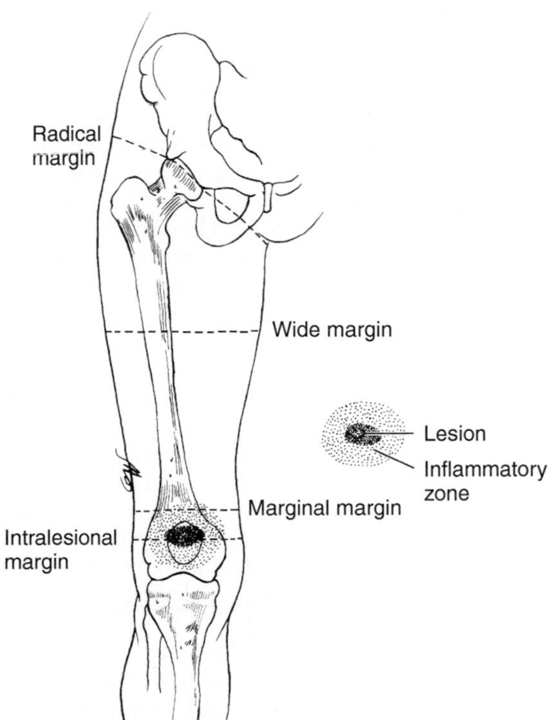

Figure 12–3. Surgical margins in tumors of the extremity.

Surgical Definitions & Techniques

Terminology for amputation level now uses an accepted international nomenclature. *Transtibial* should be used instead of below knee, and *transfemoral* instead of above knee. In the upper extremity, the terms *transradial* and *transhumeral* replace the older terms below elbow and above elbow.

Careful surgical techniques, especially in soft-tissue handling, are more critical to wound healing and functional outcome in amputation procedures than in many other surgical procedures. The tissues are often traumatized or poorly vascularized, and the risk of wound failure is high, particularly if close attention is not paid to soft-tissue technique. Flaps should be kept thick, avoiding unnecessary dissection between the skin and subcutaneous, fascial, and muscle planes. In adults, periosteum should not be stripped proximal to the level of transection. In children, however, removing 0.5 cm of the distal periosteum may help prevent terminal overgrowth. The rounding of all bone edges and the beveling of prominences are necessary for optimal prosthetic use.

Muscle loses its contractile function when the skeletal attachments are divided during amputation. Stabilizing the distal insertion of muscle can improve residual limb function by preventing muscle atrophy, providing counterbalance to the deforming forces resulting from amputation, and providing stable padding over the end of the bone. Myodesis is the direct suturing of muscle or tendon to the bone or the periosteum. Myodesis techniques are most effective in stabilizing strong muscles needed to counteract strong antagonistic muscle forces, such as in cases involving transfemoral or transhumeral amputation and in cases involving knee or elbow disarticulation. Myoplasty involves the suturing of muscle to muscle over the end of the bone. The distal stabilization of the muscle is more secure with myodesis than with myoplasty. Care must be taken to prevent a mobile sling of muscle over the distal end of the bone, which usually results in a painful bursa.

The transection of nerves always results in neuroma formation, but all neuromas are not symptomatic. Historical attempts to diminish symptomatic neuromas include clean transection, ligation, crushing, cauterization, capping, perineural closure, and end-loop anastomosis. No technique is more effective than careful and meticulous isolation, retraction, and clean transection of the nerve. This allows the cut end to retract into the soft tissues, away from the scar, pulsating vessels, and prosthetic pressure points. Ligation of a nerve is still indicated to control bleeding from the blood vessels contained within larger nerves, such as the sciatic.

Split-thickness skin grafts are generally discouraged except as a means to save a knee or elbow joint that has a stable bone and good muscle coverage. Skin grafts do best with adequate soft-tissue support and are least durable when closely adherent to bone. New prosthetic interfaces, such as silicone-based liners, can help reduce the shear at the interface and improve durability in skin-grafted residual limbs.

An open amputation is occasionally necessary to control a severe ascending infection. The term *guillotine amputation* should be avoided because it gives the impression that the limb is transected at one level through skin, muscle, and bone. Open amputations need to be performed with careful planning and forethought as to how the amputation will eventually be closed. The surgical plan must obviously consider adequate debridement of tissue necrosis and drainage of infection but must also consider the surgical flaps and tissue needed for a functional closure of the amputation to allow prosthetic fitting.

The problem of ascending infection is seen, for example, in a diabetic patient with a severe infection of the foot and cellulitis extending upward to the calf. The open amputation removes the source of infection, provides adequate drainage, and allows the acute cellulitis to resolve. After resolution, a definitive amputation and closure can be done safely. In the case of a diabetic foot infection, an open ankle disarticulation is simple, relatively bloodless, and preserves the posterior calf flap for a definitive transtibial amputation. Occasionally, it is necessary to make a longitudinal incision to drain the posterior tibial, anterior tibial, or peroneal tendon sheaths, in which case care should be taken not to violate the posterior flap of the definitive amputation. This approach often prevents having open, transected muscle bellies that can retract and become edematous—a problem that commonly occurs if an open calf-level amputation was initially performed and one that can make the definitive amputation difficult. In more severe infections or in cases in which the level of the definitive amputation will clearly be transfemoral, an open knee disarticulation has the same advantages as the open ankle disarticulation.

Postoperative Care

A. Postoperative Care and Planning

The terminal amputation allows the unique opportunity to manipulate the physical environment of the wound during healing. A variety of methods are described, including rigid dressings, soft dressings, controlled environment chambers, air splints, and skin traction. The use of a rigid dressing controls edema, protects the limb from trauma, decreases postoperative pain, and allows early mobilization and rehabilitation.

The use of an immediate postoperative prosthesis, or IPOP (Figure 12–4), is effective in decreasing the time to limb maturation and the time to definitive prosthetic fitting. In most cases involving a lower limb amputation,

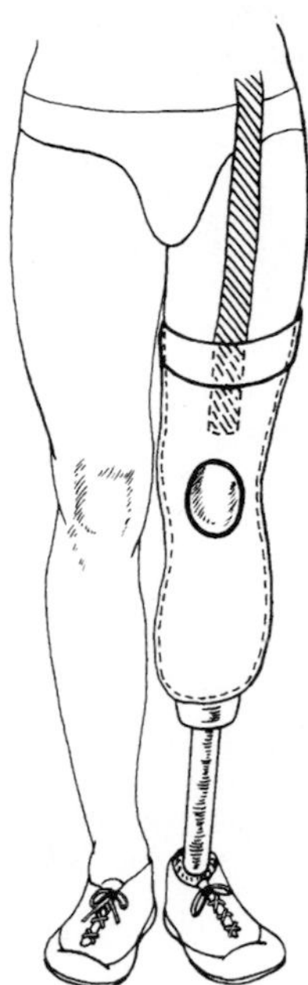

Figure 12–4. Immediate postoperative prosthetic cast for transtibial amputation.

the surgeon has the patient start with partial weight bearing if the wound appears stable after the first cast change, which usually takes place between the fifth and tenth day after surgery. Immediate postoperative weight bearing can be initiated safely in selected patients, usually young patients in whom an amputation was performed following a traumatic injury and above the zone of injury. Rigid dressings and the IPOP need to be applied carefully, but their application is easily learned and well within the scope of interested physicians. For upper extremity amputations, an IPOP can be applied immediately. Early training with an IPOP is believed to increase the long-term acceptance and use of a prosthesis. Chapter 13 offers a detailed discussion of rehabilitation.

To counsel patients adequately , some insight into the typical surgical and postoperative course can be helpful. Many patients require inpatient hospital care for 5–8 days after a transtibial amputation. Epidural or patient-controlled analgesia is usually required for pain control. Assistance with basic mobility and emotional support are also necessary. Antibiotics can minimize the risk of infection. The cast applied at the end of the surgical procedure is changed about postoperative day 5. If the wound healing is adequate, a new cast with a foot attachment is applied, and the patient can begin ambulating with approximately 30 lb of weight on the amputated extremity. Transtibial amputees are discharged to home or a nursing facility typically 5 or 8 days after surgery. Outpatient visits are scheduled weekly to change the cast, which frequently becomes loose as edema lessens, and to monitor wound healing and allow suture removal. Active and active-assisted knee range of motion (ROM) is performed between each cast. On average, approximately six casts are applied on a weekly basis until the wound heals, edema resolves, wrinkles return to the skin, and the patient is ready for prosthetic fitting. The cast and the prosthetic foot attachment are applied and aligned by either the surgeon or the prosthetist. New prefabricated, removable postoperative prosthetic systems are alternatives to the traditional casting techniques. Unfortunately, comparison trails versus traditional techniques have not been done.

Close interaction between the patient, the physical therapist, and the prosthetist is required in the first 12–18 months. The socket made for the first prosthesis must allow modifications as the residual limb continues to change shape during this time. Volume changes and mismatch between the shape of the socket and the evolving shape of the residual limb are treated with amputation socks and by adding pads to the socket or socket liner. Pads are usually needed in the region that contacts the anteromedial and anterolateral tibial flares, and posteriorly, in the popliteal region. Even with careful modifications, the prosthetic socket must be changed two or three times in the first 18 months. Because of these frequent prosthetic modifications, encouraging the patient to work with a prosthetic provider who is located close to the patient's residence can help tremendously in this rehabilitation phase. Many patients have an immediate desire to have the most advanced and high-tech components in their first prosthesis. But often these components are designed for higher activity levels than are typically achieved in the rehabilitation phase and are too rigid. Discussing how the prosthesis will evolve and be upgraded as the patient's activity increases can ease this process. A new prosthesis is typically required around month 18; the old components often can be turned into a shower leg.

B. Prevention and Treatment of Complications

1. Failure of the wound to heal properly—Problems with wound healing, especially in diabetic and ischemic limbs, occur as the result of insufficient blood supply, infection, or errors in surgical technique. Healing failure rates are difficult to interpret because they depend so much on the level of amputation selected. Low failure rates can be achieved by doing amputations at an extremely proximal level in the majority of cases, but this sacrifices the rehabilitation potential of many patients because the ability to ambulate decreases dramatically with a transfemoral amputation. Wound healing failure that necessitates reamputation at a more proximal level occurs in approximately 5–10% of cases at centers specializing in amputee treatment.

Most surgeons prefer open wound care if the wound gap is less than 1 cm wide and prefer revision surgery if the gap is wider. If the surgical edema has resolved and some atrophy has already occurred, a wedge excision of all nonviable tissue can be performed and still allow primary closure without any tension at the original level. If it is not possible to oppose the viable tissue gently without tension, bone shortening or reamputation at a more proximal level should be performed.

In patients with small local areas of wound-healing failure, successful treatment with rigid dressings and an IPOP is reported. The wounds are debrided weekly and packed open, and the IPOP is applied to allow some weight bearing. The stimulation of weight bearing can increase local circulation, decrease edema, and promote wound healing.

2. Infection—Infection without widespread tissue necrosis or flap failure may be seen after surgery, especially if active distal infection was present at the time of the definitive amputation or if the amputation was done near the zone of a traumatic injury. Hematomas can also predispose a wound to infection. In cases involving infection or hematomas, the wound must be opened, drained, and debrided. If the wound is allowed to remain open for an extended time, the flaps retract and become edematous, which makes delayed closure difficult or impossible without shortening the bone. One solution, which can be instituted after thorough debridement and irrigation, is to close only the central one third to one half of the amputation wound and to use open packing for the medial and lateral corners (Figure 12–5). This method provides coverage of the bone but also allows adequate drainage and open wound management for the edges. If the original problem was truly infection and not tissue failure, the open portions of the wound heal secondarily, and the result is still a residual limb suitable for prosthetic fitting.

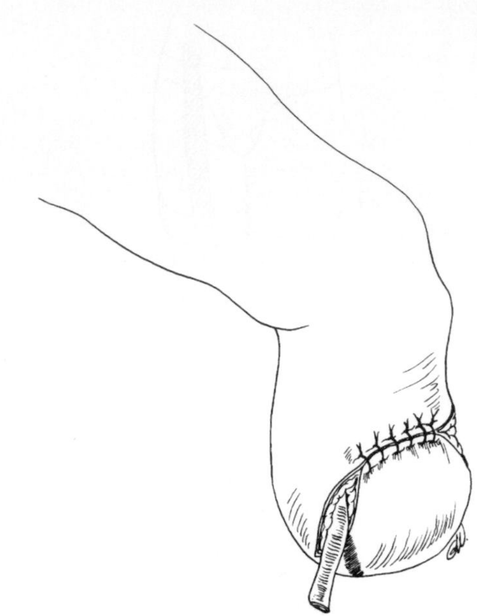

Figure 12–5. Partial closure of the infected transtibial amputation.

3. Phantom sensation—Phantom sensation is the feeling that all or a part of the amputated limb is still present. This sensation is felt by nearly everyone who undergoes surgical amputation, but it is not always bothersome. Phantom sensation usually diminishes over time, and telescoping (the sensation that the phantom foot or hand has moved proximally toward the stump) commonly occurs.

4. Pain and phantom pain—Phantom pain is defined as a bothersome, painful, or burning sensation in the part of the limb that is missing. Although from 80% to 90% of patients with acquired amputation experience some episodes of phantom pain, the episodes are often infrequent and brief. The dreaded problem of unrelenting phantom pain fortunately occurs only in a much smaller minority of patients. Surgical intervention for this problem is not very successful.

Local physical measures, including massage, cold packs, exercise, neuromuscular stimulation by external electrical currents, acupuncture, and regional sympathectomy, may under given circumstances have a place in therapy when the pain is intractable. A technique that has gained some acceptance and success is the use of transcutaneous electrical nerve stimulation (TENS), incorporated either into a prosthesis or used as an isolated unit. The TENS system can be worn by the amputee at night and even during the day with the battery pack attached to the belt or inside a pocket. We use this TENS system with moderate short-term success, but it is rare to see a patient who continues to use a TENS system for more than a year.

Pharmacologic treatment shows some success with several oral agents including gabapentin, amitriptyline, carbamazepine, phenytoin, and mexiletine. Medications can decrease the frequency of phantom pain episodes and decrease the intensity of these episodes. The appropriate use of an intravenous lidocaine challenge is predictive of a favorable response to oral mexiletine. Unfortunately, no indicators are good at predicting who will respond to treatment with gabapentin, amitriptyline, carbamazepine, or phenytoin . Psychological support can be beneficial, particularly when personality problems seem to accentuate the occurrence of pain. The individual needs patience and reassurance that the discomfort will improve with time, especially when a supportive social environment is present.

The sensations described by patients with phantom pain may be similar to the symptoms of reflex sympathetic dystrophy after an injury. Reflex sympathetic dystrophy can occur in amputated limbs and should be treated aggressively if present. Although rare, pain unrelated to the amputation can easily be overlooked. The differential diagnosis includes radicular nerve pain from proximal entrapment or disk herniation, arthritis of proximal joints, ischemic pain, and referred visceral pain.

Research has progressed in the prevention of phantom limb pain. Several authors document that the use of perioperative epidural anesthesia or intraneural anesthesia can block the acute pain associated with amputation surgery and decrease the opiate requirements in the immediate postoperative period. They also suggest that perioperative analgesia can prevent or decrease the later incidence of phantom pain, although this is difficult to document. The literature unfortunately is not conclusive on whether preemptive measures can truly reduce the frequency or severity of phantom limb pain. Some reports dispute the claims that preemptive analgesia reduces the frequency of phantom limb problems. A randomized trial by Lambert and colleagues found that perioperative epidural block started 24 hours before amputation is not superior to infusion of local anesthetic via a perineural catheter in preventing phantom pain but does give better relief in the immediate postoperative period.

5. Edema—Postoperative edema is common in patients who have undergone amputation. Rigid dressings can help reduce this problem. If soft dressings are used, they should be combined with stump wrapping to control edema, especially if the patient is a prosthetic candidate. The ideal shape of a residual limb is cylindrical, not conical. One common mistake is wrapping the stump too tightly at the proximal end, which can lead to congestion and worsening edema and also cause the residual limb to become shaped like a dumbbell. Another common mistake is not wrapping transfemoral amputations in a waist-high soft spica cast that includes the groin. If wrapped incorrectly, the limb has a narrow, conical shape, and a large adductor roll develops. Because of the difficulty in wrapping the transfemoral amputation with elastic bandages, shrinker socks with a waist belt are frequently used as a safer alternative for the transfemoral level.

Stump edema syndrome is a condition commonly caused by proximal constriction and characterized by edema, pain, blood in the skin, and increased pigmentation. The syndrome usually responds to temporary removal of the prosthesis, elevation of the residual limb, and compression.

6. Joint contractures—Joint contractures usually develop between the time of amputation and prosthetic fitting. Contractures that exist preoperatively can seldom be corrected postoperatively.

In transfemoral amputees, the deforming forces are flexion and abduction. Adductor and hamstring stabilization can oppose the deforming forces. During the postoperative period, patients should avoid propping up the residual limb on a pillow and should begin active and passive motion exercises early, including lying prone to stretch the hip.

In transtibial amputees, knee flexion contractures greater than 15 degrees can cause major prosthetic problems and failure. Long leg rigid dressings, early postoperative prosthetic fitting, quadriceps-strengthening exercises, and hamstring stretching can prevent this complication. Because contractures in below-knee amputees can seldom be corrected, their prevention is paramount.

In the upper extremity amputee, shoulder and elbow flexion contractures often follow amputation, especially with short residual limbs. Efforts should be directed at prevention, with aggressive physical therapy beginning soon after surgery.

7. Dermatologic problems—Good general hygiene includes keeping the residual limb and prosthetic socket clean, rinsed well to remove all soap residual, and thoroughly dry. Patients should avoid the application of foreign materials and be encouraged not to shave a residual lower limb. Shaving seems to increase the problems with ingrown hairs and folliculitis.

Reactive hyperemia is the early onset of redness and tenderness after amputation. It is usually related to pressure and resolves spontaneously.

Epidermoid cysts commonly occur at the prosthetic socket brim, especially posteriorly. These cysts are difficult to treat and commonly recur, even after excision. The best initial approach is to modify the socket and relieve pressure over the cyst. Warm heat, often with a warm tea bag; topical agents; and oral antibiotics can be required as local treatment.

Verrucous hyperplasia is a wartlike overgrowth of skin that can occur on the distal end of the residual limb. It is caused by a lack of distal contact and failure to remove normal keratin. The disorder is characterized by a thick mass of keratin, sometimes accompanied by fissuring, oozing, and infection. The infection should be addressed first, and then the limb should be soaked and treated with salicylic acid paste to soften the keratin. Topical hydrocortisone is occasionally helpful in resistant cases. Prosthetic modifications to improve distal contact must be made to prevent recurrences. Because the distal limb is often tender and prosthetic modifications are uncomfortable, an aggressive preventive approach is warranted.

Contact dermatitis sometimes occurs in amputees and can be confused with infection. The primary irritation type of dermatitis is caused by contact with acids, bases, or caustics and frequently results from failure to rinse detergents and soaps from prosthetic socks. Patients should be instructed to use mild soap and to rinse extremely well. Allergic contact dermatitis is commonly caused by the nickel and chrome in metal, antioxidants in rubber, carbon in neoprene, chromium salts used to treat leather, and unpolymerized epoxy and polyester resins in plastic laminated sockets. After infection is ruled out and contact dermatitis is confirmed, treatment begins and consists of removal of the irritant and use of soaks, corticosteroid creams, and compression with elastic wraps or shrinkers.

Superficial skin infections are common in amputees. Folliculitis occurs in hairy areas, often soon after the patient starts to wear a prosthesis. Pustules develop in the eccrine sweat glands surrounding the hair follicles, and this problem is often worse if the patient shaves. Hidradenitis, which occurs in apocrine glands in the groin and axilla, tends to be chronic and responds poorly to treatment. Socket modification to relieve any pressure in these areas can be helpful. Candidiasis and other dermatophytoses present with scaly, itchy skin, often with vesicles at the border and clearing centrally. Dermatophytoses are diagnosed with a potassium hydroxide preparation and treated with topical antifungal agents.

C. Lengthening of Residual Limbs

The ultimate function of an amputation depends on both the length of the bone and the quality of the soft-tissue envelope for the residual limb. Ilizarov techniques of distraction osteogenesis are applied to lengthen the tibia or ulna in amputees. Bone lengthening can be successful, but often issues of soft-tissue coverage remain. Although great success is described in a small series of congenital short transradial amputations, another author describes the pending necrosis of the skin over the tip of the lengthened ulna. Nonadherent, mobile soft tissue that can pad the distal end of the bone is vitally important to successful prosthetic fitting. Microsurgical techniques are also applied to use free tissue transfer to supply this type of coverage over bone in select patients, most often in trauma or tumor surgery. By using these techniques, the gracilis or latissimus dorsi muscle can be transferred to the end of the residual limb and covered with skin graft. The transposed tissues do not have sensation, and the bulk of the flap can lead to tremendous volume changes over the first 2 years. Lack of sensation and volume issues do complicate prosthetic fitting and function. These extraordinary techniques are probably best reserved for very select and unique circumstances.

D. Prescription of Prosthetic Limbs

For lower limb prostheses, the major advances include the development of new lightweight structural materials (see Chapter 1), the incorporation of elastic response ("energy-storing") designs, the use of computer-assisted design and computer-assisted manufacturing technology in sockets, and microprocessor control of the prosthetic knee joint. For upper limb use, new electronic technology has increased the success and durability of myoelectric prostheses. The surgeon who prescribes prosthetic limbs should have a basic understanding of the general features available to match optimally the components with the patient's specific needs.

A good prosthetic prescription specifies the socket type, suspension, shank construction, specific joints, and terminal device. The socket can be a hard socket with no or minimal interface, or it can incorporate a liner. For the transfemoral amputee, a wide variety of socket shapes are available and range from the traditional quadrilateral design to the newer narrow mediolateral design. The prosthesis is suspended from the body by straps, belts, socket contour, liners that roll on the limb and then lock to the socket, suction, friction, or physiologic muscle control.

Shank construction can be either exoskeletal or endoskeletal. The older exoskeletal type has a rigid outer shell that is hollow in the center. The endoskeletal type has a central pylon or pipe surrounded by a soft and lightweight cosmetic foam cover. In the past, exoskeletal systems were more durable; however, as materials technology has improved, so has the durability and cosmetic appearance of endoskeletal systems. The endoskeletal systems also allow more adjustment and fine tuning of alignment and are now considered structurally as durable as the older exoskeletal designs. However, the cosmetic and foam covers for the endoskeletal systems are not as durable as an exoskeletal shell. Exoskeletal systems are rarely prescribed, except for very active patients without easy access to prosthetic services or for those involved in activities that would stain, tear, or destroy the endoskeletal cover. As the public's impression of disability has evolved, many active patients now decide not to cover the prosthesis and often take pride in the high-tech look of the titanium or carbon fiber components incorporated in an endoskeletal prosthesis.

A large variety of elbow, wrist, knee, and ankle joints are now available, as well as numerous terminal devices, including hands, hooks, feet, and special adaptive equipment for sports and work. The choice of an appropriate terminal device is extremely important. For an upper extremity amputee, there is no sensation in the prosthesis, and the critical feedback of touch and proprioception is missing. Initially, a hook may be a better choice than a prosthetic hand because vision must substitute for upper extremity proprioception, and a prosthetic hand blocks vision and makes dexterous use of the terminal device difficult and clumsy. In each case, the prosthetic prescription must be individualized to ensure the most efficient system for a particular patient.

Nearly all prosthetic sockets are fabricated by forming a thermoplastic or laminate socket over a plaster mold. An exact mold of the residual limb does not make a good socket for a prosthesis. The original mold must be modified to relieve the socket over areas that cannot tolerate pressure and to indent the socket over areas that can. Test sockets of clear plastic are commonly made to visualize the blanching of the skin at troublesome areas. automated fabrication of mobility aids (AFMA) technology uses computer-assisted design and manufacturing to aid the prosthetist by digitizing the residual limb, adding the standard modifications usually applied to a mold, and allowing additional fine manipulation of the shape on the computer screen. The computer can direct the carving of the mold or fabrication of the socket. AFMA technology can decrease the time needed for the fabrication of prostheses and increase the time available for the evaluation and training of patients. The best use of AFMA is to allow fabrication of multiple sockets for one patient during the fitting process. By using computer modifications, refinements are added in each iteration, ultimately to optimize the fit and comfort of the final socket. Before AFMA, this technique was not cost effective.

Myoelectric components are exciting but should generally not be prescribed for patients until they master traditional body-powered devices and their residual limb volume is stable. Myoelectric devices are used most successfully by patients with a midlength transradial amputation. Although a long below-elbow limb has better rotation, it is less able to contain the electronics. The need for myoelectric devices is greater in patients with a more proximal upper extremity amputation, but the weight and slow speed of the myoelectric components is a deterrent for their use. Hybrid devices utilizing body power and myoelectric components can be effective. Muscles stabilized by myodesis or myoplasty techniques seem to generate a better signal for myoelectric use.

Microprocessor control systems are applied to the knee units for transfemoral amputees. The microprocessor control alters the resistance of the knee unit to flexion or extension appropriately by sensing the position and velocity of the shank relative to the thigh. The current microprocessor-controlled knee units still do not provide power for active knee extension that would assist in rising from the sitting position or in providing power to the amputee's gait and rise up stairs. The new microprocessor-controlled so-called intelligent knee units do offer superior control when walking at varied speeds, descending ramps and stairs, and walking on uneven surfaces. Patients report improved confidence and a decrease in the tendency for the knee unit to buckle. One transfemoral amputee credits this new technology for his survival by allowing him to descend 70 stories in the World Trade Center at a normal pace during the terrorist attacks.

Attal N, Rouaud J, Brasseur L et al: Systemic lidocaine in pain due to peripheral nerve injury and predictors of response. Neurology 2004;62(2):218. [PMID: 14745057]

Bone M, Critchley P, Buggy DJ: Gabapentin in postamputation phantom limb pain: A randomized, double-blind, placebo-controlled, cross-over study. Reg Anesth Pain Med 2002;2 7(5):481. [PMID: 12373695]

Bosse MJ et al: A prospective evaluation of the clinical utility of the lower-extremity injury-severity scores. J Bone Joint Surg Am 2001;83-A(1):3. [PMID: 11205855]

Boyko EJ et al: A prospective study of risk factors for diabetic foot ulcer. The Seattle Diabetic Foot Study. Diabetes Care 1999; 22(7):1036. [PMID: 10388963]

Brooks B et al: TBI or not TBI: That is the question. Is it better to measure toe pressure than ankle pressure in diabetic patients? Diabet Med 2001;18(7):528. [PMID: 11553180]

Burgess EM et al: *The Management of Lower-Extremity Amputations.* Publication TR 10-6. U.S. Government Printing Office, 1969.

Carter SA, Tate RB: The value of toe pulse waves in determination of risks for limb amputation and death in patients with peripheral arterial disease and skin ulcers or gangrene. J Vasc Surg 2001;33(4):708. [PMID: 11296321]

Ehde DM et al: Chronic phantom sensations, phantom pain, residual limb pain, and other regional pain after lower limb amputation. Arch Phys Med Rehabil 2000;81(8):1039. [PMID: 10943752]

Lambert AW et al: Randomized prospective study comparing preoperative epidural and intraoperative perineural analgesia for the prevention of postoperative stump and phantom limb pain following major amputation. Reg Anesth Pain Med 2001;26(4):316. [PMID: 11464349]

Lane JM et al: Rehabilitation for limb salvage patients: Kinesiological parameters and psychological assessment. Cancer 2001;92 (Suppl 4):1013. [PMID: 11519028]

Marks LJ, Michael JW: Science, medicine, and the future: Artificial limbs. BMJ 2001;323(7315):732. [PMID: 11576982]

Mayfield JA et al: Trends in lower limb amputation in the Veterans Health Administration, 1989–1998. J Rehabil Res Dev 2000;37(1):23. [PMID: 10847569]

Melzack R: Phantom limbs. Sci Am 1992;266:120. [PMID: 1566028]

Mertens P, Lammens J: Short amputation stump lengthening with the Ilizarov method: Risks versus benefits. Acta Orthop Belg 2001;67(3):274. [PMID: 11486691]

Misuri A et al: Predictive value of transcutaneous oximetry for selection of the amputation level. J Cardiovasc Surg (Torino) 2000;41(1):83. [PMID: 10836229]

Nikolajsen L et al: Phantom limb pain. Curr Rev Pain 2000;4(2): 166. [PMID: 10998730]

Nikolajsen L et al: Randomized trial of epidural bupivacaine and morphine in prevention of stump and phantom pain in lower limb amputation. Lancet 1997;350:1353.

Peabody TD et al: Evaluation and staging of musculoskeletal neoplasms. J Bone Joint Surg Am 1998;80(8):1204. [PMID: 9730132]

Reiber GE, Ledoux W: Epidemiology of foot ulcers and amputations in the diabetic foot: Evidence for prevention. In Williams R et al (eds): *The Evidence Base for Diabetes Care.* Wiley, 2002.

Siddle L: The challenge and management of phantom limb pain after amputation. Br J Nurs 2004;13(11):664. [PMID: 15218432]

Smith DG, Burgess EM: The use of CAD/CAM technology in prosthetics and orthotics—Current clinical models and a view to the future. J Rehabil Res Dev 2001;38(3):327. [PMID: 11440264]

Smith DG, McFarland LV, Sangeorzan BJ et al: Postoperative dressing and management strategies for transtibial amputations: A critical review. J Rehabil Res Dev 2003;40(3):213. Review. [PMID: 14582525]

Soucacos PN: Indications and selection for digital amputation and replantation. J Hand Surg [Br] 2001;26(6):572. Review. [PMID: 11884116]

Stojadinovic A et al: Amputation for recurrent soft tissue sarcoma of the extremity: Indications and outcome. Ann Surg Oncol 2001;8(6):509. [PMID: 11456050]

Waters RL et al: The energy cost of walking of amputees: Influence of level of amputation. J Bone Joint Surg AM 1976; 58:42. [PMID: 1249111]

TYPES OF AMPUTATION

UPPER EXTREMITY AMPUTATIONS & DISARTICULATIONS

Hand Amputation

Although microsurgical replantation techniques have reduced the incidence of hand amputations, for many patients replantation is still not feasible or results in failure. There is considerable controversy about the best treatment for any given hand injury, and the optimal treatment takes into consideration the injured patient's occupation, hobbies, skills, and hand of dominance. The hand is a highly visible and important part of body image. Many patients with partial hand amputations can benefit tremendously from using a cosmetic partial hand prosthesis.

A. Fingertip Amputation

Fingertip injuries occur frequently, and fingertip amputation is the most common type of amputation. The treatment of choice usually depends on the geometry of the defect and whether or not bone is exposed. Although a large variety of local flap procedures are used to cover defects of different shapes and sizes, there is also a growing understanding that allowing secondary healing of fingertip injuries is the treatment least prone to complications in adults as well as in children. Even if bone is exposed, simply rongeuring back the exposed bone proximal to the soft-tissue defect and allowing secondary healing can give excellent results. The amount of the bone that can be removed is limited because at least a third of the distal phalanx must be left intact to prevent a hook deformity of the nail.

Two problems frequently result from fingertip amputations: cold intolerance and hypersensitivity. Overall, regardless of which treatment is chosen, approximately 30–50% of patients experience these problems. One criticism of the many local flap procedures used to obtain coverage and primary wound healing is that all of them involve incising and advancing uninjured tissue, which extends the area of scarring and damages the fine branches of the digital nerves. Newer studies suggest that the incidence of cold intolerance and hypersensitivity may be lower with secondary healing than with skin grafts or local flaps.

B. Thumb Amputation

The thumb, with its unique range of motion, plays the major role in all three prehensile activities of the hand: palmar grip, side-to-side pinch, and tip-to-tip pinch. Amputation of the thumb can result in the loss of virtually all hand function. Thumb amputations can involve (1) the distal third of the thumb (ie, distal to the interphalangeal joint), (2) the middle third of the thumb (ie, from the metacarpophalangeal joint to the interphalangeal joint), or (3) the proximal third of the thumb.

Thumb amputation of the distal third allows the patient to retain a tremendous amount of thumb function. Cold intolerance and hypersensitivity are frequent problems, as noted in the previous discussion of fingertip amputations. Treatment of distal third injuries should allow secondary healing of the thumb or should use relatively uncomplicated techniques for coverage.

Thumb amputation in the middle third is more complicated. The issues here are length, stability, and sensate skin coverage. More aggressive procedures may well be warranted and may consist of cross-finger flaps, volar advancement flaps, neurovascular island flaps from the dorsal index finger (radial nerve) or volar middle finger (median nerve), bone lengthening, or web space deepening.

Thumb amputation in the proximal third has a devastating impact on hand function. Local reconstruction for this degree of loss is not generally successful. Pollicization of another digit, a toe-to-hand transfer, or other complicated surgical techniques may be indicated to restore function.

C. Digit Amputation

Isolated amputation of a lesser digit can cause a variety of functional and cosmetic problems. Digit amputations distal to the insertion of the sublimis flexor tendon retain active flexor tendon activity and maintain useful metacarpophalangeal joint flexion. The long flexor tendon should not be sewn to the extensor tendon because it limits the excursion of both tendons and definitely limits the function of the remaining digits.

Amputations proximal to the sublimis tendon insertion retain approximately 45 degrees of proximal phalanx flexion at the metacarpophalangeal joint through the action of the intrinsic muscles. This is usually enough to keep small objects from falling through the defect and to allow the residual finger to participate to some degree in grip. If the patient uses a cosmetic finger prosthesis and wears a ring to cover the proximal edge of the prosthesis, the amputation is almost unnoticeable.

The index finger participates principally in side-to-side and tip-to-tip pinch with the thumb. After an amputation of the index finger at the metacarpophalangeal joint, the middle finger assumes this important role. The residual second metacarpal can interfere with side-to-side pinch between the thumb and the middle finger, however. Converting this amputation to a ray amputation often can improve function and cosmesis, but the drawback is that it also narrows the width of the palm and can decrease grip and torque strength significantly. Surgical decisions must be individualized, but the second metacarpal should probably be retained if the patient uses hand tools extensively, as does a carpenter or machinist.

Amputation of the middle or ring finger at the metacarpophalangeal joint can make it difficult for the patient to hold small objects because they tend to fall through the defect. Full ray resection can narrow the central defect and occasionally improve function, but narrowing the palm can decrease grip and torque strength.

Amputation of the small finger at the metacarpophalangeal joint is often cosmetically unacceptable because of the abrupt and noticeable change in contour of the hand. Although converting a fifth digital amputation to a ray amputation by including the metacarpal can improve cosmesis, it also narrows the width of the palm and can decrease grip and torque strength. Surgical decisions must be based on individual factors and concerns.

D. Carpus Amputation

Amputations through the carpus are generally discouraged. Most surgeons believe the result to have no real advantages over a wrist disarticulation or transradial amputation. There are isolated reports of patients valuing the little bit of wrist flexion and extension that allows them to hold objects against their body and to stabilize objects for two-handed grasp. The flexor and extensor carpi radialis and ulnaris tendons must be reattached to provide this limited motion. The prosthetic options are less standard and generally considered to be less functional than the traditional transradial designs.

Carpus amputations should probably be considered in bilateral cases. Although rare, more patients sustaining tissue loss from ischemia are seen in the intensive care unit after prolonged resuscitations and the use of vasopressors. Without the vasopressors, these patients would die. Unfortunately, part of the body's response to these lifesaving medications can be to shunt blood flow from the distal extremities, resulting in demarcation and dry gangrene in the hands and feet. Just as in frostbite, if infection is not present, it is worthwhile to delay any surgical intervention and allow adequate time for tissue demarcation and recovery. Partial hand amputation is occasionally necessary, and if required, the carpus level should be considered.

Wrist Disarticulation

Wrist disarticulation continues to be controversial. Proponents frequently argue that it has two advantages over the shorter transradial amputation: It retains the distal radioulnar joint, which preserves more forearm rotation, and it retains the distal radial flare, which dramatically improves prosthetic suspension. Volar and dorsal fish-mouth incisions are usually best, and removal of the radial and ulnar styloids can prevent painful pressure points. Tenodesis of the major forearm motors stabilizes the muscle units and thereby improves physiologic and myoelectric performance.

Opponents of wrist disarticulation argue that prosthetic substitution after this procedure is slightly more complicated than it is after a standard transradial amputation. The prosthetic socket is more difficult to fabricate because of the bone contours. Conventional wrist units add too much length to the prosthetic arm after wrist disarticulation and therefore cannot be used. The terminal device for a wrist disarticulation also needs to be modified because of length. Myoelectric prostheses are difficult to fit because there is less space to conceal the electronics and power supply.

In spite of these prosthetic concerns, wrist disarticulation patients are often excellent upper extremity prosthetic users. Some patients with an unsatisfactory hand can gain improved function by undergoing a wrist disarticulation and using a standard prosthesis. This decision must be individualized and based on contributory factors such as severity of tissue loss, pain, functional requirements, and the patient's body image.

Transradial Amputation

The transradial amputation is extremely functional, and successful prosthetic rehabilitation and sustained use are achieved in 70–80% of patients who undergo amputation at this level. Forearm rotation and strength are proportional to the length retained. Surgical incisions are best with equal volar and dorsal flaps. A myodesis should be performed to prevent a painful bursa, facilitate physiologic muscular suspension, and allow for myoelectric prosthetic use. An extremely short transradial residual limb requires the use of a Muenster-type socket, which molds up around the humeral condyles for added suspension. Occasionally, side hinges and a humeral cuff are required to achieve suspension of the prosthesis. Both of these types of suspension preserve elbow flexion and extension but limit rotation.

The value of preserving the elbow joint cannot be overemphasized. Skin grafts and even composite grafts should be considered to retain the tremendous functional benefit of an elbow with some active motion. Even a limited range of elbow motion can be useful, and an ingeniously designed, geared step-up elbow hinge can convert a limited active range of elbow motion to an improved prosthetic ROM. Although body-powered prostheses are extremely functional at the transradial level of amputation, this level is also the most successful level at which to use myoelectric devices.

Krukenberg Amputation

The Krukenberg kineplastic operation transforms the transradial amputation stump into radial and ulnar digits that are capable of strong prehension and have excellent manipulative ability because of retained sensation on the "fingers" of the forearm. The operation should not be performed as a primary amputation.

The Krukenberg amputation can be performed as a secondary procedure in a transradial amputee who has a residual limb of at least 10 cm from the tip of the olecranon, an elbow flexion contracture of less than 70 degrees, and good psychological preparation and acceptance. In this case, the amputee can become completely independent in daily activities because of the retained sensory ability of the pincers as well as the quality of the grasping mechanism (Figure 12–6). The Krukenberg amputation traditionally was indicated for blind patients with bilateral below-elbow amputations, but it also may be indicated at least unilaterally in bilateral below-elbow amputees who are able to see and in those who have limited access to prosthetic facilities.

A conventional prosthesis can be worn over the Krukenberg forearm, and myoelectric devices can be adapted to use the forearm motion. The major disadvantage is the appearance of the arm, which many people consider grotesque and do not accept. As society continues to become more understanding and accepting of disabled individuals, concerns about appearance may diminish. Intensive preoperative preparation and counseling are mandatory.

Elbow Disarticulation

Elbow disarticulation can be a satisfactory amputation level and has the advantage of retaining the condylar flare to improve prosthetic suspension and allow for the transfer of humeral rotation to the prosthesis. The longer lever arm improves strength. The disadvantage is in the design of the prosthetic elbow hinge. An outside hinge is bulky and hard on clothing, whereas the conventional elbow unit provides a disproportionately long upper arm and short forearm. Whether the advantages of the elbow disarticulation outweigh the disadvantages remains controversial. Surgically, volar and dorsal flaps work best, and myodesis of the biceps and triceps tendons are needed to preserve the distal muscle attachments.

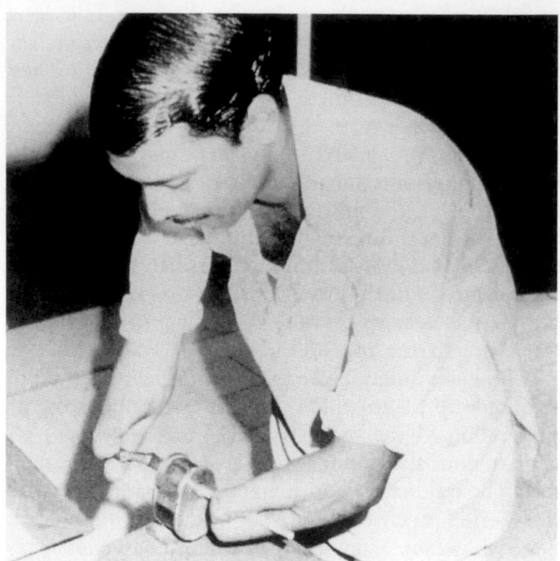

Figure 12–6. A patient with bilateral Krukenberg hands demonstrates bimanual dexterity in sharpening a pencil. (Reproduced, with permission, from Garst RJ: The Krukenberg hand. J Bone Joint Surg Br 1991;73:385.)

Transhumeral Amputation

When transhumeral amputation is performed, efforts should be made to retain as much as possible of the bone length that has suitable soft-tissue coverage. Even if only the humeral head remains and no functional length is salvageable, an improved shoulder contour and cosmetic appearance results. Myodesis helps preserve biceps and triceps strength, prosthetic control, and myoelectric signals. In most cases of transhumeral amputation, an immediate postoperative prosthesis and rigid dressings can be used successfully. Physical therapy should focus on proximal joint and muscle function. Because the terminal prosthetic device is usually controlled by active shoulder girdle motion, early prosthetic use and therapy can prevent contracture and maintain strength.

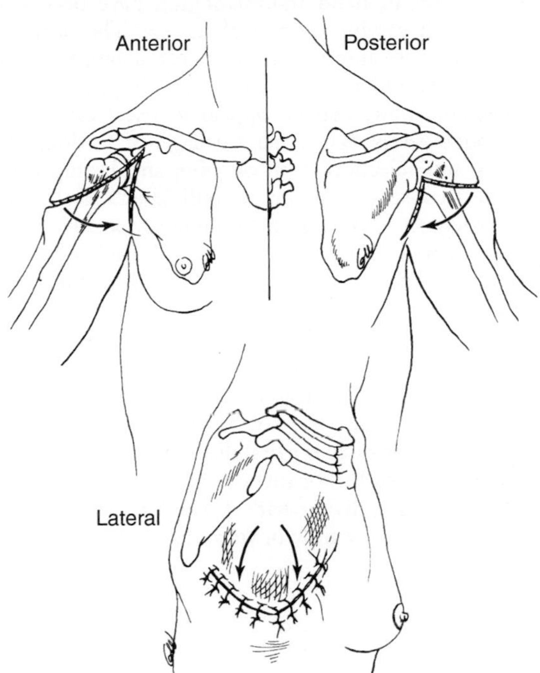

Figure 12–7. Shoulder disarticulation.

transhumeral amputation because of brachial plexus injury—one group without shoulder arthrodesis and one group with it—found a somewhat better return-to-work rate in the group without shoulder arthrodesis. Prosthetic expectations in these patients should be limited because prosthetic fitting adds weight to a dysfunctional shoulder girdle, often defeating one of the original goals of the amputation.

Shoulder Disarticulation & Scapulothoracic (Forequarter) Amputation

The performance of shoulder disarticulation (Figure 12–7) or scapulothoracic amputation (Figure 12–8) is rare. When either operation is performed, it is usually in cases of cancer or severe trauma. Either operation results in a loss of the normal shoulder contour and causes the patient difficulty because clothing does not fit well. Saving the humeral head, if possible, can improve the contour of a shoulder disarticulation tremendously. The scapulothoracic amputation, usually performed for proximal tumors, removes the arm, scapula, and clavicle. Dissection often extends into the neck and into the thorax.

Elaborate myoelectric prostheses are available for patients but are expensive, heavy, and require intensive maintenance. Body-powered prostheses are also heavy,

Prosthetic suspension traditionally was incorporated in the body-powered harness, which can be somewhat uncomfortable. Among the alternative techniques are humeral angulation osteotomy (rarely used), socket-suction suspension, and the newer elastomeric roll on locking liners. Many prosthetic options are available for the transhumeral amputee. One option is a prosthesis that is totally body powered. Another is a hybrid prosthesis that uses myoelectric control of one component (either the terminal device or the elbow device) and body-powered control of the other. The transhumeral prosthesis is heavy, often considered slow, and requires much mental concentration to use effectively. These issues lead many unilateral transhumeral amputees to choose not to wear a prosthesis at all or to wear only a lightweight cosmetic prosthesis for special occasions.

Transhumeral amputation is sometimes elected to manage a dysfunctional arm following a severe brachial plexus injury. The advantages of amputation are that it unloads the weight from the shoulder and scapulothoracic joints and eliminates the problem of having a paralyzed arm that gets in the way and hinders body function. The decision to undertake shoulder arthrodesis in combination with transhumeral amputation is controversial and should be made on an individualized basis. Investigators who compared two groups of patients with

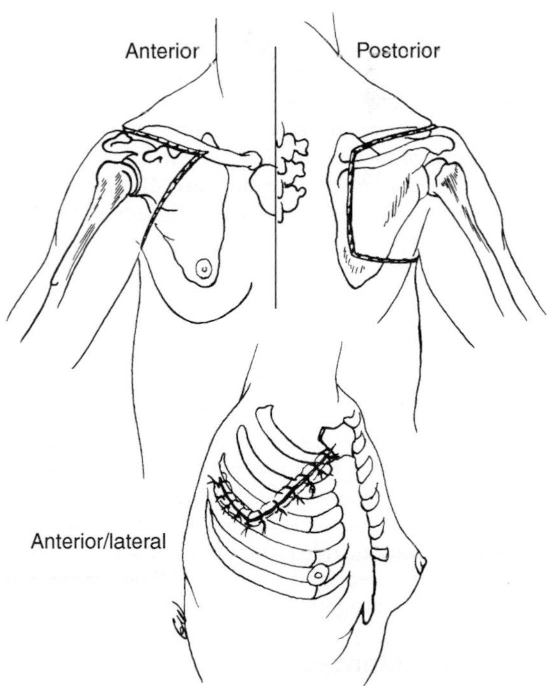

Figure 12–8. Forequarter amputation.

hard to suspend comfortably, and difficult to use. Most patients request prosthetic help for improved cosmesis and fitting of clothes. Often a simple soft mold to fill out the shoulder meets these expectations and is an alternative to a full-arm cosmetic prosthesis.

Postural Abnormalities after High Upper Extremity Amputation

Normally, the weight of the arm and the muscle activity associated with shoulder and arm function keep the shoulders appropriately level. Unilateral hypertrophy of an upper limb, including the shoulder girdle, occurs in certain occupations and is also seen in some sports. Some people are born with a degree of asymmetry of their shoulders, which is a relatively minor postural abnormality and does not require special clothing.

When the arm is removed and the clavicle and scapula remain, the muscles elevating the shoulder girdle are unopposed by both the weight of the arm and those muscles that pass across the shoulder and tend to depress the shoulder and arm. The consequence of this imbalance is an upward elevation described as "hiking" of the shoulder girdle. This high shoulder tends to accentuate the cosmetic loss, even when the individual is wearing a cosmetic shoulder filler or a cosmetic limb. Abnormal shoulder elevation can be countered by corrective exercises beginning as soon as they can be tolerated after the amputation. The wearing of a prosthesis with its dependent weight also diminishes shoulder hike. In most circumstances, the shoulder girdle elevation is inevitable; however, its degree can be minimized by appropriate physical measures.

Removal of the entire upper limb in the growing skeleton can result in a scoliosis of the spine. Muscular imbalance is considered to be the cause of the deformity. It may be seen to a slighter degree in the adult but is primarily confined to the growing skeleton. The combined postural deformity of upper dorsal spine scoliosis and elevation of the shoulder girdle produces asymmetry of the head and neck on the trunk, with the head appearing to be placed asymmetrically as the person stands.

In general, no corrective splinting or orthotic device can successfully counteract the postural changes associated with shoulder-level amputation. Neck and shoulder-girdle exercises offer the most effective prophylaxis and treatment. The postural deficits are particularly evident with forequarter amputation. Soft, light polyurethane cosmetic restoration, either as part of a cosmetic prosthesis or separately used with the empty sleeve, counters to some degree the unsightly upper body contour.

Hand Transplantation

Hand transplantation and the suppression of rejections is now technically possible. Approximately 25 documented cases of hand transplantation have been performed with varying degrees of success. The potential benefits for the amputee are certainly many, but they must be balanced against the real risks. In general, skin, muscle, and bone marrow appear to reject earlier and more aggressively than bone, cartilage, or tendon. Preventing this rejection is an ongoing and lasting issue, with real consequences for the individual's health and life expectancy. The current immunosuppressive drugs needed to prevent rejection of a composite hand transplant include toxic side effects, opportunistic infections, and increase in malignancies.

Also, the real psychological impact following hand and other organ transplantation should not be underestimated. One study examining the issues 5 years following heart transplant showed a significant increase in emotional issues such as irritability, depression, and low self-esteem. Even for a patient with no preexisting psychological issues, living with a hand transplantation, which remains constantly in view, may not be easy.

Baumeister S, Kleist C, Dohler B et al: Risks of allogeneic hand transplantation. Microsurgery 2004;24(2):98. Review. [PMID: 15038013]

Crandall RC, Tomhave W: Pediatric unilateral below-elbow amputees: Retrospective analysis of 34 patients given multiple prosthetic options. J Pediatr Orthop 2002;22(3):380. [PMID: 11961460]

Goel A et al: Replantation and amputation of digits: User analysis. Am J Phys Med Rehabil 1995;74(2):134. [PMID: 7710728]

Hatrick NC, Tonkin MA: Hand transplantation: A current perspective. ANZ J Surg 2001;71(4):245. [PMID: 11354126]

Martin C, Gonzalez del Pino J: Controversies in the treatment of fingertip amputations. Conservative versus surgical reconstruction. Clin Orthop 1998;(353):63. [PMID: 9728160]

Neusel E et al: Results of humeral stump angulation osteotomy. Arch Orthop Trauma Surg 1997;116:263. [PMID: 9177800]

Peimer CA et al: Hand function following single ray amputation. J Hand Surg [Am] 1999;24(6):1245. [PMID: 10584948]

Schatz RL, Rosenwasser MP: Krukenberg kineplasty: A case study. J Hand Ther 2002;15(3):260. [PMID: 12206329]

Waikakul S, Sakkarnkosol S, Vanadurongwan V et al: Results of 1018 digital replantations in 552 patients. Injury 2000;31(1):33. [PMID: 10716048]

Wilkinson MC et al: Brachial plexus injury: When to amputate? Injury 1993;24(9):603. [PMID: 8288380]

LOWER EXTREMITY AMPUTATIONS & DISARTICULATIONS

Foot Amputation

A. Toe Amputation

Toe amputations can be performed with side-to-side or plantar-to-dorsal flaps to use the best available soft tissue. The bone should be shortened to a level that allows adequate soft-tissue closure without tension.

In great toe amputations, if the entire proximal phalanx is removed, the sesamoids can retract and expose the keel-shaped plantar surface of the first metatarsal to weight bearing. This often leads to high local pressure, callous formation, or ulceration. The sesamoids can be stabilized in position for weight bearing by leaving the base of the proximal phalanx intact or by performing tenodesis of the flexor hallucis brevis tendon.

An isolated amputation of the second toe commonly results in severe hallux valgus deformity of first toe (Figure 12–9). This situation may be prevented by amputation of the second ray or by fusion of the first metatarsal and phalanx. In the shorter toe amputations at the metatarsophalangeal joint level, transferring the extensor tendon to the capsule may help elevate the metatarsal head and maintain an even distribution for weight bearing. Prosthetic replacement is not required after toe amputations.

B. Ray Amputation

A ray amputation removes the toe and all or some of the corresponding metatarsal. Isolated ray amputations can be durable. Multiple ray amputations, however, especially in patients with vascular disease, can narrow the foot excessively. This increases the amount of weight that must be borne by the remaining metatarsal heads and can lead to new areas of increased pressure, callous formation, and ulceration. Surgically, it is often difficult to achieve primary closure of ray amputation wounds because more skin is usually required than is readily apparent. Instead of closing these wounds under tension, it is usually advisable to leave them open and allow for secondary healing.

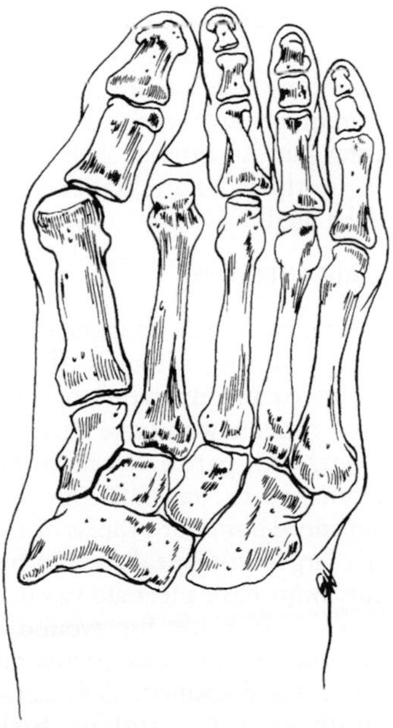

Figure 12–9. Severe hallux valgus deformity occurring after isolated second toe amputation.

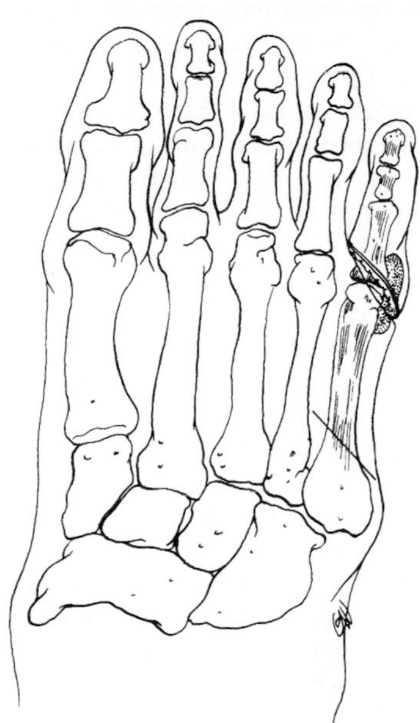

Figure 12–10. Fifth ray amputation for fifth metatarsal head ulcer.

The fifth ray amputation is the most useful of all the ray amputations. Plantar and lateral ulcers around the fifth metatarsal head often lead to exposed bone and osteomyelitis. A fifth ray amputation allows the entire ulcer to be excised and the wound to be closed primarily (Figure 12–10). In general, for more extensive involvement of the foot, a transverse amputation at the transmetatarsal level is more durable. Prosthetic requirements after ray amputations include extra-depth shoes with custom-molded insoles. The insole should include a metatarsal pad that loads the shafts of the metatarsal and unloads some of the pressure at the metatarsal heads.

C. Midfoot Amputation

The transmetatarsal and Lisfranc amputations are reliable and durable. The Lisfranc amputation is actually a disarticulation just proximal to the metatarsals where the cuneiform and cuboid bones are retained. Surgically, a healthy, durable soft-tissue envelope is more important than a specific anatomic level of amputation, so the length of bone to be removed should be based on the ability to perform soft-tissue closure without tension. A long plantar flap is preferable, but equal dorsal and plantar flaps work well, especially for transmetatarsal amputation in the treatment of metatarsal head ulcers (Figure 12–11).

Muscle balance around the foot should be carefully evaluated preoperatively, with specific attention to tightness of the heel cord and strength of the anterior tibial, posterior tibial, and peroneal muscles. Midfoot amputations significantly shorten the lever arm of the foot, so lengthening of the Achilles tendon should be done if necessary. Tibial or peroneal muscle insertions should be reattached if they are released during bone resection. For example, if the base of the fifth metatarsal is resected, the peroneus brevis tendon should be reinserted into the cuboid bone. In patients with vascular disease, this can be performed with a minimal amount of dissection to prevent further compromise of the tissues.

Postoperative casting prevents deformities, controls edema, and speeds rehabilitation. Prosthetic requirements can vary widely. During the first year following amputation, many patients benefit from the use of an ankle-foot orthosis (AFO) with a long footplate and a toe filler. To prevent an equinus deformity from developing, patients should be advised to wear the orthosis except when taking a bath or shower. Later, the use of a simple toe filler combined with a stiff-soled shoe may be adequate. Cosmetic partial foot prostheses are also available.

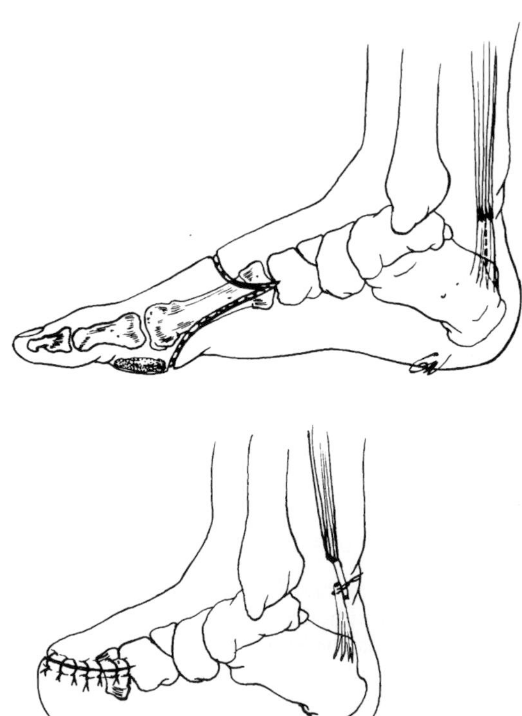

Figure 12–11. Transmetatarsal amputation with Achilles tendon lengthening.

D. Hindfoot Amputation

A Chopart amputation removes the forefoot and midfoot and saves only the talus and calcaneus. Rebalancing procedures are required to prevent equinus and varus deformities. Achilles tenotomy, transfer of the anterior tibial or extensor digitorum tendons, and postoperative casting are all usually necessary. Although tendon transfer to the talus was previously recommended, transfer to the calcaneus is now done to minimize varus positioning. Beveling the inferior, anterior surface of the calcaneus can remove a potential bone pressure point.

Two other types of hindfoot amputations are the Boyd and the Pirogoff amputations. The Boyd procedure consists of a talectomy and calcaneal-tibial arthrodesis after forward translation of the calcaneus. The Pirogoff procedure consists of a talectomy with calcaneal-tibial arthrodesis after the vertical transection of the calcaneus through the midbody and a forward rotation of the posterior process of the calcaneus under the tibia. These two types of hindfoot amputations are done mostly in children to preserve length and growth centers, prevent heel pad migration, and improve socket suspension.

Studies in which various procedures in children are compared showed that a hindfoot amputation results in better function than a Syme amputation (see section on Syme amputation) in cases in which the hindfoot is balanced and no equinus deformity has developed.

The hindfoot prosthesis requires more secure stabilization than a midfoot prosthesis to keep the heel from pistoning during gait. An anterior shell can be added to an ankle-foot prosthesis, or a posterior opening socket prosthesis can be used.

E. Partial Calcanectomy

Partial calcanectomy, which consists of excising the posterior process of the calcaneus (Figure 12–12), should be considered an amputation of the back of the foot. In selected patients with large heel ulcerations or calcaneal osteomyelitis, partial calcanectomy can be a functional alternative to transtibial amputation. The removal of the entire posterior process of the calcaneus allows for fairly large soft-tissue defects to be closed primarily. Patients must have adequate vascular perfusion and nutritional competence for wound healing to occur. As with other amputations, partial calcanectomy creates a functional and cosmetic deformity. Use of an ankle-foot prosthesis with a cushion heel is usually required to replace the missing heel and prevent further skin ulceration.

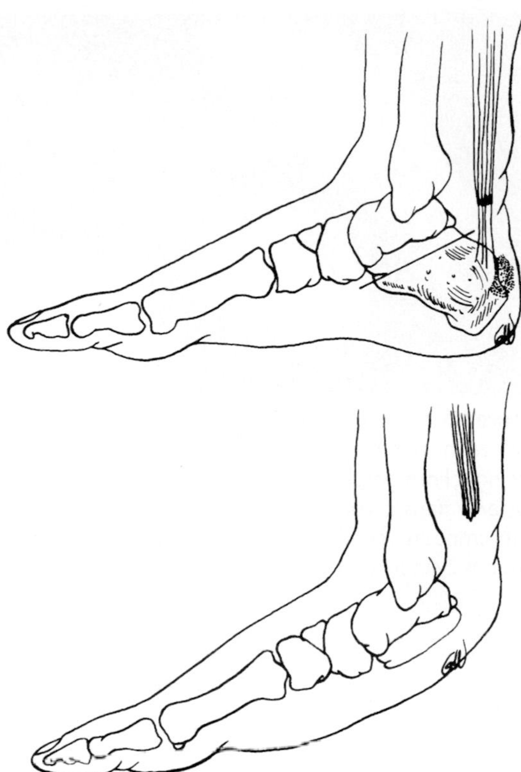

Figure 12–12. Partial calcanectomy.

Syme Amputation

In the Syme amputation, the surgeon removes the calcaneus and talus while carefully dissecting on bone to preserve the heel skin and fat pad to cover the distal tibia (Figure 12–13). The surgeon must also remove and contour the malleoli, but whether this should be done during the initial operation or 6–8 weeks later remains controversial. Proponents of the two-stage procedure argue that it can improve healing in patients with vascular disease. Opponents point out that it delays rehabilitation because the patient cannot bear weight until after the second stage of the operation. One series supports the use of the one-stage procedure, even in the presence of vascular disease or diabetes. A late complication of the Syme amputation is the posterior and medial migration of the fat pad. One of these surgical procedures can be done to stabilize the fat pad: tenodesis of the Achilles tendon to the posterior margin of the tibia through drill holes; transfer of the anterior tibial and extensor digitorum tendons to the anterior aspect of the fat pad; or removal of the cartilage and subchondral bone to allow scarring of the fat pad to bone, with or without pin fixation. Careful postoperative casting can also help keep the fat pad centered under the tibia during healing. The Syme amputation is one of the most difficult amputations to perform in terms of surgical technique and achievement of primary healing and heel pad stability.

Syme amputation should be designed to allow end bearing. Retaining the smooth, broad surface of the distal tibia and the heel pad allows direct transfer of weight from the end of the residual limb to the prosthesis. A transtibial or transfemoral amputation does not allow this direct transfer of weight. Because of the ability to end-bear, the amputee can occasionally ambulate without a prosthesis in emergency situations or for bathroom activities.

The Syme prosthesis is wider at the ankle level than is a transtibial prosthesis, and this cosmetic problem can be bothersome to some patients. The surgical narrowing of the malleolar flare and the use of new materials in the prosthesis, however, can improve the appearance of the final prosthesis. Moreover, patients can now benefit from energy-storing technology provided by the newly designed lower profile elastic response feet. Sockets do not need the high contour of a patellar-tendon bearing design because of the end-bearing quality of the residual limb. The socket can be windowed either posteriorly or medially if the limb is bulbous, or a flexible socket

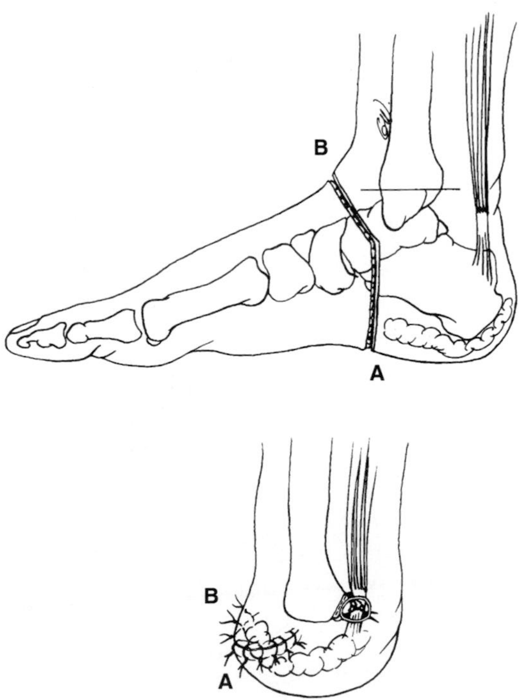

Figure 12–13. Syme amputation with tenodesis of the Achilles tendon to the distal tibia.

within a rigid frame design can be used if the limb is less bulbous. Because of the tibial flare, the socket used following Syme amputation is usually self-suspending.

Transtibial Amputation

Transtibial amputation is the most commonly performed major limb amputation. The long posterior flap technique (Figure 12–14) is now standard, and good results can be expected even in the majority of patients with vascular disease. Anterior and posterior flaps, sagittal flaps, and skewed flaps can be helpful in specific patients.

Efforts should be made to preserve as much bone length as possible between the tibial tubercle and the junction of the middle and distal thirds of the tibia, based on the available healthy soft tissues. Amputations in the distal third of the tibia should be avoided because they result in poor soft-tissue padding and are more difficult to fit comfortably with a prosthesis. The goal is a cylindrically shaped residual limb with muscle stabilization, distal tibial padding, and a nontender and nonadherent scar (Figure 12–15). The transtibial amputation is especially well suited to rigid dressings and immediate postoperative prosthetic management.

Distal tibiofibular synostosis (Ertl procedure) should be considered for the treatment of a wide trauma-induced diastasis to improve stabilization of the bone and soft tissue. The procedure is less often indicated in the treatment of patients with vascular disease. The synostosis is developed to create a broad bone mass terminally to improve the distal end-bearing property of the limb and minimize motion between the tibia and fibula. Although there is renewed interest in these techniques, true comparison of patients with osteomyoplastic techniques versus standard techniques has not been done.

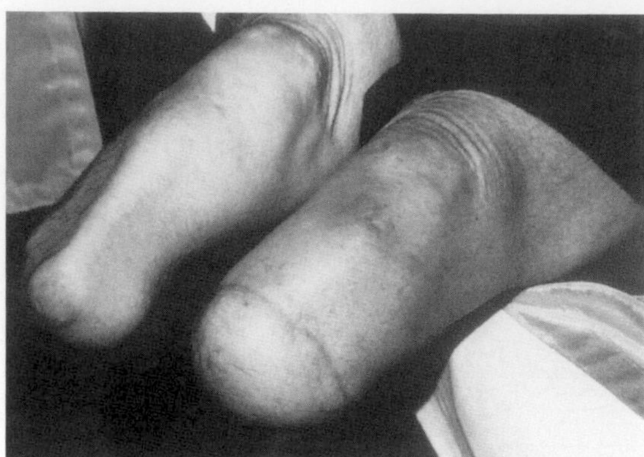

Figure 12–15. Bilateral transtibial amputations that emphasize the benefits of the long posterior flap technique. The right limb, amputated by using equal anterior and posterior flaps, is conically shaped and atrophic. The left limb, amputated by using the long posterior flap technique, is cylindrical and well padded. (Reproduced, with permission, from Smith DG, Burgess EM, Zettl JH: Fitting and Training the Bilateral Lower-Limb Amputee, in Bowker JH, Michael JW (eds): *Atlas of Limb Prosthetics Surgical, Prosthetic, and Rehabilitation Principles.* Rosemont, IL, American Academy of Orthopaedic Surgeons, 2002, pp 599–622.)

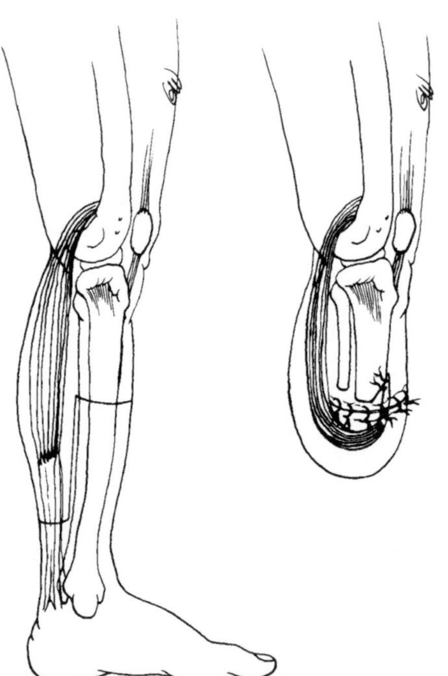

Figure 12–14. Transtibial amputation with long posterior flap technique.

A wide variety of prosthetic designs are available for the transtibial amputee. Sockets can be designed to incorporate a liner, which offers the advantages of increased comfort and accommodation of minor changes in residual limb volume. Disadvantages include increased perspiration and a less sanitary, less comfortable feeling in hot humid weather. Hard sockets are designed to have cotton or wool stump socks of an appropriate ply or thickness as the interface between the leg and the socket. Hard sockets are easier to clean and more durable than the liners are.

The Icelandic-Swedish-New York (ISNY) socket refers to the use of a more flexible socket material that is supported by a rigid frame. The flexible socket changes shape to accommodate underlying muscle contraction. This socket style can also be useful for limbs that are scarred or difficult to fit. Open-ended sockets with side joints and a thigh corset are not used much today except by patients who wore them successfully in the past and by patients with limited access to prosthetic care. The patellar tendon-bearing shape is most commonly used for the transtibial amputee. In spite of its name, the majority of the weight is borne on the medial tibial flare and laterally on the interosseus space, whereas the rest of the weight is borne on the patellar tendon area. Even the new so-called total-contact transtibial socket, which is designed to have increased contact on all areas of the residual limb, preferentially loads the tibial flare and patellar tendon regions.

Numerous types of suspension devices are available for the transtibial prosthesis. The simplest and most common is a suprapatellar strap, which wraps above the femoral condyles and patella. Sockets can be designed to incorporate a supracondylar mold or wedge to grip above the femoral condyles, but this higher profile is bulkier and less cosmetic when the patient is sitting. A waist belt and fork strap are helpful for the patient who has a very short transtibial residual limb because these devices decrease pistoning in the socket; they are also helpful for the patient whose activities require extremely secure suspension. If the patient has a limb with poor soft tissue or has intrinsic knee pain, side hinges and a thigh corset can help unload the lower leg and transfer some of the weight to the thigh.

External suspension sleeves made of latex or neoprene are still used quite frequently. Latex is more cosmetic but less durable and can be constricting. Neoprene is more durable and not as constricting but sometimes causes contact dermatitis. The newest suspension uses an elastomeric or silicone-based liner that is rolled on over the residual leg and offers an intimate friction fit. A small metal post on the distal end of the liner then locks into a catch in the prosthetic socket to suspend the socket securely to the liner. Many patients who use these elastomeric locking liners like the secure suspension and feeling of improved control of the prosthesis. The liners have the disadvantages of being less durable and requiring frequent replacement. These elastomeric locking liners can be expensive. Although elastomeric locking liners were originally touted as preventing skin problems; rashes, skin irritation, and skin breakdown remain a frequent complaint even with this new technology, however. Approximately a third of amputees cannot tolerate the forces generated at the distal part of the amputation with liners using the metal post or pin lock system. New techniques were designed to attach the elastomeric liner to the socket with vacuum pumps, clips on the side of the liner, or sealing liners and one-way socket valves to maintain a suction between the liner and the socket. Suspension must be individualized, and no system is yet proven acceptable to all amputees.

Many different designs for prosthetic feet are now available, ranging from the original solid ankle cushion heel (SACH) foot to the newer elastic response technology with a variety of keel, ankle, and pylon designs. Cost and function can vary widely, and care should be used in prescribing an appropriate prosthetic foot for an individual patient. A common error is to prescribe a foot that is either too stiff or does not get to feel flat quickly enough for an individual patient, especially in the first 12–18 months after an amputation.

Knee Disarticulation

Disarticulation through the knee joint (Figure 12–16) is indicated in ambulatory patients when a below-knee amputation is not possible but suitable soft tissue is present for a knee disarticulation. These circumstances are most commonly found in cases involving traumatic injuries. In patients with vascular disease, the blood supply is such that if a knee disarticulation would heal, a short transtibial amputation would usually heal as well. The knee disarticulation is indicated in patients who have vascular problems and are nonambulatory, especially if knee flexion contractures or spasticity are present. Although sagittal flaps or the traditional long posterior flap can be used to take advantage of the best available soft-tissue coverage, newer literature supports use of the posterior flap technique when possible. The patella is retained and the patellar tendon sutured to the cruciate stumps to stabilize the quadriceps muscle complex. The biceps tendons can also be stabilized to the

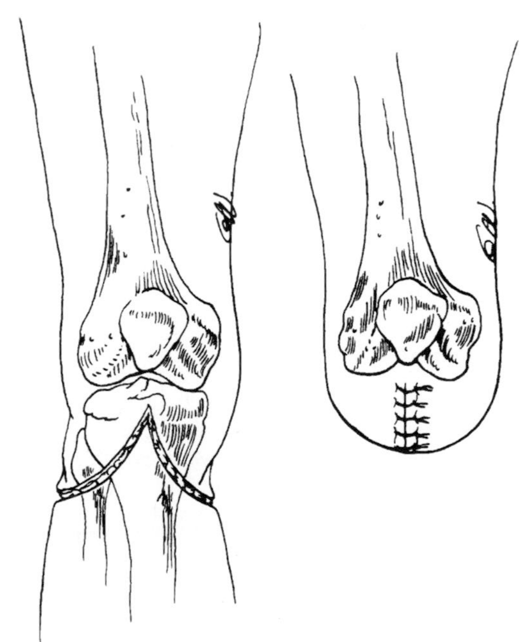

Figure 12–16. Knee disarticulation.

patellar tendon. A short section of gastrocnemius muscle can be sutured to the anterior capsule to pad the distal end. Although many techniques are described to trim the condyles of the femur, trimming is rarely necessary, and radical trimming can decrease some of the advantages of the knee disarticulation.

For ambulatory patients, the advantages of a knee disarticulation over a transfemoral amputation include improved socket suspension by contouring above the femoral condyles, the added strength of a longer lever arm, the retained muscle balance of the thigh, and, most important, the end-bearing potential to transfer weight directly to the prosthesis. In the past, the objections to a bulky prosthesis and asymmetric knee-joint level led many surgeons to abandon the practice of performing knee disarticulations. New materials allow a less bulky prosthesis to be fabricated, and the four-bar linkage knee unit, which can fold under the socket, improves the appearance of the prosthesis when the patient is sitting. The four-bar linkage knee remains the prosthetic knee of choice for a knee disarticulation. It is low profile, has excellent stability, and can incorporate a hydraulic unit for control during the swing phase of gait in patients who can walk at different cadences.

For nonambulatory patients, a knee disarticulation eliminates the problem of knee flexion contractures, provides a balanced thigh to decrease hip contractures, and provides a long lever arm for good sitting support and transfers.

The Gritti-Stokes amputation is not recommended. In this operation, the patella is advanced distally and fused by arthrodesis to the distal femur, theoretically to allow direct weight bearing. The concept behind this operation is flawed because even in normal kneeling, the weight is borne on the pretibial and patellar tendon areas and not on the patella. The added length and the asymmetry of the knee joints complicate prosthetic fitting.

Transcondylar amputation can be performed, but the end-bearing comfort and improved suspension of a transcondylar amputation appear to be diminished when compared with the true knee disarticulation.

Transfemoral Amputation

Transfemoral amputation is usually performed with equal anterior and posterior fish-mouth flaps. Atypical flaps can and should be used to save all possible femoral length in cases of trauma because the amount of function is directly proportional to the length of the residual limb.

Muscle stabilization is more important in the transfemoral amputation than in any other major limb amputation. The major deforming force is into abduction and flexion. Myodesis of the adductor muscles through drill holes in the femur can counteract the abductors, prevent a difficult adductor tissue roll in the groin, and improve prosthetic control (Figure 12–17). Without muscle stabilization, the femur commonly migrates laterally through the soft-tissue envelope to a subcutaneous location. Newer transfemoral socket designs attempt to better control the position of the femur, but they are not as effective as muscle stabilization. Even in nonambulatory patients, muscle stabilization is helpful in creating a more durable, padded residual limb by preventing migration of the femur.

An IPOP and rigid dressings are more difficult to apply and keep positioned after a transfemoral amputation than after more distal amputations. IPOP techniques do offer the advantages of early rehabilitation and control of edema and pain, and these techniques are preferred if the expertise to use them is available. The major complaints of patients with the transfemoral IPOP are the weight of the cast and the discomfort when sitting. In many cases, only a soft compressive dressing alone is used, and in these patients, the dressing should be carried proximally around the waist as a spica to better suspend the dressing and to include the medial thigh and prevent the development of an adductor roll of tissue. Proper postoperative positioning and therapy are essential to prevent hip flexion contractures.

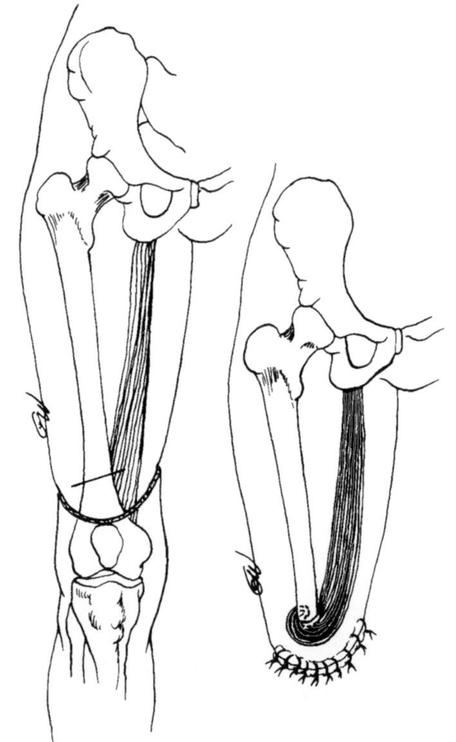

Figure 12–17. Transfemoral amputation with adductor myodesis.

The limb should be positioned flat on the bed, rather than elevated on a pillow, and hip extension exercises and prone positioning should be started early.

Suspension of the prosthesis is more complicated in transfemoral amputations than in more distal amputations because of the short residual limb, the lack of bony contours, and the increased weight of the prosthesis. The transfemoral amputation prosthesis can be suspended by suction, Silesian bandage, hip-joint and pelvic band, or by the newer elastomeric locking liners.

Traditional socket-suction suspension works when the skin forms an airtight seal against the socket. Air is forced distally through a small one-way valve when the prosthesis is donned and with each step during gait, thus maintaining negative pressure distally in the socket. No prosthetic sock or other liner is used between the hard socket and the limb because air leaks out around the sock and prevents suction from developing. Donning a socket-suction prosthesis requires skill and exertion, and patients must have good coordination, upper extremity function, and balance to perform this task. Socket-suction systems work well for average-to-long transfemoral residual limbs that have adequate soft tissues and stable shape and volume. It is usually comfortable and the most cosmetically acceptable method of socket suspension.

A Silesian bandage is a flexible strap that attaches laterally to the prosthesis, wraps back around the waist and over the contralateral iliac crest, and then comes forward to attach to the anterior proximal socket (Figure 12–18). It provides good suspension and added rotational control of the prosthesis. A Silesian bandage is commonly used to augment suction suspension for patients who have shorter-length limbs or for patients whose activities require more secure suspension than suction alone can offer.

As with the transtibial prosthesis, the newer elastomeric locking liners can provide excellent suspension and control. An elastomeric or silicone-based liner is rolled onto the leg similar to the way a condom is applied. This liner has an intimate fit with the residual limb and avoids pistoning and rotational forces. A small metal post at the distal end of the liner locks down into a catch at the bottom of the prosthetic socket to create a secure mechanical suspension. A small button must be pushed to disengage the lock and release the prosthesis. Many amputees express an improved sense of security and improved proprioception with these systems. The disadvantages continue to be the added cost, the need to replace the liners as they tear, and, rarely, developing a contact dermatitis. As discussed with transtibial amputees, approximately a third of amputees cannot tolerate the forces generated at the distal part of the amputation with liners using the metal post or pin lock system. For these patients, new methods to attach the liner to the socket must be explored.

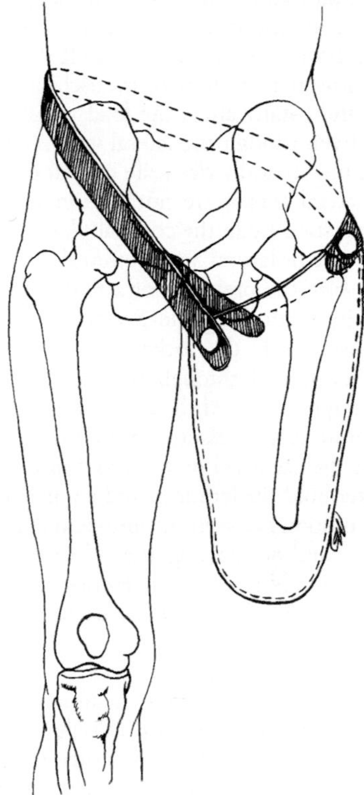

Figure 12–18. Silesian band suspension of a transfemoral prosthesis.

The hip joint and pelvic band provides extremely secure suspension and control, but the band is bulky, the least cosmetically acceptable method of suspension, and the least comfortable, especially when the patient is sitting. The pelvic band, made of metal or plastic, is thicker than a Silesian bandage. The pelvic band runs from the hip hinge, around the waist, between the contralateral iliac crest and trochanter, and back to the hip hinge. The hinge is located laterally, just anterior to the trochanter, over the anatomic axis of the hip joint. Hip joint and pelvic band suspension is indicated for very short transfemoral limbs, geriatric patients who cannot don a suction suspension, and obese patients who cannot get adequate control with suction, silicone suspension sleeves, or Silesian band suspension.

Socket design for the transfemoral amputation has changed. The traditional quadrilateral socket has a narrow anteroposterior diameter to keep the ischium positioned back and up on top of the posterior brim of the socket for weight bearing. The anterior wall of the socket is 5–7 cm higher than the posterior wall to hold the leg back on the ischial seat. Anterior pain is a frequent complaint and should be addressed by modification of the prosthetic socket in a small local area such as over the anterior superior iliac spine. If the entire anterior wall is lowered or relieved, the ischium slips inside the socket and totally alters the load transfer and pressure areas. Even though the lateral wall is contoured to hold the femur in adduction, the overall dimensions of the quadrilateral socket are not anatomic and provide poor femoral stability in the coronal plane.

Narrow mediolateral transfemoral socket designs attempt to solve the problems of a traditional quadrilateral socket by contouring the posterior wall to set the ischium down inside the socket, not up on the brim. Weight is transferred through the gluteal muscle mass and lateral thigh instead of the ischium, which eliminates the need for anterior pressure from a high anterior wall. Attention is then focused on a narrow mediolateral contour to better hold the femur in adduction and minimize the relative motion between the limb and the socket. The normal shape and normal alignment (NSNA) socket and the contoured adducted trochanteric-controlled alignment method (CAT-CAM) socket are two of the narrow mediolateral designs available.

A socket made of flexible material with a rigid frame can also be used. The flexible material allows socket wall expansion with underlying muscle contraction. A flexible socket can be made in either the traditional quadrilateral or narrow mediolateral shapes. Advantages of this type of socket include improved comfort in walking and sitting and possibly improved muscular efficiency. One drawback is that the flexible material is less durable, and cracks can result in the loss of suction suspension and skin irritation.

Prosthetic knee joints are available in many designs to address specific patient needs. The traditional standard was the single-axis constant-friction knee. The constant-friction knee is simple, durable, lightweight, and inexpensive. The friction can be set at only one level to optimize function at one cadence, and patients have difficulty when walking at different speeds.

Outside hinges were the old standard for the knee disarticulation patient, to better approximate the center of motion of the knee. Outside hinges are cosmetically poor but still available for patients who used them successfully in the past and remain satisfied with them. For new patients, other types of knee units are used.

The term *stance control knee* has replaced the term *safety knee.* It refers to a knee unit that has weight-activated friction to increase stability and resistance to buckling as more of the amputee's body weight is applied. This unit is particularly useful for patients who are older, feel less secure, and have a very short residual limb, weak hip extensors, or hip flexion contractures.

A polycentric knee provides a changing center of rotation that is located more posteriorly than other knee joints. The posterior center of rotation offers more stability during stance and the first few degrees of flexion than other knee units do. The four-bar knee is one of many polycentric knee units available.

A hydraulic or pneumatic unit can be added to most knee joints to provide superior control of the prosthesis in swing phase by using fluid hydraulics to vary the resistance according to the speed of gait. This option is useful in active amputees who walk and run at different speeds.

The variable-friction knee unit can be a less expensive way to accommodate patients who walk at different speeds. This knee changes the friction according to the degree of flexion in the knee unit and leads to an improvement in the swing phase of walking. Although a variable-friction knee is less costly and requires less maintenance than a hydraulic unit, it is not as effective in allowing the amputee to walk at different cadences.

A manual locking option can also be added to most knee units to lock the knee in full extension. Locking is helpful if the patient is blind, feels less secure, has a very short residual limb, or is a bilateral amputee.

As mentioned previously, microprocessor-controlled so-called intelligent knee units incorporate the latest technology to provide superior control of the swing and stance characteristics or the knee and respond to the amputee's speed, cadence, and accelerations. Technology has not yet advanced enough for knee units to replace the tremendous motor power lost when an amputation is done above the knee.

Specifically designed prostheses known as *stubbies* are initially recommended for bilateral knee disarticulation or transfemoral amputees, regardless of age, who have lost both legs simultaneously but are candidates for ambulation. Stubbies consist of prosthetic sockets mounted directly over rocker-bottom platforms that serve as feet. The rocker-bottom platforms have a long posterior extension to prevent the patient from falling backward, and they have a shortened anterior process that allows smooth rollover into the push-off phase of gait. These prostheses look as if the foot were positioned backward. The use of stubbies results in a lowering of the center of gravity, and the rocker bottom provides a broad base of support that teaches trunk balance, provides stability, and allows the patient to build confidence during standing and ambulation. As the patient's confidence and skills improve, periodic lengthening of the stubbies is permitted until the height becomes nearly compatible with full-length prostheses, at which time the transition is attempted. Many patients reject full-length prostheses and prefer the stability and balance afforded by the stubbies.

Hip Disarticulation

Hip disarticulation (Figure 12–19) is rarely performed. Surgically, the traditional racket-shaped incision with

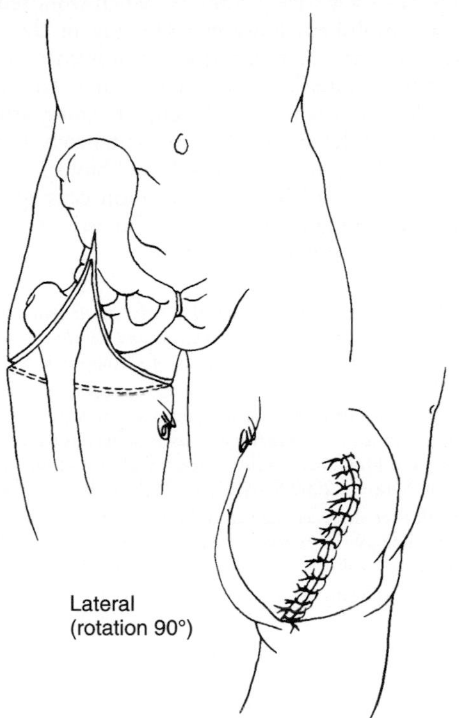

Figure 12–19. Hip disarticulation.

an anterior apex is used in patients with vascular problems and in trauma-injured patients when possible. In tumor surgery, creative flaps based on the uninvolved anatomic compartments must be designed.

Prosthetic replacement can be successful in healthy young patients who required hip disarticulation because of trauma or cancer but is generally not indicated for patients with vascular disease. The standard prosthesis is the Canadian hip disarticulation prosthesis. The socket contains the involved hemipelvis and suspends over the iliac crests. Although the hip joint and other endoskeletal components are made of lightweight materials in an effort to keep the weight to a minimum, the prosthesis is still heavy and difficult to manipulate. Ambulation with the prosthesis usually requires more energy than it would take to ambulate with crutches and a swing-through gait. For this reason, many ambulatory patients use crutches and no prosthesis. The advantage of the prosthesis is that it does allow freer use of the upper extremities.

Hemipelvectomy

Although a hemipelvectomy (Figure 12–20) is even less frequently required than a hip disarticulation, it is sometimes indicated for trauma injuries or cancer involving the pelvis. Use of a prosthesis after this procedure is extremely rare because the body weight must be transferred onto the sacrum and thorax. Special considerations for seating are usually required after hemipelvectomy.

Prosthetic Prescription following Amputation at or Above the Knee

To be considered a candidate for a high anatomic level prosthesis (knee disarticulation and higher), a patient must be able to transfer independently, rise from sitting to standing independently, and ambulate using one leg and a swing-through gait over a distance of 100 feet on the parallel bars or with a walker. Although these requirements seem extreme, they are necessary for the successful use of this heavy and complicated prosthesis. The use of a transtibial prosthesis can make it easier to transfer and to ambulate. But a current transfemoral prosthesis can make it much more difficult to rise from sitting to standing because the powerful motor force required to extend the knee is not present. High-level prosthetic devices can actually increase the energy required for walking compared with one-leg swing-through gait. Unfortunately, without the ability to meet the activity demands unas-

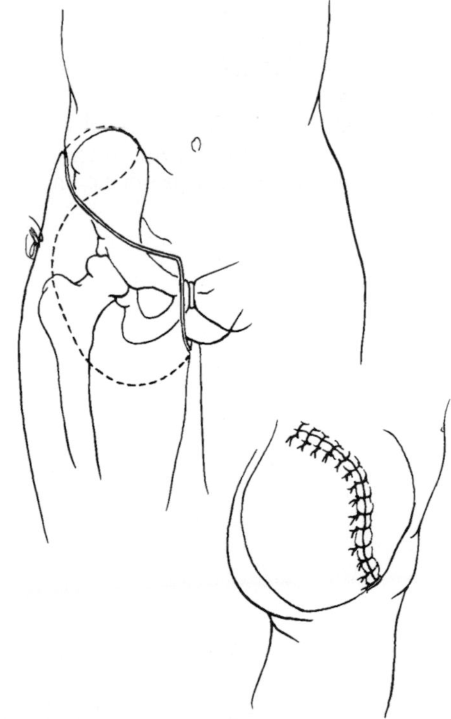

Figure 12–20. Hemipelvectomy.

sisted, a prosthesis acts as an anchor to decrease overall independence. We use these same activity requirements as a functional test before prescribing a prosthesis for all transfemoral, hip disarticulation, and hemipelvectomy amputees.

Percutaneous Direct Skeletal Attachment of Artificial Limbs

The benefits of attaching prosthetic limbs through the skin, directly to the skeleton, was envisioned for nearly 100 years. Documentation of temporary external fixation for fractures dates to Malgaigne in 1845. During and just after World War II, independent attempts were made in Germany and the United States to attach a transtibial prosthesis directly to the tibia. Four humans were fit in May 1946 by Drummer, a general surgeon in Pinneberg, Germany. The two major hurdles continue to be the bone–implant interface, and the skin–implant interface. Breakthrough work by Branemark in Gothenburg, Sweden, advanced the use of titanium and improved design implants that led to over 30 years of successful dental and maxillofacial reconstruction with prosthetic devices directly connected to the bone of the mouth and face.

The skin of the extremities posed a larger challenge to the cutaneous–implant interface. Improvements in implant design and surgical technique, however, made it possible to implant and fit thumb, forearm, and transfemoral amputees successfully. Approximately 60 amputees have undergone surgical implantation and prosthetic fitting in Sweden, the United Kingdom, and Australia.

The early results confirm the potential promise of major improvements in attachment, proprioception, and function of osseointegrated prosthetic limbs compared with socket-style prostheses. Much work remains to be accomplished, however, especially in the skin–implant interface. A tremendous improvement in the bone–implant interface led to results that far outdistance historical attempts at directly attaching artificial limbs to the skeleton. Without true cutaneous–implant integration that provides a durable and biologic barrier, however, the risk of bacterial migration causing infection and loosening continues. It is fantastic to see this dream continue and advance.

Smith DG, Michael JW, Bowker JH: *Atlas of Amputations and Limb Deficiencies: Surgical, Prosthetic, and Rehabilitation Principles,* 3rd ed. American Academy of Orthopaedic Surgeons, 2004.

Bowker JH et al: North American experience with knee disarticulation with use of a posterior myofasciocutaneous flap. Healing rate and functional results in seventy-seven patients. J Bone Joint Surg Am 2000;82-A(11):1571. [PMID: 11097446]

Branemark R et al: Osseointegration in skeletal reconstruction and rehabilitation: A review. J Rehabil Res Dev 2001;38(2):175. Review. No abstract available. [PMID: 11392650]

Gaine WJ, McCreath SW: Syme's amputation revisited: A review of 46 cases. J Bone Joint Surg Br 1996;78:461.

Gottschalk F et al: Does socket configuration influence the position of the femur in above-knee amputation? J Prosthet Orthot 1989;2:94.

Kock HJ, Friederichs J, Ouchmaev A et al: Long-term results of through-knee amputation with dorsal musculocutaneous flap in patients with end-stage arterial occlusive disease. World J Surg 2004;28(8):801. Epub accessed August 3, 2004. [PMID: 15457362]

Pinzur MS, Bowker JH, Smith DG et al: Amputation surgery in peripheral vascular disease. Instr Course Lect 1999;48:687. [PMID: 10098097]

Unruh T et al: Hip disarticulation: An eleven-year experience. Arch Surg 1990;125:791.

Rehabilitation 13

Mary Ann E. Keenan, MD, & Samir Mehta, MD

GENERAL PRINCIPLES OF REHABILITATION

In the past, rehabilitation was regarded as aftercare, but today, rehabilitation is recognized as an important part of the acute-care program. Physicians, therapists, and other health care workers in the field of orthopedics are involved in rehabilitation programs for a variety of patients, including those with congenital or acquired musculoskeletal problems (eg, bone deformities, arthritis, or fractures) as well as those with neurologic trauma or diseases that affect limb function (eg, spinal cord injury [SCI], stroke, or poliomyelitis). Rehabilitation in these patients frequently involves correcting limb deformities, increasing muscle strength, maximizing motor control, training individuals to make the most effective use of residual function, and providing adaptive equipment.

The most successful model for rehabilitation addresses the physical, emotional, and other needs of the patient and is based on a team approach. Among those frequently included in the team are physicians and nurses from various medical specialties, physical and occupational therapists, speech therapists, psychologists, orthotists, and social workers as well as the patient and members of the patient's family. The shared goal of team members is to prevent barriers to rehabilitation by (1) diagnosing accurately all current problems in the patient, (2) treating the problems adequately, (3) establishing adequate nutrition, (4) monitoring the patient for any complications that might impede progress in recovery, (5) mobilizing the patient as soon as possible, and (6) restoring function or helping the patient adjust to an altered lifestyle.

Management of Common Problems in Rehabilitation

Inadequate nutrition, decubitus ulcers, urinary tract infections, impaired bladder control, spasticity, contractures, acquired musculoskeletal deformities, muscle weakness, and physiologic deconditioning are common complications that can obstruct rehabilitation efforts and cause further loss of function in an already compromised patient. Because these problems are costly in both human and financial terms, every effort should be made to prevent them.

A. Inadequate Nutrition

Good nutritional status is the basis for avoiding many of the previously listed complications. In trauma patients, the nutritional requirements are markedly increased from the normal maintenance requirement of 30 kcal/kg/day. Most trauma patients have been receiving intravenous fluids with minimal nutritional benefit and so arrive at the rehabilitation center in various degrees of malnutrition. Patients with chronic illnesses commonly have poor appetites. Physically handicapped people expend much of their energy performing simple activities of daily living (ADLs) and may also have difficulty in obtaining and preparing adequate amounts of food. Yet another form of poor nutrition that should be noted is obesity. Inactivity leads to diminished calorie need, but boredom may result in increased consumption.

B. Decubitus Ulcers (Pressure Sores)

The combination of poor nutritional status, lack of sensation at pressure points of the body, and decreased ability to move can cause decubitus ulcers (Figure 13–1) and greatly add to the length and cost of the patient's hospital stay. The ulcer is a potential source of sepsis in an already compromised individual and often requires that a flap graft be rotated to cover the defect. After a sacral flap is rotated, the patient must remain in a prone position until the graft heals. This significantly hampers the patient's participation in a rehabilitation program because mobility and ability to interact with others are hindered. Prevention is the best treatment. The clinical rule of protecting the patient's skin is to change position every 2 hours. No cushion can completely prevent decubitus ulcers.

C. Urinary Tract Infections and Impaired Bladder Control

Urinary tract infections are a common source of sepsis and prolonged illness. An indwelling catheter is the most frequent source of contamination. In an acutely ill or multiply injured patient, an indwelling catheter may be necessary for medical reasons but should be removed as soon as possible. Urinary incontinence is not sufficient reason for continued use of an indwelling catheter. In male patients, incontinence can be managed

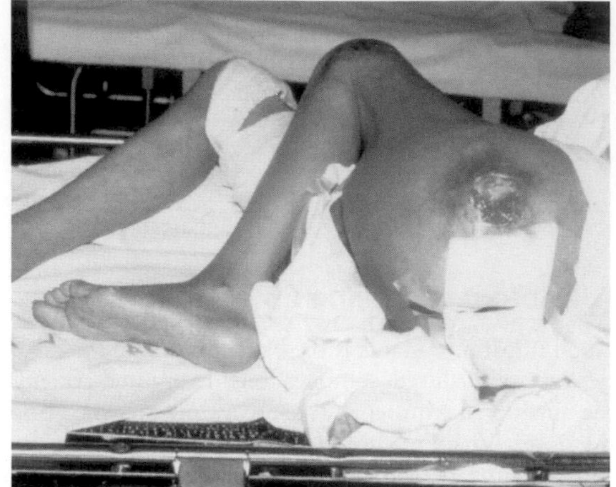

Figure 13–1. Patient with contractures and a decubitus ulcer over the greater trochanter of the femur.

with a carefully applied condom catheter. Care must be taken to inspect the penis frequently for signs of skin maceration or pressure. In female patients, diapering and frequent linen changes are necessary.

Restoring bladder function to achieve adequate reflex voiding or a balanced bladder may require the use of an intermittent catheterization program. In a balanced bladder, the volume of residual urine should not exceed a third of the volume of voided urine. In general, an intermittent catheterization program is initiated if the residual volume is greater than 100 mL or if the voided volume exceeds 400 mL. The patient is catheterized every 4 hours initially and then every 6 hours for 24 hours. Then the patient is reassessed. Good records are necessary throughout the program.

D. Muscle Weakness and Physiologic Deconditioning

During sustained exercise, the metabolism is mainly aerobic. The principal fuels for aerobic metabolism are carbohydrates and fats. In aerobic oxidation, the substrates are oxidized through a series of enzymatic reactions that lead to the production of adenosine triphosphate (ATP) for muscular contraction. A physical conditioning program can increase the aerobic capacity by improving cardiac output, increasing hemoglobin levels, enhancing the capacity of cells to extract oxygen from the blood, and increasing the muscle mass by hypertrophy.

Prolonged immobilization of extremities, bed rest, and inactivity lead to pronounced muscle wasting and physiologic deconditioning in a short period of time. Because disabled patients generally expend more energy than normal individuals in performing the routine ADLs, they must be mobilized as quickly as possible to prevent unnecessary physiologic decline. They should also be placed on a daily exercise program to maximize muscle strength and aerobic capacity.

E. Spasticity

Patients with spasticity exhibit an excessive response to the quick stretch of a muscle, which leads to hyperactive deep tendon reflexes and clonus. Spasticity must be managed aggressively to prevent permanent deformities and joint contractures.

1. Spasmolytic drugs—Drugs can be of some assistance in controlling spasticity associated with upper motor neuron diseases. Drugs are used when spasticity affects multiple large muscle groups in the body and when the spasticity is not severe.

Baclofen (Lioresal) can inhibit both polysynaptic and monosynaptic reflexes at the spinal cord level. It does, however, depress general central nervous system function. Use of oral baclofen is avoided in traumatic brain-injured patients when possible because it may cause sedation and impede cognitive recovery. Patients with attention deficits or memory disorders may be compromised by antispastic agents, such as baclofen, diazepam, and clonidine, that have sedating properties. The drug tizanidine (Zanaflex) affects the central nervous system less than other agents and may be useful. Even a drug such as dantrolene sodium, which acts peripherally, may also cause drowsiness.

Baclofen pump technology has an advantage over oral drug therapy because of the small concentrations it introduces intrathecally. The small intrathecal doses control spasticity effectively while minimizing central side effects. The pump is placed in a subcutaneous pocket in the abdominal wall. A catheter is routed subcutaneously from the intrathecal space to the pump. The pump can be refilled by injection into the reservoir chamber. The dosage and rate of administration can be easily adjusted by using a laptop computer that sends radio signals to the pump.

Dantrolene (Dantrium), another drug that can be used to control spasticity, is the drug of choice for treating clonus. Dantrolene produces relaxation by directly affecting the contractile response of skeletal muscle at a site beyond the myoneural junction. It causes dissociation of the excitation–contraction coupling probably by interfering with the release of calcium from the sarcoplasmic reticulum. Although it does not affect the central nervous system directly, it does cause drowsiness, dizziness, and generalized weakness, which may interfere with the patient's overall function. Use of dantrolene for the control of spasticity is indicated in upper motor neuron diseases, such as SCI, cerebral palsy, stroke, or multiple sclerosis. The most serious problem encountered with the use of dantrolene is hepatotoxicity. The risk appears greatest in females, in patients older than 35 years, and in patients taking other medications. When using dantrolene, the lowest effective dose should be used, and liver enzyme functions should be monitored closely. If no effect is noted after 45 days of use, the drug should be stopped.

2. Casts—Casting temporarily reduces muscle tone and is frequently used to correct a contracture. The cast is changed weekly until the problem is corrected. If a cast must be used for a prolonged period, the patient should be placed on anticoagulant therapy to prevent deep venous thrombosis.

3. Splints—Anterior and posterior clamshell splints can be used to control joint position and still allow for active and passive range of motion (ROM) of the joints in therapy. A splint applied to only one side of an extremity is not sufficient to control excessive spasticity and may result in skin breakdown from motion of the extremity against the splint. A splint can also obscure an early contracture.

4. Nerve-blocking agents—Anesthetic and phenol nerve blocks are often combined with a casting or splinting program.

Anesthetic nerve blocks are commonly used to eliminate muscle tone temporarily. They can be used diagnostically to evaluate what portion of a deformity is dynamic (occurring because of muscle spasticity) and what portion is secondary to myostatic contracture. The block can give an advanced indication of the likely results of surgical neurectomy or tendon lengthening. Repeated blocks of local anesthetics give a carryover effect to decrease muscle tone.

When muscle spasticity requires control for an extended period of time but the patient still has potential for spontaneous improvement, a phenol nerve block may be indicated. Phenol exerts two actions on the nerves. The first is a short-term effect, similar to the effect produced by a local anesthetic and directly proportional to the thickness of the nerve fibers. The second is a long-term effect that results from protein denaturation. Although this leads to wallerian degeneration of the axons, experimental studies in animals showed that the nerves regenerate with time. In patients, the direct injection of a nerve with a 3–5% solution of phenol after surgical exposure gives relief of spasticity for up to 6 months. Mixed nerves containing sensory fibers should not be injected because it could cause unwanted sensory loss or painful dysesthesia. Reduction of spasticity for up to 3 months can also be achieved by the percutaneous injection of muscle motor points with an aqueous solution of phenol after localization using a needle and nerve stimulator (Figure 13–2).

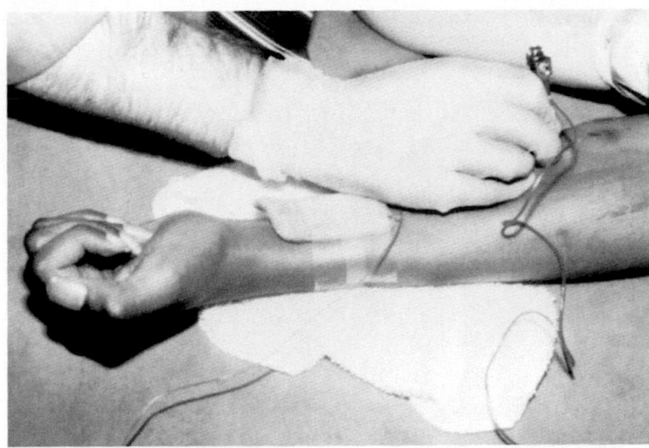

Figure 13–2. Use of a Teflon-coated needle and nerve stimulator to locate the motor points of spastic forearm muscles for phenol injection.

a. Botulinum toxin—Ordinarily, an action potential propagating down to a motor nerve to the neuromuscular junction triggers the release of acetylcholine (ACh) into the synaptic space. The released ACh causes depolarization of muscle membrane. Botulinum toxin type A is a protein produced by *Clostridium botulinum* that attaches to the presynaptic nerve terminal and inhibits the release of ACh at the neuromuscular junction. Botulinum toxin is injected directly into a spastic muscle. Clinical benefit lasts 3–5 months. Current practice is not to administer a total of more than 400 U in a single treatment session to avoid excessive weakness or paralysis. This upper limit of 400 U may be reached rather quickly when injecting a few large muscles. A delay of 3–7 days between injection of botulinum toxin A and the onset of clinical effect is typical. The patient does not see effects immediately, and usually a follow-up visit is arranged to check the result. Because botulinum toxin is the most potent biologic toxin known, and the cost is relatively high, the smallest possible dose should be used to achieve results. Most studies report side effects in 20–30% of patients per treatment cycle. The incidence of adverse effects varies based on the dosage used (ie, the higher the dose, the more frequent the adverse effects); however, the incidence of complications is not related to the total dose of botulinum toxin used. Local pain at the injection site is the most commonly reported side effect. Other adverse effects (eg, local hematoma, generalized fatigue, lethargy, dizziness, flulike syndrome, pain in neighboring muscles) are also reported.

5. Surgical procedures—If muscle spasticity is permanent and no change in muscle tone is anticipated, definitive procedures such as dorsal rhizotomy, peripheral neurectomy, tendon lengthening or release, and tendon transfer should be considered.

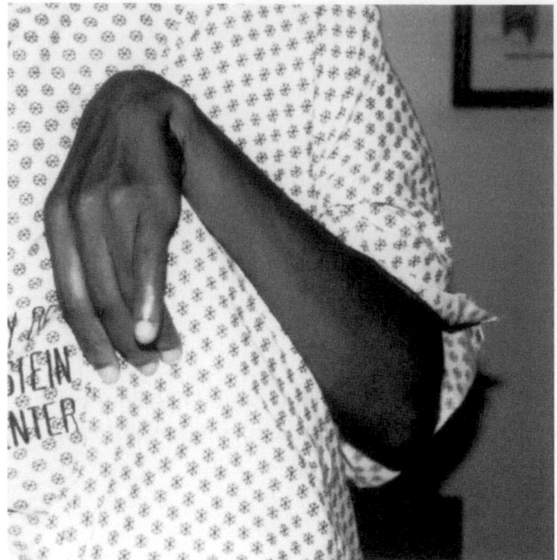

Figure 13–3. Upper extremity contractures in a patient with untreated spasticity.

F. Joint Contractures

Inactivity and uncontrolled spasticity often lead to joint contractures (Figure 13–3), which are difficult to correct and greatly extend the needed rehabilitation program. Contractures may cause difficulties in positioning an individual in a bed or chair or problems in using orthotic devices. They can also cause difficulties with hygiene and skin care and increase the risk of decubitus ulcers. Shoe wear may be rendered impossible secondary to foot deformities.

Muscle weakness is accentuated by contractures and malalignment, which cause the muscle to function at a mechanical disadvantage. Sitting and standing balance are compromised when contractural deformities displace the location of the center of gravity relative to the base of support. Functional use of the extremities is severely limited by lack of adequate joint motion. Joint contractures may require surgical release, which could further decrease function in an already compromised individual. Moreover, in children, joint contractures can lead to structural changes in the skeleton. Muscle growth lags behind skeletal growth, and this discrepancy in growth rates can cause increasing deformity with time.

To prevent contractures, exercises to maintain ROM must be performed several times daily. The patient, family members, therapists, and nursing personnel should all participate in this task.

Splinting can help maintain joints in a functional position when motor control is lacking. Splints should be removed regularly to inspect the skin condition and reassess their efficacy in maintaining the desired position.

Treatment of established contractures can be time consuming and expensive. In general, if a contracture is present for less than 3 months, it may be amenable to nonsurgical methods of correction such as serial casting or electrical stimulation of the antagonist muscles. Excessive muscle tone must be treated aggressively if present because it will only accentuate the tendency to form contractures. An anesthetic nerve block can be given to eliminate excessive tone temporarily and provide analgesia prior to manipulation of the joint and application of a cast. Each week, the cast is removed, a nerve block is given, and a new cast is applied. When the desired limb position is obtained, a holding cast is used to maintain the position for an additional week. The cast can then be bivalved and made into anterior and posterior clamshell splints, which can be removed for ROM or other activities. Another useful technique is the application of a dropout cast (Figure 13–4), which allows for further correction of the contracture while preventing the original deformity from recurring.

When contractural deformities are long standing and fixed, surgical release is indicated. Tendons, ligaments, and joint capsules are all involved. If the deformity is severe, complete correction at the time of surgery may be impossible. Neurovascular structures must be protected from excessive traction. Serial casts or dropout casts may be necessary following surgery to gain the desired limb position.

G. Other Acquired Musculoskeletal Deformities

Paralysis or weakness of trunk muscles can lead to scoliotic deformities of the spine. These deformities can impair respiratory function and tend to cause balance problems when the patient walks and sits. External support in the form of bracing or seating modifications can eliminate or minimize this tendency.

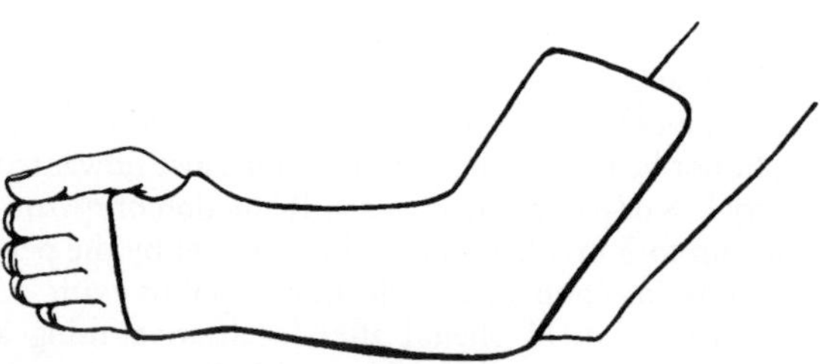

Figure 13–4. An elbow dropout cast used to increase elbow extension while preventing flexion.

Disuse and lack of muscle tone lead to osteoporosis, which in turn predisposes patients to fractures. The fractures should be treated aggressively and in a manner that maximizes function rather than prolonging immobilization.

Peripheral nerve palsy can result from pressure secondary to decreased mobility in patients confined to a bed or chair. Pressure can also result from braces, splints, and casts, and these require careful monitoring. In those patients who form heterotopic ossification, the new bone formation and the accompanying inflammation may impinge on peripheral nerves, thereby causing nerve palsy.

Evaluation of Impairment

A. Nerves

Many disabilities requiring rehabilitation result from diseases affecting the nervous system. The location and the extent of the primary lesion determine not only the degree of paralysis but also the extent to which motor control is impaired and spasticity is present. In injuries or diseases of the peripheral nerves, the damage is confined to the lower motor neurons. Normal motor control is preserved, spasticity is absent, and the magnitude of disability depends on the extent of paralysis and weakness (paresis). In pathologic conditions of the brain or spinal cord, the upper motor neurons are affected, which not only causes muscular weakness but also impairs motor control.

Motor activity can be considered as a hierarchic system of voluntary and involuntary neurologic mechanisms.

1. Voluntary muscle activity—Two types of voluntary muscle activity are clinically identifiable: selective and patterned movements. The highest level of motor activity, selective movement, depends on the integrity of the cerebral cortex. Selective movement is the ability to flex or extend one joint preferentially without initiating a mass flexor or extensor motion at other joints of the limb. Patterned movement (synergy) at a joint refers to the ability to move one joint by invoking a mass flexion or extension synergy involving movement at other joints of the limb. Patients with central nervous system disorders may have voluntary patterned movement but lack selective movement. Because most patients have mixtures of selective and patterned movement at different joints, however, the strength of each type of activity must be assessed at each joint. Patterned flexion and extension movements of the lower limb can provide sufficient motor control for ambulation, but patterned motion does not provide sufficient fine control for upper extremity function.

2. Involuntary muscle activity—Spasticity relates to two types of involuntary muscle activity: clonic and tonic responses. Each type depends on the sensitivity of the muscle spindle to the rate of stretch. If a muscle is quickly extended above the threshold of the velocity-sensitive receptors of the spindle, a phasic response may be elicited. If spasticity is severe, sudden stretch may trigger clonus, which consists of repeated bursts of phasic activity at 6–8 cycles per second. The phasic stretch response has practical clinical significance. For example, if an ankle equinus deformity is present and spasticity is severe, clonus of the triceps surae may be triggered in the stance phase each time the patient takes a step. A rigid ankle-foot orthosis (AFO) that blocks ankle motion and prevents the triceps surae from stretching may inhibit clonus, enabling the foot to be held in a neutral position. An articulated or flexible AFO that allows the ankle to move and the triceps surae to stretch may not prevent clonus from being elicited and may be less effective.

If the muscle is stretched slowly below the threshold of the velocity components of the spindle, a phasic response is not triggered, but the spindle is still capable of detecting changes in length that may generate a tonic response consisting of continuous muscle hypertonus. The tonic muscle activity during slow stretch is called **clasp-knife resistance.** This tonic activity is also of practical significance. Even if the ankle is slowly dorsiflexed for a prolonged time, hypertonus may persist in the triceps surae and restrict normal motion. Consequently, it may be necessary to differentiate spasticity from myostatic contracture by performing peripheral nerve blocks.

Patients with injury involving the brainstem may exhibit severe hypertonus that is continuously present and is called either **decorticate rigidity** or **decerebrate rigidity,** depending on the posture of the limbs. In decerebrate posturing, the patient's arms are held tightly flexed while the legs are held in extension. In decorticate posturing, both the upper and lower extremities are in rigid extension. Patients with severe muscular rigidity are at extreme risk of developing contractural deformities.

When a spastic patient is sitting or standing, labyrinthine activation increases tone in the extensor muscles of the lower extremity and also increases upper limb flexion. Consequently, patients who are examined for spasticity should be evaluated in the upright rather than supine position, to elicit the maximal stretch response. Conversely, patients who are examined for maximal ROM should be evaluated in the supine position, to minimize muscle tone and enable maximal joint range. The limb posture of patients also influences the intensity of reflex and voluntary activity.

3. Sensory perception—The final steps of sensory integration occur in the cerebral cortex, where basic sensory data are integrated into the more complex sensory phenomena. When central nervous system injury involves the cerebral cortex, the patient responds to basic modalities of touch and pain. Responses to tests of more complex aspects of sensation (such as shape, texture, and proprioception) and two-point discrimination may be impaired, however. These simple tests quickly determine the patient's ability to interpret basic sensory information. Patients with absent proprioception across the major lower joints have balance abnormalities or are unable to walk. Most patients do not routinely use an affected hand unless proprioception is intact. Patients without lesions of the cerebral cortex can generally discriminate between two points less than 10 mm apart applied simultaneously to the fingers.

B. Muscles

Manual muscle testing is often useful for evaluating an individual's ability to perform functional tasks and also documents progress made in the rehabilitation program. Several systems are currently used, but all are based on the grading system introduced by Robert Lovett in 1932. The evaluation is subjective, but the use of gravity resistance provides a measure of objective standardization (Table 13–1). A normal muscle grade as determined by manual testing does not always imply normal strength. A significant amount of weakness (a 25–30% loss of strength) must be present to be detected by this method.

C. Gait

1. Normal gait—Normal gait is the combination of postures and muscle activities that produce forward motion with minimal energy expenditure (Figure 13–5).

a. Swing phase—The swing phase (Figures 13–5 and 13–6) is divided into three equal periods: initial swing, midswing, and terminal swing. During the three-part phase, the pelvis rotates from backward to forward and the hip flexes 20–30 degrees. The knee flexes to 60 degrees initially and then extends in preparation for contact with the ground. The knee flexion is largely responsible for the foot clearing the ground during swing. Knee flexion occurs as the result of the forward momentum of the limb swinging and not as a result of hamstring contraction. The ankle joint initially plantarflexes 10 degrees and then assumes a neutral position during terminal swing so that the heel normally contacts the floor first.

The hip flexor muscles provide the power for advancing the limb and are active during the initial two thirds of the swing phase. The ankle dorsiflexors become active during the latter two thirds of the phase to ensure foot clearance as the knee begins to extend. The hamstring muscles decelerate the forward motion of the thigh during the terminal period of the swing phase.

b. Stance phase—The stance phase (Figures 13–5 and 13–7) accounts for 60% of the gait cycle and can be divided into five distinct activities: initial contact, the loading response, midstance, terminal stance, and preswing. At initial ground contact, the ankle is in neutral position, the knee is extended, and the hip is flexed. The hip extensor muscles contract to stabilize the hip because the body's mass is behind the hip joint. During the loading response, the knee flexes to 15 degrees, and the ankle plantarflexes to absorb the downward force and conserve energy by minimizing the up-and-down movement of the body's center of gravity. As the knee flexes and the stance leg accepts the weight of the body, the quadriceps muscle becomes active to stabilize the knee. In midstance, the knee is extended, and the ankle is in a neutral position. As the body's mass moves forward of the ankle joint, the calf muscles become active to stabilize the ankle and allow the heel to rise from the floor. In terminal stance, the heel leaves the floor, and the knee begins to flex as momentum carries the body forward. In the final portion of terminal stance, as the body rolls forward over the forefoot, the toes dorsiflex at the metatarsophalangeal joints. During preswing, the knee is flexed to 35 degrees and the ankle plantarflexes to 20 degrees. Because the opposite extremity is also in contact with the floor, the preswing is called the time of double-limb support.

Throughout the stance phase, the hip gradually extends and the pelvis rotates backward. During the first portion of the stance phase, the ankle dorsiflexors and hamstring muscles remain active. During the loading response and early midstance, the gluteus and quadriceps muscles become active to provide hip and knee stability. In midstance, the gastrocnemius and soleus muscles become active to stabilize the ankle joint and control the forward advancement of the tibia. This allows the heel to rise from the floor and the body weight to roll forward over the forefoot.

2. Abnormal gait—The study of movement (kinesiology) provides many important tools for evaluating patients with gait abnormalities. Among the areas of study are

Table 13–1. Muscle strength.

Grade	Strength	Description
0	Absent	Muscle does not contract.
1	Trace	Muscle contracts, but no motion is generated.
2	Poor	Muscle contraction produces movement, but muscle cannot function against gravity.
3	Fair	Muscle functions against gravity.
4	Good	Muscle can overcome some outside resistance as well as gravity.
5	Normal	Muscle can overcome resistance to motion.

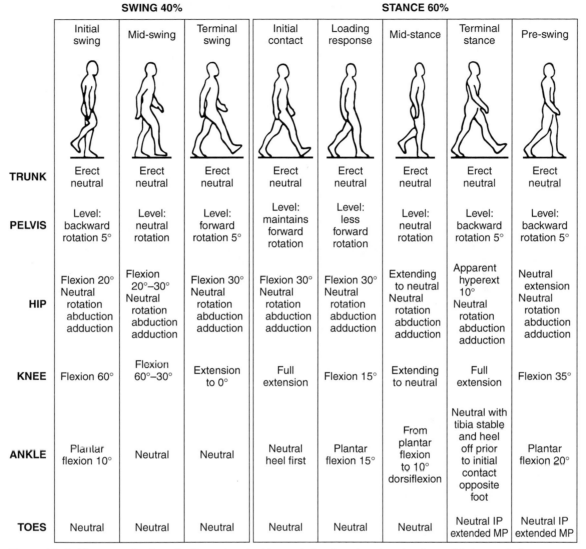

	SWING 40%			STANCE 60%				
	Initial swing	Mid-swing	Terminal swing	Initial contact	Loading response	Mid-stance	Terminal stance	Pre-swing
TRUNK	Erect neutral	Erect neutral	Erect neutral	Erect neutral	Erect neutral	Erect neutral	Erect neutral	Erect neutral
PELVIS	Level: backward rotation 5°	Level: neutral rotation	Level: forward rotation 5°	Level: maintains forward rotation	Level: less forward rotation	Level: neutral rotation	Level: backward rotation 5°	Level: backward rotation 5°
HIP	Flexion 20° Neutral rotation abduction adduction	Flexion 20°–30° Neutral rotation abduction adduction	Flexion 30° Neutral rotation abduction adduction	Flexion 30° Neutral rotation abduction adduction	Flexion 30° Neutral rotation abduction adduction	Extending to neutral Neutral rotation abduction adduction	Apparent hyperext 10° Neutral rotation abduction adduction	Neutral extension Neutral rotation abduction adduction
KNEE	Flexion 60°	Flexion 60°–30°	Extension to 0°	Full extension	Flexion 15°	Extending to neutral	Full extension	Flexion 35°
ANKLE	Plantar flexion 10°	Neutral	Neutral	Neutral heel first	Plantar flexion 15°	From plantar flexion to 10° dorsiflexion	Neutral with tibia stable and heel off prior to initial contact opposite foot	Plantar flexion 20°
TOES	Neutral	Neutral	Neutral	Neutral	Neutral	Neutral	Neutral IP extended MP	Neutral IP extended MP

Figure 13–5. The normal gait cycle. (Reproduced, with permission, from American Academy of Orthopaedic Surgeons: Home study syllabus. In Heckman JD, ed: *Orthopaedic Knowledge Update*, I. American Academy of Orthopaedic Surgeons, 1984.)

stride analysis, motion analysis (kinematics), force analysis (kinetics), and muscle activity analysis.

Three of the many specialized tools used in these studies are dynamic electromyography, force plate studies, and motion analysis. Dynamic electromyography, which records the electrical activity in multiple muscles simultaneously during functional activities, elucidates the patterns of motor control in both the upper and the lower extremities and helps in the management of spasticity and gait abnormalities. Force plate studies, which measure ground reaction forces and the fluctuations of the center of pressure, can be used to analyze gait problems and quantify balance reactions in impaired patients. Motion analysis uses multiple cameras located at different positions around the room. The cameras detect sensors placed on the patient and create a three-dimensional model of the patient moving through space.

Muscle strength can be accurately measured using torque, which can be correlated with joint position. Joint stiffness can also be assessed by measuring torque while moving the joint through a passive arc of motion. Joint powers can be calculated by multiplying joint moment times angular velocity.

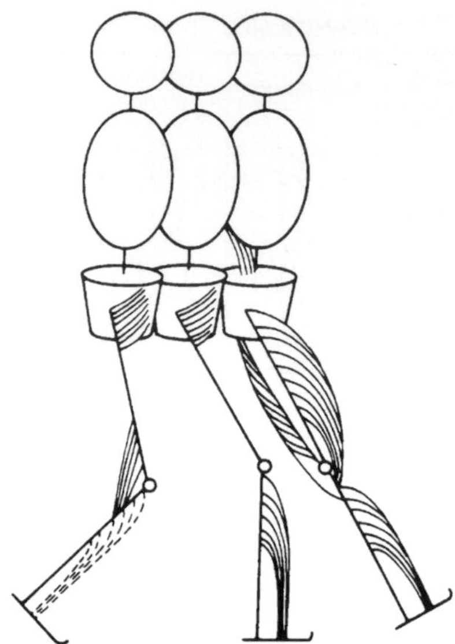

Figure 13–6. Swing phase of gait. (Reproduced, with permission, from American Academy of Orthopaedic Surgeons: Home study syllabus. In Heckman JD, ed: *Orthopaedic Knowledge Update*, I. American Academy of Orthopaedic Surgeons, 1984.)

Measurement of velocity, stride length, cadence, and single- and double-limb support times can be combined with dynamic electromyography, force plate studies, and joint goniometric recordings to present a complete analysis of gait dysfunction. These studies can also be used to assess the influence of surgery, orthotic corrections, or prosthetic design on gait characteristics.

D. Oxygen Consumption and Aerobic Capacity

Perhaps the most important measurement for understanding the difficulties faced by disabled people comes from oxygen consumption studies. Oxygen consumption indicates the energy required to perform an activity. Measuring an individual's maximal aerobic capacity is the single best indicator of the level of physical fitness.

1. Effects of disease and aging on energy expenditure—Cardiorespiratory disease, anemia, muscle atrophy, and any other condition that restricts oxygen uptake causes a decrease in the maximal aerobic capacity. Even in a healthy person, 3 weeks of bed rest decreases maximal aerobic capacity by up to 30%.

During normal walking, the rate of energy expenditure by adults varies from approximately 30% to 45% of the maximal aerobic capacity, with the higher percentage used in people over 60. Because of the decline in maximal aerobic capacity with age, an older person is more susceptible than a person under 50–60 years of age to the penalties of a gait disability.

2. Effects of exercise on energy expenditure—When exercise is performed at less than 50% of an individual's maximal aerobic capacity, the exercise can be continued for prolonged periods because the ATP needed for muscle contraction is provided by aerobic pathways. Anaerobic pathways of ATP production, which do not use oxygen, increasingly come into play when exercise is performed at work rates exceeding approximately 50% of maximal aerobic capacity. The amount of energy that can be delivered by anaerobic metabolism is limited, and fatigue ensues because of the accumulation of lactate in the muscle. Consequently, the normal ADLs and working that must be performed throughout an 8-hour day, including walking, are performed below anaerobic threshold.

3. Effects of musculoskeletal impairment on energy expenditure—Gait abnormalities that interfere with efficient, coordinated limb movement can increase energy demand. Some affected patients respond to this increased demand by working harder, which increases the output of physiologic energy and is reflected in the higher-than-normal heart rate and oxygen consumption rate. Rather than increasing the rate of energy expenditure, however, most patients slow their gait velocity in an effort to keep the power requirement from exceeding normal limits.

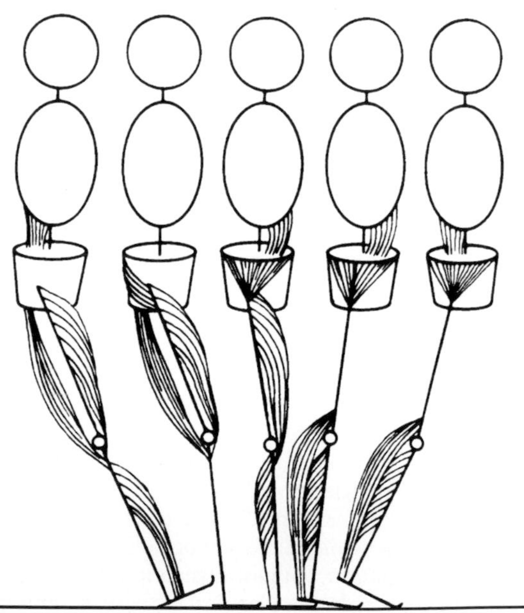

Figure 13–7. Stance phase of gait. (Reproduced, with permission, from American Academy of Orthopaedic Surgeons: Home study syllabus. In Heckman JD, ed: *Orthopaedic Knowledge Update*, I. American Academy of Orthopaedic Surgeons, 1984.)

Among amputees, patients progressively walk slower at increasingly more proximal amputation levels. Younger patients with traumatic or congenital amputations walk faster than older dysvascular amputees because of their greater maximal aerobic capacity. Patients with limited joint movement or with arthritis and painful joints also reduce their gait velocity. The heart rate and energy expenditure rate do not exceed normal in any of these groups of patients if crutches are not required.

Patients requiring crutches and exerting considerable force to support the body often have high heart rates and energy expenditure rates. A swing-through, crutch-assisted gait in a paraplegic or a patient who has a fracture and is unable to bear weight on one leg requires strenuous physical exertion, which is why few paraplegics use swing-through gait and why older patients with fractures can ambulate for only short distances. Even patients who use a reciprocal gait pattern, such as patients with low lumbar paraplegia resulting from SCI or myelodysplasia, use their arms for considerable exertion. Consequently, these types of patients may also be restricted ambulators in the community.

Patients with hip and knee flexion deformities caused by fixed or dynamic contractures require increasing muscle effort not only to walk but also to maintain an upright posture because the center of gravity during stance passes farther away from the axis of rotation of the joint. The fact that knee flexion greater than 30 degrees significantly increases the energy expenditure rate even in otherwise normal persons points to the importance of preventing and correcting contractures.

Children who have cerebral palsy and diplegia and who walk in a crouch gait may have energy expenditure rates that are above the anaerobic threshold. This is why these children are restricted ambulators who frequently discontinue walking when they mature and their maximal aerobic capacities decrease.

Use of Orthoses

Orthotic (brace) prescription plays a vital role in rehabilitation. The physician must understand the functional needs of the patient and provide the orthotist with an exact prescription that specifies the materials, type of joints, joint position, and ROM. Brace prescriptions should not be left to the discretion of the patient and orthotist.

A temporary orthosis may be used in an early stage of illness until a definitive, custom-fitted orthosis is fabricated. Definitive orthoses for the lower extremity are the below-knee ankle-foot orthosis (AFO) and the above-knee knee-ankle-foot orthosis (KAFO).

The bichannel adjustable ankle-locking (BiCAAL) type of AFO is commonly applied as the first orthosis following stroke, head trauma, spinal injury, or other condition that causes extensive muscle imbalance about the foot and ankle (Figure 13–8). A rigid ankle is useful in controlling plantarflexion spasticity, stabilizing the ankle in a flaccid limb, and correcting a dynamic varus deformity (inversion of the foot). The adjustable ankle joint mechanism enables the clinician to determine the optimal ankle position in the acute period following onset of illness when the neurologic picture and orthotic requirement are changing. Once neurologic recovery stabilizes, a plastic (polypropylene) orthosis often becomes the treatment of choice (Figure 13–9).

The use of plastic materials in lower extremity orthotics is now widespread. Orthoses fabricated from plastics are lighter, more comfortable, and more attractive. A plastic AFO can be rigid or can be flexible, allowing motion at the ankle. Polypropylene is presently the most practical plastic material. Skillful fitting is critical because of the close skin and bone contact.

A. Ankle-Foot Orthosis

1. Types—Of several currently available orthoses classified as limited-motion ankle joint orthoses, two are commonly used: the conventional metal, double-upright, single-adjustable ankle joint with dorsiflexion spring assist (Klenzak) and the molded plastic posterior shells made

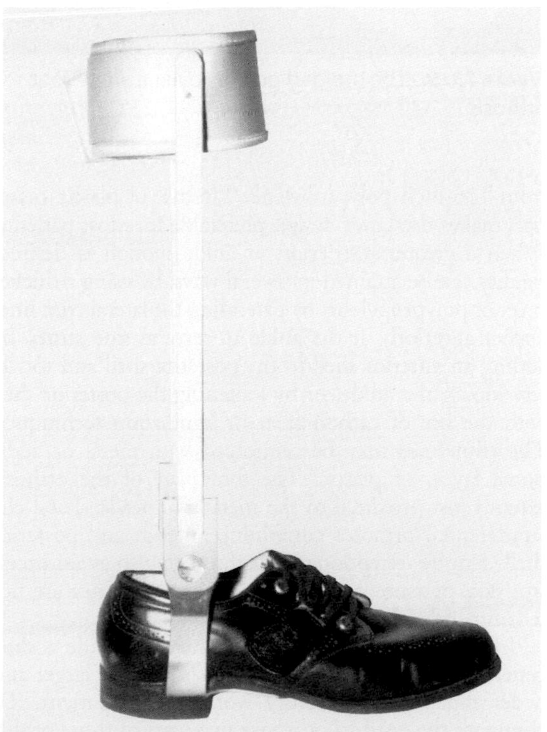

Figure 13–8. The bichannel adjustable ankle-locking (BiCAAL) type of ankle-foot orthosis.

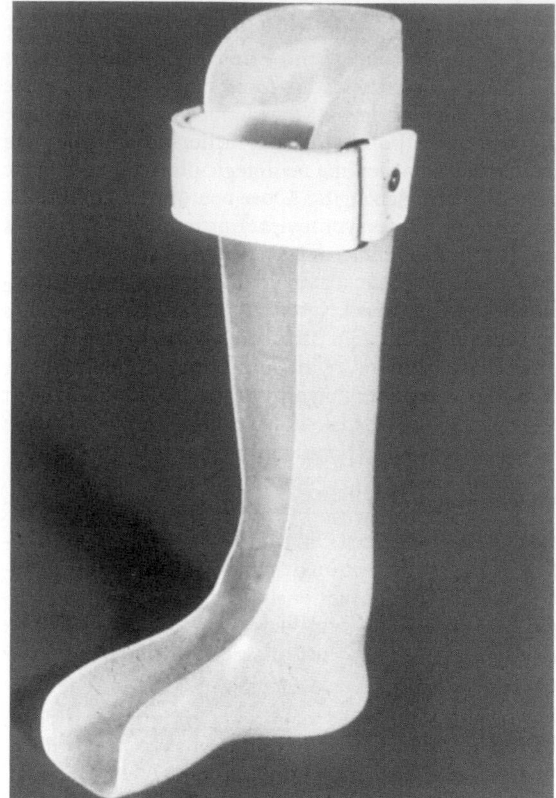

Figure 13–9. The molded polypropylene ankle-foot orthosis.

from 116-inch polypropylene. The use of plastic materials makes the latter design preferable for most patients. When a greater restriction of ankle motion is desired, rigidity can be attained in several ways: by using a thicker sheet of polypropylene, by extending the lateral trim lines farther anteriorly at the ankle to serve as side struts, by adding an anterior shell to the posterior shell and totally enveloping the ankle, or by stiffening the posterior shell with the use of carbon fiber or lamination techniques. The trim lines may be reinforced with metal or additional layers of plastic. The foot plate of the orthosis extends just proximal to the metatarsal heads. Total circumferential orthoses combining anterior and posterior shells require exceptionally careful fitting to avoid excessive skin pressure over bony prominences. They are not recommended for routine use.

Insertion of a polypropylene orthosis inside a shoe generally requires a shoe size that is a half size larger and wider than that previously worn by the patient. To eliminate the need to purchase two pairs of shoes of different sizes, an inlay can be inserted in the shoe of the sound limb to prevent excessive looseness once a shoe is fitted on the polypropylene side. The ankle position of the polypropylene orthosis should be assessed with the patient wearing his or her shoe with the normal heel height.

2. Indications—The primary requirement for orthotic support is that all joints must be passively capable of being positioned in adequate alignment. An orthosis cannot correct a fixed bony deformity or fixed joint contracture.

a. Inadequate dorsiflexion for foot clearance during swing—An AFO is indicated for inadequate toe clearance (footdrop) during the midswing phase of gait. This problem may result from inadequate ankle dorsiflexion caused by weakness of the dorsiflexors or by the inability of dorsiflexors to overcome spasticity of the triceps surae. A lightweight, flexible polypropylene orthosis is indicated if inadequate dorsiflexion is the only problem at the ankle. A flexible orthosis can also be used for a mild swing-phase varus deformity (foot inversion). A rigid orthosis is needed in patients who have excessive plantarflexion resulting from severe spasticity and in patients who initiate a strong extensor pattern activity prior to heel strike.

b. Inadequate dorsiflexion for initial contact—A patient with inadequate dorsiflexion from any cause contacts the ground with the forefoot or with the foot flat and the tibia extended backward. This problem is commonly combined with varus deformity, and weight bearing is on the lateral edge of the foot. The results are a backward thrust to the limb, which decreases forward momentum and produces excessive hyperextension forces on the knee, which leads to knee instability in the patient who is a functional walker. A rigid AFO in the neutral position provides heel strike for the patient who has full-knee extension and allows the tibia to rotate forward during stance.

c. Medial-lateral subtalar instability during stance—Varus deformity is more common than valgus deformity. The patient walks on the lateral border of the foot and is hesitant to accept weight on the leg. A rigid orthosis can correct the varus deformity unless spasticity is severe. To correct a mild varus deformity, a limited ankle orthosis may be used. No orthosis is effective in controlling the severe spastic varus deformity.

d. Inadequate tibial stability during stance—Some patients have inadequate strength or control of the plantarflexors for maintenance of normal tibial position and alignment during stance. Early after midstance, this problem is manifested by excessive dorsiflexion and accompanying knee flexion. Whether or not the limb collapses during weight bearing depends on the amount of quadriceps muscle control and strength. Patients with sufficient proprioception learn to compensate by locking the knee in hyperextension as the foot contacts the floor, which keeps the knee from buckling. A rigid orthosis that prevents both dorsiflexion and plantarflexion is indicated to provide vertical tibial alignment during midstance. Its use prevents tibial collapse forward during terminal stance as a substitution for adequate calf control.

A knee extension thrust, caused by inadequate calf control as described earlier, may result also from severe plantarflexion tone or fixed equinus deformity resulting from contracture. At foot strike, the forefoot strikes the floor first, resulting in a knee extension or hyperextension thrust. A rigid AFO with a plantarflexion block prevents the development of knee instability and pain.

A T-strap (a leather T-shaped strap attached to the brace at the ankle and applied around the ankle to hold the foot from either an inverted or everted position) is usually not desirable for correction of severe varus deformity in patients fitted with metal orthoses. If a T-strap is applied with sufficient force to provide significant control to prevent foot twisting, it usually causes excessive pressure over the lateral malleolus in the patient with severe spasticity. This problem can be treated better by the use of a split anterior tibial tendon transfer or by the addition of a lateral wedge and flare to the shoe of the nonsurgical candidate.

B. Knee-Ankle-Foot Orthosis

A KAFO may be used if quadriceps muscle weakness or hamstring muscle spasticity is present. A knee immobilizer may be used as a training aid before having a KAFO fabricated. A KAFO is more difficult to don than a below-knee brace, and most patients with a central nervous system disease such as stroke or cerebral palsy have difficulty walking with a KAFO. Consequently, if hamstring spasticity rather than quadriceps spasticity necessitates external support to align the knee in extension, it is preferable to perform hamstring tenotomy or tendon lengthening, thereby eliminating the need for knee support.

Most patients with lower extremity quadriceps paresis resulting from SCI lack sufficient proprioception to walk with a free-knee mechanism (unlocked knee joint mechanism).

When a KAFO is prescribed for quadriceps paresis, it is necessary to determine if the knee will be locked while walking or if it will be freely movable to allow knee flexion in swing. When a KAFO is prescribed because of knee instability or because of varus or valgus instability, a polycentric joint (a joint in which the center of rotation moves following the anatomic instantaneous center of rotation) permits flexion extension movement but blocks medial and lateral angulation. A posterior stop added to the knee mechanism prevents excessive hyperextension.

If proprioception is intact, as is the case with poliomyelitis, even patients with considerable quadriceps weakness may be able to walk with an unlocked knee using an offset knee joint. This is accomplished by careful orthotic alignment. The center of rotation of the orthosis is positioned anterior to the center of rotation of the knee. As long as the patient can fully extend the knee in the swing stage preparatory to limb loading, the resulting movement caused by vertical loading acts to extend the knee against the posterior stop, thereby locking the knee in extension. This requires at least fair (grade 3) hip flexor strength (see Table 13–1) to provide sufficient forward momentum of the leg to position the knee in full extension.

The substitution of plastic components, such as a pretibial shell, has led to significantly improved fit and reduced weight in KAFOs.

Esquenazi A. Evaluation and management of spastic gait in patients with traumatic brain injury. J Head Trauma Rehabil 2004; 19(2):109. [PMID: 15247822]

Hebela N, Smith DG, Keenan MA: What's new in orthopaedic rehabilitation. J Bone Joint Surg Am 2004;86-A(11):2577. [PMID: 15523043]

Hsu JD: Rancho Los Amigos Medical Center. A unique orthopaedic resource and teaching institution. Clin Orthop 2000; 374:125. [PMID: 10818973]

Kaelin DL, Oh TH, Lim PA et al: Rehabilitation of orthopedic and rheumatologic disorders. 4. Musculoskeletal disorders. Arch Phys Med Rehabil 2000;81(3 Suppl 1):S73. [PMID: 10721764]

Pearson OR, Busse ME, van Deursen RW et al: Quantification of walking mobility in neurological disorders. QJM 2004;97(8): 463. [PMID: 15256604]

Schmalz T, Blumentritt S, Jarasch R: Energy expenditure and biomechanical characteristics of lower limb amputee gait: The influence of prosthetic alignment and different prosthetic components. Gait Posture 2002;16(3):255. [PMID: 12443950]

Ulkar B, Yavuzer G, Guner R et al: Energy expenditure of the paraplegic gait: Comparison between different walking aids and normal subjects. Int J Rehabil Res 2003;26(3):213. [PMID: 14501573]

SPINAL CORD INJURY

Trauma to the spinal cord causes dysfunction of the cord, with nonprogressive loss of sensory and motor function distal to the point of injury. Approximately 400,000 people have spinal cord damage in the United States, and the incidence rate is estimated to be 10,000 per year. The leading causes of SCI are motor vehicle accidents, gunshot wounds, falls, sports (especially diving) injuries, and water injuries.

Patients are generally categorized into three groups. The first consists predominantly of younger individuals who sustained their injury from a motor vehicle collision or other high-energy traumatic accident. The second consists of individuals over 50 years of age with cervical spinal stenosis caused by congenital narrowing or spondylosis. Patients in this second group often sus-

dorsiflexors (tibialis anterior); L5, long toe extensors (extensor hallucis longus); and S1, ankle plantarflexors (gastrocnemius, soleus). In an individual with no deficit, the total possible LEMS is 50 points. The LEMS at 30 days is used to predict the chance of successful ambulation in incomplete tetraplegics, incomplete paraplegics, and complete paraplegics. All individuals with a LEMS of at least 20 and an incomplete injury are expected to be community ambulators 1 year after injury.

American Spinal Injury Association, International Medical Society of Paraplegia: *International Standards for Neurological Classification of Spinal Cord Injury* (revised). American Spinal Injury Association, 2000.

Banovac K et al: Prevention of heterotopic ossification after spinal cord injury with indomethacin. Spinal Cord 2001;39:370. [PMID: 11464310]

Bracken MB: Methylprednisolone and acute spinal cord injury: An update of the randomized evidence. Spine 2001;26(Suppl 24):S47. [PMID: 11805609]

Bracken MB, Holford TR: Neurological and functional status 1 year after acute spinal cord injury: Estimates of functional recovery in National Acute Spinal Cord Injury Study II from results modeled in National Acute Spinal Cord Injury Study III. J Neurosurg Spine 2002;96(3):259. [PMID: 11990832]

Burns AS, Ditunno JF: Establishing prognosis and maximizing functional outcomes after spinal cord injury: A review of current and future directions in rehabilitation management. Spine 2001;26:S137. [PMID: 11805621]

Hebela N, Smith DG, Keenan MA: What's new in orthopaedic rehabilitation. J Bone Joint Surg Am 2004;86-A(11):2577. [PMID: 15523043]

Hurlbert RJ: Methylprednisolone for acute spinal cord injury: An inappropriate standard of care. J Neurosurg Spine 2000; 93(1):1. [PMID: 10879751]

Keith MW, Hoyen H: Indications and future directions for upper limb neuroprostheses in tetraplegic patients: A review. Hand Clin 2002;18(3):519, viii. [PMID: 12474601]

Kirshblum SC, O'Connor KC: Levels of spinal cord injury and predictors of neurologic recovery. Phys Med Rehabil Clin North Am 2000;11(1):1, vii. [PMID: 10680155]

Lee TT, Green BA: Advances in the management of acute spinal cord injury. Orthop Clin North Am 2002;33(2):311. [PMID: 12389277]

Little JW et al: Neurologic recovery and neurologic decline after spinal cord injury. Phys Med Rehabil Clin North Am 2000; 11(1):73. [PMID: 10680159]

Macciocchi SN, Bowman B, Coker J et al: Effect of co-morbid traumatic brain injury on functional outcome of persons with spinal cord injuries. Am J Phys Med Rehabil 2004;83(1):22. [PMID: 14709971]

McKinley WO, Seel RT, Gadi RK et al: Nontraumatic vs. traumatic spinal cord injury: A rehabilitation outcome comparison. Am J Phys Med Rehabil 2001;80(9):693. [PMID: 11523972]

Nockels RP: Nonoperative management of acute spinal cord injury. Spine 2001;26(24 Suppl):S31. [PMID: 11805606]

Pollard ME, Apple DF: Factors associated with improved neurologic outcomes in patients with incomplete tetraplegia. Spine 2003;28:33. [PMID: 12544952]

Salisbury SK, Choy NL, Nitz J: Shoulder pain, range of motion, and functional motor skills after acute tetraplegia. Arch Phys Med Rehabil 2003;84:1480. [PMID: 14586915]

Van der Putten JJ et al: Factors affecting functional outcome in patients with nontraumatic spinal cord lesions after inpatient rehabilitation. Neurorehabil Neural Repair 2001;15:99. [PMID: 11811258]

von Wild KR: New development of functional neurorehabilitation in neurosurgery. Acta Neurochir Suppl (Wien) 2003;87:43. [PMID: 14518522]

Waters RL, Sie IH: Spinal cord injuries from gunshot wounds to the spine. Clin Orthop 2003;408:120. [PMID: 12616048]

STROKE

Stroke (cerebrovascular accident or brain attack) occurs when thrombosis, embolism, or hemorrhage interrupts cerebral oxygenation and causes the death of neurons in the brain. This leads to deficits in cognition and in motor and sensory function.

In the United States, where cerebrovascular accidents are the leading cause of hemiplegia in adults and the third leading cause of death, 2 million people have permanent neurologic deficits from stroke. The annual incidence of stroke is 1 in 1000, with cerebral thrombosis causing nearly three fourths of the cases. More than half of stroke victims survive and have an average life expectancy of approximately 6 years. Most survivors have the potential for significant function and useful lives if they receive the benefits of rehabilitation.

Neurologic Impairment & Recovery

Infarction of the cerebral cortex in the region of the brain supplied by the middle cerebral artery (MCA) or one of its branches is most commonly responsible for stroke. Although the middle cerebral artery supplies the area of the cerebral cortex responsible for hand function, the anterior cerebral artery supplies the area responsible for lower extremity motion (Figure 13–11). The typical clinical picture following middle cerebral artery stroke is contralateral hemianesthesia (decreased sensation), homonymous hemianopia (visual field deficit), and spastic hemiplegia with more paralysis in the upper extremity than in the lower extremity. Because hand function requires relatively precise motor control, even for activities with assistive equipment, the prognosis for the functional use of the hand and arm is considerably worse than for the leg. Return of even gross motor control in the lower extremity may be sufficient for walking.

Infarction in the region of the anterior cerebral artery causes paralysis and sensory loss of the opposite lower limb and to a lesser degree the arm. Patients who have cerebral arteriosclerosis and suffer repeated bilateral infarctions are likely to have severe cognitive impairment that limits their general ability to function even when motor function is good.

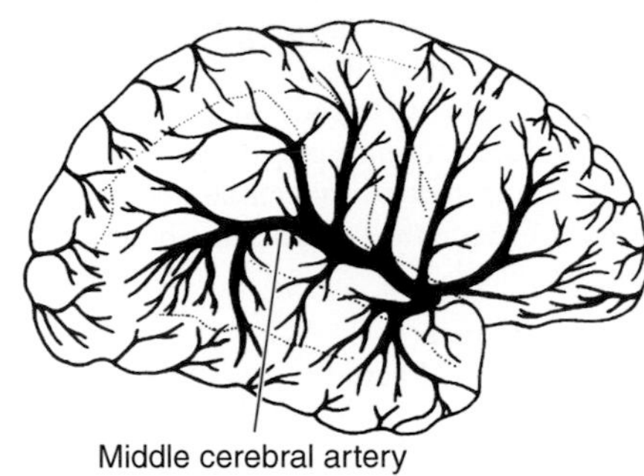

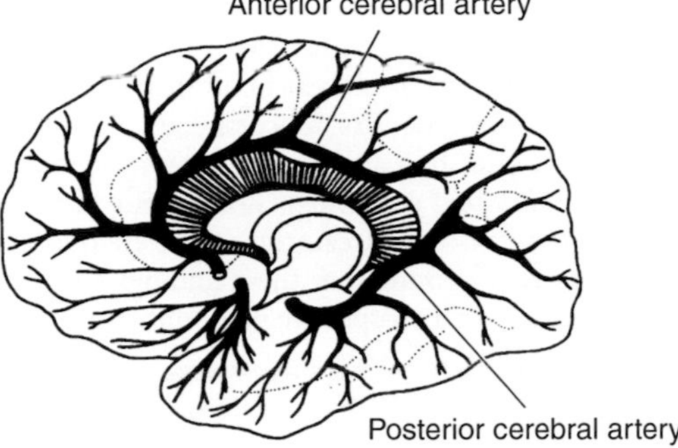

Figure 13–11. Cerebral artery circulation.

After stroke, motor recovery follows a fairly typical pattern. The size of the lesion and the amount of collateral circulation determine the amount of permanent damage. Most recovery occurs within 6 months, although functional improvement may continue as the patient receives further sensorimotor reeducation and learns to cope with disability.

Initially after a stroke, the limbs are completely flaccid. Over the next few weeks, muscle tone and spasticity gradually increase in the adductor muscles of the shoulder and in the flexor muscles of the elbow, wrist, and fingers. Spasticity also develops in the lower extremity muscles. Most commonly, there is an extensor pattern of spasticity in the leg, characterized by hip adduction, knee extension, and equinovarus deformities of the foot and ankle (Figure 13–12). In some cases, however, a flexion pattern of spasticity occurs, characterized by hip and knee flexion.

Whether the patient recovers the ability to move one joint independently of the others (selective movement) depends on the extent of the cerebral cortical damage. Dependence on the more neurologically primitive patterned movement (synergy) decreases as selective control improves. The extent to which motor impairment restricts function varies in the upper and lower extremities. Patterned movement is not functional in the upper extremity, but it may be useful in the lower extremity, where the patient uses the flexion synergy to advance the limb forward and the mass extension synergy for limb stability during standing.

The final processes in sensory perception occur in the cerebral cortex, where basic sensory information is integrated to complex sensory phenomena such as vision, proprioception, and perception of spatial relationships, shape, and texture. Patients with severe parietal dysfunction and sensory loss may lack sufficient perception of space and awareness of the involved segment of their body to ambulate. Patients with severe perceptual loss may lack balance to sit, stand, or walk. A visual field deficit further interferes with limb use and may cause patients to be unaware of their own limbs.

Management

A. Acute Management

Medical intervention in the treatment of a stroke is most effective when initiated within 3 hours from the onset of symptoms. However, pharmacologic intervention may play a role, although limited, if administered within 24 hours of onset.

1. Thrombolytics

a. Tissue plasminogen activator (t-PA) (**also known as recombinant t-PA or recombinant tissue-type plasminogen activator [rt-PA]**)—The efficacy of intravenous t-PA was established in two randomized double-blind placebo-controlled studies published in combination by the National Institute of Neurological Disorders and Stroke (NINDS). At 3 months after stroke, approximately 12% more patients in the t-PA group experienced a cure of symptoms relative to those who did not receive

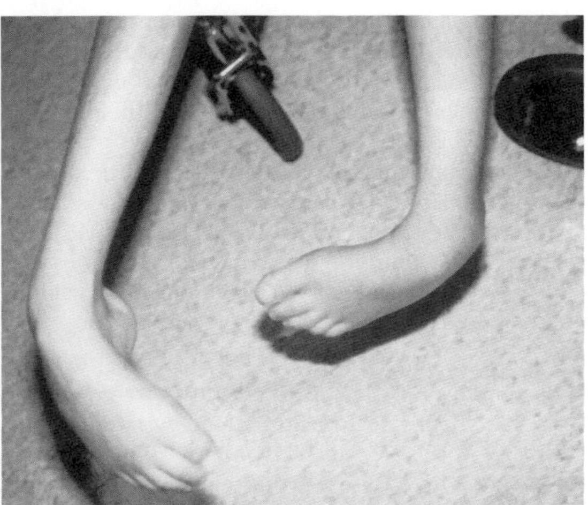

Figure 13–12. Equinovarus deformities of the feet in a patient with spasticity.

it. The risk of intracerebral hemorrhage in the t-PA group was 6% (50% of which were fatal), compared to 0.6% in the placebo group. Despite the differences in hemorrhage rates, there were no differences in mortality (17% in the t-PA group versus 21% in the placebo group).

Key points about the administration of thrombolytic agents include the following:

1. They must be administered within 3 hours of symptom onset. Patients who wake up with symptoms or those who cannot describe accurately the time of their symptom onset are timed to when they were last known to be well.
2. An imaging study of the head (CT scan or MRI) must be performed prior to treatment to rule out hemorrhage as a cause of symptoms.
3. Blood pressure should be lower than 185 systolic and 110 diastolic. Agents such as labetalol may be used to lower the blood pressure for the purposes of treatment.
4. Blood must be tested for platelet count (should be over 100,000); international normalized ratio (INR) (many recommend under 1.6); partial thromboplastin time (PTT) (many recommend less than 40); and glucose (should be 50–400).

b. Prourokinase (also known as recombinant prourokinase, or r-pro-UK)—This intraarterial therapy requires the involvement of a skilled interventionist. The time window is 6 hours from symptom onset. In addition, and in contrast to the NINDS t-PA study, patients with a CT scan showing over a third involvement of the MCA territory as seen on CT scan are not eligible for treatment. The absolute percentage increase in patients with slight or no disability at 3 months was 15% in the prourokinase group compared with the placebo group. The hemorrhage rate in the prourokinase group was 10% versus 2% in subjects who received placebo. No difference was noted, however, in mortality (25% in the prourokinase group versus 27% in the placebo group).

This therapy may be especially useful for patients who arrive later than 3 hours from symptom onset and who have less than a third involvement of the MCA territory on initial scan.

2. Antiplatelet agents

a. Aspirin—The Chinese Acute Stroke Trial (CAST) and the International Stroke Trial (IST) are two large studies evaluating the use of aspirin (160–300 mg/d) within 48 hours of ischemic stroke symptom onset. Compared to no treatment, there was approximately a 1% absolute reduction in stroke and death in the first few weeks. At further time points (eg, 6 months), there was a similar absolute reduction of approximately 1% in death or dependence.

b. Abciximab—An ongoing phase III study of the efficacy of abciximab (ReoPro) in acute stroke is being conducted. A phase II study of 400 patients found an 8% absolute reduction in poor outcomes at 3 months ($P < 0.05$). Symptomatic intracranial hemorrhage occurred in 3.6% of patients on abciximab and in 1.0% of patients on placebo.

3. Anticoagulants

a. Warfarin—No studies have evaluated use of warfarin for the acute treatment of stroke.

b. Heparin and heparinoids—At this time, only one randomized trial showed benefit for heparins or heparinoids in acute ischemic stroke. In that study, no benefit was seen at 10 days or 3 months, only at 6 months. Other large studies failed to find benefit of heparin or heparinoids, either intravenous or subcutaneous, at 3 months. An exploratory post hoc analysis of one intravenous low molecular randomized study suggested benefit in patients with severe large vessel (eg, carotid) atherosclerosis; however, the authors conclude that these findings need to be properly evaluated in a prospective randomized trial.

4. Neuroprotectants—Various classes of neuroprotectants were tested and include calcium channel antagonists, potassium channel openers, glutamate antagonists, antiadhesion molecules, N-methyl-D-aspartate (NMDA) receptor antagonists and modulators, α-amino-3-hydroxy-5-methylisoxazole-4-propionic acid (AMPA) receptor antagonists, membrane stabilizers, growth factors, and glycine site antagonists. At this time, no neuroprotectant shows efficacy in the treatment of acute stroke.

B. Lower Extremities

1. Hemiplegia—To walk independently, the hemiplegic patient requires intact balance reactions, hip flexion to advance the limb, and stability of the limb for standing. If a patient meets these criteria and has acceptable cognition, the orthopedic surgeon can restore ambulation in most cases by prescribing an appropriate lower extremity orthosis and an upper extremity assistive device such as a cane. Surgery to rebalance the muscle forces in the leg can greatly enhance ambulation.

Except for the correction of severe contractures in nonambulatory patients, surgical procedures should be delayed for at least 6 months to allow spontaneous neurologic recovery to occur and the patient to learn how to cope with the disability. After this time, surgery may safely be performed to improve usage in the functional limb.

In the nonfunctional limb, surgery may be performed to relieve pain or correct severe hip and knee flexion contractures caused by spasticity. Most severe contractural deformities in the nonfunctional limb, however, are the result of an ineffective program of daily passive ROM, splinting, and limb positioning.

Most hemiplegics with motor impairment have hip abductor and extensor weakness. A quad cane (cane with four feet to provide more stability) or a hemi-walker is prescribed to provide better balance. Because of paralysis in the upper extremity, the hemiplegic patient is unable to use a conventional walker.

2. Limb scissoring—Scissoring of the legs caused by overactive hip adductor muscles is a common problem. This gives the patient an extremely narrow base of support while standing and causes balance problems. When no fixed contracture of the hip adductor muscles is present, transection of the anterior branches of the obturator nerve denervates the adductors and allows the patient to stand with a broader base of support. If a contracture of the adductors occurs, surgical release of the adductor longus, adductor brevis, and gracilis muscles should be performed (Figure 13–13).

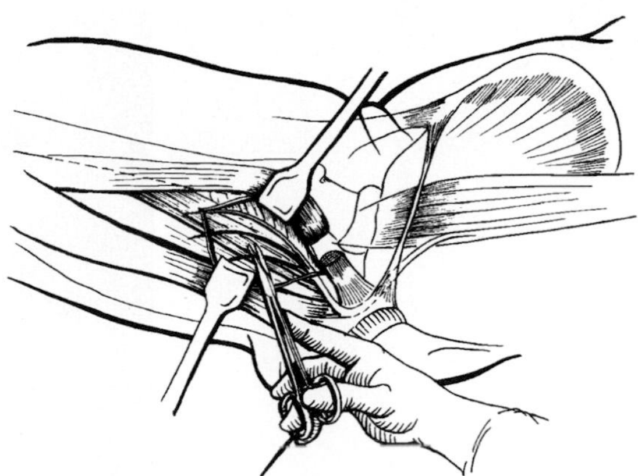

Figure 13–13. Release of the hip adductor tendons and neurectomy of the anterior branches of the obturator nerve to correct the problem of limb scissoring. (Illustration by Anthony C. Berlet. Reproduced, with permission, from Keenan MAE et al: *Manual of Orthopaedic Surgery for Spasticity*. Raven, 1993.)

3. Stiff-knee gait—Patients with a stiff-knee gait are unable to flex the knee during the swing phase of gait. The deformity is a dynamic one meaning that it only occurs during walking. Passive knee motion is not restricted, and the patient does not have difficulty sitting. Usually the knee is maintained in extension throughout the gait cycle. Toe drag, which is likely in the early swing phase, may cause the patient to trip. Thus, balance and stability are also affected. The limb appears to be functionally longer. Circumduction of the involved limb, hiking of the pelvis, or contralateral limb vaulting may occur as compensatory maneuvers.

A gait study with dynamic electromyography (EMG) should be done preoperatively to document the activity of the individual muscles of the quadriceps. Dyssynergic activity is commonly seen in the rectus femoris from preswing through terminal swing throughout the gait cycle. Abnormal activity is also common in the vastus intermedius, vastus medialis, and vastus lateralis muscles. If knee flexion is improved with a block of the femoral nerve or with botulinum toxin injection of the quadriceps, the rationale for surgical intervention is strengthened. Any equinus deformity of the foot should be corrected prior to evaluation of a stiff-knee gait because equinus causes a knee extension force during stance. Because the amount of knee flexion during swing is directly related to the speed of walking, the patient should be able to ambulate with a reasonable velocity to benefit from surgery. Hip flexion strength is also needed for a good result because the forward momentum of the leg normally provides the inertial force to flex the knee. In the past a selective release of the rectus femoris or rectus and vastus intermedius was done to remove their inhibition of knee flexion. On average, a 15-degree improvement in peak knee flexion was seen after surgery. Transfer of the rectus femoris to a hamstring tendon not only removes it as a deforming muscle force; it also converts the rectus into a corrective flexion force. This procedure provides improved knee flexion over selective release. When any of the vasti muscles are involved, they can be selectively lengthened at their myotendinous junction (Figure 13–14) and knee flexion improves.

4. Knee flexion deformity—A knee flexion deformity increases the physical demand on the quadriceps muscle, which must continually fire to hold the patient upright. Knee flexion often leads to knee instability and causes falls. It is most often caused by spasticity of the hamstring muscles. A KAFO can be used to hold the knee in extension on a temporary basis as a training aid in physical therapy. Such an orthosis, however, is difficult for the stroke patient to don and wear for permanent usage.

Surgical correction of the knee flexion deformity is the most desirable treatment. Hamstring tenotomy (Figure 13–15) eliminates the dynamic component of the deformity and generally results in a 50% correction of the contracture at the time of surgery. The residual joint contracture is then corrected by serial casting done weekly after surgery. Hamstring function posterior to the knee joint is not necessary for ambulation. In fact, ambulation may only be feasible in patients with knee flexion deformities of greater than 30 degrees if a hamstring release is done.

5. Equinus or equinovarus foot deformity—Surgical correction of an equinus deformity is indicated when the foot cannot be maintained in the neutral position with the heel in firm contact with the sole of the shoe in a well-fitted, rigid AFO. Despite a wide variety of surgical methods designed to decrease the triceps surae spasticity, none is more effective than Achilles tendon

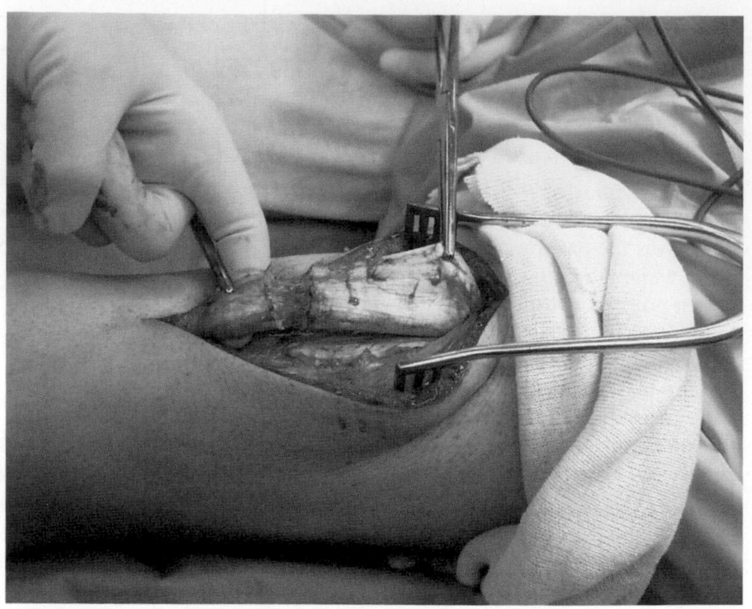

Figure 13–14. Selective lengthening of the rectus femoris tendon to correct a stiff-knee gait abnormality.

lengthening. In this procedure, triple hemisection tenotomy is performed via three stab incisions, with the most distal cut based medially to alleviate varus pull of the soleus muscle (Figure 13–16).

An anesthetic block of the posterior tibial nerve can be a valuable tool in preoperative assessment of the patient with equinus deformity because it demonstrates the potential benefits of Achilles tendon lengthening if the deformity is a result of increased muscle tone.
Surgical release of the flexor digitorum longus and brevis tendons at the base of each toe (Figure 13–17) is done prophylactically at the time of Achilles tendon lengthening because increased ankle dorsiflexion following heel cord tenotomy increases tension on the long toe flexor and commonly leads to excessive toe flexion (toe curling). The flexor hallucis longus and flexor digitorum longus tendons can be transferred to

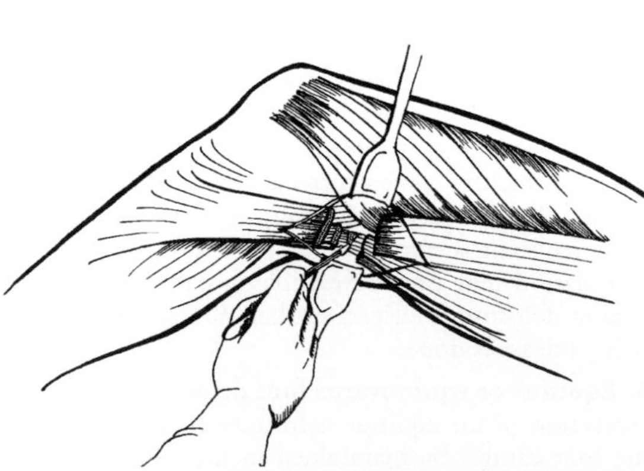

Figure 13–15. **Distal release of the hamstring tendons to correct a knee flexion contracture.** (Illustration by Anthony C. Berlet. Reproduced, with permission, from Keenan MAE et al: *Manual of Orthopaedic Surgery for Spasticity*. Raven, 1993.)

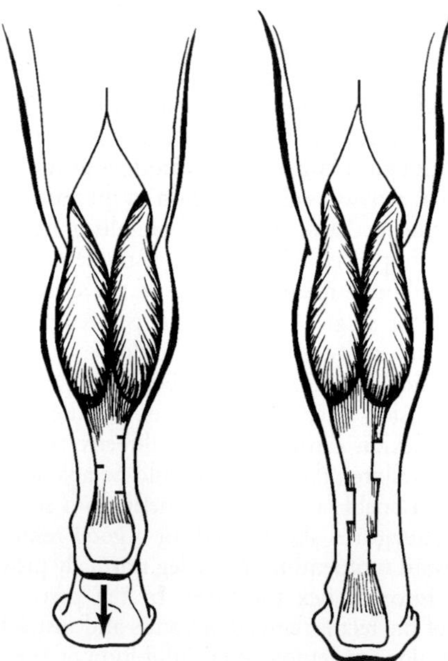

Figure 13–16. **Hoke triple hemisection Achilles tendon lengthening to correct an equinus foot deformity.** (Illustration by Anthony C. Berlet. Reproduced, with permission, from Keenan MAE et al: *Manual of Orthopaedic Surgery for Spasticity*. Raven, 1993.)

the os calcis to provide additional support to the weakened calf muscles.

Surgical correction of varus deformity is indicated when the problem is not corrected by a well-fitted orthosis. It is also indicated to enable the patient to walk without an orthosis when varus deformity is the only significant problem. The tibialis anterior, tibialis posterior, extensor hallucis longus, flexor hallucis longus, flexor digitorum, and soleus pass medial to the axis of the subtalar joint and are potentially responsible for varus deformity. EMG studies demonstrate that the peroneus longus and peroneus brevis are generally inactive, and the tibialis posterior is also usually inactive or minimally active.

The tibialis anterior is the key muscle responsible for varus deformity, and in most patients, this can be confirmed by visual examination or palpation while the patient walks. A procedure known as the split anterior tibial tendon transfer (Figure 13–18) diverts the inverting deforming force of the tibialis anterior to a corrective force. In this procedure, half of the tendon is transferred laterally to the os cuboideum. When the extensor hallucis longus muscle is overactive, it can be transferred to the middorsum of the foot as well.

Treatment of equinovarus deformity consists of simultaneously performing the Achilles tendon lengthening procedure and the split anterior tibial tendon transfer. At surgery, the tibialis anterior is secured and held sufficiently taut to maintain the foot in a neutral position. After healing, 70% of patients are able to walk without an orthosis.

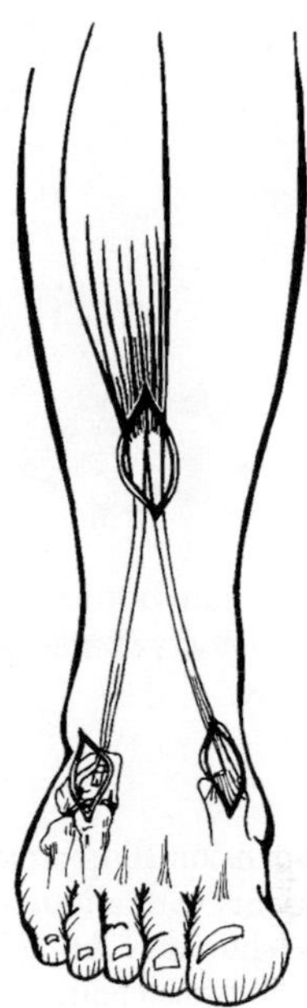

Figure 13–18. **Split anterior tibial tendon transfer to correct a spastic varus foot deformity.** (Illustration by Anthony C. Berlet. Reproduced, with permission, from Keenan MAE et al: *Manual of Orthopaedic Surgery for Spasticity.* Raven, 1993.)

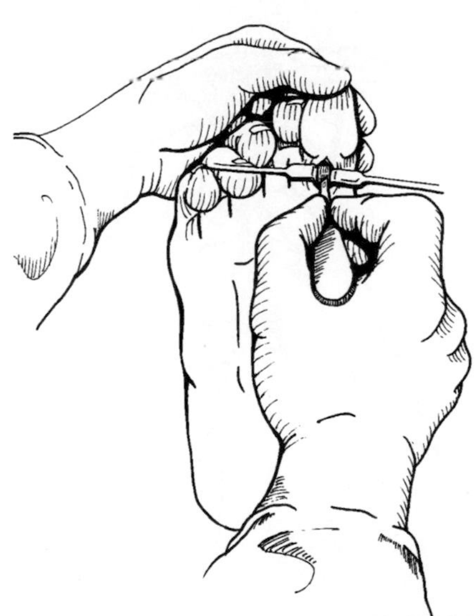

Figure 13–17. **Release of the flexor digitorum longus and brevis tendons to correct the problem of toe curling.** (Illustration by Anthony C. Berlet. Reproduced, with permission, from Keenan MAE et al: *Manual of Orthopaedic Surgery for Spasticity.* Raven, 1993.)

C. Upper Extremities

1. Spasticity—The first objective in treating the spastic upper extremity is to prevent contracture. Severe deformities at the shoulder, elbow, and wrist are seen in the neglected or noncompliant patient. Assistive equipment can be used to position the upper extremity, to aid in prevention of contractures, and to support the shoulder. Positioning extends spastic muscles but does not subject them to sudden postural changes that trigger the stretch reflex and aggravate spasticity. Brief periods should be scheduled when the upper extremity is not suspended and time can be devoted to ROM therapy and hygiene.

Most hemiplegics do not use their hand unless some selective motion is present at the fingers or thumb. Thumb opposition begins with opposition of the thumb to the side of the index finger (lateral or key pinch) and proceeds by circumduction to oppose each fingertip. In most stroke patients with selective thumb–finger extension, proximal muscle function is comparatively intact. Hence, orthotic stabilization of proximal joints is rarely necessary in the patient with a functional hand.

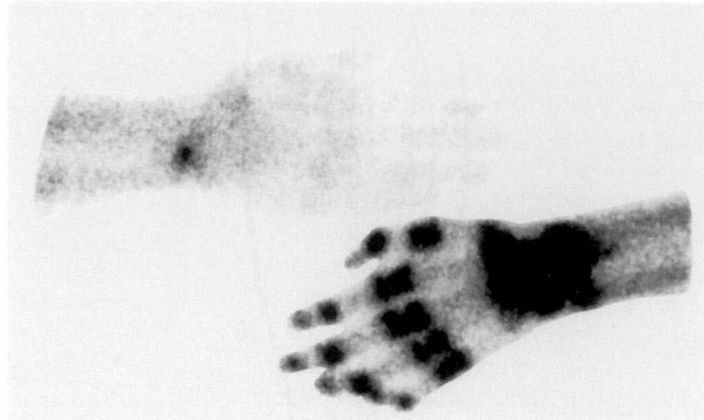

Figure 13–19. Technetium bone scan showing the periarticular increase in activity characteristic of reflex sympathetic dystrophy.

An overhead suspension sling attached to the wheelchair is used for patients with adductor or internal rotator spasticity of the shoulder. An alternative is an arm trough attached to the wheelchair.

It is usually not possible to maintain the wrist in neutral position with a WHO when wrist flexion spasticity is severe or when the wrist is flaccid. With minimal to moderate spasticity, either a volar or dorsal splint can be used. The splint should not extend to the fingers if the finger flexor spasticity is severe because slight motion and sensory contact of the fingers or palm may elicit the stretch reflex or grasp response, causing the fingers to jack-knife out of the splint.

2. Shoulder or arm pain—The hemiplegic shoulder deserves special attention because it is a common source of pain. A variety of different factors contribute to the painful shoulder: reflex sympathetic dystrophy, inferior subluxation, spasticity with internal rotation contracture, adhesive capsulitis, and degenerative changes about the shoulder. If early ROM exercises are performed and the extremity is properly positioned with a sling to reduce subluxation, severe or chronic pain at the shoulder can usually be prevented or minimized.

The classic clinical signs of reflex sympathetic dystrophy (swelling and skin changes) may not be apparent in the hemiplegic patient. If the patient complains that the arm is painful and no cause is apparent, a technetium bone scan assists in establishing the diagnosis (Figure 13–19). Treatment should be instituted immediately, and the patient should be given positive psychological reinforcement. The use of narcotics must be avoided. Treatment options include the use of medications such as corticosteroids, amitriptyline, or gabapentin (Neurontin), physical therapy, or nerve blocks (stellate ganglion blocks, brachial plexus blocks, or Bier IV regional blocks). Each of these techniques is successful with some patients; however, none is reliable for all patients.

3. Shoulder contracture—Contracture of the shoulder can cause pain, hygiene problems in the axilla, and difficulty in dressing and positioning. Shoulder adduction and internal rotation are caused by spasticity and myostatic contracture of four muscles: the pectoralis major, the subscapularis, the latissimus dorsi, and the teres major.

When the deformity is not fixed, lengthening of the pectoralis major, latissimus, and teres major at their myotendinous junction provides satisfactory correction of the deformity. In a nonfunctional extremity, surgical release of all four muscles (Figure 13–20) is usually necessary to resolve the deformity. Release of the subscapularis muscle is performed without violating the glenohumeral joint capsule. The joint capsule should not be opened because instability or intraarticular adhesions may result. A

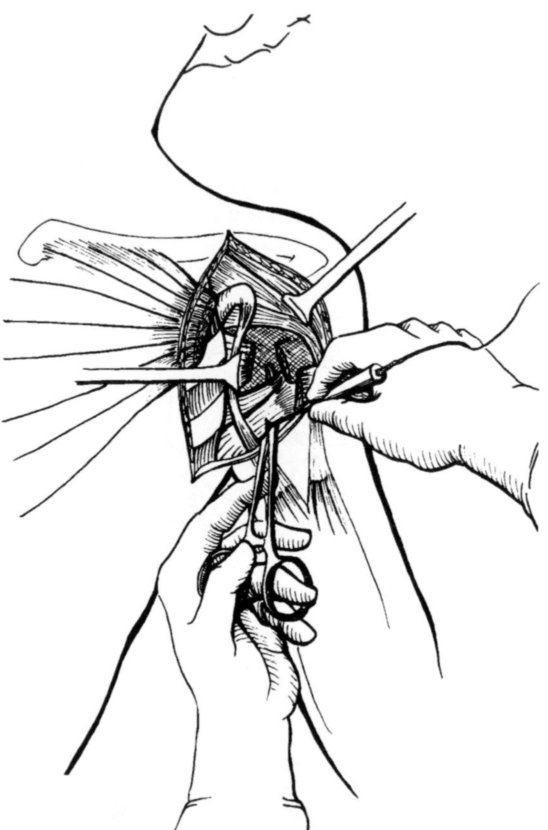

Figure 13–20. Release of the pectoralis major, subscapularis, latissimus dorsi, and teres major to correct an internal rotation and adduction contracture of the shoulder. (Illustration by Anthony C. Berlet. Reproduced, with permission, from Keenan MAE et al: *Manual of Orthopaedic Surgery for Spasticity*. Raven, 1993.)

Z-plasty of the axilla may be needed if the skin is contracted. After the wound heals, an aggressive mobilization program is instituted. Gentle ROM exercises are employed to correct any remaining contracture. Careful positioning of the limb in abduction and external rotation is necessary for several months to prevent recurrence.

4. Elbow flexion contracture—Persistent spasticity of the elbow flexors causes a myostatic contracture and flexion deformity of the elbow. Frequent accompanying problems include skin maceration, breakdown of the antecubital space, and compression neuropathy of the ulnar nerve.

Surgical release of the contracted muscles and gradual extension of the elbow corrects the deformity and decreases the ulnar nerve compression. The brachioradialis muscle and biceps tendon are transected. The brachialis muscle is fractionally lengthened at its myotendinous junction by transecting the tendinous fibers on the anterior surface of the muscle while leaving the underlying muscle intact (Figure 13–21). Complete release of the brachialis muscle is not performed unless a severe contracture was present for several years. An anterior capsulectomy is not needed and should be avoided because of the associated increased stiffness and intraarticular adhesions that occur postoperatively. Anterior transposition of the ulnar nerve may be necessary to further improve ulnar nerve function.

Approximately 50% correction of the deformity can be expected at surgery without causing excessive tension on the contracted neurovascular structures. Serial casts or dropout casts can be used to obtain further correction over the ensuing weeks.

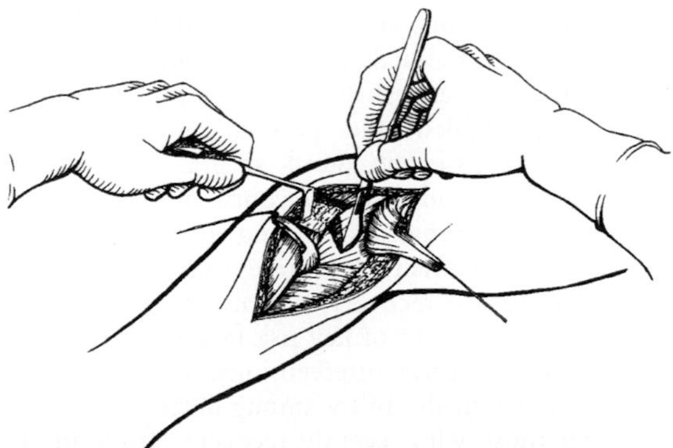

Figure 13–21. Surgery of the brachioradialis muscle, biceps tendon, and brachialis muscle to correct an elbow flexion contracture in a nonfunctional arm. (Illustration by Anthony C. Berlet. Reproduced, with permission, from Keenan MAE et al: *Manual of Orthopaedic Surgery for Spasticity*. Raven, 1993.)

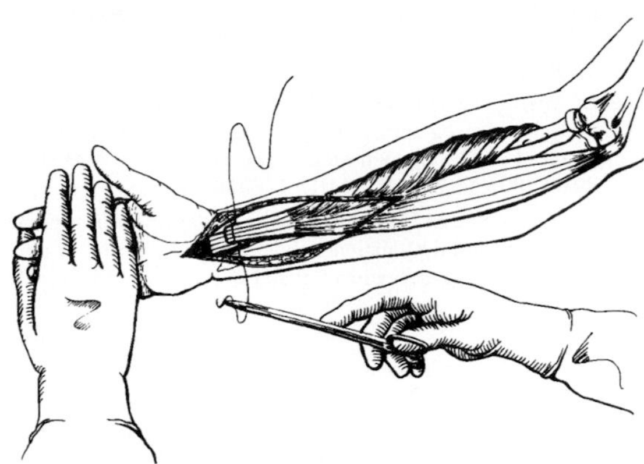

Figure 13–22. The superficialis-to-profundus tendon transfer to correct a severe clenched-fist deformity in a nonfunctional hand. (Illustration by Anthony C. Berlet. Reproduced, with permission, from Keenan MAE et al: *Manual of Orthopaedic Surgery for Spasticity*. Raven, 1993.)

5. Clenched-fist deformity—A spastic clenched-fist deformity in a nonfunctional hand causes palmar skin breakdown and hygiene problems. Recurrent infections of the fingernail beds are also common.

Adequate flexor tendon lengthening to correct the deformity cannot be attained by fractional or myotendinous lengthening without causing discontinuity at the musculotendinous junction. Transection of the flexor tendons is not recommended because any remaining extensor muscle tone may result in an unopposed hyperextension deformity of the wrist and digits. The recommended procedure is a superficialis-to-profundus tendon transfer (Figure 13–22), which provides sufficient flexor tendon lengthening with preservation of a passive tether to prevent a hyperextension deformity. The wrist deformity is corrected by release of the wrist flexors. A wrist arthrodesis is done to maintain the hand in a neutral position and to eliminate the need for a permanent splint. Because intrinsic muscle spasticity is always present in conjunction with severe spasticity of the extrinsic flexors, a neurectomy of the motor branches of the ulnar nerve in the Guyon canal should be routinely performed along with the superficialis-to-profundus tendon transfer to prevent the postsurgical development of an intrinsic plus deformity.

After surgery, the wrist and digits are immobilized for 4 weeks in a short arm cast extended to the fingertips.

Botte MJ, Bruffey JD, Copp SN et al: Surgical reconstruction of acquired spastic foot and ankle deformity. Foot Ankle Clin 2000;5(2):381. [PMID: 11232236]

Fuller DA, Keenan MA, Esquenazi A et al: The impact of instrumented gait analysis on surgical planning: Treatment of spastic equinovarus deformity of the foot and ankle. Foot Ankle Int 2002;23(8):738. [PMID: 12199388]

Gardner MJ, Ong BC, Liporace F et al: Orthopedic issues after cerebrovascular accident. Am J Orthop 2002;31(10):559. [PMID: 12405561]

Keenan MA, Fuller DA, Whyte J et al: The influence of dynamic polyelectromyography in formulating a surgical plan in treatment of spastic elbow flexion deformity. Arch Phys Med Rehabil 2003;84(2):291. [PMID: 12601663]

Keenan MA, Mehta S: Neuro-orthopedic management of shoulder deformity and dysfunction in brain-injured patients: A novel approach. J Head Trauma Rehabil 2004;19(2):143. [PMID: 15247824]

Mayer NH: Choosing upper limb muscles for focal intervention after traumatic brain injury. J Head Trauma Rehabil 2004; 19(2):119. [PMID: 15247823]

Pollock A, Baer G, Pomeroy V et al: Physiotherapy treatment approaches for the recovery of postural control and lower limb function following stroke. Cochrane Database Syst Rev 2003;2:CD001920. [PMID: 12804415]

Vuagnat H, Chantraine A: Shoulder pain in hemiplegia revisited: Contribution of functional electrical stimulation and other therapies. J Rehabil Med 2003;35:49. [PMID: 12691333]

GERIATRIC ORTHOPEDICS

General Principles

A major challenge facing society is the aging of the population. By 2020, 52 million Americans will be older than 65 years. By 2040, 68 million people will be older than 65 years. Both the absolute numbers and proportion of elderly people is increasing dramatically. People are living longer and have higher expectations for a good quality of life. Despite this trend, proportionally less disability occurs among the elderly now than in the past.

Although the passage of time, chronological age, is the convenient measure used, it is not necessarily the most precise marker of aging. A more sensitive marker would be to consider the person's functional age, but this is often difficult to define and measure. Age 65 is generally considered the beginning of old age.

The young elderly are those individuals 65 to 75 years of age. These people are usually functionally intact. They have isolated orthopedic problems, such as mild osteoporosis, osteoarthrosis, overuse injuries (sports), and occasionally cancer.

The frail very elderly are those persons older than 80 years. These people tend to have multiple musculoskeletal impairments such as advanced osteoporosis, generalized muscle weakness, multiple organ diseases, and dementia.

1. Disability

The leading causes of death in the elderly are heart disease, malignant neoplasms, and cerebrovascular disease. The overall leading causes of disability in the elderly are cancer, heart disease, dementia, and musculoskeletal disorders. The leading causes of disease-related disability before death are arthritis, hypertension, hearing impairment, heart disease, and orthopedic conditions. Despite the increasing incidence of disability with aging, only 5% of Americans live in nursing homes.

When evaluating the elderly, five functional domains of disability need to be considered:

1. *Physical ADLs* include activities such as bathing, dressing, eating, and walking.
2. *Instrumental ADLs* are home management tasks such as shopping, meal preparation, money management, using the telephone, and performing light housework.
3. *Cognitive functioning* is particularly important in the elderly. Dementia is one of the four leading causes of disability in the elderly and a principal reason for institutionalization.
4. *Affective function* is important. Secondary depressions are common in the elderly, and suicide is a more frequent cause of death in the elderly than in the young.
5. *Social functioning* is less of a problem. Only 1% of the elderly rate their social interactions as inadequate.

Disability in basic ADLs is common among community-dwelling older persons, with prevalence rates ranging from 7% in those 65 to 74 years of age to 24% in those 85 years of age or older. Restricted activity, defined as staying in bed for at least half a day and/or cutting down on usual activities because of an illness, injury, or other problem, is common among community-living older persons, regardless of risk for disability, and it is usually attributable to several concurrent health-related problems. Although disability in older persons is often thought to be progressive or permanent, previous research shows it is a dynamic process, with individuals moving in and out of states of disability. To set realistic goals and plan for appropriate care, disabled older persons, along with their families and clinicians, need accurate information about the likelihood and time course of recovery. Prevention of functional decline and disability includes not only management of acute episodes of disability and promotion of recovery, but also ongoing evaluation and management of key risk factors for disability and use of preventive interventions. The high likelihood of recurrent disability among older persons suggests that those who recently recovered from an episode of disability are an important target population for preventive interventions. Although some interventions designed to prevent recurrent disability may be disease specific (eg, anticoagulation after embolic stroke), others may be broadly applicable regardless of the specific precipitant of disability (eg, exercise-based programs).

2. Challenges for the Orthopedic Surgeon

When working with the elderly, the orthopedic surgeon becomes a member of a multidisciplinary team. The people making up this team include internists, geriatricians, rehabilitation specialists, psychiatrists, psychologists, social workers, nutritionists, skin care specialists, physical and occupational therapists, and the so-called young elderly children of the patient. Osteoporosis, fractures, arthritis, foot disorders, stroke, and amputations are the most frequent causes of musculoskeletal impairment.

3. Osteoporosis

Osteoporosis is an age-related disorder characterized by decreased bone mass and increased fracture risk in the absence of other recognizable causes of bone loss. Osteoporosis can occur either as a primary disorder or secondary to other diseases.

A. Primary Osteoporosis

Primary osteoporosis, the most common form of the disease, occurs in people from 51 to 65 years of age with a female-to-male ratio of 6:1. Primary osteoporosis can be further subdivided into two types. Type I, postmenopausal osteoporosis, results from decreased circulating levels of estrogen. It is seen in postmenopausal women and affects the majority of persons older than 70 years. Bone loss is rapid. There is swift trabecular bone loss up to 8% per year. Type I osteoporosis causes primarily trabecular bone loss with only 0.5% cortical bone loss per year. Fractures occur in locations of trabecular bone loss such as the distal radius and vertebrae. The cause of primary osteoporosis is a changing hormonal milieu.

Type II, senile osteoporosis, is a consequence of aging. It causes a more global bone loss affecting cortical and cancellous bone such as in the femoral neck. Type II osteoporosis is seen in persons older than 70 years. The female-to-male ratio is 2:1. The bone loss occurs in both the trabecular and cortical bone and averages 0.3–0.5% per year. Fractures occurring as the result of type II osteoporosis typically involve the hip, pelvis, humerus, tibia, and vertebral bodies. The causes of senile osteoporosis are those seen with aging and include calcium deficiency, decreased vitamin D, and increased parathormone activity.

B. Secondary Osteoporosis

Secondary osteoporosis results from a variety of causes. The most common are chronic or prolonged corticosteroid use and endocrine disorders. The endocrine disorders associated with osteoporosis are hyperthyroidism; hyperparathyroidism; diabetes, Cushing disease, and euplastic disorders.

Prevention Strategies

Restoration of bone is difficult. It is therefore imperative to maximize peak bone mass during skeletal growth and then to maintain it during maturity. This requires adequate dietary calcium and vitamin D intake. The recommended amounts for adults are 1200 mg/day of calcium and 400 mg of vitamin D. For postmenopausal women, 1500 mg/day of calcium is recommended. Impact exercise is effective in maintaining bone mass. It is also important to avoid those factors that promote osteoporosis such as the use of tobacco products and excessive alcohol consumption.

Diagnosis

Osteoporosis is a clinical diagnosis often made following a fracture. Radiographic findings include osteopenia (seen with more than 30% mineral loss); loss of horizontal trabeculae in vertebral bodies; thoracic wedge fractures; lumbar spine endplate fractures; stress fractures of the pelvis; and fractures of humerus, wrist, hip, supracondylar femur, tibial plateau. Quantification of bone mass is done for confirmation and follow-up. Dual-energy x-ray absorptiometry (DEXA) is used to quantify bone mass. The following criteria for diagnosis are based on the DEXA scan:

Normal: within 1 standard deviation (SD) of young adult reference

Osteopenia: between 1.0 and 2.4 SD below reference

Osteoporosis: 2.5 or more SD below reference

Severe osteoporosis: 2.5 plus one or more fragility fractures

Treatment

Calcium alone does not prevent bone loss during the early postmenopausal period, but adequate daily calcium replacement is helpful. In late menopause (more than 6 years), calcium replacement does reduce bone loss. Weight-bearing exercise is also useful in maintaining bone mass.

Newer treatments using bisphosphonates show promise in treating osteoporosis. The bisphosphonates are a class of compounds similar to pyrophosphate that are readily adsorbed by bone mineral surfaces. Once bound, they inhibit the bone absorption activity of osteoclasts. Two bisphosphonates currently are available for clinical use: alendronate sodium (Fosamax) and risedronate sodium (Actonel).

Only approximately a third of women in the United States diagnosed with osteoporosis during the 1990s were offered treatment for the condition. Fewer than 2% of the women 60 years and older were diagnosed with osteoporosis, but the rate increased from 1.2% in 1993 to 2.7% in 1997. Overall, 36% of women diagnosed with osteoporosis were prescribed calcium, vitamin D, or drugs to treat the disease, but this also increased, from 20% in 1993 to 55% in 1997.

Exercise

The ability to walk safely is vital for independent living. Both strength and endurance determine the capacity for independent movement. Muscle strength is associated with the capacity to perform ADLs. A reduction in strength with age is attributed to these factors:

1. a loss of muscle mass because of smaller and fewer fibers;
2. a loss of motor neurons (anterior horn cells);
3. changes in muscle architecture;
4. a defect in the excitation-contraction mechanism; and
5. psychosocial changes leading to reduced capacity to activate motor units.

Strength training can lead to major functional improvements in the elderly. The plasticity of the motor system to adapt to a training load appears to be maintained into the 10th decade of life. Strength training has no effect on the central determinants of aerobic capacity such as maximum heart rate, blood pressure hemoglobin concentration, and blood volume.

Aerobic exercise does lead to increased endurance and functional capacity. Endurance is the time a person can maintain either a static force or a power level involving a combination of concentric or eccentric muscular contractions. The stress that exercise imposes on a person and the tolerance or endurance for that exercise intensity depends on how much energy is needed to perform the task in relation to the person's maximal capacity. With training, activities become easier to perform. The person has increased endurance for submaximal exercise. Improvements in movement can lower the energy cost of an activity.

4. Arthritis

Osteoarthritis is very prevalent in the elderly. Total joint arthroplasty has dramatically improved the mobility and quality of life for the elderly. A variety of studies confirm the appropriateness and effectiveness of both total hip and total knee arthroplasty in the elderly with low complication rates. The elderly patient is more likely to require the use of an upper extremity assistive device for ambulation following joint replacement.

5. Fractures

A. General Considerations

One of the most compelling reasons to determine the etiology of a fracture and provide appropriate treatment is that a previous low-energy fracture is among the strongest risk factors for new fractures. Specifically, patients with a low-energy fracture of the wrist, hip, proximal humerus, or ankle have nearly a two- to fourfold greater risk for future fractures than individuals who have never experienced a fracture. Furthermore, up to half of patients with a prior vertebral fracture experience additional vertebral fractures within 3 years, many within the first year. Indeed, compared to individuals with no history of fracture, a patient with a prior vertebral fracture has nearly a fivefold increased risk of future vertebral fractures and up to a sixfold increased risk of hip and other nonvertebral fractures. Taken together, these data indicate that patients with a history of any type of prior fracture have a two- to sixfold increased risk of subsequent fractures compared to those without a previous fracture.

These findings emphasize that optimal care of fragility fracture patients includes not only management of the presenting fracture, but also evaluation, diagnosis, and treatment of the underlying cause(s) of the fracture, including low bone density or other medical conditions. In this regard, supplementation with calcium and vitamin D lowers fracture risk in the elderly. In addition, several pharmacologic agents reduce the risk of future fracture by as much as 50% in patients with existing fractures. Nonpharmacologic interventions, such as fall prevention programs and individually tailored exercise programs, reduce falls among the elderly, which may decrease the incidence of fractures. In addition, trochanteric padding dramatically reduces hip fractures among those at highest risk. Thus, initiating interventions soon after a fragility fracture occurs may significantly reduce the incidence and severity of subsequent fractures.

In the elderly, fractures result from low-energy injuries. Falls in the home most frequently result in fractures of the hip, distal radius, pelvis, proximal humerus, and ribs. Approximately 90% of fractures of the pelvis, hip, and forearm result from a fall. Only 3–5% of falls result in fractures.

Many of the risk factors for fracture are also risk factors for falls. Risk factors can be divided into categories. Risk factors associated with aspects of aging include primary osteoporosis, impaired vision or balance; gait abnormalities; and loss of muscle and fat padding the bones. Environmental risk factors consist of uneven surfaces; slippery surfaces; obstacles such as throw rugs, pets, and steps; poor lighting; and lack of railings or other supports for balance. Fall prevention programs include home safety measures such as the installation of safety bars in the bathtub and shower, elimination of heavily waxed floors and slippery rugs, and the use of rubber sole shoes with low wide heels that provide more stability.

Genetic factors are seen in both gender and race. Women sustain more fractures than men. Whites have more fractures than African Americans. Illnesses commonly associated with fractures include stroke, syncope, hypotension, secondary osteoporosis, Parkinson disease, dementia, and paraparesis. The use of medications such as benzodiazepines, tricyclic antidepressants, antipsychotics, corticosteroids, and barbiturates are connected with fractures. Lifestyle factors include exercise, nutrition, alcohol or other substance abuse, immobilization, and shoe style.

Other factors contribute to the risk of traumatic fractures occurring in falls. The first is the orientation of the fall. A fall that happens while standing still or walking very slowly imparts little or no forward momentum so the point of impact is near the hip. Gait velocity slows with aging, putting the hip more at risk of injury in a fall. Protective responses during a fall decrease with age. Local shock absorbers, muscle and fat, that surround the bone decrease with age. Bone strength is less secondary to the osteoporosis associated with aging.

B. Hip Fractures

Fractures of the hip are classified by location and severity. The basic considerations are whether the fracture occurs in the intracapsular or extracapsular area and the stability of the fracture pattern. Intracapsular fractures occur along the neck of the femur. When they are displaced, the blood supply to the femoral head is likely disrupted, which increases the possibility of osteonecrosis.

Treatment of hip fractures is operative whenever possible. The nonoperative treatment of hip fractures is very occasionally chosen for patients at high medical risk. It is sometimes recommended for demented nonambulatory patients. The nonoperative treatment of a hip fracture involves months of bed rest and sometimes traction. It requires excellent nursing care to avoid decubitus ulcers and respiratory dysfunction. Fracture malunion, limb-length inequality, pain, and higher mortality rates are common with nonoperative care. The chances for eventual ambulation are only 55% compared with 76% for patients treated operatively.

The basic principles of treatment of hip fractures are well established. Nondisplaced fractures of the femoral neck are usually treated with multiple pins or screws. Displaced fractures of the femoral neck are usually treated with a hemiarthroplasty because of the high incidence of avascular necrosis. Stable intertrochanteric fractures are generally treated with a sliding screw and side plate system. Unstable intertrochanteric fractures may require additional measures to gain adequate medial support. In very osteoporotic bone, it may be necessary to add methyl methacrylate bone cement to gain sufficient fixation and stability. When a patient is known to have severe arthritis, a primary total hip arthroplasty may be performed.

The postoperative rehabilitation of the elderly patient is critical to a successful outcome. Non–weight-bearing ambulation is extremely difficult and more often impossible for elderly patients. Every effort should be made in the operative treatment to gain enough stability of the fracture to allow weight bearing as tolerated. The patient should be mobilized on the first or second day after surgery to prevent the many complications of immobility. Pain management is important to allow mobilization, but oversedation of the elderly patient needs to be avoided. When a prosthesis was inserted, dislocation must be avoided. The elderly patient may not remember the precautions. Use of elevated chairs and toilet seats helps avoid the excessive hip flexion associated with posterior dislocation. A knee immobilizer splint while in bed prevents knee flexion that in turn results in flexion of the hip. It is prudent occasionally to place the patient in a hip brace, which limits flexion and adduction while soft-tissue healing occurs.

C. Fractures of the Pelvis

A common pelvic classification is based on whether or not the ring of the pelvis is disrupted because this indicates the amount of energy involved with the initial trauma. A fracture that does not disrupt the pelvic ring such as a pubic ramus fracture is a low-energy injury. Formerly, pelvic fractures were associated with high-energy trauma, were displaced, and occurred in patients less than 40 years old. With the aging of America, now more than 50% of fractures occur in those older than 60 years, with a preponderance occurring in women. The majority of pelvis fractures in the elderly are low-energy injuries and can be treated nonoperatively with analgesia and bed rest. Early mobilization is desirable to prevent the complications of immobility. Full weight bearing is allowed. A walker or other assistive device is useful to decrease pain and increase stability during walking. Stool softeners are often helpful. Fractures of the coccyx and sacrum are treated in a similar manner.

D. Fractures of the Distal Femur

The management of distal femur fractures in the elderly patients must be individualized. Advanced age in itself is not a contraindication to surgery. The objects of surgical treatment of the distal femur are anatomic reduction and stable fixation. In the presence of severe osteopenia, stable fixation is difficult. The addition of methyl methacrylate or long-stem knee replacement can help with stability. Occasionally, a postoperative cast brace is needed to supplement the internal fixation.

E. Fractures of the Forearm

Most fractures of the distal radius (Colles fracture) can be treated by closed reduction and casting. Significant loss of radial height and dorsal comminution can occur in osteoporotic bone even after lower energy injuries. In this situation, most surgeons would agree that external fixation and bone grafting of the fracture are warranted to obtain and maintain a more anatomic reduction. Early ROM exercises for both the shoulder and the fingers should be encouraged to avoid stiffness.

F. Fractures of the Proximal Humerus

Fractures of the proximal humerus account for 4–5% of all fractures and occur most commonly in the elderly. Humeral fractures in the elderly are minimally displaced 80% of the time. In these cases, sling immobilization is used to control pain. Pendulum exercises are begun early to prevent excessive stiffness in the shoulder. Limited external rotation of the shoulder predisposes to a future spiral fracture of the humerus during dressing. In unstable and markedly displaced fractures of the humeral head, a hemiarthroplasty can be considered. If coexisting severe osteoarthritis of the glenohumeral joint is present, a total shoulder arthroplasty can be considered.

6. Stroke

Stroke is a common cause of disability in the elderly. This topic was covered in detail earlier in this chapter.

7. Foot Disorders

The foot tends to widen with age as the transverse arch support weakens and abnormal bony alignments of the foot become common. Surgical reconstruction of foot deformities may be contraindicated in the frail elderly patient, particularly because of peripheral vascular disease. Nonoperative treatment consists of active and passive ROM exercises of the foot to maximize flexibility. Strengthening exercises of the lower extremity can be useful to improve the overall gait pattern. The patient should try to optimize body weight to eliminate excessive forces on the foot. Functional orthoses of a semirigid material with little or no posting may improve the foot position and provide symptomatic relief. Accommodative orthoses of a soft material may also be used. These soft orthoses are designed to control foot posture and eliminate areas of pressure, but they are not intended to correct the foot position. Orthoses are used in combination with soft extra-depth shoes that provide more clearance for deformities of the toes. Flat shoes are helpful for forefoot deformities because they prevent the foot sliding forward in the shoe. A shoe with a low heel is desirable for patients with a severe pronation deformity because the Achilles tendon is commonly tight. Placing the heel cord on stretch only increases the pronation forces on the foot.

8. Amputation

The majority of amputations done in a civilian population are of the lower extremity. Most amputations are done in the sixth decade of life or later, so this is largely a problem of the elderly. The issues associated with amputation are discussed in Chapter 12.

Chao EY, Inoue N, Koo TK et al: Biomechanical considerations of fracture treatment and bone quality maintenance in elderly patients and patients with osteoporosis. Clin Orthop 2004;(425):12. [PMID: 15292783]

Gehlbach SH et al: Recognition of osteoporosis by primary care physicians. Am J Public Health 2002;92:271. [PMID: 11818304]

Gill TM, Allore HG, Holford TR et al: Hospitalization, restricted activity, and the development of disability among older persons. JAMA 2004;292(17):2115. [PMID: 15523072]

Hardy SE, Gill TM: Factors associated with recovery of independence among newly disabled older persons. Arch Intern Med 2005;165(1):106. [PMID: 15642885]

Hooven F, Gehlbach SH, Pekow P et al: Follow-up treatment for osteoporosis after fracture. Osteoporos Int 2005;16:296–301. [PMID: 15221208]

Lorich DG, Geller DS, Nielson JH: Osteoporotic pertrochanteric hip fractures: Management and current controversies. Instr Course Lect 2004;53:441. [PMID: 15116633]

Phillips FM: Minimally invasive treatments of osteoporotic vertebral compression fractures. Spine 2003;28(Suppl 15):S45. [PMID: 12897474]

Stromsoe K: Fracture fixation problems in osteoporosis. Injury 2004;35(2):107. [PMID: 14736465]

Tosi LL, Kyle RF: Fragility fractures: The fall and decline of bone health. Commentary on "Interventions to improve osteoporosis treatment following hip fracture" by Gardner et al. J Bone Joint Surg Am 2005;87-A(1):1. [PMID: 15634807]

BRAIN INJURY

Brain injury resulting from trauma to the head is a leading cause of death and disability. Head injury is at least twice as common in males as in females and occurs most often in people 15–24 years of age. Approximately half of the injuries result from motor vehicle accidents. In the United States, 410,000 new cases of traumatic brain injury can be expected each year, with each case presenting a challenge to the team of health care providers involved in providing emergency treatment and long-term management.

Neurologic Impairment & Recovery

The Glasgow Coma Score (Table 13–3) is frequently used to evaluate eye opening, motor response, and verbal response of patients with impaired consciousness. Analysis of scores from patients in several countries sheds light on the chances for survival and neurologic recovery. According to the data, approximately 50% of patients with impaired consciousness survived.

Table 13–3. The Glasgow Coma Score.

Response	Description	Numerical Value
Eye opening	Spontaneous response	4
	Response to speech	3
	Response to pain	2
	No response	1
Motor response	Obeying response	6
	Localized response	5
	Withdrawal	4
	Abnormal flexion	3
	Extension	2
	No response	1
Verbal response	Oriented conversation	5
	Confused conversation	4
	Inappropriate words	3
	Incomprehensible sounds	2
	No response	1

Adapted, with permission, from: Teasdale G, Jennett B: Assessment of coma and impaired consciousness. A practical scale. Lancet 1974;2:81.

Six months after injury, moderate or good neurologic recovery was seen in 82% of patients with initial (24-hour) Glasgow scores of 11 or higher, 68% of patients with initial scores of 8–10, 34% with initial scores of 5–7, and 7% with initial scores of 3 or 4. Age was an important factor related to neurologic outcome, with 62% of patients younger than 20 years and 46% of patients between 20 and 29 years of age showing moderate or good recovery.

The incidence of good recovery declines not only with advancing age but also with advancing duration of coma. Patients recovering from coma within the first 2 weeks of injury have a 70% chance of good recovery. The recovery rate drops to 39% in the third week and to 17% in the fourth week. Decerebrate or decorticate posturing indicates a brainstem injury and is indicative of a poor prognosis.

Management

The rehabilitation process has three distinct phases: the acute injury period, the subacute period of neurologic recovery, and the residual period of functional adaptation. Health care workers from a variety of disciplines are involved in each phase.

A. Phases of Patient Care and Rehabilitation

1. Acute injury phase—The initial phase of rehabilitation begins as soon as the patient reaches the acute-care hospital. Brain injury is frequently the result of a high-velocity accident. Diagnosis is problematic because multiple injuries are common, resuscitation and other lifesaving efforts make a complete examination difficult, and the patient who is comatose or disoriented cannot assist in the history or physical examination.

Under the circumstances, three important principles should be followed. The first is to make an accurate diagnosis based on a thorough examination. Fractures or dislocations are missed in 11% of patients, and peripheral nerve injuries are missed in 34%. The second is to assume that the patient will make a good neurologic recovery. Basic treatment principles should not be waived on the erroneous assumption that the patient will not survive. The third principle is to anticipate uncontrolled limb motion and lack of patient cooperation. The patient often goes through a period of agitation as neurologic recovery progresses. Traction and external fixation devices are best avoided for extremity injuries. Open reduction and internal fixation of fractures and dislocations diminishes complications, requires less nursing care, allows for earlier mobilization, and results in fewer residual deformities.

2. Subacute phase of neurologic recovery—During the subacute phase, when the patient is generally in a rehabilitation facility, spontaneous neurologic recovery occurs. During this recovery period, which may last from 12 to 18 months, spasticity is frequently present, and heterotopic ossification may develop. Management is aimed at preventing limb deformities, maintaining a functional arc of motion in the joints, and meeting both the physical and the psychological needs of the patient.

3. Residual phase or period of functional adaptation—When neurologic recovery reaches a plateau, the third phase of rehabilitation begins. Medical and surgical management is aimed at correction of residual limb deformities and excision of heterotopic ossification while specialists from various disciplines continue moving toward the goals planned for the individual patient.

B. The Team Approach to Patient Care and Rehabilitation

Members of the rehabilitation team are involved in setting short-term goals, which are meant to be accomplished by the time of discharge from the rehabilitation program, and long-term goals, which will take an extended period of time to achieve. The identification of needs and the setting of goals are performed independently by health care workers from each discipline.

The team members then meet to discuss their goals and draw up a coordinated plan.

1. Medical management—General medical goals are usually straightforward. Because most patients with traumatic brain injuries are younger persons, chronic premorbid illnesses are uncommon. Prevention and treatment of infections are important goals, especially while shunts, tubes, and catheters are in place. If seizures are present, controlling them without causing sedation is vital.

In patients with decreased ROM in a joint, the cause of the problem should be explored. Possible causes include increased muscle tone, pain, myostatic contracture, periarticular heterotopic ossification, an undetected fracture or dislocation, and lack of patient cooperation secondary to diminished cognition. Peripheral nerve blocks with local anesthetics are useful in distinguishing between severe spasticity and fixed contractures.

Phenol blocks or botulinum toxin injections are used to decrease spasticity only during the period of potential neurologic recovery. The rationale for phenol injection is that by the time the nerve regenerates, the patient will have recovered more control of the affected muscle.

The technique for administering the phenol block depends on the anatomic accessibility and composition of the nerve; the direct injection of a peripheral nerve gives the most complete and long-lasting block. If a peripheral nerve has a large sensory component, however, direct injection is not recommended because loss of sensation is undesirable and some patients may develop painful hyperesthesia. In some cases, it is necessary to dissect surgically the individual motor branches of a nerve that runs to a muscle and inject each branch separately. In other cases, the motor points of the muscles can be localized using a needle electrode and nerve stimulator and then injected. Motor point injections do not completely relieve spasticity but can be helpful in reducing muscle tone. The duration of motor point blocks is approximately 2 months, and the blocks can be repeated as necessary.

Botulinum toxin is injected directly into the muscle belly. The onset of action is delayed but lasts for approximately 3 months. The injections can be repeated as needed and do not result in any scarring of the muscle. The limitation of botulinum toxin is the total dose tolerated at a given time and its high cost relative to phenol.

2. Nursing care—Nursing goals concentrate on basic bodily needs such as nutrition, hygiene, and handling of secretions. Removal of tubes at the earliest possible time is a desirable goal.

Tracheostomy tubes are commonly used in patients with brain injury. General principles of care include changing an uncuffed tube as soon as possible to prevent pressure necrosis of the trachea, adding mist if necessary to provide moisture to the artificial airway, establishing suctioning procedures to prevent trauma and infection, and eliminating the dressing once the tracheostomy incision is healed because the dressing can be a source of infection. The size of the tube is gradually reduced, and the tube is then plugged to tolerance. When continual plugging is tolerated for 3 consecutive days, the tube can be removed.

Feeding tubes are also commonly used. If oral feeding is not anticipated in the near future, a percutaneous endoscopic gastrostomy tube is recommended. If oral feeding is anticipated soon, a nasogastric tube is inserted, cleaned daily, and changed once a week. Instituting and carrying out an oral feeding program requires the combined efforts of the nursing and physical therapy staffs. Head and trunk control are necessary to provide alignment of swallowing structures. The presence of a cough reflex indicates some measure of laryngeal control and the ability to clear the airway. The presence of a swallowing reflex indicates inherent coordination of swallowing structures. The gag reflex, although protective, is not necessary for functional swallowing. Oral feeding should be started with thickened liquids and pureed foods, which provide more oral stimulus and allow time to initiate swallowing. Thin liquids are more easily aspirated.

The ability to inhibit voiding is generally a cognitive function. Restoring continence in the brain-injured patient requires a consistent routine with repeated instructions and positive feedback. Bowel programs should be initiated as soon as the patient begins taking nourishment via the gastrointestinal tract. Again, a consistent routine is most successful.

3. Cognitive and neuropsychological management—The return of cognitive abilities follows the same sequence of stages that normal cognitive development follows, with each new level of cognitive function stemming from the previous level. Table 13–4 shows the eight levels. Cognitive and behavioral management focuses on providing stimulation for patients with a level II or III response; providing structure for patients with a level IV, V, or VI response; and encouraging community activities for patients with a level VII or VIII response.

Memory loss and diminished cognitive function are frequently the most pervasive limitations to overall function. Cognitive retraining is an essential part of the rehabilitation process at every stage. As cognition increases and the patient becomes more aware of the injury, he or she also becomes increasingly aware of the possible consequences of the injury and requires counseling and psychological support.

4. Speech therapy—After traumatic brain injury, patients may have temporary or permanent physical handicaps that prevent them from communicating effectively. In communicating with nonverbal patients, a variety of methods and devices can be used, ranging from yes-and-no signals to communication boards and electronic devices. Patients need to acquire at least a minimal level of attentional, memory, and organiza-

Table 13–4. Cognitive function.

Level	Description
I	No response
II	Generalized response
III	Localized response
IV	Confused, agitated response
V	Confused, inappropriate response
VI	Confused, appropriate response
VII	Automatic, appropriate response
VIII	Purposeful, appropriate response

Adapted from Malkmus D et al: *Rehabilitation of the Head-Injured Adult. Comprehensive Cognitive Management*. Professional Staff Association of Rancho Los Amigos Hospital, Inc: Downey, CA. 1980.

tional skills to facilitate use of such communication devices. In verbal patients, language disorders may be present because of an underlying cognitive disruption following head trauma. The most frequent residual language disorders are those seen in the areas of work retrieval and auditory processing. Language therapy in patients with these long-term disorders should be directed toward reorganization of the cognitive process.

5. Physical therapy—Areas of concern in physical therapy include patient positioning, mobility, and performance of daily activities. Making it possible for bedridden patients to sit can significantly improve the quality of life and greatly enhance the opportunities to interact with other people. In some patients, casts or orthotic devices may be required to maintain the desired limb positions. Aggressive joint ROM exercises are necessary to prevent contractures.

Among the factors that influence whether a patient can walk are limb stability, motor control, good balance reactions, and adequate proprioception. Equipment and devices to aid in movement (canes, walkers, wheelchairs, etc.) should always be of the least complex design to accomplish the goal and should be chosen on the basis of the individual patient's cognitive and physical level of function.

In developing appropriate exercises and activities for a patient, the physical therapist should consider factors such as the joint ROM, muscle tone, motor control, and cognitive functions of the patient. Even the confused and agitated patient may respond to simple, familiar functional activities such as washing the face and brushing the teeth. Patients with higher cognitive function should be encouraged to carry out hygiene, grooming, dressing, and feeding activities.

6. Surgical management of residual musculoskeletal problems—After neurologic recovery stabilizes, surgical procedures may be indicated to correct residual limb deformities and to excise heterotopic ossification.

a. Correction of limb deformities in the lower extremities—In functional lower limbs, surgery is most often directed at correcting the equinovarus deformity of the foot (see Figure 13–12). The procedures needed for correction of the deformity are determined by clinical evaluation combined with laboratory assessment using dynamic polyelectromyography (poly-EMG). Commonly several procedures are done simultaneously: lengthening of the Achilles tendon (see Figure 13–16), release of the flexor digitorum longus, flexor hallucis longus and flexor brevis tendons (see Figure 13–17), a split anterior tibial tendon transfer (see Figure 13–18), and transfer of the flexor digitorum longus tendon to the heel. The object of surgery is to provide a plantigrade foot for standing and walking, and the surgery is highly successful in this goal. Seventy percent of patients are able to ambulate without a brace after surgery.

A stiff-knee gait is a common deformity that causes the patient to hike the pelvis and circumduct the leg for clearance of the foot during the swing phase of walking. Inappropriate activity in the quadriceps muscle at this time prevents knee flexion. If the vasti muscles of the quadriceps muscle are firing out of phase, the affected head or heads can be lengthened surgically (see Figure 13–14) to allow knee flexion while retaining quadriceps function. Transfer of the rectus femoris muscle to the sartorius or gracilis muscle provides active knee flexion during swing.

In nonfunctional lower limbs, surgery commonly consists of releasing contractures of the hips and knees.

b. Correction of limb deformities in the upper extremities—In functional upper limbs, surgery is frequently needed to correct problems of the wrist, fingers, and thumbs. If active hand opening is restricted by flexor spasticity, lengthening of the extrinsic finger flexors (Figure 13–23) weakens the overactive flexors and improves hand function while preserving the ability of the patient to grasp objects. In cases in which spastic thenar muscles cause thumb-in-palm deformity, a procedure consisting of proximal release of the thenar muscles (Figure 13–24) corrects the problem while preserving function of the thumb. In some patients, adequate placement of the hand for functional activities is impaired by elbow spasticity, although triceps function is generally normal. In these patients, lengthening the elbow flexors (Figure 13–25) enhances the ability to extend the elbow smoothly while preserving active flexion.

In nonfunctional upper limbs, common procedures consist of releasing various contractures and performing neurectomies to eliminate muscle spasticity. The problems of shoulder contracture, elbow contracture, and clenched-fist deformity are discussed in the section on

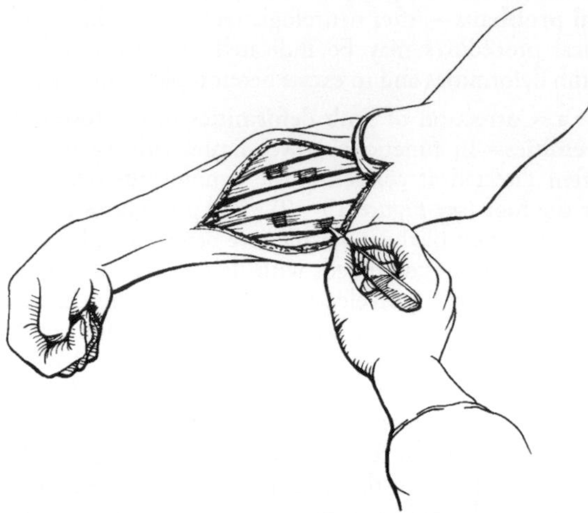

Figure 13–23. **Lengthening of the extrinsic finger flexors to correct the problem of flexor spasticity and improve hand function while preserving the ability to grasp objects.** (Illustration by Anthony C. Berlet. Reproduced, with permission, from Keenan MAE et al: *Manual of Orthopaedic Surgery for Spasticity.* Raven, 1993.)

stroke (see previous discussion), and the surgical procedures used in their treatment are shown in Figures 13–20, 13–21, and 13–22.

c. **Excision of heterotopic ossification**—Surgical measures for treatment of this problem are discussed later in this chapter.

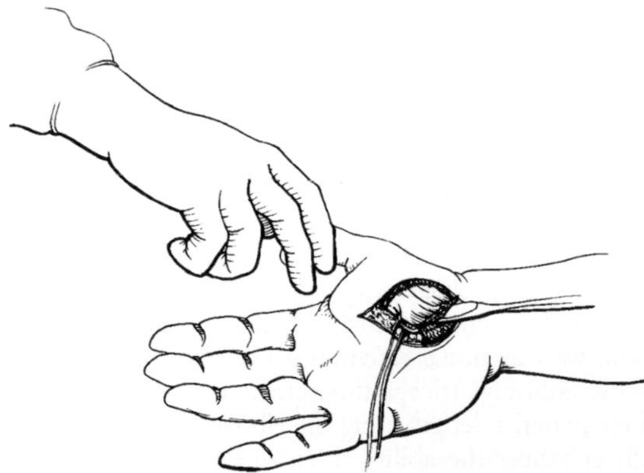

Figure 13–24. **Proximal release of the thenar muscles to correct a thumb-in-palm deformity while preserving function of the thumb.** (Illustration by Anthony C. Berlet. Reproduced, with permission, from Keenan MAE et al: *Manual of Orthopaedic Surgery for Spasticity.* Raven, 1993.)

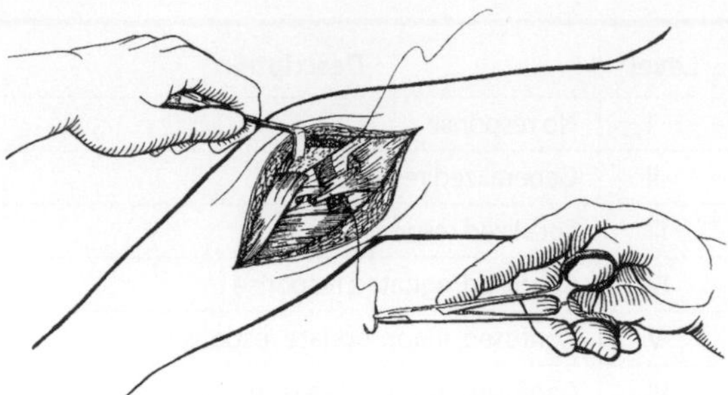

Figure 13–25. **Lengthening of the elbow flexors to correct flexor spasticity and improve movement of the elbow.** (Illustration by Anthony C. Berlet. Reproduced, with permission, from Keenan MAE et al: *Manual of Orthopaedic Surgery for Spasticity.* Raven, 1993.)

d. **Occupational therapy and social services**—Before patients are released from the hospital or rehabilitation facility, both they and their families must be informed about social service agencies, support groups, and special programs that can be of help. Social adjustment and the resumption of occupational pursuits and leisure activities depend on the recovery of mental factors first, personality status second, and physical factors third. Physical factors are more responsive to rehabilitation than are mental, personality, or social factors. Mental impairment, however, interferes the most with independence in ADLs.

7. **Inpatient rehabilitation**—Changes in the rules governing inpatient rehabilitation hospitals and units, particularly the implementation of the new prospective payment system for inpatient rehabilitation facilities by the Centers for Medicare & Medicaid Services (CMS), complicate the admission of patients with rehabilitation goals to an inpatient setting.

Physicians generally agree on the circumstances that justify a medical or surgical patient's hospitalization. In addition, in some cases an admission to a rehabilitation hospital or to the rehabilitation service of a short-term hospital can be justified on essentially the same medical or surgical grounds. In other cases, however, a patient's medical or surgical needs alone may not warrant inpatient hospital care, but hospitalization may nevertheless be necessary because of the patient's need for rehabilitative services.

Patients needing rehabilitative services require a hospital level of care if they need a relatively intense rehabilitation program that requires a multidisciplinary coordinated team approach to upgrade their ability to function (eg, patients with traumatic brain injury or SCI after corrective extremity surgery). Two basic requirements must be met for inpatient hospital stays for rehabilitation care to be covered:

1. The services must be reasonable and necessary (in terms of efficacy, duration, frequency, and amount) for the treatment of the patient's condition; and
2. It must be reasonable and necessary to furnish the care on an inpatient hospital basis, rather than in a less intensive facility such as a skilled nursing facility (SNF), or on an outpatient basis.

To meet the requirements just cited, the following basic components must be met:

1. Close medical supervision by a physician with specialized training or experience in rehabilitation;
2. The patient requires the 24-hour availability of a registered nurse with specialized training or experience in rehabilitation;
3. The general threshold for establishing the need for inpatient hospital rehabilitation services is that the patient must require and receive at least 3 hours a day of physical and/or occupational therapy; and
4. A multidisciplinary team (usually includes at minimum a physician, rehabilitation nurse, and one therapist).

Banovac K, Sherman AL, Estores IM et al: Prevention and treatment of heterotopic ossification after spinal cord injury. J Spinal Cord Med 2004;27(4):376. [PMID: 15484668]

Botte MJ, Bruffey JD, Copp SN et al: Surgical reconstruction of acquired spastic foot and ankle deformity. Foot Ankle Clin 2000;5(2):381. [PMID: 11232236]

Dahners LE, Mullis BH: Effects of nonsteroidal anti-inflammatory drugs on bone formation and soft-tissue healing. J Am Acad Orthop Surg 2004;12(3):139. [PMID: 15161166]

Esquenazi A et al: Dynamic polyelectromyography, neurolysis, and chemodenervation with botulinum toxin A for assessment and treatment of gait dysfunction. Adv Neurol 2001;87:321. [PMID: 11347237]

Gardner MJ, Ong BC, Liporace F et al: Orthopedic issues after cerebrovascular accident. Am J Orthop 2002;31(10):559. [PMID: 12405561]

van Kuijk AA, Geurts AC, van Kuppevelt HJ: Neurogenic heterotopic ossification in spinal cord injury. Spinal Cord 2002; 40(7):313. [PMID: 12080459]

HETEROTOPIC OSSIFICATION

Heterotopic ossification is commonly detected 2 months after traumatic brain injury or SCI and is characterized by increasing pain and decreasing ROM about a joint. The problem affects adults but is virtually unheard of in children. Although the cause of heterotopic ossification is unknown, a genetic predisposition is suspected. Unidentified humoral factors that enhance osteogenesis are demonstrated in the sera of patients with brain injury. Other contributing factors include soft-tissue trauma and spasticity.

Clinical Findings

Clinically significant heterotopic ossification is seen in 20% of adults with traumatic brain injuries or spinal cord injuries and may affect one joint or multiple joints. The overall rate of joint ankylosis is 16%. In affected patients, the bone forms in association with spastic muscles, and the alkaline phosphatase level is elevated. Bone scans may aid in early diagnosis, and the diagnosis is most commonly confirmed by radiographs.

In 27% of patients with heterotopic ossification, shoulder involvement is found inferomedial to the glenohumeral joint. Although ankylosis of the joint in these cases is unusual, motion may be sufficiently restricted to require surgical resection. Elbow involvement is seen in 26% of patients with heterotopic ossification and in 89% of those who suffered a fracture or dislocation about the elbow. When ossification forms posterior to the elbow joint, pressure neuritis of the ulnar nerve is common. Anterior transposition of the ulnar nerve is frequently required to prevent entrapment, and this procedure also facilitates later bone resection. Joint ankylosis is a common complication in patients with elbow involvement. Hip involvement is seen in 44% of patients who form ectopic bone. Bilateral hip involvement and joint ankylosis are common in these patients. Heterotopic ossification in the knee joint is less common but significantly impedes both flexion and extension of the joint.

Management

A. Early Measures

Aggressive treatment of spasticity is necessary because this problem appears to play an etiologic role in mechanically stimulating bone formation. To eliminate spasticity in the muscle groups adjacent to the bone formation, phenol blocks are administered. To prevent the deposition of calcium crystals in the collagen matrix of the periarticular connective tissue, etidronate disodium (Didronel) is used. When the heterotopic bone is detected very early, the use of intravenous etidronate sodium, 300 mg for 3 days, followed by oral therapy is very effective. The recommended dosage is 20 mg/kg/day orally in a single dose, and the drug should be taken on an empty stomach for proper absorption. Antiinflammatory medications are also used to control the intense inflammatory reaction that occurs during the formation of heterotopic bone. The most commonly documented medication is indomethacin, 75–150 mg daily, but in theory, other medications are equally effective. Physical therapy is aimed at providing gentle ROM to the joint to prevent ankylosis. Forceful joint manipulation is not advised because it can cause fractures or soft-tissue damage with contracture formation.

B. DEFINITIVE TREATMENT

Surgical excision is the definitive treatment for heterotopic ossification. To prevent recurrence of the problem, excision should be delayed until the heterotopic bone is fully mature. A true bone cortex should be visible radiographically. The serum alkaline phosphatase level does not need to be normal. If the patient has voluntary motion about the joint, surgical excision predictably results in an increased ROM. Following surgery, a single dose of radiation therapy (800 rads) and oral etidronate therapy for 6 weeks is used to prevent recurrence. Physical therapy is continued after surgery.

Banovac K, Sherman AL, Estores IM et al: Prevention and treatment of heterotopic ossification after spinal cord injury. J Spinal Cord Med 2004;27(4):376. [PMID: 15484668]

Burd TA et al: Indomethacin compared with localized irradiation for the prevention of heterotopic ossification following surgical treatment of acetabular fractures. J Bone Joint Surg Am 2001;83-A:1783. [PMID: 11741055]

Dahners LE, Mullis BH: Effects of nonsteroidal anti-inflammatory drugs on bone formation and soft-tissue healing. J Am Acad Orthop Surg 2004;12(3):139. [PMID: 15161166]

Kaplan FS, Glaser DL, Hebela N et al: Heterotopic ossification. J Am Acad Orthop Surg 2004;12(2):116. [PMID: 15089085]

van Kuijk AA, Geurts AC, van Kuppevelt HJ: Neurogenic heterotopic ossification in spinal cord injury. Spinal Cord 2002; 40(7):313. [PMID: 12080459]

Viola RW, Hastings H II: Treatment of ectopic ossification about the elbow. Clin Orthop 2000;(370):65. [PMID: 10660703]

RHEUMATOID ARTHRITIS

Rheumatoid arthritis (RA) is a systemic disease that affects connective tissue and results in chronic inflammatory synovitis. The cause of the disease remains unknown. An infectious agent, perhaps viral, is suspected to be the initiating factor. A genetic predisposition may also be a factor.

Immune mechanisms are involved, as evidenced by the presence of large numbers of lymphocytes in the synovial tissue and by the presence of rheumatoid factor (IgM antibodies) in the serum and synovial fluid of 80% of patients. The antigen-antibody reactions activate the complement system and attract neutrophils to the joint fluid. The immune complexes are then phagocytized, and lysosomal enzymes are released into the synovial fluid. These enzymes and the inflammatory synovial pannus are in part responsible for the destruction of articular cartilage and periarticular structures. Tendons are also directly invaded by the inflammatory synovium and may attenuate and rupture. Ligaments and joint capsules become weakened by the chronic inflammatory process and may become stretched by repeated joint effusions (Figure 13–26).

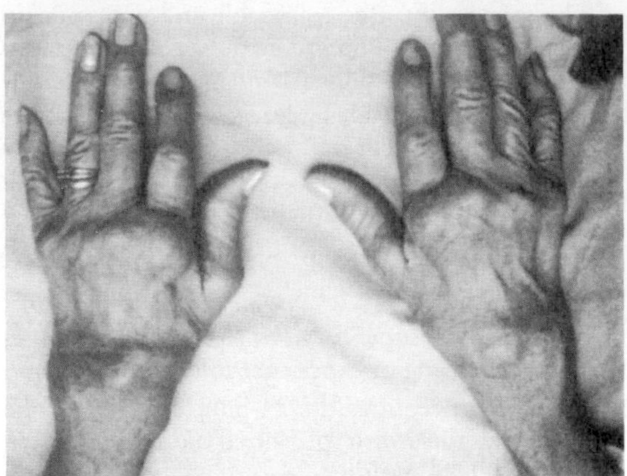

Figure 13–26. Chronic synovitis of the joints and extensor tendons in a patient with rheumatoid arthritis.

The erosion of articular cartilage is greatly enhanced by the superimposition of mechanical derangements on a joint weakened by chronic inflammation and enzymatic deterioration. Osteoporosis results from the hyperemia of inflammation. Disuse of limbs secondary to pain, weakened muscle action, and mechanical derangements enhances the osteoporosis.

Clinical Findings

RA affects synovial joints, bones, muscles, fasciae, ligaments, and tendons. Because it is a systemic disease, it can also affect internal organs. The diagnosis is made primarily on clinical grounds and supported by radiographic and laboratory data (Table 13–5). RA is two or three times more common in women than men. The disease is seen in some children but has increasing prevalence with increasing age up to the seventh decade. Rheumatic complaints are responsible for the largest share of chronic disability in the United States.

The clinical course of RA is variable with respect to the extent and intensity of the disease. The time course of the disease, measured in months and years, is progressive. Several factors affect the course of disease and are associated with a poor prognosis. These factors include insidious onset, symmetric disease, presence of rheumatoid factor in the serum, and presence of rheumatoid nodules, which occur in patients with rheumatoid factor. In patients under 40 years of age, with RA, females have a worse prognosis than males. Eosinophilia of 5% or greater is associated with an increased incidence of vasculitis, pleuropericarditis, pulmonary fibrosis, and subcutaneous nodules.

The multisystem nature of RA and its variable clinical pattern make it difficult to devise a precise system for describing the overall functional ability of the patient. The most commonly employed scale is the functional classification devised by the American Rheumatism Association (Table 13–6).

Table 13–5. American Rheumatism Association criteria for diagnosing and categorizing rheumatoid arthritis.

Category	Description
Classic rheumatoid arthritis	Presence of 7 of the following findings: (1) morning stiffness,[a] (2) pain on motion of 1 joint[a] (3) swelling of 1 joint[a] (4) swelling of an additional joint[a] (5) symmetric swelling of joints, (6) presence of subcutaneous nodules, (7) presence of rheumatoid factor in the serum, (8) poor results in the mucin clot test of synovial fluid, (9) characteristic roentgenographic changes, (10) characteristic histopathologic findings in the synovial fluid, and (11) characteristic histopathologic findings in nodule biopsies.
Definite rheumatoid arthritis	Presence of 5 of the above findings.
Probable rheumatoid arthritis	Presence of 3 of the above findings.

[a]Finding must be present for at least 6 weeks.

Management

A. The Team Approach to Patient Care and Treatment

Optimal management requires an interdisciplinary team approach involving many specialists, including a liaison nurse, rheumatologist, orthopedic surgeon, physical therapist, occupational therapist, psychologist, and social worker. The patient and members of his or her family are also important members of the team. Because the disease is an ongoing and progressive process, the goal of management is to prevent deformities and maintain function for the patient over a lifetime.

1. Nursing care and patient education—The liaison nurse functions as the coordinator of the team. The nurse provides the critical link between the inpatient medical and surgical management of the disease and the continuation of treatment in the outpatient environment.

Much of the responsibility for patient education in the daily care of the disease rests with the nurse, who explains the techniques for protecting joints; advises patients about the need to perform exercises for maintaining joint ROM and optimizing failing muscle strength; cautions patients that exercising too vigorously can damage weakened joints and ligaments; and reminds patients that because the disease tends to decrease their physical activity, they will need regular periods of rest during the day and good nutrition to maximize their general health and to prevent obesity.

2. Medical and surgical management—The rheumatologist is commonly the team leader and in charge of medical management, which is directed toward the control of synovitis, the relief of pain, and the prevention or treatment of other organ involvement by the disease. The medications used for treatment include aspirin, nonsteroidal antiinflammatory drugs (NSAIDs), corticosteroids, immunosuppressive drugs, and suppressive agents. A local injection of corticosteroids can be useful in controlling an acute inflammatory process in a specific joint. Corticosteroids can also be used systemically but are generally avoided because of undesirable side effects. Agents that produce suppression or remission of arthritis inclumde gold salts, antimalarial drugs, and penicillamine. Immunosuppressive drugs or total lymphoid irradiation can also be used to suppress immune reactions. The most important measure to treat RA successfully is the use of disease-modifying antirheumatic drug (DMARDs), which can retard or prevent disease progression and, thus, joint destruction and subsequent loss of function. Until the full action of DMARDs takes effect, antiinflammatory or analgesic medications may be required as bridging therapy to reduce pain and swelling. DMARDs can be classified into xenobiotic and biologic agents. Methotrexate (MTX) and sulfasalazine (SSZ) are the most active xenobiotic compounds in terms of frequency of remissions and time to onset of action and provide the best risk-benefit ratios. MTX alone or in combination with other agents is now the standard of care for moderate-to-severe RA.

Table 13–6. American Rheumatism Association classification of function in patients with rheumatoid arthritis.

Class	Description
I	Complete function; able to perform usual duties without handicap.
II	Adequate function for normal activities, despite handicap of pain or limited range of motion in one or more joints.
III	Limited function; able to perform few or none of the duties of usual occupation or self-care.
IV	Largely or wholly incapacitated; bedridden or confined to a wheelchair; able to perform little or no self-care.

The recognition of TNF-α and IL-1 as central proinflammatory cytokines led to the development of biologic agents that block these cytokines or their effects. The first such biologics were the TNF blockers etanercept and infliximab. These agents are expensive. Consensus statements do not recommend their use until at least one xenobiotic DMARD, usually MTX, was administered without sufficient success. A new addition to the biologics is anakinra (interleukin-1 receptor antagonist [IL-1RA]). IL-1RA occupies the IL-1 receptor without triggering it and prevents receptor binding of IL-1.

The orthopedic surgeon should be involved early in the course of the patient's disease and not merely be called on when medical management fails to be effective. A knowledge of biomechanics, gait dynamics, and energy requirements can be useful in preserving function for the patient. The orthopedist can often recommend orthotic supports, walking aids, and shoe wear that minimize unwanted stress on joints and maximize strength.

In selected situations, early surgical intervention may prevent excessive deterioration of joint structure and function. Synovectomy is effective in preventing tendon rupture in the hand, whereas arthroscopic synovectomy of the knee and shoulder show promise for preventing joint destruction. Fusion of an unstable cervical spine can prevent the disastrous effect of a SCI.

Most surgical procedures are reconstructive. Because relief of pain is the most consistent result of reconstructive surgery, pain is the primary indication for surgery. Restoration of motion and function and the correction of deformity are additional indications for surgical intervention but are more difficult goals to achieve. Preoperative assessment is a painstaking process. In addition to performing a physical examination and reviewing radiographic findings, the surgeon must attempt to elicit sufficient information from the patient, family, and therapists to ascertain which deformities are causing the greatest functional losses. The patient can only tolerate a finite number of surgical procedures, and these must be carefully staged to obtain the maximal result.

For further discussion of medical and surgical treatment, see the section Management Approaches Based on the Area of Disease Involvement.

3. Physical therapy—The physical therapist uses modalities such as heat and ultrasound to decrease joint stiffness and relieve pain. An exercise program is essential for preserving the functional abilities of the patient. The exercise should gently put all joints through their full arc of motion to maintain this range.

Patients with joint effusions and synovitis automatically assume positions that minimize intraarticular pressure and therefore minimize pain. These positions are usually not optimal for function and can result in flexion deformities. An abnormal position may be reversible if discovered early. Daily joint ROM exercises are central to preventing unwanted contractures.

Muscles weakened by the concomitant myopathy need strengthening but are susceptible to damage from overuse or from an excessively vigorous exercise program. Orthotics may be indicated to support weakened ligaments and provide a means of joint protection and support for functional activities such as walking. Upper extremity walking aids may be useful to give the patients additional support. These aids often require modification to meet the specific needs of the individual. Forearm troughs allow the patient to use the entire arm for support when the hands and wrists are weak or deformed. They are also useful for protecting the hands from excessive stress. A rolling walker, which does not require the patient to lift the walker for advancement, may be useful in patients with limited strength.

4. Occupational therapy—The occupational therapist evaluates and instructs the patient in modified techniques for performing ADLs, such as grooming, dressing, and meal preparation. Because of the weakness and deformities imposed by the arthritis, adaptive equipment and alternative methods are commonly needed. Modifications in clothing, such as larger fasteners for ease of manipulation, Velcro strips at seams or on shoes, and front openings, can all facilitate dressing. Upper extremity splints can be used to provide joint protection and stabilization and to prevent further deformity from occurring. The splints must be lightweight and easily donned by the patient.

5. Psychological counseling—It is not uncommon for patients or their family members to have feelings of anxiety, denial, anger, or depression. The psychologist provides assistance in dealing with these feelings and coping with alterations in lifestyle and self-image. Comprehensive care involves an understanding of how patients respond to weakness, fatigue, altered physical appearance, progressive disability, diminished independence, and the financial burdens of chronic illness. Coping skills are needed to deal with these problems as well as with pain, which becomes an everyday occurrence and may interfere with both intellectual and emotional functioning.

6. Social services—A variety of modifications in lifestyle accompany chronic illness with RA. Occupational changes may be necessary, or the patient may no longer be able to work at all. Additional assistance may be needed in the home for housework and the preparation of meals. In more advanced stages, the patient may require help for personal care. Transportation needs become more complex, and the patient finds it increasingly difficult to leave the home. The social worker becomes an invaluable team member in helping families with the numerous practical arrangements required for everyday existence and for locating financial aid to help defray the mounting costs.

B. Management Approaches Based on the Area of Disease Involvement

Orthopedic surgery is frequently necessary for patients with RA affecting the cervical spine or extremities.

1. Cervical spine—Depending on the study and diagnostic criteria, involvement of the cervical spine is found in anywhere from 6.4% to 90% of patients with RA. Three forms of cervical spine involvement are seen.

The first and most common form is atlantoaxial instability (Figure 13–27), which results from erosion of the transverse and alar ligaments. These ligaments normally function to maintain the odontoid process of the axis within the anterior third of the atlas ring, where the two bones articulate with each other. Disruption of the transverse and alar ligaments results in excessive motion between C1 and C2. Forward flexion of the head causes anterior subluxation of the atlas on the axis and possible impingement of the spinal cord or occlusion of the vertebral arteries. This is best seen in lateral flexion and extension radiographs of the cervical spine.

The second form of cervical spine involvement is subaxial instability (Figure 13–28), which may lead to subluxation of two or more cervical vertebrae below the level of C2. If subluxation is severe or its appearance is sudden, it can exert sufficient pressure on the spinal cord to cause permanent quadriparesis. If subluxation occurs slowly over a long time, however, as commonly happens, the spinal cord is able to adapt to the pressure, so that a severe degree of deformity occurs before clinical symptoms appear.

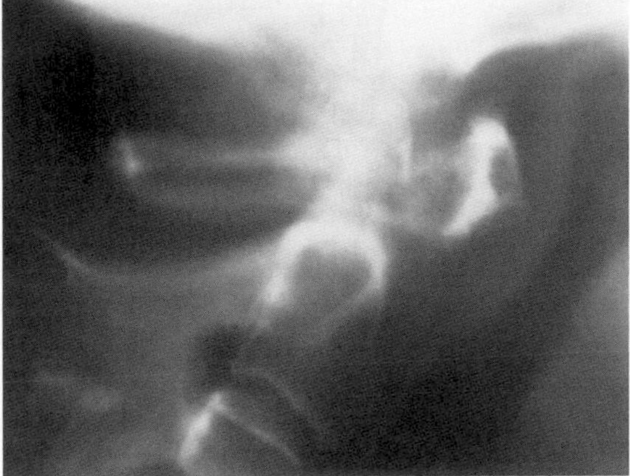

Figure 13–27. Tomogram of the upper cervical spine, showing atlantoaxial instability in a patient with rheumatoid arthritis.

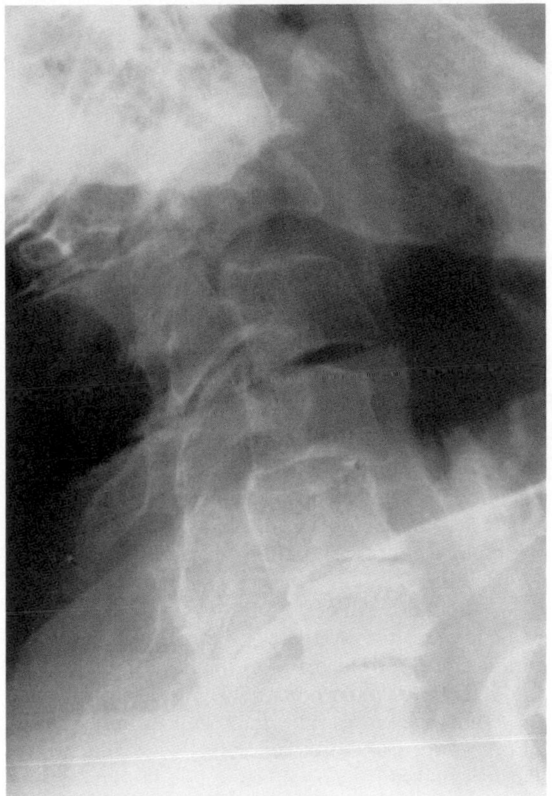

Figure 13–28. Radiograph of the cervical spine, showing multiple levels of subaxial instability in a patient with rheumatoid arthritis.

The third and least common form of cervical spine involvement is superior migration of the odontoid process of C2 resulting from severe degrees of bone erosion. This form of involvement is reported in from 3.8% to 15% of patients with RA. As the dens migrates proximally, radiographic detail is lost because of the overlapping of bony structures. CT scanning is most useful in elucidating the exact nature of the involvement and can show rotational instability caused by asymmetric bone erosions (Figure 13–29).

Orthotic supports are useful in controlling the patient's symptoms. Posterior cervical fusion is indicated when the spinal cord is at risk of damage. The most common level of fusion is C1 to C2, supplemented by wire fixation. If the subluxation is irreducible or if severe osteoporosis is present, fusion to the occiput may be necessary. Occasionally, it is useful to supplement the bone graft with polymethyl methacrylate fixation.

In patients with severe erosive disease of the cervical spine and proximal migration of the odontoid

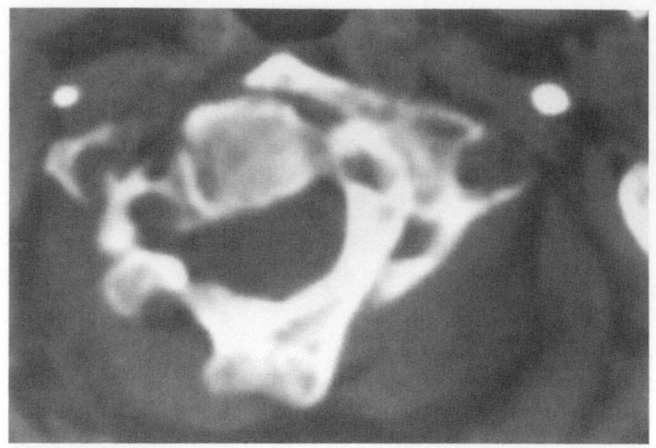

Figure 13–29. CT scan showing rotational instability of C1 on C2 in a patient with advanced psoriatic arthritis.

process, a rotational deviation of the larynx may occur, making intubation impossible except with the use of a flexible fiber optic scope (Figure 13–30). Because cervical spine disease often presents difficulties in endotracheal intubation at the time of surgery, the stability of the cervical spine should be assessed preoperatively in all patients with RA. Lateral flexion-extension radiographs taken within 1 year of surgery are sufficient to detect significant instability problems. Use of the flexible fiber optic bronchoscope for such problems is valuable. Among the indications for fiber optic intubation in patients with arthritis are an unstable cervical spine on flexion and extension; limited mobility of the cervical spine; and impaired motion of the temporomandibular joints, with or without associated micrognathia.

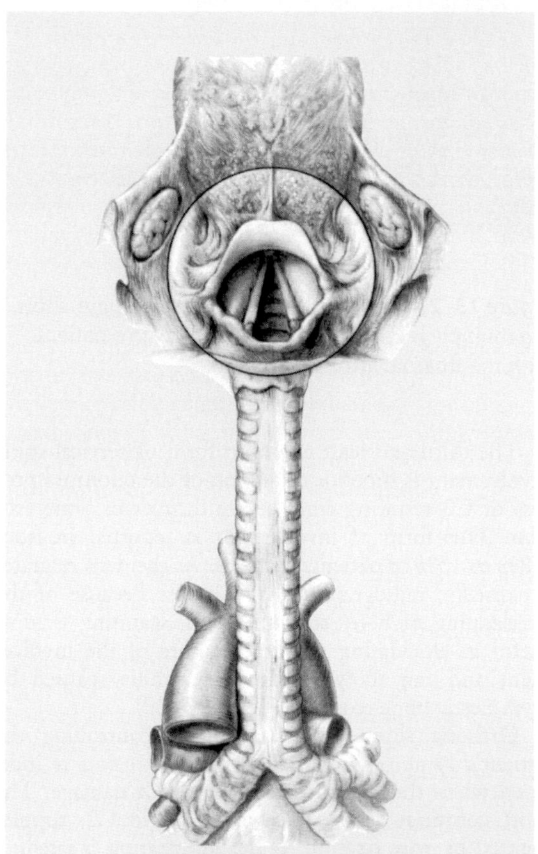

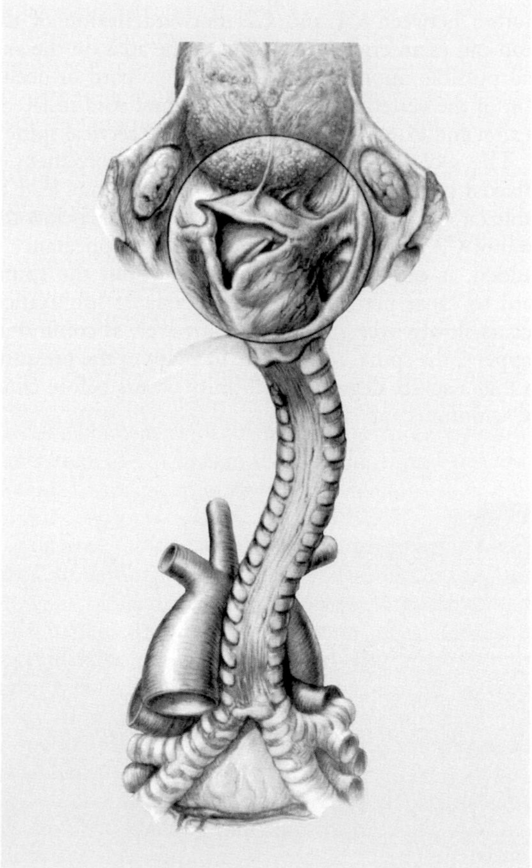

Figure 13–30. *Left*: Diagram showing the normal relationship of the trachea and larynx. The insert shows the view seen through the fiber optic bronchoscope. *Right*: Diagram showing the triple-plane rotational deviation of the larynx noted secondary to cervical spine disease in inflammatory arthritis. (Illustrations by Ted Bloodhart. Reproduced, with permission, from Keenan MA et al: Acquired laryngeal deviation associated with cervical spine disease in erosive polyarticular arthritis. Anesthesiology 1983;58:441.)

2. Lower extremities

a. Hips—Total joint replacement has vastly improved the quality of life for patients with RA. Special problems exist in this group of patients, however, and must be considered before total hip arthroplasty is performed. Because osteoporosis is pronounced, fracture can occur easily during surgery. Protrusio acetabuli, another common problem, may require bone grafting. The risk of infection is increased in this population, and wound healing may also be delayed, especially if the patient has been taking systemic corticosteroids. In patients under the 60 years, excess femoral anteversion may be present and distort the anatomy. Moreover, the small size of the bone may require a special prosthesis. Despite these problems, total joint arthroplasty remains the treatment of choice for the arthritic hip.

b. Knees—Knee pain is common and may be the result of a valgus deformity of the hindfoot, which places excessive stress on the knee proximally. Mild medial knee pain can be relieved with the use of an AFO to correct the valgus deformity. Knee pain may also be caused by the presence of a joint effusion, which increases the intraarticular pressure and thereby increases the pain. When patients attempt to minimize pain by placing the knee in 30 degrees of flexion, this encourages the formation of flexion contractures.

Arthroscopic evaluation of the rheumatoid knee demonstrates the importance of the meniscus in the degeneration of the knee. The synovium directly invades the body of the meniscus and tears it. The mechanical derangement resulting from the torn meniscus then causes rapid deterioration of the articular surfaces, which were rendered abnormal by the action of enzymes. Synovectomy of the joint line and partial meniscectomy are easily accomplished under arthroscopic control and may have a role in preventing articular damage in the rheumatoid knee.

Total knee arthroplasty is effective in restoring knee alignment and motion and relieving pain. When a valgus deformity is present, serial releases of the soft tissue should be performed to realign the limb prior to cutting the bone for insertion of the prosthetic components. The lateral retinaculum, popliteal tendon, proximal iliotibial band, posterolateral capsule, and lateral collateral ligament can be released in this sequence to provide soft-tissue balance. A flexion deformity is corrected at the time of arthroplasty by releasing the posterior capsule from the femur or by removing additional bone from the distal femur in severe cases.

c. Feet—Forefoot involvement is common in RA. Clawtoe deformities with plantar subluxation of the metatarsal heads result in painful callosities on the plantar surface of the forefoot. These problems are usually accompanied by a hallux valgus deformity. Skin ulcerations may form over bony prominences. Forefoot pain prevents the patient from transferring body weight over the foot during terminal stance, which results in an awkward gait with a shortened step length. Extra-depth shoes with wide toe boxes and molded pressure-relieving inserts may be sufficient to relieve pain and improve gait. When the deformities are marked, resection of the metatarsal heads in conjunction with arthroplasty or fusion of the metatarsophalangeal joint of the great toe is indicated.

Hindfoot involvement is also common and results in a planovalgus or pronation deformity. A longitudinal arch support or similar shoe insert is not sufficient to hold the hindfoot in alignment. When the deformity is supple, an AFO with a well-molded arch support can control the position of the heel and subtalar joint during gait. This also reduces the valgus thrust on the knee joint. If the deformity is fixed, a triple arthrodesis aligns the hindfoot.

3. Upper extremities

a. Shoulders—In patients with RA, shoulder involvement is common but is generally insidious in onset or episodic in nature. Because the pain is not constant early in the course of the disease, shoulder involvement is often not appreciated until a significant amount of destruction occurs. The shoulders must be examined regularly to detect early loss of motion and function.

Arthroscopy provides a useful tool in examining the shoulder and assessing the integrity of the glenoid labrum, rotator cuff, and biceps tendon. Arthroscopy can also be used to perform synovectomy of the shoulder joint.

Normally, the glenohumeral joint has more motion than any other joint. This motion is rotation, and it is facilitated by the shallow shape of the glenoid labrum. The rotator cuff muscles, which are central to the normal functioning of the shoulder, provide stability to the humeral head and also provide rotation. If the rotator cuff ruptures, the humeral head rides upward and is subjected to abnormal muscle forces as the patient attempts to compensate for the loss of motion. This results in the rapid deterioration of the glenohumeral joint. Normally, the anterior portion of the deltoid muscle provides forward elevation of the humerus. This is the position of function and the most common arc of motion for activities involving the upper extremity. The tendon of the long head of the biceps muscle serves to stabilize the humeral head against riding upward and also to reduce subacromial impingement. Whenever surgery of the shoulder is performed, it is important to preserve the deltoid muscle fibers and their attachments as well as the intraarticular portion of the biceps tendon.

The subacromial bursa is often involved with the inflammatory response of RA and may become thickened. The inflammatory process may cause a decrease in nutrition of the rotator cuff tendons and lead to attrition of the tendons with or without rupture of the rotator cuff. Subacromial bursitis can be treated by local injection of a corticosteroid preparation. When the inflammation subsided, the patient is begun on a program of gentle ROM exercises.

Repair of a ruptured rotator cuff is often possible and should be performed. If the rupture is detected early, excessive damage to the glenohumeral joint can be avoided. If extensive joint damage is already present, repair or reconstruction of the rotator cuff is done at the time of prosthetic arthroplasty of the glenohumeral joint. Preoperative radiographic evaluation should include axillary radiographs to assess the glenoid alignment. The glenoid labrum is often eroded asymmetrically, and the prosthetic component must be accurately aligned to ensure optimal function and to minimize the abnormal forces that might lead to prosthetic loosening. In patients with total shoulder replacement, pain is effectively alleviated. Shoulder function depends on the integrity of the soft tissues and on muscle function. Resurfacing of the glenoid should be reserved for those patients with an intact rotator cuff. If the rotator cuff is destroyed, humeral hemiarthroplasty is the preferred surgical treatment. A careful postoperative therapy program is essential for maximizing shoulder function.

b. Elbows—The elbow joint consists of three separate articulations: radiocapitellar, ulnotrochlear, and radioulnar. These articulations allow the hand to rotate 180 degrees around the longitudinal axis of the forearm. The function of the hand depends on being placed in space as necessary for use. The elbow is the most important joint for positioning the hand. Unlike the shoulder or wrist, if the elbow is fused, the functional loss is great. The goal of treatment is to maintain a painless arc of motion.

Olecranon bursitis is common in patients with RA. The usual treatment consists of aspirating the bursa and injecting a corticosteroid preparation. Rarely, chronic bursitis develops and requires surgical excision of the bursa.

Subcutaneous rheumatoid nodules are common along the extensor surface of the ulna. The nodules are often sensitive to pressure when the arm is resting on any surface, and they may interfere with the use of forearm troughs on walking aids. If they are bothersome, the nodules should be excised surgically. The patient should be advised, however, that nodules can recur.

Radiocapitellar arthritis is often the predominant feature of elbow involvement and can cause marked pain and a decrease in motion. The pain is most pronounced with pronation and supination of the forearm.

When the joint destruction is severe, prosthetic arthroplasty is indicated. Elbow prostheses fall into two basic categories: semiconstrained and unconstrained. An unconstrained design is less likely to loosen. The shoulder should be evaluated carefully prior to prosthetic elbow arthroplasty. A patient with limited shoulder motion exerts greater forces on the elbow in an effort to compensate for the decrease in shoulder function.

c. Wrists and hands—In patients with RA, evaluating the wrist and hand deformities and developing a rational treatment plan can be a complex task for the surgeon. Many joints, tendons, and ligaments are involved in a linked system of structure and function. Treatment can be divided into three categories: nonsurgical treatment, preventive surgery, and reconstructive or salvage surgery. Nonoperative treatment consists of resting inflamed joints; exercising joints for short periods of time but frequently and gently to maintain motion; using resting or dynamic splints to alleviate pain and prevent deformity; and judiciously using local corticosteroid injections for control of synovitis.

(1) Tendons—Dorsal tenosynovitis is common. It is of significance because it often results in rupture of the extensor tendons either from attrition or from direct invasion of the inflamed synovial tissue into the tendon substance. Tenosynovectomy should be performed in patients whose synovitis has persisted for 4–6 months despite medical treatment. Recurrence of the synovitis is rare following synovectomy, and the procedure prevents extensor tendon rupture.

Rupture of an extensor tendon can result from attenuation of the tendon caused by chronic inflammation, friction against abnormal bony surfaces, ischemia secondary to interference with the normal circulation to the tendon, or direct invasion of the tendon by synovium. The most common tendons to rupture, listed in order of frequency, are the extensors of the fifth finger, the extensors of the ring finger, and the long extensor of the thumb (the extensor pollicis longus). Surgical repair by tendon transfer is more successful when fewer tendons are involved. Therefore, prompt diagnosis and treatment are essential for a successful outcome. For a single tendon rupture in the fifth and ring fingers, a side-to-side repair using the adjacent extensor tendon is advised. The tendon of the index finger extensor can be transferred to repair a rupture of the thumb extensor tendon or a rupture of two finger tendons. For more complex ruptures, tendon transfer from the wrist extensors or from the superficial flexor muscles of the fingers may restore function.

Synovitis in the flexor tendon sheaths is characterized by crepitation that is palpable in the palm during finger flexion and extension. Triggering of the fingers may result from the inflamed synovial tissue catching on the flexor pulleys with motion. Carpal tunnel syndrome may also occur as a result of swelling within the carpal canal, which causes pressure on the median nerve. Early treatment consists of local corticosteroid injection to reduce the inflammation, application of a splint, and medical management of the underlying synovitis. Persistent synovitis may require carpal tunnel release and synovectomy. Rupture of the flexor tendons is rare.

(2) Wrist joints—The wrist joint is a frequent site of synovitis and may begin to show radial deviation and volar subluxation. The radioulnar joint is commonly inflamed and painful. Early treatment consists of splinting for support and medical control of the synovitis. Dorsal synovectomy of the extensor compartments is indicated when medications do not control the synovitis adequately. Dorsal synovectomy prevents rupture of the extensor tendons. Radial deviation of the carpus can be corrected by transfer of the extensor carpi radialis longus tendon to the extensor carpi ulnaris.

When the wrist becomes unstable, several choices of surgical treatment are available. If the deformity is mild, bone stock can be preserved and motion maintained by a limited carpal fusion. The lunate and scaphoid bones are fused to the distal radius to prevent further displacement of the carpus. The distal ulna can be fused to the distal radius to provide a platform to support the wrist. A segment of the ulna is removed just proximal to the fusion to allow for pronation and supination of the forearm. If the intercarpal joints are severely affected by the arthritis, the base of the capitate bone can be removed and a tendon spacer inserted to preserve motion at the intercarpal row.

Another option is to perform a prosthetic arthroplasty of the wrist. More bone stock is removed with this procedure, but revision is still possible in the event of fracture of the prosthesis. Several designs of total joint prosthesis are available for the wrist.

Fusion of the wrist joint provides a stable pain-free joint and remains a reasonable surgical choice for selected patients. Because fusion may interfere with personal hygiene tasks, it is advisable to avoid fusing both wrist joints.

(3) Metacarpophalangeal and carpometacarpal joints—Finger and wrist deformities commonly occur together in a collapsing zigzag pattern. The wrist deviates in a radial direction, and the fingers then drift ulnarward at the metacarpophalangeal joint level. When both deformities are present, the wrist must be realigned prior to correcting the finger deformities, or the ulnar deviation of the fingers recurs.

Ulnar deviation and volar subluxation of the fingers at the metacarpophalangeal joint level are common. With ulnar deviation, the extensor tendons move into the valleys between the metacarpal heads. This condition can be confused with extensor tendon rupture. If the joint surfaces are preserved, function can be improved by a synovectomy, soft-tissue release of the volar capsule, and realignment of the extensor tendons. If the joint surfaces are destroyed, then a total wrist arthroplasty can be considered. If the joints are unstable because of ligament loss, it may be necessary to reconstruct the radial collateral ligament using a portion of the volar plate to provide a stable pinch. Tightness of the intrinsic tendons commonly occurs in conjunction with the subluxation of the metacarpophalangeal joints. To correct this problem, a release of the intrinsic tendons is performed along with the arthroplasty. Dynamic splinting of the fingers, which maintains alignment while allowing motion, is used continuously for 6 weeks following surgery and then for an additional 6 weeks at night.

Flexion of the metacarpophalangeal joint with extension of the interphalangeal joint in the thumb is the equivalent of a boutonnière deformity. The reverse deformity can also be seen, with extension of the metacarpophalangeal joint and flexion of the interphalangeal joint. An adduction deformity of the metacarpal bone places increased stress on the metacarpophalangeal joint and produces lateral instability and hyperextension. Adduction of the thumb occurs when the carpometacarpal joint shifts radially. Derangements of the carpometacarpal joint can be treated by fusion or by arthroplasty. Interposition arthroplasty is desirable to maintain motion and can be performed using a Silastic spacer or soft tissue.

(4) Interphalangeal joints—Continued synovitis gradually attenuates the capsular and ligamentous structures and results in tendon imbalance. In the fingers, this will be seen as either a flexion or an extension deformity.

Flexion deformity results from rupture or attenuation of the central slip of the extensor mechanism, with gradual volar displacement of the lateral bands. As the lateral bands shift in the volar direction, a hyperextension deformity of the distal interphalangeal joint results. This flexion malalignment, called a **boutonnière,** or **buttonhole, deformity,** interferes with the ability to grasp large objects but does not usually impede the pinch function used for picking up small items. Interposition arthroplasty using a Silastic spacer gives unpredictable results. Fusion of the interphalangeal joints gives dependable results when the boutonnière deformity is fixed. In the index and long fingers, stability for pinch is required for good function and is more important than a large arc of motion. In the ring and small fingers, motion is more important for a functional grasp. When arthroplasty is considered, the ring and fifth fingers are usually selected.

Hyperextension deformities, or swan-neck deformities, can be either primary or secondary. Primary deformities are caused by stretching of the volar plate from synovitis or rupture of the flexor digitorum superficialis tendon. Secondary deformities are characterized by flexion of the metacarpophalangeal joints, with tightness of the intrinsic muscles proximally and presence of a mallet deformity distally. This hyperextension deformity interferes with picking up small objects but does not cause much difficulty with grasping larger objects. If the deformity is treated early and is secondary to intrinsic muscle tightness, a release of the intrinsic tendons corrects the imbalance. If the deformity is seen late and is rigid, joint fusion or arthroplasty is indicated.

Derangements of the distal interphalangeal joints are either mallet deformities secondary to rupture of the extensor tendon or lateral deformities from loss of capsular and ligamentous support. When the deformities interfere with function, fusion of the joint is indicated.

Abboud JA, Beredjiklian PK, Bozentka DJ: Metacarpophalangeal joint arthroplasty in rheumatoid arthritis. J Am Acad Orthop Surg 2003;11(3):184. [PMID: 12828448]

Belt EA et al: Outcome of ankle arthrodesis performed by dowel technique in patients with rheumatic disease. Foot Ankle Int 2001;22:666.

Berger RA et al: Long-term follow-up of the Miller-Galante total knee replacement. Clin Orthop 2001;388:56. [PMID: 11451133]

Chen AL, Joseph TN, Zuckerman JD: Rheumatoid arthritis of the shoulder. J Am Acad Orthop Surg 2003;11(1):12. [PMID: 12699368]

Dionne RA et al: Analgesia and COX-2 inhibition. Clin Exp Rheumatol 2001;19:S63. [PMID: 11695255]

Gordon P et al: A 10-year prospective followup of patients with rheumatoid arthritis 1986–96. J Rheumatol 2001;28:2409. [PMID: 11708411]

Johnstone BR: Proximal interphalangeal joint surface replacement arthroplasty. Hand Surg 2001;6:1. [PMID: 11677661]

Kauffman JI, Chen AL, Stuchin S et al: Surgical management of the rheumatoid elbow. J Am Acad Orthop Surg 2003;11(2): 100. [PMID: 12670136]

King JA, Tomaino MM: Surgical treatment of the rheumatoid thumb. Hand Clin 2001;17:275. [PMID: 11478050]

Nelissen RG: The impact of total joint replacement in rheumatoid arthritis. Best Pract Res Clin Rheumatol 2003;17(5):831. [PMID: 12915160]

Shen FH, Samartzis D, Jenis LG et al: Rheumatoid arthritis: Evaluation and surgical management of the cervical spine. Spine J 2004;4(6):689. [PMID: 15541704]

POLIOMYELITIS

Poliomyelitis is caused by an enterovirus that attacks the anterior horn cells of the spinal cord. Infection can lead to a variety of clinical findings, ranging from minor symptoms to paralysis. The last major epidemics in the United States occurred during the early 1950s. Because of effective immunization programs, acute poliomyelitis has now become rare in the United States and other developed nations of the world. Nevertheless, orthopedic surgeons today are frequently called on to treat patients with postpoliomyelitis syndrome.

Classification

Four stages of poliomyelitis are recognized.

A. Acute Poliomyelitis

All of the anterior horn cells are attacked during the acute stage, which accounts for the diffuse and severe paralysis seen with the initial infection. The anterior horn cells control the skeletal muscle cells of the trunk and limbs. Clinically, the infection is characterized by the sudden onset of paralysis and the presence of fever and acute muscle pain, often accompanied by stiff neck. Paralysis of the respiratory muscles is life-threatening in the acute stage. When the shoulder muscles are involved, respiratory compromise should be suspected because of the close proximity of the anterior horn cells controlling each in the spinal cord. Mechanical support of ventilation may be required.

A variable number of anterior horn cells survive the initial infection. The treatment in the acute stage of the disease consists of providing the needed respiratory support, decreasing muscle pain, and performing regular ROM exercises to prevent the formation of joint contractures.

B. Subacute Poliomyelitis

Anterior horn cell survival, axon sprouting, and muscle hypertrophy occur in the subacute phase and provide three mechanisms for regaining strength. An average of 47% (range of 12–94%) of the anterior horn cells in the spinal cord survive the initial attack. Because cell survival occurs in a random fashion, the distribution of paralysis is variable and depends on which anterior horn cells were destroyed. Each anterior horn cell innervates a group of muscle cells. When a group of muscle cells is orphaned, as it were, by the death of the anterior horn cell that supports it, a nearby nerve cell can sprout additional axons and adopt some of the orphaned cells. By means of this process, a motor unit (defined as a nerve cell and the muscle cells it innervates) can expand greatly. Moreover, muscle cells in the unit enlarge, and this hypertrophy provides additional strength for the patient.

C. Residual Poliomyelitis

It is only after 16–24 months following onset that the ultimate extent of poliomyelitis can be determined and procedures to restore lost function and provide structural stability can be instituted.

D. Postpoliomyelitis Syndrome

Patients who had acute poliomyelitis during childhood often complain of increased muscle weakness 30–40 years later. This weakness is not a result of infectious spread of the earlier disease but, rather, is caused by the overuse of muscles that were originally affected, whether or not they were known to have been affected at the onset of the disease. Studies show that a muscle must lose from 30% to 40% of its strength for weakness to be detected using manual muscle testing. Studies of gait also demonstrate that the ADLs require more muscle strength and stamina than were previously appreciated. The traditional program, which encouraged patients to work harder to regain strength and was based on the concept of "no pain, no gain," proved detrimental because it encouraged chronic overuse of muscles and resulted in further deterioration of function.

The diagnosis of postpoliomyelitis syndrome is based on a history of poliomyelitis; a pattern of increased muscle weakness that is random and does not follow any nerve root or peripheral nerve distribution; and the presence of additional symptoms such as muscle pain, severe fatigue, muscle cramping or fasciculations, joint pain or instability, sleep apnea, intolerance to cold, and depression. No pathognomonic tests for the syndrome are currently available. Electromyography can demonstrate the presence of large motor units resulting from the previous axon sprouting. This finding is supportive but not diagnostic of poliomyelitis.

Management

A. Acute Poliomyelitis

When the shoulder muscles are involved, respiratory compromise should be suspected, and mechanical support of ventilation should be instituted. Other measures are aimed at decreasing muscle pain and preventing complications. Regular ROM exercises prevent the formation of joint contractures.

B. Subacute Poliomyelitis

During the subacute stage, which may last as long as 24 months, the emphasis is on preventing deformities and preserving function. Splints and braces are often helpful for maintaining joint position and supplementing function.

C. Residual Poliomyelitis

Patients with compromised function of the diaphragm can be taught glossopharyngeal breathing. This method, in which air is swallowed into the lungs, provides sufficient air exchange for the patient to perform light activities in the sitting position. Mechanical support of ventilation may still need to be continued while the patient sleeps. It is during the residual stage that orthopedic surgery is commonly performed to restore lost function and provide structural stability. If the patient is still growing, it is important to prevent the formation of skeletal deformities that result from muscle imbalance. Before any surgery that requires general anesthesia or significant sedation is performed, the vital capacity should be assessed to determine the patient's need for respiratory support.

D. Postpoliomyelitis Syndrome

Treatment is directed at preserving current muscle strength and preventing further weakness from occurring. Generally, strength cannot be restored in a muscle that was weakened by poliomyelitis. Some gain in strength can be seen, however, when chronic overuse is corrected.

General management strategies consist of modifying lifestyle to prevent chronic overuse of weak muscles; instituting a limited exercise program that incorporates frequent rest periods to prevent disuse atrophy and weakness; providing lightweight orthotic support of the limbs to protect joints and substitute for muscle function; and performing orthopedic surgery to correct limb or trunk deformities.

Specific management strategies depend on the areas of disease involvement.

1. Spine—Back pain is a common complaint and usually results from postural strain caused by excessive lumbar extension in patients who have weak or paralyzed hip extensor muscles. Neck pain, like back pain, is a common complaint associated with slowly increasing weakness. Both complaints can be treated by the use of external supports. Patient education is imperative because many patients are reluctant to don braces again, after having passed decades without using them. Patients should be instructed in methods to relieve excess strain on the neck muscles and prevent further deterioration. Tilting the seat of a chair 10 degrees backward is often sufficient to relieve the fatigue of the posterior cervical muscles from supporting the head.

Paralysis of the cervical spine musculature can result in the inability to maintain the head erect and can interfere with the performance of a vast number of functions, including ambulation. Surgical fusion of the cervical spine corrects the problem.

Scoliosis is common in patients with muscle imbalance caused by paralysis. The condition is particularly pronounced in patients with leg-length discrepancies. External supports can be used to hold the spine in position, but these often interfere with respiration if the patient depends on the use of accessory muscles for breathing. Posterior spinal fusion may be needed to control the spine adequately. After fusion is performed, prolonged immobilization must be avoided. Segmental spine fixation may be helpful.

2. Lower extremities—Full ROM of the hip and knee joints is needed for function. Contractures should be corrected when possible to permit more effective bracing. In iliotibial band contractures, which are common deformities, the hip assumes a position of flexion, external rotation, and abduction; the knee assumes a valgus alignment; and the tibia is externally rotated on the femur. Release or lengthening of the iliotibial band corrects the deformity.

A patient with flailing lower extremities can stand using crutches and a KAFO with the knees locked in extension and the ankles in slight dorsiflexion by hyperextending the hips and using the strong anterior hip capsule for support. Flexion contractures of the hips or knees prevent this alignment. If trunk support and upper extremity strength are adequate, the patient could ambulate with a swing-through gait for short distances. This gait has high energy demands. With time, the posterior knee joint capsule becomes stretched, and the knee develops a recurvatum deformity that is painful and can lead to arthritic degeneration of the knee. A KAFO protects the knee and provides improved stability for walking. If there is fair (grade 3) strength in the hip flexor muscles (see Table 13–1) and passive full-knee extension, then the knee joints can be left unlocked for walking. In this case, a posteriorly offset knee joint is used to stabilize the knee, and ankle dorsiflexion is limited to minus 3 degrees of neutral dorsiflexion to provide a hyperextension moment to the knee for stability. Thus, at stance phase, the net ankle plantarflexion locks the knee in hyperextension, restrained by posterior capsular static structures.

Quadriceps muscle strength is not essential for ambulation. A strong gluteus maximus and good calf strength can substitute by keeping the knee locked in extension. If the calf strength is inadequate to control the forward motion of the tibia in mid to late stance, an AFO is needed. It is not necessary to fix the ankle in mild plantarflexion to provide knee stability, and such a position could cause a recurvatum deformity in any case. An equinus position of the foot inhibits forward momentum and limits step length by preventing body weight from rolling over the forefoot prior to contact of the contralateral extremity with the ground. When good hamstring function is present, the biceps femoris and the semitendinosus can be transferred anteriorly to the quadriceps tendon to provide dynamic knee stability.

Muscle imbalances in the foot can lead to deformity. When muscle imbalances exist, tendon releases or transfers should be considered prior to the development of fixed deformities.

Equinus contracture of the ankle is a common problem and results in genu recurvatum. Accommodating the equinus posture by using an elevated heel places excessive stress on the calf muscles to control the leg. A surgical procedure to lengthen the Achilles tendon is frequently needed to correct the equinus contracture of the ankle and to permit adequate bracing.

A cavus foot deformity causes forefoot equinus, which also limits bracing. If no fixed bony abnormalities are present, then release of the plantar fascia is sufficient to correct the deformity. If the cavus deformity is caused by bony abnormalities, then a closing wedge osteotomy is needed. A triple arthrodesis of the hindfoot can also be used to correct deformities and provide a stable base of support.

The long-standing muscle imbalances, patterns of muscle substitution, and resulting joint and ligament strains often lead to degenerative arthritis. Total joint replacement can be performed, but several special considerations are needed. In patients with postpoliomyelitis syndrome, osteoporosis is common because of prolonged lack of muscle action on the bone. Joint contractures must be corrected at the time of surgery to prevent excessive forces on the prosthetic components because these forces might lead to loosening of the prosthesis. Weak muscles must be supported with the appropriate orthoses after surgery. The rehabilitation program is lengthy because it takes an extended period to regain joint motion and muscle function. Continuous passive motion devices and frequent joint ROM must be used to gain joint mobility after surgery. Because the hip joint is difficult to brace, there must be at least fair (grade 3) strength (see Table 13–1) in the hip extensors, abductors, and flexors to provide stability to the hip after surgery. Surgery can be expected to weaken the surrounding muscles, which must be taken into account before total hip arthroplasty is undertaken to prevent chronic dislocation.

3. Upper extremities

a. Shoulders—The shoulder is important for placing the hand in the desired position for use. The shoulder totally depends on muscle strength for active mobility. In patients who use a wheelchair, weak muscles about the shoulder can be made more functional with the use of mobile arm supports on the wheelchair. These supports allow the patient a greater arc of motion with less muscle strength. Shoulder stability is more important in the ambulatory patient who requires upper extremity aids. A glenohumeral fusion may be helpful if the patient has sufficient strength in the scapulothoracic muscles. When the shoulder is fused, scapulothoracic motion is maintained, allowing use of the extremity for tabletop activities. Glenohumeral fusion does restrict the ability of the patient to position the hand for bathroom hygiene, so it is undesirable to perform the procedure on both shoulders.

Preservation of shoulder strength should be a priority of treatment. Rotator cuff tears are a common problem in postpolio patients. Surgical repair of the torn rotator cuff should be done when possible. In large tears that cannot be repaired, arthroscopic debridement offers significant relief of pain. Shoulder weakness is found in 95% of patients with postpoliomyelitis syndrome and correlates closely with the amount of lower extremity weakness present. Patients with weak legs use their arms to push up from a chair and pull themselves up stairs. They also lean heavily on upper extremity aids while walking. It is therefore important to remove as many unnecessary strains from the shoulders as possible with the use of elevated seats, motorized lift chairs, elevators or motorized stair chair glides, and optimal lower extremity bracing. In minimally ambulatory or nonambulatory patients, an electric wheelchair or motorized scooter should be prescribed to prevent excessive strain on the shoulder muscles caused by propelling a manual wheelchair.

b. Elbows—The elbow requires sufficient flexor strength to lift an object against gravity for function. A mobile arm support can maximize the effectiveness of the muscle strength for the patient. Tendon transfers, such as those involving the deltoid and biceps muscles, may also be useful in restoring active flexion.

c. Wrists and hands—Opponens paralysis is common in the hand and results in a 50% loss of hand function. A splint used during the acute and recovery phases is useful in preventing an adduction contracture. Opponens function can be restored by tendon transfer. The most common muscle transferred is the flexor digitorum superficialis of the ring finger.

Paralysis of the intrinsic muscles of the hand interferes with function. A lumbrical bar orthosis prevents hyperextension of the metacarpophalangeal joints and allows the long extensors to extend the fingers and open the hand. Surgical capsulodesis to limit metacarpophalangeal joint extension accomplishes the same result.

Paralysis of the finger flexors and extensors can be overcome with the use of a flexor hinge orthosis if wrist extensor function is present. Tendon transfers can provide the same result, allowing the tenodesis effect to provide grasp and pinch functions.

Bruno RL: Paralytic vs. "nonparalytic" polio: Distinction without a difference? Am J Phys Med Rehabil 2000;79(1):4. [PMID: 10678596]

Chasens ER, Umlauf MG: Post-polio syndrome. Am J Nurs 2000;100(12):60. [PMID: 11202787]

Dhillon MS, Sandhu HS: Surgical options in the management of residual foot problems in poliomyelitis. Foot Ankle Clin 2000;5(2):327. [PMID: 11232234]

Gandevia SC, Allen GM, Middleton J: Post-polio syndrome: Assessments, pathophysiology and progression. Disabil Rehabil 2000;22(1-2):38. [PMID: 10661756]

Giori NJ, Lewallen DG: Total knee arthroplasty in limbs affected by poliomyelitis. J Bone Joint Surg Am 2002; 84-A(7):1157. [PMID: 12107315]

Klein MG et al: Changes in strength over time among polio survivors. Arch Phys Med Rehabil 2000;81:1059. [PMID: 10943755]

Klein MG et al: The relationship between lower extremity strength and shoulder overuse symptoms: A model based on polio survivors. Arch Phys Med Rehabil 2000;81:789. [PMID: 10857526]

Sunnerhagen KS, Grimby G: Muscular effects in late polio. Acta Physiol Scand 2001;171(3):335. [PMID: 11412146]

CEREBRAL PALSY (Static Encephalopathy)

Cerebral palsy is a nonprogressive and nonhereditary disorder of impaired motor function. The onset may be prenatal, perinatal, or postnatal. An exact cause is not always known, but the impairment is sometimes associated with prematurity, perinatal hypoxia, cerebral trauma, or neonatal jaundice. In the United States, more than 500,000 people are affected by cerebral palsy. The degree of neurologic impairment is severe in a third of patients and mild in approximately a sixth.

Classification

Because of the diversity of neurologic findings seen in patients with cerebral palsy, a classification system is essential. The disease can be classified by the types of movement disorder and by the patterns of neurologic deficit.

A. Types of Movement Disorder

Three types of disorder are seen.

1. Spastic disorders—These are characterized by the presence of clonus and hyperactive deep tendon reflexes. Patients with spastic movement can be helped by orthopedic intervention.

2. Dyskinetic disorders—Among the conditions classified as dyskinetic disorders are athetosis, ballismus, chorea, dystonia, and ataxia. For practical purposes, these conditions are grouped together because they are not amenable to surgical correction.

3. Mixed disorders—These usually consist of a combination of spasticity and athetosis with total body involvmement.

B. Patterns of Neurologic Involvement

1. Monoplegia—With single-limb involvement, the disorder is usually spastic in nature. Because monoplegia is rare, it is advisable to test the patient before making the diagnosis. The stress of performing an activity such as running at a fast pace often uncovers spasticity in another limb.

2. Hemiplegia—Spasticity affects the upper and lower extremities ipsilaterally. Equinovarus posturing is common in the lower extremity. The upper extremity is usually held with the elbow, wrist, and fingers flexed and the thumb adducted. The major problem interfering with upper extremity function, however, is a loss of proprioception and stereognosis. Surgery for the upper extremity is aimed at making the hand assistive and at improving cosmesis. An arm that is involuntarily held in severe flexion while the patient walks can present a major social disadvantage for the patient.

3. Paraplegia—In paraplegia, neurologic deficits involve only the lower extremities. Because paraplegia is rare in patients with spastic cerebral palsy, the existence of a high spinal cord lesion that could also be responsible for the neurologic findings must be ruled out. Bladder problems coexist with spastic paralysis that affects the lower extremities and is secondary to spinal cord damage.

4. Diplegia—Spastic diplegia, seen in 50–60% of cerebral palsy patients in the United States, is the most common neurologic pattern. It is characterized by major involvement in both lower extremities with only minor incoordination in the upper extremities. Findings in the lower extremities include marked spasticity, particularly about the hips, hyperactive deep tendon reflexes, and a positive Babinski sign. The hips are commonly held in a position of flexion, adduction, and internal rotation secondary to the spasticity. The knees are in the valgus position and may have excessive external rotation of the tibia. The ankles are held in the equinus position, with a valgus attitude of the feet. Speech and intellectual functions are usually normal or only slightly impaired. Esotropia and visual perception problems are common.

5. Total body involvement—Sometimes referred to as quadriplegia, total body involvement is characterized by impairments affecting all four extremities, the head, and the trunk. Sensory deficits are typical, and speech and swallowing are commonly impaired. The most serious deficit is often the inability to communicate with others. Although mental retardation is found in approximately 45% of patients, intelligence is often masked by communication dysfunction. Ambulation is not usually a goal because the equilibrium reactions of affected patients are severely impaired or absent. Sitting may require braces or adaptive supportive devices. Scoliosis, contractures, and dislocated hips are common orthopedic problems and may interfere with sitting.

Management

Because cerebral palsy in children is discussed elsewhere (see Chapter 11), the following discussion concentrates on the needs of the adult with cerebral palsy.

A. Special Considerations in Adult Patients

1. Musculoskeletal problems—Long-standing deformities may be rigid. Bony deformities are common and may preclude surgery for soft-tissue rebalancing unless concomitant osteotomies are done. In comparison with the young patient, the adult patient has a greater body mass to support and therefore has increased energy demands. Spastic muscles are weak and frequently further compromised by the chronic overuse of muscles to compensate for contractural deformities.

2. Mobility—The patient who can sit independently has good balance and may propel a wheelchair. It may be easier to propel the wheelchair backward, using the feet to push. A self-propped sitter may require some external support to remain erect, whereas a propped sitter needs a straight spine and flexible hips to remain erect with support.

Ambulation can be divided into four categories: community ambulation, household ambulation, physiologic ambulation (exercise), and wheelchair ambulation. A patient categorized as a community ambulator is able to maneuver independently and safely around obstacles normally encountered in the community. Orthotics or upper extremity walking aids may be required. A household ambulator is able to walk independently for short distances but requires assistance to negotiate obstacles such as stairs or curbs and requires a wheelchair for long distances. A physiologic ambulator is someone who is capable of walking for short distances with assistance or walks as a means of exercise but finds it impractical to walk for normal activities. The energy requirements for walking determine the category to which a patient belongs and also determine the types of equipment that are recommended. It is unreasonable to expect patients to expend all their energy in merely transporting themselves from one location to another.

B. Treatment of Patients with Lower Extremity Problems

1. Hips—An adduction and internal rotation deformity of the hip is sometimes seen during ambulation. Release of the hip adductor tendons (see Figure 13–13) may be needed to correct this tendency.

A crouch gait and lumbar lordosis are evidence of hip flexion deformity. In patients with cerebral palsy, gait studies with dynamic poly-EMG demonstrated dysphasic activity of the iliopsoas, which is the main hip flexor muscle. Gait studies with poly-EMG should be undertaken to evaluate the activity of the iliopsoas and pectineus and to aid in surgical decision making. If release of the iliopsoas is indicated, the tendon is cut distally and allowed to retract proximally to the point where it reattaches to the anterior hip capsule (Figure 13–31). Release of the pectineus muscle is often also necessary.

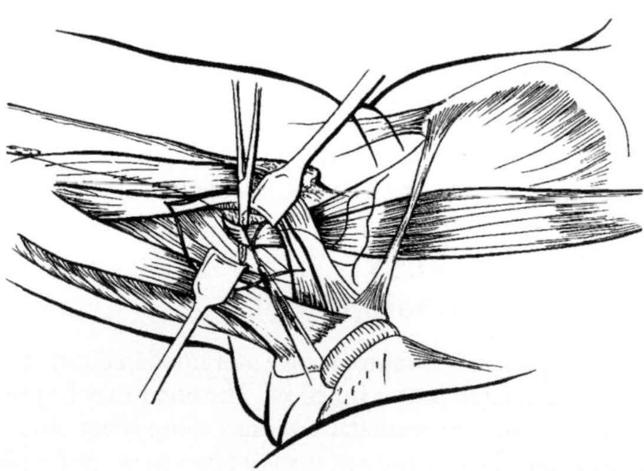

Figure 13–31. **Release of the iliopsoas tendon from its insertion on the lesser trochanter of the femur to correct a hip flexion deformity.** (Illustration by Anthony C. Berlet. Reproduced, with permission, from Keenan MAE et al: *Manual of Orthopaedic Surgery for Spasticity*. Raven, 1993.)

2. Knees—Correction of a knee flexion deformity in a patient with a crouch gait may be necessary. Attention should first be paid to the hip deformity. Weakness of the gastrocnemius and soleus muscles and inability to maintain the position of the tibia may also contribute to a crouch posture and should be considered prior to performing any knee surgery. Gait electromyograms are useful in determining which muscles are responsible for the abnormal posture. Release of the offending hamstring tendons (see Figure 13–15) or hamstring lengthening may be useful.

3. Feet—Equinus posturing of the ankle is common. If no fixed contracture is present, an AFO controls the position of the foot. If the deformity is the result of an equinus contracture, Achilles tendon lengthening (see Figure 13–16) should be performed to bring the foot to a neutral position. The foot should be held in a short leg walking cast for 6 weeks following surgery. An AFO is then used to maintain the position of the foot and support the tibia during walking.

Equinovarus posturing of the ankle is also common. Although the anterior tibial muscle is the primary varus force in patients with stroke or traumatic brain injuries, it is equally likely that the posterior tibial muscle may be causing equinovarus posturing in patients with cerebral palsy. Therefore, in order to find the cause and make the correct decision concerning surgery, it is important to make dynamic EMG recordings while the patient walks.

If the anterior tibial muscle is overactive, Achilles tendon lengthening should be accompanied by a split anterior tibial tendon transfer (see Figure 13–18). If the posterior tibial muscle is overactive, it is advisable to lengthen the posterior tendon. If the EMG studies show that the posterior tibial muscle is active only during the swing phase of gait, it may be more logical to transfer the posterior tendon through the interosseous membrane to the dorsum of the foot, rather than performing a split anterior tibial tendon transfer. After surgery is performed, a short leg cast that allows weight bearing is worn for 6 weeks, and the leg is then supported with an AFO. If hallux valgus subsequently develops, management consists of correcting the subtalar deformity and realigning the first digital ray.

A pes cavus deformity of the foot is occasionally seen in patients with spasticity of the intrinsic muscles. If the problem is detected early, it can be corrected by plantar fasciotomy and release of the flexor origins from the os calcis. If the problem is detected late and a concomitant bony deformity is present, a wedge osteotomy of the midtarsal bones should be performed.

C. Treatment of Patients with Upper Extremity Problems

Function of the upper extremities depends on a variety of factors, including cognition, intact sensation, and the ability to place the hand in space. The amount of spasticity present also affects the ability to control movement of the arm and hand. Surgery can influence hand placement and modify spasticity, but a successful outcome requires the ability to cooperate with postoperative therapy programs. Mental impairment, motion disorders, and poor sensation are relative contraindications to surgery in the functional arm and hand.

1. The functional upper extremity—In patients with problems involving the functional hand, treatment begins with careful clinical evaluation of motor and sensory deficits. Dynamic EMG is extremely useful in determining which muscles should be lengthened or transferred to improve function. The least severely involved hands exhibit a minor degree of spasticity in the flexor carpi ulnaris and a resulting mild flexion deformity of the wrist. In this case, all that is required to improve hand function and position is surgical lengthening of the flexor carpi ulnaris tendon.

In some patients, release of objects from the hand is a problem. In this case, the synergistic action of the finger extensors and wrist flexors causes difficulty with finger extension when the wrist is extended. This resembles the tenodesis effect seen in paralytic hands, but the mechanism is a dynamic one. Selective lengthening of the overactive finger flexors (see Figure 13–23) improves hand function.

Transfer of a wrist flexor to a wrist extensor should be done with caution. Often a patient flexes the wrist to adjust the dynamic balance between the finger flexors and extensors. Holding the wrist in extension can rob the patient of this important method of compensation.

The thumb-in-palm deformity is treated by proximal release of the thenar muscles (see Figure 13–24) and lengthening of the flexor pollicis longus tendon. Distal release of the thenar muscles is not recommended because it may cause a hyperextension deformity of the metacarpophalangeal joint of the thumb.

2. The nonfunctional upper extremity—Surgery may be indicated in the nonfunctional upper extremity to prevent skin breakdown, to improve hygiene or cosmesis, or to make dressing easier. The problems of shoulder contracture and elbow contracture are discussed in the section on stroke, and the surgical procedures used in their treatment are shown in Figures 13–20 and 13–21. Patients who have a flexed wrist with flexed fingers and a thumb-in-palm deformity should be treated because severe wrist flexion can cause median nerve compression against the proximal edge of the transverse carpal ligament. An arthrodesis of the wrist in neutral position, combined with a superficialis-to-profundus tendon transfer (see Figure 13–22), reliably corrects the wrist deformity and also improves skin care. Management of the thumb deformity consists of lengthening the flexor pollicis longus tendon, fusing the interphalangeal joint, and performing a proximal release of the thenar muscles (see Figure 13–24).

D. Treatment of Patients with Total Body Involvement

Patients with total body involvement are rarely functional ambulators, although they may transfer from one position to another either independently or with assistance. They frequently have a combination of spasticity and motion disorders such as athetosis, and they spend most of their time in a chair. Flexible hips and a straight spine are needed for functional sitting.

Occasionally, knee flexion deformities require distal hamstring release or lengthening to allow for greater flexibility in positioning the patient. Rigid extension contractures of the knee are sometimes seen and interfere with sitting tolerance. Lengthening of the quadriceps tendon (Figure 13–32) allows the knee to flex.

Foot deformities in the spastic patient are extremely common and require treatment to allow shoe wear and to prevent skin breakdown. Sitting balance is improved when the feet can be positioned on the leg support of a wheelchair.

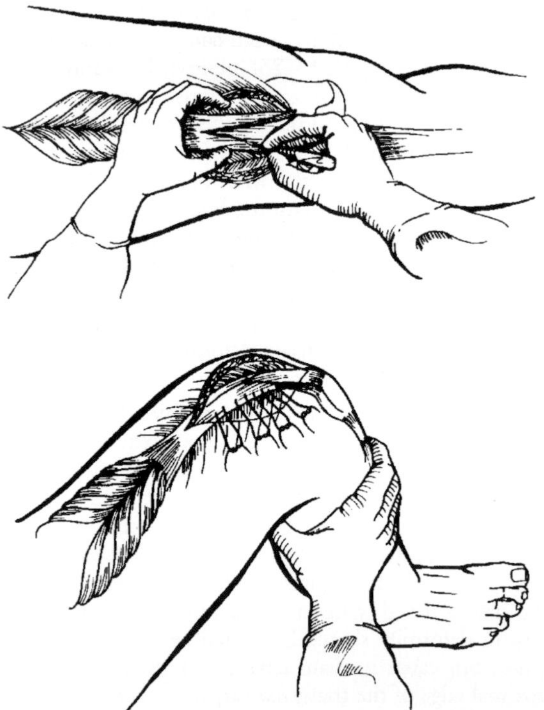

Figure 13–32. The dV-Y incision (*top*) and lengthening (*bottom*) of the quadriceps tendon to correct a rigid extension contracture of the knee and allow improved sitting. (Illustration by Anthony C. Berlet. Reproduced, with permission, from Keenan MAE et al: *Manual of Orthopaedic Surgery for Spasticity.* Raven, 1993.)

The spine is of major concern in patients with total body involvement because scoliosis is common. Adaptive seating or orthotics are useful in supporting the spine and helping the patient maintain an erect posture while seated. Spinal fusion with instrumentation is indicated for treatment of progressive scoliosis. Obliquity of the pelvis greatly interferes with sitting. When this problem is present, fusion should include the sacrum.

Buckon CE, Thomas SS, Piatt JH Jr et al: Selective dorsal rhizotomy versus orthopedic surgery: A multidimensional assessment of outcome efficacy. Arch Phys Med Rehabil 2004; 85(3):457. [PMID: 15031833]

Johnston TE, Finson RL, McCarthy JJ et al: Use of functional electrical stimulation to augment traditional orthopaedic surgery in children with cerebral palsy. J Pediatr Orthop 2004;24(3):283. [PMID: 15105724]

Koman LA: Cerebral palsy: Past, present, and future. J South Orthop Assoc 2002;11(2):93. [PMID: 12741589]

Moran CG, Tourret LJ: Recent advances: Orthopaedics. BMJ 2001; 322(7291):902. [PMID: 11302907]

Pfister AA, Roberts AG, Taylor HM et al: Spasticity in adults living in a developmental center. Arch Phys Med Rehabil 2003; 84(12):1808. [PMID: 14669188]

Sussman MD, Aiona MD: Treatment of spastic diplegia in patients with cerebral palsy. J Pediatr Orthop B 2004;13(2):S1. [PMID: 15076595]

Tilton AH: Management of spasticity in children with cerebral palsy. Semin Pediatr Neurol 2004;11(1):58. [PMID: 15132254]

Wren TA, Rethlefsen S, Kay RM: Prevalence of specific gait abnormalities in children with cerebral palsy: Influence of cerebral palsy subtype, age, and previous surgery. J Pediatr Orthop 2005;25(1):79. [PMID: 15614065]

NEUROMUSCULAR DISORDERS

The neuromuscular disorders represent a diverse group of chronic diseases characterized by the progressive degeneration of skeletal musculature, which results in weakness, atrophy, joint contractures, and increasing disability. These disorders are best classified as motor unit diseases because the primary abnormality may involve the motor neuron, the neuromuscular junction, or the muscle fiber. Two broad categories are considered. Myopathies are diseases of the muscle fibers. Neuropathies are disorders in which muscle degeneration is seen secondary to lower motor neuron disease. Most of the neuromuscular disorders are hereditary (Table 13–7), although point mutations may result in spontaneous cases. Early diagnosis is important not only for initiation of appropriate therapy but also for genetic counseling. Treatment programs are aimed at symptomatic and supportive care. Appropriate orthopedic intervention can significantly increase the functional capacity of patients with neuromuscular disorders.

Table 13–7. Classification of the more commonly encountered neuromuscular disorders.

Disorder	Inherited	Creatine Phosphokinase Level	Electromyographic Pattern	Nerve Conduction	Biopsy Pattern
Muscular dystrophies					
Duchenne (pseudohypertrophic) type	Yes	Markedly elevated	Myopathic	Normal	Myopathic
Facioscapulohumeral type	Yes	Normal or elevated	Myopathic	Normal	Myopathic
Limb-girdle type	Yes	Elevated	Myopathic	Normal	Myopathic
Spinal muscular atrophy					
Werdnig-Hoffmann and Kugelberg-Welander types	Yes	Normal or slightly elevated	Neuropathic	Normal	Neuropathic
Hereditary motor and sensory neuropathies					
Type I (Charcot-Marie-Tooth disease)	Yes	Normal	Neuropathic	Markedly decreased	Neuropathic
Type II	Yes	Normal	Neuropathic	Decreased or normal	Neuropathic
Type III	Yes	Normal	Neuropathic	Decreased	Neuropathic
Type IV	Yes	Normal	Neuropathic		Neuropathic
Type V	Yes	Normal	Neuropathic	Normal	Neuropathic
Myopathies					
Central core, nemaline, mini-core, mitochondrial, myo-tubular, and other types	Often	Often normal	Normal or mildly myopathic	Usually normal	Myopathic
Poliomyelitis	No		Neuropathic	Normal	Neuropathic
Guillain-Barré syndrome	No	Normal	Neuropathic	Slow in acute phase	Neuropathic
Polymyositis	No	Normal or elevated	Myopathic	Normal	Myopathic
Myotonic diseases	Usually	Usually normal	Diagnostic	Normal	
Myasthenia gravis	Sometimes		Diagnostic		

Data compiled by Irene Gilgoff, MD, Rancho Los Amigos Medical Center, Downey, CA.

Diagnosis

A. History and Physical Examination

A careful genetic history is important. The clinical history and physical examination delineates the onset and pattern of muscle involvement. Neuropathies generally present with distal involvement. Muscle fasciculation and spasticity are common, and muscle atrophy is in excess of the weakness. Myopathies usually display weakness of the proximal limb musculature initially. Fasciculations and spasticity are not seen. The weakness is more pronounced than the atrophy. Disorders of neuromuscular transmission, such as myasthenia gravis, present with fatigue and ptosis.

B. Muscle Enzyme Studies

Serum levels of muscle enzymes are elevated in myopathies but normal in neuropathies. The enzymes studied include creatine phosphokinase (CPK), lactate dehydrogenase (LDH), aldolase, aspartate aminotransferase (AST, SGOT), and alanine aminotransferase (ALT, SGPT). CPK levels are the most elevated in the Duchenne type of muscular dystrophy and less elevated in the more slowly progressive disease forms. In Duchenne-type muscular dystrophy, the highest enzyme levels are seen at birth and during the first few years of life, before the disease is clinically apparent. As the disease progresses and the muscle mass deteriorates, the enzyme levels decrease.

C. Electromyography and Nerve Conduction Studies

EMG and nerve conduction studies differentiate between primary muscle diseases and neuropathies (see Table 13–7). EMG is useful in differentiating among muscle diseases, peripheral nerve disorders, and anterior horn cell abnormalities. A myopathic pattern on EMG is characterized by (1) increased frequency, (2) decreased duration, and (3) decreased amplitude of action potentials. In addition, increased insertional activity, short polyphasic potentials, and a retained interference pattern are evident. A neuropathic pattern on EMG is characterized by the opposite constellation of findings: (1) decreased frequency, (2) increased duration, and (3) increased amplitude of action potentials. In addition, frequent fibrillation potentials, a group polyphasic potential, and a decreased interference pattern can be seen. In myasthenia gravis and the myotonic diseases, the patterns on EMG are diagnostic. In myasthenia gravis, the fatigue phenomenon is exhibited. In myotonia, the EMG is characterized by positive waves and trains of potentials that fire at high frequency and then wax and wane until they slowly disappear.

D. Muscle Biopsy

To gain the maximal amount of information from muscle biopsy, the clinician should choose a muscle that has mild to moderate involvement and was not recently traumatized by electrodes during EMG. Muscle biopsy can be used to differentiate myopathy, neuropathy, and inflammatory myopathy. The biopsy, however, cannot be used to determine prognosis. Histochemical staining further distinguishes the congenital forms of myopathy.

Histologically, myopathies are characterized by muscle fiber necrosis, fatty degeneration, proliferation of the connective tissue, and an increased number of nuclei, some of which have migrated from their normal peripheral position to the center of the muscle fiber.

Neuropathies display small, angulated muscle fibers. Bundles of atrophic fibers are intermingled with bundles of normal fibers. There is no increase in the amount of connective tissue.

Biopsy findings in polymyositis include prominent collections of inflammatory cells, edema of the tissues, perivasculitis, and segmental necrosis with a mixed pattern of fiber degeneration and regeneration.

Dietz FR, Mathews KD: Update on the genetic bases of disorders with orthopaedic manifestations. J Bone Joint Surg AM 1996;78:1583. [PMID: 88765869]

Esquenazi A et al: Dynamic polyelectromyography, neurolysis, and chemodenervation with Botulinum toxin A for assessment and treatment of gait dysfunction. In Ruzicka E et al, eds: *Advances in Neurology: Gait Disorders,* Vol. 87. Lippincott Williams & Wilkins, 2001.

Roberts A, Evans GA: Orthopedic aspects of neuromuscular disorders in children. Curr Opin Pediatr 1993;5:379.

1. Duchenne-Type Muscular Dystrophy

Duchenne-type muscular dystrophy, which is also called **pseudohypertrophic muscular dystrophy,** is a progressive disease that affects males. It is inherited in an X-linked recessive manner and has its onset in early childhood. Generally, affected children have a normal birth and developmental history. But by the time they reach 3–5 years of age, sufficient muscle mass has been lost to impair function.

Clinical Findings

Early signs of disease include pseudohypertrophy of the calf, which is the result of the increase in connective tissue; planovalgus deformity of the feet, which is secondary to heel cord contracture; and proximal muscle weakness. Muscle weakness in the hips may be exhibited by the Gower sign, in which the patient uses the arms to support the trunk while attempting to rise from the floor. Other signs are hesitance when climbing stairs, acceleration during the final stage of sitting, and shoulder weakness.

Weakness and contractures prevent independent ambulation in approximately 45% of patients by 9 years of age and in the remainder by 12 years of age. It is common for patients to have difficulty first in rising from the floor, next in ascending the stairs, and then in walking. Cardiac involvement is seen in 80% of patients. Findings generally include posterobasal fibrosis of the ventricle and electrocardiographic changes. In patients with a decreased level of activity, clinical evidence of cardiomyopathy may not be obvious. Pulmonary problems are common in the advanced stages of the disease and are found during periodic evaluations of pulmonary function. Mental retardation, noted in 30–50% of patients, is present from birth and not progressive.

Management

Efforts are made to keep patients ambulating for as many years as possible to prevent the complications of obesity, osteoporosis, and scoliosis. The hip flexors, tensor fasciae latae, and triceps surae develop ambulation-limiting contractures. With progressive weakness and contractures, the base of support decreases and the patient cannot use normal mechanisms to maintain upright balance. The patient walks with a wide-based gait, hips flexed and abducted, knees flexed, and the feet in equinus and varus position. Lumbar lordosis becomes exaggerated to compensate for the hip flexion contractures and weak hip extensor musculature.

Equinus contractures of the Achilles tendon occur early and are caused by the muscle imbalance between the calf and pretibial muscles. Initially, this problem can be managed by heel cord stretching exercises and night splints. A KAFO may be needed to control foot position and substitute for weak quadriceps muscles. Stretching exercises and pronation can be employed to treat early hip flexion contractures.

Surgical intervention is directed toward the release of ambulation-limiting contractures. Early postoperative mobilization is important to prevent further muscle weakness. Anesthetic risks are increased in these patients because of their limited pulmonary reserve and because the incidence of malignant hyperthermia is higher than normal in patients with muscle disease.

The triceps surae and tibialis posterior are the strongest muscles in the lower extremity of the patient with muscular dystrophy. These muscles are responsible for equinus and varus deformities. Management that consists of releasing the contracted tensor fasciae latae, lengthening the Achilles tendon, and transferring the tibialis posterior muscle anteriorly is indicated and prolongs walking for approximately 3 years. Postoperative bracing is required.

Scoliosis is common in nonambulatory patients confined to a wheelchair. Adaptive seating devices that hold the pelvis level and the spine erect are useful in preventing deformity. Alternatively, a rigid plastic spinal torso orthosis may be used for support. When external support is not effective, scoliosis develops rapidly. Spinal fusion is occasionally indicated. Blood loss during surgery is high, and the incidence of pseudarthrosis is increased. Postoperative immobilization is to be avoided; therefore, segmental spinal stabilization is often the preferred technique of internal stabilization.

Fractures in patients with myopathies occur secondary to osteoporosis from the inactivity and the loss of muscle tension. No abnormalities of bone mineralization are present. The incidence of fracture increases with the severity of the disease. Most fractures are metaphyseal in location, show little displacement, cause minimal pain, and heal in the expected time without complication.

Bentley G et al: The treatment of scoliosis in muscular dystrophy using modified Luque and Harrington-Luque instrumentation. J Bone Joint Surg Br 2001;83:22. [PMID: 11245532]

Biggar WD, Klamut HJ, Demacio PC et al: Duchenne muscular dystrophy: Current knowledge, treatment, and future prospects. Clin Orthop 2002;401:88. [PMID: 12151886]

Do T: Orthopedic management of the muscular dystrophies. Curr Opin Pediatr 2002;14(1):50. [PMID: 11880734]

Sussman M: Duchenne muscular dystrophy. J Am Acad Orthop Surg 2002;10(2):138. [PMID: 11929208]

Yamashita T et al: Prediction of progression of spinal deformity in Duchenne muscular dystrophy: A preliminary report. Spine 2001;26:E223. [PMID: 11389405]

2. Spinal Muscular Atrophy

Spinal muscular atrophy is a neuropathic disorder in which fewer anterior horn cells are present in the spinal cord congenitally. The severe infantile form of the disease is called **Werdnig-Hoffmann paralysis.** The disorder is inherited in an autosomal-recessive pattern.

Approximately 20% of patients with spinal muscular atrophy are ambulatory, and 1% are totally dependent. Fractures are common in these patients and occur secondary to decreased mobility and function.

The goal of orthopedic intervention is to prevent collapse of the spine and contractures. Orthotic support is often needed to stabilize the spine. In the nonambulatory patient, adaptive seating devices or orthotics may be used. If collapse of the spine occurs, spinal fusion is indicated.

Bentley G et al: The treatment of scoliosis in muscular dystrophy using modified Luque and Harrington-Luque instrumentation. J Bone Joint Surg Br 2001;83:22. [PMID: 11245532]

Frugier T, Nicole S, Cifuentes-Diaz C et al: The molecular bases of spinal muscular atrophy. Curr Opin Genet Dev 2002;12(3): 294. [PMID: 12076672]

Hopf CG, Eysel P: One-stage versus two-stage spinal fusion in neuromuscular scolioses. J Pediatr Orthop B 2000;9(4):234. [PMID: 11143465]

Iannaccone ST, Burghes A: Spinal muscular atrophies. Adv Neurol 2002;88:83. [PMID: 11908238]

Iannaccone ST, Smith SA, Simard LR: Spinal muscular atrophy. Curr Neurol Neurosci Rep 2004;4(1):74. [PMID: 14683633]

Nicole S, Diaz CC, Frugier T et al: Spinal muscular atrophy: Recent advances and future prospects. Muscle Nerve 2002; 26(1):4. [PMID: 12115944]

Noordeen MH et al: Blood loss in Duchenne muscular dystrophy: Vascular smooth muscle dysfunction? J Pediatr Orthop B 2001;8:212. [PMID: 10399127]

3. Charcot-Marie-Tooth Disease

Charcot-Marie-Tooth disease is the most common of the hereditary degenerative myopathies. It is generally inherited in an autosomal-dominant pattern. EMG studies show a neuropathic pattern, and the nerve conduction velocity of the involved nerves is markedly decreased. Muscle enzyme levels are normal. Clinical onset of the disease is between 5 and 15 years of age.

The peroneal muscles are affected early in the course of the disease. For this reason, Charcot-Marie-Tooth disease is sometimes referred to as **progressive peroneal muscular atrophy.** The intrinsic muscles of the feet and hands are affected later. Patients usually present with progressive clawtoe and cavus deformities of the feet. In the skeletally immature patient, release of the plantar fascia is done to correct the cavus deformity. This is often combined with transfer of the extensor digitorum longus tendon to the neck of the metatarsal and fusion of the proximal interphalangeal joints of the toes to correct the clawtoe deformities. If the tibialis posterior muscle is active during swing phase, it can be transferred through the interosseous membrane to the lateral cuneiform bone. Triple arthrodesis is often necessary in the adult to correct the deformity.

The intrinsic minus hand deformity causes difficulty in grasping objects. An orthosis with a lumbrical bar to hold the metacarpophalangeal joints flexed improves hand use. A capsulodesis of the volar portion of the metacarpophalangeal joints accomplishes the same objective. To restore active intrinsic muscle function in the hand, the flexor digitorum superficialis tendon of the ring finger can be divided into four slips and transferred through the lumbrical passages to the proximal phalanx.

Aktas S, Sussman MD: The radiological analysis of pes cavus deformity in Charcot Marie Tooth disease. J Pediatr Orthop B 2000;9:137. [PMID: 10868366]

Borg K, Ericson-Gripenstedt U: Muscle biopsy abnormalities differ between Charcot-Marie-Tooth type 1 and 2: Reflect different pathophysiology? Exerc Sport Sci Rev 2002;30:4.

Guyton GP, Mann RA: The pathogenesis and surgical management of foot deformity in Charcot-Marie-Tooth disease. Foot Ankle Clin 2000;5(2):317. [PMID: 11232233]

Olney B: Treatment of the cavus foot. Deformity in the pediatric patient with Charcot-Marie-Tooth. Foot Ankle Clin 2000;5(2): 305. [PMID: 11232232]

Smith AG: Charcot-Marie-Tooth disease. Arch Neurol 2001;58: 1014. [PMID: 11405820]

Schwend RM, Drennan JC: Cavus foot deformity in children. J Am Acad Orthop Surg 2003;11(3):201. [PMID: 12828450]

PARKINSON DISEASE

A. Epidemiology

Parkinson disease (PD) is a progressive neurodegenerative disorder associated with a loss of dopaminergic nigrostriatal neurons. PD is recognized as one of the most common neurological disorders, affecting approximately 1% of individuals older than 60 years. The incidence and prevalence of PD increase with age. The average age of onset is approximately 60 years. Onset in persons younger than 40 years is relatively uncommon.

B. Pathophysiology

The major neuropathologic findings in PD are a loss of pigmented dopaminergic neurons in the substantia nigra and the presence of Lewy bodies. The loss of dopaminergic neurons occurs most prominently in the ventral lateral substantia nigra. Approximately 60–80% of dopaminergic neurons are lost before clinical symptoms of PD emerge.

C. History

Onset of PD is typically asymmetric, with the most common initial finding being an asymmetric resting tremor in an upper extremity. Approximately 20% of patients first experience clumsiness in one hand. Over time, patients notice symptoms related to progressive bradykinesia, rigidity, and gait difficulty. The initial symptoms of PD may be nonspecific and include fatigue and depression.

D. Physical Examination

The three cardinal signs of PD are resting tremor, rigidity, and bradykinesia. Of these cardinal features, two of three are required to make the clinical diagnosis. Postural instability is the fourth cardinal sign, but it emerges late in the disease, usually after 8 years or more.

E. Medical Care

The goal of medical management of PD is to provide control of signs and symptoms for as long as possible while minimizing adverse effects. Medications (eg, levodopa) usually provide good symptomatic control for 4–6 years. After this, disability progresses despite best medical management, and many patients develop long-term motor complications including fluctuations and dyskinesia. Additional causes of disability in late disease include postural instability (balance difficulty) and dementia.

F. Neurosurgical Care

When medical management is exhausted, neurosurgical interventions include deep brain stimulation, thalamotomy, pallidotomy, and fetal cell transplantation.

G. Orthopedic Care

Treatment of orthopedic problems in patients with PD can be problematic and include failure of fixation or prosthetic dislocation. Despite successful pain relief, the functional results of total joint arthroplasty in patients with Parkinson disease are poor, especially in patients older than 65 years, and complications are more frequent. Success in terms of pain relief and no further need for intervention can be obtained with appropriate medical management of the PD after orthopedic intervention.

Gauggel S, Rieger M, Feghoff TA: Inhibition of ongoing responses in patients with Parkinson's disease. J Neurol Neurosurg Psychiatry 2004;75(4):539. [PMID: 15026491]

Tabamo RE, Fernandez HH, Friedman JH et al: Spinal surgery for severe scoliosis in Parkinson's disease. Med Health R I 2000;83(4):114. [PMID: 10821012]

Weber M, Cabanela ME, Sim FH et al: Total hip replacement in patients with Parkinson's disease. Int Orthop 2002;26(2):66. [PMID: 12078878]

BURNS

More than 2 million people sustain burns of sufficient severity each year in the United States to require medical attention. Of these, 50,000 individuals remain hospitalized for more than 2 months, attesting to the serious nature of their injuries.

Thermal burns affect the skin most directly but can also involve the underlying muscles, tendons, joints, and bones. Scar contractures cause the greatest limitation to later function and the greatest deformity. Rehabilitation efforts ideally should begin when the patient first enters the hospital, immediately following acute resuscitation and continuing through the reconstruction process.

Classification

Burn wounds are traditionally classified as first, second, or third degree, depending on the depth of the damage. Currently, it is thought to be more useful to simply divide burns into two categories: partial thickness (involving part of the dermis) and full thickness (involving the entire dermis).

First-degree burns damage only the epidermis. They cause erythema, minor edema, and pain. The skin surface remains intact, and healing occurs uneventfully in 5–10 days, without residual scar formation.

Second-degree burns involve the epidermis and a variable amount of the underlying corium. The depth of damage to the corium determines the outcome of healing. In the more superficial second-degree burns, blister formation is prominent and occurs secondary to the osmotic gradient formed by particles in the vesicle fluid. Superficial second-degree burns heal in 10–14 days, with minimal scarring. Deep dermal burns are characterized by either a reddish appearance or by the presence of a white tissue that is barely perceptible and adheres to the underlying viable dermis. These wounds may advance to a full-thickness loss if infection occurs. They heal with a fragile epithelial covering. Healing occurs over 25–30 days, and dense scar formation is common.

Third-degree burns are full-thickness injuries that damage the epidermis and the entire corium. Because of the loss of pain receptors, which are normally found within the corium, pain is absent. The burns have a thick leathery surface of dead tissue.

Management

A. Techniques for Maintaining Functional Position

Burn scars contract and become rigid, so it is critical to maintain the head, trunk, and extremities in a functional position. Contractures, if allowed to form, severely limit later function. The location of the burns determines which techniques are useful in preventing deformity.

To prevent deformities of the neck and jaw in patients with burns of the neck or upper torso, molded splints should be applied early to maintain the head and neck in a neutral position or in slight extension. Patients with burns in the shoulder region are at risk for contractures characterized by a protracted scapula with an adducted arm. Placing a roll between the scapulae and providing support with a firm mattress help prevent scapula protraction. To keep the arms abducted 75–80 degrees and the shoulder flexed 20–30 degrees, axillary foam pads are used and can be held in position with a figure-of-8 wrapping, which maintain the glenohumeral joint in a functional position. Untreated contractures not only limit limb motion but also can result in joint subluxation from extremes in positioning.

When the burns involve the torso, the goal is to maintain a straight spine in the face of contracting scar tissue. Burns involving only one side of the trunk sometimes result in scoliosis. This should be corrected by scar excision and splinting. If left uncorrected, the scoliosis becomes structural, with resultant bony changes. Burns in the groin area tend to cause flexion and adduction contractures of the hip. To prevent this, the patient should be positioned with the hips extended and in 15–20 degrees of abduction. If the patient is lying on a soft mattress, mild flexion deformities of the hips may be masked. Daily pronation is useful in maintaining the extension range of the hips.

Regardless of the location of burn wounds on the extremities, the knees and elbows tend to develop flexion contractures. Custom-molded thermoplastic splints can be applied over dressings or skin grafts to maintain the extremities in extension. The splints should be removable to allow for daily wound care. Burns in the ankle area result in equinus contractures with inversion of the foot. Splints can be used here also to maintain the foot in a neutral position, but care must be taken to ensure the splint is holding the foot adequately and not merely obscuring a deformity. Custom-molded splints applied to the anterior and posterior surfaces in a clamshell fashion are more effective in maintaining the desired position. They also assist in the control of edema and can be removed for wound care and motion exercises. Burns on the dorsum of the foot cause hyperextension deformities of the toes. Early grafting and toe traction are useful.

Burns of the hands present special problems. Scar contracture results in a flexion deformity of the wrist and a clawhand position similar to that seen with loss of the intrinsic musculature. The hand should be splinted with the wrist in neutral or in a slightly extended position. The metacarpophalangeal joints should be flexed 60–75 degrees and the interphalangeal joints extended. The thumb should be held with the metacarpal in abduction and flexion, the metacarpophalangeal joint in mild flexion, and the interphalangeal joint in the extended position.

B. Skeletal Traction and External Suspension

In patients with circumferential burns on an extremity, the use of skeletal traction or external fixators and suspension is efficacious and has several advantages. It permits access to all surfaces, elevates the limb to decrease edema, and maintains the extremity in the desired position while allowing joint motion. Traction can be used to correct contractures. In addition, traction still allows for daily hydrotherapy. Generally, traction is only employed for a 2-week period because longer use may result in a pin tract infection with formation of sequestra.

Special splints are fabricated for use in the hand. The traction frame is secured proximally with a pin inserted through the distal radius. Pins are also placed through the distal phalanges of the fingers and thumb by drilling through the nail bed from the dorsal to the volar surface. Traction is applied to the fingers in the desired direction by attaching rubber bands from the distal pins to the outrigger frame. The frame can be modified for use in the foot to apply traction to the toes. In this case, the traction frame is secured proximally with a pin inserted through the calcaneus.

C. Pressure Dressings

Consistent pressure of 25 torr applied evenly aids in the prevention of hypertrophic scar formation and contracture. Elastic wraps applied over splints are used early after the injury and following grafting because they can be adjusted for changes in the amount of edema present. Later, when the amount of swelling shows little fluctuation, custom elastic garments are employed. Pressure must be continued for as long as the scar tissue is biologically active. When the skin is soft and flat and returns to normal color, the pressure can be discontinued. Pressure dressings should be employed for a minimum of 6 months and may be necessary for as long as a year. The daily application of lanolin relieves the dryness of grafted skin or substitutes for the loss of sebaceous gland secretions in deep burns.

D. Mobilization

Early motion is desirable for burned and uninvolved extremities. Splints should be removed frequently to allow for ROM exercises. If the patient is being treated with skeletal traction, motion exercises can be performed on the extremities. If the patient is receiving hydrotherapy for the burn wounds, the motion exercises are facilitated with the extremities supported in the fluid environment.

Patients with burns of the lower extremities can begin to stand or walk before skin grafts are performed, provided the legs are wrapped with elastic supports to control edema. Ambulation should be resumed after skin grafting as soon as the grafts are stable. Early mobilization not only preserves joint motion but also decreases the incidence of sequelae such as osteoporosis, physiologic deconditioning, muscle atrophy, and heterotopic ossification.

E. Treatment of Special Problems

1. Fractures—If fractures occurred at the time of the burn, they can be treated with the use of skeletal traction or external supports such as splints. Diagnosis may be delayed if the fractures do not result in any obvious deformity. If fractures occur secondary to disuse osteoporosis, they are usually minimally displaced and heal uneventfully. Pathologic fractures are less common with early mobilization.

2. Osteomyelitis—Osteomyelitis is not a common complication, despite the high incidence of sepsis associated with burns. Prolonged exposure of bone sometimes results in the formation of a tangential sequestrum in the devitalized cortex. Exposed bone surfaces can be drilled to promote the formation of a granulation tissue bed for skin grafting without an increased risk of infection. The prolonged use of pins for skeletal traction causes infection in 5% of patients who require traction. The use of threaded traction pins minimizes the motion of the pin in the bone. Pins should be removed as soon as possible.

3. Exposed joints—Children and adolescents with exposed joint surfaces may retain some function after healing, but adults often develop joint ankylosis or deformities that require arthrodesis at a later date. To maintain the joint in the desired position, traction can be used. The joint should be irrigated with hypochlorite solution daily and debrided as necessary. The exposed bone surfaces can be drilled to promote the formation of granulation tissue. When the bed of tissue covers the joint, skin grafting is performed.

4. Heterotopic ossification—Periarticular bone formation is seen in 2–3% of patients with severe burns. Although the cause is unknown, predisposing factors include full-thickness burns involving more than 30% of the body surface, prolonged immobilization, and superimposed trauma. The location of the heterotopic bone is not determined by the distribution of the burns. Ossification can occur in any of the major joints. In adults, the elbow is the joint most frequently affected; the hip is rarely affected. In children, the hip and elbow are common sites; the shoulder is an uncommon site.

Heterotopic bone can continue to form as long as open granulating wounds are present. If joint ankylosis does not occur, the ossification gradually diminishes after the burns heal. In children, it may disappear completely. If joint ankylosis occurs, surgical resection is indicated and usually restores a functional arc of motion, particularly when the heterotopic bone is in a single plane and the articular surface is not violated. When the heterotopic bone is present in multiple planes, the problem may recur after resection. Early mobilization of patients with burns decreases the incidence and severity of heterotopic ossification.

Edgar D, Brereton M: Rehabilitation after burn injury. BMJ 2004;329(7461):343. [PMID: 15297346]

Goldberg DP et al: Reconstruction of the burned foot. Clin Plast Surg 2000;27:145. [PMID: 10665363]

James J: The treatment of severe burns of head, hands and feet. Trop Doct 2001;31:178. [PMID: 11444349]

Luce EA: The acute and subacute management of the burned hand. Clin Plast Surg 2000;27:49. [PMID: 10665355]

Prakash V, Bajaj SP: A new concept for the treatment of postburn contracture of the elbow. Ann Plast Surg 2000;45:339. [PMID: 10987541]

Silverberg R et al: Gait variables of patients after lower extremity burn injuries. J Burn Care Rehabil 2000;21:259. [PMID: 10850909]

Tilley W et al: Rehabilitation of the burned upper extremity. Hand Clin 2000;16:303. [PMID: 10791175]

Index

Note: Page numbers in **boldface** type indicate a major discussion. Page numbers followed by *b* indicate boxed material; page numbers followed by *f* indicate figures; and page numbers followed by *t* indicate tables.